PEDIATRIC NEUROSURGERY

2nd EDITION

Surgery of the Developing Nervous System

SECTION OF PEDIATRIC NEUROSURGERY OF THE
AMERICAN ASSOCIATION OF NEUROLOGICAL SURGEONS

Robert L. McLaurin, M.D.
Department of Neurosurgery
Children's Hospital Medical Center
Cincinnati, Ohio

Luis Schut, M.D.
Division of Neurosurgery
Children's Hospital of Philadelphia
Philadelphia, Pennsylvania

Joan L. Venes, M.D.
Pediatric Neurosurgery
University of Michigan
Ann Arbor, Michigan

Fred Epstein, M.D.
Department of Neurosurgery
New York University Medical Center
New York, New York

1989
W.B. SAUNDERS COMPANY
Harcourt Brace Jovanovich, Inc.

Philadelphia   London   Toronto   Montreal   Sydney   Tokyo

W. B. SAUNDERS COMPANY
Harcourt Brace Jovanovich, Inc.

The Curtis Center
Independence Square West
Philadelphia, PA 19106

Library of Congress Cataloging-in-Publication Data

Pediatric neurosurgery.

Bibliography:

1. Nervous system—Surgery.   2. Children—Surgery.
3. Pediatric neurology.   I. McLaurin, Robert L. II.
American Association of Neurological Surgeons.
Section of Pediatric Neurosurgery.   [DNLM:
1. Neurosurgery—in infancy and childhood.
WL 368 P372]
RD593.P383 1989   617'.48'0088054   88-11636
ISBN 0-7216-2748-X

Editor: Martin Wonsiewicz
Designer: Maureen Sweeney
Production Manager: Bill Preston
Manuscript Editor: Gina Scala
Illustration Coordinator: Lisa Lambert
Indexer: Dorothy Stade

Pediatric Neurosurgery: Surgery of the Developing Nervous System   ISBN 0-7216-2748-X

© 1989 by W. B. Saunders Company. Copyright 1982 by W. B. Saunders Company. Copyright under the Uniform Copyright Convention. Simultaneously published in Canada. All rights reserved. This book is protected by copyright. No part of it may be reproduced, stored in a retrieval system, or transmitted in any form or by any means, electronic, mechanical, photocopying, recording, or otherwise, without written permission from the publisher. Made in the United States of America. Library of Congress catalog card number 88-11636.

Last digit is the print number: 9   8   7   6   5   4   3   2   1

CONTRIBUTORS

Martin H. Adson, M.D.
North Memorial Hospital and Private Practice, Minneapolis, Minnesota.

Jeffrey C. Allen, M.D.
Associate Professor in Neurology and Pediatrics, New York University Medical Center and Attending, New York University Medical Center, Bellevue Hospital, New York, New York.

Louis C. Argenta, M.D.
Professor and Chairman, Department of Plastic and Reconstructive Surgery, Bowman Gray School of Medicine. Attending, Baptist Hospital of North Carolina, Bowman Gray School of Medicine, Winston-Salem, North Carolina.

Alex Berenstein, M.D.
Professor, Department of Radiology, New York University Medical Center. Director, Surgical Neuroangiography, New York University Medical Center. Attending, New York University Medical Center, Bellevue Hospital, New York, New York.

Rudy P. Briner, M.D.
Chief Resident, Division of Neurosurgery, The University of Texas Medical Branch, Galveston, Texas.

Derek A. Bruce, M.D., M.B., Ch.B.
Clinical Associate Professor, University of Texas Southwestern Medical School. Director, Pediatric Neurosurgical Institute, Humana Advanced Surgical Institutes, Humana Medical City Hospital, Dallas, Texas.

William R. Cheek, M.D.
Assistant Professor, Neurosurgery and Pediatrics, Baylor College of Medicine. Chief, Neurosurgery Service, Texas Children's Hospital and St. Luke's Episcopal Hospital, Houston, Texas.

D. Ryan Cook, M.D.
Professor of Anesthesiology and Pharmacology, University of Pittsburgh School of Medicine. Chief of Anesthesiology, Children's Hospital of Pittsburgh, Pittsburgh, Pennsylvania.

Kerry R. Crone, M.D.
Assistant Professor, University of Cincinnati Medical Center, Children's Hospital Medical Center. Assistant Attending Staff, Pediatric Neurosurgery, Children's Hospital Medical Center, and Neurological Surgery, Good Samaritan Hospital; Active Medical Staff, University of Cincinnati Hospital; Courtesy Staff, Neurological Surgery, The Christ Hospital, Bethesda Hospital, and Jewish Hospital, Cincinnati, Ohio.

Patricia K. Crumrine, M.D.
Associate Professor of Pediatrics and Neurology, University of Pittsburgh School of Medicine. Staff Pediatric Neurologist, Director of Electroencephalography, Director of Seizure Clinic, Children's Hospital of Pittsburgh, Pittsburgh, Pennsylvania.

Richard M. Dasheiff, M.D.
Associate Professor of Neurology and Psychiatry, University of Pittsburgh School of Medicine. Director, University of Pittsburgh Epilepsy Center, Pittsburgh, Pennsylvania.

Ann-Christine Duhaime, M.D.
Instructor in Neurosurgery, University of Pennsylvania School of Medicine, Philadelphia, Pennsylvania.

Charles C. Duncan, M.D.
Associate Professor of Neurosurgery and Pediatrics, Section of Neurosurgery, Yale University School of Medicine. Attending and Chief of Pediatric Neurosurgery, Yale–New Haven Hospital, New Haven, Connecticut.

Michael S. B. Edwards, M.D.
Associate Professor in Residence, Departments of Neurological Surgery and Pediatrics, School of Medicine, University of California. Director, Division of Pediatric Neurosurgery, Department of Neurological Surgery, School of Medicine, University of California, San Francisco, California.

Howard M. Eisenburg, M.D.
Professor of Surgery/Neurosurgery and Professor of Pediatrics, University of Texas Medical Branch. Chief of Neurosurgery, University of Texas Medical Branch Hospitals, Galveston, Texas.

Fred J. Epstein, M.D.
Professor and Director, Division of Pediatric Neurosurgery, New York University Medical Center. Attending, New York University Medical Center, Bellevue Hospital, Manhattan Veterans Hospital, St. Vincent's Medical Center, New York, New York.

Barry N. French, M.D., F.R.C.S.(C.), F.A.C.S.
Co-Director, Sutter Neuroscience Center, Sutter General Hospital, Sacramento, California.

Arno H. Fried, M.D.
Assistant Professor of Neurosurgery, University of Pennsylvania Medical School. Attending Neurosurgeon, The Children's Hospital of Philadelphia, Philadelphia, Pennsylvania.

Anthony E. Gallo, Jr., M.D.
Professor of Neurological Surgery and Head, Pediatric Neurosurgical Section, Oregon Health Sciences University. Attending Staff, Oregon Health Sciences University Hospitals and Veterans' Administration Hospital; Courtesy Staff, St. Vincent Hospital, Bess Kaiser Hospital, and Kaiser Sunnyside Hospital, Portland, Oregon.

John C. Godersky, M.D.
Associate Professor of Neurosurgery, University of Iowa School of Medicine. Attending, University of Iowa Hospitals and Clinics, Iowa City, Iowa.

E. Bruce Hendrick, M.D., B.Sc.(Med.), F.R.C.S.(C.)
Professor of Surgery (Neurosurgery), University of Toronto Medical School. Associate Chief of Surgery and Senior Neurosurgeon, The Hospital for Sick Children, Toronto, Ontario.

Harold J. Hoffman, M.D., B.Sc.(Med.), F.R.C.S.(C.), F.A.C.S.
Professor of Surgery, University of Toronto. Neurosurgeon-in-Chief, The Hospital for Sick Children, Toronto, Ontario.

Roger J. Hudgins, M.D.
Attending Pediatric Neurosurgeon, Scottish Rite Children's Hospital, Atlanta, Georgia.

Alan R. Hudson, M.B., Ch.B., F.R.C.S.E., F.R.C.S.(C.)
Professor and Chairman, Division of Neurosurgery and Deputy Chairman, Department of Surgery, University of Toronto. Attending, St. Michael's Hospital, Toronto, Ontario.

Robin P. Humphreys, M.D., F.R.C.S.(C.), F.A.C.S.
Associate Professor, Departments of Surgery and Anatomy, Faculty of Medicine, University of Toronto. Associate Surgeon-in-Chief, Hospital for Sick Children; Consulting Neurosurgeon, Hugh MacMillan Medical Centre, North York General Hospital, Women's College Hospital, Toronto, Ontario.

Hector E. James, M.D.
Clincal Professor of Neurosurgery and Pediatrics, University of California San Diego School of Medicine. Attending, Children's Hospital of San Diego, University Hospital Medical Center, San Diego, California.

Dennis L. Johnson, M.D.
Associate Professor of Neurological Surgery and Child Health and Development, George Washington University. Associate Neurosurgeon, Department of Neurosurgery, Children's Hospital National Medical Center, Washington, D.C.

David M. Klein, M.D.
Associate Professor of Neurosurgery, State University of New York at Buffalo. Chief, Department of Neurosurgery, Children's Hospital of Buffalo, Buffalo, New York.

David D. Kline, M.D.
Professor and Chairman, Department of Neurosurgery, Louisiana State University. Staff, Oschner Clinic, Charity Hospital, New Orleans, Louisiana.

Sanford J. Larson, M.D., Ph.D.
Professor, Department of Neurosurgery, Medical College of Wisconsin. Chairman, Department of Neurosurgery, Medical College of Wisconsin and Affiliated Hospitals, Milwaukee, Wisconsin.

John P. Laurent, M.D.
Clinical Assistant Professor, Department of Neurosurgery, Baylor College of Medicine. Active Staff, Texas Children's Hospital, Houston, Texas.

Ronald J. Lemire, M.D.
Professor, Department of Pediatrics, University of Washington School of Medicine, Seattle, Washington. Director of Inpatient Services, Children's Hospital and Medical Center, Seattle, Washington.

Luke Lin, M.D.
Chief, Section of Neuroradiology, Department of Radiology, Western Pennsylvania Hospital, Pittsburgh, Pennsylvania.

Susan E. Mackinnon, M.D., F.R.C.S.(C.)
Associate Professor, Division Plastic Surgery, University of Toronto. Sunnybrook Medical Centre, Toronto, Ontario.

Anthony Marmarou, Ph.D.
Professor in Neurosurgery, Medical College of Virginia, Virginia Commonwealth University, Richmond, Virginia.

J. Gordon McComb, M.D.
Professor of Neurosurgery, University of Southern California School of Medicine. Head, Division of Neurosurgery, Children's Hospital of Los Angeles, Los Angeles, California.

David C. McCullough, M.D.
Professor of Neurological Surgery and Child Health and Development, George Washington University. Chairman, Department of Neurosurgery, Children's Hospital National Medical Center, Washington, D.C.

Robert L. McLaurin, M.D.
Professor of Surgery (Neurosurgery), University of Cincinnati. Attending Staff and Director, Division of Neurosurgery, Children's Hospital and Cincinnati General Hospital; Attending Staff and Consultant, Our Lady of Mercy Hospital; Attending Staff, Good Samaritan Hospital, Cincinnati, Ohio.

David G. McLone, M.D., Ph.D.
Professor of Surgery (Neurosurgery), Northwestern University Medical School. Division Head, Pediatric Neurosurgery, Children's Memorial Hospital, Chicago, Illinois.

John Mealey, Jr., M.D.
Professor of Surgery (Neurosurgery), Indiana University Medical Center. Attending, Indiana University Hospital, James Whitcomb Riley Hospital for Children, Robert Long Hospital, Wishard Memorial Hospital; Consultant, Indianapolis Veterans Administration Hospital, Indianapolis, Indiana.

Arnold H. Menezes, M.D.
Professor of Neurological Surgery, University of Iowa School of Medicine. Professor of Neurological Surgery, University of Iowa Hospitals and Clinics, Iowa City, Iowa.

Laura R. Ment, M.D.
Associate Professor of Pediatrics and Neurology, Yale University School of Medicine. Attending, Yale–New Haven Hospital, New Haven, Connecticut.

Thomas H. Milhorat, M.D.
Professor and Chairman, State University of New York, Health Science Center. Neurosurgeon-in-Chief, Kings County Hospital Center and University Hospital, Brooklyn; Director of Neurosurgery, Long Island College Hospital; Regional Chairman of Neurosurgery, Long Island Hospital, Brooklyn, New York.

Thomas P. Naidich, M.D.
Professor of Radiology, Northwestern University Medical School, Chicago, Illinois. Director of Neuroradiology, Baptist Hospital of Miami, Miami, Florida.

Mark S. O'Brien, M.D., F.A.C.S., F.A.A.P.
Professor of Surgery, Associate Professor of Pediatrics, Emory University School of Medicine. Chief, Neurosurgical Section, Henrietta Egleston Hospital for Children, Atlanta, Georgia.

Eileen M. Ogle, B.S.N., P.A.-C.
Lecturer, Yale University School of Medicine, Section of Neurosurgery. Physician Assistant, Yale–New Haven Hospital, New Haven, Connecticut.

Roger J. Packer, M.D.
Associate Professor of Neurology and Pediatrics, University of Pennsylvania School of Medicine. Senior Attending Neurologist, Children's Hospital of Philadelphia, Director, Neuro-Oncology Program, Children's Hospital of Philadelphia, Philadelphia, Pennsylvania.

Jogi V. Pattisapu, M.D.
Chief, Section of Neurosurgery, St. Christopher's Hospital for Children; Assistant Professor of Neurosurgery, Temple University School of Medicine, Philadelphia, Pennsylvania.

Joseph Piatt, Jr., M.D.
Fellow, Division of Neurosurgery, Hospital for Sick Children, Toronto, Ontario. Neurosurgical Section, Madigan Army Medical Center, Tacoma, Washington.

Antonio Prats, M.D.
Chief Resident in Neurosurgery, Grady Hospital and Emory University, Atlanta, Georgia.

Matthew R. Quigley, M.D.
Instructor in Neurosurgery (Clinical), University of Pittsburgh. Attending Staff, West Penn Hospital, Pittsburgh, Pennsylvania.

Corey Raffel, M.D., Ph.D.
Assistant Professor, Department of Neurological Surgery, University of Southern California. Assistant Staff Neurosurgeon, Children's Hospital of Los Angeles, Los Angeles, California.

Anthony J. Raimondi, M.D.
Professor of Surgery, Northwestern University Medical School, Chicago, Illinois.

Donald H. Reigel, M.D., F.A.C.S.
Chief, Division of Neurosurgery, The Western Pennsylvania Hospital, Pittsburgh, Pennsylvania. Somerset Community Hospital, Somerset, Pennsylvania.

Harold L. Rekate, M.D.
Chief, Pediatric Neurosurgery, Barrow Neurological Institute, Phoenix, Arizona; Clinical Associate Professor of Neurosurgery, University of Arizona School of Medicine, Phoenix, Arizona; Adjunct Associate Professor, Systems Engineering, Case Western Reserve University, Cleveland, Ohio. Attending in Pediatric Neurosurgery, Children's Health Center of St. Joseph's Hospital and Phoenix Children's Hospital, Phoenix, Arizona.

Kenneth L. Renkens, Jr., M.D.
Chief Resident, New England Medical Center, Boston, Massachusetts.

Lucy Balian Rorke, M.D.
Clinical Professor of Pathology, Clinical Professor of Neurology, University of Pennsylvania School of Medicine. Neuropathologist, The Children's Hospital of Philadelphia, Philadelphia, Pennsylvania.

Fernando Rueda-Franco, M.D.
Professor of Neurosurgery, University of Mexico. Chief, Department of Neurosurgery, Instituto Nacional de Pediatria, Mexico City, Mexico.

Luis Schut, M.D.
Professor of Neurosurgery and Pediatrics, University of Pennsylvania School of Medicine. Chief, Neurosurgical Services, Children's Hospital of Philadelphia, Philadelphia, Pennsylvania.

R. Michael Scott, M.D.
Associate Professor, Harvard Medical School. Director, Division of Pediatric Neurosurgery, The Children's Hospital of Boston, Boston, Massachusetts.

Kenneth Shapiro, M.D.
Humana Hospital–Medical City Dallas, Children's Medical Center, Dallas, Texas.

Joseph R. Siebert, Ph.D.
Research Assistant Professor, Department of Pathology, School of Medicine, University of Washington. Research Associate, Department of Laboratories, Children's Hospital and Medical Center, Seattle, Washington.

Wendy R. K. Smoker, M.D.
Associate Professor of Radiology, University of Utah. Clinical Director of Radiology-MRI, Department of Radiology, University of Utah, Salt Lake City, Utah.

Bruce B. Storrs, M.D.
Assistant Professor of Surgery (Neurosurgery), Northwestern University. Attending, Children's Memorial Hospital, Salt Lake City, Utah.

Leslie N. Sutton, M.D.
Assistant Professor of Neurosurgery, University of Pennsylvania School of Medicine. Associate Neurosurgeon, Children's Hospital of Philadelphia, Philadelphia, Pennsylvania.

Richard B. Towbin, M.D.
Professor, Radiology and Pediatrics, Wayne State University School of Medicine. Assistant Chief and Staff Radiologist, Children's Hospital of Michigan; Attending Radiologist, Detroit University Health Center and Harper-Grace Hospitals, Detroit, Michigan.

Joan L. Venes, M.D.
Associate Professor of Surgery, University of Michigan Hospitals. Chief, Pediatric Neurosurgery, Ann Arbor, Michigan.

John K. Vries, M.D.
Assistant Professor of Neurological Surgery, University of Pittsburgh School of Medicine. Director of Surgery, University of Pittsburgh Epilepsy Center, Presbyterian-University Hospital, Children's Hospital of Pittsburgh, Pittsburgh, Pennsylvania.

Steven L. Wald, M.D.
Assistant Professor, University of Vermont College of Medicine. Attending Neurosurgeon, Medical Hospital of Vermont, Burlington, Vermont.

Marion L. Walker, M.D.
Associate Professor of Surgery (Neurosurgery), Associate Professor of Pediatrics, University of Utah. Chairman, Division of Pediatric Neurosurgery, Primary Children's Medical Center; Chairman, Section of Pediatric Neurosurgery, University of Utah Health Sciences Center, Salt Lake City, Utah.

Josef Warkany, M.D., D.Sc.
Professor Emeritus of Research Pediatrics, University of Cincinnati College of Medicine. Professor Emeritus of Research Pediatrics, Cincinnati Children's Hospital, Cincinnati, Ohio.

Jeffrey H. Wisoff, M.D.
Assistant Professor, Division of Pediatric Neurosurgery, New York University Medical Center. Assistant Attending, New York University Medical Center, Bellevue Hospital, Manhattan Veterans Hospital, St. Vincent's Medical Center, New York, New York.

FOREWORD

Pediatric neurosurgery has undergone explosive expansion during the past decade. This growth resulted from increased understanding of pathophysiology associated with lesions affecting the developing nervous system, awareness of pathologic entities that were previously undefined, and the application of newer diagnostic and therapeutic techniques. As a consequence of these factors, the editors of the first edition of *Pediatric Neurosurgery*, published in 1982, concluded that a more up-to-date account of this specialty was needed. Again under the auspices of the Pediatric Section of the American Association of Neurological Surgeons, this volume has been developed.

The nucleus of contributors remains unchanged, although each chapter has been revised to reflect recent progress. New authors have been added to fill gaps resulting from expansion of knowledge in this specialty. Several examples may be cited. A chapter devoted to cysticercosis of the nervous system was added to the section on infection, since this particular disease, once nearly unknown in the United States, has increasingly appeared owing to our mobile population. The author of the chapter, Dr. Rueda-Franco, is recognized world-wide as an expert in that field. Dr. David McLone has reviewed the entity of tethered cord and Chiari deformities in much greater depth than was possible in the prior edition. Dr. Michael Scott, an authority on ischemic vascular disease in children, has amplified the material relating to that disorder, including the management of patients with moyamoya disease. A chapter concerned with the latest advances in neuro-oncology by Dr. Roger Packer complements the section devoted to tumors of the nervous system. Noteworthy also is the addition of a discussion by Dr. Anthony Gallo concerning biomedical ethics as applied to pediatric neurosurgical entities.

Technical advances have also been recorded. Dr. Bernstein and colleagues have discussed the newer developments in interventional neuroradiology, a technique that has expanded the diagnostic and therapeutic capabilities relating to several disease entities. Improved techniques applied to tumor removal, craniofacial deformities, and epilepsy surgery have been added. The applications of stereotaxis to pediatric neurosurgery have been introduced.

The above examples of enhanced coverage of the field of pediatric neurosurgery, while not exhaustive, provide an indication of the need for continual updating of relevant information. The editors believe that this volume fulfills that need and that it will be of interest to neurosurgeons, neurologists, and those who care for infants and children with disease or injury affecting the nervous system.

The editors express gratitude to the numerous authors who have contributed generously to this effort and to the publishers who have patiently encouraged its completion.

ROBERT L. MCLAURIN, M.D.

To Donald Darrow Matson, M.D.

Although Donald Darrow Matson was not the founder of pediatric neurosurgery, he was its undisputed champion for nearly two decades until his premature death in 1969. It is with the deepest admiration and respect that this volume is dedicated to his memory by those who have attempted to expand the frontiers that he originally explored.

Donald Matson was born in 1913 at Fort Hamilton, New York. His college education was obtained through a scholarship at Cornell University, and his medical education continued at Harvard. Except for a three-year distinguished period of service in the armed forces and a year as chief neurosurgical resident at Duke University, he remained at Harvard for the rest of his career.

The major part of his neurosurgical training was obtained at Peter Bent Brigham and Children's Hospitals, where he developed an interest in pediatrics under the guidance of Dr. Franc Ingraham. Dr. Matson was invited to join Dr. Ingraham after completing his medical training. This alliance resulted in an impressive productivity of laboratory investigation and clinical progress relating to pediatric neurosurgery. One of the by-products of their work was a textbook published in 1954, *Neurosurgery of Infancy and Childhood*. Following Dr. Ingraham's retirement, Dr. Matson became the first Ingraham Professor of Neurosurgery at Harvard, a chair he held until his death.

In addition to his dedication to pediatric neurosurgery, he was equally committed to teaching and the improvement of neurosurgical training. He was a superb teacher himself, not didactic, but rather he set forth a method of approaching, investigating, and resolving clinical problems. Although his knowledge was not overwhelming, his ability to reach the correct diagnostic and therapeutic answers was uncanny. Dr. Matson's interest in neurosurgical training was not confined to his own program; throughout his term on the American Board of Neurological Surgery he attempted to exert an impact on all programs to improve standards of training and medical care.

Dr. Matson's experience in pediatric neurosurgery was eloquently recorded in his volume, *Neurosurgery of Infancy and Childhood* (2nd ed.), published in 1969, the year of his death. This textbook has remained the most complete and influential work in the field. The authors of this book, therefore, humbly dedicate this effort to the principle of excellence in pediatric neurosurgery which Donald Matson so clearly defined.

ROBERT L. MCLAURIN, M.D.

To Kenneth Shulman, M.D.

Kenneth Shulman was born on September 6, 1928. He was first introduced to medicine while working in the family drugstore where his father was a pharmacist.

Ken Shulman graduated from Clark University, with Honors, in 1952, and from Washington University School of Medicine, with Honors, in 1954. He received his neurosurgical training at the Neurological Institute in New York City, under the guidance of J. Lawrence Pool, M.D. Dr. Shulman first became seriously interested in the evolving subspecialty of pediatric neurosurgery toward the end of his residency training, and he spent 3 months with Dr. Donald Matson at the Children's Hospital in Boston, Massachusetts. In 1961 Dr. Shulman became the director of the pediatric neurosurgical service at New York University Medical Center, where he spent 3 years. From 1964 to 1967 he was the Director of Pediatric Neurosurgery at the Children's Hospital of Philadelphia. He returned to New York in 1967 at the Albert Einstein College of Medicine where he ultimately became Professor and Chairman of the Department of Neurological Surgery.

One of Dr. Shulman's accomplishments was his early research, which reflected his complete commitment to pediatric neurosurgery. He also was a leader in the organization and establishment of the Pediatric Section of the American Association of Neurological Surgeons, of which he was President pro-tem from 1971 to 1972 and Chairman from 1975 to 1976. More recently, he supervised a large laboratory complex within his department that was investigating intracranial pressure, brain tissue pressure, and brain edema and its biomechanics.

Dr. Shulman had a brilliant mind as well. He was capable of expressing his thoughts succinctly and thereby imparting knowledge to all who either worked with him or attended his many lectures. His gift for poetic and philosophical thought brought an additional dimension to his scientific contributions. Most of all, he was a sensitive and compassionate human being who was admired, respected, and regarded with affection by everyone who had the opportunity to know him.

With Dr. Shulman's death we have lost a teacher, colleague, and friend; yet we are all the better for having been associated with him. It is in the spirit of friendship and respect that we acknowledge the masterful and talented contributions he made to pediatric neurosurgery and to the publication of this volume.

FRED EPSTEIN, M.D.

CONTENTS

PART I DEVELOPMENTAL ABNORMALITIES

1. **Normal Development of the Central Nervous System** 1
   Ronald J. Lemire, M.D.,
   Joseph R. Siebert, Ph.D.,
   and Josef Warkany, M.D.

2. **Abnormal Development of the Central Nervous System** 9
   Barry N. French, M.D.

3. **Spina Bifida** 35
   Donald H. Reigel, M.D.

4. **Myelomeningocele: Outcome and Late Complications** 53
   David G. McLone, M.D., Ph.D.,
   and Thomas P. Naidich, M.D.

5. **The Tethered Spinal Cord** 71
   David G. McLone, M.D., Ph.D.,
   and Thomas P. Naidich, M.D.

6. **Encephalocele, Dermoid Sinus, and Arachnoid Cyst** 97
   Hector E. James, M.D.

7. **Craniosynostosis** 107
   John P. Laurent, M.D.,
   and William R. Cheek, M.D.

8. **Craniofacial Surgery** 120
   Harold J. Hoffman, M.D.,
   and Corey Raffel, M.D., Ph.D.

9. **Anomalies of the Craniocervical Junction** 142
   Steven L. Wald, M.D.,
   and Robert L. McLaurin, M.D.

10. Medical Ethics: The Resolution of Moral Dilemmas in the
    Management of Children with Severe Congenital Anomalies............ 151
    Anthony E. Gallo, Jr., M.D.

PART II HYDROCEPHALUS AND INTRACRANIAL HYPERTENSION

11. Cerebrospinal Fluid Formation and Absorption 159
    J. Gordon McComb, M.D.

12. Circulation of the Cerebrospinal Fluid..................................... 170
    Thomas H. Milhorat, M.D.

13. Hydrocephalus: Etiology, Pathologic Effects, Diagnosis, and
    Natural History 180
    David C. McCullough, M.D.

14. Treatment of Hydrocephalus.. 200
    Harold L. Rekate, M.D.

15. Ventricular Shunts: Complications and Results........................... 219
    Robert L. McLaurin, M.D.

16. Acquired Problems of the Newborn 230
    Charles C. Duncan, M.D.,
    Laura R. Ment, M.D.,
    and Eileen Ogle, P.A.-C.

17. Mechanisms of Intracranial Hypertension in Children 238
    Kenneth Shapiro, M.D.,
    and Anthony Marmarou, Ph.D.

18. Treatment of Intracranial Hypertension 245
    Derek A. Bruce, M.D.

PART III TRAUMA

19. Management of Scalp Injuries.. 255
    Louis C. Argenta, M.D.,
    and Martin H. Adson, M.D.

20. Skull Fractures... 263
    John Mealey, Jr., M.D.

21. Concussion and Contusion Following Pediatric Head Trauma........... 271
    Derek A. Bruce, M.D.,
    and Luis Schut, M.D.

22. **Post-traumatic Hematomas** 277
    Robert L. McLaurin, M.D.,
    and Richard B. Towbin, M.D.

23. **Late Complications of Head Injury** 290
    Howard M. Eisenburg, M.D.,
    and Rudy P. Briner, M.D.

24. **Spinal Cord Injury** 298
    Arnold H. Menezes, M.D.,
    John C. Godersky, M.D.,
    and Wendy R. K. Smoker, M.D.

25. **Peripheral Nerve Injuries in Children** 318
    Alan R. Hudson, M.B.,
    David D. Kline, M.D.,
    Joseph Piatt, Jr., M.D.,
    Susan E. Mackinnon, M.D.,
    and Harold J. Hoffman, M.D.

PART IV NEOPLASMS

26. **Introductory Survey of Pediatric Brain Tumors** 335
    Lucy Balian Rorke, M.D.,
    and Luis Schut, M.D.

27. **Cerebellar Astrocytomas** 338
    Leslie N. Sutton, M.D.,
    and Luis Schut, M.D.

28. **Medulloblastomas and Primitive Neuroectodermal Tumors of the Posterior Fossa** 347
    Michael S. B. Edwards, M.D.,
    and Roger J. Hudgins, M.D.

29. **Brainstem Tumors in Childhood: Surgical Indications** 357
    Fred J. Epstein, M.D.,
    and Jeffrey H. Wisoff, M.D.

30. **Tumors of the Fourth Ventricle: Ependymomas, Choroid Plexus Papillomas, and Dermoid Cysts** 366
    E. Bruce Hendrick, M.D.,
    and Corey Raffel, M.D., Ph.D.

31. **Tumors of the Cerebral Hemispheres in Children** 373
    Marion L. Walker, M.D.,
    Arno H. Fried, M.D.,
    and Jogi V. Pattisapu, M.D.

32. **Intraventricular Tumors** 383
   Anthony J. Raimondi, M.D.

33. **Optic Nerve Gliomas and Other Tumors Involving the Optic Nerve and Chiasm** 391
   David C. McCullough, M.D.,
   and Dennis L. Johnson, M.D.

34. **Craniopharyngiomas** 399
   Harold J. Hoffman, M.D., B.Sc.(Med.),
   and Corey Raffel, M.D., Ph.D.

35. **Pineal Region Tumors** 409
   Derek A. Bruce, M.D., Ch.B.,
   Luis Schut, M.D.,
   and Leslie N. Sutton, M.D.

36. **Metastatic Tumors** 417
   Mark S. O'Brien, M.D.,
   and Antonio Prats, M.D.

37. **Pediatric Skull Tumors** 421
   Donald H. Reigel, M.D.,
   Matthew R. Quigley, M.D.,
   and Luke Lin, M.D.

38. **Intramedullary Tumors of the Spinal Cord** 428
   Fred J. Epstein, M.D.,
   and Jeffrey H. Wisoff, M.D.

39. **Extramedullary Spinal Tumors** 443
   David M. Klein, M.D.

40. **Phakomatoses: Surgical Considerations** 453
   Luis Schut, M.D.,
   Ann-Christine Duhaime, M.D.,
   and Leslie N. Sutton, M.D.

41. **Postsurgery Management of Children with Brain Tumors** 463
   Roger J. Packer, M.D.

42. **Management of Recurrent Disease** 472
   Jeffrey C. Allen, M.D.

PART V INFECTIONS

43. **Suppurative Cranial and Intracranial Infections** 479
   William R. Cheek, M.D.,
   and John P. Laurent, M.D.

44. **Spinal Infections** 490
    William R. Cheek, M.D.,
    and John P. Laurent, M.D.

45. **Neurocysticercosis** 494
    Fernando Rueda-Franco, M.D.

PART VI VASCULAR DISEASES

46. **Strokes in Children** 501
    Kenneth L. Renkens, Jr., M.D.,
    and R. Michael Scott, M.D.

47. **Arteriovenous Malformations of the Brain** 508
    Robin P. Humphreys, M.D.

48. **Hemophilia and Other Coagulopathies** 517
    Kerry R. Crone, M.D.,
    and Robin P. Humphreys, M.D.

49. **Interventional Neuroradiology** 524
    Jeffrey H. Wisoff, M.D.,
    Alex Berenstein, M.D.,
    and Fred J. Epstein, M.D.

PART VII MISCELLANEOUS DISEASES

50. **Epilepsy Surgery in Childhood** 535
    John K. Vries, M.D.,
    Patricia K. Crumrine, M.D.,
    and Richard M. Dasheiff, M.D.

51. **Hemispherectomy for Intractable Epilepsy** 549
    Harold J. Hoffman, M.D., B.Sc.(Med.),
    and Corey Raffel, M.D., Ph.D.

52. **Movement Disorders and Spasticity** 556
    Sanford J. Larson, M.D., Ph.D.

53. **Stereotaxic Procedures in Children** 561
    Bruce B. Storrs, M.D.

54. **Pediatric Neuroanesthesia and Intensive Care** 565
    D. Ryan Cook, M.D.

INDEX 587

I Developmental Abnormalities

1
NORMAL DEVELOPMENT OF THE CENTRAL NERVOUS SYSTEM

Ronald J. Lemire, M.D.
Joseph R. Siebert, Ph.D.
Josef Warkany, M.D.

METHODS OF STUDYING HUMAN CENTRAL NERVOUS SYSTEM DEVELOPMENT

The study of the development of the human central nervous system (CNS) has been from a descriptive viewpoint, utilizing individual specimens or large collections of embryos and fetuses. While each specimen represents an important contribution, thus far it has not been possible to study human neural developmental processes either in vivo or by explanation. Therefore, the descriptions of the human central nervous system must reference important experimental studies in animals if the dynamic processes of development are to be fully understood.[4] Most such studies have been done in amphibians, although information has also been obtained from rodents, nonhuman primates, and avians.

This chapter concentrates on human CNS development but also includes experimental information derived from embryologic studies. Early CNS development is emphasized, as most structural anomalies arise during the first few months of gestation.

It is not practical to discuss human CNS development without including information about surrounding structures such as the cranium, vertebral column, and meninges. The intimate relationship of these structures with the brain and the spinal cord are clinically apparent to neurosurgeons. Developmental anomalies frequently include those of the brain-skull or the spinal cord–vertebral column variety. Interposed between the structures in the two aforementioned anatomic sets are the meninges, which are developmentally and functionally related to both.

STAGES OF EMBRYONIC GROWTH

The timing of development in the human embryo is based on 23 morphologic stages, each of which encompasses two to three days.[3, 12, 14, 19] These stages include the period from fertilization to approximately 60 gestational days of age. While many important studies of the development of the human CNS occurred prior to this staging method, fre-

---

The authors wish to acknowledge the help of Marjorie Clausing with manuscript preparation.

quently information can be correlated closely. Many of the specific landmarks in the development of the early neural tube are correlated with these stages. Table 1-1 depicts these developmental stages as correlated with both crown-rump (CR) length and the approximate gestational age.

Interfacing the stages of human development with those in animals is problematic, but some accurate correlations are available. In this regard, it is important to stress that a large portion of the information on the "process" of CNS development has been derived from teratologic studies in rodents and avians. For example, the closure of the human embryonic neural tube can be related to stages 8 through 12 morphologically, but the mechanism by which this closure occurs cannot be studied dynamically. In rodents, the process can be followed by in vitro embryo transplantation and can be altered by subjecting these embryos to teratogenic agents. Numerous experimental studies have subsequently confirmed these findings and have greatly contributed to our understanding of the process in humans. Therefore, it is not important that staging in nonhuman subjects correlate directly with that in humans from a numeric standpoint, but that the differences are taken into account by tabular comparisons.

FETAL AND POSTNATAL GROWTH

To date, staging of fetal growth has not been done, and most references are based on the CR length of the fetus. While this approach permits discrepancies, it is the most practical method, even though fetal foot-length correlations are more accurate. During the last three months of gestation and after birth, the reference is shifted to gestational weeks again. Later, days, weeks, months, and years are emphasized.

The main concept in CNS development is that, like other developmental processes, it is a continuum. Among the major organ systems in the body, it is one of the first to be recognized in the embryo and one of the last to finish significant development after birth. Eventually, it will be important to establish some type of staging system for human fetuses. As will be seen later, there are stages for spinal cord development, but these stages are isolated and may not be relevant to other organ systems. The task of a complete staging of fetuses may be insurmountable, and, therefore, it is probably best to consider crown-rump, crown-heel, and foot lengths as sufficient for description in chapters such as the present one. These measurements can be roughly equated with gestational age and can be accurate, at least in terms of a week or two. Previous publications on human CNS development have provided resources of information, whether or not relating to the newer stages.[1, 9, 13, 18]

EARLY CNS DEVELOPMENT

Induction and Experimental Studies

It is not known how the human CNS is induced, but studies on experimental animals have provided some clues about the process in general.[4] The chordomesoderm (notochord and mesoderm), underlying the presumptive neural plate, appears to be instrumental in activating the ectoderm, both initially to form the neural plate and then to transform it into various structures. In chicken embryos, regular indentations of the overlying neural plate by the notochord have been demonstrated. The ratio of neuroectodermal cells to mesodermal cells is important in determining the type of structure that will develop. When there is an increase in the ratio of neuroectoderm to mesoderm, more rostral structures develop, whereas an increase in the mesoder-

Table 1-1. STAGES OF HUMAN EMBRYONIC DEVELOPMENT

Stage	Gestational Age (days)	Crown-Rump (CR) Length (mm)	Selected External Features
1	1	—	Fertilization
2	2–3	—	Two-cell to 16-cell stage
3	4–5	—	Blastocyst
4	5–6	—	Blastocyst attaches to uterine wall
5	7–12	0.1–0.2	Implantation
6	13–15	0.2	Primitive streak
7	15–17	0.4	Notochordal process
8	17–19	1.0–1.5	Neural plate; neurenteric canal
9	19–21	1.5–2.5	One to three somites; neural folds
10	22–23	2–3.5	Four to 12 somites; first fusion of neural folds
11	23–26	2.5–4.5	Thirteen to 20 somites; anterior neuropore closes
12	26–30	3–5	Twenty-one to 29 somites; posterior neuropore closes
13	28–32	4–6	Arm and leg limb buds
14	31–35	5–7	Optic cup; lens invagination
15	35–38	7–9	Cerebral vesicles; hand develops
16	37–42	8–11	Retinal pigment; foot develops
17	42–44	11–14	Finger rays
18	44–48	13–17	Toe rays; nipples appear
19	48–51	16–18	Trunk straightening; limbs extend straight
20	51–53	18–22	Elbows bent
21	53–54	22–24	Vascular plexus on head is half the distance to normal position
22	54–56	23–28	Hands overlap
23	56–60	27–31	Hands erect; scalp plexus near vertex

mal component causes differentiation of caudal structures. The mechanism by which the induction occurs is not known, but evidence exists that both cellular contact and diffusion of cellular material may be important.

Cellular Kinetics

The developing neural tube is generally divided into ependymal, mantle, and marginal layers, with cellular division taking place mainly in the ependyma (the germinal layer). The early neural tube consists entirely of germinal cells arranged in a pseudostratified epithelium. The nuclei of these cells move freely through the cytoplasm, from periphery to central canal, a "to-and-fro" cycle that has four general phases:

M Phase. In the mitotic phase the nucleus is located at the luminal surface.

G1 Phase. The G stands for "gap." In this first gap, daughter nuclei are moving back toward the periphery, and thymidine incorporation is beginning.

S Phase. Nuclei are located peripherally, thymidine is continuing to be incorporated, and most of the synthesis of DNA occurs.

G2 Phase. The second gap phase has some thymidine incorporation and DNA synthesis. Now, the nuclei are moving back toward the lumen.

The generation time for the entire cycle to be completed varies according to species and also regions of the brain.[4] In humans, neuroblasts differentiate from these germinal cells shortly after neural tube closure and then migrate into the mantle layer. Glioblasts probably originate in the same manner. Some small cells are found in the subependymal zone, which is formed between the mantle layer and the germinal cell layer (the ependymal layer). These cells do not participate in the interkinetic cell cycle but can divide and may become small neurons. The importance of the interkinetic cell cycle is that, in a sense, it predisposes to future development of the cellular layers of the brain and the spinal cord. Waves of cells that are generated from this region migrate into different layers and cell groups. If some teratologic event should occur at a critical time during cell division or migration, it is easy to visualize the adverse consequences. Therefore, this mechanism must be considered, in addition to other possible causes (e.g., anoxia and vascular disturbances), in investigating the pathogenesis of such problems as microcephaly.

Neurulation in Animals

Neurulation is the process by which the neural plate folds into a tube. Because neurulation occurs very early, it is vitally important to the developing embryo. Although this process has been well studied, many of its mechanisms remain unclear. Controversy exists as to whether the neuroepithelium, the surrounding mesoderm, or both are responsible for the processes of neurulation: Are the effective factors within the neuroepithelium related to cell division, to a differential water gradient, to differential contractile tensions across the neural plate, or to contractile filaments? Interaction between neuroepithelium and mesoderm has been suggested by some studies, and more recently, with the help of the scanning electron microscope, cytoplasmic blebs, short microvilli, microfilaments, cytoplasmic threads, and lamellipodia all have been identified as factors that may be involved in the process of neurulation.[5]

Neurulation in Humans

Discussion of neurulation in human embryos can be related to the staging system previously discussed (Table 1-1), and then correlations made with the estimated gestational age and CR length.[9, 15] The primary orientation of the embryo arises in stage 6, when the primitive streak and Hensen's node are present. Shortly thereafter (stage 7), a cellular process (the notochord) is found extending rostrally from Hensen's node. It was previously mentioned that the notochord is thought to play a role in induction of the neural plate, and the neural plate is in contact with the notochord in stage 8. This is, perhaps, the first definable period of neurulation, from the standpoint of morphology alone. Over the following ten days, one of the most critical phases of embryonic development occurs: the formation and closure of the neural tube. Somites (lateral mesodermal condensations) begin to appear in stage 9, and the neural folding process begins. The embryo is 1.5–2.5 mm in CR length and about 20 days old. Over the next two days, when there are six to seven somites, fusion of the neural folds occurs (stage 10). The initial site of fusion is at the level of the third or fourth somite, which correlates with the future rhombencephalon (hindbrain) region.

After the initial fusion occurs, there are unfused rostral and caudal neural folds. The time at which these become known as the anterior and posterior neuropores, respectively, is somewhat arbitrary. Fusion continues caudally near the most recently formed somite. By the early part of stage 11 (13 to 15 somites), the younger embryos have fused neural folds, to the level of the colliculi rostrally. Closure of the anterior neuropore is completed during this stage, around the 25th day of gestation. The primordia of the thalamus and corpus striatum distort the final opening and may be involved in the process closure. Following this, the only contact between the neuroectoderm and the amniotic cavity is through the posterior neuropore.

Neurulation is completed during stage 12 (CR

Table 1–2. STAGES RELATING TO NEURULATION IN HUMAN EMBRYOS

Stage	CR Length (mm)	Gestational Age (days)	Somites	Neurulation Event	Non-Neurulation CNS Development
7	0.5	15–17	—	Hensen's node	—
8	1.0–1.5	17–19	—	Neural plate	—
9	1.5–2.5	19–21	1–3	Neural folds	Otic primordium
10	2.0–3.5	22–23	4–12	First fusion	Optic primordium; anterior pituitary
11	2.5–4.5	23–26	13–20	Anterior neuropore closes	Optic evagination
12	3–5	26–30	21–29	Posterior neuropore closes	Many cranial nerve nuclei

length, 3–5 mm; gestational age, 26–30 days). The final site of closure has now been determined, and it is the future midsacral level. There are 21 to 29 somites by stage 12, and if one subtracts the four somites that are incorporated into the occipital bone, and 20 from the cervical and thoracic vertebrae, a rough correlation can be made regarding the closure site. Two important factors should be noted at this time. First, there is no longer contact between the amniotic fluid and the neuroectoderm. Second, more segments of spinal cord and vertebrae need to be formed. Table 1–2 summarizes the events regarding neurulation in the human embryo and other aspects of neural tube development that are occurring during this same period.

Postneurulation Development of the Caudal Neural Tube

When the posterior neuropore closes during stage 12, there are approximately 25 segments of neural and vertebral development. While this actually is a simplified statement of a complex developmental process, it is intended to call attention to the fact that the spinal cord and the spinal column still have more segmentation to acquire. Because neurulation has been completed, the additional lengthening must take place by a different process, which is poorly understood in humans.[2, 6, 7]

The notochord and the caudal end of the neural tube blend into an undifferentiated group of cells, called the caudal cell mass. This cellular mass can differentiate in many ways, and some cells are destined to become spinal cord. The manner in which the tail elongates and the new cord is formed has been described in nonhuman subjects experimentally and in humans. In some manner, vacuoles appear and cells orient around them. These vacuoles eventually coalesce and then make contact with the existing spinal cord, causing elongation of the neural tube. This growth occurs during stages 13 through 20 and results in numerous accessory lumens. The overall process of elongation of the caudal neural tube is referred to as canalization (or secondary neurulation).

The third phase of caudal neural tube development overlaps with canalization. Too many segments are formed and sometime around stages 18 through 20, a regression of the more caudal segments occurs. This phenomenon, termed retrogressive differentiation, results in the formation of the filum terminale, conus medullaris, and its cavity, the ventriculus terminalis. The ascent of the caudal end of the spinal cord continues throughout gestation.

LATER DEVELOPMENT OF THE NEURAL TUBE

Cerebral Cortex

Following closure of the anterior neuropore in stage 11, there is an interval before the first indication of differentiation of the telencephalon in human embryos. Some comparative indicators of brain and spinal cord development during the embryonic stage are shown in Table 1–3. In stage 15, bilateral cerebral vesicles appear; their connections with the existing neural tube later become termed the foramina of Monro. The midline lamina terminalis forms a keel for these enlarging structures, and by stage 17, areas that will become frontal and parietal lobes are identifiable. Primordia of the occipital pole are present in stage 19; primordia of the temporal pole appear in stage 23. These areas have no resemblance to the final form, as the main differentiation of cerebral cortex takes place throughout gestation, especially during the middle third.[9]

Development of other structures also takes place at this time. During stage 16, the primordium of the corpus striatum arises, and in stage 18, the wall of the cerebral vesicle begins to differentiate into mantle layer. The first indication of cortical gray matter is when neuroblasts migrate from the ependymal zone into this mantle layer in stage 22. Four defined cell layers are present by the end of the embryonic period, stage 23. These do not correspond to the adult layers and include (1) the innermost ependymal layer, (2) the mantle layer, (3) a layer of cells (the "intermediate" layer) that have migrated to form the primordium of the cortical cellular layer, and (4) the marginal veil of His, a relatively acellular layer. When the CR length of the fetus is 46 mm, the intermediate layer subdivides into two layers, a fiber layer and an inner nuclear layer (spongioblasts and neuroblasts). When CR length is 95 mm, primordia of three of

Table 1–3. SELECTED FEATURES OF CENTRAL NERVOUS SYSTEM DEVELOPMENT DURING THE EMBRYONIC STAGES

Stage	Characteristic Features in Development	
	Brain	*Spinal Cord*
7–8	Neural plate and groove	Neural plate, primitive pit
9	Neural folds, three rhombomeres	Neural folds
10	Optic primordium; fusion of rhombencephalic folds; cranial flexure	Spinal cord–brain demarcation
11	Anterior neuropore closes; acousticofacial complex; optic vesicle; primordium of corpus striatum	Posterior neuropore opens
12	Roof of hindbrain thins; cerebellar plate	Anlage of spinal ganglia; posterior neuropore closes
13	Three divisions of trigeminal nerve; pontine flexure; olfactory placode	Caudal cell mass begins differentiation; marginal zone appears; cervical flexure
14	Oculomotor nerve; hypothalamic sulcus; roots of cranial nerves V to X	Motor roots from C1 to S2 present; spinal ganglia migrate ventrally
15	Cerebral vesicles appear; striatal ridge; cranial nerve IV decussate	Dorsal and ventral roots blend to form spinal nerves; sulcus limitans; meninx primitiva
16	Infundibulum; subthalamic nucleus	Lumbar and brachial plexuses defined; anlage of denticulate ligaments
17	Frontal and parietal lobe areas; choroid fissure closes; posterior commissure	Three major subdivisions of brachial plexus defined; denticulate ligaments
18	Choroid plexus in fourth ventricle; superior and inferior colliculi; caudate nucleus	First indications of obliteration of central canal; primordium of ventriculus terminalis
19	Choroid plexus in lateral ventricle; putamen; occipital pole area present; first fibers in internal capsule	Major subdivisions of brachial plexus similar to adult
20	Tentorium begins laterally; nerve fiber layer in retina	Retrogressive differentiation begins; dura mater differentiating
21	Choroid plexus in third ventricle	Neuroblasts and glioblasts can be classified; spinal ganglia surrounded by dura mater
22	Anlage of dentate nucleus; superior colliculus	Dura mater in lumbar region
23	Temporal pole area present	Spinal ganglia lie within intervertebral foramina; first indication of filum terminale; anlage of Clark's column

With permission from Lemire RJ: Embryology of the skull. *In* Cohen MM, Jr. (ed): Craniosynostosis: Diagnosis, Evaluation and Management. New York, Raven Press, 1986.

the final cell layers are present: precursors of layers IV, V, and VI. Obviously, the differentiation of the cytoarchitecture of the cerebral cortex is very complex and has regional variations.

The external surfaces of the developing brain can provide some clues as to gestational age. Because of the fissures and sulci, most of the cortical surface becomes buried once development of the gyri begins. The timing of such development has not yet been determined with the precision of embryonic staging, and some morphologic variability exists between specimens that are supposedly the same age. Therefore, rather than centering on a given gyrus or sulcus, the viewer may assess the overall pattern in ascertaining an approximate age. While there will not be further discussion in the present chapter about important factors involved in these morphologic variations, a normal spurt of growth of the brain may be a major influence on form as well as function.

Other changes within the forebrain (prosencephalon) can be identified specifically in the young fetus. For example, the internal capsule fibers, first present at stage 19, have almost completely separated the caudate nucleus from the lentiform nucleus when the fetal CR length is 70 mm. The separation of cellular areas, fiber tracts, and nuclear groups takes place over a long period, yet myelination is a relatively late event, beginning in the fourth or fifth gestational month and continuing for several years after birth. While the diencephalon is developing independently, there are obvious interrelationships with the forebrain that must take place. Development of these deep nuclei is intimately involved in the overall pattern of this region. Each aspect of fetal CNS development is a dynamic process that does not yet conveniently fit into stages such as are found in the embryo.

Cerebellum

In the developing embryo, the anlage of the cerebellum can be found when the pontine and cervical flexures begin to form during stage 13. Although the rhombencephalon constitutes a significant portion of the early embryonic brain, it is not until stage 14 that the cerebellar plates can be identified. At the end of this period, the cerebellum is very primitive; most of its growth takes place during the fetal period. This can been seen by looking at the timing of the appearance of various portions of the midline vermis (Table 1–4). The sequential growth of the cerebellum throughout fetal life has been studied extensively, and fairly accurate assessments of developmental age can be made grossly and histologically.

Table 1-4. APPEARANCE OF LOBULES AND FISSURES IN THE CEREBELLAR VERMIS

Structure	CR Length (mm)	Estimated Gestational Age (days)
Anterior medullary velum	60	70
Lingula	105	92
Precentral fissure	105	92
Central lobule	105	92
Preculminate fissure	78	80
Culmen	78	80
Primary fissure	72	75
Declive	130	105
Posterior superior fissure	130	105
Folium	130	105
Horizontal fissure	132	106
Tuber	132	106
Prepyramidal fissure	87	87
Pyramis	105	92
Secondary fissure	105	92
Uvula	105	92
Posterolateral fissure	45	62
Nodulus	105	92
Posterior medullary velum	127	102

SPINAL CORD

Early development of the spinal cord was previously discussed as it relates to neural tube closure and postneurulation differentiation of the caudal neural tube. Obviously, the spinal cord undergoes many further changes throughout gestation to reach the newborn form. There has been an attempt[10] to provide an approach to this development, which is shown in Table 1-5.

Cranium and Vertebral Column

The development both of the brain and cranium and of the spinal cord and vertebrae is known in considerable detail.[8] Precursor cells form, differentiate, and migrate within biochemically complex matrices, simultaneously exerting biomechanical force on, and absorbing the biomechanical forces of, neighboring tissues. All this occurs within intricate genetic and environmental milieux. However, despite the burgeoning knowledge of development at individual levels, the interaction of events often goes unrecognized. This situation is especially true for craniocerebral and axial morphogenesis.

Major occurrences in cranial development include membrane formation (22 to 38 days, stages 10 through 15) and chondrification (37 to 54 days, stages 16 through 21). Ossification begins at 54 days (stage 22) and is completed during the first years of postnatal life. By the end of the embryonic period, the chondrocranium is well developed and is joined with partly chondrified nasal, orbital, and otic tissues.[11] The skull resembles a fetal one, except that the brain is covered by endochondral and membranous bone in rostral areas only. When CR length is 50 mm, the head manifests several adult characteristics: The cerebri, dura mater, and skin are intact, as are major components of the vasculature. During the fetal period, some 110 ossification centers in the skull coalesce to form 45 bones; additional fusion results ultimately in 32 adult bones.[17]

With regard to the axial skeleton, early growth and segmentation of the sclerotomes precede formation of the primitive vertebrae and intervertebral discs in connective tissue. Chondrification begins in the seventh week of gestation; four centers in the body and arches join, producing the cartilaginous vertebrae. After birth, the configuration of the spine is closely related to posture: As the infant becomes able to hold its head erect, the cervical curve develops. The lumbar curvature is a consequence of upright posture and bipedality. Important events in the development of the cranium and vertebral column are shown in Tables 1-6 and 1-7.

Table 1-5. POSTNEURULATION DEVELOPMENT OF THE SPINAL CORD

Length (mm)	Age (days)	Spinal Cord Development
4-7	25-29	Lateral walls thicken; dorsoventral axis of central canal greater than lateral; groups of cells in basal lamina begin to differentiate; marginal zone present
7-14	29-35	Sulcus limitans divides ependymal zone into two symmetric halves; marginal zone present in several areas
13-22	35-41	Sulcus limitans more ventrally placed; first indication of obliteration of central canal in dorsal part
21-26	41-49	Neuroblasts and glioblasts can be classified in the basal lamina; contralateral funiculi not yet fused in medial plane
26-38	49-57	Marginal zone around entire spinal cord, with some glial cells migrating into it; first groups of large motor neurons in basal lamina
38-55	57-67	Ependymal zone much thinner; central canal small and pentagonal
55-75	67-77	Increase in marginal zone greater than increase in mantle zone; thin glial layer is first indication of posterior median septum
75-105	77-91	Greater volume of white matter than gray matter; first myelin formation by electron microscopy, first synapses
105-145	91-112	Posterior columns more flattened and elongated; myelin sheaths visible through light microscope
145-180	112-140	Fetal spinal cord has similar shape and ultrastructural features of postnatal spinal cord
180-265	140-189	Thoracic spinal cord over 60 percent white matter
265-340	189-full term	All cells in gray and white matter can be classified
340	Newborn	—

With permission from Lemire RJ, Loeser JD, Leech RW, et al: Normal and Abnormal Development of the Human Nervous System. New York, Harper & Row, 1975.

Table 1–6. SELECTED EVENTS IN THE EMBRYONIC DEVELOPMENT OF THE CRANIUM AND VERTEBRAL COLUMN

Stage	CR Length (mm)	Cranium	Vertebral Column
10	2–3.5	Membrane formation begins	Vertebrae appear
11	2.5–4.5	Early formation of cranium: neural crest development; otic plate marks future temporal bone; occipital segments form	Sclerotomic fissure in occipital region contributes to atlas (stages 10–12)
12	3–5	Sphenoid, occipital borders appear	Membrane formation continues
13	4–6	Mesoderm coalesces in parachordal region; vessels form in mesoderm	Verebral anlage from meninx primitiva; early rib formation
14	5–7	Meninx primitiva visible	Cells of sclerotomes (perichordal sheath) form about notochord
15	7–9	Cranium is separate from vertebral column; perichordal sheath about notochord; mesenchymal syncytium forms in otic region	Spinal ganglia differentiate; "closure membrane" begins to form over dorsal neural tube
16	8–11	Membranous formation nearly complete; calvaria present; ethmoidal, orbitotemporal processes appear; chondrification begins in basisphenoid, basiocciput	Notochord flexed; anlage of intervertebral discs and vertebral bodies
17	11–14	Semicircular ducts form (stages 17–23); orbital roof forms in membrane	Bodies start to chondrify; dens visible
18	13–17	Portions of auditory ossicles form in precartilage; vomeronasal organs first appear	Cartilage appears in arches; cervical, lumbar regions flex
19	16–18	Most cranial foramina appear; septum and walls of nasal cavity present; craniopharyngeal canal patent	Pedicles chondrify
20	18–22	Trabecular (ethmoidal) cartilages join basisphenoid; dura mater present	Atlantooccipital articulation (stages 19–20)
21	22–24	Parietal and mastoid plates fuse with exoccipital bone and squamous portions of parietal bone	Closure membrane stratified
22	23–28	Early ossification of zygomatic arch, palate, frontal bone, vomer	Coccygeal curve complete
23	27–31	Chondrification complete; major components of sphenoid complete; semicircular ducts formed; crista galli present	Neural arch tips oriented medially

Table 1–7. SELECTED EVENTS IN THE FETAL AND POSTNATAL DEVELOPMENT OF THE CRANIUM AND VERTEBRAL COLUMN

Age	Body Length	Cranium	Vertebral Column
Fetal Period[a]			
55–60	33	Nasal capsule completes chondrification; head achieves essential fetal configuration	Ossification begins in cervical, thoracic vertebrae
55–60	40	Fusion of palatal shelves	Ossification of lumbar vertebrae starts
65	50	Basiocciput ossifies	Dorsal arches joined in thoracic, lumbar regions
65–75	55–65	Ossification of zygoma, interparietal, and supraoccipital components of occipital bone	Ossification of sacral vertebrae begins
85	90	Ossification of frontal, temporal (squamous portion), and exoccipital bones	
90–150	100–200	Ossification proceeds in auditory bones	Ossification of vertebral column continues
112	140	Numerous ossification centers appear in sphenoid and coalesce	Ossification of vertebral column continues
140	185	Parietal bones ossified	
Postnatal Period[b]			
Birth	50	Multiple components persist in temporal and occipital bones; orbital roof intact; maxilla, palatine, and malar bones are united	Anterior and posterior notches visible; three primary ossification centers
1 yr	73	Ethmoidal centers appear	Ossification of coccyx; cervical curve is apparent
2 yr	87	Ossification of cribriform plate unites ethmoid bone	Spine twice its birth length (sacrum excluded); lumbar curve develops
3–7 yr	95–122	Fusion of basilar, condylar, and squamous components of occipital bone is complete	Annular cartilages ossify

a, body length in mm (crown-rump length); age in days
b, body length in cm (crown-heel length)

Table 1-8. SELECTED FEATURES IN THE EMBRYONIC DEVELOPMENT OF THE MENINGES

Stage	CR Length (mm)	Age (days)	Developmental Features
9	1.5–2.5	19–21	Neural crest
10	2–3.5	22–23	Increased neural crest; somites begin; sclerotomic cells migrate ventromedially
11	2.5–4.5	23–26	Pia mater beginning in medulla oblongata region; 13–20 somites
12	3–5	26–30	Pia mater found in regions of mesencephalon; 21–29 somites
13	4–6	28–32	Meninx primitiva distinguishable from vertebrae; vascularization around cephalic neural tube
14	5–7	31–35	Mesenchyme around telencephalon; primordium of tentorium cerebelli
15	7–9	35–38	Meninx primitiva around brain; vessels surround neural tube
16	8–11	37–42	Cellular sheath of notochord contributes to tentorium cerebelli
17	11–14	42–44	First indication of denticulate ligament; dural limiting membrane forming
18	13–17	44–48	Stratification of pia mater; continuation of meninx primitiva
19	16–18	48–51	Anlage of falx cerebri; dura mater differentiates
20	18–22	51–53	Stratification of closure membrane
21	23–28	54–56	Transverse and sigmoid sinuses within dura; dura mater in lumbar region
22	27–31	56–60	Dura mater complete around cord; cisternae are present

Meninges

The meninges are of equal importance in the consideration of CNS development relating to neurosurgical interests. Transposed between the CNS and its bony coverings, these membranes serve in both support and functional manners. The origin of the meninges is somewhat uncertain, but contributions from the neural crest and paraxial mesoderm seem to exist. Their history and specific early development have recently been summarized and expanded.[8] Table 1–8 presents selected features of meningeal development.

References

1. Bartelmez GW, Dekaban AS: The early development of the human brain. Contrib Embryol 37:13, 1962.
2. Bolli P: Sekundäre Lumenbildungen im Neuralrohr und Rückenmark menschlicher Embryonen. Acta Anat 64:48, 1966.
3. Heuser CH, Corner GW: Developmental horizons in human embryos. Description of age group X, 4 to 12 somites. Contrib Embryol 36:29, 1957.
4. Jacobson M: Developmental Neurobiology, 2nd ed. New York, Plenum Press, 1978.
5. Karfunkel P: The mechanisms of neural tube formation. Int Rev Cytol 38:245, 1974.
6. Kunitomo K: The development and reduction of the tail and the caudal end of the spinal cord. Contrib Embryol 8:161, 1918.
7. Lemire RJ: Variations in development of the caudal neural tube in human embryos (Horizons XIV–XXI). Teratology 2:361, 1969.
8. Lemire RJ: Embryology of the skull. In Cohen MM, Jr. (ed): Craniosynostosis: Diagnosis, Evaluation, and Management. New York, Raven Press, 1986, pp 105–129.
9. Lemire RJ, Loeser JD, Leech RW, et al: Normal and Abnormal Development of the Human Nervous System. Hagerstown, Harper & Row, 1975.
10. Malínský J, Malínská J: Developmental stages of prenatal spinal cord in man. Folia Morphol (Praha) 18:228, 1970.
11. Müller F, O'Rahilly R: The human chondrocranium at the end of the embryonic period, proper, with particular reference to the nervous system. Am J Anat 159:33, 1980.
12. O'Rahilly R: Developmental Stages in Human Embryos, Part A: Embryos of the First Three Weeks (Stages 1 to 9). Washington, DC, Carnegie Institution of Washington, 1973.
13. O'Rahilly R, Gardner E: The timing and sequence of events in the development of the human nervous system during the embryonic period proper. Z Anat Entwicklungsgesch 134:1, 1971.
14. O'Rahilly R, Müller F: The first appearance of the human nervous system at Stage 8. Anat Embryol 163:1, 1981.
15. O'Rahilly RO, Müller F: The normal and abnormal development of the nervous system in the early human embryo. J Pediatr Neurosci 2:89, 1986.
16. O'Rahilly R, Müller F: The meninges in human development. J Neuropathol Exp Neurol 45:588, 1986.
17. Sperber GH: Craniofacial Embryology. Bristol, Wright PSB, 1981.
18. Streeter GL: The development of the nervous system. In Keibel F, Mall FP (eds): Manual of Human Embryology, vol 11. Philadelphia, JB Lippincott, 1912, pp 1–156.
19. Streeter GL: Developmental Horizons in Human Embryos. Age Groups XI–XXIII, Embryology Reprint, vol 11. Washington, DC, Carnegie Institution of Washington, 1951.

2
ABNORMAL DEVELOPMENT OF THE CENTRAL NERVOUS SYSTEM

Barry N. French, M.D.

The neurosurgeon is called upon to treat a variety of abnormalities of the brain and spinal cord originating during the prenatal period. The commonly encountered malformations of the brain and spinal cord are listed in Table 2–1. Although many malformations of the brain occur, they are often of academic interest, being untreatable, but for accompanying hydrocephalus. The Arnold-Chiari and Dandy-Walker malformations are exceptions, to a limited extent.

This chapter is designed for the practicing neurosurgeon and does not attempt to detail conditions such as anencephaly, holoprosencephaly, and other similar conditions. Neurosurgeons encounter the treatable malformations and should be familiar with their basic embryology and its derangement. A host of theories have been proposed to explain the disordered development that occurs in these conditions, but each theory must be assessed against a background of what is truly known, as opposed to what is only theorized, about normal embryogenesis. Some theories are simplistic and fail to address all the abnormalities that occur in a malformation. For example, the open forms of spina bifida display abnormal embryogenesis throughout the central nervous system. Simple theories that explain only the open spine are inadequate.

The purposes of this chapter are three: to review the normal processes occurring in the development of the central nervous system; to describe the morphology of a variety of embryogenic malformations; and to review and analyze the many theories of their causation.

Table 2–1. EMBRYONIC ABNORMALITIES OF THE BRAIN AND SPINAL CORD

Arnold-Chiari malformation
Dandy-Walker malformation
Spina bifida aperta
  Myeloschisis
  Myelomeningocele
  Hemimyelomeningocele
  Hydrosyringomyelomeningocele
  Spinal meningocele
Occult spinal dysraphism
  Spinal dermal sinus
  Tethered cord syndrome
  Lumbosacral lipoma
  Lipomyelomeningocele
  Diastematomyelia
  Neurenteric cyst
  Combined anterior and posterior spina bifida

EMBRYOLOGIC TERMINOLOGY

The neurosurgeon who reads the embryologic literature meets an unfamiliar terminology used to describe the age of the developing conceptus.[41]

Embryologists divide the intrauterine period of development into the embryonic and the fetal periods. During the embryonic period, which constitutes approximately the first 52 days (seven weeks), the basic tissues and the primitive organs and organ systems are formed. The fetal period, which covers the next seven months of gestation, involves the sophisticated development of the primitive tissues and organs that emerged in the embryonic period. The embryologist, rather than stating the gestational age of development in days or months, generally uses the term horizon, or stage, for the embryonic period or employs the crown-rump (CR) length of the embryo. The CR length is used well into the fetal period, but in the later fetal period, the crown-heel (CH) measurement is generally recorded.

Streeter divided the embryonic period into a timetable of 23 "horizons" defined by Roman numerals, with each horizon described by specific morphologic features of the organ systems.[65] O'Rahilly and Gardner detailed the earlier phases and elected to employ the term "stage" in preference to "horizon," using Arabic numbers to designate each stage.[48] The end of the embryonic period was arbitrarily defined by Streeter as the appearance of marrow formation in the humerus, generally correlating with a CR length of 30 mm and a gestational age ranging from 50 to 62 days. The horizon, or stage, method of dating the development of the embryonic period is preferred, because embryos of similar morphologic development may have a marked variability in gestational age or CR length, owing to simple difficulties in measurement, anatomically incomplete embryos, or inaccurate menstrual cycle data.

The origins of the malformations in the open and closed forms of spinal dysraphism, Arnold-Chiari malformation, and Dandy-Walker malformation occur in the embryonic period, with developments in the fetal period modifying and complicating their eventual anatomic and clinical appearances. More simply put, the embryonic abnormality is primary, but certain secondary events later in development, before and after birth, alter the appearance of the malformation and its clinical presentation.

NORMAL EMBRYOLOGY OF THE CENTRAL NERVOUS SYSTEM

Coordination of Development

The cellular migrations that occur in the embryonic period are well described; however, the mechanisms that coordinate developmental processes such as the interaction between different tissues, the migrations of cell populations, the regulated proliferation of cells, and the control of cellular death are poorly understood. Certain tissues in early embryonic development influence adjacent tissues and are called inductors, or organizers. Human inductors are unknown, but in the avian embryo, the primitive streak, the notochord, and the paraxial mesoderm act as primary organizers of the central nervous system.[47] For instance, primitive streak tissue transplanted to another area of the embryonic disc influences the formation of a neural plate; similarly, transplanted notochordal tissue causes a localized neural tube to form. The chemical mediators that control induction are poorly understood in the experimental situation, and not at all in human development. Indeed, once the major primary inductors have outlined the central nervous system, a series of secondary inductions occurs, as in the development of the optic vesicle that ultimately forms the eye.

Abnormalities of these complex and poorly understood embryonic areas may contribute to many of the central nervous system anomalies that confront the neurosurgeon. Thus, while simple or easily understood mechanical explanations for complicated embryonic anomalies may be attractive, such explanations should always be weighed against the essential complexities of embryonic development.

The development of certain regions of the nervous system during normal embryogenesis has to be discussed in a sequential manner, whereas in reality, the formation of all the components of the nervous system occurs in a parallel way.

Formation of the Embryonic Disc

The Bilaminar Embryo. The first two weeks of development after fertilization (embryonic stages 1 to 5) consist of implantation of the conceptus into the uterine wall and development of a bilaminar, or two-layered, embryo. The union of sperm and egg creates the single-celled zygote, and subsequent repeated cell divisions form the 12 to 16 cells of the morula, which enters the uterus. A cavitation within the morula creates two cellular groups: the outer trophoblast, which contributes to the formation of the placenta, and a group of centrally located cells, the internal cell mass, which gives rise to the embryo. During stage 5, at 7 to 12 days of development, this structure, now called the blastocyst, implants into the uterine wall.

As development proceeds, the internal cell mass separates from the overlying trophoblast to create a slitlike amniotic cavity that progressively enlarges and ultimately contains the embryo. Simultaneously, the internal cell mass becomes a flattened and circular embryonic disc with two cell layers, the so-called bilaminar embryo. The outer layer adjacent to the amniotic cavity is the epiblast, which gives rise to all or nearly all the cells of the embryo. The inner layer adjacent to the primary yolk sac is the hypoblast, which is actually displaced laterally and does not contribute to the embryonic cellular development.

During stage 6, at 13 to 15 days of development, the hypoblastic cells near the future rostral end of the embryo form a thickened circular area called the prochordal plate, at the future site of the mouth (Fig. 2–1). The prochordal plate is important not only because it is an organizer of the head region but also because the outer and inner layers of the bilaminar embryo are fused at this site. The cephalic growth of the future notochord is limited by this fusion of tissue layers because the interposition of mesoderm is prevented in later development.

The Trilaminar Embryo. Gastrulation is the process that converts the embryo from two layers to three, by interposition of a mesoblastic layer between the epiblast and the hypoblast. In actual fact, some cells of the mesoblastic layer invade and displace the early hypoblastic cells. Thus, the epiblast is the eventual source of all three layers of the trilaminar embryo—the outer embryonic ectoderm; the middle, intraembryonic mesoderm; and the inner embryonic entoderm.

At the end of stage 6, usually at 15 days of development, a longitudinal orientation of the embryo becomes evident, and the process of gastrulation begins. A linear thickening, called the primitive streak, appears in the epiblast, in the midline of the caudal aspect of the embryonic disc (Fig. 2–1). The primitive streak is the site and source of the majority of migrating cells that form the middle and inner layers of the embryo. The interval between the primitive streak, caudally, and the prochordal plate, rostrally, marks the future posterior midline of the embryo. At the caudal end of the primitive streak is an area of fusion of the two cell layers, similar to the rostral prochordal plate. This site is the circular cloacal membrane, which is the future location of the anus and urogenital structures.

Cellular proliferation increases the length of the primitive streak, and a thickening forms at its rostral end, called variously the primitive knot or node or Hensen's node (Fig. 2–1). Simultaneously, a longitudinal central depression called the primitive groove develops along the streak and deepens somewhat at the level of Hensen's node to form the primitive pit. Cells from the epiblast move into the primitive streak and groove, separate from the epiblast, and migrate rostrally between the epiblast and hypoblast to form the mesoblast, thus creating the earliest stage of the trilaminar embryo (Fig. 2–2). The epiblast (ectoderm) is destined to form the central nervous system (neuroectoderm) and the epidermis (cutaneous ectoderm). The mesoblast (mesoderm) forms the skeleton, striated and smooth muscles, connective tissues, blood vessels, blood cells, bone marrow, and the reproductive and excretory organs. The hypoblast (entoderm) is the source of the epithelial linings of the respiratory and digestive tracts and the glandular cells of the liver and pancreas.

The primitive streak is the source of intraembryonic mesoderm until approximately the fourth week of development, and then it rapidly regresses in size and importance. During its functional lifetime, the embryo increases in length fivefold, predominantly by the complex development of the embryo rostral to the primitive streak. The primitive streak occupies the sacrococcygeal area by this time and normally disappears in later development. Occasionally, cells persist and produce a tumor called a sacrococcygeal teratoma, which may contain a variety of tissue types reflecting the pleuripotential nature of primitive streak cells. These tumors present at birth and must be differentiated by the neurosurgeon from a sacral meningocele or a form of occult spinal dysraphism because their management is quite different.[27, 28]

Development of the Notochord

During embryonic stage 7, at days 16 and 17 of development, some of the mesoblastic cells migrate in the midline rostral to Hensen's node between the ectoderm and entoderm all the way to the prochordal plate, to create the rodlike notochordal process, around which the skull base and vertebral column ultimately form (Fig. 2–2). The intraembryonic mesoderm that is originating simultaneously from the primitive streak cannot cross the midline but extends to the left or right sides of the midline and eventually condenses alongside the midline notochordal process. The development of the notochord itself extends through several of the later embryonic stages, in concert with developments of the overlying neuroectoderm, to be discussed later.

Initially, the notochordal process is a solid core of cells until an extension of the primitive pit at

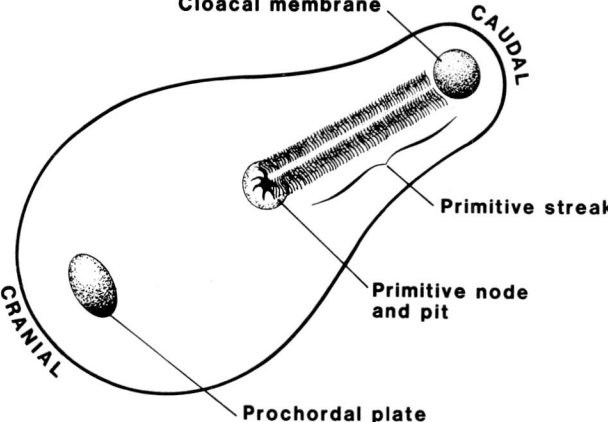

Figure 2–1. Embryonic stage 6 (13 to 15 days) bilaminar embryo showing the cranial and the caudal areas of fusion at the future mouth (prochordal plate) and the future anus (cloacal membrane). Primitive streak and pit formed for the process of gastrulation, which converts the embryo from two to three layers. The areas of fusion define the cranial and the caudal ends of the embryo.

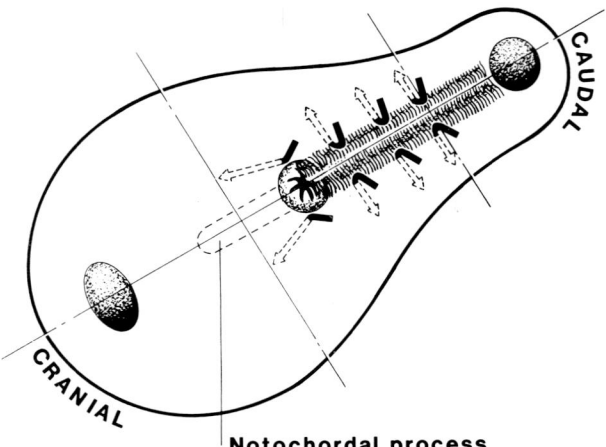

Figure 2–2. Embryonic stage 7 (16 to 17 days) showing the cells of the epiblast migrating into the primitive groove and passing cranially and laterally to form the mesoblast (gastrulation). Cells passing from Hensen's node cranially in the midline between the epiblast and hypoblast form the notochordal process around which the future vertebral column will organize. The trilaminar embryo is forming.

Hensen's node burrows into the notochordal process, converting it into a hollow cylinder of cells surrounding a central cavity called the notochordal canal (Fig. 2–3). A complex series of steps now occurs to form the notochord itself, and several embryonic anomalies of importance to the neurosurgeon are attributed to aberrations in this sequence—diastematomyelia, neurenteric cyst, and combined anterior and posterior spina bifida. The hollow notochordal process fuses with the adjacent entoderm ventrally, and the two cellular layers degenerate along the length of the fusion (Fig. 2–4). The notochordal canal then opens into the yolk sac, and the cells of the notochordal process form a longitudinally grooved notochordal plate in the roof of the yolk sac. This process is called intercalation of the notochord into the entoderm. At the caudal end of the notochordal plate, where the primitive pit first extended into the notochordal process as the notochordal canal, a communication called the neurenteric canal now extends directly through the dorsoventral thickness of the embryo. Temporarily, the amniotic cavity is in communication with the yolk sac.

Subsequently, the cranial end of the notochordal plate infolds to form a solid cord of cells called the notochord, and the process of infolding or excalation of the notochord proceeds to the level of Hensen's node (Fig. 2–5). As the notochord reforms, the entoderm once again becomes a continuous layer ventrally, and the neurenteric canal ceases to exist. The notochord is the structure around which the mesoderm condenses to form the vertebral column. In the early stages, the notochord induces the overlying ectoderm to form the neural plate, from which the central nervous system develops. In the adult, the only remnants of the notochord are represented by the nucleus pulposus of the intervertebral discs.

The development of the notochord, entoderm, neurenteric canal, and neural plate during the processes of intercalation and excalation of the notochord represents the probable stages at which aberrations lead to three of the forms of occult spinal dysraphism: the neurenteric cyst, diastematomyelia

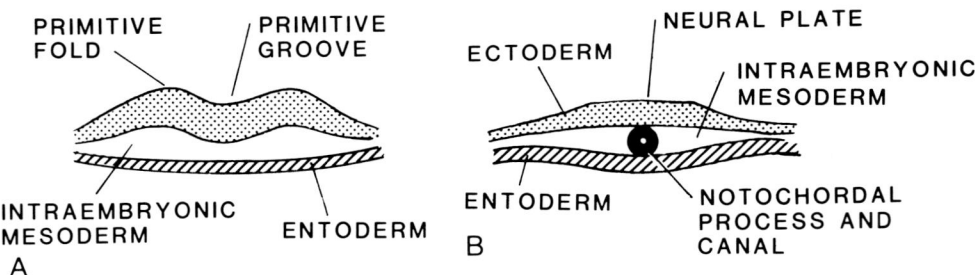

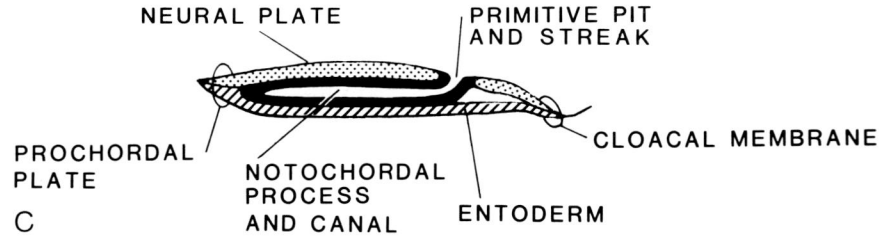

Figure 2–3. Cross sections (A and B) and longitudinal section (C) through the stage 7 (16 to 17 days) trilaminar embryo shown in Figure 2–2. A, Cross section through the primitive streak showing the primitive folds and groove into which the cells pass to form the intraembryonic mesoderm during gastrulation. B, Cross section through the level of the hollow notochordal process showing early induction of the overlying ectoderm to form the neural plate. The notochordal process is in contact with both the ectoderm and the entoderm. C, Midline sagittal section showing the hollow notochordal process extending up to the cranial area of fusion at the prochordal plate.

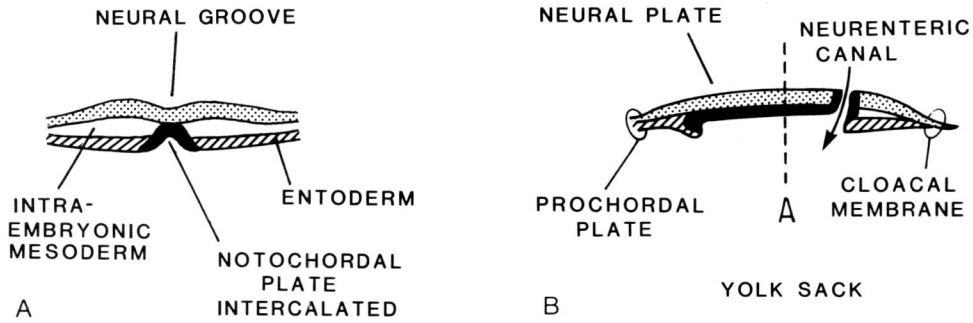

Figure 2–4. Embryonic stage 7 (16 to 17 days). *A*, Cross section cranial to Hensen's node shows intercalation of the notochordal canal through the entoderm into the yolk sac. The neural groove is forming dorsally. *B*, Midline sagittal section along the fully intercalated notochordal process shows the amniotic cavity is in communication with the yolk sac through the neurenteric canal at Hensen's node.

with septum, and combined anterior and posterior spina bifida.[6, 9, 10, 27, 28, 46, 63]

Formation of the Neural Tube

The neural tube is the primordium of the entire central nervous system and forms by a process called neurulation, during embryonic stages 8 to 12, at gestational age 18 to 27 days. It is during these developmental stages or soon afterwards that the most severe and most frequent open forms of cranial and spinal dysraphism occur.

In the later stages of embryonic development occur the processes by which the caudal neural tube (canalization) and the filum terminale and cauda equina (regression) form. Aberrations during these processes contribute to some types of occult spinal dysraphism, including lumbosacral lipoma, lipomyelomeningocele, and the tethered cord syndrome.

Neurulation. The ectoderm that overlies the notochordal process rostral to Hensen's node begins to proliferate in response to the notochordal tissue and the adjacent mesoderm and forms the neural plate. A longitudinal central depression called the neural groove develops along the length of the neural plate as the edges of the plate heap up to form the neural folds (Fig. 2–6A). The neural folds in the cephalic region are always larger and anticipate the location of the future brain. The mid-dorsal region of the embryo, which corresponds to the area of the future upper cervical spinal cord, is relatively precocious in its development. The earliest developmental steps advance here and precede similar progress in the neural plate and adjacent tissues in the caudal regions.

While the notochord and the neural plate are developing, the paraxial mesoderm on either side of the notochord is thickening to form bilateral paramedian longitudinal mesodermal rods. Condensations of cells occur within the mesodermal rods, creating the paired segments of mesoderm called somites, which first develop during stage 9 (days 20 and 21) at the level of the future occipital bone, just short of the rostral end of the notochord. Subsequent pairs form in a rostral-caudal sequence until about 30 to 35 pairs are formed by day 30. The maximum number of somite pairs is debatable, but as many as 42 to 44 pairs may be formed as follows: occipital, 4; cervical, 8; thoracic, 12; lumbar, 5; sacral, 5; and sacrococcygeal, 8 to 10. The first occipital and caudal five to seven coccygeal pairs regress.[47]

At stage 10 (days 22 to 23), the neural groove deepens, and the neural folds meet in the dorsal midline to form first the neural tube (Fig. 2–6B through E). Initially, closure occurs at the level of the third or fourth somite, at the future cervicomedullary junction, and then extends cephalically and caudally simultaneously. By the end of stage 10, the neural tube has formed from the optic plate region of the rhombencephalon (hindbrain) through the future cervical spinal cord to the level of the

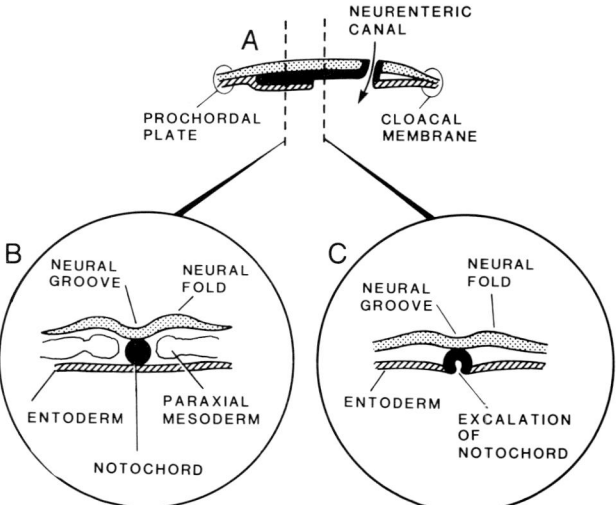

Figure 2–5. Embryonic stage 7 (17 days) showing excalation of the notochordal process and formation of the solid notochord. *A*, Midline sagittal section shows that excalation proceeds in a rostrocaudal direction, with eventual obliteration of the neurenteric canal. *B*, Cross section through the cranial embryonic disk shows the notochord as a solid cylinder of cells. The neural groove has deepened and thickened laterally to form the neural folds. *C*, Cross section shows intercalation as a process of infolding of the notochordal process that draws the entoderm to the midline, with complete re-formation of an intact entodermal layer.

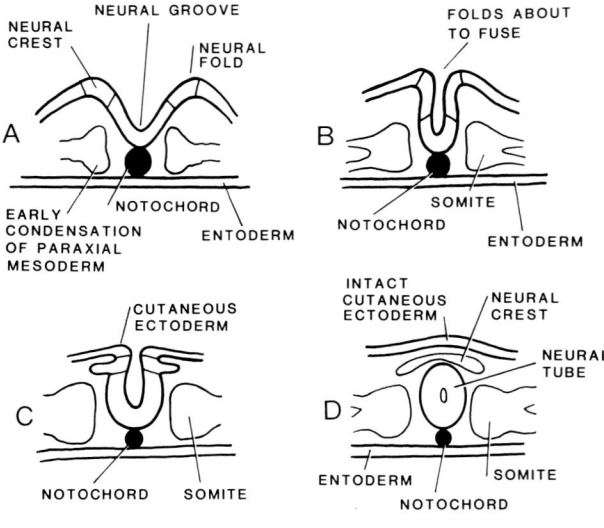

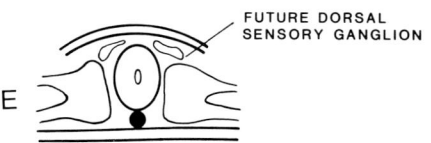

Figure 2–6. Embryonic stages 8 through 12 (18 to 27 days) in cross section showing the process of neurulation, which transforms the neural plate into the neural tube buried beneath a continuous layer of cutaneous ectoderm (A through E). The paraxial mesoderm condenses to form paired segmental blocks called somites, from which the vertebral bodies form. If the embryo were sectioned along its length in the early stages of neurulation, all these steps would be seen, with the advanced step (E) in the cervicomedullary area.

twelfth somite, which is the most caudal somite formed in stage 10. Thereafter, caudal neural tube closure keeps pace with the level of the most distal somite formed in each embryonic stage (Fig. 2–7).

The ectoderm that is continuous with the lateral edge of the neural folds is destined to form the epidermis. As the folds close in the midline, the cutaneous ectoderm is similarly drawn medially and fuses along the midline (Fig. 2–6C and D). Shortly thereafter, the cutaneous ectoderm separates from the neural tube, and ultimately, mesoderm interposes itself to form dermal appendages and muscle and skeletal structures. Abnormal persistent adhesion of the cutaneous ectoderm to the neural tube has been implicated in the creation of congenital dermal sinuses and the intraspinal inclusion tumors of the epidermoid and dermoid varieties.

During stage 11 (days 24 and 25), the future thoracic spinal cord forms caudally, while cephalically, the neural tube completes its closure at the rostral opening, the anterior neuropore, at the level of the future lamina terminalis. Finally, during stage 12 (days 26 and 27), the caudal aspect of the neural tube closes at the level of the posterior neuropore, which is at the level of spinal cord segments L1 or L2, with a range of error of two segments above or below (T11 to L4).[41] In other words, the process of neurulation only accounts for the lumbar spinal cord segments, and the more caudal cord develops by a different process, called canalization. Cutaneous ectoderm completely covers the neural tube by the end of neurulation.

Canalization of the Tail Bud. The process of formation of the neural tube caudal to that formed by neurulation occupies embryonic stages 13 through 20 (days 28 to 48).[33, 41] Caudal to the posterior neuropore is the undifferentiated caudal cell mass of the primitive streak, extending into the tail fold (Fig. 2–8). Under an intact covering of cutaneous ectoderm, the caudal cell mass develops vacuoles around which the cells assume a neural appearance. Subsequently, the vacuoles coalesce to form the neural tube, which then fuses with the rostral neural tube formed by neurulation (Fig. 2–9A, B, C). The ventriculus terminalis, which marks the level of the future conus medullaris, becomes identifiable during stages 18 to 20 (days 43 to 48). The process of canalization is less precise than that of neurulation, with abnormalities such as central canal forking or duplication in the region of the conus medullaris, ventriculus terminalis, and filum terminale quite common.[39, 40, 43] Forms of occult

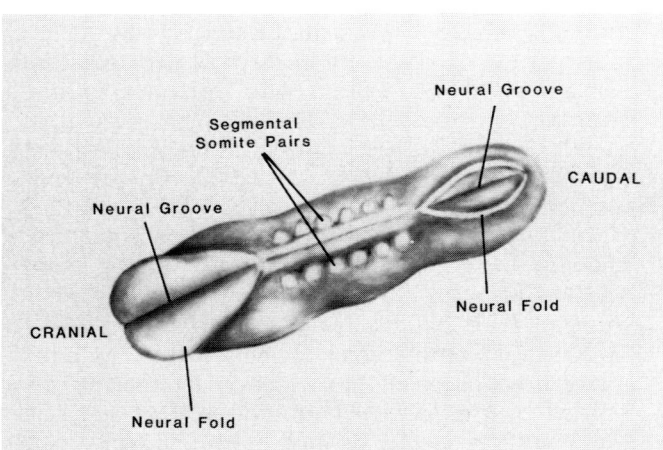

Figure 2–7. Embryonic stage 10 (22 to 23 days) in dorsolateral view, showing the closed neural tube, sex somite pairs, and open cranial and caudal neural grooves. Neural tube closure keeps pace with somite formation from stage 11 onward. Just caudal to the posterior neuropore is the undifferentiated cell mass of the primitive streak, extending into the future tail fold. Cross sections of this stage at various levels would show all the steps of neurulation seen in Figure 1–6.

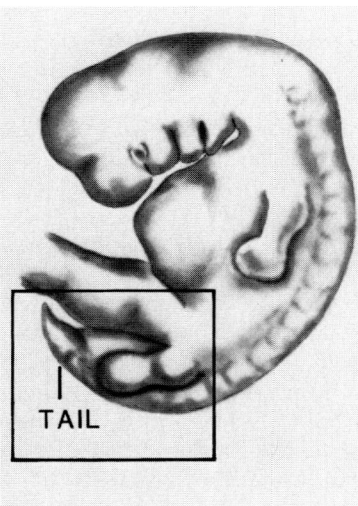

Figure 2–8. Embryonic stage 15 (34 to 36 days) showing the tail process, within which the formation of the neural tube occurs by canalization under intact epithelial ectoderm.

spinal dysraphism such as lumbosacral lipoma and lipomyelomeningocele probably have their origin during the process of canalization of the tail bud. Some authors debate the importance of this process in human embryogenesis, but the concept merits discussion.

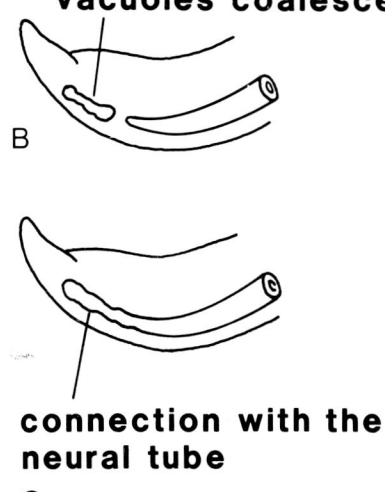

Figure 2–9. Canalization of the tail bud (28 to 48 days) may form the neural tube caudal to the midlumbar area by a process of vacuolization (A), coalescence (B), and fusion of the distal neural tube to the proximal neural tube formed by neurulation (C). (With permission from Lemire RJ, Loesser JD, Leech RW, et al.: Normal and Abnormal Development of the Human Nervous System. New York, Harper & Row, 1975.)

Regression. The processes by which the filum terminale and cauda equina are formed from that portion of the neural tube formed by canalization and by which the conus medullaris eventually comes to lie at its adult level opposite the L1–L2 intervertebral disc space are termed regression, or retrogressive differentiation.[38, 65] These processes begin as early as embryonic stages 18 to 20 (days 43 to 48) and extend throughout the fetal period and on into the early postnatal period (Fig. 2–10).

The ventriculus terminalis is a localized dilatation of the central canal in the conus medullaris and can be identified in stages 18 to 20, at which time it lies opposite the level of the developing C2 level (vertebrae 32). In other words, in the early developmental stages, the spinal cord and the vertebral body levels correspond segment for segment.

As the process of regression begins, an epidermal cell rest known as the coccygeal medullary vestige remains at the level of the tip of the coccygeal vertebral segments. Between this and the ventriculus terminalis, the caudal neural tube regresses and forms the fibrous band called the filum terminale, first identifiable during embryonic stage 23 (day 52). After approximately nine weeks of development, the ventriculus terminalis "ascends" within the spinal canal, by the simultaneous occurrences of regression and of disproportionate growth of the vertebral column relative to the neural tube. Rapid ascent occurs between 9 and 18 weeks of development, at which time the conus medullaris may have reached the level of the L4 vertebral body. Thereafter, ascent slows such that the conus medullaris is at the level of the L3 vertebral body by birth and at the adult level by as early as two months postnatally.[2] Of course, the spinal nerve roots, which early in development exit directly opposite their segmental spinal cord level of origin, become elon-

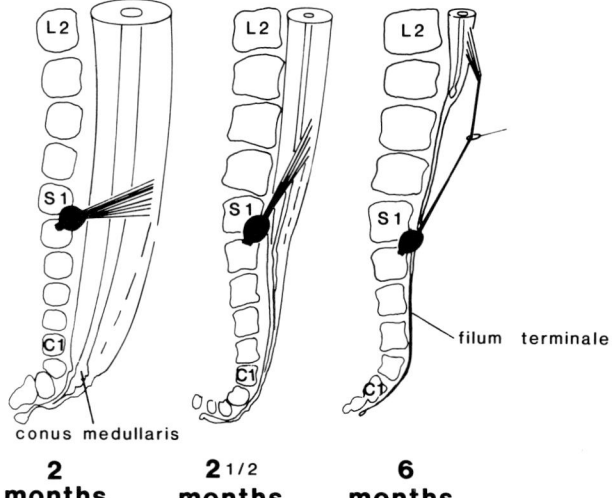

Figure 2–10. Formation of the cauda equina and filum terminale (8 to 25 weeks) during the processes of regression and disproportionate elongation of the vertebral column compared with that of the spinal cord. The conus medullaris "ascends" as a result. (After Streeter GL: Factors involved in the formation of the filum terminale. Am J Anat 25:1, 1919.)

gated as the conus medullaris ascends, thus creating the cauda equina.

Abnormalities of the process of regression may account for the form of occult spinal dysraphism known as the tethered cord syndrome, owing to a thick filum terminale or to bands and adhesions. Any of the processes that prevent the normal separation of neuroectodermal structures from those structures derived from the mesoderm or cutaneous ectoderm may prevent or impair ascent of the conus medullaris and so may tether the developing spinal cord at an abnormally low level early in development.

Formation of the Brain, with Particular Reference to the Cerebellum

The reader is referred to specialized texts concerning the complex development of the brain, but a brief review of the early development of the cephalic neural tube and cerebellum is important to an understanding of the so-called Arnold-Chiari malformation occurring in association with the open forms of spinal dysraphism and the Dandy-Walker malformation.[41, 47]

Early Formation of the Brain. By embryonic stage 10 (days 22 and 23), the cephalic neural folds distinguish the future brain from the slender tube of the future spinal cord. Two constrictions divide the developing brain into three areas: the prosencephalon (forebrain), mesencephalon (midbrain), and rhombencephalon (hindbrain). The divisions become more prominent as the anterior neuropore closes at approximately day 25. By 35 days, the prosencephalon has divided into the telencephalon (future cerebral hemispheres) and the diencephalon, while the rhombencephalon has formed the metencephalon (future pons) and the myelencephalon (future medulla oblongata).

Both cerebral hemispheres, which grow from the telencephalon, contain a cavity, the lateral ventricle. The lateral, third and fourth ventricular cavities are continuous with the central canal of the spinal cord in this early stage. Only subsequent normal development obliterates this communication at the site of the future obex. This fact is quite important to the understanding of hydrosyringomyelia, as it develops in the Arnold-Chiari malformations.

The embryo begins to develop a convex dorsal curve and eventually assumes the shape of the letter C by a process of flexion. The first to form is the cephalic (mesencephalic) flexure, at 20 days, between the prosencephalon and mesencephalon, and by 28 days, the cervical flexure forms between the rhombencephalon and the spinal cord. Both these curves are convex dorsally. At approximately 30 days, the pontine flexure forms a curve that is convex ventrally.

Early Formation of the Cerebellum. The ventrally convex pontine flexure of the rhombencephalon is established at the future level of the trigeminal nerve during days 28 to 39 (five weeks). The pons and cerebellum form from the apex and rostral limb of the flexed rhombencephalon, called the metencephalon, while the caudal limb, called the myelencephalon, forms the medulla oblongata. The pontine flexure probably forms because of an intrinsic differential growth within the rhombencephalon and is quite different in formation from the earlier cephalic and cervical flexures. Somewhat akin to bending a hollow rubber tube at an acute angle, the concave dorsal surface buckles laterally, carrying the alar plates, or rhombic lips, laterally with it and making the lumen of the rhombencephalon the widest portion of the neural tube. The cavity destined to become the fourth ventricle becomes rhomboidal, or diamond-shaped, as a result of the buckling. Also, the rhombic roof is attenuated and is transversely creased during the buckling phenomenon. Within this transverse crease, called the plica choroidea, the choroid plexus eventually forms by six weeks, with the lateral edges of the crease corresponding to the foramina of Luschka. The crease divides the thinned rhombic roof into the area membranacea superior and the area membranacea inferior. The cerebellum develops rostral to the transverse crease and to the area membranacea superior, which eventually forms the posterior medullary velum. The rostral rhomboid roof is more active histologically than the inert-looking caudal rhombic roof or the area membranacea inferior. The caudal roof extends from the plica choroidea to the cervical spinal cord in the area of the future obex. Eventually, the roof attenuates and perforates, to form the midline foramen of Magendie.

The cells in the laterally lying alar plates rostral to the area membranacea superior proliferate extensively during days 34 to 42, to form the thickened, paired rhombic lips, which are the precursors of the cerebellum and which ultimately fuse in the midline at approximately eight weeks of development. The most primitive portions of the cerebellum, the flocculus and nodulus, form the earliest, at the level of the vestibular nuclei.

The cerebellum lies within the fourth ventricle of the rhombencephalon during the first two months of development, and the choroid plexus is essentially dorsal to the cerebellum. Brocklehurst noted that a meshwork of mesenchymal cells and blood vessels surround the dorsal aspect of the rhombencephalon where the roof plate is thin or deficient.[11] However, during the third month, the cerebellum enlarges rapidly and begins to bulge extraventricularly. The sagittal structure of the cerebellum alters as the central portions undergo this rapid proliferation and the cerebellum mushrooms dorsally. The relative inactivity of the roof of the fourth ventricle ventral to the rapidly enlarging cerebellar vermian lobules causes the roof to buckle in a fashion similar to that of a kernel of popcorn exploding and inverting a part of its shell.[41] As a result of this process of involution, the nodulus of the vermis, the posterior medullary velum, the adjacent choroid plexus, and the foramen of Magendie all become tucked in and hidden from view under and between the cerebellar tonsils, by approximately three and one-half months of development. The primitive cerebellum develops rapidly, with formation of the lobules and fissures between one and one-half and four months of gestation.

Formation of the Choroid Plexus and Cerebrospinal Fluid Flow. The choroid plexus first appears in the fourth ventricle at days 43 to 44, in the lateral ventricles at days 45 to 46, and in the third ventricle at days 48 to 49. The relationship of the developing choroid plexus and the perforation of the rhombic roof to form the foramen of Magendie is important to a critical evaluation of the so-called hydrodynamic theory proposed by Gardner as an explanation for a variety of congenital malformations.[30] The rhombencephalic roof protrudes from the dorsal surface of the embryo and becomes attenuated during days 28 to 33. However, the caudal rhombencephalic roof, or the area membranacea inferior, does not perforate to form the foramen of Magendie until approximately days 47 to 48 or even until eight or nine weeks of development.[11, 52] In this same stage, the choroid plexus cells develop the appearance of secretory epithelium and first produce extraventricular cerebrospinal fluid, which helps to open up the loose meshwork of mesenchymal cells surrounding the brain to create the subarachnoid space. The opening up process begins in the cisterna magna and spreads to other basal areas and then over the hemispheres and spinal cord.

Which comes first, perforation or cerebrospinal fluid formation, is argued. Brocklehurst's histologic studies of the roof of the fourth ventricle suggest that perforation of the caudal roof is due to active differentiation occurring prior to the ability of the choroid plexus to form cerebrospinal fluid rather than a bursting of the roof in response to an increase in the intraventricular cerebrospinal fluid pressure.[11]

The central canal of the spinal cord is obliterated normally after birth, by the cellular proliferation within the spinal cord, and thus, the ventricular system terminates at the obex in the caudal floor of the fourth ventricle. The disturbed embryology of the caudal cerebellum in the spina bifida–Arnold-Chiari malformation complex frequently alters this normal course of events, so that the central canal remains patent and enlarged to the point of causing the development of symptomatic hydrosyringomyelia.

Formation of the Vertebrae

The vertebral unit is composed of a vertebral body and posterior elements (pedicles, transverse processes, laminae, and spinous process) and is separated from the other units by the intervertebral discs. Cells originating from the medial portion of the somites form the vertebral units in three stages: a period of membrane formation, from stages 11 to 16 (days 22 to 39); a period of cartilage formation, from stages 17 to 23 and on into the early fetal period (days 40 to 64); and a period of bone formation, which overlaps the later portions of the period of cartilage formation and carries on throughout the fetal period to well beyond birth. The notochord is an important influence on the formation of the vertebral bodies, whereas the neural tube appears to direct formation of the posterior elements.[4]

Membrane Formation Period. The notochord, which is in contact with the neuroectoderm above and the entoderm below during stages 10 and 11 (days 22 to 25), is flanked by the somites. Each somite is divided into a medial half (sclerotome), which ultimately forms the vertebral structures, and a lateral half (myotome), which develops into the supporting musculature. Cells from the sclerotome portion migrate medially to form a perichordal tube, after the notochord separates from the neural tube and the entoderm. This process occurs first in the cervical segments and then proceeds rostrally and caudally. The vertebral bodies ultimately form from the perichordal tube of mesoderm, and other sclerotomic cells migrate dorsally to surround eventually the neural tube, forming the posterior elements.

Cartilage Formation Period. The vertebral body that does form is not from the segmental somites at its level; rather, the segmental arrangement is altered. The sclerotome cells that condense around the notochord to outline a vertebral body originate from adjacent sclerotome pairs. On each side of the notochord, cells from the caudal half of the sclerotome above condense with cells from the rostral half of the sclerotome below. Thus, each vertebral body is composed of portions of four somites. Later, the intervening sclerotome cells form the annulus fibrosus of the intervertebral disc, and the notochord persists as the nucleus pulposus. The notochord within the future vertebral body regresses. Chondrification begins first in the vertebral body and later in a separate center in each neural arch. The centra and arches are chondrified by 47 days of development, but the arches remain incomplete dorsal to the neural tube. Arch closure is progressive, and by 64 days, the arches are complete in the thoracic and upper lumbar regions but remain open in the upper cervical and lower lumbar areas. These are common sites where arches fail to close completely, leaving a simple spina bifida.

Bone Formation Period. Endochondral ossification centers develop in the centra and in each of the neural arch processes and the costal processes. The neural arch processes extend dorsally and medially to form the laminae, and with fusion and further dorsal prolongation, the spinous process is formed. The ventral extension of each arch fuses with the vertebral body; the lateral extension forms the transverse process, with which the rib articulates. The shafts of the ribs are formed by extension of their primary ossification centers. Thus, any process that interferes with development and growth of the vertebral unit may be associated with malformations such as aplasia or fusion of one or more ribs, hemivertebrae, fused vertebrae, or anterior or posterior spina bifida.

The formation of the sacrococcygeal vertebrae deserves special attention. As already mentioned, a maximum of 42 to 44 somite pairs may be formed, with the caudal seven to eight pairs formed in the embryonic tail. The neural tube extends to the level of the most distal somite pair and even beyond, into the tip of the so-called nonvertebrated tail, which does not contain somites. The period of regression that must involve the caudal neural tube also involves these terminal somites. The sacrum is formed at somite levels 25 through 29, and the coccygeal segments usually consume the thirtieth to thirty-fifth pairs. All the remaining somite pairs have regressed by the end of stage 17 (42 days).

Formation of the Skull

The skull, or neurocranium, is divided into two sections. The skull base (occipital, sphenoid, ethmoid, and petrous temporal bones), which is formed by endochondral ossification, and the cranial vault, which is formed by the membranous process. The latter process does not involve a cartilaginous phase. A brief review of the formation of the skull base is pertinent to one of the theories of the origin of the Arnold-Chiari malformation proposed by the Marin-Padillas.[45]

The notochord separates from the neural tube in the cervical and cranial areas during stage 12 (days 26 to 27), and subsequent prechordal and parachordal mesodermal condensations form nearly all the major bones of the skull base. The rostral tip of the notochord marks the junction between the occipital bone and the sphenoid bone. The first chondrification begins during stage 17 (40 to 44 days) in the basiocciput and the body of the sphenoid. The occipital bone has four endochondral ossification centers, which create the clivus, the occipital arch around the foramen magnum, and the supraoccipital part of the occipital bone, which is that portion below the inion and the superior nuchal line. The occipital bone above the superior nuchal line is termed the interparietal occipital bone, and it is formed by the membranous process, as are all of the bones of the cranial vault. These two portions of the occipital bone unite in approximately the third month. The other three bones of the skull base are the sphenoid bone; ethmoid bone, including the crista galli, cribriform plate, ethmoidal labyrinth, and the cartilaginous nasal septum; and the petrous portion of the temporal bone. The endochondral skull base appears to have its own intrinsic growth potential and, in contrast to the passive intramembranous bone of the cranial vault, is subject to abnormal osseous development independent of the influence of the overlying neural structures. This is particularly true of the bones around the foramen magnum, which are malformed in occipitoatlantal fusion and platybasia, or basilar impression.

SPINA BIFIDA APERTA AND THE ARNOLD-CHIARI MALFORMATION

Spina Bifida Aperta

The subtypes of spina bifida aperta listed in Table 2–1 refer to those open forms of spinal dysraphism most familiar to neurosurgeons.[27] The anatomy of the open defect fits well with a process disordering the normal development already described. At the open area, the neural malformation is exposed on the surface, and, obviously, the other tissue layers that were to close in the midline over neural tissue are separated. The skin is deficient but is in continuity with the edge of the neural plaque, through an intervening layer of modified epithelium and arachnoid called the zona epithelioserosa. The dura is splayed widely open, with its lateral margins ballooned over the edges of the open pedicles and hypoplastic lamina that form the spina bifida. The dura lies gently adherent to the underlying fascia covering the paraspinous muscles and fuses laterally to the edge of the skin defect.

The spina bifida varies in its extent, depending on whether the posterior elements at the T12–L1 level are normally formed. If T12 and L1 are involved, the entire lumbar and sacral spine is also bifid, regardless of the level of the neurocutaneous lesion; if the T12 and L1 posterior elements are normal, the posterior spina bifida may be localized to the lumbar or to the sacral spine and correlates closely with the level of the neurocutaneous malformation.[3] As a consequence of the time during embryonic development that the neural defect forms, the spinal cord is always abnormally low in myelomeningocele and is tethered to the surrounding tissues.

The subtypes of spina bifida aperta reveal fascinating clinical and pathologic variations, which should be explained by any theory of abnormal embryology that addresses this deformity.[23]

Myeloschisis. In myeloschisis, the neural tube at the site of the defect is totally open, with no evidence of the central canal having been formed. It is commonly found at the thoracolumbar junction and is associated with a posterior spina bifida of the entire lumbar and sacral spines.

Myelomeningocele and Hemimyelomeningocele.

In myelomeningocele and hemimyelomeningocele, a central canal has been formed, although it may be partially open to a variable degree on the dorsal surface of the neural plaque. These forms seem to be more commonly found in the lumbar and sacral regions, in contrast to a myeloschisis. The hemimyelomeningocele is a special variation that involves a diastematomyelia with septum. One hemicord is found in its own bony spinal canal, and usually, the ipsilateral lower limb has a better level of function than does the limb supplied by the adjacent hemicord, which is exposed on the surface as a "hemimyelomeningocele." This form is different from the diastematomyelia with or without septum that may occur above the open neural plaque area.

Hydrosyringomyelomeningocele. The hydrosyringomyelomeningocele is a rare form, commonly found in the cervical or thoracic areas and often misinterpreted as a meningocele because the patient's neurologic function is usually normal. The malformation appears to be a herniation of a dilated central canal and dysplastic neural tissue between the dorsal columns of a fused spinal cord through a localized posterior spina bifida. The dysplastic neural tissue in the wall of the sac differentiates this lesion from a benign meningocele.

Spinal Meningocele. Spinal meningocele is rare. This form, by definition, means that the patient is neurologically normal, and it usually involves only an outpouching of the meninges, with a normally formed spinal cord located safely within the spinal canal. This is not to say that nerve roots cannot be adherent to the neck of the meningeal sac and cannot be endangered by cavalier dissection, or that the spinal cord is not tethered abnormally low by intraspinal anomalies, but, at least at birth, the neural structures function normally. In this simpler form, the incidence of the Arnold-Chiari malformation and of hydrocephalus is less than in the complex forms.

Any theory offered to explain the formation of these forms of spina bifida aperta should also explain frequently found associated malformations such as the Arnold-Chiari malformation; diastematomyelia (without septum) located above the plaque (found in approximately one quarter of cases in autopsy studies); and hydrosyringomyelia of the proximal cord (found in 43 percent of cases). Other minor malformations are frequently found as well.[27]

Arnold-Chiari Malformation

Whether the eponym "Arnold-Chiari" is applied properly to this malformation, in a historical sense, has been debated. The term has been used in the clinical setting for years, although some authors refer to this malformation occurring in 90 percent of all infants with spina bifida aperta as the Chiari type II anomaly.[17, 27] In any event, the anomaly has a number of variable but key features: the inferior cerebellar vermis and fourth ventricle are displaced caudally or are prolonged into the upper cervical spinal canal; the cervicomedullary junction is caudally displaced or prolonged below the level of the foramen magnum into the upper cervical spinal canal; the medulla oblongata is often kinked dorsally over the upper cervical spinal cord; the upper cervical nerve roots run a cephalad course; and hydrosyringomyelia and hydrocephalus frequently occur, as well as other anatomic variations listed in Table 2-2.[27]

However, in infants with spina bifida aperta, there is a gradation of severity of the anatomic abnormalities, which is described well by Emery and MacKenzie, but the degree of severity does not correlate directly with the anatomic level of the spinal lesion.[25] A number of the more minor degrees of Arnold-Chiari malformation occur with the caudal lumbar or sacral myelomeningocele. Occasionally, no Arnold-Chiari malformation develops with the hydrosyringomyelomeningocele. The influence of the hydrodynamic effects of hydrocephalus may modify some features of the malformation, including the degree of caudal displacement of the brainstem and cerebellum, the molding of the collicular plate, the shape and size of the aqueduct, the presence of the cerebellar "tower," and the development of hydrosyringomyelia.

Embryologic Timing of Development of Spina Bifida Aperta and Arnold-Chiari Malformation

The anatomic and pathologic variations in spina bifida aperta and Arnold-Chiari malformation imply

Table 2–2. ANOMALIES ASSOCIATED WITH THE ARNOLD-CHIARI–SPINA BIFIDA COMPLEX

Cerebellum	Caudal displacement of vermis and fourth ventricle; cerebellum smaller than normal
Brainstem	Caudal displacement of pons, medulla, and cervicomedullary junction with kink; displaced basilar and vertebral arteries; stretching of lower cranial nerves
Cervical and lower spinal cord	Compression of upper segments; hydrosyringomyelia
Midbrain	Tectal "beak"; aqueduct stenosis and forking
Cerebral hemispheres and third ventricle	Polymicrogyria; cortical heterotopia; enlarged massa intermedia; Meynert's commissure; hydrocephalus
Meninges	Hypoplasia of falx cerebri; low-set tentorium with enlarged incisura; low position of torcula and lateral sinuses; thick, adhesive leptomeninges at foramen magnum
Skull and cervical spine	Craniolacunia; enlarged foramen magnum; small posterior fossa; scalloped petrous bone; enlarged upper cervical spinal canal

Table 2–3. TIME OF OCCURRENCE OF MALFORMATIONS OF THE BRAIN AND SPINE

Malformation	Gestational Age (days)
Neurenteric cyst; diastematomyelia with septum; combined spina bifida	16–17
Congenital dermal sinus	22–48
Myeloschisis	26–27 or 28+
Arnold-Chiari malformation	28–39+
Myelomeningocele; lumbosacral lipoma; lipomyelomeningocele	28–48
Tethered cord syndrome; spinal meningocele	43–fetal period
Dandy-Walker malformation	60+

that the causative multifactorial teratogenic events may occur at any time from near the end of neurulation, at 28 days, to some period after neurulation, when the less complex anomalies, such as the spinal meningocele, probably form (Table 2–3).

In general, the earlier the event occurs during the development of the nervous system, the higher the neuroanatomic level of the spinal lesion and the more severe are the associated anomalies. For example, an insult occurring just prior to or just after closure of the posterior neuropore, at 28 days, is likely to cause a myeloschisis at the thoracolumbar junction, a posterior spina bifida of the entire lumbosacral spine, and, probably, a more severe degree of the Arnold-Chiari malformation and other brain anomalies. This latter assumption has yet to be pathologically proved, although clinical experience suggests that the higher the spinal lesion, the greater is the incidence of hydrocephalus and the lower the intellectual achievements.

In contrast, an insult occurring after closure of the posterior neuropore is associated with a lower lumbar or sacral myelomeningocele in which the spinal cord already has developed through the neural tube stage, the posterior spina bifida may be localized, and the spinal cord may be formed normally below the level of the open lesion, in occasional patients. Clinical experience indicates that the frequency of hydrocephalus and Arnold-Chiari malformation is less in the later-occurring lower lesions and that intellectual development may be normal (Fig. 2–11). Indeed, in spinal meningocele, the neural tube development is virtually normal, and the meninges, posterior elements of the spine, and the skin are the main participants in the lesion.

The pathologic material studied in spina bifida aperta suggests that the spinal lesion may develop just before or just after neurulation and may create a myeloschisis at a higher level, or that it may involve the lower regions of the spine where the neural tube has formed, either by neurulation or canalization, in which case a myelomeningocele is created. Such a lower lesion could form early in the second month of development, if these observations are valid. The embryologic timing of the occurrence of the Arnold-Chiari malformation is not clear.

The terms prolongation, displacement, and herniation are used interchangeably to describe the caudal location of the cerebellar vermis and brainstem, as compared to normal individuals. Prolongation implies that the structures are abnormally lengthened and are, thereby, in an abnormal location; displacement, or herniation, implies some active process forcing the structures into their abnormal location. Both factors, a primary embryologic malformation and a secondary active displacement may, in fact, play a part in the evolution of the malformation.

For example, in the Arnold-Chiari malformation, the choroid plexus of the fourth ventricle is frequently found external to the ventricle and matted over the cervicomedullary junction; the anatomic divisions of the vermis are plastered out over the upper cervical cord area, rather than being "tucked up" within the fourth ventricle; and the brainstem does appear to be truly elongated. These anatomic variations could have their origin in the failure of the pontine flexure to form normally from the twenty-eighth to the thirty-ninth day of gestation, leading to an elongated brainstem. The normal growth of the midportion of the cerebellum during the third month ultimately leads to the caudal vermis and choroid plexus tucking in under the cerebellar tonsils. A failure of this process could lead to the persistent extraventricular position of the vermis and choroid plexus seen pathologically. Once this anatomic malformation is created, the normal processes of cerebrospinal fluid circulation

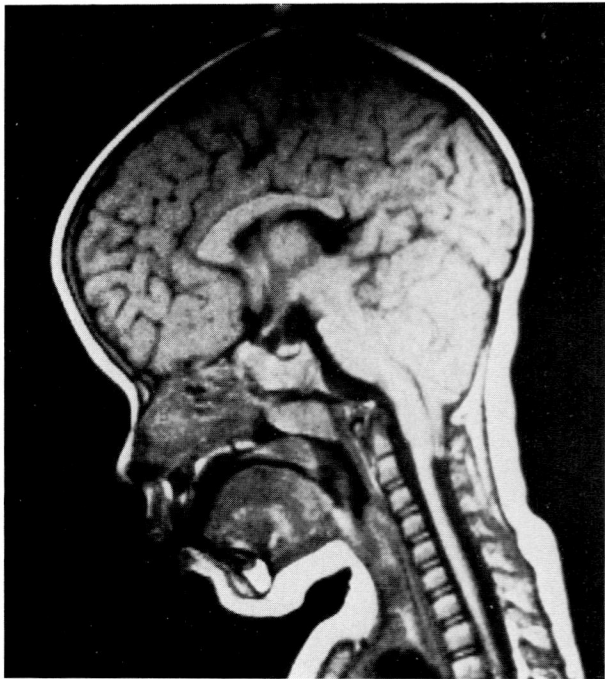

Figure 2–11. Nuclear magnetic resonance imaging scan of a child with spina bifida–Arnold-Chiari complex. Note the cervicomedullary "kink" at the C2 to C3 level, overlying tongue of cerebellar vermis, slit fourth ventricle, elongated brainstem, "beaking" of the collicular plate region, and enlarged massa intermedia. The spinal cord is normal, with no evidence of hydrosyringomyelia.

may be disturbed. This could lead to an embryonic hydrocephalus and a directing of the outflow of cerebrospinal fluid of the fourth ventricular into the central canal, since formation of the foramen of Magendie is impaired. A persistent hydromyelia could follow. The hydrocephalus could also cause an increase in the extent of prolongation or herniation of the cerebellar tissues into the upper cervical spine and could push the tentorium further inferiorly, to decrease the size of the posterior fossa (Fig. 2–12).

In other words, a primary embryonic malformation could, in itself, lead to secondary hydrodynamic factors important in increasing the severity of the anatomic malformation. The earlier in gestation the causative event acts, the more likely these normal embryogenic steps are to be disturbed and to lead to a higher, anatomically more primitive spinal lesion and an increase in the occurrence of associated malformations. The later in gestation the event occurs, the more likely these critical steps are to be initiated normally, resulting in a lower, more developmentally advanced spinal lesion and a less frequent occurrence and lesser severity of the associated malformations.

THEORIES OF ABNORMAL EMBRYOGENESIS OF SPINA BIFIDA APERTA AND THE ARNOLD-CHIARI MALFORMATION

Unfortunately, no single theory proposed satisfactorily explains all of the pathologic variations witnessed clinically in spina bifida aperta or the Arnold-Chiari malformation. The theories that have been offered attempt to explain the mechanisms for the malformations but do not stipulate the cause that initiates those mechanisms. This is understandable, since the etiology of spina bifida aperta is multifactorial, with both genetic and environmental interactions involved.[67] The theories fall into five general groups, with one additional theory reserved for the Arnold-Chiari malformation: (1) developmental arrest; (2) overgrowth; (3) hydrodynamic mechanisms; (4) neuroschisis; (5) neuroectodermal-mesodermal spatial dyssynchrony; and (6) the outmoded traction theory, suggested as a cause of the Arnold-Chiari malformation. Woven into all these theories is the question of whether the spinal defect develops before the neural tube closes or after it has closed and becomes covered with cutaneous ectoderm. The fact that the cutaneous ectoderm is in continuity with the exposed neuroectoderm has been used as proof that the neural tube never closed; however, experimental work suggests that a closed neural tube covered by cutaneous ectoderm can reopen and develop continuity with the edges of the split cutaneous ectoderm.[62] The presence of

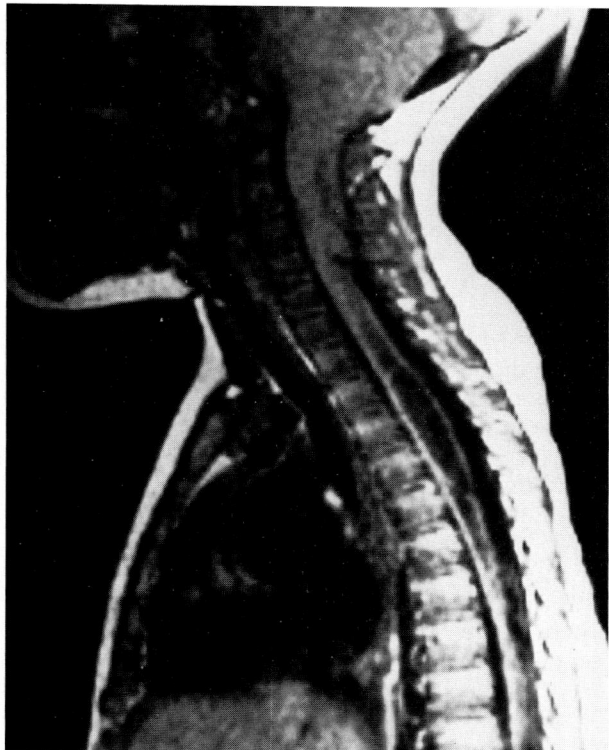

Figure 2–12. Nuclear magnetic resonance imaging scan of a child with spina bifida–Arnold-Chiari complex with displacement of the cervicomedullary junction to the C4 level, prominent dorsal "kink" of the brainstem over the cervical spinal cord, and marked hydrosyringomyelia. The degree of malformation is quite marked compared with the mild Arnold-Chiari malformation shown in Figure 2–11.

a central canal in many human specimens indicates that neurulation did occur before the neural plaque became exposed, and thus reopening of fused cutaneous ectoderm to expose the neurulated cord must occur in many forms.[23] In addition, the sacral myelomeningocele may involve spinal cord created by canalization under intact cutaneous ectoderm. Thus, opening of this intact ectoderm layer must occur in the lower lesions, if the mechanism of canalization is valid in the human.

Developmental Arrest

This theory proposes that myeloschisis is a simple failure of the neural plate to close because of an arrest of normal development, with subsequent secondary changes in the surrounding tissue.[72] However, not all open lesions are in the form of a myeloschisis, and the theory does not adequately explain the neurulated types. Indeed, the occurrence of open lesions at levels of the spinal cord formed by canalization under intact cutaneous ectoderm is not addressed. Such lesions must involve breakdown of the cutaneous layer to expose the neural tissue.

Developmental arrest of the brainstem was invoked as a cause of the Arnold-Chiari malformation by Daniel and Strich[22] in 1958 and was expanded later by other authors.[24, 58, 59] If the pontine flexure that develops at the level of the pons at stages 13 to 16 (days 28 to 39) were to fail to form, then the pons and medulla would be abnormally elongated into the future cervical spinal canal. When the cervical flexure straightens during the second month, the elongated brainstem could bulge dorsally over the upper cervical spinal cord that is fixed by the dentate ligaments and could thus create the "kink." Failure of the vermis of the cerebellum and the adjacent choroid plexus to become tucked up within the fourth ventricle, as normally occurs during the rapid development of the central cerebellum during the third month, would create the elongated tail of caudal vermis and matted choroid plexus found over the cervicomedullary junction. The caudal displacement of the cerebellum and brainstem causes the foramen magnum to be enlarged and the posterior fossa to be small and permits the tentorium to migrate to an abnormally low position.

While the theory of developmental arrest has been expanded to explain the malformations of the Arnold-Chiari complex, it is deficient in describing all the subtypes of the open spinal lesions, the associated spinal cord anomalies, and the associated cerebral anomalies.

In 1981, a new theory was offered by Marin-Padilla and Marin-Padilla.[45] The explanation for the spinal lesion has yet to be presented in as detailed a fashion for the Arnold-Chiari malformation, but it would involve the same basic mechanism. A primary mesodermal deficiency is the cause of all the neural developmental abnormalities. Their theory for the Arnold-Chiari malformation is an extension from observations in pregnant hamsters treated with vitamin A. A primary paraxial mesodermal insufficiency results in underdevelopment of the occipital bone, particularly the basal portion. As a result, the posterior fossa is short and small and is therefore inadequate to contain the developing cerebellum and brainstem. Also, the skull base is flattened, compared with that of a normal person. The overall consequence is that the cerebellum must grow toward the foramen magnum, the pontine flexure is reduced, and the angle of the cervical flexure is increased. The mesodermal abnormality might affect an embryo before, during, or after closure of the neural folds and, thus, might explain all varieties of cranial and spinal dysraphism, open and closed. No experimental embryo had displacement of the cerebellum below the foramen magnum because that displacement is attributed to the postnatal growth of the cerebellum or possibly to the development of hydrocephalus, a secondary factor.

Several problems exist in applying this experimental model to the human situation as the Marin-Padillas do: (1) The model demonstrates a tendency toward, but not the full expression of, the Arnold-Chiari malformation; (2) which dysgenesis comes first, neural or mesodermal, is not proved; (3) the Arnold-Chiari malformation has been shown to exist in human embryos as early as 16 to 18 weeks of development, with and without hydrocephalus[1, 12, 36, 49]; (4) the cerebellum has been shown to be smaller than normal at all postnatal ages in the Arnold-Chiari malformation, suggesting the small posterior fossa may be a secondary phenomenon;[69] and (5) the flattening of the nasion-sella-basion angle may be a secondary occurrence in the second half of gestation, according to human embryo examination.[36]

Overgrowth

This theory suggests that an overgrowth of the neural plate prior to neurulation everts the neural folds and prevents their fusion. Thus, an open neural tube lesion in the form of a myeloschisis is created. The theory was proposed in 1881 by Lebedeff from observations in chicken embryos and was adopted by Cleland in 1883 to explain some forms of spina bifida aperta in humans.[18] More recently, the theory has been associated with observations in human embryos by Patten,[55, 56] by Lemire and coworkers,[42] and by Osaka and colleagues.[49] Debate exists as to whether overgrowth is the primary cause of, or is a secondary reaction to, either the failure of fusion or a reopening of a fused neural tube.

The same objection holds for this theory as for the theory of arrested development. The occurrence of open lesions at levels of the cord formed by canalization under intact cutaneous ectoderm and the occurrence of lesions with a central canal indicating neurulation are not addressed. Such lesions must involve an opening of the cutaneous layer to expose the neural tube, which may or may not then open as a myeloschisis or remain partially or totally closed as a myelomeningocele.

In 1957, Barry and coworkers reported an increase in the volume of the cerebellum and brainstem in two human fetuses of 17 weeks and 18 weeks of development, with evidence of the Arnold-Chiari malformation.[1] They noted that the posterior fossa was abnormally small and the tentorium was inferiorly situated. An overgrowth of the cerebral hemispheres was believed responsible for displacing the tentorium caudally and causing a diminution in the volume of the posterior fossa. They proposed that the too large cerebellum and brainstem in a too small posterior fossa led to caudal herniation and kinking of the cervicomedullary junction. Hydrocephalus was present in only one of the specimens. Thus, overgrowth of the cerebellum and brainstem, along with overgrowth of the cerebrum, was invoked as a cause for the Arnold-Chiari malformation.

The fact that the cerebellum is smaller than normal in later life in children with spina bifida aperta was attributed rather vaguely to changes in differential growth in the second half of gestation. No other authors studying the problem have suggested that the posterior fossa structures were overgrown, and certainly not the cerebral hemispheres.[12, 26] The cerebellum in infants with the Arnold-Chiari malformation weighs uniformly less than normal at all ages.[69] Thus, the overgrowth theory can be abandoned as an explanation for the Arnold-Chiari malformation.

Hydrodynamic Mechanisms

Although the hydrodynamic theory is associated with W. J. Gardner, many authors have espoused earlier but less expansive theories or alternative hydrodynamic mechanisms.[13, 15, 25, 30, 68] Gardner's monograph, "The Dysraphic States from Syringomyelia to Anencephaly," details the historical development of the hydrodynamic theories through Morgagni and Chiari and his own concept that all dysraphic states can be explained by a series of mechanical steps consequent to the inadequate escape of fluid from the neural tube during the embryonic period, or from the subarachnoid space during later development.[30] The essential features of the theory depend to a great deal upon the developmental chronology of the rhombencephalic roof, through which communication with the primitive subarachnoid space first occurs.

As already mentioned, the rhombencephalic roof is divided by a transverse fissure, the plica choroidea, into a superior and an inferior portion. The choroid plexus develops in the fissure. The area membranacea superior develops between the cerebellum above and the plica choroidea below and is destined to thicken to form the posterior medullary velum. The area membranacea inferior forms between the plica choroidea above and the obex region below and later perforates to form the foramen of Magendie. Initially, the attenuated roof of the rhombencephalon begins to bulge as early as days 28 to 34, soon after the closure of the posterior neuropore, presumably as a result of the accumulation of a proteinaceous material within the neural tube, even before the formation of cerebrospinal fluid. After formation of the choroid plexus in the fourth ventricle during days 43 and 44 of development, a so-called physiologic hydrocephalus and hydromyelia develop, according to W. J. Gardner. The semipermeable membrane of the area membranacea superior is the first route of escape for fluid into the primitive subarachnoid space. With subsequent development, the area membranacea superior thickens, the area membranacea inferior opens to form the foramen of Magendie, and a defined anatomic communication is created between the fourth ventricle and the subarachnoid space.

Early reports suggested that patency is achieved by 12 to 16 weeks of development, but Brocklehurst[12] and Padget[52] have observed open foramina in human embryos at developmental stages as early as eight or nine weeks. W. J. Gardner suggests that either too rapid an accumulation of fluid or too little an escape through the rhombencephalic roof can cause an overdistension of the neural tube to a degree that a rupture occurs at some site. An extensive rupture at the cranial end of the neural tube can cause anencephaly; a rupture at the lower end causes a myeloschisis. Various stages and complexities of rupture can create virtually any of the open or occult dysraphic malformations.

According to Gardner, the Arnold-Chiari malformation forms because of an unequal competition between the pulsating choroid plexus in the fourth ventricle and that in the lateral ventricles. He applies two mechanical theories. The Bering effect attributes the ventricular cerebrospinal fluid pulse wave to the arterial pulsation within the choroid plexus; the law of Laplace finds the distending tension (T) in a cylindric vessel of any given pressure (P) directly proportional to the radius (R), or $T = P \times R$. The choroid plexus of the fourth ventricle forms first at six weeks of development but is rapidly exceeded in size by that in the lateral ventricles a few days later. The Bering effect is more pronounced in the lateral ventricles and results in the cerebral hemispheres gradually encroaching posteriorly to cause the migration of the tentorium to its final resting place. In the event of a caudal neural tube rupture for reasons just explained, the Bering effect of the small fourth ventricle choroid plexus is completely dissipated, and the Bering effect of the lateral ventricles is relatively enhanced, producing a marked posterior migration of the tentorium. As a result, the posterior fossa is small, and the hindbrain and cerebellum are forced, or herniated, out of the posterior fossa into the upper cervical spinal canal. The subsequent impairment of cerebrospinal fluid circulation by this herniation leads to the hydrocephalus above, with further compression on the midbrain, perhaps leading to aqueductal stenosis and the usual midbrain tectal malformation.

Gardner's theory has been criticized on several points. Those who believe that myeloschisis forms because of a failure of the neural tube to close dismiss it out of hand. Others point to the fact that fetal myeloschisis has been found even before evidence of choroid plexus formation and have not found embryonic hydrocephalus in young embryos with myeloschisis.[1, 42, 49] If cerebrospinal fluid production is required to produce the overdistension necessary for rupture of the neural tube, then the theory is deficient. However, Gardner believes that excessive proteinaceous fluid found within the neural tube before choroid plexus formation is sufficient to rupture the tube.

Anencephaly or craniorachischisis are extensive lesions, and one would suspect that the initial point of rupture would decompress the distending forces within the neural tube and limit the extent of the lesion. Even more basic is the belief that the roof plate of the rhombencephalon is burst by the secretory pressure of the cerebrospinal fluid in a physiologically distended neural tube. Brocklehurst suggests that a sequential developmental process of the roof plate results in the foramen opening, rather than a mechanistic blowout.[11]

These criticisms of Gardner's theory on the cause of spina bifida aperta and the Arnold-Chiari malformation should not be interpreted to mean that hydrodynamic mechanisms are not important to the pathologic evolution or the clinical manifestations of spinal dysraphism. It is quite clear that active hydrocephaly can contribute to the clinical presentation of the Arnold-Chiari malformation and to the evolution of hydrosyringomyelia.[27]

Neuroschisis

Dorcas Padget developed a theory of spinal dysraphism that postulates a reopening of the closed neural tube, based on observations in monkey and human embryos.[50-52] A cleft develops in the dorsal midline of the closed neural tube, permitting the proteinaceous material within to escape into the surrounding mesoderm and to elevate the overlying cutaneous ectoderm. Padget likened the elevation to a dermatologic blister and named the embryonic lesion a neuroschistic bleb. The future of the bleb varies from total healing to creation of an adhesion between cutaneous and neuroectoderm (congenital dermal sinus) or to rupture through the cutaneous ectoderm, resulting in an open spinal lesion. The edges of the cutaneous ectoderm become fused secondarily to the everted edges of the neural plate, thus converting the lesion into one having the appearance of the "never closed" neural tube lesion, which fits in with the prevailing theory of nonclosure. Bleb formation can occur at any level of the neural tube and at any site around the circumference, thus explaining some of the ventral lesions as well as the forms of cranial dysraphism.

Padget also explained the Arnold-Chiari malformation as a sequel to a neural cleft, which allows fluid to escape from the neural tube. Embryonic microcephaly results, and the cerebellar primordia prematurely approximate and fuse in a posterior fossa already small. Subsequent development of the cerebellum in the too small posterior fossa leads to herniation into the upper cervical spinal canal. Hydrocephalus follows this obstruction at the level of the fourth ventricle or is due to aqueduct stenosis caused by folding and fusion at the level of the midbrain due to microcephaly. Support for the theory of primary embryonic microcephaly with secondary hydrocephalus is provided by the frequent clinical observation that infants with myelomeningocele may have a normal head circumference despite marked hydrocephalus. The head becomes microcephalic after successful shunting.

Objections to this theory are few, as it is a relatively recent proposal. Osaka and associates observed neuroschistic lesions in both normal embryos and those with myeloschisis but could not relate the lesions to neural tube defects.[49] They suggested that the neuroschistic lesion could even be an artifact of handling.

Neuroectodermal-Mesodermal Spatial Dyssynchrony

Jennings and coworkers studied a 130-day-old fetus in detail and presented a new theory invoking an abnormally low origin for the transition zone between the brain and the cervical spinal cord.[36] Normally, the zone develops at the point of initial fusion of the neural folds adjacent to the third and fourth somites, which happens to be the site of the foramen magnum. They postulate that the initial area of fusion of the neural folds is displaced caudally below the third to fifth somite pairs. Essentially, this displaces the area of formation of the cervicomedullary junction into the future cervical spinal canal. Since the initial closure of the neural folds initiates a progressive "flow" of closure distally, this wave of closure may precede sufficient maturation of the caudal tissues. The closure of the posterior neuropore might remain uncompleted, creating a caudal neuroschisis. As the authors state, "This hypothesis links the initial site of fusion of the neural folds with the establishment of a cervicomedullary junction relative to the appropriate mesodermal support structures."

The theory is similar to Daniel and Strich's suggestion that the pontine flexure fails to form.[22] In the latter, the brainstem is displaced caudally and develops in the upper cervical spine; the cause is the elongation of the brainstem. In the theory proposed by Jennings and associates, the cause is more complex and involves a displacement of the site of formation of the cervicomedullary junction into the spine primarily. Evaluation of this theory will depend on examination of future early gestational specimens.

Traction

The traction theory, described by Penfield and Coburn, suggests that the fixation of the spinal cord to the skin at a low level prevented upward migration of the spinal cord during early development.[60] Thus, the cerebellum and brainstem were pulled down into the cervical spinal canal as the vertebral column elongated. Objections to the theory are incontrovertible:[27] (1) The traction force caused by the fixation of the spinal cord low in the spinal canal is dissipated within five segments above the fixation; (2) the spinal cord is tethered low in the spinal canal in occult spinal dysraphism, and yet the Arnold-Chiari malformation is not found; (3) the dorsal aspects of the pons, medulla, and upper cervical cord are displaced more than the ventral portions, which would not be the case in traction from below; (4) the anatomy of the dorsal kink can be explained only by the structures being displaced from above rather than pulled down from below; (5) the Arnold-Chiari malformation is absent in some cases of low lumbar or sacral myelomeningoceles, in which traction forces might be expected to be maximal, and has been reported in a patient with normal lower spine and spinal cord; (6) the malformation may be seen in embryos before the spinal cord ascends to a great degree; and (7) experimental tethering of the spinal cord in animals has failed to produce the malformation.[1, 15, 24-27, 33, 49, 57] Thus, the traction theory is an outdated historical theory that should not be invoked as an explanation for the occurrence of the Arnold-Chiari malformation.

CHIARI I MALFORMATION AND HYDROSYRINGOMYELIA

The Arnold-Chiari malformation associated with spina bifida aperta that has been discussed to this point is considered an embryologically more complex abnormality affecting widespread areas of the central nervous system. Its origin in time must be early, at or soon after the closure of the posterior neuropore, at 28 days of gestation, and the formation of the pontine flexure, between 28 and 39 days. This form has been referred to as the "Chiari II" malformation.[16]

On the other hand, the anatomically simpler Arnold-Chiari malformation associated with hydrosyringomyelia involves only the caudal cerebellum and the obex. The vermis is generally normal, and it is the elongated tonsils that project below the level of the foramen magnum over the dorsal cervical spinal cord. The brainstem is not elongated, the cervicomedullary junction is at the foramen magnum, the nerve roots run a more horizontal course, and the remainder of the brain is normal. The volume of the posterior fossa is normal. The spine is also normal, but for scoliosis; hydrocephalus rarely develops; and clinical presentation is delayed into the first decade or adulthood. Embryologically, the origin has to be later in gestation, prior to the time the caudal vermis and tonsillar area are "tucking up" into their normal relationship, by three and one-half months of development. This form has been referred to as the "Chiari I" malformation (Fig. 2–13).

However, the continuum of "severities" of the Arnold-Chiari malformation in these entities is also clear. Some patients with spina bifida aperta have no Arnold-Chiari malformation, some have a profound caudal brainstem malformation. The majority

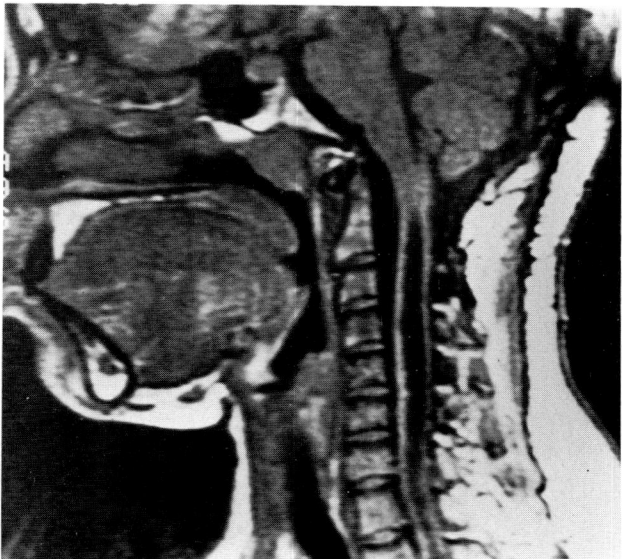

Figure 2–13. Adolescent experiencing loss of temperature and pain sensation in one upper extremity, in whom there was no evidence of spina bifida. Mild Arnold-Chiari malformation (Chiari type I) with marked hydrosyringomyelia extending almost to the cervicomedullary junction. Note the normal fourth ventricle and the lack of displacement of the vermis on the midline sagittal scan. The tonsils were displaced asymmetrically to the C1 and C2 levels, lateral to the plane of this scan, and the obex was patent into the syrinx.

have a malformation between the extremes. The simpler Arnold-Chiari malformation associated with hydrosyringomyelia may present early or late in life, with or without the spinal cord syrinx and, occasionally, with some suggestion of mild caudal brainstem displacement, observed at operation. The categorization of the Arnold-Chiari malformation as "I" or "II" is too simplistic.

DANDY-WALKER MALFORMATION

The Dandy-Walker malformation is a developmental abnormality of the rostral embryonic roof of the rhombencephalon associated with a varying degree of hypoplasia of the cerebellar vermis and the medial aspects of the cerebellar hemispheres. The fourth ventricle forms a large cavity and may act as an expansile cyst, and the exit foramina may or may not be atretic. The cystic expansion enlarges the posterior fossa and is associated with elevation of the tentorium cerebelli and lateral sinuses onto the parietal bones. Hydrocephalus and other neuroanatomic and systemic abnormalities occur frequently. For example, agenesis of the corpus callosum occurs in 30 percent of patients (Fig. 2–14).

The time of occurrence in embryonic development seems clear. The paired alar plates lie above the area membranacea inferior and proliferate actively from five weeks to eight weeks, at which time they fuse in the midline. The foramen of

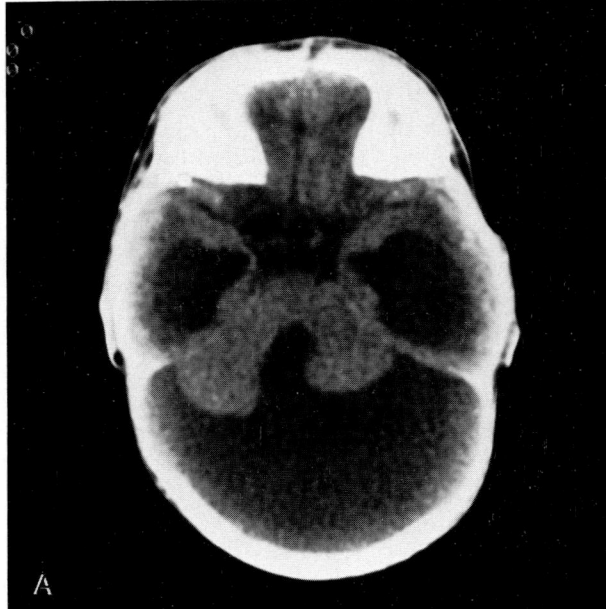 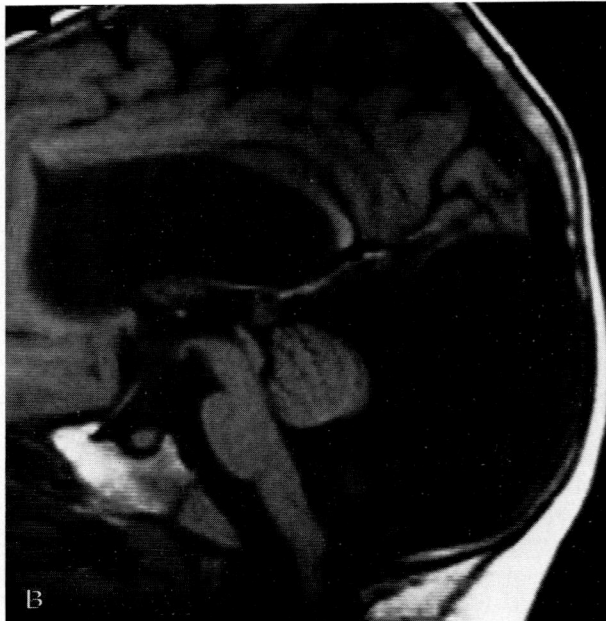

Figure 2–14. Dandy-Walker malformation in an infant with hydrocephalus. A, The CT scan shows prominent temporal horn enlargement and a large cystlike area in the markedly enlarged posterior fossa. The vermis and both cerebellar hemispheres are hypoplastic, with the fourth ventricle open to the "cyst." Contrast material in the ventricles did not enter the posterior fossa "cyst" because of occlusion at the level of the cerebral aqueduct. B, Nuclear magnetic resonance imaging scan of Dandy-Walker malformation showing the hypoplasia of the corpus callosum, profound vermal hypoplasia, and huge posterior fossa. Compare the upwardly displaced tentorium in this child with the inferiorally displaced tentorium in the Arnold-Chiari malformation in Figure 2–11.

Magendie may open anytime from seven to nine weeks of development, which "decompresses" the fourth ventricle. The interplay between the evolution of the alar plates and the timing of permeability of the area membranacea superior and perforation of the area membranacea inferior to form the foramen of Magendie is crucial to the development of a Dandy-Walker malformation.

An element of confusion and overlap occurs with the posterior fossa extra-axial arachnoid cyst associated with a normal-sized but compressed fourth ventricle and hydrocephalus and with the fourth ventricular ependymal cyst that expands the fourth ventricle.

Abnormal Embryology

The development of this embryonic abnormality is based on the normal cerebellar embryology already discussed. Four main theories have been proposed to explain the disturbed formation of the rhombic roof and corpus cerebelli: (1) congenital atresia of the foramina of Magendie and Luschka; (2) dysraphism of the corpus cerebelli; (3) neuroschisis; and (4) hydrodynamic mechanisms.

Congenital Atresia of the Foramina of Magendie and Luschka. In 1914, Dandy and Blackfan reported a patient with hydrocephalus presumed to be due to inflammatory obstruction of the foramina of Magendie and Luschka. A greatly dilated fourth ventricle separated the lateral lobes of the cerebellum.[20] In 1917, they reported a similar patient with congenital closure of the foramina and postulated that an intrauterine inflammatory process had caused a condition resembling that reported in 1914.[21] In 1921, Dandy reviewed congenital occlusion of the foramina of Magendie and Luschka as a specific cause of hydrocephalus and concluded that ". . . this type of hydrocephalus results from the failure of these foramina to develop, rather than a secondary closure after development."[19]

In 1942, Taggart and Walker also stated that congenital atresia of the foramina of Magendie and Luschka was the primary factor producing the dilated fourth ventricle with secondary maldevelopment of the cerebellar vermis and hydrocephalus.[66]

However, in 1955, Gibson found the foramina of Luschka open in some cases.[32] He also found remnants of the vermis in the cyst wall and hypothesized that the vermis was compressed and distorted rather than absent. Thus, midline fusion of the corpus cerebelli might have occurred normally at eight weeks of development, with later secondary compression by the expanded fourth ventricle.

The finding of open fourth ventricular outlets has been confirmed by several authors and suggests that a primary failure of opening of these outlets is not the entire cause of the Dandy-Walker malformation. However, delayed opening could precipitate changes that affect cerebellar development, and certainly, an expansile cyst could create secondary damage beyond the initial embryonic insult.

Dysraphism of the Corpus Cerebelli. In 1954, Benda applied the eponym "Dandy-Walker syndrome," thus ignoring the contribution of Blackfan and of Taggart.[7, 8] He believed that atresia of the foramina was not the essential feature, although it might well be present, and considered the malformation to be a failure of fusion of the corpus cerebelli, comparable to myeloschisis. He did not address the problem of the lack of cranium bifidum in the vast majority of such patients.

Neuroschisis. Padget suggested that a neuroschistic cleft and bleb formation involving the roof of the fourth ventricle in the region of the corpus cerebelli without rupture of the cutaneous ectoderm might produce adhesions with the inner dural layer and might inhibit complete development of the vermis.[18, 53] Thus, failure of normal cerebellar development is the cause of the Dandy-Walker malformation rather than impaired perforation of the caudal membranous roof at the site of the foramen of Magendie.

Hydrodynamic Mechanisms. Two somewhat similar theories postulate that an abnormal distention of the fourth ventricle leads to maldevelopment of the cerebellar vermis. In 1959, Brodal and Hauglie-Hanssen reported a strain of hydrocephalic mice with changes similar to the Dandy-Walker malformation.[14] Prior to the expected time of perforation of the foramina, some undetermined process increased the intraventricular pressure and caused the area membranacea superior to bulge, which impaired development of the vermis and displaced the primitive choroid plexus caudally.

Gardner considers that delayed permeability of the area membranacea superior leads to an increase in physiologic embryonic encephalohydromyelia and causes the area membranacea superior to bulge and form an incipient Dandy-Walker malformation.[30, 31] The bulging coincides with the development of the posterior choroid plexus but occurs before the appearance of the anterior choroid plexus. The interplay between the distending forces created by the posterior and anterior primitive choroid plexuses determines the size of the posterior fossa and the final position of the tentorium and venous sinuses. If the earlier developing posterior choroid plexus produces excessive distending forces, then a dilated fourth ventricle, a large posterior fossa, and a high location of the tentorium result. The opposite situation results in the Arnold-Chiari malformation.

W. J Gardner also described a variant of the Dandy-Walker malformation that he calls the Dandy-Walker cyst. He suggested that the ependymal layer of the rhombic roof is more permeable to ventricular fluid than is the outer layer of the glia and pia, with the result that ventricular fluid pumped through the ependymal layer may accumulate to form a true cyst, or so-called "arachnoid cyst," between the two layers. This loculated cyst between the layers of the rhombic roof distends the fourth ventricle and may bulge between the spread cerebellar hemispheres into the enlarged aqueduct.

Gardner believes that noncommunication between the lateral ventricles and an "enlarged fourth ventricle" containing high-protein fluid in a suspected Dandy-Walker malformation is, in reality, a Dandy-Walker cyst.[61, 66]

E. Gardner and coworkers concluded that the Dandy-Walker malformation and the Arnold-Chiari malformation are different and separate disorders, since the only major pathologic feature that they have in common is hydrocephalus, which is a frequent result of any teratogenic insult to the central nervous system.[29] Not even hydrocephalus can be used as a unifying concept, as both the Arnold-Chiari and the Dandy-Walker malformations may occur without hydrocephalus.[27]

OCCULT SPINAL DYSRAPHISM

Classification

Occult spinal dysraphism is an entity composed of a variety of malformations of embryonic development, varying from the very simple to the very complex.[27, 35] The major subtypes are listed in Table 2–1. Spinal dermal sinus and the neurenteric cyst have special clinical features, whereas the other types generally present with one or more features of a cutaneous malformation, a neuromusculoskeletal syndrome, sphincter disturbance, spinal curvature, and, occasionally, back or leg pain.

The infant may have a neurologic deficit at birth, resulting from a primary embryologic myelodysplasia, or may be normal. In either case, a new deficit or progression of an existing one may occur in the first or second decade because of the secondary effects of tethering or compression. A brief description of the clinical and pathologic abnormalities in each type is appropriate before discussing the abnormal embryology that might contribute to the lesions.

Congenital Spinal Dermal Sinus. A congenital spinal dermal sinus is an epithelium-lined tract that may occur anywhere along the posterior midline of the spine. It forms a potential communication between the skin surface and the deeper tissues. The tract may end in the subcutaneous tissues, on the bone, in the epidural or subdural space, or in the neural tissues, with the intraspinal extension often expanding into a dermoid or epidermoid inclusion tumor. The posterior elements may be normal radiologically, although usually a minor degree of posterior spina bifida is present. The vertebral bodies are virtually always normal. If the tract attaches to the neural elements and the normal degree of ascent of the conus medullaris has occurred during early development, the cutaneous opening may be lower than the ultimate termination of the tract on the spinal cord by two or three segments. On occasion, the tract itself may act as a tethering agent to prevent the normal extent of upward migration, resulting in a low-lying conus medullaris. Spinal dermal sinus exhibits the special presentation of meningitis in the very young and spinal cord or cauda equina compression by tumor in the older child.

Tethered Cord Syndrome. The tethered cord syndrome can be defined as an abnormally low conus medullaris tethered by one or more forms of intradural abnormalities such as a short, thickened filum terminale, fibrous bands or adhesions, or a totally intradural lipoma fixing the neural elements to the caudal dural sac. The pathologic feature that distinguishes this from congenital dermal sinus, lumbosacral lipoma, and lipomyelomeningocele is the lack of continuity between the visible cutaneous lesion, if there is any, and the intradural pathologic condition. Important clinically are the facts that cutaneous manifestations are present in only approximately 50 percent of the patients and that scoliosis is as frequent an occurrence as in diastematomyelia with septum. Posterior spina bifida is usually present, but the vertebral bodies are usually normal. The syndrome has been known by a variety of terms over the years, such as the tethered conus, tight filum terminale, filum terminale syndrome, and meningocele manque.[27]

Lumbosacral Lipoma and Lipomyelomeningocele. The lumbosacral lipoma and lipomyelomeningocele are quite related, with the latter a more complex lesion. The pathologic hallmark is a subcutaneous lipoma overlying the lumbar or sacral region that extends through a defect in the fascia and posterior elements to merge with the neural elements, which are invariably tethered low in the spinal canal (Fig. 2–15). The feature that justifies differentiating the two lesions is that, in the simpler form, the neural elements are within the spinal canal; in the complex lipomyelomeningocele, the spinal cord herniates out of the spinal canal to enter the subcutaneous lipoma. Thus, the complex lesion is somewhat akin to the open forms in which the neural tissues are exposed at skin level; hence, the term "lipomyelomeningocele." In addition, a meningocele component may be present in the lipomatous mass itself. The bony anomalies are more complex with lipomas than with the dermal sinus or the tethered cord syndrome. Frequently, the vertebral bodies are malformed by scalloping of their posterior margins, the interpedicular distance is more likely to be widened, and hemivertebrae or hypoplasia of the iliac wing may occur. An important factor in treatment is that compression of the neural elements may be a cause of a neurologic deficit as well as tethering. The compression may be due to the intraspinal fat itself, usually by the portion extending under intact posterior elements. In the lipomyelomeningocele, the last intact neural arch may compress the exiting spinal cord at the point of its angulation around the arch.

Diastematomyelia. Diastematomyelia is a fascinating pathologic entity already mentioned as a part of spina bifida aperta, especially in the spinal

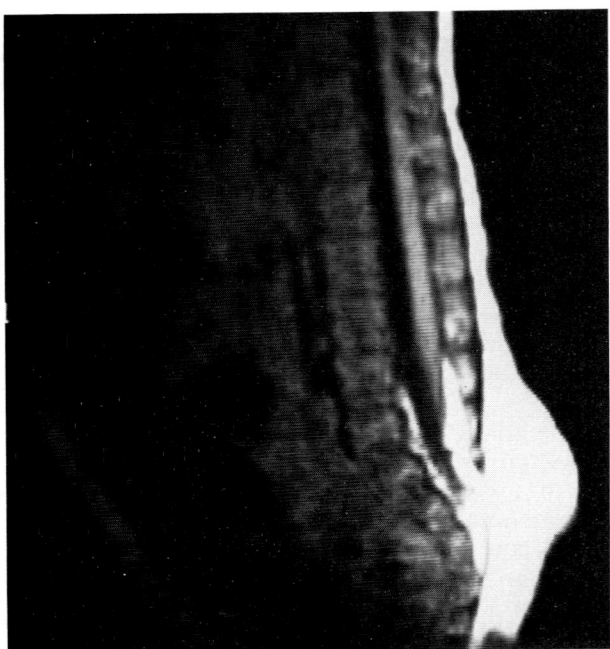

Figure 2–15. Nuclear magnetic resonance imaging scan of a lumbosacral lipoma with spinal cord tethered to the level of L5. Note the continuity of lipoma from the subcutaneous to the intraspinal fusion with the conus medullaris.

cord proximal to the neural plaque. In that area, there is usually no structural element between the hemicords, and the hemicords are located in a single dural sac. The infrequent form of hemimyelomeningocele is an exception, however. In occult spinal dysraphism, the division of the spinal cord into two, more or less, equal halves is commonly associated with a midline septum of fibrous tissue, cartilage, or bone separating the hemicords, each of which is located in a separate dural sac. The conus medullaris is usually low in the spinal canal, with the transfixing septum located between T7 and T12 in 25 percent of patients and between L1 and L4 in 67 percent.[27] Scoliosis is a common clinical manifestation that is no doubt related to the vertebral anomalies that are more complex than those in the other forms of occult dysraphism just discussed. Vertebral body anomalies occur often, especially in those patients with scoliosis, and posterior spina bifida is virtually always present near the level of the septum.

Neurenteric Cyst. The neurenteric cyst occurs in an intramedullary or intradural extramedullary location ventral to the spinal cord in the cervicodorsal region of the spine. The neurenteric cyst may present with an associated congenital thoracic cyst or an enteric duplication with vertebral body defects and a compressive intraspinal lesion at the cervicodorsal level. The embryologic origin of these lesions seems to be related to entoderm development, which explains an associated intrathoracic or intra-abdominal cyst, and the frequent malformation of the vertebral bodies. In rare cases, a transvertebral communication between the intraspinal cyst and the cyst anterior to the spine may be found. The posterior elements are virtually always normal, and no cutaneous manifestations are seen.

Combined Anterior and Posterior Spina Bifida. Finally, the very rare combined anterior and posterior spina bifida is mentioned only to give evidence of the potential validity of some of the theories of abnormal embryology. These rare instances of a longitudinal division of the vertebral bodies forming an anterior cleft and a posterior spina bifida at the same level usually occur in the cervicodorsal or lumbar areas of the spine. The higher lesions are associated with severe anomalies in other organ systems and are of pathologic interest only. The lower lesions have been reported rarely in living children and usually involve prolapse of intestinal duplications through the anterior and posterior vertebral defects to the back. The neural elements are either open and exposed as in a myeloschisis, or they are closed. In the latter case, a diastematomyelia rings the enteric structure, and the enteric duplication may appear as a skin-covered swelling that can mimic a meningocele or lipoma. Rarely, the enteric duplication may open onto the back and drain meconium.

Pathogenesis of the Clinical Presentation

The pathogenesis of the clinical presentation in occult spinal dysraphism is usually the product of one or more factors such as true myelodysplasia, traction, compression, and, rarely, inflammation in congenital spinal dermal sinus complicated by meningitis. True myelodysplasia (i.e., an embryologic malformation of the neural structures) may be seen in all types but is a source of neurologic deficit at birth more often in lipomyelomeningocele, lumbosacral lipoma, and diastematomyelia.

The source of neurologic deficits after birth, whether new or progressive, is usually compression or the traction phenomenon. Compression is caused more frequently in the lipomatous malformations by the lipoma itself, is caused by the last intact vertebral arch in lipomyelomeningocele, or, rarely, by the septum in diastematomyelia. Traction results in any situation in which the neural elements are fixed at a lower-than-normal level when the spinal cord and spine are symmetric in length. The normal ascent of the conus medullaris during regression of the tail bud is prevented, and the spinal cord is stretched. Although the stretching or tethering itself may not create a neurologic deficit, the day-to-day repetitive incremental trauma of stretching occurring during normal spinal movements in active children can produce neurologic deficits. Ischemia of the stretched caudal spinal cord appears to play a part in the neurologic dysfunction, and Yamada and coworkers show that release of the tether can improve oxidative metabolism within the caudal spinal cord.[73]

Theories of Abnormal Embryogenesis of Occult Spinal Dysraphism

Occult spinal dysraphism in its many subtypes would appear to form in the earliest embryonic stages, as evidenced by the intimate cutaneous-neural (congenital dermal sinus) and enteric-neural (neurenteric cyst) communications, abnormal neurulation (diastematomyelia), and abnormal canalization and regression of the tail bud (tethered cord syndrome, lumbosacral lipoma, lipomyelomeningocele) (Table 2–1).

The theories offered to explain these malformations involve five basic mechanisms: (1) abnormal separation of tissue layers; (2) abnormal neurulation; (3) abnormal formation of the notochord; (4) abnormal formation of the neurenteric canal; and (5) abnormal canalization and regression of the tail bud. Except for the latter mechanism, they are variations on a theme and focus only on which feature is the primary cause. The theories are more easily discussed by separating the malformations into three groups: (1) congenital dermal sinus; (2) tethered cord syndrome, lumbosacral lipoma, and lipomyelomeningocele; and (3) diastematomyelia, neurenteric cyst, and combined anterior and posterior spina bifida.

Congenital Dermal Sinus

The spinal dermal sinus can occur at any level of the spine and is rarely, if ever, associated with complicated vertebral abnormalities unless it is related to one of the more complex forms of occult dysraphism such as diastematomyelia with septum. The more common simple forms probably represent adhesion between the neural tube and the cutaneous ectoderm at the time when separation of these layers should occur, just after neurulation or canalization of the tail bud (Fig. 2–16). The mechanism was popularized by Walker and Bucy in 1934.[71] The misplaced ectodermal cells can then develop into the inclusion epidermoid or dermoid tumor. Since the communication may be small, the mesoderm can condense in a virtually normal fashion around the neuroectodermal adhesion, resulting in only a minor degree of posterior spina bifida.

Padget proposed the neuroschisis theory as a cause of the adhesion that causes a congenital dermal sinus.[50] The neuroschistic bleb that forms between the neural tube and the cutaneous ectoderm largely heals, leaving the neural tube to develop normally but creating an adhesion between skin and cord, and thus, the sinus.

Tethered Cord Syndrome, Lumbosacral Lipoma, and Lipomyelomeningocele

These malformations involve the caudal spinal cord and, very probably, are related to some abnormality of canalization of the caudal cell mass, regres-

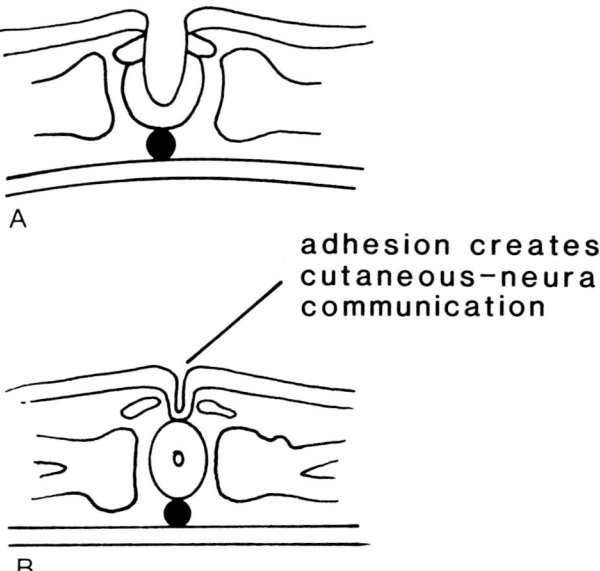

Figure 2–16. Possible genesis of the congenital spinal dermal sinus. A, The neural folds approximate, fuse, and draw the cutaneous ectoderm to the midline, where separation normally occurs. B, An adhesion between cutaneous ectoderm and the neural tube could create a sinus of ectoderm-derived tissue. The mesodermal migrations may occur virtually normally and may leave little malformation of the surrounding bone.

sion of the neural tube, and ascent of the conus medullaris. From day 28 to day 48 of development, abnormal canalization is likely to cause lumbosacral lipoma and lipomyelomeningocele. Abnormal regression, starting as early as 43 to 48 days of development and continuing to the postnatal period, would be related to the tethered cord syndrome.

Few theories of causation have been advanced, and none has been advanced in great detail. Since canalization occurs in the caudal cell mass of pleuripotential cells under intact cutaneous ectoderm, it is not unrealistic to believe that abnormal inductive influences on these cells of mesodermal nature may form fat and other tissues in conjunction with those cells destined to form the neural tube. Subsequent development of both tissues results in a dorsal subcutaneous lipoma fused to the caudal spinal cord in varying degrees of intimacy.

In the complex lipomyelomeningocele, the spinal cord is drawn out of the confines of the spinal canal, the fusion is intimate, and the potential for primary myelodysplasia with congenital neurologic deficit is high. The simpler lipoma fuses with the spinal cord within the canal and may produce no functional impairment of neural development. In both instances, the lipoma traverses several tissue planes extending from the subcutaneous plane through fascia, bone, dura, and arachnoid-pia. If the area of fusion is broad, the condensing mesodermal elements are disordered, which explains the high incidence of bone malformation. Tethering of the spinal cord low in the spinal canal results, and ascent of the conus medullaris is prevented, setting the stage for postnatal neurologic deficit from traction.

In the tethered cord syndrome, the process of canalization has usually occurred normally, but regression is abnormal, leading to various abnormalities such as lipoma of the filum terminale, an abnormally thick and short filum terminale, or a variety of bands and adhesions between neural structures and the dura. These intradural tethering lesions impair ascent of the conus medullaris and have the same potential for later postnatal neurologic deficit.

These mechanisms would not explain spinal cord lipomas at the higher levels of the spine unassociated with spina bifida or cutaneous anomalies. That embryologic abnormality should involve a misplacement of pleuripotential cells in the mesodermal condensations alongside the notochord and under the neural plate prior to neurulation that ultimately form fat.

Diastematomyelia, Neurenteric Cyst, and Combined Anterior and Posterior Spina Bifida

These forms of occult spinal dysraphism involve the higher levels of the spine and are often associated with malformation of the vertebral bodies. In neurenteric cysts and combined spina bifida, the enteric structures may also be abnormal and may even communicate, to a variable degree, through the anterior spina bifida with the spinal canal and the spinal cord. The primary abnormality must involve the neural tissue itself, the mesoderm, the notochord, or the entoderm, and since all are abnormal to some degree, each has been implicated in one or more theories. Some theories are expansive and describe all three malformations, whereas others are limited to a description of only one malformation. Four origins have been theorized: (1) abnormal separation of tissue layers; (2) abnormal neurulation; (3) abnormal formation of the notochord; and (4) abnormal formation of the neurenteric canal.

Abnormal Separation of Tissue Layers. Beardmore and Wiglesworth[5] and McLetchie and coworkers[46] reviewed the theories regarding abnormal fusion of tissue layers as these hypotheses relate to the neurenteric cyst. A primary adhesion could develop between the ectoderm and entoderm in the midline prior to the formation of the notochord, perhaps akin to the type of fusion that marks the future mouth at the prochordal plate and anus at the cloacal membrane (Fig. 2–17A). Subsequently, the notochord cells extending rostrally split around the adhesion, forming a split notochord (Fig. 2–17B). Further development of the tissues and persistence of the adhesion result in an entoderm to neuroectoderm band. Evidence that adhesions can occur in this area is supported by Patten's observation of an area of fusion between the notochord and the neural tube in an embryo of six weeks development.[54]

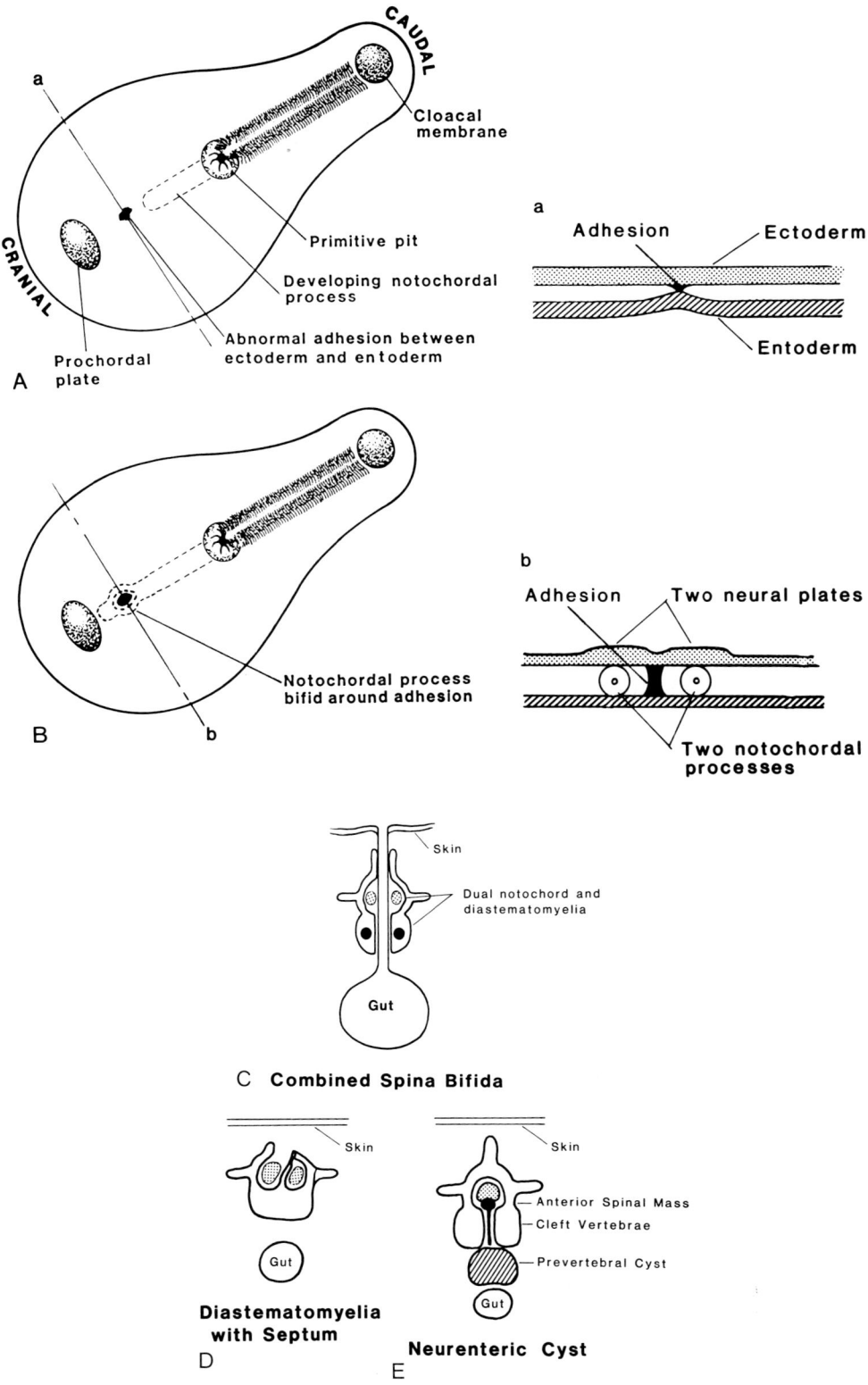

Figure 2–17. Split notochord theory. A, An adhesion between the ectoderm and entoderm of the two-layered embryonic disk may occur cranial to the developing notochordal process; a, cross-sectional view. B, The notochordal process is forced to divide around the adhesion, creating two notochordal processes. Two neural plates may be induced as shown in cross section (b), which ultimately could form an area of diastematomyelia. C, An enterocutaneous fistula may penetrate through a vertebral body cleft, diastematomyelia, and posterior spina bifida to create a combined anterior-posterior spina bifida. The theories invoking an abnormality of the neurenteric canal are attractive (see Figure 2–4B). D, Healing of the anterior portions of the fistula could lead to diastematomyelia with septum, which is usually accompanied by posterior element and vertebral body abnormalities. E, Healing of the posterior and midportions of the fistula could lead to neurenteric cyst, vertebral body anomalies, and various enteric malformations.

This abnormal communication has a variable potential in its ultimate expression, depending upon the degree of healing. The adhesion impairs the formation of the vertebral bodies around the split notochord and can lead to hemivertebrae or midline cleft formation. An enteric-neural fistula, an enteric diverticulum with abnormal vertebral body formation, or a localized cyst can form anterior to the spine, intraspinally, or in both locations (Fig. 2–17E).

Abnormal adhesions can develop between the notochord and the entoderm during the process of intercalation and excalation of the notochord from the yolk sac, but the neural malformations are not explained on this basis alone.[70] The adhesion theory was not extended to explain diastematomyelia or combined spina bifida, as some later authors have done with similar theories. Such an elaboration of the theory would seem justified.

Abnormal Neurulation. Abnormalities of neurulation have been invoked to explain diastematomyelia with septum for many years. All but one of the theories are limited to diastematomyelia and do not explain neurenteric cyst. In 1940, Herren and Edwards suggested that diastematomyelia was due to a "twinning" in which the neural folds turned inward excessively and fused with the neural plate ipsilateral to the neural groove rather than with one another across the midline.[34] Subsequently, two neural tubes formed, and the mesoderm migrated between the neural tubes to form the separate dural envelopes and the septum. They offered no explanation for the behavior of the neural folds themselves.

In the same year, Lichtenstein suggested that the mesoderm created the midline septum primarily and split the neural plate with subsequent secondary formation of the separate neural tubes.[44]

Several authors have indicated mechanisms for abnormal neurulation as a primary phenomenon. In 1949, Kapsenberg and Van Lookeren Campagne[37] suggested that overgrowth of the neurectoderm similar to that observed in spina bifida aperta by Patten[55] might explain diastematomyelia. Since the overgrown neural folds and plate cannot bend sufficiently to meet in the midline, each fold fuses with the plate on its own side, thus forming two separate neural tubes.

Padget suggested that the theory of neuroschisis could explain the malformation if neuroschistic blebs formed simultaneously dorsally and ventrally to the neural tube and each half tube then fused with itself to create separate neural tubes.[50]

Gardner postulated that hydrodynamic overdistension of the embryonic neural tube ruptures the roof and floor plates simultaneously, with two neural tubes forming as a result.[30]

In each theory, the mesoderm passively fills in the space between the neural tubes secondarily, to form the separate dural sheaths and septum. None of the theories, except for W. J. Gardner's, explain the mechanism for the vertebral body anomalies. In addition, each theory attributes the primary role in the creation of this malformation to the neural tube. This mechanism does not fit comfortably with the fact that the notochord and the mesoderm function as important inductors of neural tube formation. Gardner alone extends his theory to suggest that overdistension of the neural tube may also cause the notochord to split to create a neuroectoderm-entoderm communication, thus explaining the neurenteric cyst.

Abnormal Formation of the Notochord. Abnormal formation of the notochord is an attractive theory for these malformations, since the notochord is important in inducing the formation of the neural tube and provides the framework for vertebral body development. In 1943, Saunders described a primary split in the notochord as being responsible for combined spina bifida but did not expand the description to other forms of occult spinal dysraphism.[63] In 1960, Bentley and Smith[9] and Smith[64] separately reviewed the split notochord syndrome and were of the opinion that diastematomyelia, neurenteric cyst, combined spina bifida, and congenital dermal sinus all could be explained.

A primary split at a variable level and extent develops in the notochord for reasons not stated, and thus a gap opens between the two parts of the notochord under the neural plate. The spinal cord develops in two halves. Through this gap, the entoderm herniates and adheres to the cutaneous ectoderm covering the dorsal embryo. If the hernia ruptures, a fistula from amniotic sac to yolk sac will exist, passing between the two halves of the notochord and spinal cord (Fig. 2–17C). The extent of the healing process determines what type of lesion remains. If the entire hernial sac remains, true combined spina bifida occurs; if only the very dorsal portion persists and the remainder heals, a congenital dermal sinus may result; if the dorsal and ventral portions heal, a diastematomyelia may form (Fig. 2–17D); if only the ventral portion remains, a form of neurenteric cyst may develop (Fig. 2–17E).

The notochord theory is attractive because it explains all the types of occult spinal dysraphism, except for those resulting from abnormal canalization and regression of the caudal tail bud. However, congenital dermal sinuses are located frequently below the level of the spinal cord formed by neurulation, and spinal cord malformations or vertebral body malformations are rare, suggesting that the simpler theories of cutaneous ectodermal-neuroectodermal adhesion are a more probable explanation than persistence of the posterior remnant of a fistula between the yolk sac and the amniotic cavity.

Abnormal Formation of the Neurenteric Canal. The neurenteric canal is the passageway that temporarily penetrates the caudal embryo to join the dorsal amniotic sac with the ventral yolk sac during the formation of the notochord at stage 8 (days 18 and 19). It ceases to exist as the process of excalation of the notochord from the yolk sac is completed and the entoderm becomes a continuous layer once again. The dorsal opening of the canal is at the level of Hensen's node, and at this early stage, no somites have yet formed. Two theories involving abnormal development of the neurenteric canal have been offered as explanations for combined spina bifida, diastematomyelia with septum, neurenteric cyst, and congenital dermal sinus.

In 1923, Bell reviewed the early concepts that abnormal persistence of the neurenteric canal could give rise to anterior spina bifida at any level of the spine and thereby create lesions of the neurenteric cyst variety.[6] Even at this time, some authors discredited this notion as a cause of any abnormalities in the cervicothoracic area, since the neurenteric canal is believed to be located at the caudal end of the embryo. However, those authors favoring the theory applied, to the human situation, the embryonic development noted in amphibian embryos, in which the neurenteric canal migrates craniocaudally. In that case, arrest of closure of the neurenteric canal at different times could cause lesions at any level of the vertebral column. Bremer, writing in 1952, agreed that the final resting place for Hensen's node, through which the neurenteric canal was located, was the coccygeal tip.[10] Thus, any abnormal enteric-neural communications proximal to the coccyx must be due to "an ectopic or an accessory canal."

Subsequent herniation of the entodermal layer through the persistent canal creates the fistula that divides the vertebral bodies and the spinal cord. Healing to a varying degree may create any of the types of occult dysraphism, as discussed for the split notochord syndrome (Fig. 2–17C through E).

The differences between the split notochord syndrome, described by Bentley and Smith in 1960,[9] and the accessory neurenteric canal theory, described by Bremer in 1952,[10] are minor, with the former suggesting that the notochord is at fault and the latter suggesting that an "extra" neurenteric canal was responsible. Bremer's theory is less attractive because the mechanism for the so-called "accessory neurenteric canal" is difficult to describe embryologically. The true neurenteric canal is created during the complicated process of notochord formation at the caudal end of the embryo, and it never divides the neural plate or the notochord longitudinally; the accessory canal must divide both and thus fails its comparison to the true canal, except in the communication between the amniotic cavity and yolk sac.

SUMMARY

The theories of abnormal embryogenesis suggested as explanations for the various forms of spina bifida aperta and occult spinal dysraphism appear in some instances all too encompassing, as in Gardner's hydrodynamic theory or Padget's neuroschisis theory, or too limited, as in the theory of arrested development proposed by Daniel and Strich for the Arnold-Chiari malformation, or just too speculative in many cases. The observation of a completed defect does not allow one to venture backward in development to a specific time and cause with any accuracy. Perhaps several different causes striking different tissues at different times can set up a series of aberrations that lead to morphologically similar mature anomalies. The ability of developmental processes to heal themselves, as shown experimentally, may obscure the true mechanism and timing of occurrence, although the final morphologic expression may be dramatic. Since the study of human embryogenesis in the experimental laboratory is ethically unacceptable although technically feasible, the elucidation of the mechanisms of these neural defects will be long in coming.

References

1. Barry A, Patten BM, Stewart BH: Possible factors in the development of the Arnold-Chiari malformation. J Neurosurg 24:285, 1957.
2. Barson AJ: The vertebral level of termination of the spinal cord during normal and abnormal development. J Anat 106:489, 1970.
3. Barson AJ: Spina bifida: The significance of the level and extent of the defect to the morphogenesis. Dev Med Child Neurol 12:129, 1970.
4. Barson AJ: Differentiation, growth and disorders of development of the vertebrospinal axis. In Davis JA, Dobbins J (eds): Scientific Foundations of Paediatrics. London, William Heinemann Medical Books, 1974, pp 577–586.
5. Beardmore HE, Wiglesworth FW: Vertebral anomalies and alimentary duplications. Pediatr Clin North Am 5:457, 1958.
6. Bell HH: Anterior spina bifida and its relation to a persistence of the neurenteric canal. J Nerv Ment Dis 57:445, 1923.
7. Benda CE: Dysraphic states. J Neuropathol Exp Neurol 18:56, 1953.
8. Benda CE: The Dandy-Walker syndrome or the so-called atresia of the foramen of Magendie. J Neuropathol Exp Neurol 13:14, 1954.
9. Bentley JFR, Smith JR: Developmental posterior enteric remnants and spinal malformations: The split notochord syndrome. Arch Dis Child 35:76, 1960.
10. Bremer JL: Dorsal intestinal fistula: Accessory neurenteric canal; diastematomyelia. Arch Pathol 54:132, 1952.
11. Brocklehurst G: The development of the human cerebrospinal fluid pathway with particular reference to the roof of the fourth ventricle. J Anat 105:467, 1969.
12. Brocklehurst G: A quantitative study of a spina bifida foetus. J Pathol 99:205, 1969.
13. Brocklehurst G: Spina Bifida for the Clinician. London, William Heinemann Medical Books, 1976, pp 1–195.
14. Brodal A, Hauglie-Hanssen E: Congenital hydrocephalus with defective development of the cerebellar vermis (Dandy-Walker syndrome). Clinical and anatomical findings in two cases with particular reference to so-called atresia of the foramina of Magendie and Luschka. J Neurol Neurosurg Psychiatry 22:99, 1959.
15. Cameron AH: The Arnold-Chiari and other neuro-anatomical malformations associated with spina bifida. J Pathol Bacteriol 73:195, 1957.
16. Carmel PW: Management of the Chiari malformations in childhood. Clin Neurosurg 30:385, 1983.
17. Carmel PW, Markesbery WR: Early descriptions of the Arnold-Chiari malformation: The contribution of John Cleland. J Neurosurg 37:543, 1972.
18. Cleland J: Contribution to the study of spina bifida, encephalocele and anencephalus. J Anat Physiol 17:257, 1883.
19. Dandy WE: The diagnosis and treatment of hydrocephalus

due to occlusions of the foramina of Magendie and Luschka. Surg Gynecol Obstet 32:112, 1921.
20. Dandy WE, Blackfan KD: Internal hydrocephalus: An experimental clinical and pathological study. Am J Dis Child 8:406, 1914.
21. Dandy WE, Blackfan KD: Internal hydrocephalus. Am J Dis Child 14:424, 1917.
22. Daniel PM, Strich SJ: Some observations on the congenital deformity of the central nervous system known as the Arnold-Chiari malformation. J Neuropathol Exp Neurol 17:255, 1958.
23. Emery JL, Lendon RG: The local cord lesion in neurospinal dysraphism (meningomyelocele). J Pathol 110:83, 1973.
24. Emery JL, Levick RK: The movement of the brain stem and vessels around the brain stem in children with hydrocephalus and the Arnold-Chiari deformity. Dev Med Child Neurol (Suppl) 11:49, 1966.
25. Emery JL, MacKenzie N: Medullo-cervical dislocation deformity (Chiari II deformity) related to neurospinal dysraphism (meningomyelocele). Brain 96:155, 1973.
26. Emery JL, Naik D: Spinal cord segment lengths in children with meningomyelocele and the "Cleland-Arnold-Chiari" deformity. Br J Radiol 41:287, 1968.
27. French BN: Midline fusion defects and defects of formation. In Youmans JR (ed): Neurological Surgery, 2nd ed. Philadelphia, WB Saunders Co., 1982, pp 1236–1380.
28. French BN: The embryology of spinal dysraphism. Clin Neurosurg 30:295, 1983.
29. Gardner E, O'Rahilly R, Prolo D: The Dandy-Walker and Arnold-Chiari malformations. Arch Neurol (Chicago) 32:393, 1975.
30. Gardner WJ: The Dysraphic States from Syringomyelia to Anencephaly. Amsterdam, Excerpta Medica, 1973, pp 1–201.
31. Gardner WJ: Hydrodynamic factors in Dandy-Walker and Arnold-Chiari malformations. Child's Brain 3:200, 1977.
32. Gibson JB: Congenital hydrocephalus due to atresia of the foramen of Magendie. J Neuropathol Exp Neurol 14:244, 1955.
33. Goldstein F, Kepes JJ: The role of traction in the development of the Arnold-Chiari malformation: An experimental study. J Neuropathol Exp Neurol 25:654, 1966.
34. Herren RY, Edwards JE: Diplomyelia (duplication of the spinal cord). Arch Pathol 30:1203, 1940.
35. James CCM, Lassman LP: Spina Bifida Occulta. New York, Grune and Stratton, 1981, pp 1–230.
36. Jennings MT, Clarren SK, Kokich VG, et al: Neuroanatomic examination of spina bifida aperta and the Arnold-Chiari malformation in a 130-day human fetus. J Neurol Sci 54:325, 1982.
37. Kapsenberg JG, Van Lookeren Campagne JA: A case of spina bifida combined with diastematomyelia, the anomaly of Chiari and hydrocephaly. Acta Anat 7:366, 1949.
38. Kunitomo K: The development and reduction of the tail and of the caudal end of the spinal cord. Contrib Embryol 8:161, 1918.
39. Lemire RJ: Variations in development of the caudal neural tube in human embryos (Horizons XIV–XXI). Teratology 2:361, 1969.
40. Lemire RJ: Embryology of the central nervous system. In Davis JA, Dobbins J (eds): Scientific Foundations of Paediatrics. London, William Heinemann Medical Books, 1974, pp 547–564.
41. Lemire RJ, Loeser JD, Leech RW, et al: Normal and Abnormal Development of the Human Nervous System. New York, Harper & Row, 1975, pp 1–421.
42. Lemire RJ, Shepard TH, Alvord EC, Jr.: Caudal myeloschisis (lumbosacral spina bifida cystica) in a five millimeter (Horizon XIV) human embryo. Anat Rec 152:9, 1965.
43. Lendon RG, Emery JL: Forking of the central canal in the equinal cord of children. J Anat 106:499, 1970.
44. Lichtenstein BW: Spinal dysraphism, spina bifida and myelodysplasia. Arch Neurol Psychiatry 44:792, 1940.
45. Marin-Padilla M, Marin-Padilla TM: Morphogenesis of experimentally induced Arnold-Chiari malformation. J Neurol Sci 50:29, 1981.
46. McLetchie NGB, Purves JK, Saunders RL de CH: The genesis of gastric and certain intestinal diverticula and enterogenous cysts. Surg Gynecol Obstet 99:135, 1954.
47. Moore KL: The Developing Human, 3rd ed. Philadelphia, WB Saunders Co., 1982, pp 1–479.
48. O'Rahilly R, Gardner E: The timing and sequence of events in the development of the human nervous system during the embryonic period proper. Z Anat Entwicklungsgesch 134:1, 1971.
49. Osaka K, Tanimura T, Hirayama A, et al: Myelomeningocele before birth. J Neurosurg 49:711, 1978.
50. Padget DH: Spina bifida and embryonic neuroschisis—a causal relationship. Definition of the postnatal conformations involving a bifid spine. Johns Hopkins Med J 128:233, 1968.
51. Padget DH: Neuroschisis and human embryonic maldevelopment: New evidence on anencephaly, spina bifida and diverse mammalian defects. J Neuropathol Exp Neurol 29:192, 1970.
52. Padget DH: Development of so-called dysraphism, with embryologic evidence of clinical Arnold-Chiari and Dandy-Walker malformations. Johns Hopkins Med J 130:127, 1972.
53. Padget DH, Lindenberg R: Inverse cerebellum morphogenetically related to Dandy-Walker and Arnold-Chiari syndromes: Bizarre malformed brain with occipital encephalocele. Johns Hopkins Med J 131:228, 1972.
54. Patten BM: Fusion of notochord to neural tube in a human embryo of the sixth week. Anat Rec 95:307, 1946.
55. Patten BM: Overgrowth of the neural tube in young human embryos. Anat Rec 113:381, 1952.
56. Patten BM, Embryological stages in the establishing of myeloschisis with spina bifida. Am J Anat 93:365, 1953.
57. Peach B: Arnold-Chiari malformation with normal spine. Arch Neurol 10:497, 1964.
58. Peach B: The Arnold-Chiari malformation: Morphogenesis. Arch Neurol 12:527, 1965.
59. Peach B: Arnold-Chiari malformation: Anatomic features of 20 cases. Arch Neurol 12:613, 1965.
60. Penfield W, Coburn DF: Arnold-Chiari malformation and its operative treatment. Arch Neurol Psychiatry 40:328, 1938.
61. Raimondi AJ, Samuelson G, Yarzagaray L, et al: Atresia of the foramina of Luschka and Magendie. The Dandy-Walker cyst. J Neurosurg 31:202, 1969.
62. Rokos J: The pathogenesis of spina bifida and related malformations. In Smith WT (ed): Recent Advances in Neuropathology. Glasgow, Churchill Livingstone, 1979, pp 225–245.
63. Saunders RL de CH: Combined anterior and posterior spina bifida in a living neonatal human female. Anat Rec 87:255, 1943.
64. Smith JR: Accessory enteric formations: A classification and nomenclature. Arch Dis Child 35:87, 1960.
65. Streeter GL: Factors involved in the formation of the filum terminale. Am J Anat 25:1, 1919.
66. Taggart JK Jr., Walker AE: Congenital atresia of the foramens of Luschka and Magendie. Arch Neurol Psychiatry 48:583, 1942.
67. Thompson MW, Rudd NL: The genetics of spinal dysraphism. In Morley TP (ed): Current Controversies in Neurosurgery. Philadelphia, WB Saunders Co., 1976, pp 126–146.
68. Van Hoytema GJ, van den Berg R: Embryological studies of the posterior fossa in connection with the Arnold-Chiari malformation. Dev Med Child Neurol (Suppl) 11:61, 1966.
69. Variend S, Emery JL: The weight of the cerebellum in children with myelomeningocele. Dev Med Child Neurol (Suppl 29) 15:77, 1973.
70. Veeneklaas GMH: Pathogenesis of intrathoracic gastrogenic cysts. Am J Dis Child 83:500, 1952.
71. Walker AE, Bucy PC: Congenital dermal sinuses; a course of spinal meningeal infection and subdural abscesses. Brain 57:401, 1934.
72. Warkany J: Morphogenesis of spina bifida. In McLaurin RL (ed): Myelomeningocele. New York, Grune & Stratton, 1977, pp 31–39.
73. Yamada S, Zinke DE, Sanders D: Pathophysiology of "tethered cord syndrome." J Neurosurg 54:494, 1981.

3
SPINA BIFIDA

Donald H. Reigel, M.D.

Spina bifida is the most common central nervous system birth defect encountered by the pediatric neurosurgeon. Although archaeologic observations reveal the presence of spina bifida for 3000 years, the person who first used the term "spina bifida" remains unknown.[39] Traditionally, spina bifida was defined by characteristic developmental abnormalities of the vertebrae and spinal cord. More recently, associated profound changes in the cerebrum, brainstem, and peripheral nerves and their continuing complications from these abnormalities have been appreciated. The expressions of spina bifida range from the minimum of an absent spinous process to multiple vertebral anomalies with marked changes in spinal cord anatomy and function. Spina bifida's associated multisystem abnormalities contribute to its widely accepted identity as the most complex developmental defect compatible with life.

The ongoing debate over the ethics and technique of primary closure has gradually moved on to the recognition of a variety of delayed neurologic and systemic complications of spina bifida. Clearly, awareness of these complications has led to improved, microsurgical neural tube reconvolution and anatomic closure. Marked advances in neuroimaging techniques have produced a more precise definition and understanding of hydrocephalus, cerebrospinal fluid shunt failure, and other treatable associated neuroanatomic abnormalities. Our increased understanding of the continuum of multidisciplinary care required for the developing child with spina bifida has enhanced the prognosis for a rewarding and meaningful life for each patient.

TERMINOLOGY

Spina Bifida Occulta. This term refers to anatomic abnormalities of the vertebrae identified on spine x-ray films. The spinous process of one or more vertebrae is absent, along with minor amounts of the vertebral arch (failure of fusion of the posterior arch). This change may be found in 20 to 30 per cent of the general population and is most frequently seen on incidental x-ray films at the L-5 and S-1 level. Usually, the central nervous system, cauda equina, and peripheral nervous system are not involved.

The overlying skin and the neurologic examination are normal. However, when spine x-ray films demonstrating these changes are obtained because of the presence of a skin abnormality, such as dimples, sinus tracts, hypertrichosis, or capillary hemangiomas, suspicion of an occult intraspinal lesion increases. These abnormalities, including epidermoid and dermoid tumors, lipomas, disastematomyelia, dural bands, and tethered spinal cord, are grouped under the terms *occult spinal dysraphism*, *occult spinal lesions*, and *meningocele manqué*.[142]

The high frequency of spina bifida occulta has led many to question the significance of its relationship to back pain, enuresis, and scoliosis.[24, 37, 160] In recent studies of patients treated in emergency rooms (which excluded those with spine abnormalities, back pain, and enuresis), a 22 per cent incidence of spina bifida occulta was discovered, and the incidence progressively declined with increasing age.[11] The high incidence, with or without associated problems, has not permitted conclusions about the clinical significance of uncomplicated spina bifida occulta. Indeed, many have placed little emphasis upon the isolated finding and have suggested that the diagnosis not even be described in the x-ray report. Perhaps of more overriding concern is the question of whether spina bifida occulta is related to the overall spectrum of expressions of spina bifida and, therefore, deserves special consideration in genetic counseling.[30, 115] Data pertinent to this point are incomplete, and at this time, the increased association of spina bifida occulta with occult intraspinal lesions is the most important consideration.

Meningocele. Meningocele designates a skin- or membrane-covered cystic midline mass usually found over the lumbodorsal area. It is most commonly found at the time of birth, and patients with meningocele comprise about 10 per cent of all patients with spina bifida.[53] The dorsal half of one or more vertebrae is absent, and the contents of the bulge are limited to cerebrospinal fluid, meninges, and skin. However, tissue discarded at the time of operative treatment frequently shows histologic evidence of ganglion cells, aberrant peripheral nerve, and, occasionally, tissue suggestive of spinal cord. Similar to the situation with spina bifida occulta, a high index of suspicion must be maintained regarding associated occult intraspinal lesions, either at the site of the meningocele or at a removed location.[146] Generally, the remainder of the central nervous system is not involved, and the prognosis for development is excellent. Hydrocephalus is associated with meningocele, but much less frequently than the 80 to 90 per cent incidence expected with myelomeningocele.

Myelomeningocele. Including spina bifida cystica and spina bifida aperta, this form of spina bifida is associated with severe neurologic change and is identified at birth by a posterior midline mass covered by a membrane that may or may not incorporate nervous tissue and leak cerebrospinal fluid. Vertebral anomalies include (1) absence of the spinous process and lamina, (2) reduction in the anterior-posterior size of the vertebral body, (3) increased interpedicle distance, (4) decreased height of the pedicle, and (5) large laterally extending transverse processes. Often, adjacent transverse processes fuse and surround the exiting peripheral nerve. The midline mass is most frequently located in the thoracolumbar area and contains cerebrospinal fluid, meninges, cauda equina, and abnormal spinal cord (neural plaque) (Fig. 3–1). Several abnormalities of the cerebrum and cerebellum have been described, in addition to the Arnold-Chiari malformation, which is present in all patients with myelomeningocele. Depending upon the series reported, at least 75 per cent of patients develop hydrocephalus. Clinical examination reveals sensory and motor changes distal to the anatomic level of the lesion that produce varying degrees of anesthesia, weakness of the lower extremities, and urine and fecal incontinence. Orthopedic deformity and other system anomalies are also commonly present.

Spina bifida cystica refers to either meningocele or myelomeningocele[67] whereas *spina bifida aperta* (open) implies that the lesion communicates with the environment.

Neural Plaque. Neural plaque indicates the dorsal neural tissue contained within a myelomeningocele, consisting of spinal cord (usually abnormal conus medullaris). A midline groove may be visualized; this is the anterior half of the neural groove that is, embryologically, the central canal of the spinal cord. Often, cerebrospinal fluid exits from the proximal portion of this groove—the distal intact central canal (Fig. 3–2).

Lipomeningocele, Lipomyelomeningocele, Lipomyeloschisis,[85] and Lipomyelolipoma.[19] These refer to the lipomatous content of the spina bifida lesion. The lipoma may be extradural, intradural, or both, with lipoma invading the dorsal spinal cord or conus medullaris, with associated envelopment of the cauda equina (Fig. 3–3). Naidich and coworkers have described the embryologic and radiographic and surgical anatomy of these lesions, which aids immensely in surgical consideration.[85]

Anterior Meningocele. This term most commonly refers to a pelvic mass or, rarely, a thoracic mass that communicates with the spinal subarachnoid space through a small opening in the anterior vertebral column. The content of the mass is primarily cerebrospinal fluid; however, a variety of tumors such as teratomas, lipomas, neurofibromas, and dermoids have been associated with anterior meningocele. This lesion is probably also the result of abnormal development of the distal neural tube.

Spinal Dysraphism. This is a generic term describ-

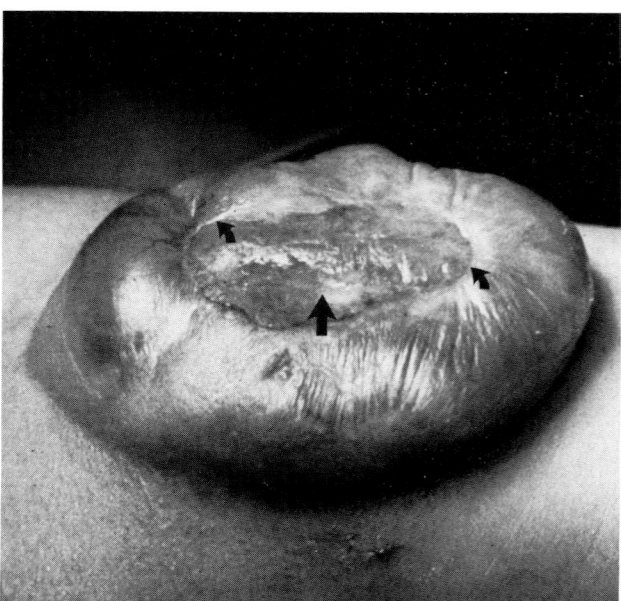

Figure 3–1. Thoracolumbar myelomeningocele showing the neuroplaque (straight arrow) and the white line that defines the junctional zone of the arachnoid, dura, and skin (curved arrows).

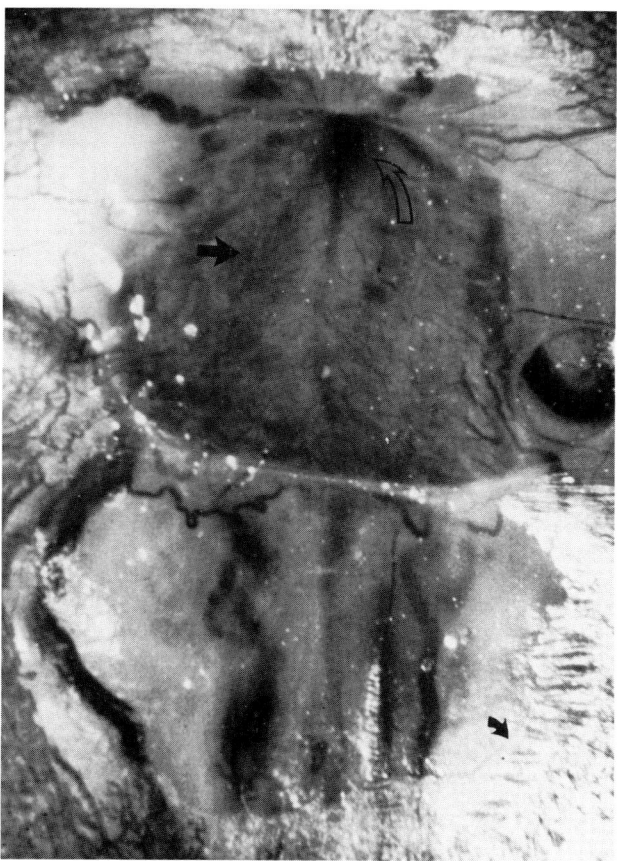

Figure 3–2. External appearance at lumbar myelomeningocele. The open arrow points to the central canal, the solid straight arrow identifies neuroplaque, and the curved black arrow indicates junctional zone.

ing pathologic conditions that occur because of improper development (fusion) of the posterior neuropore. These conditions express themselves as abnormalities of ectodermal, mesodermal, and neuroectodermal tissues of the fetus.[64] The term frequently encompasses all of the conditions associated with spina bifida.

Rachischisis. Rachischisis describes a condition of the fetus in which the brain and spinal cord are dorsally exposed to the environment. This lesion results from complete lack of closure of the neural groove and occurs at about 15 to 23 days of gestation.[62] This rare anomaly is incompatible with survival.

Arnold-Chiari Malformation. This term denotes a congenital anomaly of the hindbrain that is almost always associated with myelomeningocele. The medulla oblongata and pons are posteriorly bowed and elongated, frequently extending into the rostral cervical spinal canal, along with the cerebellar vermis. Abnormalities of the posterior skull, dura, medulla oblongata, pons, midbrain, cerebellum, cerebral hemispheres, cisterns, and ventricles have been described.[87–89]

INCIDENCE AND EPIDEMIOLOGY

Spina bifida occulta is relatively common in our society, with incidence rates reportedly as high as 30 per cent.[11] The incidence for open spina bifida (meningocele or myelomeningocele) is approximately 1 per 1000 live births.[48, 70] However, there are marked geographic variations, with the incidence reaching 4 to 5 per 1000 live births in regions of Ireland.[25] Similarly, within continents, incidence gradients have been observed from east to west in the United States, and from southeast to northwest in the British Isles.[26, 141] Since the 1940's, there has been a decreasing incidence, but during the past decade, the incidence has been relatively stable.[130] Analysis of sex ratios indicates a significantly higher incidence among females.[122]

The rates of incidence are also much lower in blacks and Asians than in whites.[26] The incidence of spina bifida does seem to increase with poverty level and poor nutrition. However, these observations have not led to meaningful etiologic information, and reported clusters, at this time, have been explained by chance.[130] Studies of variations with season, maternal age, and parity do not seem to provide meaningful clues regarding etiology.[17, 57, 143] The fact that open spina bifida has been reported

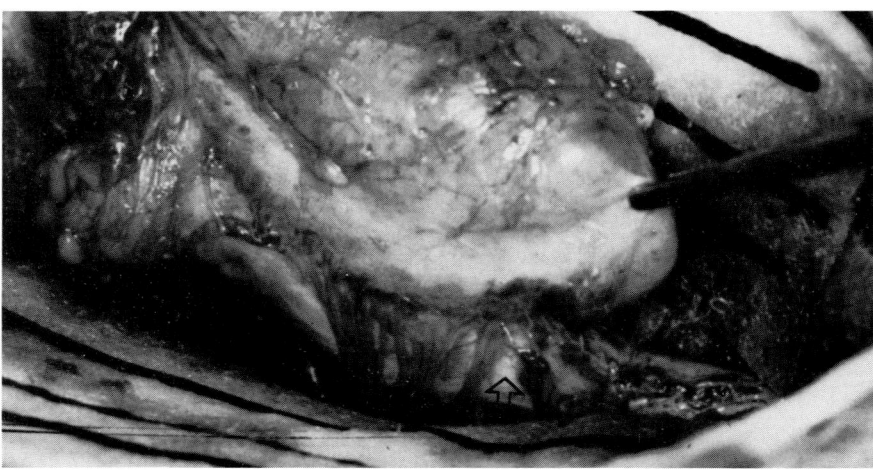

Figure 3–3. Lipomyelomeningocele. The open arrow points to spinal cord anterior to large lipoma contiguous with conus.

to be 13 times more common in spontaneously aborted fetuses than in full-term infants leads one to question what the true risk of neural tube defects may be with conception for any given parent.[95]

GENETICS

There is a familial tendency, or predisposition, to the occurrence of spina bifida.[144] The occurrence statistics do not fit mendelian transmission, although neural tube defects attributable to single genes have been described.[30, 145] Multifactorial inheritance[141] is strongly supported by environmental factors, familial tendency, declining risk with increasing distance of relatives, and the fact that when one or more siblings are affected there is a marked increase in risk for subsequent siblings to be affected. In North America, the risk of having a child with spina bifida is about 0.1 to 0.2 per cent. If there is one sibling with spina bifida, the risk of a subsequent child having spina bifida increases to about 5 per cent, and if there are two, the risk increases to approximately 12 to 15 per cent.[33] Studies of monozygotic and dizygotic twins, consanguinity studies, and environmental studies have produced little further information to elucidate genetic inheritance.[52, 141]

The known tendency of neural tube defects to recur in families suggests several possible genetic mechanisms, including a recessive gene, a dominant gene with reduced penetrance, a recessive X-linked gene, cytoplasmic inheritance, and polygenic inheritance. On the basis of pedigree analysis, Jorde and colleagues proposed that spina bifida cystica and spina bifida occulta may be related to an autosomal dominant trait with a 75 per cent penetrance.[46] However, further analysis will be required to test this thesis. It may be that there is a genetic and a nongenetic form of spina bifida.

Regardless of the genetic forms of inheritance, genetic counseling should be offered to all parents and close relatives of children with spina bifida. A detailed listing of facilities offering these services may be obtained from the National Foundation of the March of Dimes.[8]

ETIOLOGY

Interest in identifying etiologic factors in spina bifida has been driven by the goal of prevention. The incidence variation with season, geography, ethnic class, social group, parity, and maternal age has fueled the search for an environmental factor. This search was exemplified by the theory of Renwick that a teratogenic substance existed in blighted potatoes that caused anencephaly and spina bifida.[113, 141] Subsequent trials of potato avoidance and evaluation of exposure patterns failed to produce convincing evidence to support the potato blight teratogen.[21, 91] Since that time, numerous teratogens have been suggested, including valproic acid, phenytoin, trimethadione, haloperidol, alcohol, viral infections, local anesthetics, triamcinolone, infectious diseases, hydroxyurea, hypervitaminosis, dextromethorphan, and maternal fever.* Despite the abundance of teratogens suggested for spina bifida, conclusive supporting data for a causal factor continues to be missing. Further review of teratogens affecting neural tube development is available from the literature search conducted by the Environmental Teratology Information Center, done at the request of the Teratology Society.[29]

Numerous nutritional deficiency states, including folic acid and zinc deficiencies, have also been suggested as etiologic factors. Recently, it was reported that periconceptual vitamin supplementation was associated with a statistically significant reduction in neural tube defects when compared with an unsupplemented group.[51, 90, 119, 133] Although this observation was ascribed to folic acid deficiency and effective supplementation, many have questioned other possible mechanisms or deficiencies. Furthermore, these studies are weakened by the absence of randomized control groups, multivitamin administration, small numbers, poor compliance, and failure to consider social class, ethnicity, and maternal history. Thus, the data are inconclusive, and a larger, randomized placebo study in populations with high incidences is required.

EMBRYOLOGY

In 1886, Von Recklinghausen proposed that failure of the embryonic neural plate to close, forming the neural tube, at about 26 to 28 days of gestation led to myelomeningocele.[151] Most researchers now agree that the embryonic origin of spina bifida stems from a sequence of abnormalities originating from this point in fetal development.[156] Some of the various forms of spina bifida may be related to ensuing abnormal development of the neural tube, separation of superficial ectoderm, and migration of the mesoderm toward the cleavage space between superficial ectoderm and neuroectoderm.[76] Malformations arising during this period have been termed neurulation defects, and those following this period (about 30 days) have been termed postneurulation defects. The neurulation defects lead to cranioschisis, anencephaly, and myelomeningocele, whereas the postneurulation defects probably lead to skin-covered variants of spina bifida, such as meningocele, sinus tracts, and diastematomyelia.[61] The sequence of events leading to a neural tube open beyond the time of embryonic closure currently includes three possibilities:

1. Patten observed overgrowth of the dorsal caudal neural plate in chicken and human embryos

---

*References 45, 54, 56, 58, 59, 78, 80, 103, 115, 121, 139

and suggested that this was the primary event preventing neural tube closure.[100-102] Whether overgrowth is the primary event or secondary to fusion failure remains to be determined.

2. Gardner proposed overdistention of the neural tube by cerebrospinal fluid as a distending force leading to rupture of the caudal neural sac and thus producing spina bifida.[36, 157]

3. Padget suggested the appearance of a cleft in the neural tube that permitted a "bleb" of proteinaceous material to protrude into the surrounding mesodermal and ectodermal tissues, leading to changes in all three embryonic tissue derivatives.[96-99]

McLone and associates have been able to produce myelomeningoceles in laboratory chicken embryos by altering incubator temperatures and have succeeded in preventing neural tube closure in mice by the addition of tunicamycin to in vitro culture media. They have also been able to show distention and rupture of the neural tube in mouse embryos by producing vitamin A poisoning in pregnant mice. Therefore, they believe that both failure of primary closure and secondary rupture of the neural tube may be causes of myelomeningocele.[76]

PATHOLOGY

Although the pathologic abnormalities observed at the site of the neural plaque may be most obvious, additional changes are frequently found throughout the entire central and peripheral nervous systems. Furthermore, there may be congenital defects in other systems such as the genitourinary and the cardiovascular. The variations and combinations are numerous, and awareness of this potential contributes to more comprehensive understanding and treatment from the health care team and parents.

Brain

Lobar agenesis, polymicrogyria, holoprosencephaly, and cerebellar dysplasia and necrosis are commonly observed.[148] In addition, defects of cellular migration such as heterotopias, schizencephaly, and gyral anomalies have been described.[161] Agenesis of the corpus callosum, cysts of the septum pellucidum, midline lipoma, and arachnoid cysts have also been observed.[134] Hydrocephalus and associated anomalies of the aqueduct and cerebrospinal fluid pathways occur at a very high frequency.

Spinal Cord

The most common site of spinal cord lesions is the distal thoracic, lumbar, or sacral area. Over 85 per cent of meningoceles and myelomeningoceles are found at these levels. Approximately 10 per cent are detected in the thoracic area, and an additional 5 per cent are found in the cervical area.[67] Occasionally, more than one lesion is observed, and as many as three have been reported.[146]

In about one third of patients, the neural plaque has an appearance like that of an open book, with the midline neural groove and caudal central canal visible at the rostral aspect of the lesion (Fig. 3–2). The anterior columns of the spinal cord are frequently intact, whereas there are varying degrees of destruction of the dorsal columns and the internuncial pathways.[27] Since the neural plaque represents a splaying out of the neural tube, the dorsal roots exit from what appears to be the lateral anterior half of the spinal cord, and the ventral roots exit from the medial anterior neural plaque. In addition, the angle of exit of the nerve roots is more tangential than that of the rostral nerve roots. In approximately one third of the patients, the spinal cord rostral to the lesion shows diplomyelic changes, and about 40 per cent of patients have hydromyelia or syringomyelia.[27] These studies do not reveal the incidence of hydrocephalus, and therefore, it is possible that a high frequency of uncontrolled hydrocephalus could artificially inflate the figures for occurrence of hydromyelia.

The arachnoid forming the cystic wall of the lesion is adherent to the neural plaque, dura, and skin. Intradural and extradural lipoma, dermoid, epidermoid, squamous cell carcinoma, histiocytoma, enterogenous cyst, and teratoma have been observed with myelomeningocele.[18, 42, 79]

Neuronal counts in the lumbosacral spinal cords of children with myelomeningoceles have demonstrated reductions related to the degree of cord damage or of deformity present. Rostral spinal cord segments contain normal numbers of neurons.[63] Studies of the peripheral nervous systems of newborn children with myelomeningoceles have demonstrated reductions in the size of peripheral nerves. However, preservation of some or all the fibers of nerves distal to the plaque has been demonstrated.[105]

In patients with spina bifida, there is a high incidence of congenital malformations of other systems. A study of 434 patients with spina bifida demonstrated an average of 2.2 associated defects per patient.[14] Skeletal anomalies are the most frequent, with clubfeet and hip dislocation being the most common. Table 3–1 lists generally associated anomalies.

NEUROPHYSIOLOGY

In the past, it was commonly thought that the motor lesion of myelomeningocele was at the level

Table 3–1. SYSTEMIC ANOMALIES ASSOCIATED WITH SPINA BIFIDA

Skeletal	Gastrointestinal	Pulmonary	Craniofacial	Cardiovascular	Genitourinary
Clubfeet	Inguinal hernia	Tracheoesophageal fistula	Synostosis	Ventriculoseptal defect (VSD)	Hydronephrosis
Hip dislocation	Meckel's diverticulum	Situs inversus	Cleft palate	Atrial-septal defect (ASD)	Hydroureter
Rib anomalies	Malrotation		Strabismus	Patent ductus	Horseshoe kidney
Kyphoscoliosis	Omphalocele		Low-set ears	Coarctation	Undescended testes
Pectus excavatum	Imperforate anus		Hypertelorism		Hydrocele
Syndactyly					Malrotation, exstrophy

of the anterior horn cell. However, clinical observations have revealed upper motor neuron lesions in patients with functioning isolated distal cord segments.[134] Stark and Drummond have demonstrated that neural plaque stimulation results in involuntary contraction of 80 to 100 per cent of paralyzed muscles of the lower extremities.[135] The magnitude of contraction was similar to that observed following peripheral nerve stimulation of normal infants. Absence of fibrillation potentials further led Stark and Drummond to conclude that paralysis associated with myelomeningocele was secondary to an upper motor neuron lesion. They postulated that the lesion was either within the plaque itself or just rostral to the plaque.[135] The etiology of the upper motor neuron lesion remains undetermined. Possible explanations include abnormal development and change occurring in the neural plaque before, during, or after birth.

Somatosensory evoked potential studies of newborn children with myelomeningoceles have demonstrated intact sensory pathways to and from the neural plaque. In two of seven patients studied, afferent integrity through the plaque was observed.[109] Therefore, interference with afferent conduction appears to be located at the level of the neural plaque.

The observation of functioning motor and sensory systems within the neural plaque provides further support for meticulous protection and preservation of the neural plaque during early care of the patient with myelomeningocele. Furthermore, these findings, coupled with Lendon's observation of normal neuronal populations in the rostral spinal cord,[63] have provided the background data to justify cauda equina reconstruction, as described by Epstein and coworkers, in which proximal intercostal nerves are anastomosed to nerve roots distal to the lesion.[28] Early electromyographic observations have indicated reinnervation of muscle groups within the lower extremities. This exciting technique offers the possibility of bypassing the afferent and efferent interruption that occurs at the level of the plaque but requires further investigation and long-term study.[28, 63]

HISTORY OF TREATMENT

It is not known who first used the term spina bifida. It is known that neural tube defects of the sacrum have been identified in skeletons from the fifth millennium B.C.[39] The first description of a child with spina bifida was made by Peter Van Forest in 1587,[31, 39] and Tulp provided the first accurate anatomic illustrations of spina bifida in 1641.[39, 147] In 1761, Morgagni related the clinical changes to the spinal cord lesion, and it was Lebedeff who in 1881 first suggested failure of the neural tube to close.[39, 55, 83] In 1886, Von Recklinghausen classified the anatomic types of spina bifida and discussed treatment that included surgery.[152]

Although operative treatment for spina bifida may have occurred as early as 1610, when Forestus ligated a sac,[32] significant attempts to treat the lesion surgically did not occur until the twentieth century. Since the report of Fraser that of 131 patients operated upon, 63 per cent were discharged between 1898 and 1923, and 23 per cent were still alive in 1929,[34] there has been a steady succession of reports indicating continuously improving results with operative treatment. With the advent of aseptic surgical technique and antibiotics, an increasing number of surgeons began to consider operative closure of spina bifida. Care in selecting candidates for surgery was exercised, and often, extensive paralysis and hydrocephalus were contraindications to surgery. Operative delay was recommended in order to permit epithelialization of the lesion.[44, 82] While these measures led to a marked reduction in operative mortality, infection and hydrocephalus were still the leading causes of death in the child with spina bifida.

With the introduction of antibiotics, cerebrospinal fluid shunts, modern pediatric anesthesia, and improved neonatal care came new hope and enthusiasm for children with spina bifida as exemplified by Matson, by Nulsen and Spitz, and by Sharrard and coworkers.[67, 92, 129] These improvements in care resulted in an unprecedented number of survivors with spina bifida. However, many early survivors had significant physical and mental disabilities.

Care and support systems were not prepared for the continuum of associated problems such as a chronic urinary tract infection, reduced intellect, intractable shunt infections, unrelenting scoliosis, and psychosocial maladjustment. This led to a second wave of pessimism and the advancement of the concept of selecting ideal children for treatment while permitting (if not actively supporting) others who might not be expected to achieve an acceptable quality of life to die without treatment.[66]

The criteria for no treatment included extensive paralysis, severe hydrocephalus, kyphosis, and associated major anomalies. Proponents of these criteria reported that death uniformly followed selection. Contrary to the original reports, numerous investigators found that significant numbers of the children selected for no treatment survived. These discussions catapulted the care of children with spina bifida into the center of an international medical ethics debate.[9] Frequently, the rhetoric was based on disproportionately small experiences and scientific analysis. However, since 1959, four studies of treatment results of unselected newborns have been completed. McLone analyzed these studies[73, 75] and found that if selected patient populations and unselected patient populations are compared on the basis of continence, renal function, ambulation, mortality, and I.Q., the results are distinctly better for current unselected series than for the highly selected series reported by Lorber.[66, 73, 75] Quite simply, the results of treatment and comprehensive continuing care are of such high quality that they have led most treatment centers to provide aggressive multidisciplinary care from infancy to adulthood. The outlook and potential for rewarding, meaningful existence now extends to all patients with spina bifida and puts the selection discussion to rest because it cannot be supported on the basis of clinical experience or ethical principles.

Thus, it is clear that the potential for a high quality of life has been documented and should give comfort to neurosurgeons, who have seen the operative mortality of primary closure go down to zero per cent and the survival rate for the first two years of life exceed 95 per cent. Nonetheless, despite these very favorable survival statistics, two recent studies report that 35 per cent of 69 and 24 per cent of 58 children died within six months when treatment was withheld.[20, 40] The justification for no treatment in these reports was not the quality of life of the infant but the opportunity of making a decision and the quality of life for the parents. It is the experience of most large centers that families can cope, that financial support is available, and that increasing comprehensive programs for educational and psychosocial enrichment offer excellent opportunities for the child with spina bifida and the family.[35] We can now assure Father McCormick that infants with spina bifida will survive in relative comfort and will be able to experience our caring and love.[68]

CLINICAL ASSESSMENT

Prenatal

Meningocele and myelomeningocele are usually evident at birth. With advances in prenatal diagnosis, such as alpha-fetoprotein analysis, amniocentesis, and ultrasound imaging, increased numbers of fetuses with spina bifida are being identified during intrauterine life. This has led to parents consulting with the neurosurgeon during pregnancy. Often, these sessions include social workers, obstetricians, and neonatologists in order fully to prepare the parents and to plan for timely delivery, usually by cesarean section. Most pediatricians and neurosurgeons now agree that prompt closure of the open lesion is associated with decreased mortality and morbidity rates. When prenatal diagnosis has been made and the parents have been prepared and informed, the baby should be taken as soon as possible to the operating room after delivery. Ultrasonography of the brain and general pediatric evaluation are completed promptly, preferably in the delivery room.

Postnatal

Initial Examination

Infants are usually transferred with the mother. This system of child-maternal transfer leads to complete participation of the parents in health care and to early acceptance of and bonding to the mother. Routine intensive neonatal care is started immediately, and oral intake is withheld. Normothermia is rigorously maintained by continuous temperature monitoring. Lesions are covered with sterile, saline-moistened, nonadherent dressings, and the patient is kept in the prone or lateral decubitus position in order to protect exposed neural tissue. The initial evaluation includes prompt assessment of the infant's general pediatric condition and the degree of neurologic deficit or the functional level.

With the aid of the neonatologist or the pediatrician, the possibility of associated cardiopulmonary, genitourinary, and gastrointestinal conditions that would interfere with early operation is ruled out. Occasionally, delivery is complicated by unexpected abnormal fetal presentation or hydrocephalus. Thus, initial observation should include a search for trauma. After general neurologic examination of the newborn infant is completed, the size and location of the lesion is noted. The rostral level of spinal cord involvement provides a general estimate of the level of the spinal cord lesion. The sensory-motor examination of a child with myelomeningocele is complicated by the presence of numerous normal and abnormal reflexes and possibly an element of spinal cord shock.[73, 134, 135] Understanding this phenomenon is mandatory for the protection of parents and medical staff from developing an overly optimistic or pessimistic opinion about the motor potential of the child. Such understanding is also important for the surgeon, since the disappearance of reflex activity following the operation may be misinterpreted as a significant loss of function, or conversely, the appearance of motion that was previously absent may be falsely credited to operative treatment. Light pressure stimulation, motion, and sound may elicit abnormal reflex activities in the lower extremities that may have no bearing upon future appearance of volitional motor function.

The sensory examination requires that the child be relaxed and quiet or even sleeping. The cutaneous dermatomes are stimulated sharply distally to proximally, until one identifies the dermatome that produces facial or upper extremity response characteristic of pain perception. Some have advocated that dermatomal somatosensory evoked potentials be used to evaluate and follow sensory function in children with myelomeningocele, and have suggested that these potentials may help to identify more precisely the future sensory level.[118]

The motor examination is also done with the child at rest and begins with sharp or painful stimulation of the torso or upper extremities, with observation for voluntary motion below the level of the lesion. Hip flexion requires the innervation of L1-3, and adduction requires innervation of L2-4, as does knee extension. Hip abduction, hip extension, and knee flexion require the presence of L5-S2. Plantar flexion and intrinsic muscle action of the feet require the preservation of the sacral roots.[124] Orthopedic deformities may also provide clues to the motor level. Patients with levels above T12, for example, often have flaccid hips and feet, whereas patients with lesions below L1-2 have flail feet. Sharrard has described the limb and spinal deformities associated with neurologic deficit in detail.[124, 125, 127, 128] Additional aid in identifying the sensory level may come in the future with the application of somatosensory evoked potentials.

Bladder Dysfunction

Over 90 per cent of patients with myelomeningocele have a form of neurogenic bladder. It is extremely difficult to predict the type of bladder dysfunction an infant will display at the time of neonatal examination. Because of the presence of abnormal reflexes, anal wink and tone cannot be used as a reliable indication of perineal sensation. One is left with observing for the presence of spontaneous voiding and the nature of the urinary stream. It will be easy to perform Credé's maneuver on those children with lower motor neuron defect (approximately 30 per cent), and they often remain dry. However, in those patients with sphincter or bladder spasticity, Credé's maneuver may be extremely difficult to perform and may lead to ureteral reflux and subsequent infection. Reliable determination of bladder function may not be possible for months after the operation. The important fact is that the high incidence of neurogenic bladder be recognized and that appropriate steps be taken to ensure that the bladder is intermittently and completely emptied. Usually, bowel incontinence is associated with bladder incontinence, and, generally, lower motor neuron lesions produce anal relaxation and prolapse. As the child develops, bladder and bowel training programs offer the possibility of achieving continence.

Dealing with Parents

Once the initial evaluation of the infant is completed, it is recommended that early repair of all lesions be performed unless there are overriding pediatric complications or death is imminent (less than 1 per cent). Clearly, the parents always make the final decision concerning surgery, but it is the neurosurgeon's responsibility to provide current factual data on the natural untreated course and the prognosis with aggressive prompt management. Since less than 5 per cent of pregnant patients currently are forewarned and prepared as a result of prenatal diagnosis, the majority of couples will experience immense emotional turmoil and sadness. Their primary worries are related to prognosis for intellectual development, ambulation, and survival. The parents should be given the current data that 90 per cent or more of newborn children with myelomeningocele will survive, 80 per cent or more will have normal intelligence, and 85 per cent will walk with or without some form of assistance. Extreme caution should be exercised regarding predicting motor function of the lower extremities, and one should repeatedly emphasize that surgery will not restore function but will preserve existing function. Furthermore, most parents must be repeatedly reminded that there is no therapy available to restore neural function. The neurosurgeon will find it necessary to teach the parents about hydrocephalus, which develops in 80 to 90 per cent of infants with spina bifida and to explain the meaning of neurogenic bowel and bladder. Today, it can be expected that 80 per cent of patients will become socially continent with the use of drugs and clean intermittent catheterization. At the present time, it is difficult to predict the patients who will have complete independence.

One must be continually cognizant of the fact that these are devastated parents with dashed dreams and that the responsibility of "caring" surgeons is to provide the facts and repeatedly to teach the parents about the problem, the proposed treatment, and the support systems. Especially in the case of first-born children so affected, parents experience self-doubt and fears of inadequacy, along with profound guilt. It is helpful to assure the parents that these feelings are not unique to the parents of children with spina bifida but that all parents feel guilt when their children are ill or injured. They also experience a natural universal doubt about parental competency. Assure the parents that they can cope, and introduce them to the team concept of continuing care and compassion of the entire multidisciplinary health care team. Finally, the parents are seeking guidance and help, and the neurosurgeon who has negative personal opinions about meaningful life for children with spina bifida will convey hesitancy, tentativeness, and doubt, which will only impair quality care and further unsettle the parents. The care team should assure the parents that it has confidence in them and in the prospects for a rewarding existence for their child. This requires a continuing commitment, through all phases of life, to the well-being of the child and the family. Given this approach, most parents request aggressive management and care.

Most people now believe that closure is not a surgical emergency and that a limited period of time should be used to inform and counsel the parents.[149] Simultaneously, the pertinent members of the multidisciplinary team including nurses, social workers, orthopedists, urologists, and therapists begin to participate in the care of the child and the family.

If the lesion is open and draining cerebrospinal fluid and surgery cannot be performed within 24 hours, or if the lesion is closed and surgery cannot be performed in 48 hours, surgery should be delayed until three negative, consecutive 24-hour cultures are obtained from the surface of the lesion. The lesion can usually be sterilized with good local care. If signs of sepsis or ventriculitis develop, treat with external ventricular drainage and systemic and intrathecal antibiotics until sterilization of the cerebrospinal fluid and lesion is achieved.[117]

OPERATIVE TECHNIQUE

The purposes of surgery are to preserve intellectual, motor, and sensory function by restoring the spinal cord to its normal cerebrospinal fluid environment and to prevent central nervous system infection. Meningitis and ventriculitis produce intellectual and developmental delay.[74] An additional purpose is to restore the normal contour of the back, which contributes to ease of care and future bracing.

The operative technique for primary closure of myelomeningocele has been described by many; modern methods include the use of the microscope and kyphectomy.[2, 72, 106] The general guidelines for closure include protection and preservation of exposed neural tissue, reconvolution of the spinal cord within the spinal canal, and a five-layer closure. Potentially neurotoxic scrubs and topical antibiotics are avoided. The five-layer closure begins with the reconvolution of the spinal cord by closing the pia-arachnoid and continues with sequential closure of the dura, iliocostal fascia, subcutaneous tissue, and skin. The operating microscope and microinstruments are used for reconvolution of the spinal cord while avoiding all forms of traction. Magnification leads to preservation of the vascular supply of the neural plaque, and the use of bipolar cautery is mandatory to avoid unnecessary neural trauma.

The child is placed in the prone position on bilateral, firm chest rolls so that the abdomen is suspended freely and femoral pulsation is maintained. The initial incision follows the circumferential white line formed by the junction of the arachnoid and the skin (Figs. 3–4A and B and 3–5). This leads to isolation of the neural plaque and the immediately rostral spinal cord. At this point, one may observe arachnoidal adhesions to the ventral, lateral intradural surface, and these are lysed by sharp dissection.

Following isolation of the neural plaque and arachnoid investment, the dura is isolated. To identify the dura, the skin defect is extended rostrally in the midline in order to observe the inferior aspect of the most caudal intact lamina and, immediately beneath it, the intact dorsal dura (Fig. 3–6). With the normal rostral dura thus identified, the dura is then isolated by dissecting laterally and inferiorward in the epidural space to the caudal margin of the defect (Fig. 3–4C and D). The caudal defect is extended in the midline in order to identify the termination of the defect and the inferior dorsal dural surface.

With the use of the operating microscope, dural remnants, fat, and excess arachnoid are now sharply dissected free from the circumference of the neural plaque. Inclusion of these tissues in the intradural repair may lead to subsequent intraspinal lipoma and epidermoid tumor.[107] Magnification is required at this point because it is the area of the alar plate or dorsal root entry zones. The medial aspect of the plaque represents the basilar plate, or area of the anterior horn cells. The lateral arachnoidal edges are now approximated in the midline with 7–0 suture, thus reconstituting the neural plaque to a tubular structure resembling the remainder of the spinal cord (Fig. 3–4E). The interior of this tube is the continuation of the central spinal canal.

The dura is then approximated in the midline, thus restoring the continuity of the dural sac to a tubular structure surrounding the reconstituted spinal cord (Fig. 3–4F).

Every effort should be made to make the dural sac patulous and water-tight. Constriction at any point could contribute to ischemia of the neural plaque, subsequent tethering, or both. Some have advocated plastic and other forms of dural substitute in order to maintain a patulous intradural space. Unfortunately, many of these also carry the risk of arachnoiditis and secondary tethering.

The lumbodorsal fascia is identified at its attachment to the posterior iliac crest and sacrum. The fascia is bilaterally incised and dissected free from

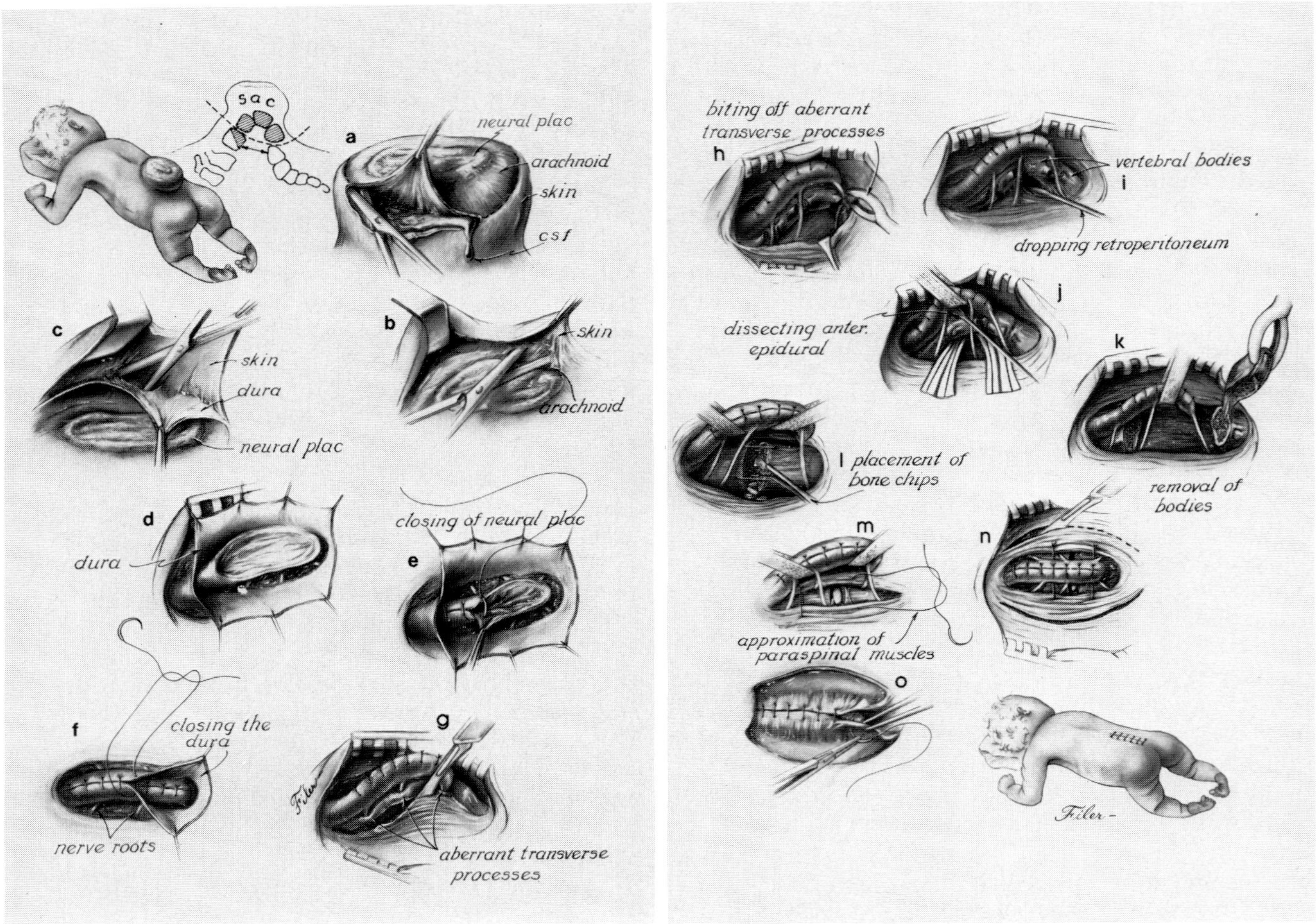

Figure 3–4. Diagrammatic illustration of technique for closure of myelomeningocele. (With permission from Reigel DH: Kyphectomy and myelomeningocele repair. *In* Ransohoff J [ed]: Modern Technics in Surgery. Neurosurgery, Vol. 13. Mt. Kisco, NY, Futura Publishing Co., 1979, pp 1–9.)

the posterior iliac crest and the underlying sacrospinalis muscle (Fig. 3–4N). The sacral attachment of the fascia is not disturbed. Attenuated fascia may be protected by including some of the superficial fibers of the sacrospinalis muscle. The lateral edges of the fascial flaps are then folded medially and sutured in the midline over the dorsal dural surface (Fig. 3–4O). Again, attention must be given to avoid constriction of the dural sac.

The subcutaneous tissue is closed in the midline, and the skin margins are then sharply incised to form a vertical midline incision. With closure of the skin, the five-layer closure is completed.

Recently, there has been increasing interest in a variety of myocutaneous reconstructive procedures designed to obtain full-thickness skin covering for large myelomeningocele defects.[7, 10, 22, 60, 69, 84, 162] These procedures, while obtaining excellent skin coverage, have the potential to interfere significantly with muscle function of the upper torso and shoulders, which is vital for daily activities and ambulation. Furthermore, such procedures extend the operation and increase the risk for significant blood loss. In a recent series of 358 consecutive patients with myelomeningocele, we were able to obtain primary skin coverage in all patients without the use of flaps.[111] There were no dehiscences, and the average blood loss was 29 cc.

Approximately 15 per cent of patients with myelomeningocele have thoracolumbar kyphosis (Figs. 3–4A and 3–7). The width of the vertebral bodies is increased, and they may actually protrude posterior

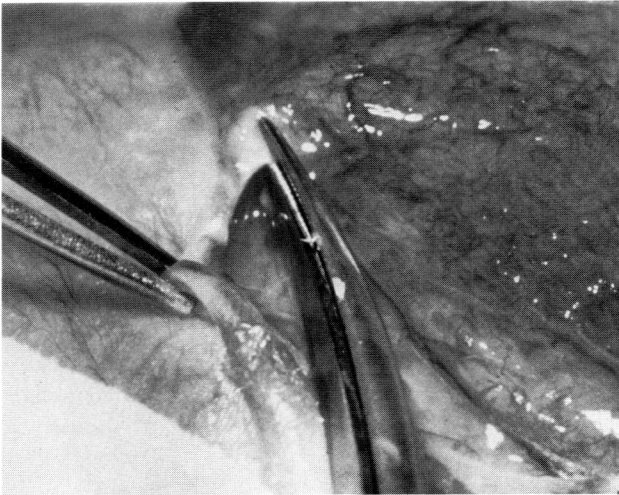

Figure 3–5. Operative photograph demonstrating the line of incision along the junctional zone.

Figure 3–6. Intraoperative photograph demonstrating the rostral skin incision (curved arrow), the last normal lamina (reversed arrow), the intact dorsal dural sac overlying spinal cord (large straight arrow), and the point of dural dissection (small straight arrow).

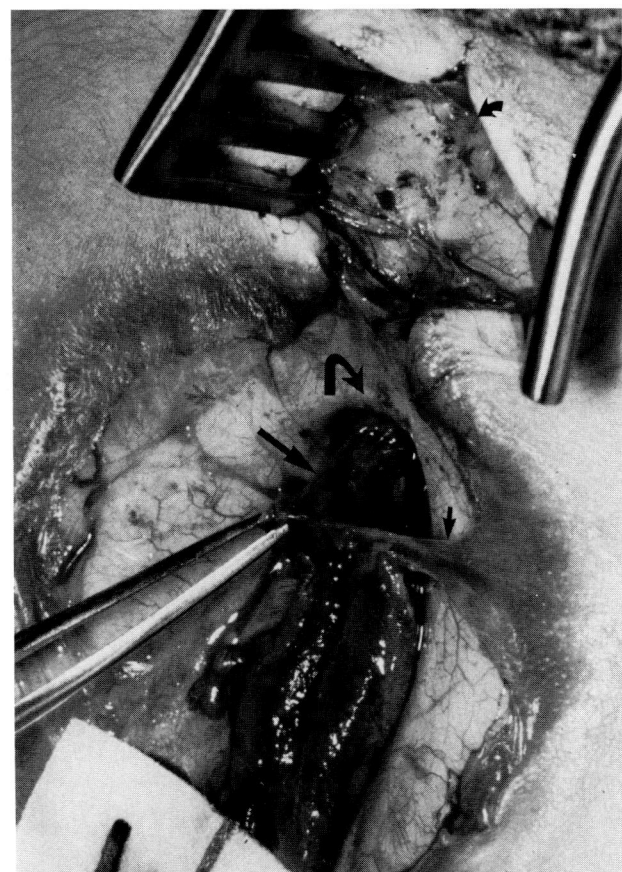

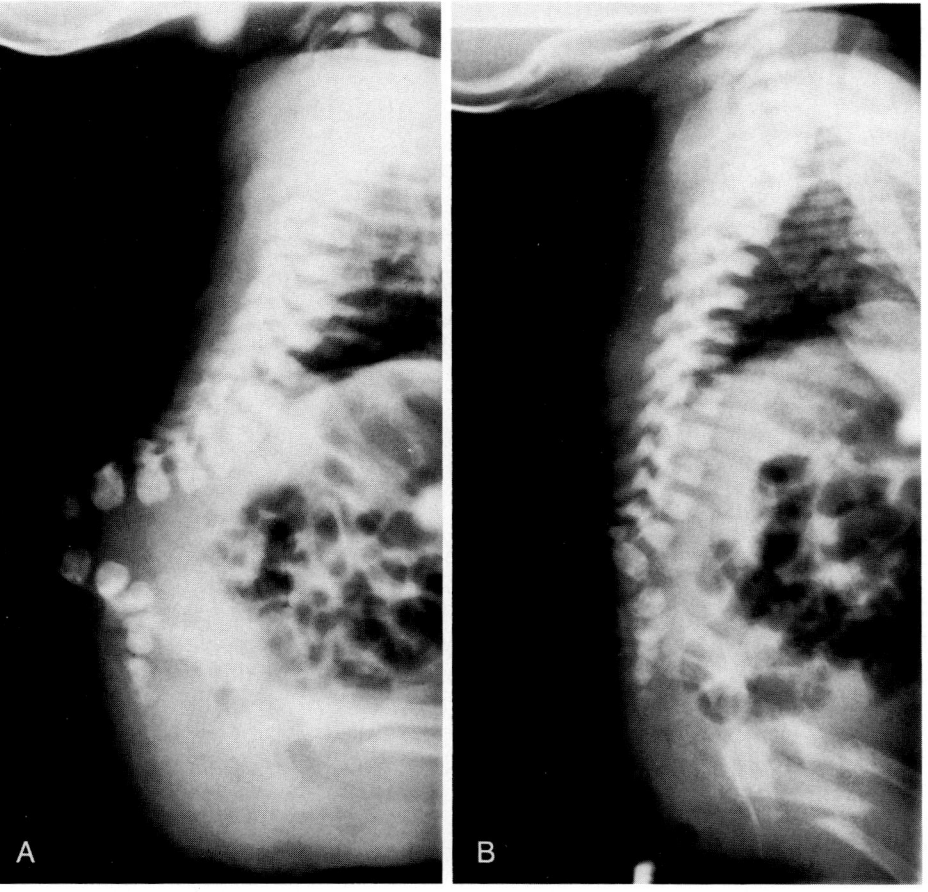

Figure 3–7. *A*, X-ray film of lumbar kyphosis, prekyphectomy, at birth. *B*, Postoperative x-ray film following kyphectomy and primary closure.

to the dermal surface of the back. With growth and development, the natural course of this defect is progressive angulation and deformity. The presence of kyphosis complicates early repair in that it is difficult to obtain adequate subcutaneous tissue and skin coverage over the defect, which causes skin necrosis and, in turn, postoperative infection and ventriculitis. However, even in the presence of adequate skin coverage, the progression of the underlying kyphosis leads to the recurring complication of skin ulceration and vertebral angulation. Bracing becomes difficult, ambulatory capacity declines, and, ultimately, life expectancy is reduced because of associated progressive cardiopulmonary complications.

Primary spinal osteotomy for kyphosis associated with myelomeningocele was proposed by Sharrard in 1968.[126] He was able partially to correct the deformity and obtain good skin coverage. The author has found that kyphectomy can be done safely at birth, during the time of primary operation, and that it enables one to obtain good skin coverage and vertebral alignment, leading to reduced hospitalization time and early ambulation (Fig. 3–4H through M).[108]

POSTOPERATIVE MANAGEMENT

Following surgery, the infant is returned to the Isolette, with no restriction on positioning. Every effort should be made to have the mother hold the baby within the first postoperative day. As soon as bowel sounds are present, routine feeding is started. Prophylactic antibiotics are not used.

The wound is observed closely for signs of infection and wound breakdown. If an early, meticulous, five-layer closure has been achieved, it is unlikely that superficial infection or necrosis will be followed by meningitis and attendant ventriculitis. However, cellulitis and wound breakdown will delay insertion of a cerebrospinal fluid shunt for hydrocephalus. If wound infection develops, the patient should be treated with appropriate local drainage, surgical scrubs, and high-dose systemic antibiotics selected on the basis of cultures and sensitivity studies. If ventriculitis develops in the presence of hydrocephalus, prompt clearing of the infection and control of the hydrocephalus can be achieved with the use of external ventricular drainage and the addition of intrathecal antibiotics.[117] Meticulous closure, as described, is associated with significant reduction in the incidence of postoperative cerebrospinal fluid leak or fistula. When fistulas do occur, most will close spontaneously. In the rare event that a fistula does not spontaneously close, secondary closure is performed immediately. External ventricular drainage of hydrocephalus has been proposed to control leaks, but it predisposes to secondary infection, with meningitis and ventriculitis. Insertion of a shunt is ill-advised in the presence of cerebrospinal fluid leaks, since the incidence of infection may be increased because of the failure to recognize early infection at the site of the leak.

Although the etiology of hydrocephalus associated with myelomeningocele has been ascribed to aqueductal stenosis, many surgeons have noted exacerbation of hydrocephalus following repair of myelomeningocele. Perhaps as few as 15 per cent of patients with myelomeningocele are born with signs of hydrocephalus, but 80 per cent or more will develop them in early infancy.[137] One explanation is that the hydrocephalus may be aggravated by a shift in the brainstem after repair, which produces changes in the aqueduct or the Arnold-Chiari malformation, leading to further alterations in the cerebrospinal fluid flow pathways. Aqueductal stenosis may be a secondary phenomenon of hydrocephalus rather than the primary cause.[77, 159] It is doubtful that the sac serves as a site of absorption and that its removal aggravates the hydrocephalus.

For those patients with signs of hydrocephalus at birth, obtain ultrasound brain scans before transfer to the operating room. With the verification of significant hydrocephalus, we insert a ventriculoperitoneal shunt prior to closure of the myelomeningocele. The experience of the author and colleagues with shunt insertion before repair is recent and consists of 15 patients. The morbidity (i.e., infection) has not exceeded our previous experience, and the length of hospitalization has been significantly reduced, to approximately five days in the absence of complication.

The onset of hydrocephalus after closure may be indicated by intermittent short periods of apnea, decreased spontaneous activity, and poor feeding patterns. The onset of hydrocephalus can usually be verified by serial examinations, transcephalic impedance, and ultrasonography.[110, 116] Marked hydrocephalus may be present with only minimal cranial enlargement. These children should only rarely be discharged without a computerized tomographic (CT) scan.[137] As soon as clinical suspicion is high that progressive hydrocephalus is present, a CT scan should be performed. If clinical examination indicates the absence of wound infection, and there are no signs and symptoms of meningitis or ventriculitis, insertion of a ventriculoperitoneal shunt is recommended because of its described advantages over ventriculoatrial shunts.[114, 136] We do not predispose a child to porencephaly by ventricular taps preoperatively for cerebrospinal fluid culture. In the rare event that cultures and analysis of cerebrospinal fluid obtained at the time of shunt insertion indicate ventriculitis, externalize the shunt and treat with systemic and intrathecal antibiotics. McLaurin[71] has demonstrated successful treatment with only high-dose intravenous and intrathecal antibiotics.

RESULTS AND TREATMENT

The operative mortality rate is approaching zero, and 95 per cent or greater survival rates for the first two years of life have been reported.[4, 73, 111] In a recent review of the primary closure of 358 consecutive myelomeningoceles, the average blood loss was 29 cc, and postoperative ileus (3 per cent), wound effusion (2.7 per cent), and pneumonia (6.3 per cent) were infrequent complications. Wound infection occurred in 12 per cent, but there were no dehiscences.[111] In this recent series, the incidence of cerebrospinal fluid leak was a surprising 17 per cent. However, the leak was rarely associated with infection, spontaneously closed, and was thought to be increased because of special efforts to obtain a patulous dural closure in order to prevent tethered spinal cord. A total of 18 per cent of patients developed ventriculitis, and all were promptly and successfully treated with external drainage and intrathecal and systemic antibiotics.[117] Prophylactic antibiotics have had no significant effect upon the frequency of ventriculitis. The risk of postoperative ventriculitis is increased for patients with delayed primary operations and remote sources of infection such as the urinary tract. The most common cause for early demise is pulmonary infection often related to the Arnold-Chiari malformation and ventriculitis.[43]

Although the prognosis for intellectual development is difficult to determine for any given infant, it now appears that, in the absence of ventriculitis and intracerebral hemorrhage, children with myelomeningocele, with or without hydrocephalus, will have IQ test results within the normal range.[74, 104, 123] However, of those with myelomeningocele and a history of cerebrospinal fluid shunt infections, only 31 per cent will have IQ test results within the norm. There is no correlation between degree of hydrocephalus and the presence of lacunar skull deformity.[23, 65] Despite these encouraging observations, discussion of prognosis for intellectual development must be tempered by other emerging findings that children with myelomeningocele have significant disturbance in hand function, perhaps related to neurologic change, incoordination, delayed hand dominance, and delayed use of the hands for balance during crucial developmental phases. Furthermore, significant problems with visual perception and eye-hand coordination have been documented in this group of patients.[123] All these findings may partially account for the frequently reported verbal-performance discrepancies in IQ testing. Additionally, memory deficits have now been documented for children with myelomeningocele.[23, 123] Therefore, an early awareness of these possible impairments may lead to improved family counseling and educational opportunity for the child.

For parents of the newborn child with myelomeningocele, concerns about ambulation are superseded only by those about intelligence. Improved recognition and treatment of tethered spinal cord, with reduction in the incidence of scoliosis and maintenance of motor function; orthopedic care of extremity deformity; and appropriate orthosis when required means that more than 80 per cent will be ambulatory.[73, 111, 112]

The management of urinary incontinence has been markedly improved with the advent of pharmacologic treatment of neurogenic bladder and the introduction of nonsterile intermittent catheterization. Continence (staying dry for three to four hours) rates of 85 per cent are now possible.[1, 6, 41, 47, 49, 120, 158] For the small percentage of patients who remain incontinent, the artificial sphincter holds promise.[15] Intelligent and comprehensive management of urinary incontinence contributes significantly to the development of social relationships.

Frequently, parents inquire about the patient's sexual development and activity. The sacral (S2–4) innervation is required for erection and ejaculation. An individual's ability in these areas is highly variable, and with certain lesions, reflex erection and ejaculation is possible.[153] Shurtleff and Sousa have indicated that 18 per cent of patients of a group of 60, aged 16 to 24, were sexually active.[131] Counseling has been urged for all these patients.

It is clear that one of the major handicaps imposed upon children with myelomeningocele is that of psychosocial problems originating within themselves, their families, and society. These forms of stress can be reduced by bringing the child into the educational mainstream, personal and family counseling, improved understanding of the patient's potential, and increased public awareness of spina bifida.

MENINGOCELE

In addition to the routine assessment described with myelomeningocele, other recommended methods include preoperative ultrasonography,[86] metrizamide myelography with CT, and nuclear magnetic resonance (NMR) imaging to identify dermoid tumor, diastematomyelia, lipoma, or tethered spinal cord. After complete evaluation, surgery is recommended to prevent infection and to restore continuity of the back. Delaying surgery until the child is older predisposes the patient to irreversible neurologic deficit and psychologic trauma. Therefore, surgery at the time of diagnosis is encouraged, which is usually at birth. Then, the child can begin a healthy normal development process with the parents and family.

The operative technique follows the guidelines described for myelomeningocele. The neck of the dural sac is often significantly smaller than the sac and may be surprisingly narrow. Occasionally, nerve roots or the filum terminale may be involved within the sac. Nerve roots should be replaced and the filum terminale sectioned. The spinal cord is normal. Excessive dura is excised, and the remainder is closed in the midline. The fascia and skin closures are similar to those for myelomeningocele. The postoperative management requires all the same precautions and observations as with the child with myelomeningocele. However, the incidence of hydrocephalus is markedly reduced, and the prognosis for normal development is very good.

Anterior Sacral Meningocele

This form of meningocele extends anteriorly into the presacral retroperitoneal space and usually communicates with the sacral subarachnoid space through a narrow anterior sacral defect. The natural course of this meningocele is one of progressive enlargement of the intrapelvic sac, secondary to hydrostatic pressure of cerebrospinal fluid. The sacral canal also may be enlarged secondary to lipoma, dermoid tumor, teratoma, or intrasacral meningocele. The lesion is probably more common in females than in males and is often associated with other pelvic organ anomalies such as bicornate uterus, vaginal septation, rectovaginal fistula, duplication of the kidneys, changes in the ureter, and imperforate anus.

These patients may appear with chronic constipation, obstetric complications, or pelvic masses.[5, 94, 150] Incontinence, recurrent urinary tract infection, headache, dysmenorrhea, dyspareunia, and radicular pain may also alert one to this diagnosis. The mass may be palpable by abdominal, rectal, or pelvic examination. The differential diagnosis includes most pelvic tumors. Plane x-ray films of the sacrum show the posterior aspect of the pelvis to be intact and the classic "scimitar" (sickle-shaped) sacrum.[132] Intravenous pyelography and ultrasonography may identify changes in the kidneys, ureter, and bladder. The diagnosis is established by metrizamide myelography. Ultrasonography, computerized tomography, and NMR imaging may also assist in elucidating the diagnosis.[86, 155]

Generally, sacral laminectomy has been primarily recommended because it permits visualization of the intraspinal contents and direct anterior suture of the opening into the sacral canal. With aspiration of the meningocele and the obliteration of the dural communication, the pelvic mass disappears. Occasionally, dural graft may be required to close the meningocele.[5] Rarely, because of intrameningocele neural structures, a delayed anterior abdominal operation may be required to obliterate the meningocele.[3] Barring complications such as infection, the results of surgical treatment should be gratifying.

Anterolateral Meningocele

These meningoceles appear at the thoracic and lumbar levels, protrude through enlarged intervertebral foramina, and are often associated with vertebral scalloping and scoliotic deformity. This form of meningocele is often associated with neurofibromatosis, Marfan's syndrome, or both.[93, 140] Myelography, CT scanning, and NMR imaging enable establishment of the diagnosis and exclusion of neoplasm. Operative treatment in collaboration with the orthopedist is designed to obliterate the meningocele and ensure spinal stability.

DELAYED COMPLICATIONS

Even with improved care and prognosis, it has become evident that spina bifida is a dynamic birth defect of the entire central nervous system and that optimal development of the child requires serial examinations of all systems for delayed complications. These complications include esotropia, auditory deficits, swallowing disorders, apnea, cranial nerve dysfunction, seizure, cervical medullary compression, kyphoscoliosis, hydromyelia, intraspinal tumor, tethered spinal cord, urinary tract change, nutrition and growth disturbances, psychosocial adjustment problems, and skin breakdown. Early recognition of the potential onset of these complications often leads to their prevention or the interruption of their progression. Aggressive identification and treatment of these problems leads to enhanced development and performance. These delayed problems are discussed in detail in Chapter 4.

Prenatal Diagnosis

Open neural-tube defects permit fetal protein (alpha-fetoprotein) to enter amniotic fluid and the maternal blood stream. Elevations of alpha-fetoprotein reach peaks at about 16 to 18 weeks following the last menstrual period.[38]

Separate collaborative studies in the United States and the United Kingdom have shown maternal serum alpha-fetoprotein assays to be an effective way of screening for identification of the fetus with an open neural tube defect.[38, 81, 154] This method has an accuracy of 60 to 70 per cent. Mothers with positive serum alpha-fetoprotein screenings should be considered for amniotic fluid assay and serial ultrasonography studies.[81] Genetic counseling helps identify couples at high risk for a fetus with open neural tube defect (i.e., those with affected second- or third-degree relatives). Amniocentesis for alpha-fetoprotein and serial ultrasonography should also be recommended for this group. Examination of amniotic fluid for alpha-fetoprotein carries an accuracy of 90 to 95 per cent. A total of 5 to 20 per cent of neural tube abnormalities are the closed type, and elevated alpha-fetoprotein is not detected.[13] Factors such as errors in gestational age, twins, placental bleeding, and malformations (i.e., omphalocele and gastroschisis) may lead to false-positive results. Serial ultrasonography has a high accuracy (80 per cent) and may help define the false-positive or false-negative result.[16] An elevated level of acetylcholinesterase in the amniotic fluid is specific in the range of 99 per cent for open neural tube defects (without epithelial coverage) and may further help differentiate neural tube defects from other abnormalities.[12]

Screening programs may lead to early intrauterine diagnosis, which will provide the parents with the opportunity to decide whether to prepare effectively for a child with spina bifida or to terminate the pregnancy. Greater availability of nondirective genetic counseling and the widespread use of screening techniques can only benefit society. Neurosurgeons should be prepared to inform the parents and relatives of children with spina bifida and the rapidly growing population of young adults with spina bifida of genetic counseling, screening, and diagnostic centers.

CONCLUSIONS

The prognosis for newborn infants with myelomeningocele is better at this time than at any time in history. New operative methods of closure of the neural plaque and initial kyphectomy preserve existing neural function and reduce the incidence of wound breakdown and infection. The development of new shunting systems and diagnostic tools such as ultrasonography and computerized tomography have enabled critical determination of shunt function, leading to earlier revision and, thus, preventing irreversible pathologic and functional change of the brain. Multimodality neuropsychologic testing has confirmed normal intellectual performance in many of these children. Intermittent, clean catheterization and pharmacologic treatment of the neurogenic bladder have drastically reduced the incidence of unrelenting urinary tract infection and renal failure. Early recognition and treatment of tethered spinal cord have reduced the incidence of delayed neurologic deterioration and scoliosis. Advances in selection and the technique of orthopedic procedures and improved orthotics have led to most children with myelomeningocele being able to achieve ambulation. The quality of the patient's life and the prognosis appear to be directly related to comprehensive health care. Advances in community understanding and interaction have enabled children with spina bifida to attain social acceptance, educational opportunities, and a rewarding life. The conclusions make the question of selection for treatment a matter only of historical interest.

References

1. Action Committee of Myelodysplasia, Section of Urology: Current approaches to evaluation and management of children with myelomeningocele. Pediatrics 63:663, 1979.
2. Amacher L: The microsurgical anatomy of lumbar rachischisis. Adv Ophthalmol 37:197, 1978.
3. Amacher AL, Drake CG, McLachlin AD: Anterior sacral myelocele. Surg Gynecol Obstet 126:986, 1968.
4. Ames MD, Schut L: Results of treatment of 171 consecutive myelomeningoceles—1963 to 1968. Pediatrics 50:466, 1972.
5. Anderson TM, Burke BL: Anterior sacral meningocele. A presentation of three cases. JAMA 237:39, 1977.
6. Awad SA, Downie J, Kiruluta H: Pharmacologic treatment of disorders of bladder and urethra: A review. Can J Surg 22:515, 1979.
7. Bannister CM: A method of repair of myelomeningoceles. Br J Surg 59:445, 1972.
8. Birth Defects. Genetic Services International Directory, 8th ed. The National Foundation–March of Dimes, 1986.
9. Black PM: Selective treatment of infants with myelomeningocele. Neurosurgery 5:334, 1979.
10. Blaiklock CR, Demetriou EL, Rayner CRW: The use of a latissimus dorsi myocutaneous flap in the repair of spinal defects in spina bifida. Br J Plast Surg 34:358, 1981.
11. Boone D, Pansons D, Lochman SM, et al: Spina bifida occulta: Lesion or anomaly? Clin Radiol 36:159, 1985.
12. Brock DJH, Barron L, Von Heyningen V: Prenatal diagnosis of neural tube defects with monoclonal specific for acetylcholine esterase. Lancet 125:391, 1981.
13. Brock DJH, Sutcliffe RG: Alpha-fetoprotein in the antenatal diagnosis of anencephaly and spina bifida. Lancet 2:197, 1972.
14. Brown SF: Congenital malformations associated with myelomeningocele. J Iowa Med Soc 65:101, 1975.
15. Burch DM: The artificial sphincter to correct sphincter incontinence in the myelodysplastic child. In: McLaurin RL (ed): Spina Bifida—A Multidisciplinary Approach. New York, Praeger Publishers, 1986, pp 277–280.
16. Campbell S: Early prenatal diagnosis of neural tube defects by ultrasound. Clin Obstet Gynecol 20:351, 1977.
17. Carter CO, Evans KA: Spina bifida and anencephalus in greater London. J Med Genet 10:209, 1973.
18. Chadduck WM, Uthman EO: Squamous cell carcinoma and meningomyelocele. Neurosurgery 14:601, 1984.
19. Chapman PH, Beyerl B: The tethered spinal cord, with particular reference to spinal lipoma and diastematomyelia. In: Hoffman HJ, Epstein F (eds): Disorders of the Developing Nervous System: Diagnosis and Treatment. Boston, Blackwell Scientific Publishers, 1986, p 119.
20. Charney EB, Miller SC, Sutton LN, et al: Management of the newborn with myelomeningocele: Time for a decision-making process. Pediatrics 75:58, 1985.
21. Clarke CA, McKendrick OM, Sheppard PM: Spina bifida and potatoes. Br Med J 3:251, 1973.
22. Cruz NI, Ariyan S, Duncan CC, et al: Repair of lumbosacral myelomeningoceles with double Z-rhomboid flaps. J Neurosurg 59:714, 1983.
23. Cull C, Wyke MA: Memory function of children with spina bifida and shunted hydrocephalus. Dev Med Child Neurol 26:177, 1984.
24. Eckstein HB: Neuropathic bladder. In: Williams DI (ed): Urology in Childhood. Berlin, Springer Verlag, 1974, p 250.
25. Elwood JH: Major central nervous system malformations notified in Northern Ireland, 1964–1968. Dev Med Child Neurol 14:731, 1972.
26. Elwood JM, Elwood JH: Epidemiology of Anencephalus and Spina Bifida. New York, Oxford University Press, 1980.
27. Emery JL, Lendon RG: Clinical implications of cord lesions in neurospinal dysraphism. Dev Med Child Neurol 14:45, 1972.
28. Epstein F, Spielholz N, Battista A, et al: Delayed cauda equina reconstruction in meningomyelocele. Neurosurgery 6:540, 1980.
29. ETIC Search Subject, Neural Tube Environmental Teratology Information Center (F Jordan), PO Box 12233, NIEHS, Maildrop 18-01 Research Triangle Park, North Carolina, 27709.
30. Fineman RM, Jorde LB, Martin RA, et al: Spinal dysraphia

as an autosomal dominant defect in four families. Am J Med Genet 12:457, 1982.
31. Forest P Van: Observationum Medicinalium libri tres, de capitis et cerebre morbis ac symptomatis. Leiden, Ex Off Plantiniana Raphelemgii, 1587.
32. Forestus: Obs Chir, Libri V, Lib III, Obs VII, 1610.
33. Fraser F: Genetic counseling in some common paediatric diseases. Am J Hum Genet 26:636, 1974.
34. Fraser J: Spina bifida. Edinburgh Med J 36:284, 1929.
35. Freeman JM: Early management and decision making for treatment of myelomeningocele: A critique. Pediatrics 73:564, 1984.
36. Gardner WJ: Etiology and pathogenesis of the development of myelomeningocele. In: McLaurin RL (ed): Myelomeningocele. New York, Grune & Stratton, 1977, pp 3–30.
37. Gillespie HW: The significance of congenital lumbosacral anomalies. Br J Radiol 22:270, 1949.
38. Globus MS, Loughman WD, Epstein CJ, et al: Prenatal genetic diagnosis in 3000 amniocenteses. N Engl J Med 300:157, 1979.
39. Gool JB, Gool JD: A Short History of Spina Bifida. Netherlands, Society for Research into Hydrocephalus and Spina Bifida, 1986.
40. Gross HR, Cox A, Tatyrek R, et al: Early management and decision making for the treatment of myelomeningocele. Pediatrics 72:450, 1983.
41. Hannigan KF: Teaching intermittent self-catheterization to young children with myelodysplasia. Dev Med Child Neurol 21:365, 1979.
42. Helle TL, Hanbery JW, Becker DH: Meningeal malignant fibrous histiocytoma arising from a thoracolumbar myelomeningocele. J Neurosurg 58:593, 1983.
43. Holinger PC, Holinger LD, Reichert TJ, et al: Respiratory obstruction and apnea in infants with bilateral abductor vocal cord paralysis, meningomyelocele, hydrocephalus, and Arnold-Chiari malformation. Pediatrics 92:368, 1978.
44. Ingram FD, Swan H: Spina bifida and cranium bifidum: I: A survey of five hundred forty-six cases. N Engl J Med 228:559, 1943.
45. Janerich DT: Influenza and neural-tube defects. Lancet 2:551, 1971.
46. Jorde LB, Fineman RM, Martin RA: Epidemiology and genetics of neural tube defects: An application of the Utah Genealogical Data Base. Am J Phys Anthropol 62:23, 1983.
47. Kaplan WE: Clear intermittent catheterization. In: McLaurin RL (ed): Spina Bifida: A Multidisciplinary Approach. New York, Praeger Publishers, 1986, pp 274–276.
48. Khoury MJ, Erickson JD, James LM: Etiologic heterogeneity of neural tube defects: Clues from epidemiology. Am J Epidemiol 115:538, 1982.
49. Lapides J, Diokno AC, Lowe BS, et al: Follow-up of unsterile intermittent self-catheterization. J Urol 111:184, 1974.
50. Lassman LP, James CCM: Meningocele manqué. Child's Brain 3:1, 1977.
51. Laurence KM: In prevention of neural tube defects by improvement in maternal diet and preconceptional folic acid. Supplementation in Prevention of Physical and Mental Congenital Defects, Part B: Epidemiology, Early Detection and Therapy and Environmental Factors. Prog Clin Biol Res 163:383, 1985.
52. Laurence KM, Carter CO, David PA: Major central nervous system malformations in South Wales II: Pregnancy factors, seasonal variation, and social class effects. Br J Prev Soc Med 22:212, 1968.
53. Laurence KM, Tew BJ: Natural history of spina bifida cystica and cranium bifidum cysticum. Arch Dis Child 46:127, 1971.
54. Layde PM, Edmonds LD, Erickson JD: Maternal fever and neural tube defect. Teratology 21:105, 1980.
55. Lebedeff A: Uber che Enstehurg der Anencephalie and Spina Bifida dei Vogelin and Menschen. Virchows Arch Pathol Anat Physiol 86:263, 1881.
56. Leck I: Maternal hyperthermia and anencephaly. Lancet 1:671, 1978.
57. Leck I: The geographical distribution of neural tube defects and oval clefts. Br Med J 40:309, 1984.
58. Leck I, Hay S, Witte JJ, et al: Malformations recorded on birth certificates following A2 influenza epidemics. Public Health Rep 84:971, 1969.
59. Lee H, Nagele RG: Neural tube defects caused by local anesthetics in early chick embryos. Teratology 31:119, 1985.
60. Lehrman A, Owen MP: Surgical repair of large meningomyeloceles. Ann Plast Surg 12:501, 1984.
61. Lemire RJ: Neural tube defects: Clinical correlations. Clin Neurosurg 30:165, 1983.
62. Lemire RJ: Causes of neural tube defects. In: McLaurin RL (ed): Spina Bifida: A Multidisciplinary Approach. New York, Praeger Publishers, 1986, pp 2–7.
63. Lendon RG: Neuron population in the lumbosacral cord of myelomeningocele children. Dev Med Child Neurol 20:82, 1969.
64. Lichtenstein BW: Spina dysraphism (spina bifida and myelodysplasia). Arch Neurol Psychiatry 99:792, 1940.
65. Lonton AD: The relationship between intellectual skills and the computerized axial tomograms of children with spina bifida and hydrocephalus. Z Kinderchir 28:368, 1977.
66. Lorber J: Results of treatment of myelomeningocele: An analysis of 524 unselected cases with special references to possible selection for treatment. Dev Med Child Neurol 13:279, 1971.
67. Matson DD: Neurosurgery of Infancy and Childhood, 2nd ed. Springfield, IL, Charles C Thomas, 1969.
68. McCormick RA: To save or let die. JAMA 229:172, 1974.
69. McDevitt NB, Gillespie RP, Woosley RE, et al: Closure of thoracic and lumbar dysraphic defects using bilateral latissimus dorsi myocutaneous flap transfer with extended gluteal fasciocutaneous flaps. Child's Brain 9:394, 1982.
70. McLaughlin JF, Shurtleff DB: Management of the newborn with myelodysplasia. Clin Pediatr 18:463, 1979.
71. McLaurin RL: Treatment of infected ventricular shunts. Child's Brain 1:306, 1975.
72. McLone DG: Technique for closure of myelomeningocele. Child's Brain 6:65, 1980.
73. McLone DG: Treatment of myelomeningocele and arguments against selection. Clin Neurosurg 33:359, 1986.
74. McLone DG, Czyzewski D, Raimondi AJ, et al: Central nervous system infarctions as a limiting factor in the intelligence of children born with myelomeningocele. Pediatrics 70:338, 1982.
75. McLone DG, Dices L, Kaplan WE, et al: Concepts in the management of spina bifida. In: Humphreys RP (ed): Concepts in Pediatric Neurosurgery, Vol. 5. Basel, S Karger, 1985.
76. McLone DG, Suna J, Collins JA, et al: Neurulation: Biochemical and morphological studies on primary and secondary neural tube defects. In: Humphreys R (ed): Concepts in Pediatric Neurosurgery, Vol. 4. Basel, S. Karger, 1983, pp 15–19.
77. McMillan JJ, Williams B: Aqueduct stenosis: Case review and discussion. J Neurol Neurosurg Psychiatry 40:521, 1977.
78. Michejda M, Hodgen GD: Induction of neural-tube defects in nonhuman primates in prevention of physical and mental congenital defects, Part B: Epidemiology, early detection and therapy and environmental factors. Prog Clin Biol Res 163:243, 1985.
79. Mickle JP, McLennan JE: Malignant teratoma arising within a lipomyelocele. J Neurosurg 43:761, 1975.
80. Miller P, Smith DW, Shepard TH: Maternal hyperthermia as a possible cause of anencephaly. Lancet 1:519, 1978.
81. Milunsky A, Alpert E, Neff RK, et al: Prenatal diagnosis of neural tube defects. IV. Maternal serum alpha-fetoprotein screening. Obstet Gynecol 55:60, 1980.
82. Moore JE: Spina bifida with a report of 385 cases treated by excision. Surg Gynecol Obstet 1:137, 1905.
83. Morgagni J-B: De sedibus et causis morborum per anatomen indagatis Libri V; Ex Typographia Remondiona, Venice, 1761.

84. Mustarde JC: Meningomyelocele: The problem of skin cover. Br J Surg 53:36, 1966.
85. Naidich TP, McLone DG, Mutluer S: A new understanding of dorsal dysraphism with lipoma (lipomyeloschisis): Radiologic evaluation and surgical correction. AJR 140:1065, 1983.
86. Naidich TP, McLone DG, Shkolnik A, et al: Sonographic evaluation of caudal spine anomalies in children. AJNR 4:661, 1983.
87. Naidich TP, Publowski RM, Naidich JB: Computed tomographic signs of Chiari II malformation. II. Midbrain and cerebellum. Radiology 134:391, 1980.
88. Naidich TP, Publowski RM, Naidich JB: Computed tomographic signs of Chiari II malformation. III. Ventricles and cisterns. Radiology 134:657, 1980.
89. Naidich TP, Publowski RM, Naidich JB, et al: Computed tomographic signs of the Chiari II malformation. Part I: Skull and dural partitions. Radiology 134:65, 1980.
90. Nevin NC: The role of periconceptional vitamin supplementation in the prevention of neural tube defects, Part B: Epidemiology, Early Detection and Therapy and Environmental Factors. Prog Clin Biol Res 163:389, 1985.
91. Nevin NC, Merrett JD: Potato avoidance during pregnancy in women with a previous infant with either anencephaly or spina bifida. Br J Prev Soc Med 29:111, 1975.
92. Nulsen FE, Spitz EB: Treatment of hydrocephalus by direct shunt from ventricle to jugular vein. Surg Forum 2:399, 1951.
93. O'Neill P, Whetmore WJ, Booth AE: Spinal meningoceles in association with neurofibromatosis. Neurosurgery 13:82, 1983.
94. Oren M, Lorber B, Lee SH, et al: Anterior sacral meningocele: Report of five cases and review of the literature. Dis Colon Rectum 20:492, 1977.
95. Osaka K, Tanimiwa T, Hivayama A, et al: Myelomeningocele before birth. J Neurosurg 49:711, 1978.
96. Padget DH: Spina bifida and embryonic neuroschisis—a causal relationship. Definition of the postnatal conformations involving a bifid spine. Johns Hopkins Med J 123:233, 1968.
97. Padget DH: Neuroschisis and human embryonic maldevelopment: New evidence on anencephaly, spina bifida and diverse mammalian defects. J Neuropathol Exp Neurol 29:192, 1970.
98. Padget DH: Development of so-called dysraphism; with embryologic evidence of clinical Arnold-Chiari and Dandy-Walker malformations. Johns Hopkins Med J 130:127, 1972.
99. Padget DH, Lindenberg R: Inverse cerebellum morphogenetically related to Dandy-Walker and Arnold-Chiari syndromes: Bizarre malformed brain with occipital encephalocele. Johns Hopkins Med J 131:228, 1972.
100. Patten BM: Embryological stages in the development of spina bifida and myeloschisis. Anat Rec 94:487, 1946.
101. Patten BM: Overgrowth of the neural tube in young embryos. Anat Rec 113:381, 1952.
102. Patten BM: Embryological states in the establishment of myeloschisis with spina bifida. Am J Anat 93:365, 1953.
103. Paulson RB, Sucheston ME, Hayes TG, et al: Teratogenic effects of valporate in the CD-1 mouse fetus. Arch Neurol 42:980, 1985.
104. Raimondi AJ, Soare P: Intellectual development in shunted hydrocephalic children. Am J Dis Child 127:664, 1974.
105. Ralis J, Ralis HM: Morphology of peripheral nerves in children with spina bifida. Dev Med Child Neurol 109:101, 1972.
106. Reigel DH: Kyphectomy and myelomeningocele repair. Modern techniques in surgery. Neurosurgery 13:1, 1979.
107. Reigel DH: Tethered spinal cord. In: Humphreys RP (ed): Concepts in Pediatric Neurosurgery, Vol. 4. Basel, S Karger, 1983, pp 142–164.
108. Reigel DH: Indications for and techniques of kyphectomy. In: McLaurin RL (ed): Spina Bifida: A Multidisciplinary Approach. New York, Praeger Publishers, 1986, pp 140–145.
109. Reigel DH, Dallmann DE, Scarff TB, et al: Intraoperative evoked potential studies of newborn infants with myelomeningocele. Dev Med Child Neurol 18:42, 1977.
110. Reigel DH, Dallmann DE, Scarff TB, et al: Transcephalic impedance measurement during infancy. Dev Med Child Neurol 19:295, 1977.
111. Reigel DH, McLone DG: Myelomeningocele: Operative treatment and results. In: Marlin AE (ed): Concepts in Pediatric Neurosurgery, Vol. 8. Basel, S Karger, 1987.
112. Reigel DH, Stanitski C, Solomon H, et al: The relationship of scoliosis and kyphosis to tethered spinal cord. Pediatr Neurosci (in press).
113. Renwick JH: Hypothesis: Anencephaly and spina bifida are usually preventable by avoidance of a specific but unidentified substance present in certain potato tubers. Br J Prev Soc Med 26:67, 1972.
114. Robertson JS, Maraqa MI, Jennett B: Ventriculoperitoneal shunting for hydrocephalus. Br Med J 2:289, 1973.
115. Rudd LN: Genetics. In: Hoffman HJ, Epstein F (eds): Disorders of the Developing Nervous System: Diagnosis and Treatment. Boston, Blackwell Scientific Publications, 1986, p 47.
116. Sauerbrei EE, Harrison PB, Ling E, et al: Neonatal intracranial pathology demonstrated by high-frequency linear array ultrasound. JCU 9:33, 1981.
117. Scarff TB, Nelson P, Reigel DH: External drainage for ventricular infection following cerebrospinal fluid shunts. Child's Brain 5:129, 1978.
118. Scarff TB, Toleikis JR, Bunch WH, et al: Dermatomal somatosensory evoked potentials in children with myelomeningocele. Z Kinderchir 28:384, 1979.
119. Scharah CJ, Wild S, Hartley R, et al: The effect of periconceptional supplementation on blood vitamin concentrations in women of recurrence risk for neural tube defect. Br J Nutr 49:203, 1983.
120. Scott FB, Bradley WE, Timm GW: Treatment of urinary incontinence by an implantable prosthetic sphincter. Urology 1:252, 1973.
121. Seller MJ: The cause of neural tube defects: Some experiments and a hypothesis. J Med Genet 20:164, 1983.
122. Sever LE, Saunders M, Monsen R: An epidemiologic study of neural tube defects in Los Angeles County. I. Prevalence at birth based on multiple sources of case ascertainment. Teratology 25:315, 1982.
123. Shaffer J, Wolfe L, Friedrich W, et al: Developmental expectations: Intelligence and fine motor skills. In: Shurtleff DB (ed): Myelodysplasias and Exstrophies: Significance, Prevention, and Treatment. New York, Grune & Stratton, 1986, pp 359–372.
124. Sharrard WJW: The mechanism of paralytic deformity in spina bifida. Dev Med Child Neurol 4:310, 1962.
125. Sharrard WJW: The segmental innervation of the lower limb muscles in man. Ann R Coll Surg Engl 35:106, 1964.
126. Sharrard WJW: Spinal osteotomy for congenital kyphosis in myelomeningocele. J Bone Joint Surg 50:466, 1968.
127. Sharrard WJW: Neuromotor evaluation of the newborn. In: American Academy of Orthopaedic Surgeons: Symposium on Myelomeningocele. St. Louis, CV Mosby, 1972, pp 26–40.
128. Sharrard WJW: Assessment of the myelomeningocele child. In: McLaurin RL (ed): Myelomeningocele. New York, Grune & Stratton, 1977, pp 389–410.
129. Sharrard JW, Zachary RB, Lorber J, et al: A controlled trial of immediate and delayed closure of spina bifida cystica. Arch Dis Child 38:18, 1963.
130. Shurtleff DB, Lemire RJ, Warkany J: Embryology, etiology, and epidemiology. In: Shurtleff DB (ed): Myelodysplasias and Exstrophies: Significance, Prevention, and Treatment. New York, Grune & Stratton, 1986, pp 39–64.
131. Shurtleff DB, Sousa JC: The adolescent with myelodysplasia: Development, achievement, sex and deterioration. In: McLaurin RL (ed): Myelomeningocele. New York, Grune & Stratton, 1977, pp 809–835.

132. Silvis RS, Riddle LR, Clark GG: Anterior sacral meningocele. Am Surg 22:554, 1956.
133. Smithells RW, Sheppard S, Schorah CJ: Possible prevention of neural-tube defects by periconceptional vitamin supplementation. Lancet 1:647, 1980.
134. Stark GD, Baker GCW: The neurological involvement of the lower limbs in myelomeningocele. Dev Med Child Neurol 9:732, 1967.
135. Stark GD, Drummond M: The spinal cord lesion in myelomeningocele. Dev Med Child Neurol 13:1, 1971.
136. Stark GD, Drummond MB, Poneprasert S, et al: Primary ventriculo-peritoneal shunts in treatment of hydrocephalus associated with myelomeningocele. Arch Dis Child 49:112, 1974.
137. Stein SC, Schut L: Hydrocephalus in myelomeningocele. Child's Brain 5:413, 1979.
138. Stein S, Schut L, Borns P: Lacunar skull deformity (Lückenschädel) and intelligence in myelomeningocele. J Neurosurg 41:10, 1974.
139. Strassburg MA, Saunder G, Wang S: A correctional study of neural tube defects and infectious diseases. Public Health (London) 97:275, 1983.
140. Stroud RD, Eisenberg HM: Anterior sacral myelocele in association with Marfan's syndrome. Radiology 99:653, 1971.
141. Thompson MW, Rudd NL: The genetics of spinal dysraphism. In: Morley TP (ed): Current Controversies in Neurosurgery. Philadelphia, WB Saunders, 1976, pp 126–146.
142. Till K: Occult spinal dysraphism. The value of prophylactic surgical treatment. Recent Progress in Neurological Surgery. Amsterdam, Excerpta Medica ICS, no. 320, 1973, pp 61–66.
143. Till K: Paediatric Neurosurgery. London, Blackwell, 1975.
144. Toriello HV, Higgins JV: Occurrence of neural tube defects among first-, second-, and third-degree relatives of probands: Results of a United States study. Am J Med Genet 15:601, 1983.
145. Toriello HV, Warran ST, Lindstrom JA: Brief communication: Possible X-linked anencephaly and spina bifida—report of a kindred. Am J Med Genet 6:119, 1980.
146. Tryfonas G: Three spina bifida defects in one child. J Pediatr Surg 8:75, 1973.
147. Tulp N: Observationum medication libri tres (3rd ed.) cum aetieis figuris; Apud Ludovicam Elzevirium, Amsterdam, 1641.
148. Variend S, Emery JL: The pathology of the central lobes of the cerebellum in children with myelomeningocele. Dev Med Child Neurol 16:99, 1974.
149. Venes JL: Letters to the Editor. Pediatrics 74:948, 1984.
150. Vogel EH: Anterior sacral meningocele as a gynecologic problem: Report of a case. Obstet Gynecol 36:766, 1970.
151. Von Recklinghausen F: Virchows Arch Pathol Anat 105:243, 1886.
152. Von Recklinghausen F: Untersuchungen ubev che Spina Bifida. Arch Pathol Anat 105:243, 1886.
153. Wabrek AJ: Myelodysplasia and interpersonal and sexual aspects. In: McLaurin RL (ed): Spina Bifida: A Multidisciplinary Approach. New York, Praeger Publishers, 1986, pp 332–340.
154. Wald NJ, Cuckle H, Brock JH, et al: Maternal serum alpha-fetoprotein measurement in antenatal screening for anencephaly and spina bifida in early pregnancy (Report of United Kingdom collaborative study on alpha-fetoprotein in relation to neural tube defects). Lancet 1:1323, 1977.
155. Walpert SM, Scott RM, Carter BL: Computed tomography in spinal dysraphism. Surg Neurol 8:199, 1977.
156. Warkany J: Morphogenesis of spina bifida. In: McLaurin R (ed): Myelomeningocele. New York, Grune & Stratton, 1977, pp 31–35.
157. Weed LH: The development of cerebrospinal spaces in pig and in man. Cont Embryol Carnegie Inst 5:1, 1971.
158. Whitehead WE, Parker LH, Masek BJ, et al: Biofeedback treatment of fecal incontinence in myelomeningocele. Dev Med Child Neurol (in press).
159. Williams B: Is aqueduct stenosis the result of hydrocephalus. Brain 96:399, 1973.
160. Wynne-Davies R: Congenital vertebral anomalies: Etiology and relationship to spina bifida cystica. J Med Genet 12:280, 1975.
161. Yakolev PI, Wadsworth RC: Schizencephalies. J Neuropathol Exp Neurol 5:116, 1946.
162. Zook EG, Dzenitis AJ, Bennett JE: Repair of large myelomeningoceles. Arch Surg 98:41, 1969.

4
MYELOMENINGOCELE: OUTCOME AND LATE COMPLICATIONS

David G. McLone, M.D., Ph.D.
Thomas P. Naidich, M.D.

More children are crippled by myelomeningocele than by polio, muscular dystrophy, or traumatic paraplegia. As a consequence, many physicians must confront this disease and help determine the proper management of the affected child and family. Until recently, there has been little solid information about the long-term prognosis for children with myelomeningocele. The medical, social, and ethical issues provoked heated debate.

Within the last decade, significant new data have emerged to provide the physician with a scientific basis for guiding patient management.[27] There is now a growing consensus that children with myelomeningocele should be treated aggressively and that such treatment benefits many, but not all, affected children. It seems clear that no criteria can predict successfully the children for whom there will be a favorable long-term result.[2, 24, 25, 27] So-called "selection criteria"[19] are simply invalid.

It seems equally clear that the physician must avoid making a decision about treating the child based solely upon a personal bias about what constitutes an "acceptable" quality of life. The authors' experience with over 1000 families indicates that the family's view often differs from the physician's. Rather, the physician must review *current* knowledge regarding the outcome and late complications of myelomeningocele and must make this information available to the family to assist the parents in deciding these issues for their child.[24] To that end, this chapter presents our experience with the outcome and late complications of treating a large population of children with myelomeningocele and addresses a few of the remaining controversies.

HISTORICAL PERSPECTIVE

The medical and social problems facing the patient with myelomeningocele are not new. Hippocrates and the Arabic physicians knew this lesion. Aristotle "resolved" the social problem by recommending infanticide. Tulpius,[51] De Ruysch,[8] and Morgagni[31] first noted the relationship of paralyses of the legs to the sac and advised against ligation. Trowbridge,[50] 150 years later, continued to recommend ligation, although all his patients died with fever. Morton[32] treated the back with an iodide sclerosing solution that was later found to be more hazardous than doing nothing or performing minimal surgical repair.

From the early 1900's onward, steady progress was made toward closure of the back without infection. Individual patients began to survive. Laurence[18] reviewed the effect of closing the myelomeningocele by deflating the sac with a wide-bore needle and then laying on a skin graft. He detailed the natural history of spina bifida cystica and documented the poor outcome in children not treated for hydrocephalus.

Hippocrates and Galen described children with large heads, but Vesalius[53] was the first to note the large accumulation of water within the ventricular system of the brain.

In the early 1900's, Dandy and Blackfan[7] produced hydrocephalus in a dog by plugging the aqueduct. Later, Dandy demonstrated that the choroid plexus produced cerebrospinal fluid (CSF) and performed choroid plexectomies to treat hydrocephalus.[6] In 1952, Holter[30] and Nulsen and Spitz[39] initiated modern management of hydrocephalus by developing one-way shunt valves for the controlled drainage of CSF.

OUTCOME

Survival

Between 1947 and 1956, 89 percent of English children born with a myelomeningocele died before the age of six months. In 1964, Laurence[18] reviewed the outcome of 407 children cared for at a large children's hospital just before effective shunting devices became available. In this group, the myelomeningocele was repaired in only 160 of the 407 children (39 percent). Seventy-three percent of the children had clinical evidence of hydrocephalus. Intracranial infection was the single most common cause of death. In Laurence's study, a newborn infant with myelomeningocele had a 29 percent chance of living to the age of 12 years. Infants who survived four months had a 51 percent chance of living to be 12 years old. Those who survived to the age of one year had a 77 percent chance of surviving to the age of 12 years. The mortality rate began to level off at about 48 months. Similar leveling of the mortality rate has also been observed in recent studies of children treated aggressively.[27] It may be a natural part of the disease.

During the period from the middle of the 1950's to 1985, effective methods were developed for treating hydrocephalus. As patient survival rates improved, Lorber[19] applied "selection" criteria to divide children with myelomeningocele into two groups: one with poor prognosis and the other with good prognosis. Long-term follow-up of Lorber's selected series indicates that the overall mortality rate of the two groups approached 70 percent, mostly because of the selection process itself.[20] The mortality rate in the group with a bad prognosis was nearly 100 percent. The mortality rate in the group with a good prognosis, selected to be the "best" possible survivors, was 14 percent.

McLone and coworkers[27] treated all patients with myelomeningocele, without applying any "selection" criteria at all. The overall mortality rate for the initial cohort of 100 *un*selected patients followed for 8 to 12 years after closure of the back was 15 percent. Survival curves for the second cohort of 100 children are identical to those for the first group. These studies document that 2 percent of the children did not survive to leave the hospital, despite initial closure of the back and shunting procedures (Fig. 4–1). A total of 10 percent died by the end of the *third* year, and a total of 14 percent died by the end of five years. Death was unusual after 48 months, when the mortality curves leveled off. The commonest cause of death was hindbrain dysfunction, with stridor, apneic spells, and reflux aspiration. Eleven of the deaths in the first cohort of 100 patients were from hindbrain dysfunction (11 percent). Death was caused by central nervous system (CNS) infection in 1 percent. Two children died prior to discharge from the hospital (2 percent). One additional patient died after 48 months from

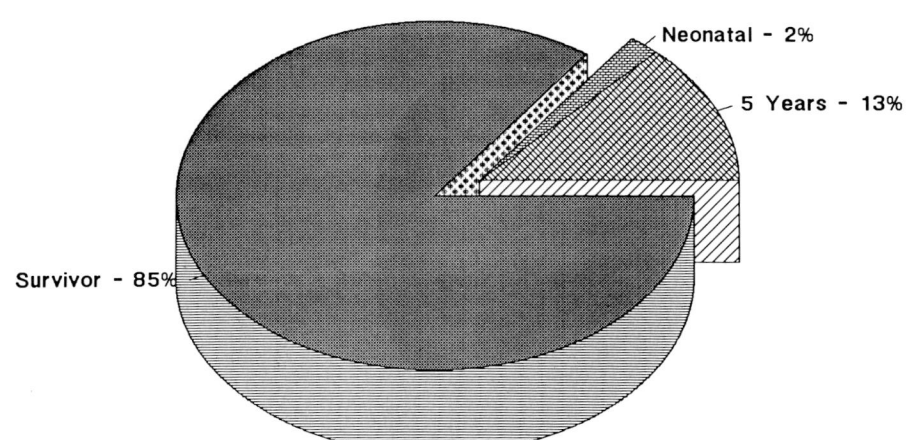

Figure 4–1. Mortality rate in a cohort of 100 children followed prospectively from 8 to 12 years. Of the 100, 2 percent died prior to discharge from the hospital. During the remaining 12 years, 13 additional children died.

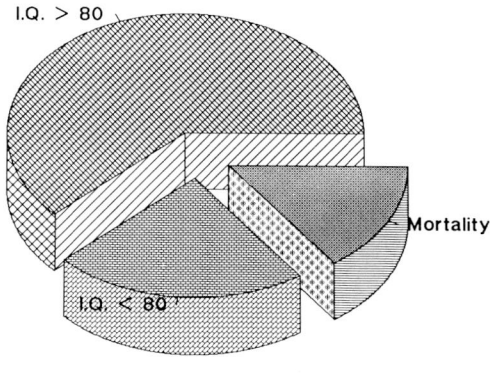 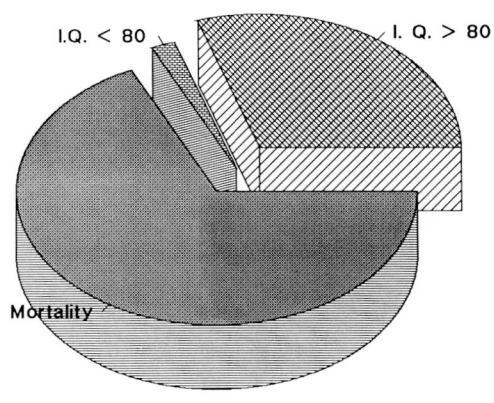

Figure 4–2. A and B, Pie graphs comparing intelligence quotients above and below 80 as well as mortality. Nonselected series (A) versus selected series (B). (A reproduced with permission from McLone DG, Dias L, Kaplan WE, et al.: Concepts in Pediatric Neurosurgery, 5. Basel, S. Karger, 1985. B reproduced with permission from Lorber J, Salfield S: Results of selective treatment of spina bifida cystica. Arch Dis Child 56:822, 1981.)

complications during a urologic procedure at another hospital.

In evaluating the selection process, one must weigh the differences in mortality rates (68 percent versus 15 percent) and in the number of children who survived with and without certain problems. Only 29 of 100 children in a selected series,[20] versus 62 children in a nonselected series,[27] survived with an intelligence quotient (IQ) higher than 80. However, 22 children survived with an IQ lower than 80 in the nonselected series, versus only two in the selected group. A similar situation results when one looks at ambulation. Figures 4–2 and 4–3 summarize the results of the selected versus the nonselected series in these two areas.

The mortality rate in *un*selected patients with myelomeningocele is not statistically different from the survival rate in Lorber's best "selected" cases. For this reason, most major centers now treat nearly all newborn children with myelomeningocele. Only the small number of children who are already agonal at birth (approximately 1 to 2 percent) are cared for without surgery. This number will probably decrease with time as obstetric ultrasonography and fetal surgery improve.

Hindbrain Dysfunction

Nearly all children with myelomeningocele have occasional problems from hindbrain dysfunction. Thirty-two percent of the first 100 had serious

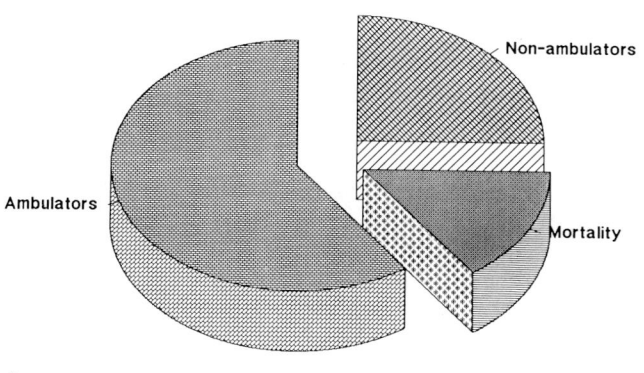 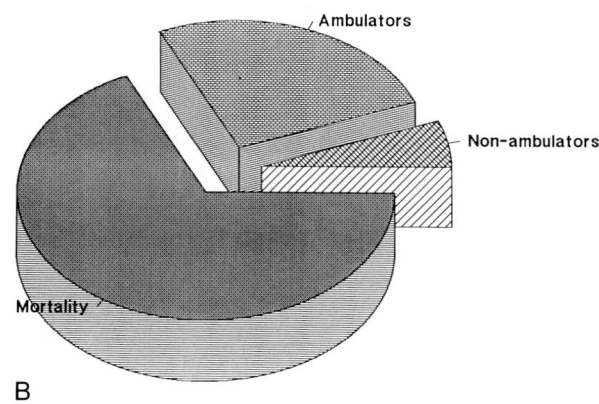

Figure 4–3. A and B, Pie graphs comparing ambulation as well as mortality. Nonselected series (A) versus selected series (B). (A reproduced with permission from McLone DG, Dias L, Kaplan WE, et al.: Concepts in Pediatric Neurosurgery, 5. Basel, S. Karger, 1985. B reproduced with permission from Lorber J, Salfield S: Results of selective treatment of spina bifida cystica. Arch Dis Child 56:822, 1981.)

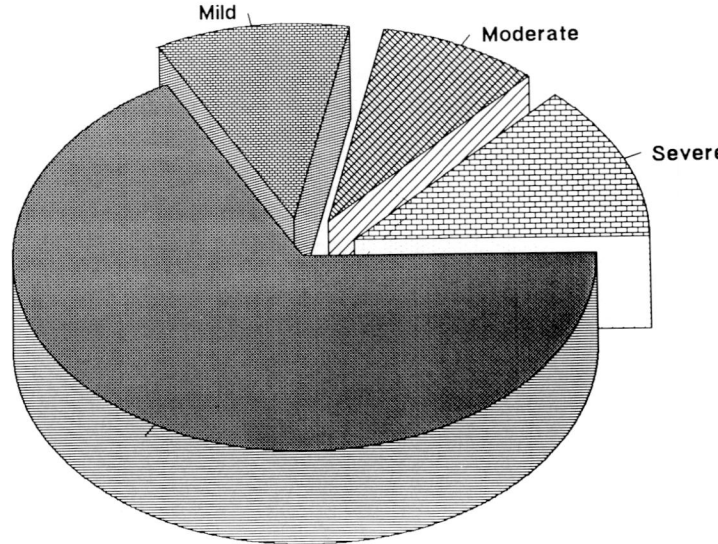

Figure 4–4. Pie graph of children born with myelomeningoceles shows the percentage of children with significant hindbrain dysfunction. Ten percent had mild dysfunction, with stridor; 9 percent had moderate dysfunction, with stridor and periodic apnea; 13 percent had severe dysfunction, with periodic apnea and gastroesophageal reflux.

sequelae of such dysfunction (Fig. 4–4).[23, 27] Eleven percent died of hindbrain dysfunction. Representing 73 percent of all deaths in the myelomeningocele group, hindbrain dysfunction is now the major cause of death in children with myelomeningocele.

In the *first* cohort of 100 patients, 13 patients suffered severe problems (apnea, cyanosis, gastric reflux with aspiration) during the neonatal period and required repeated hospitalizations and surgical procedures to manage the sequelae. One of the 13 children was born with vocal cord paralysis. The other 12 developed problems in the neonatal period. Four of the 13 underwent posterior cervical decompression to treat progressive respiratory pauses and apnea.[3] Two of these four died. One still requires a tracheostomy, and one has recovered. Of these 13 patients, 11 ultimately died (85 percent).

Thus, of the 32 children with significant hindbrain dysfunction, four were treated surgically. Two of the four died—a 50 percent operative mortality rate. Of the remaining 28 patients, nine died—a 32 percent *non*operative mortality. Of the 19 survivors, one required a tracheostomy, and 18 have recovered. In this group of 32 children with serious hindbrain dysfunction, managed as described, the overall mortality rate was 34 percent (11 of 32 patients).

Hoffman and colleagues[15] and Park and coworkers[41] reported a 38 percent mortality rate in a series in which they operated on all neonates with similarly serious hindbrain dysfunction. The mortality rates reported by these authors are not significantly different from those arrived at by the authors. Indeed, our data indicate that many children who would have been operated upon by the authors survive well without surgery. The natural history of hindbrain dysfunction in the neonate appears to be one of gradual improvement over time in those children who survive the acute problems. For that reason, the authors feel that it is best to temporize as much as possible in these newborn children and to operate only when no other course is possible.

Hydrocephalus

In Laurence's[18] study of the natural history of myelomeningocele (1964), hydrocephalus was evident *clinically* in 73 percent of children. Shunting was attempted in 53 of 407 patients (13 percent) but probably was not effective in any case. Eight of the 53 children (15 percent) had arrest of the hydrocephalus.

In McLone's study[27] of an initial cohort of 100 children, 80 percent of the children showed clinical evidence of hydrocephalus requiring shunting. In 20 percent, shunting was not performed. However, in this group, not all children were evaluated radiologically. In a second cohort of 100 children, routine ultrasonography of the head detected ventricular dilatation in 95 percent. Shunts were required in 90 percent of the 100 children; in 10 percent shunts were not performed. In a third cohort of nearly 100 patients, a pattern similar to the second 100 has emerged. Thus, it would appear that approximately 10 percent of myelomeningocele patients will not require shunt diversion of CSF.

The criteria used for deciding to place the initial shunt were (1) rapid, progressive enlargement of ventricular size or head circumference; (2) stridor, apnea, or gastroesophageal reflux attributed to hindbrain dysfunction from Chiari II malformation; (3) continued leakage of CSF at the closure site; (4) evidence of developmental delay; and (5) cosmetically unpleasant head shape.

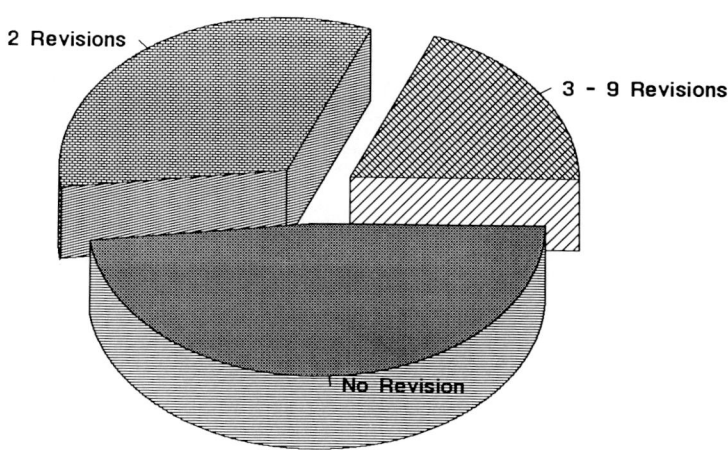

Figure 4–5. Pie graph of children born with myelomeningoceles who required a shunt and were followed for six years. A total of 48 percent did not require a shunt revision, 32 percent had one or two revisions, and 20 percent had three or more revisions.

Shunt revisions were required in 52 percent of the patients by six years of age.[27] No attempt was made to perform elective shunt lengthening as the child grew. Instead, adequate length was placed in the peritoneal cavity at the initial insertion. Nearly half (48 percent) of all the children reached the sixth year of life without any shunt revision. Another one third of the children had only one or two revisions by the sixth year. The remaining 20 percent required between three to nine revisions (Fig. 4–5).

In the entire cohort of 285 patients, 264 (93 percent) developed ventricular enlargement. Of the 264 with enlarged ventricles, 245 (93 percent) had shunts performed. Thus, 86 percent of the entire group received shunts. The size of the ventricles varied after shunting: Forty percent showed slit ventricles; 20 percent had ventricles of normal size; and 40 percent had enlarged ventricles (Fig. 4–6). IQ did not correlate with ventricular size, except in the extreme case.[48] There were no differences in IQ among any of the groups based on ventricular size until the ventricles were 4+ dilated after shunting (less than 1 cm of cortical mantle). Only 14 percent of surviving children with 4+ ventricles have IQs above 80, whereas 70 percent of all other children have IQs above 80. The shunt revision rate in children with slit ventricles is twice that of the other groups combined.

Infection

In Laurence's study (1964),[18] intracranial infection was the single most common cause of death. Analysis of that study reveals that most children with CNS infection became infected via the unrepaired myelomeningocele. In the authors' experience, the incidence of ventriculitis is affected by the speed with which the myelomeningocele is repaired. It has been 7 percent in those repaired within 48 hours of birth and 37 percent in those repaired after

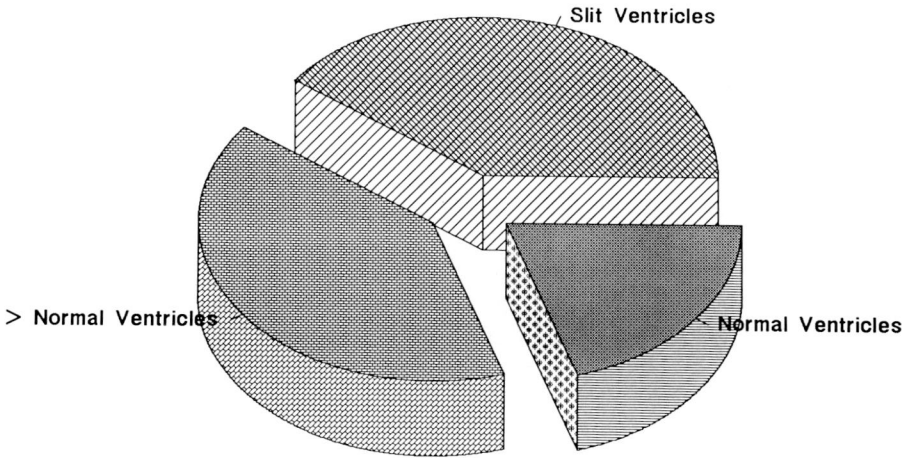

Figure 4–6. Pie graph of 264 children with myelomeningoceles and a shunt for hydrocephalus shows the distribution of ventricular size following the shunt insertion: slit ventricles, 40 percent; larger-than-normal ventricles, 40 percent; and normal-sized ventricles, 20 percent.

48 hours. However, recent studies have not shown any increase in neurologic defects caused by delay in closing the back, although delay did cause a significant increase in the mortality rate.[5]

Since it has become routine practice to close the myelomeningocele within 48 hours and to use antibiotics to control infection, the incidence of CNS infection has declined. The overall incidence of *shunt* infection in the first cohort was 12 percent.

Intelligence Quotient (Fig. 4–2)

In Laurence's study, half the children who survived with moderate to severe hydrocephalus had IQs above 85. Several children were well above average. In the past decade, a number of studies have claimed a significant reduction in IQ when the myelomeningocele is associated with hydrocephalus severe enough to require a shunt. Soare and Raimondi[47] evaluated 173 unselected children with myelomeningocele. The mean IQ of those with myelomeningocele alone was 102. The mean IQ of children with myelomeningocele and hydrocephalus was 87, a significant difference. Put differently, 87 percent of those with myelomeningocele alone had IQs higher than 80, whereas only 63 percent of those with myelomeningocele and hydrocephalus had IQs above 80. Allowing for the heterogeneity of patient populations, differences in treatment regimens, and variations in the tests used to evaluate IQ, it appears to be valid to conclude that IQ can be expected to be significantly lower when the myelomeningocele is associated with hydrocephalus. However, there was an uncontrolled variable that affected the results.

In 1974, Hunt and Holmes[16] reported that CNS infection dramatically lowered the IQ of patients with shunts and hydrocephalus compared with those of patients who required no shunt or who remained infection-free despite shunting. Therefore, McLone and associates[26] made a complete survey of 167 of the original 173 patients in the Soare-Raimondi study to determine the age of onset and the duration of any infection, the causative organism, and the severity of the process as judged by CSF protein level, glucose level, and cell count. The patients were then grouped as (1) those without shunts, (2) those with shunts without CNS infection, and (3) those with shunts with infection. Only the patients with shunts suffered CNS infection.

As previously reported, the mean IQ of those not requiring a shunt was 102. The mean IQ of those patients who did receive shunts but remained free of infection was 95. This is not significantly different from the IQ of the group without shunts. Those children who received shunts and then developed a CNS infection had a mean IQ of only 73. This is significantly different from the other two groups.

Put differently, of those who did not require a shunt, 87 percent had IQs higher than 80. Of those with shunts with CNS infections, only 31 percent had IQs higher than 80. Thus, our data indicate that hydrocephalus alone is not a significant limiting factor in the ultimate intellectual growth of the child. CNS infection is. Control of shunt infection must be a major concern for all physicians treating patients with myelomeningocele.

Children from the first and second cohorts of 100 are now old enough for reliable intelligence testing. A total of 73 percent of the survivors of the first cohort of 100 children have IQs higher than 80.[27] Since 90 percent of Lorber's series[20] of selected patients showed IQs higher than 80, application of selection criteria would appear to result in a significant increase in the IQs of surviving patients. However, it is essential to take into account the difference between the mortality rates of the two series. In Lorber's series, only 29 of 100 children survived with IQs higher than 80 (Fig. 4–2). In our series, 62 of 100 children survived with IQs higher than 80. This is more than twice as many. Expressed another way, application of Lorber's selection criteria means that for every surviving child with an IQ higher than 80, one child with a potential IQ above 80 was allowed to die.

IQ is not the sole predictor of performance. Studies[1] have demonstrated that as many as one half of children with myelomeningocele may have some learning disability. The severity of the learning disability in these first two cohorts has yet to be determined.

The impact of the shunt procedure and the subsequent control of hydrocephalus on the child's ultimate intelligence is difficult to determine. We know from Laurence's paper that half of the survivors of untreated, moderate to severe hydrocephalus have average or above-average intelligence. Treatment of the hydrocephalus increases patient survival, protects vision, and may preserve intelligence in the other half of children who are destined to be retarded. Our results suggest that it is more important to prevent progression of the hydrocephalus than to achieve a specific "normal" ventricular size. It is also evident that complications of the shunt procedure inflict retardation on a number of children. Shunt infection can reduce intelligence. Early aggressive shunting can produce "slit" ventricles and create difficulty in maintaining a functioning shunt in this population. Alternatively, delay in shunting until after the cranial sutures close and the intracranial volume becomes fixed increases the risk of subdural hematoma following shunting.

Routine assessment of the child's intellectual function is valuable not only in projecting future competitiveness but also as a baseline for shunt function. The authors have seen a number of children with subtle shunt malfunctions that were discovered on medical psychologic evaluation.

Urinary Continence

Prior to 1975, many children with myelomeningocele underwent a series of urinary-diversion procedures in an effort to minimize the loss of renal function from infection. The consequences of these procedures and the odor of urine made these children social pariahs. Since 1975, introduction of clean intermittent catheterization (CIC) and pharmacotherapy has permitted these children to develop "social" continence of urine. That is, they can avoid incontinence in social situations and can behave like other children by maintaining a schedule of self-catheterization (or parent-performed catheterization) in the bathroom. These children will not have normal neuromuscular control of urination, but they can have normal social behavior.

In our series,[27] nearly 85 percent of the 6- to 10-year-old population have been able to achieve such social continence of urine. Urinary diversions are now rare. More than 100 patients from our total clinic population have undergone reimplantation procedures ("undiversions") during the last ten years. A small number of selected children have been treated with artificial sphincters. As a result, these children no longer exude the objectionable odor of urine. The children are accepted by their peers, and they are placed in regular schools in the mainstream of education.

Motor and Sensory Function

Most children with myelomeningocele are born with a neurologic deficit. In the authors' series, 37 percent of patients with myelomeningocele showed significant motor recovery shortly after surgical closure of the back. This motor improvement provides active function across a joint that was previously nonfunctional. This improvement persists throughout the follow-up period (Fig. 4–7). In our experience, delay in closing the myelomeningocele for more than 72 hours after birth decreases motor function in a small percentage of children. Other studies have not documented any increase in the neurologic deficits in patients who survive delayed closure.[5]

Community Ambulation and Schooling

Patients are designated "community ambulators" if they can move about the community without resorting to wheelchairs. Because of their motor deficits, many patients require reciprocal braces, canes, and walkers to assist them in maintaining the erect posture necessary for becoming community ambulators. However, as these children become older the increase in their body weight may exceed the increase in their motor strength, so they face greater difficulties in walking. Many ultimately become wheelchair bound.

As adults, most myelomeningocele patients with thoracic-level function require the use of wheelchairs to be mobile. In spite of this, the authors do not agree with placing these children into a wheelchair immediately. Rather, we start them in the erect position and then "graduate" them into wheelchairs if necessary. Electing to use a wheelchair must not be seen as failure. Rather, the children choose to use the wheelchair in order to conserve energy for other activities of daily living. That these patients are able to move about the community to accomplish their business is socially more important than whether they do so by brace or by wheelchair.

Complete ambulation data are available on 80 of 85 survivors of the first cohort of 100 patients with myelomeningocele. Ambulation was precluded in 13 children with severe CNS involvement in the form of significant mental retardation, hypotonia, or both. These children are unlikely to be competitive and independent. In the children without such CNS involvement, the community ambulation rate is 89 percent. This represents 75 percent of all surviving children and 60 percent of the original cohort of 100. Community ambulation was achieved by 100 percent of those patients with sacral and lower lumbar myelomeningoceles. Community ambulation was achieved by 63 percent of those with higher lesions. Use of the reciprocating brace has markedly increased the number of children with thoracic-level function who ambulate. However, it is probable that the number of ambulators with thoracic-level function will decrease with time and that the wheelchair will become the preferred method of locomotion for such patients in the community.

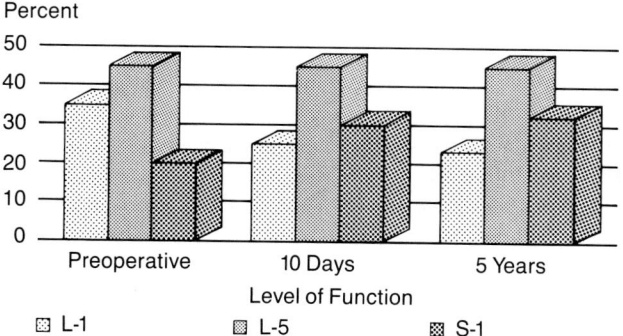

Figure 4–7. Bar graph shows the preoperative motor function level in newborn children with myelomeningoceles compared with the levels ten days after closure of the back and five years into follow-up.

Competitive Individuals

An IQ of 80 or higher makes it probable that the child can compete successfully in society as an adult and can become a self-supporting citizen. Individuals with IQs lower than 80 are unlikely to be competitive. Our data indicate that approximately 25 percent of unselected myelomeningocele children will survive in a noncompetitive condition. Mental retardation, hindbrain dysfunction, and hypotonia are the most common causes of inability to compete successfully.

Attempts to assess the competitive independence of the adult population have only now been undertaken. Of 71 adults living in the Chicago area, 80 percent live with relatives, but 82 percent are independent in activities of daily living. Thirty percent finished, or are in, college, but only 32 percent are employed full time. Preliminary returns from a national questionnaire show high rates of employment and ambulation. However, in this preliminary data, only one third of those responding had hydrocephalus. This skewing reflects the fact that in the past, the least affected individuals survived best. Those individuals with the most severe problems have died or have been lost in the recesses of our society.

The adult survivor presents the medical community with a new challenge. Our medical and surgical colleagues who treat principally adult patients usually have not been exposed to the growing population of young adolescents prior to seeing them for the first time as young adults. Thus, they may lack the special expertise developed by those of us who "grew up" with these patients.

It is also obvious that besides addressing the medical needs of these individuals, major efforts should be directed toward job training and employment.

LATE COMPLICATIONS

It was long assumed that gradual deterioration in neurologic function was the natural history for children with myelomeningocele. This assumption has been proved wrong. It is now quite clear that neurologic deterioration should not occur, at least into adulthood, *provided* that late complications of myelomeningocele are sought and treated diligently.

It is too soon to state with certainty what the outcome will be beyond childhood, since we must wait to determine the long-term effects of such things as clean intermittent catheterization on the urethral mucosa, the effects of repeated trauma to joints that lack sensation, and the life expectancy of a patient with a shunt. The number of independent adults who have reached middle age is not sufficient to produce a clear picture of the probable outcome and complications that will be faced by the children we treat today.

However, the major late complications in patients with myelomeningocele include the Chiari II malformation, tethering by scarring of the spinal cord to the closure, and hydromyelia leading to scoliosis, spasticity, and loss of function.

Chiari II Malformation

In a few patients, the hindbrain dysfunction associated with the Chiari II malformation (Fig. 4–8) continues to present problems through childhood and into adolescence and early adulthood.[9, 13, 17, 40] Pain at the base of the skull and neck posteriorly, nystagmus, weakness in the upper extremities, lower cranial nerve symptoms, and hypotonia or spasticity are common features of this problem. Early recognition and treatment can preserve function and occasionally can prevent sudden death.[49] Posterior cervical decompression is much more likely to be effective in correcting symptoms in this age group than in newborns.

In a number of children, late progressive scoliosis and spasticity insidiously rob the children of function. This scoliosis develops proximal to the level of the myelomeningocele and is not associated with vertebral anomalies. The role that the Chiari II malformation and cervical compression plays in this late deterioration is not clear. Hall and colleagues[11, 12] demonstrated that the hydromyelia communicated with the ventricular system, and they advocated the establishment of a functioning ventricular shunt to manage the hydromyelia. A shunt malfunction is the first problem to be ruled out and certainly must be done prior to cervical decompression. Resolution of the neurologic deterioration with cervical decompressive laminectomy[30] and plugging of the obex[40, 41] has been reported. This procedure is based on the hydrodynamic theory proposed by Morgagni[31, 40] and modified by Gardner.[10] In Park's series, the condition of 8 of 12 children improved following cervical decompression and plugging of the obex, and the condition of the other four remained unchanged.

Although Park stated that "hydromyelia and compression of the brain stem are solely or concurrently responsible,"[40] and Hoffman[13] felt that "although investigations . . . will show the malformation, they are not essential" and that "myelography is unnecessary because all of these infants have the malformation," the magnetic resonance imaging (MRI) findings may not correlate well with the clinical manifestations. Many children with progressive scoliosis, spasticity, or both have little evidence of hindbrain compression and no hydromyelia. One unfortunate child in our series is quadriparetic and ventilator dependent and has almost no evidence of a Chiari II malformation or hydromyelia. The authors also see segmental hydromyelia and syringomyelia (Fig. 4–9) and occasional holocord hydromyelia that do not appear to communicate with the ventricular system. When this occurs, the origin of the fluid and the hydrodynamics of this lesion are difficult to explain.

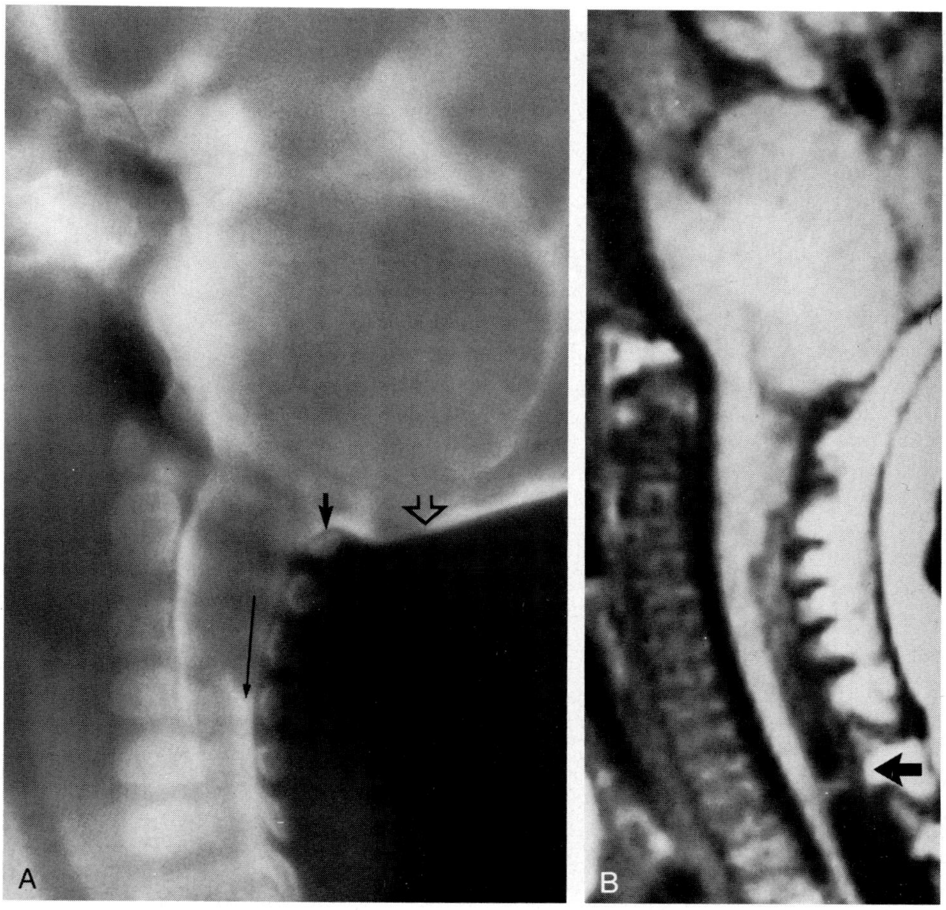

Figure 4–8. *A,* A water-soluble contrast-enhanced cisternogram shows the edge of the foramen magnum (open arrow), the cerebellum sitting on the arch of C1 (short arrow), and the vermian peg down to C4 (long arrow). *B,* A magnetic resonance image of a Chiari type II malformation showing a vermian peg extended to lower cervical levels (arrow).

When scoliosis fails to respond to a shunt revision, the authors perform a cervical decompression and plug the obex if there is MRI evidence of hindbrain compression and hydromyelia. Our results have been mixed but best in children with evidence of hindbrain dysfunction, upper extremity involvement, or both (Table 4–1).

Hydromyelia

Hydromyelia signifies dilatation of the central canal of the spinal cord, just as hydrocephalus signifies dilatation of the ventricles of the brain (Fig. 4–10). In patients with myelomeningocele, CSF has been shown to pass from the ventricles to the central canal via the iter of the central canal at the level of the obex. Thus, hydromyelia may be the consequence of untreated or inadequately treated hydrocephalus.[11, 12]

The most common symptoms of hydromyelia include rapidly progressive scoliosis, weakness of the upper extremities, spasticity, and an ascending motor loss in the lower extremities.

In patients with myelomeningocele, the incidence of hydromyelia has been reported to vary from 50 to 80 percent.[4, 21] This wide variation probably re-

Table 4–1. LATE COMPLICATIONS

Signs and Symptoms
Pain in neck
Pain in closure site
Pain in pelvis
Pain in legs
Decreased tone in upper extremities
Weakness in upper extremities
Hypotonia
Spasticity
Scoliosis
Loss of function in lower extremities
Change in bladder and bowel patterns
Causes
Shunt malfunction (untreated hydrocephalus)
Chiari II compression
Encysted fourth ventricle
Syringobulbia
Hydromyelia with or without shunt malfunction
Arachnoid cyst
Tethered spinal cord
Inclusion dermoid tumor
Diagnosis
History and physical examination
Medical psychology evaluation
Physical therapy evaluation
Muscle test
Ultrasonography
Spine x-ray films
Myelography
CT scans
Magnetic resonance imaging

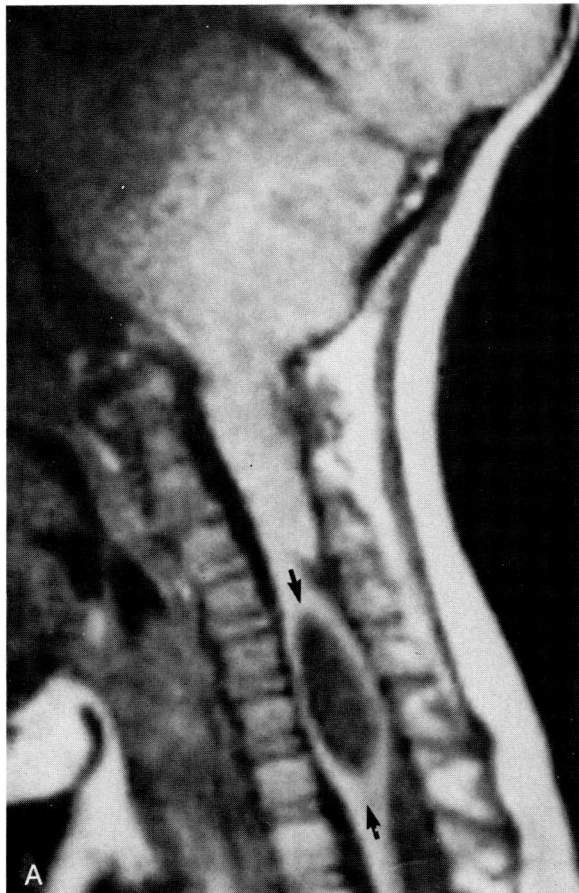 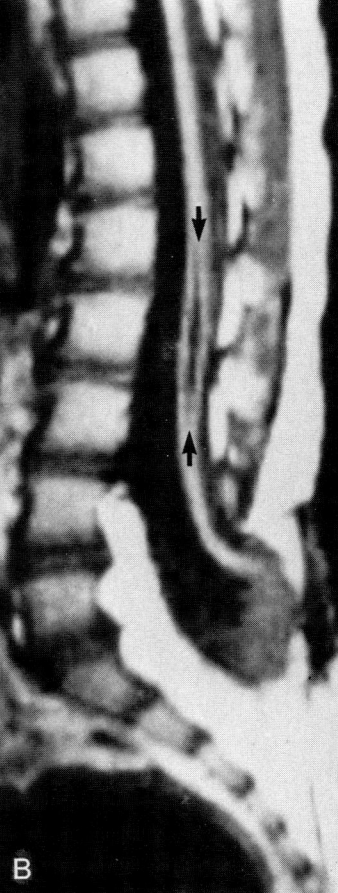

Figure 4–9. Magnetic resonance images of two children with segmental hydromyelia (syringomyelia?) (arrows). *A* also shows a Chiari type II malformation. In *B*, the terminal spinal cord appears tethered into the myelomengingocele repair.

flects the degree to which hydrocephalus was controlled, the difficulty in making the diagnosis accurately prior to computed tomography (CT) and MRI, and the diligence with which the diagnosis was sought. In our series, CT and MRI demonstrate that hydromyelia is present in 40 percent of the cases studied.

Several methods are available to investigate the causes of late deterioration of spinal cord function.[33–35, 37, 38] For the head,[36] CT scanning will probably be replaced by MRI. In patients with symptomatic hydromyelia, even when the head scan is unchanged from previous examinations, it must be determined that the shunt is actually working properly before other forms of therapy are undertaken. The authors have several cases in which the shunt was revised in the face of an unchanged CT scan, resulting in dramatic improvement or stabilization of the scoliotic curve. MRI has limited value in patients with severe scoliosis, because the spinal cord images move in and out of the plane of the MRI cut. Therefore, in this group, we currently favor use of mini-myelogram with CT for determining the presence of either a tethered cord or hydromyelia (Fig. 4–11).

Kyphoscoliosis has been reported to be present in 90 percent of patients with myelomeningocele.[42, 46] It is very often progressive in patients with retethering of the cord by scar and in those with hydromyelia. Therefore, kyphoscoliosis should be viewed as a symptom of an underlying problem. Hydromyelia must be sought specifically in any patient with very rapidly progressive scoliosis. In these patients, effective treatment of the hydromyelia often permits the curvature to return (nearly) to the original severity. It is hoped that by aggressive treatment of tethered cord and hydromyelia the incidence of kyphoscoliosis can be reduced to less than 20 percent.

Once it is determined that hydromyelia persists despite a functioning shunt, if hindbrain compression is present by MRI, posterior cervical decompression is indicated. The authors prefer posterior cervical decompression, opening of the fourth ventricle, and plugging of the obex, placement of a shunt from the fourth ventricle to the subarachnoid space, or both. Venes and associates[52] have advocated placing a catheter into the fourth ventricle at the time of decompression to bypass the central canal of the spinal cord. Ten of 14 patients showed improvement after this procedure.[52] If this procedure failed or in the absence of clinical or MRI

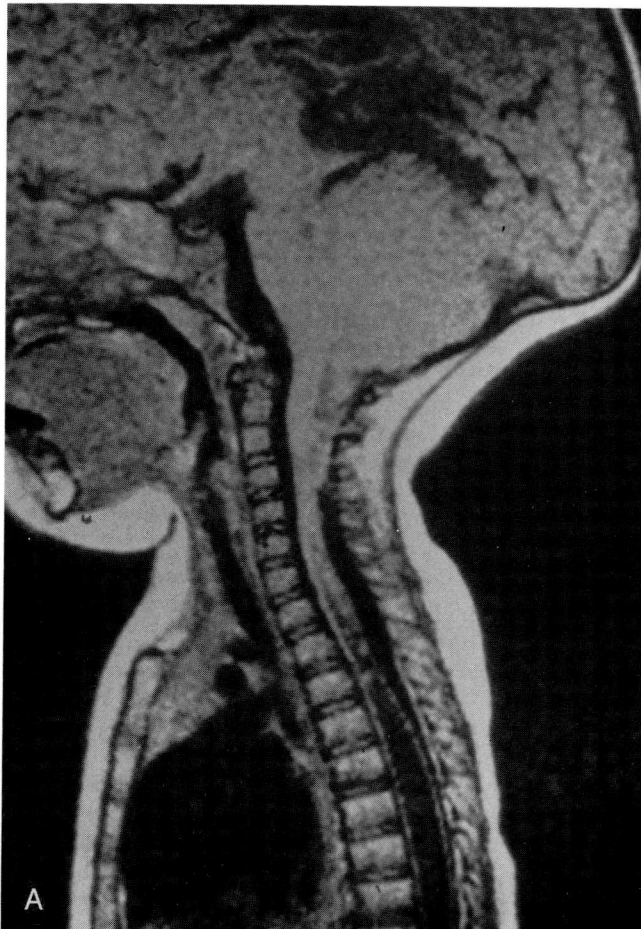
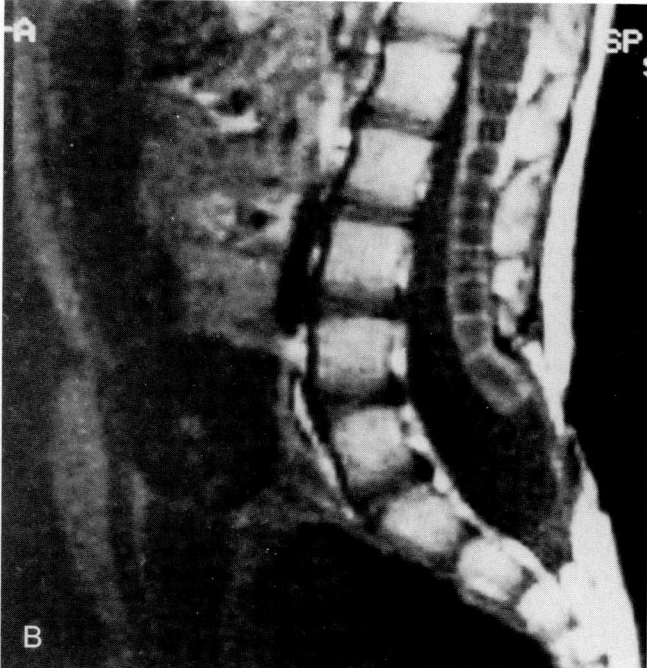

Figure 4–10. Magnetic resonance images show severe hydromyelia. In A, it is associated with the Chiari type II malformation. B shows the common haustral pattern in the hydromyelia cavity and a distal spinal cord that appears tethered.

evidence of hindbrain compression, we would place a central canal–to–pleural cavity shunt with a flushing device over a rib.

Aggressive treatment of hydromyelia in children with myelomeningocele who are experiencing the onset of scoliosis at levels rostral to the myelomeningocele should be done early in the scoliotic process. The authors were able to improve or stabilize the curve in 80 percent of the patients.

In a child with a thoracic-level myelomeningocele, it is difficult to know whether the kyphosis is treatable and whether the progression of kyphosis can be arrested. Because the laminae are widely everted in spina bifida, the paraspinal muscles that

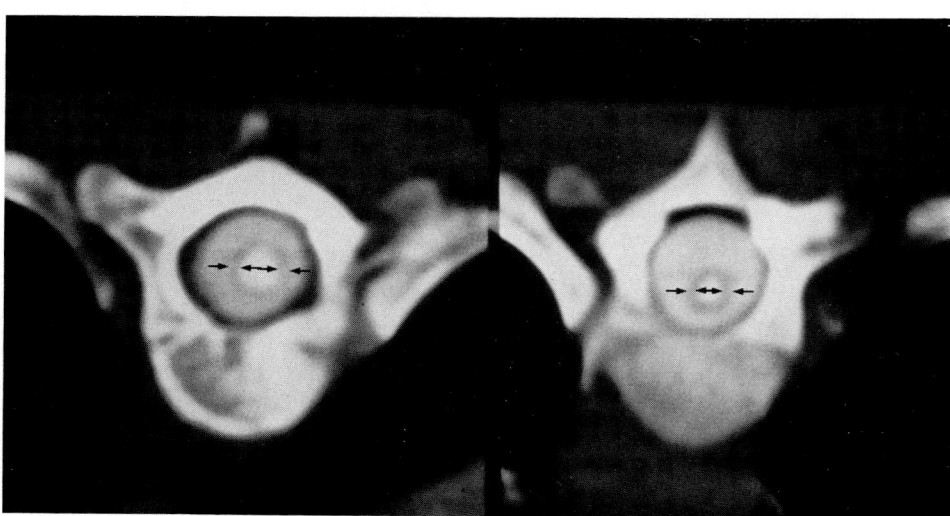

Figure 4–11. A delayed CT myelogram reveals the target sign of water-soluble contrast material in the hydromyelia cavity surrounded by a thin spinal cord (arrows).

develop along the laminae come to lie in an abnormal position lateral to—or even ventral to—the spinal canal. As a result, the spinal extensor muscles come to serve as spinal flexors. They no longer oppose the pull of the psoas but augment it. This abnormal, unstable relationship may lead to progressive "jackknife" kyphosis requiring spinal fusion. Reigel has suggested that early kyphectomy and untethering[43] of the spinal cord can slow or even arrest this process.

Progressive lordosis is often associated with a tethered cord. In the absence of a vertebral anomaly, thoracic or upper lumbar scoliosis in a child with a lesion at the level of the low lumbar or sacral spine is almost invariably the result of a treatable lesion. Most often, the cause is hydromyelia; less often, it is tethered cord.

Retethering of the Spinal Cord

Limitation of movement of the distal end of the spinal cord can produce a variety of symptoms referable to deterioration of spinal cord function. (A full discussion of this problem is contained in Chapter 5.) This fixation, or tethering, of the end of the spinal cord allows intermittent "bow-stringing" of the spinal cord between the normal cephalic attachment and the point of the tether. Yamada and colleagues[54] have supplied data that support the concept that the spinal cord stretches under tension, that the distal cord vasculature is attenuated by this stretching, and that the distal spinal cord consequently suffers intermittent ischemia that results in myelomalacia. The authors believe that the middle and upper levels of the spinal cord are compressed anteriorly against the apices of the curved vertebral column and deteriorate from chronic cord compression (Fig. 4–12).

The most common symptoms of cord tethering in patients with myelomeningocele are subtle atrophy, pain, progressive orthopedic foot deformities, ascending motor loss, and scoliosis (Fig. 4–13).[14, 28, 43] Commonly, the pain radiates into the legs, especially with exercise. Pain, sensory loss, and motor loss often do not follow dermatomal patterns. The children may exhibit lordosis and a bent-knee posture on standing.[43] In children previously doing well, hip dislocation may be the first sign of neurologic deterioration. Bladder and bowel dysfunction or a change in catheterization pattern may signal an urgent situation requiring immediate attention.

In addition to these signs of cord tethering, patients with myelomeningocele often exhibit subtle changes in muscle tone, usually spasticity and muscle functional loss.[29] These changes are often insidious and will be picked up only by a scheduled routine of close follow-up observation. Routine muscle function examinations have proved very useful for early detection of this problem. Other investigators have reported that routine somatosensory evoked potentials reliably detect early spinal cord deterioration.[43]

The authors have operated upon and followed closely 49 cases of retethering of the spinal cord after primary repair of the myelomeningocele (Fig. 4–14). Three of these 44 cases were part of the first cohort of 100 patients, suggesting that the incidence of retethering is at least 3 percent in myelomeningoceles repaired by our technique (Fig. 4–15).[22] We believe that the incidence of retethering is probably related to the type of initial repair that is performed. "Tight" closure that restricts the underlying neural elements is a serious hazard to the child, for both immediate ischemic cord damage and for later retethering of the spinal cord. "Loose," or "patulous," closure provides a generous CSF compartment in which the spinal cord may float away from the surgical scar. In addition, when it is possible to roll the neural placode into a tube, by use of pial-pial sutures, one can sequester the raw tissue of the neural placode deep to the glistening pia of the "remade" cord and reduce the raw surface most likely to scar to a vertical mid-dorsal suture line. In

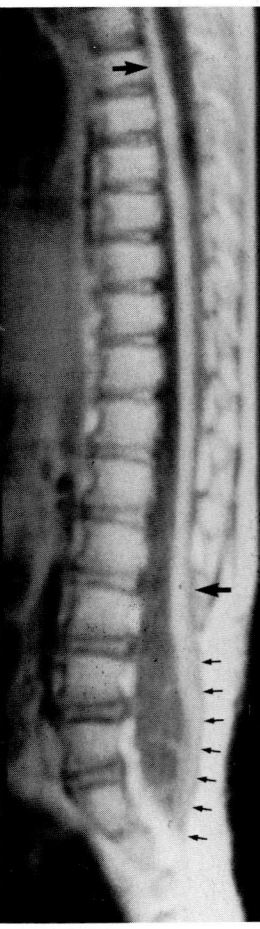

Figure 4–12. A magnetic resonance image of a child with a tethered cord at the myelomeningocele repair site (small arrows). Note that the spinal cord is held against the tangents of the spinal curvature (large arrows).

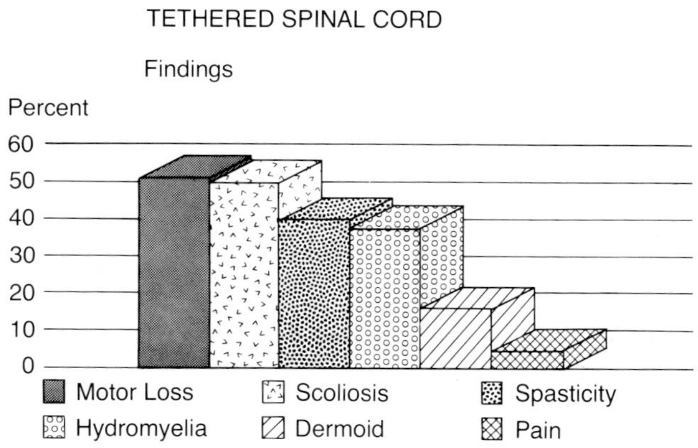

Figure 4–13. A bar graph shows the percentage of some common findings seen in children with a tethered spinal cord at the myelomeningocele repair site.

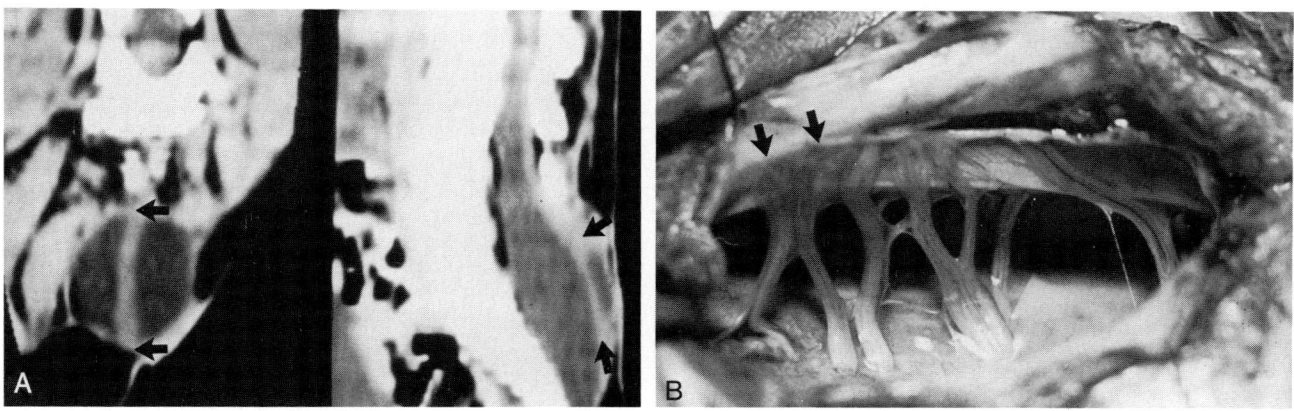

Figure 4–14. A, A re-formatted CT scan shows a previously repaired myelomeningocele tethered proximally and distally (arrows) but free in between. B, An operative photograph of the same patient shows the proximal point of tethering (arrows).

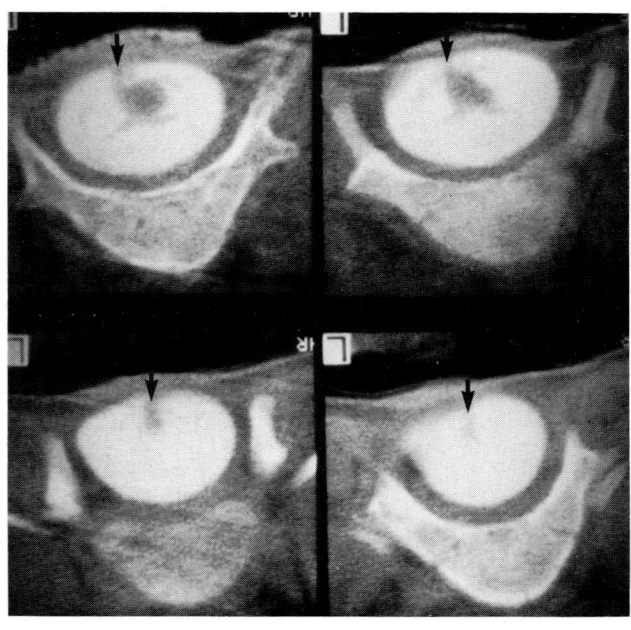

Figure 4–15. A water-soluble contrast-enhanced CT myelogram shows a myelomeningocele closed by pial-to-pial suture that has become tethered by a thin adhesion along the placode closure line (arrows). (With permission from McLone DG, et al.: Central nervous system infections as a limiting factor in the intelligence of children with myelomeningocele. Pediatrics 70:338, 1982.)

our experience, both factors help reduce the incidence of rescarring.[44]

Of the 49 patients with retethering of the cord, 38 percent had associated hydromyelia, and 16 percent had an inclusion (epi)dermoid tumor. Fifty percent of the children presented with progressive scoliosis; 51 percent had motor loss; 40 percent had spasticity. Pain was the principal symptom in two children.

Following release, 53 percent had improvement in their scoliosis, 14 percent were stable, and 33 percent progressed (Fig. 4–16). Sixty-four percent had improvement, or decrease, in their spasticity, while 36 percent remained stable. Bladder and bowel function improved in 25 percent, and pain was relieved in 100 percent of the patients. Motor improvement was noted in 57 percent; however, the condition of three children worsened. One of these children was significantly weaker in his legs after release but had a marked improvement in his scoliosis. We are hoping to develop better methods of managing spasticity.

Other Causes

It must be stressed again that subtle shunt malfunction can mimic any of these conditions and can cause all the signs of deterioration mentioned previously. Therefore, it is essential to establish first that the shunt is indeed functioning properly. Other treatable causes of late deterioration in neurologic function include syringobulbia, inclusion (epi)dermoid tumors, arachnoid cysts, undetected thick filum terminale, and diastematomyelia.

Syringobulbia presents clinically essentially in the same manner as late manifestations of the Chiari II malformation. Although syringobulbia is not reported in other series,[4, 41] the authors have now seen three cases. MRI demonstrates the lesion well (Fig. 4–17), and intraoperative ultrasonography localizes[44] the cavity within the brainstem. We have managed syringobulbia with laser fenestration and by placing a small tube from the cavity to the subarachnoid space. Dramatic, almost immediate, improvement has occurred in the children managed by this method.

Arachnoid cysts produce symptoms very similar to those of a tethered cord. MRI is less effective in identifying the lesion than the mini-myelogram (Fig. 4–18). Once the cyst is identified the outer membrane is totally or partially removed and the cavity is communicated with the subarachnoid space.

Diastematomyelia and a thick filum terminale are the result of incomplete evaluation of the child at the time of the initial repair of the myelomeningocele. Again, the symptoms are those of a tethered cord. Plain spine x-rays usually suggest the presence of a diastematomyelia. CT with myelography or MRI should delineate both of these problems.[38] The treatment is the same as in either of these lesions in the absence of a myelomeningocele. In addition it is usually necessary to untether the distal spinal cord at the closure site.

The signs and symptoms of an inclusion (epi)dermoid are difficult to separate from tethered cord because the two are almost invariably associated (Fig. 4–19).

CONCLUSION

In summary, late deterioration is not uncommon in children with myelodysplasia. Most, possibly all, of this deterioration is preventable or correctable. It is not simply the natural history of this disease. Only through close follow-up by trained observers can these problems be anticipated and discovered early. Regularly scheduled evaluations of intellec-

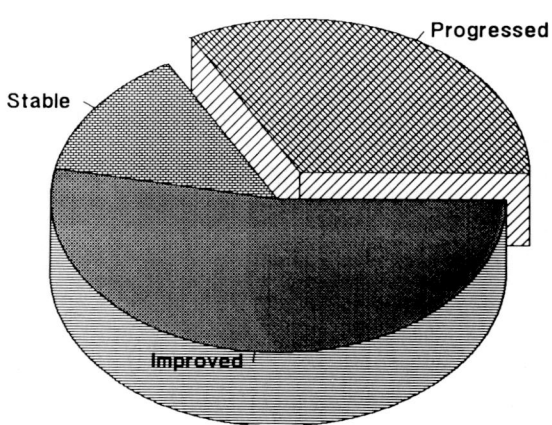

Figure 4–16. A pie graph shows the effect of release of a tethered spinal cord on scoliosis in children with a myelomeningocele.

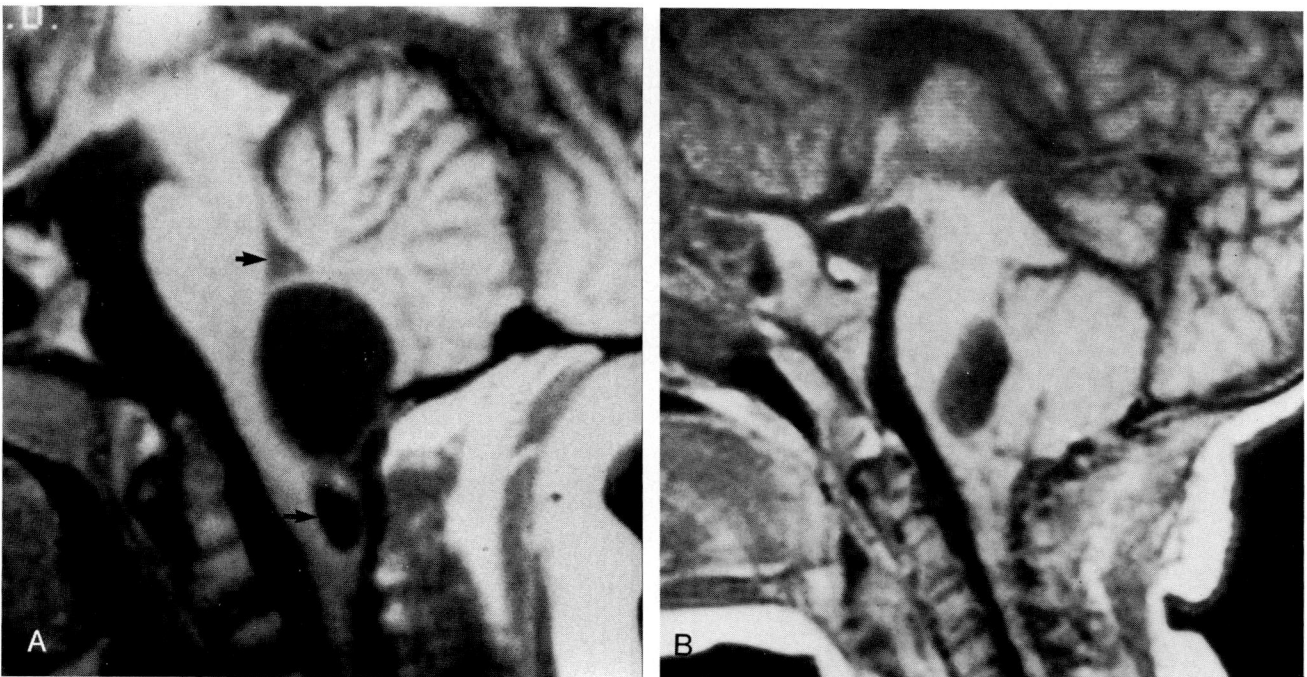

Figure 4–17. Magnetic resonance images of two children with Chiari type II malformations and syringobulbia. *A* also shows the proximal and distal fourth ventricle (arrows).

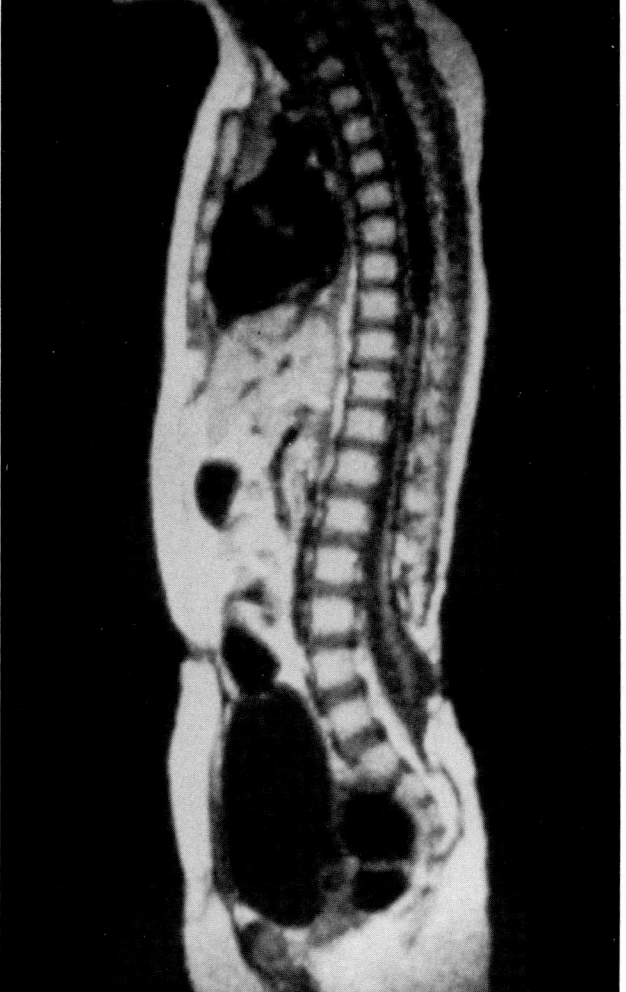

Figure 4–18. A magnetic resonance image of a large arachnoid cyst that was initially thought to be hydromyelia.

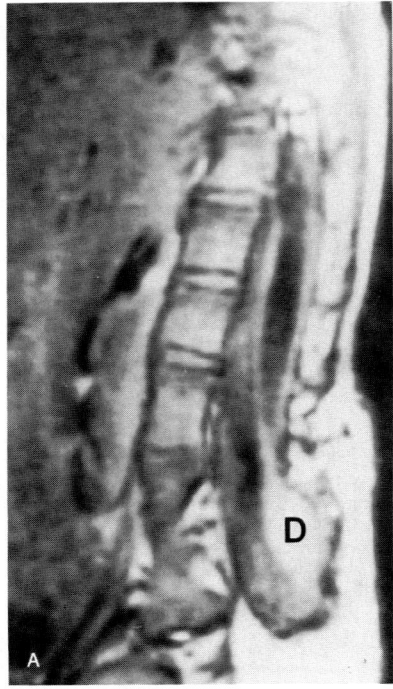
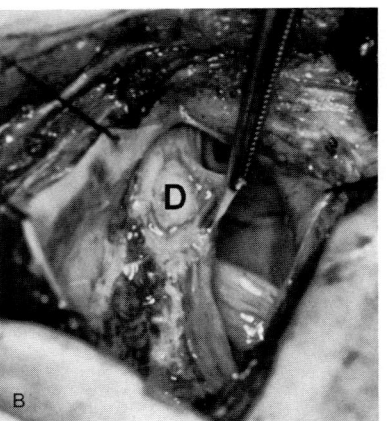

Figure 4–19. *A*, Magnetic resonance image of a child with hydromyelia, a tethered cord, and an inclusion dermoid tumor (D). *B*, An operative photograph shows an inclusion dermoid tumor (D) within the repaired myelomeningocele.

tual, musculoskeletal, and urinary systems are essential. When the observer is familiar with the signs and the symptoms of the various causes of deterioration and utilizes ultrasonography, myelography, CT, and MRI, the most probable cause can be identified, and a treatment plan outlined.

A not infrequent problem is that either the Chiari II malformation or a tethered cord cannot be excluded or both are contributing to the problem. In these cases, the authors have done cervical decompressions and have untethered the spinal cord during the same operation. If the child's condition precludes a double procedure, we would do cervical decompression first.

Analysis of our data on the *un*selected population of all children with myelomeningocele indicates the following.

1. *Survival*. Two percent will die during the initial hospitalization, and 15 percent will die by the age of ten years. The mortality rate appears to flatten out by age four years.

2. *Morbidity*. A total of 32 percent will exhibit serious hindbrain dysfunction, and 34 to 38 percent of this group will die of the dysfunction. Hindbrain dysfunction is the cause of 75 percent of all myelomeningocele deaths.

3. *Hydrocephalus*. A total of 93 percent will have ventricular dilatation, and 86 percent will require shunting. Until at least the age of six, 48 percent will need no revision. Prior to age six, 32 percent will require one to two revisions. Before the age of six years, 20 percent will need multiple revisions.

4. *Infection*. A total of 25 percent will experience one shunt infection during follow-up from 1 to 12 years.

5. *Intelligence*. Twenty-seven percent of survivors will have IQs lower than 80. A total of 73 percent of survivors will have IQs higher than 80, and 27 percent will have IQs higher than 100. Up to one half of myelomeningocele patients may suffer other learning disabilities.

6. *Urinary Continence*. Nearly 85 percent achieve social continence of urine by scheduled clean intermittent catheterization.

7. *Motor Function*. Nearly 100 percent have some motor deficit, and 37 percent gain function after the initial repair.

8. *Community Ambulation*. A total of 68 percent of survivors will achieve community ambulation as pre-adolescents, and 32 percent will use wheelchairs.

9. *Competitive Individuals*. Seventy percent are potentially competitive.

10. *Late Complications*. A total of 3 percent develop retethering of the spinal cord at the initial closure site, and 40 percent develop hydromyelia.

Physicians who enter into the care of the infant born with a myelomeningocele must be familiar with the current state of treatment and the current outcome. They must make this information available to the family of the affected infant to help them decide what is best for their child. No valid criteria exist for predicting the outcome of the individual child. The precise functional level of treated children becomes evident only over time. It is certain that not all children with myelomeningocele can be treated. A few are born dying. Others respond poorly to therapy.

We believe that it is proper to treat all viable newborns with myelomeningocele aggressively, by closure of the back within 48 hours, shunting as needed, revising the shunts as required, and diligently seeking and treating any late complications such as hindbrain compression, tethering of the spinal cord, hydromyelia, and dermoid tumors in order to maintain the child in the best possible condition.

Optimal care of the patient with myelomeningocele requires a comprehensive, coordinated plan of treatment. Because children with myelomeningocele suffer many problems, care of these patients requires a multidisciplinary team composed of a pediatric neurosurgeon, an orthopedic surgeon, a urologic surgeon, and a neuroradiologist interested in pediatric problems. All these individuals should be involved in the care of the infant from the beginning, and thereafter.

References

1. Agnes P, McLone DG: Learning disabilities in children with a myelomeningocele. Personal communication, 1987.
2. Ames M, Schut L: Diagnosis and treatment. Results of treatment of 171 consecutive myelomeningoceles—1962 to 1968. Pediatrics 50:466, 1972.
3. Caldarelli M, Di Rocco E, McLone DG: Chiari II Malformation: Clinical Manifestations and Indications for Decompression. In: McLaurin R (ed): Proceedings of the Second Symposium on Spina Bifida. New York, Praeger Publishing, 1986, pp 174–181.
4. Cameron AH: The Arnold-Chiari and other neuro-anatomical malformations associated with spina bifida. J Pathol Bacteriol 73:195, 1957.
5. Charney EB, Weller SC, Sutton LN, et al: Management of the newborn with myelomeningocele: Time for a decision-making process. Pediatrics 75:58, 1985.
6. Dandy WE: Extirpation of the choroid plexus of the lateral ventricles in communicating hydrocephalus. Ann Surg 68:569, 1918.
7. Dandy WE, Blackfan KD: International hydrocephalus: An experimental, clinical and pathological study. Am J Dis Child 8:406, 1914.
8. DeRuysch F, Morgagni GB: Considerations generales et observations particulaires sur le spina bifida. J Med 27:162, 1806.
9. Fernbach SK, McLone DG: Derangement of swallowing in children with myelomeningocele. Pediatr Radiol 15:311, 1985.
10. Gardner WJ: Hydrodynamic mechanisms of syringomyelia: Its relationship to myelocele. J Neurol Neurosurg Psychiatry 28:247, 1965.
11. Hall PV, Campbell RL, Kalsbeck JE: Meningomyelocele and progressive hydromyelia. Progressive paresia in myelodysplasia. J Neurosurg 43:457, 1975.
12. Hall PV, Lindseth RE, Campbell RL, et al: Myelodysplasia and developmental scoliosis. A manifestation of syringomyelia. Spine 1:48, 1956.
13. Hoffman HJ, Hendrick EB, Humphreys RP: Manifestations and management of Arnold-Chiari malformations in patients with myelomeningocele. Child's Brain 1:255, 1975.
14. Hoffman HJ, Hendrick EB, Humphreys RP: The tethered spinal cord: Its protean manifestations, diagnosis and surgical correction. Child's Brain 2:145, 1976.
15. Hoffman HJ, Park TS, Hendrick EB, et al: Manifestazioni e trattamento della malformazione di Arnold-Chiari nel bambino con Mielomeningocele. In: DiRocco M, Caldarelli M (eds): Mielomeningocele. Rome, Casa del Libro Editrice, 1983, pp 251–260.
16. Hunt GM, Holmes AE: Some factors relating to intelligence in treated hydrocephalic children. Am J Dis Child 127:664, 1974.
17. Ishak B, McLone DG, Seleny F: Autonomic dysfunction associated with Arnold-Chiari malformation. Child's Brain 7:146, 1981.
18. Laurence KM: The natural history of spina bifida cystica: Detailed analysis of 407 cases. Arch Dis Child 39:41, 1964.
19. Lorber J: Results of treatment of myelomeningocele. An analysis of 524 unselected cases, with special reference to possible selection for treatment. Dev Med Child Neurol 13:279, 1971.
20. Lorber J, Salfield S: Results of selective treatment of spina bifida cystica. Arch Dis Child 56:822, 1981.
21. MacKenzie NG, Emery JL: Deformities of the cervical cord in children with neurospinal dysraphism. Dev Med Child Neurol 13:58, 1971.
22. McLone DG: Technique for closure of myelomeningoceles. Child's Brain 6:65, 1980.
23. McLone DG: Results of treatment of children born with a myelomeningocele. Clin Neurosurg 30:407, 1983.
24. McLone DG: The handicapped newborn: Diagnosis, prognosis and outcome—the neonatal view. Issues in Law and Medicine, Vol. 1, no. 2, May 1986.
25. McLone DG: Arguments against selection. Clin Neurosurg 34:359, 1986.
26. McLone DG, Czyzewski D, Raimondi A, et al: Central nervous system infections as a limiting factor in the intelligence of children with myelomeningocele. Pediatrics 70:338, 1982.
27. McLone DG, Dias L, Kaplan WE, et al: Concepts in the management of spina bifida. In: Humphreys RP (ed): Concepts in Pediatric Neurosurgery, 5. Basel, S Karger, 1985, pp 97–106.
28. McLone DG, Naidich TP: Spinal dysraphism: Experimental and clinical. In: Holtzman RNN, Stein BM (eds): The Tethered Spinal Cord. New York, Thieme-Stratton Inc., 1985, pp 14–28.
29. McLone DG, Naidich TP: Myelodysplasia and tethered spinal cord. In: Tachdjian MO (ed): Pediatric Orthopedics. New York, Praeger Publishing, 1986, pp 164–173.
30. Milhorat TH: Hydrocephalus: Historical notes, etiology and clinical diagnosis. In: McLaurin RL (ed): Pediatric Neurosurgery. New York, Grune & Stratton, 1982, p 200.
31. Morgagni GB: The Seats and Causes of Disease Investigated by Anatomy. London, R. Miller and J. Cadell, 1969.
32. Morton M: Spina bifida aperta, treatment by injection. Br Med J 1:381, 1875.
33. Naidich TP, Harwood-Nash DC, McLone DG: Radiology of spinal dysraphism. Clin Neurosurg 30:341, 1983.
34. Naidich TP, Maravilla K, McLone DG: The Chiari II malformation. In: McLaurin RL (ed): Proceedings of the Second Symposium on Spina Bifida. New York, Praeger Publishing, 1986, pp 164–173.
35. Naidich TP, McLone DG: Myelocele and myelomeningocele. In: McLaurin RL (ed): Proceedings of the Second Symposium on Spina Bifida. New York, Praeger Publishing, 1986, pp 119–128.
36. Naidich TP, McLone DG: The investigation of hydrocephalus by computed tomography. In: Little JR (ed): Clinical Neurosurgery. Baltimore, Williams & Wilkins, 1984, pp 527–539.
37. Naidich TP, McLone DG, Fulling KH: The Chiari II malformation: Part IV. The hindbrain deformity. Neuroradiology 25:179, 1983.
38. Naidich TP, McLone DG, Harwood-Nash D: Dysraphism. In: Newton TH, Potts DG (eds): Modern Neuroradiology, Vol. 1. Computed Tomography of the Spine and Spinal Cord. San Francisco/New York, Clavadel Press, 1982, pp 299–355.
39. Nulsen FE, Spitz EB: Treatment of hydrocephalus by direct heart shunt from ventricle to jugular vein. Surg Forum 2:399, 1952.
40. Park TS, Cail WS, Maggio WM, et al: Progressive spasticity

and scoliosis in children with myelomeningocele. J Neurosurg 62:367, 1985.
41. Park TS, Hoffman HJ, Hendrick EB, et al: Experience with surgical decompression of the Arnold-Chiari malformation in young infants with myelomeningocele. Neurosurg 13:147, 1983.
42. Piggott H: The natural history of scoliosis in myelodysplasia. J Bone Joint Surg (Br) 62:54, 1980.
43. Reigel DH: Tethered spinal cord. In: Humphreys RP (ed): Concepts in Pediatric Neurosurgery, Vol. 4. Basel, S Karger, 1983, pp 142–164.
44. Reigel D, McLone DG: Spina bifida. In: Mustarde JC, Jackson IT (eds): Plastic Surgery in Infancy and Childhood. London, Churchill Livingstone, 1988 (in press).
45. Shkolnik A, McLone DG: Intraoperative real-time ultrasonic guidance of intracranial shunt tube placement in infants. Radiology 144:573, 1982.
46. Shurtleff DB, Goiney R, Gordon LH, et al: Myelodysplasia: The natural history of kyphosis and scoliosis. A preliminary report. Dev Med Child Neurol 18:126, 1976.
47. Soare PL, Raimondi AJ: Intellectual and perceptual motor characteristics of treated myelomeningocele children. Am J Dis Child 131:199, 1977.
48. Storrs BB, McLone DG: Ventricular size and intelligence in myelodysplastic children. In: Marlin AE (ed): Concepts in Pediatric Neurosurgery, Vol. 8. Basel, S Karger, 1988, pp. 51–56.
49. Tomita T, McLone DG: Acute respiratory arrest: A complication of malfunction of the shunt in children with myelomeningocele and Arnold-Chiari malformation: A report of three cases. Am J Dis Child 137:142, 1983.
50. Trowbridge A: Three cases of spina bifida, successfully treated. Boston Med Surg J 1:753, 1828.
51. Tulpius N: Obs. Med. Lib. III Cap. XXIX, XXX. 1641:229.
52. Venes JL, Black KL, Latack JT: Preoperative evaluation and surgical management of the Arnold-Chiari II malformation. J Neurosurg 64:363, 1986.
53. Vesalius A: DeCorporis Humani Fabrica. Basileau, Joannis Oporini, 1543.
54. Yamada S, Schreider S, Ashwal S, et al: Pathophysiologic mechanisms in the tethered spinal cord syndrome. In: Holtzman RNN, Stein BM (eds): The Tethered Spinal Cord. New York, Thieme-Stratton Inc., 1985.

5
THE TETHERED SPINAL CORD

David G. McLone, M.D., Ph.D.
Thomas P. Naidich, M.D.

For many years children with cutaneous stigmas in the midline of the back and congenital anomalies of the spine were seen to suffer gradual deterioration in spinal cord function.[2, 3, 86, 92] This progressive deficit was interpreted as the natural history for these children. Insidious deterioration in spinal cord function was also observed in a second group of children with no visible stigmas of spinal disease. This group was thought to be distinct from the first. However, the common factor in these two groups of children has recently been shown to be the presence of a low-lying terminal end of the spinal cord, with limitation of the movement ("tethering") of the spinal cord in the cephalocaudal plane. The specific reason for the limitation of motion varied from patient to patient.

Until recently, many physicians have not regarded these data as proof that tethering of the spinal cord produces neurologic dysfunction. Phrases such as "I don't believe in tethered cord!" were frequently offered at national meetings. Well-meaning surgeons continued to perform cosmetic procedures on the cutaneous manifestations of these lesions without addressing the intraspinal pathologic condition. Others corrected the orthopedic deformities alone, although these deformities were the result of primary neurologic dysfunction.

With time, larger series of children treated earlier in life began to appear.[13, 16, 38, 65] These series documented that untethering the spinal cord of an asymptomatic patient *prevents* the otherwise expected urologic and orthopedic complications; late surgery offers stabilization of the deficits present in most patients and a significant reversal of symptoms in a few patients.[13, 16, 38, 65]

In the past, the term "tethered spinal cord" was commonly considered to be interchangeable with the term "tight filum terminale." Also, tethered cord was thought to occur primarily with spina bifida occulta. More recently, tethered spinal cord has come to signify a pathologic fixation of the spinal cord in an abnormal caudal location, so that the cord suffers mechanical stretching, distortion, and ischemia with daily activities, growth, and development.[80] Such tethering can be caused by many conditions, including tight filum terminale, spinal lipoma, dermoid tumor, diastematomyelia, repaired myelomeningocele, and arachnoiditis.[80] Hydromyelia has proved to be a common accompaniment of spinal cord tethering.[68]

This chapter reviews some of the important observations published on tethered cord, the embryology of the spinal cord, and the authors' theories on the embryopathies that lead to fixation of the spinal cord. Methods of diagnosis and management of the various lesions are discussed.

DEVELOPMENT OF THE MAMMALIAN SPINAL CORD

Understanding congenital lesions is best achieved with a knowledge of normal embryology and fetal development. This knowledge of the developmental sequence is necessary for interpreting the relationships of mature structures. Likewise, an understanding of the structure of a congenital lesion affords insight into the time and the stage of development at which the sequence was altered. It is important to remember that the relationship of primitive cell layers limits the form that the embryopathy can take.

By day 17, ectodermal cells have migrated into the primitive pit and have advanced cephalically, in the midline, to create a column of cells that is situated between the ectoderm and the entoderm. This column of cells, called the notochordal process, extends from Hensen's node caudally to the prochordal plate cephalically. The primitive pit then deepens and invaginates into the previously solid notochordal process, lengthening it into a hollow notochordal canal. This quickly fuses with the entoderm. At the points of fusion, breakdown of cells opens the notochordal canal to the yolk sac. As a result, there is a transient communication from the amnion through the notochordal canal to the yolk sac. This is the neurenteric canal of Kovalevsky (Fig. 5–1). Soon thereafter, the notochordal canal undergoes complex changes that close the communication with the yolk sac, re-establish complete layers of entoderm and of ectoderm, and re-form a solid core of tissue designated the true notochord. The entoderm then ultimately forms gut. The notochord induces formation of the neural plate and guides formation of the vertebral bodies. The ectoderm forms spinal cord and skin.

The greatest portion of the spinal cord, essentially all of the *functional* spinal cord, forms by an orderly sequence of steps designated *neurulation*. This mechanism establishes the brain, the cervical and thoracic segments of the spinal cord, and the upper portion of the lumbar enlargement. The smaller, distal portion of the spinal cord forms by a far-less-well-organized sequence of agglomeration of cells, vacuolation, and involution that is designated canalization and retrogressive differentiation. This process establishes the distal conus medullaris and the filum terminale.

Initially, the immature spinal cord extends to the distal end of the tail fold of the embryo. In a full-term infant, the tip of the spinal cord typically lies at the L2–3 interspace (98 percent) or overlies the L3 vertebra (1.2 percent of cases).[7] By three months postpartum, the tip of the conus medullaris is nearly at the adult level of the L1–2 interspace. This "ascent" of the cord results from both retrogressive differentiation and disproportionately greater growth of the vertebral column (Fig. 5–2).

Formation of the vertebrae proceeds along with formation of the neural elements. By day 17, mesodermal cells at the cephalic end of the embryo form a thick mass of *paraxial mesoderm* situated lateral to the notochord and ventrolateral to the neural plate. This paraxial mesoderm forms bilaterally symmetric longitudinal columns of solid mesoderm. By day 20, these columns begin to segment into paired blocks called *somites*. Somites first form in the future occipital region. Then, they continue to form as the embryo lengthens until, ultimately, 42 to 44 pairs are formed: 4 occipital, 8 cervical, 12 thoracic, 5 lumbar, 5 sacral, and 8 to 10 coccygeal. Later, the first occipital and the last five to seven coccygeal pairs disappear.

The ventromedial portion of each somite differentiates into a sclerotome that will form the cartilage, bone, and ligament of the vertebral column, as follows: During the fourth week of development, the notochord separates from the ectoderm and the entoderm. Cells from the sclerotomes then migrate medially, surround the notochord, and form a dense longitudinal column of mesenchyme about the notochord. After the neural tube closes and

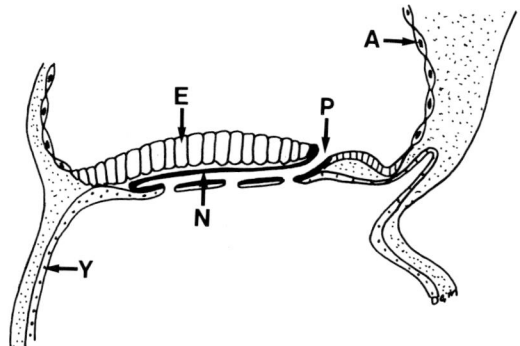

Figure 5–1. A cephalocaudal section through an 18-day-old embryo, showing the notochordal process (N) and the primitive pit (P) leading to the neurenteric canal. Note ectoderm (E), wall of the yolk sac (Y), and amnion (A).

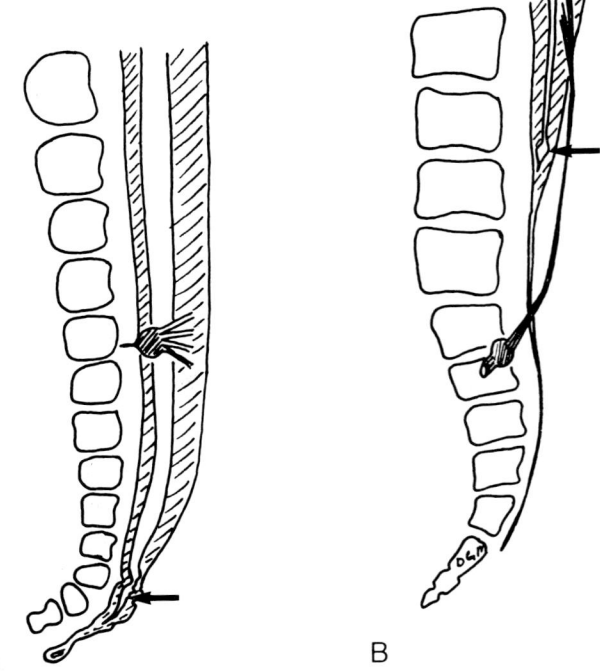

Figure 5–2. A schematic drawing of the embryonic spinal cord (A) and the spinal cord of a fetus nearly full-term (B). Note the change in level of the terminal ventricle (arrow) and the marked change in length and direction of the dorsal root as the cauda equina and filum terminale form.

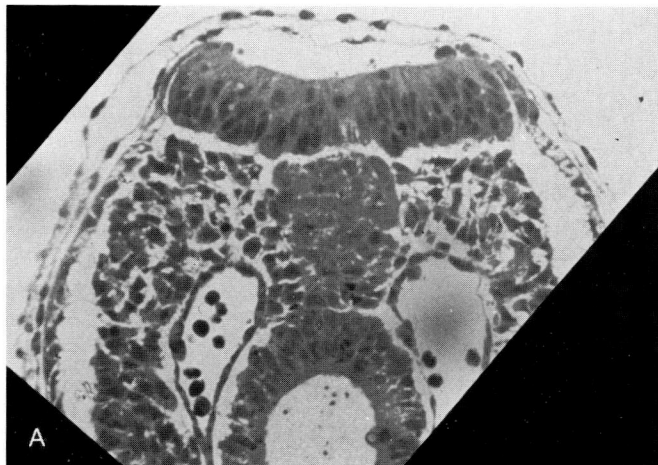

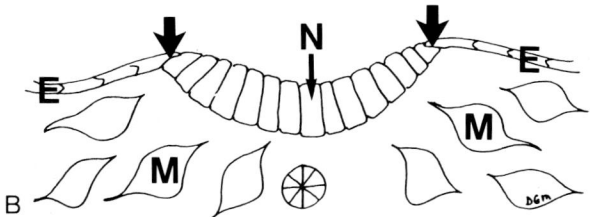

Figure 5–3. A, Transverse section of an embryo, showing the neural plate. B, Schematic drawing demonstrates the ectoderm (E) junction (large arrows) with the neural plate (N). Below is the notochord and mesenchyme (M).

separates from the superficial ectoderm, cells from the sclerotomes also migrate dorsal to the neural tube, between future cord and future skin, to establish the precursors of the neural arches of the vertebrae. Migration of sclerotomic cells ventrolaterally forms the costal processes and ribs. These elements then undergo a complex resegmentation, chondrify, and ossify, creating the spinal column. These diverse processes will be addressed in greater detail in the following sections.

Neurulation

Normal Neurulation. By the end of the third week, the notochord induces formation of a slipper-shaped plate of ectodermal cells in the midline, just cephalic to Hensen's node. This *neural plate* is directly contiguous laterally with the superficial ectoderm from which it differentiated (Fig. 5–3). During the next days, the lateral portions of the neural plate elevate to form the neural folds, while the midline portion remains depressed as the ventral neural groove (Fig. 5–4). Progressive elevation and rolling over causes the left and the right neural folds to approximate each other and fuse together in the midline. This process forms a neural tube (future spinal cord) with a central channel (future central canal of the spinal cord) (Fig. 5–5). The folds first meet and fuse in the future cervical region. Thereafter, the entire process proceeds both cranially and caudally as a "wave," such that the level of fusion corresponds to the level of the most recently formed somite. At approximately 23 days' and 25 days' gestation, respectively, the cephalic and caudal ends of the neural tube close at the anterior and posterior neuropores.

Immediately following fusion of the neural folds into the neural tube, the two portions of superficial ectoderm then fuse together in the midline, dorsal to the neural tube, to establish the integrity of the superficial ectoderm (future skin). Only then does the superficial ectoderm of each side separate from the neural ectoderm in a process designated disjunction. As mesenchyme migrates dorsally between the neural tube and the skin, the entire cord becomes buried beneath a thick layer that ultimately forms the meninges, neural arches, and paraspinal muscles.

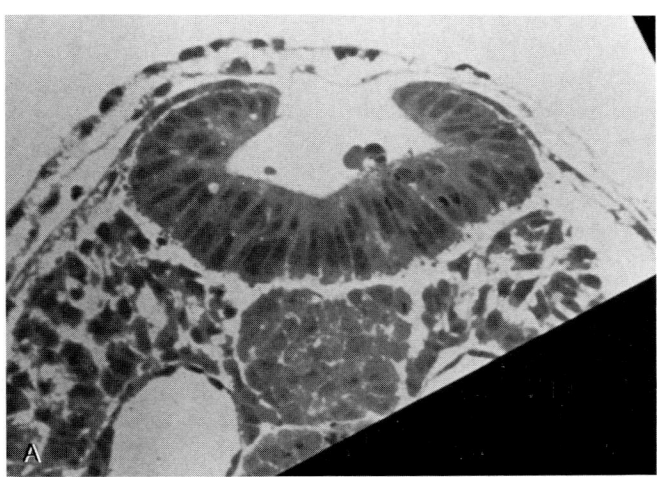

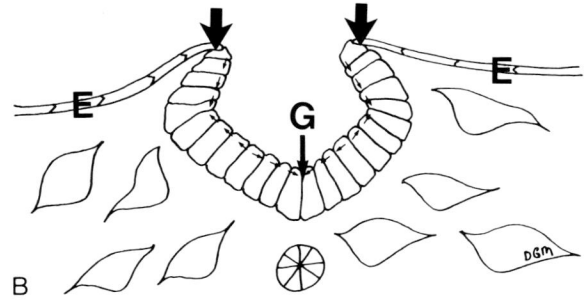

Figure 5–4. A, Transverse section of an embryo, showing the neural folds. B, Schematic drawing demonstrates the ectoderm (E) junction (large arrows) with neuroectoderm forming the neural groove (G). Small arrows represent actin filaments.[102]

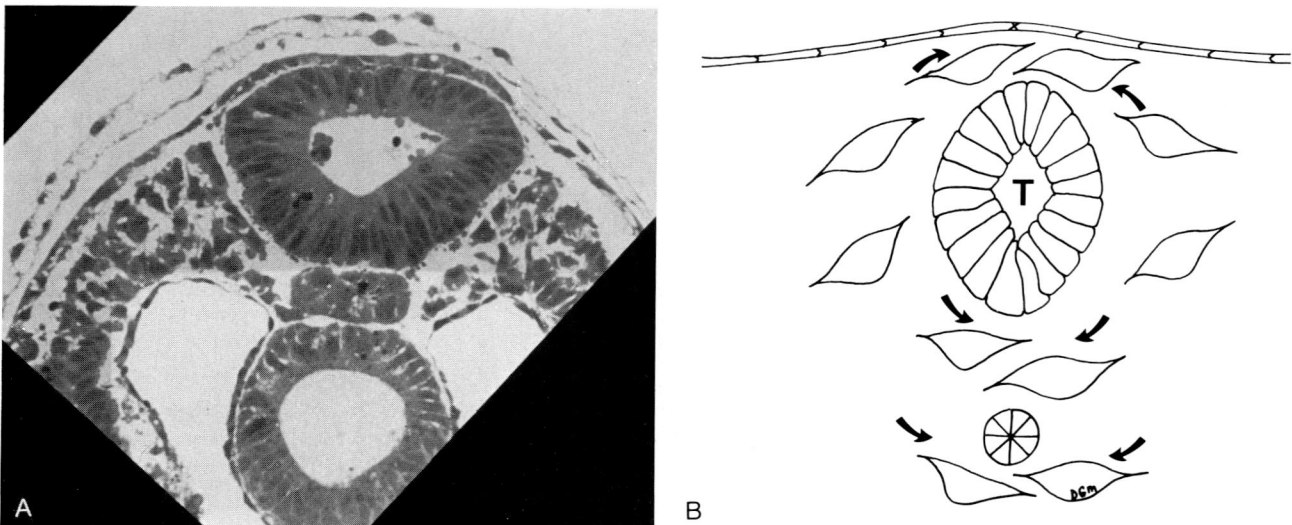

Figure 5–5. A, Transverse section of an embryo, showing the neural tube. B, Schematic drawing demonstrates the neural tube (T) separated from the superficial ectoderm, and the mesenchyme now has access to the dorsal and ventral surfaces of the neural tube (curved arrows).

Caudal Regression

Normal Canalization and Retrogressive Differentiation. After neurulation is complete, on approximately day 25, the distal spinal cord has yet to be formed. The caudal end of the neural tube and the caudal end of the notochord remnants of Hensen's node blend into a large aggregate of undifferentiated cells (the *caudal cell mass*) that extends into the tail fold, adjacent to the distal end of the developing hindgut and the mesonephros. This juxtaposition of developing genitourinary, notochordal, and neural structures within the tail fold appears to account for the common concurrence of distal vertebral, neural, anorectal, renal, and genital anomalies.

Within the caudal cell mass, small vacuoles form, coalesce, and eventually connect with the central canal of the spinal cord above, "canalizing" the caudal cell mass (Fig. 5–6). Since vacuoles form at many sites and link up variably, accessory central canals are commonly observed in the distal cords of embryos (35 percent) and, occasionally, in otherwise normal adults.

As the vacuoles form, groups of cells orient themselves around the vacuoles and differentiate toward glial cells. By this method, the distal spinal cord and the canal of the cord elongate far into the tail fold. The most cephalic portion of this distal spinal cord forms the tip of the conus medullaris. The major portion of the distal spinal cord involutes to form the filum terminale. A portion of the lumen persists into adulthood as the terminal ventricle that lies within the distalmost conus or the proximal filum terminale.

The process of involution of the distal spinal cord

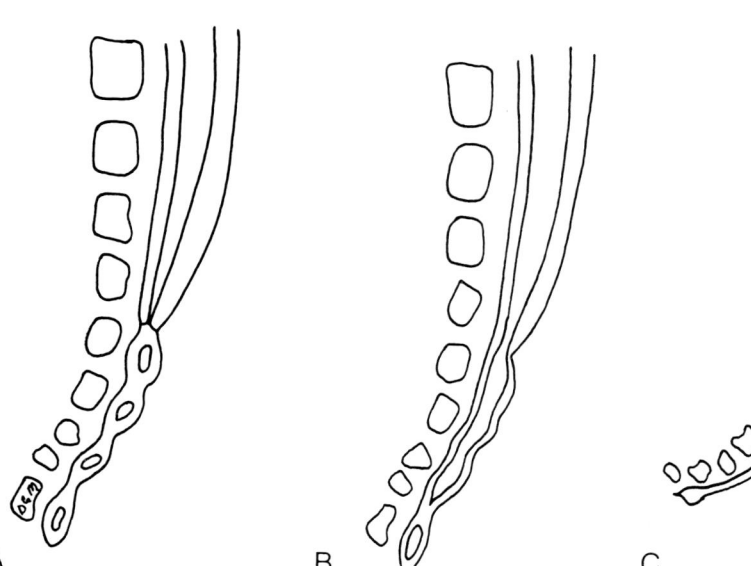
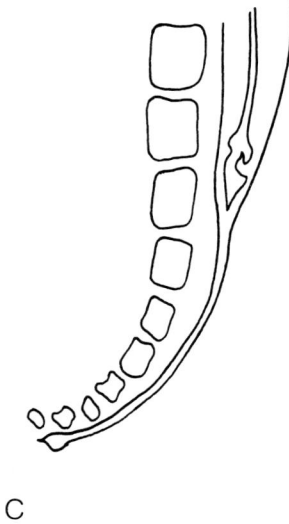

Figure 5–6. A schematic drawing showing vacuoles and coalescence of the caudal cell mass *(A)*, canalization *(B)*, and the formation of the filum terminale and the terminal ventricle *(C)*.

is designated *retrogressive differentiation*. It begins even before canalization is complete. The embryonic tail disappears first. The lumen distal to future C2 becomes progressively narrower than the lumen above. The cells surrounding the narrowing distal lumen differentiate less completely than do those above and then involute further to leave only the pial-ependymal strand, designated filum terminale. A small portion of the distalmost involuting spinal cord frequently remains within the connective tissue dorsal to the last two vertebrae for long periods of time, as the coccygeal medullary vestige.

After the distal spinal cord involutes into the filum terminale, the newly formed conus medullaris lies opposite C2 or C3. Thereafter, the spinal cord does not shorten further. Rather, it elongates with growth. The vertebral column also elongates with growth—faster than the spinal cord. Thus, all further "ascent"[7] of the spinal cord results from *disproportionate* longitudinal growth of the vertebrae; the bones grow away from the spinal cord.

At this point, it is sufficient to understand that the caudal spinal column also forms by a less-well-organized process than that responsible for the more cephalic portions of the spine above. The caudal cell mass formed by notochord, mesoderm, and neural tissue simply segments into somites to form the sacral, coccygeal, and tail vertebrae. Retrogressive differentiation then leads to reduction of most of these segments, with loss of the tail.

EMBRYOPATHIES

Deranged Neurulation

Several common forms of dysraphism appear to result from deranged neurulation.

Myelomeningocele

Myelomeningoceles (myeloceles) are a form of spina bifida in which a focal segment of spinal cord appears as a flat plate of neural tissue that is exposed to view in the midline of the back. Such an anatomic derangement could result from either a primary failure of neurulation or a secondary disruption and splitting of a normally formed spinal cord.[61]

If the neural folds fail to roll up and fuse into a tube, they persist instead as a flat plate of neural tissue (Fig. 5–7). Because the tube does not close, the superficial ectoderm does not separate from the neural ectoderm and remains in a lateral position. Therefore, the skin that develops from the ectoderm is also lateral in position, leaving a midline defect. Mesenchyme cannot migrate between the neural tube and the superficial ectoderm, so it remains in an abnormal lateral position. Therefore, the bony, cartilaginous, muscular, and ligamentous elements

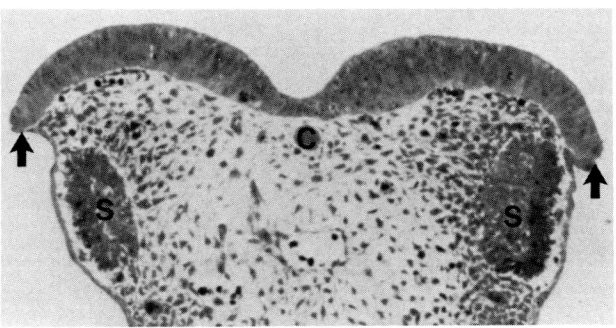

Figure 5–7. Transverse section of an embryo, showing failure of the neural tube to close. Note the persistence of a junction with ectoderm (arrows). Also note that the somites (S) are lateral and ventral to the notochord (C).

that develop from the mesenchyme also remain in abnormal lateral positions. They are deficient in the midline. Since the laminae and muscles develop in an abnormal lateral position, they appear bifid and "everted." The unfused neural plate is exposed to view in the midline of the back, at the site of midline deficiency of skin, bone, cartilage, muscle, and ligament. This state is designated myelocele or myelomeningocele. Together, myelocele and myelomeningocele are the commonest form of spinal dysraphism.

In myelocele and myelomeningocele, the exposed surface of the neural plate appears as a raw, reddish, vascular, oval plate in the midline of the back (Fig. 5–8). The raw surface represents the interior of what should have been the closed spinal cord. A midline groove runs down the center of this plate. This groove is the residuum of the ventral neural groove and is directly continuous with the central canal of the normally formed cord above (and sometimes below) the plate.

The neural plate is surrounded on all sides by thin membranes representing the skin and the arachnoid. The size of this membranous ring varies. When the subarachnoid space is small, the membranous ring is narrow, and the neural plate lies flush with the back. This situation is designated myelocele (Fig. 5–8). When the subarachnoid space is very large, the membranous ring is wide, and the neural plate is elevated far above the skin surface. This condition is designated myelomeningocele (Fig. 5–9). In both myelocele and myelomeningocele, the neural plate and the membranous ring are surrounded by normal skin. With time, the membranous ring and the neural plate may become partially epithelialized by cells that grow medially from the skin margins to cover the midline defect.

Deep to the surface, the *ventral* face of the neural plate represents the neural tissue that should have formed the entire outer circumference of the spinal cord. The two ventral nerve roots arise from the ventral surface, just to each side of the midline sulcus. The left and right dorsal roots also arise

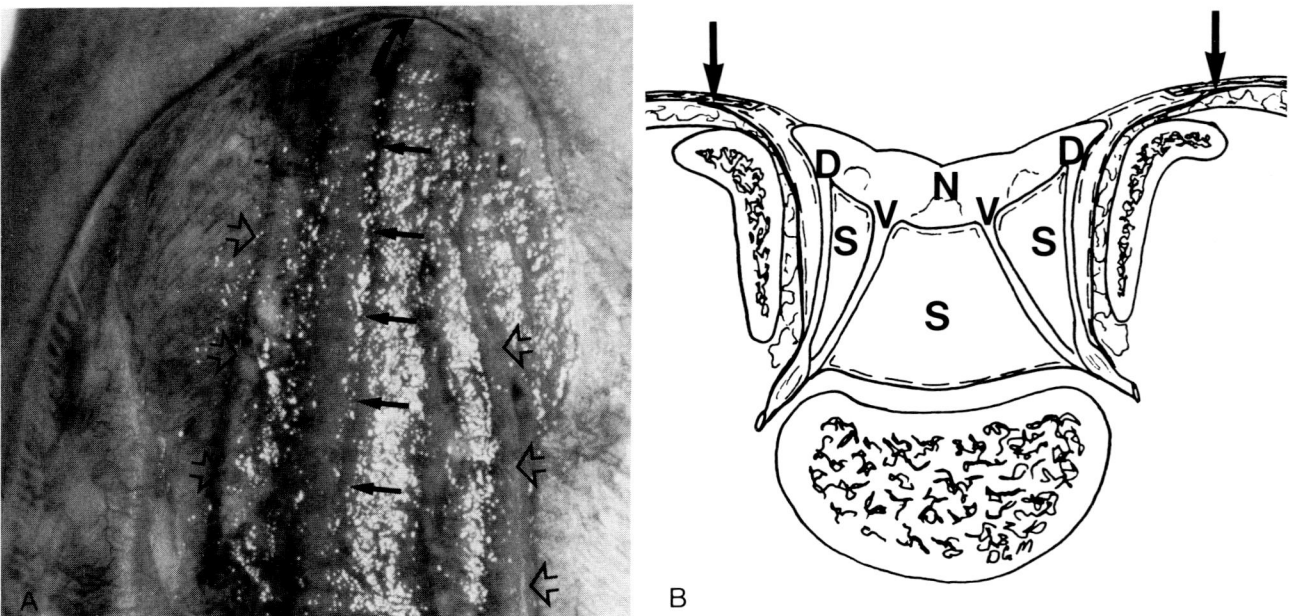

Figure 5–8. *A,* Myelocele form of dysraphism, showing the ventral sulcus (straight black arrows), the entrance to the central canal (curved arrow), and the dorsal root entry zone (open arrows) of the neural placode. *B,* Schematic drawing of a transverse section shows the neural placode (N), dura mater skin junction (arrows), subarachnoid space (S), and dorsal (D) and ventral (V) roots.

from the ventral surface of the neural plate, lateral to the corresponding ventral roots. These roots traverse the subarachnoid space and exit via the neural foramina, in the usual fashion.

The pia-arachnoid membrane continues medially over the ventral surface of the neural plate and around the entire subarachnoid space as one continuous sheet. This membrane is given the name pia mater where it is contiguous with neural tissue, and the name arachnoid mater where it is separate from the neural tissue. The dura mater lies peripheral to the arachnoid and becomes lost in the margins of the skin defect dorsally. Because the neural plate and meninges are anchored to the skin surface, the spinal cord is tethered and is relatively immobile.

The exact abnormality of embryogenesis that creates myelomeningocele is unknown. Two basic theories of its pathogenesis have been proposed: (1) the neural tube fails to close properly,[98] and (2) the once-closed neural tube ruptures open.[29] Experimental data suggest that both mechanisms may lead to myelomeningocele.[61, 63]

Nonclosure. The best data strongly suggest that

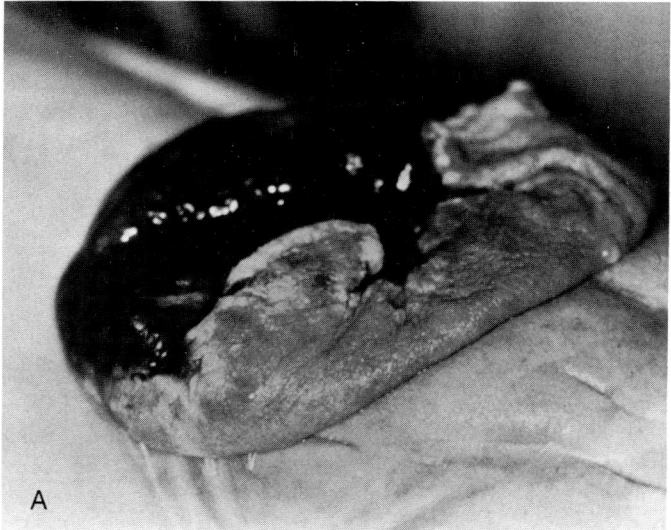
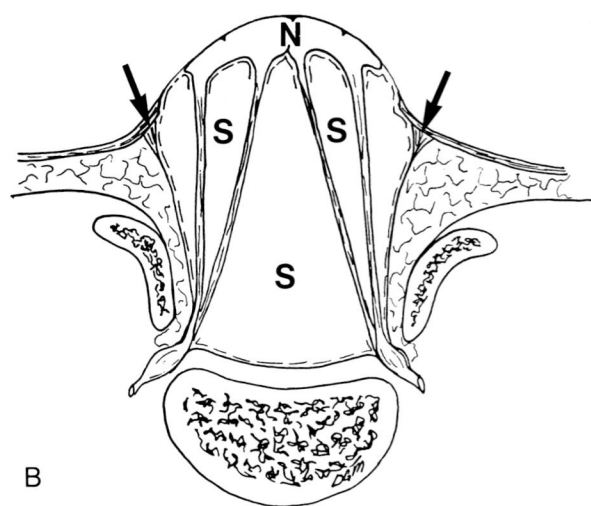

Figure 5–9. *A,* Large myelomeningocele with the neural tissue spread over the surface. The basic relationships are the same, only distended over a large CSF sac. *B,* Schematic drawing shows the neural placode (N), dura mater skin junction (arrows), and subarachnoid space (S).

myelomeningocele represents a disturbance in the closure of the neural placode at or before the time the embryo reaches 3 to 5 mm (crown-rump length), leaving the neural tissue in its embryonal, plaque-like state. The authors' experiments with neurulating mouse embryos explanted into in vitro culture indicate that addition of toxins such as tunicamycin interferes with the normal formation of glycosaminoglycans (GAGs) and prevents the neural tube from closing. This creates spina bifida.[61] Hydrocephalus and the Chiari II deformity at the cervicomedullary junction do not develop in the embryonic period but appear later, during fetal life.[73] How they form is also unknown.

Reopening. Also in the authors' laboratory, addition of vitamin A to the same in vitro culture of a mouse embryo had no apparent effect on the developing embryo. However, injection of vitamin A into the pregnant mouse before and during the period of neurulation caused neural tube defects in some embryos and a remarkable increase in the volume of the neural tube in other embryos. In these latter embryos, the central canal appeared grossly distended. Light microscopy of the sectioned embryos documented marked distention of the neural tube. The neuroepithelia showed evidence of toxicity, with multiple intracellular inclusions.

In this experimental arrangement, the two portions of the neural tube that appeared to be the most thinned were the ventral and the dorsal sulci. In some embryos, the ventral sulcus of the neural tubes gaped. Since the ventral neural tube is normally never open, vitamin A–induced distention of the central canal must have caused the spinal cord to rupture.[61] The results of the vitamin A study support the postulate advocated by Padget[103] and by Gardner[29] and provide the first experimental evidence that the neural tube did, in fact, close and then reopen secondarily because of distention and rupture.

Other theories of the origin of myelomeningocele probably reflect secondary phenomena.[24, 29]

The studies of Osaka and colleagues[73] of the incidence and distribution of myeloschisis in 92 human embryos and four human fetuses document that, in utero, diffuse myeloschisis is common (13 percent), cervical myeloschisis is frequent (29 percent), and holoprosencephaly is commonly associated with myeloschisis (20 percent). Those embryos with diffuse myeloschisis, focal cervical myeloschisis, and concomitant holoprosencephaly will most probably be extruded by spontaneous abortion. Thus, the increased frequency of lumbosacral myelomeningocele in newborns does not indicate a greater occurrence of myelomeningocele in the lumbosacral area. Rather, it reflects the milder nature of lumbosacral myelomeningoceles, which permits fetuses affected with this relatively infrequent form to live to full term.

Lipomyelomeningocele

Spinal lipomas are distinct collections of fat and connective tissue that are at least partially encapsulated and that have a definite connection with the spinal cord.

A number of theories have been proposed to explain their occurrence. Chiari and von Recklinghausen noted that fat cells may appear normally in the pia-arachnoid and suggested that lipomas might represent overgrowth of cells already present.[92] Conceivably, spinal lipomas might also result from fatty differentiation of the perivascular mesenchyme, which normally invades the spinal cord during embryonal vascularization, or from overgrowth of embryonic rests of ectodermal origin.

McLone and associates[62] suggested that spinal lipomas arise by focal, premature disjunction of neuroectoderm from cutaneous ectoderm, at the stage immediately preceding closure of the neural tube. Such premature disjunction would allow paraxial mesenchyme access to the dorsal surface of the yet-unclosed neural ectoderm (Fig. 5–10). Such mesenchyme, in contact with the dorsal neural surface, might impede or prevent closure of the neural tube in the midline dorsally, accounting for the association of lipoma with partial dorsal mye-

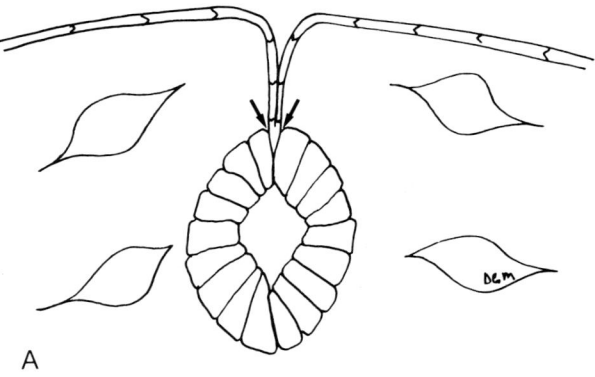

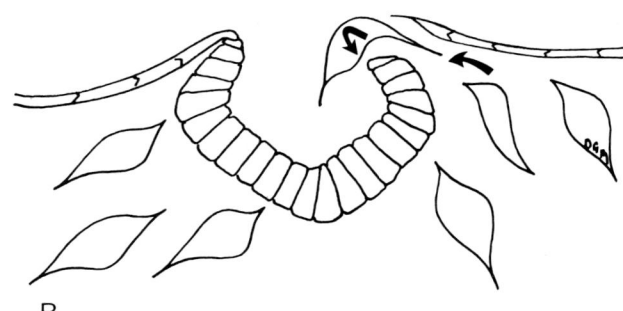

Figure 5–10. Schematic drawings of problems that could arise if the disjunction of the neural tube from superficial ectoderm were delayed (A) or premature (B). A, Delayed disjunction (arrows) would result in a dermal sinus. B, Premature disjunction (curved arrows) would allow a lipoma to form in the neural groove.

loschisis. In partial dorsal myeloschisis, the spinal cord is split in the midline, dorsal to the central canal. The dorsal columns are splayed laterally, exposing the interior of the cord. This interior represents the dorsal surface of the neural plate that rolled up into a cord. It is postulated that this dorsal surface of the neural ectoderm can only induce the adjacent mesenchyme to form fat. Thus, the lipoma forms dorsal in the cord, between the splayed dorsal columns. The ventral surface of the neural ectoderm (which would have formed the exterior of the neural tube) would still induce the surrounding mesenchyme to form normal pia-arachnoid and dura.[57, 59, 89] Thus, the dura, pia-arachnoid, and subarachnoid space form ventral to the neural plate. The junction of neural tissue, pia-arachnoid, and dura would necessarily lie at the lateral edge of the unclosed neural tube. The lipoma would be bounded laterally by pia-arachnoid and dura. Since lipoma and arachnoid form separately in relation to the two different surfaces of the neural plate, no lipoma would be found within the subarachnoid space. However, lipoma could readily extend upward from the cleft into the central canal of the contiguous portion of normal spinal cord, bulge the canal, and appear to protrude through the thinned lateral wall of the spinal cord. Such protrusions would remain covered by pia-arachnoid. Variable expansion of the subarachnoid space ventral to the cord might influence the presence and the degree of any associated myelocele or myelomeningocele, as postulated by Warkany and coworkers.[98]

Dermal Sinus

Dorsal dermal sinuses are thin, usually midline, epithelium-lined tubes that pass inward from the skin of the back toward the spinal canal and spinal cord. These dermal sinuses appear to result from focal, incomplete separation of the cutaneous ectoderm from the neuroectoderm, at the fourth week of fetal development.[67] If the superficial ectoderm fails to separate from the neural ectoderm at one point, a focal segmental adhesion is created (Fig. 5–10). As the spinal cord becomes buried beneath the surface by the developing spinal column and as different rates of growth between neural and spinal tissues lead to "ascent" of the cord, the local "spot-weld" is drawn out into an elongated epithelial tube that still connects the spinal cord segment with the appropriate segment of the skin. Thus, the dorsal dermal sinus appears to be an example of delayed or incomplete disjunction.

The incidence of dermal sinuses is highest in the lumbosacral region, which is the site of the posterior neuropore and one of the last portions of the neural folds to fuse into a tube.

Dermoid and epidermoid tumors usually arise from focal expansion of the dermal sinus. They may also arise from congenital rests or may be acquired as iatrogenic lesions resulting from implantation of viable dermal and epidermal elements by spinal needles not provided with trocars.[30, 94] Such implants may be single or multiple, subcutaneous, intradural, or intramedullary and may give rise to daughter lesions.[18]

Diastematomyelia

Diastematomyelia signifies a sagittal clefting of the spinal cord, conus medullaris, filum terminale, or all three into two, not necessarily symmetric hemicords. The cleft may be short or very long. Diastematomyelia occurs mostly in females (80 percent overall; up to 94 percent in some series). In most patients, cutaneous nevi and especially large patches of silky hair overlie the site of the diastematomyelia.

The genesis of diastematomyelia is not known. Theories center on (1) primary abnormalities in the extraneural tissue, causing secondary splitting of the cord, and (2) primary abnormalities of the neural tissue, inducing secondary changes in the surrounding bone and soft tissue.

1. The most tenable of the first group of theories is Bremer's[12] concept of a persistent accessory neurenteric canal. The normal neurenteric canal (canal of Kovalevsky) is a transient connection from the yolk sac (future intestinal cavity) through the primitive knot (Hensen's node) to the amnion (dorsal surface of the embryo, represented by the external surface of the neural groove). The neural tissue associated with the normal neurenteric canal comes to lie at the tip of the coccyx. Some authorities suggest that there may also be accessory neurenteric canals.[33] If the canal of Kovalevsky (or an accessory canal) were to persist, the neural plate would be cleft focally, perhaps leading to formation of paired hemicords at that site. Persistence of an accessory neurenteric canal that traversed the notocord and the neural plate would explain the concurrence of the multiple segmentation anomalies, hemivertebrae, butterfly vertebrae, spina bifida, skin lesions, cleft dura and cord, and midline cysts and tumors that are associated with diastematomyelia. Alternatively, if, as they migrate cephalically, the notochordal cells encounter an obstruction such as a midline adhesion between the ectoderm and entoderm, then the notochordal cells might migrate leftward or rightward around the adhesion, or to both sides of the adhesion. As a result, the notochord could develop with a focal left-sided or right-sided notch, or a central "doughnut hole." Since the notochord guides formation of the vertebrae, these alterations in the notochord would create, respectively, a local unilateral vertebral agenesis (i.e., hemivertebrae) or ring vertebrae (i.e., butterfly vertebrae) with posterior spina bifida.

2. The most interesting of the second group of theories suggests that as the lateral edges of the neural plate approach the midline dorsally, prelim-

inary to fusing into a single tube, they may curl too far ventrally, touch the ventral portion of the plate, and form two (not necessarily symmetric) neural tubes, one to each side of the midline.[36] The two tubes could lie close together or migrate laterally. The mesenchyme would then migrate inward to surround the tubes. If the distance between the tubes were small, the mesenchyme between the tubes might be induced to form only pia, creating a narrow diastematomyelia with both hemicords lying within a single arachnoidal and dural tube. If the distance between the tubes were greater, the mesenchyme between the tubes might be induced to form arachnoid, dura, and bone, creating a widely split diastematomyelia with two hemicords within separate arachnoidal and dural tubes, separated by an osteocartilaginous spur. All other bony changes would similarly be secondary to induction by anomalously developed neural tissue.

Diastematomyelia could also represent an abortive form of twinning. The occurrence of diastematomyelia with multiple bony spurs in a Siamese twin supports this concept, in at least some cases.

Deranged Retrogressive Differentiation

Terminal Myelocystocele

Terminal myelocystoceles are a special form of occult spinal dysraphism and hydromyelia in which the distal end of the tethered spinal cord is ballooned into a terminal cyst.[64] Terminal myelocystoceles develop at the tail end of the embryo, from an originally undifferentiated aggregate of cells, the caudal cell mass. This mass includes remnants of Hensen's node, the primitive streak, the notochord, and other cells destined to become distal spinal cord. In early embryogenesis, these cells are juxtaposed to those destined to form hindgut and the urogenital system, probably accounting for the frequent concurrence of anomalies in these different systems.

The detailed embryogenesis of the distal end of the normal spinal cord is reviewed carefully by Kunitomo,[48] Streeter,[91] Friede,[26] and Lemire and associates.[50, 51]

Based on the authors' understanding of this normal embryogenesis, we postulate that the anatomic arrangements observed in terminal myelocystocele probably arise as follows: (1) For unknown reasons, cerebrospinal fluid (CSF) is unable to exit from the early neural tube. (2) After canalization occurs, this cerebrospinal fluid is vented into the terminal ventricle. (3) The terminal ventricle dilates. (4) The expanding terminal ventricle bulges into and disrupts the dorsal *mesenchyme*, but not the superficial *ectoderm*. (5) As a result, the posterior elements of the spine fail to develop (spina bifida), but the lesion remains situated deep to an intact skin cover. (6) As the terminal ventricle balloons into a cyst, it distends the arachnoid lining of the distal spinal cord, forming a meningocele. (7) The bulge of the cyst prevents ascent of the cord, producing tethered cord. (8) After formation of the arachnoid, progressive distention of the distalmost spinal cord causes it to bulge caudally, below the end of the meningocele, into the extra-arachnoid space, where it is covered by fat. (9) The cyst also bulges cephalically, to expand the distal spinal cord. This produces trumpetlike flaring of the distal spinal cord. (10) Disruption of the caudal motor segments produces symptoms that may be present at birth or may appear later and be progressive. Myelocystoceles are commonly but not invariably associated with exstrophy of the bladder.

Lesions such as terminal myelocystocele, because they occur in the intragluteal fold, must be differentiated from the sacral coccygeal teratoma. Ultrasonography can usually do this easily in the neonatal unit.

Tight Filum Terminale Syndrome

Tight filum terminale syndrome is a form of occult spinal dysraphism in which the spinal cord is tethered by an abnormally short, abnormally thick filum terminale, and by no other pathologic condition. Normally, the neural tube becomes atrophic beyond the forty-second somite. Lengthening of the filum terminale with subsequent growth of the organism is the result of degeneration of the primitive conus medullaris and intrinsic increase in the length of the nerve fibers.[44] Failure of involution of the terminal cord, failure of lengthening of the nerve fibers, or both could result in the tight filum terminale syndrome.

Other Embryopathies

Embryonic Deformation and Caudal Suppression (Caudal Regression Syndrome)

The term "caudal regression syndrome" has been used to describe a spectrum of anomalies of the lower extremities, genitourinary system, anorectal area, and lumbosacral spine.[9] These include sirenomelia (fusion of the lower extremities), agenesis of the lumbosacral spine, anal atresia, malformations of the external genitalia, and renal aplasia. Caudal regression syndrome suggests that these anomalies are associated with embryopathies of the caudal cell mass and the process of retrogressive differentiation. In fact, retrogressive differentiation is the process by which the coccygeal segments and the filum terminale are formed. The portions of the child affected by this syndrome are principally those segments that develop in conjunction with the final stages of neurulation. Therefore, the authors postulate an alternative explanation and prefer the term "embryonic deformation and caudal suppression."

The syndrome appears to result from disturbances of the caudal mesodermal axis prior to the fourth week of gestation.[45] The degree of derangement is variable, causing the wide spectrum of pathologic conditions observed.

Complete absence of the rump may be produced in chickens by subjecting developing eggs to high temperature[20] or by injecting insulin and other sulfur-containing molecules into the yolk sac of incubated eggs.[74] In these animals, the degree of tail suppression depends upon the precise period of gestation at which the insult is offered.

Lack of vertebrae in patients with lumbosacral agenesis might be secondary to nondevelopment of the lower portions of the notochord and spinal cord. Experimental studies in vertebrates have shown that if a portion of the neural tube is extirpated and the notochord is left intact, vertebral bodies develop, but vertebral arches do not.[39] If the notochord is removed but the neural tube is preserved, vertebral arches develop without distinct bodies.

In chicken embryos, it is known that the development and maintenance of muscle depend upon a trophic influence from the nervous tissue. The aplasia, hypoplasia, and immaturity of the gluteal, paraspinal, and distal extremity musculature observed in human patients with caudal suppression syndrome probably arise on a similar basis.[39] Additional embryologic data are summarized by Pang and Hoffman.[74]

Heredity appears to play a limited role in this syndrome. Although some strains of laboratory mice exhibit hereditary sacrococcygeal agenesis as an autosomal recessive gene,[27] there are few reports of familial caudal regression syndrome. The karyotype studies of affected infants are usually normal.[6, 74, 81]

At the junction of the superficial ectoderm and the neural plate, a group of specialized cells forms the neural crest. The neural crest cells later migrate from this junctional site to a position lateral to the closed neural tube. Neural crest cells will become the dorsal root ganglia and the dorsal roots. They will also contribute the myelin sheaths of the peripheral nervous system.

Other important structures throughout the embryo also depend upon the integrity and migration of the neural crest cells. As they migrate, the neural crest cells induce the formation of the myotomes. Thus, the absence of a dorsal root would result in the absence of one of these specific myotomes, which would then prevent formation of the corresponding ventral root.

Another possible mechanism proposed by McLone and Stevens[58] involves constriction of the embryo. During the fourth week of embryogenesis, the embryo lies in a position of marked extension. As the neural tissue grows rapidly, the position of the embryo must change to marked flexion. During this period, a deficiency in the size of the amniotic cavity could restrict or prevent the change in position from extension to flexion, so that the embryo becomes compressed or even hyperextended. Since the process of neurulation has normally been completed by this time, the upper portion of the spinal cord that forms by neurulation would remain essentially intact. Less commonly, extreme hyperextension might impair the process of neurulation in the distalmost neural tube. In either case, the majority of the spinal cord would be intact. Only the filum terminale, the distal conus medullaris, and, perhaps, the immediately contiguous portion of the distal neurulated spinal cord would be deficient.

At the time that these events occur, the neural crest and the somites are forming the dorsal roots and the vertebral bodies. If the embryo were constricted and compressed at this time, the paraspinous somites and the neural crest cells could be forced to coalesce, resulting in a group of anomalous vertebral forms: (1) Portions of one or more vertebral bodies might be absent at various levels, or (2) other portions could coalesce with adjacent vertebral bodies to form single vertebrae or bony bars reducing the number of vertebrae present (Fig. 5–11).

It is also probable that constriction of the embryo is responsible for agenesis or dysgenesis of the sacrum and the coccyx. Duhamel[21] theorized that sacral anomalies occurred as an extension of the process of involution and resorption of the tail and its vertebral segments. The authors believe otherwise. The sacrum is formed in association with the process of neurulation, not with the process of canalization and retrogressive differentiation. Once neurulation is complete, caudal regression would not affect these portions of the spinal cord and

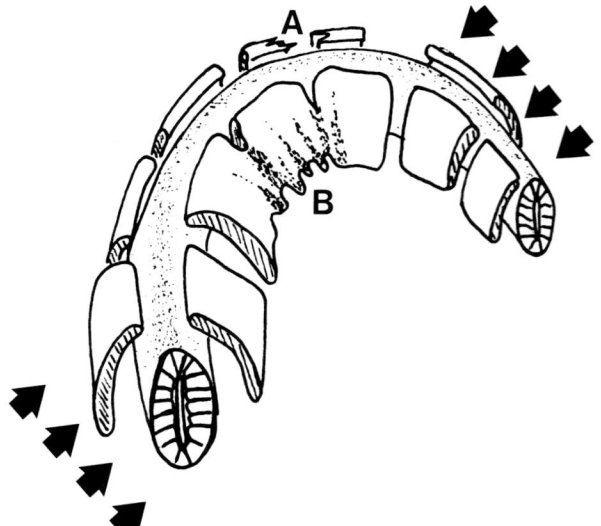

Figure 5–11. A schematic drawing showing the proposed mechanism of embryonic deformation and caudal suppression. Constraints (arrows) placed on the embryo cause somites and neural crest to fragment (A) or coalesce (B), leading to absence of nerve roots and to vertebral bars.

vertebrae. Better terms for this group of anomalies might be embryonic deformation syndromes or caudal suppression syndromes resulting from constraint of the growth of the developing embryo.

Dorsal Enteric Fistula and Neurenteric Cyst

The dorsal enteric fistula is a complete patent fistula from the mesenteric (dorsal) surface of the gut through the mesentery and prevertebral tissue, through the vertebral bodies, spinal canal, and spinal cord, and through bifid laminae to an ostium in the middle of a myelocele or in the midline of the skin of the back. This exceptionally rare fistula is believed to represent persistence of a patent notochordal canal (canal of Kovalevsky) (Fig. 5–1).

Incomplete forms of this fistula are more common than the complete fistula and are believed to explain neurenteric cysts and associated segmentation anomalies of the spine. With variable degrees of repair of the defect in the embryo, *portions* of a dorsal enteric fistula might persist as (1) diverticula or patent duplications arising from the mesenteric border of the gut and extending into the mesentery or through the diaphragm to the mediastinum; (2) persistent cords between the gut and vertebrae; (3) enteric-lined cysts in the mesentery, mediastinum, spinal canal, and midline of the back; (4) anterior spina bifida, posterior spina bifida, or both; (5) diastematomyelia; (6) neurenteric cysts; or (7) various combinations of these. Such a mechanism could also be an alternative pathogenesis for the dorsal dermal sinuses, discussed earlier as resulting from the failure of separation of cutaneous ectoderm from neural ectoderm.

Neurenteric cysts most commonly arise at the cervicothoracic junction or at the conus medullaris. They may lie anterior or posterior to the spinal cord or between the two hemicords of a diastematomyelia. Neurenteric cysts may be lightly or densely adherent to the cord and dura, and they may be isolated or may freely communicate with large mesenteric or mediastinal cysts.

PATHOPHYSIOLOGY

The narrowed appearance of the tethered spinal cord prior to surgical release and the retraction of the proximal segment following release suggest that mechanical traction on the spinal cord may be one mechanism accounting for cord dysfunction in patients with tethered cord. The observation that the length of the intracord segments is increased immediately rostral to the point of tethering further implicates spinal cord stretching in the pathogenesis of cord dysfunction associated with tethering. The authors have observed that flexion and extension of the pelvis are associated with further attenuation and relaxation of the spinal cord, respectively. This observation helps explain the postural changes seen in these patients and suggests that intermittent stretching of the spinal cord may occur with normal sitting, standing, and daily activities, leading to worsening deficit. Breig[11] has demonstrated that the cervical cord becomes attenuated with flexion. The distal cord becomes attenuated with flexion of the pelvis. Breig[11] suggested that symptoms occur whenever a mechanical factor interferes with normal elongation of the spinal cord. It seems probable that tethering of the spinal cord limits the normal elongation of the spinal cord that occurs with body motions and an increase in stature.

Reigel[80] has also observed that multiple peripheral nerves are often stretched and distorted around the distal spinal cord and the sac. Dysfunction of these nerves may help account for weakness, orthopedic deformity, and pain.

The blood vessels overlying the tethered spinal cord often appear thin and attenuated. These become dilated and hyperemic following release of the cord.[80] These observations suggest that any process leading to lengthening or stretching of the cord such as pelvic flexion, cervical flexion, growth and development, and change in curvature of the vertebral column may lead to intermittent but chronic, repetitive ischemia or to progressive ischemia with resulting spinal cord dysfunction. Yamada and coworkers[100, 101] have suggested that there is mitochondrial anoxia within the conus medullaris of patients with tethered spinal cords. In the cat, tethering of the cord produced changes in redox activity of cytochrome aa_3.[100] The slow rate of progression of neurologic symptoms further supports the concept of vascular insufficiency as a factor in cord dysfunction. In addition, stretching may reduce the blood supply to peripheral nerves and could lead to pain and weakness.

Somatosensory Evoked Potentials. Reigel[80] was able to obtain serial somatosensory evoked potentials (SSEP) by peroneal nerve stimulation in 40 patients who subsequently underwent operations for tethered cord syndrome. The evoked responses from the lower extremities were frequently asymmetric. Serial studies over a 6- to 12-month period preceding surgery demonstrated an increase in the latency and a reduction in the amplitude of the evoked response with time, suggesting progressive dysfunction.

Postoperatively, 33 of the 40 patients exhibited a decrease in the latency of the response.

CLINICAL FEATURES OF THESE ANOMALIES

Signs and Symptoms

Cutaneous Signs and Symptoms

Those lesions in which the neural tissue is hidden by an intact skin cover are designated occult spinal dysraphism. This group comprises a heterogeneous collection of lesions including dorsal dermal sinus, spinal lipoma, tight filum terminale syndrome, anterior sacral meningocele, neurenteric cyst, and diastematomyelia. The common feature among these lesions is that the spinal cord may be cleft, is tethered in an abnormally low position, or both. Cutaneous stigmas such as skin dimple, skin tags, hemangiomatous nevi, and patchy hypertrichosis frequently signal the presence of a hidden pathologic condition of the spine and spinal cord (Fig. 5–12). A pit or dimple attached to the tip of the coccyx is usually "benign" and almost never is associated with a tract into the central nervous system. Storrs and Walker[90] have reported cases of small presacral teratomas associated with these dimples. Therefore, in children with these stigmas, the authors recommend a digital rectal examination and ultrasonography of the presacral area.

Neuro-orthopedic Deformity

Seventy-five percent of patients with occult spinal dysraphism have one or more orthopedic deformities. The most common signs and symptoms reported by the patient or the family are changes in gait, weakness, deformity, and pain.[37, 41, 42] Gait change and weakness occur with equal frequency among those whose sensory and motor function extend to the lumbar or to the sacral level. Increasing spasticity is often found in association with gait change. The most common orthopedic deformities are varus, valgus, and cavus changes of the foot (Fig. 5–13). Recurrent hip dislocation and rotational changes of the lower extremities occur in 27 percent of the children and are associated predominantly with lumbar sensory and motor levels. A unique observation in patients with tethered spinal cord is the development of progressive change in posture consisting of flexion of the knees, increased lumbar lordosis, and a wide-based gait. Physical examination demonstrated such postural change in 30 percent of the patients, predominantly those with sacral sensory and motor levels.

It is now evident that tethering of the spinal cord plays a role in the etiology of scoliosis.[46] In our series, 60 percent of scoliotic patients with tethered cords had improvement, or arrest of the progression, of scoliosis following surgical release of their spinal cords. To date, most of these patients have not required spinal fusion to stabilize their curvatures. A few of the patients had spinal fusions at the time of the spinal cord release, because of the magnitude of the pre-existing curvature. None of these patients suffered any neurologic complication from the spinal fusion. In the remaining patients, the scoliosis progressed despite release of the tethered spinal cords. It may be that in these patients, operative treatment was performed too late to alter favorably the course of their scoliosis. Thus, releasing the tethered spinal cord early in the progression of scoliosis may arrest the process and may lead to reversal of the abnormal curvature. Prolonged follow-up is necessary to determine whether early release of the tethered cord is adequate treatment for scoliosis of neuromuscular origin. Scoliosis developing according to concurrent hemivertebrae, bony bars, and other segmentation anomalies is not expected to respond to a single untethering of the spinal cord.

Sensory Loss and Pain

The loss of sensation in the lower body is often vague and subjective. The loss as determined by the examiner is usually asymmetric and may not follow dermatomes. The authors have seen patients with "stocking" sensory loss in the legs. The loss of sensation may go unnoticed until revealed by an ulcer or callus on the foot. Loss of sensation over the perineum is a common early finding.

Pain is a frequent manifestation of a tethered spinal cord, and, like sensory loss, is often vague and difficult for the child to localize. The pain often radiates into the anterior thigh or even up the spine. Pain in the perineum and genitals is a common symptom. Flexion of the neck on the trunk can often reproduce the pain, and lordotic posture and bent knees can prevent the pain. Fortunately, of all the problems presented by tethered spinal cord, pain is the most likely to be relieved by untethering of the cord.

Urologic Dysfunction

Urologic abnormalities are commonly missed in the infant and the young child. Problems are usually discovered during the evaluation of the child for other signs of tethered cord. Ultrasonography or magnetic resonance imaging (MRI) may demonstrate a large bladder, and a cystometrogram will reveal abnormal function.

Failure of the child to become trained, enuresis, bladder infections, and stress incontinence become obvious as the child approaches school age. We continue to be amazed to see children followed for years for these problems, while cutaneous markers of occult dysraphism on the child's back are ignored.

SPECIFIC LESIONS

Myelomeningocele[34, 35]

These lesions are discussed in Chapter 4.

Lipomyelocele and Lipomyelomeningocele

Spinal lipomas are perhaps the most common type of occult spinal dysraphism and account for some 35 percent of skin-covered lumbosacral masses. There are several forms of spinal lipoma.

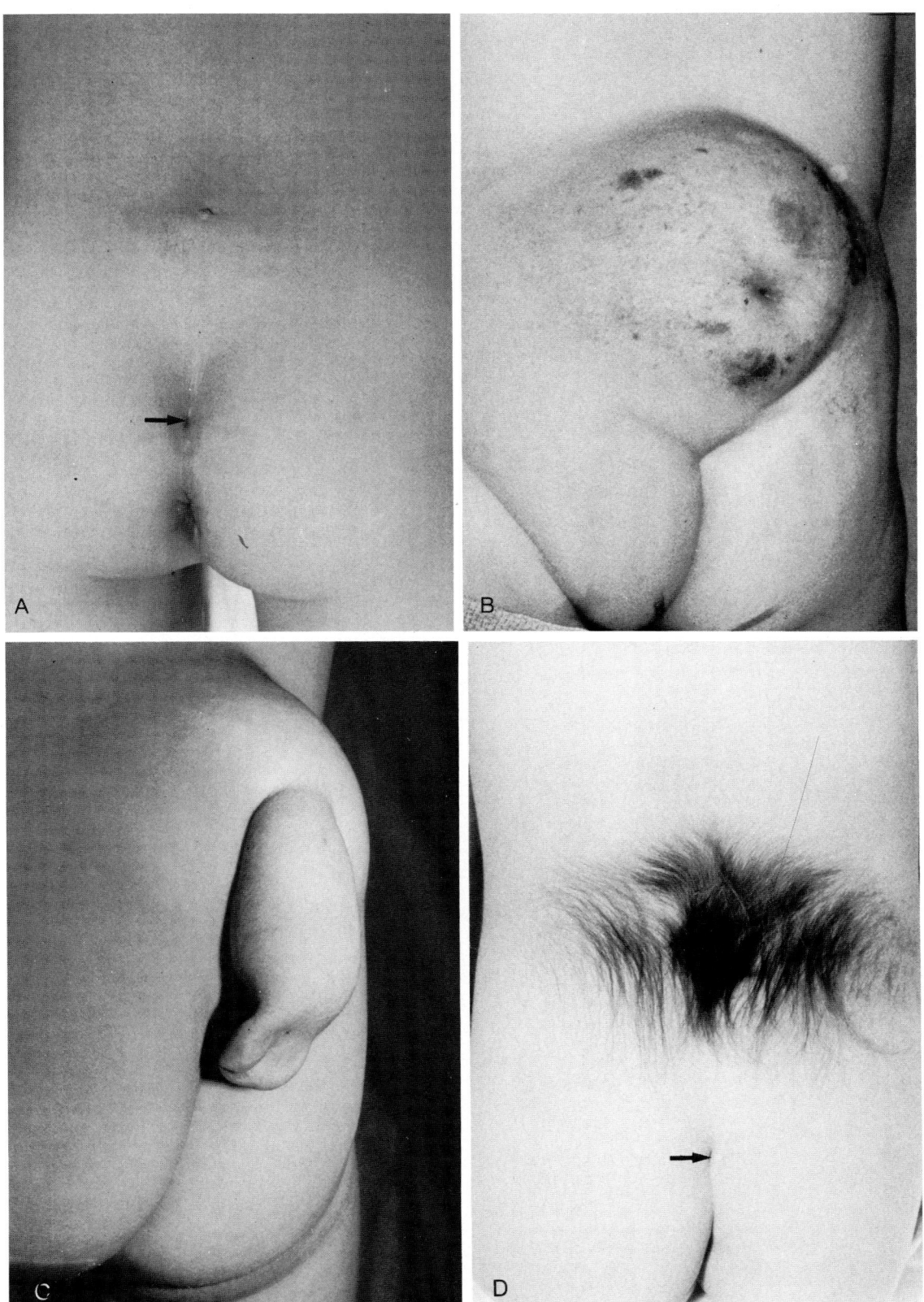

Figure 5–12. The lumbosacral area of the backs of four children. A, A dermal sinus with a faint hemangioma; B, lipomyelomeningocele with a dermal sinus, freckles, and nevi; C, lipomyelomeningocele with an appendage; and (D) a hairy patch over diastematomyelia. Note that A and D also have a "benign" pit, or dimple, over the coccyx (arrows).

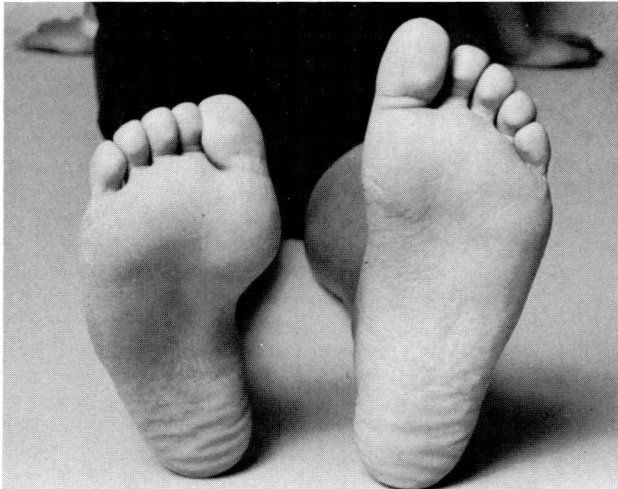

Figure 5–13. A child with occult spinal disease with a typical short foot with talipes cavus.

Spinal Lipomas with Intact Dura (Subpial Lipomas)

Intradural lipomas are a small group of juxtamedullary tumors that form subpial masses of fat, usually in relation to the cervical and thoracic spinal cords (Fig. 5–14).[2] They constitute approximately 4 percent of the lipomas in our series.[65] In this group, the spinal canal is usually nearly normal, with narrow spina bifida or segmentation anomalies. The canal itself may be expanded by the mass. The dura is thinned but intact and is displaced peripherally by the combined mass of cord and lipoma. The lipoma typically lies dorsal or dorsolateral within the cord and can cause high-grade stenosis or block. Often, the upper or lower pole of the lipoma protrudes outward from the surface of the cord.

Spinal Lipomas with Deficient Dura (Lipomyelocele and Lipomyelomeningocele)

The most common forms of spinal lipoma (84 percent) are associated with definite defects in the dura, through which the lipoma may extend from the spinal cord to the subcutaneous tissue (Fig. 5–15).[22, 49, 62, 83, 95, 97] In patients so affected, the subcutaneous component of the lipoma typically forms a large skin-covered, lumbosacral mass that lies cephalad to the intergluteal crease. The subjacent spinal canal usually shows a wide spina bifida. Sacral anomalies and segmentation anomalies[56] are present in nearly 50 percent of patients.

The spinal cord beneath the lipoma is cleft dorsally (partial dorsal myeloschisis) and very closely resembles the neural plate of a myelomeningocele. The dura that normally forms a complete tube around the spinal cord is deficient in the dorsal midline, deep to the lipoma.[16, 65] The medial edges of the dural defect are not just free margins of a tube. Rather, the dura appears to attach to the edges of the neural plate, just dorsal to the entry

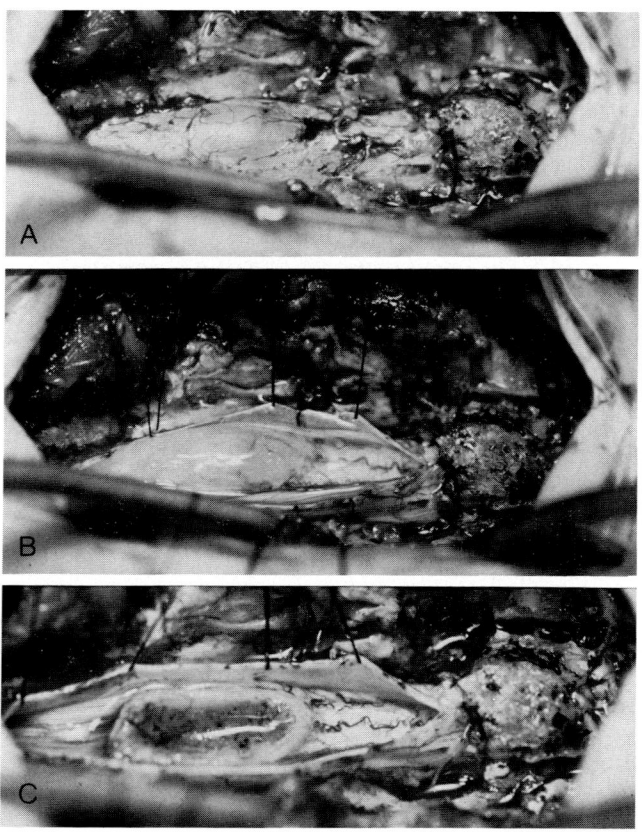

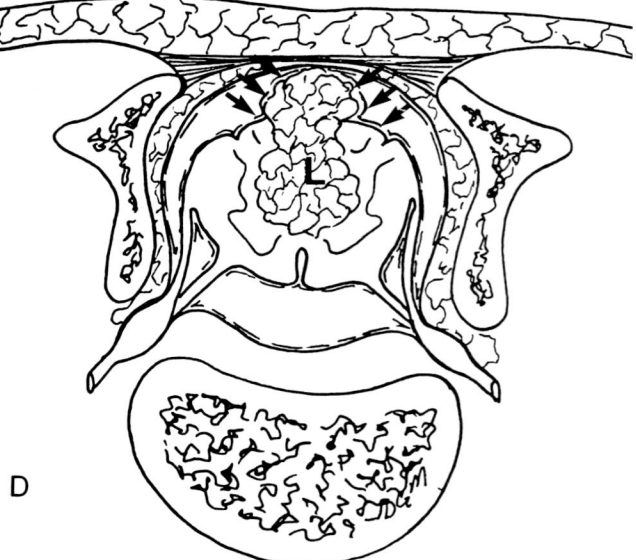

Figure 5–14. An intradural lipoma at the conus medullaris. *A,* Intact dura mater. *B,* After the dura was opened. *C,* After laser vaporization of most of the subpial lipoma. *D,* Schematic drawing shows the relationship of the lipoma (L) to the dorsal spinal cord and the pial covering (arrows).

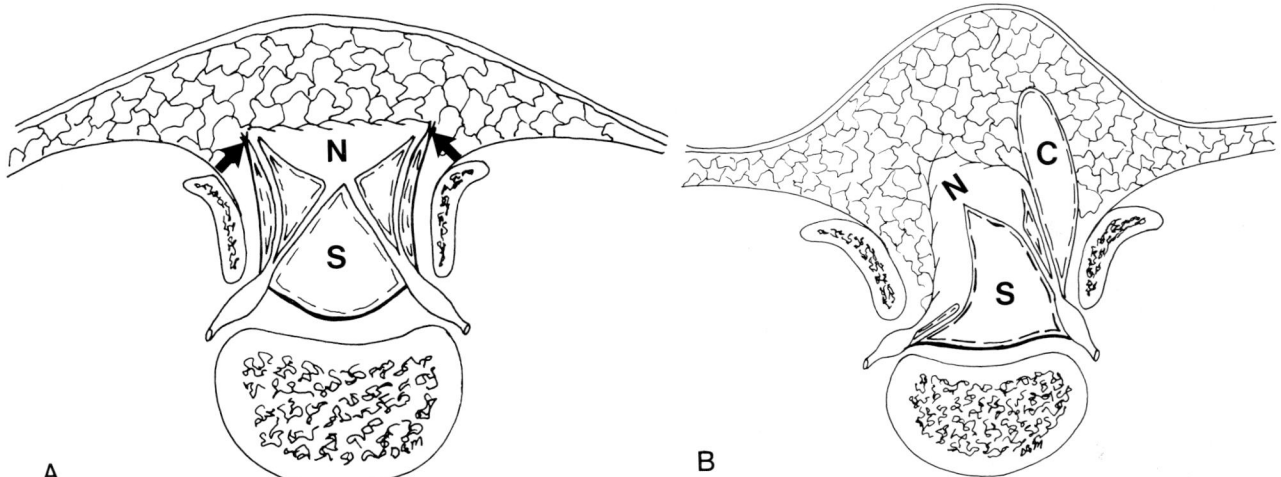

Figure 5–15. Schematic drawings of a lipomyelomeningocele, showing the neural placode (N), the junction of the dorsal root entry zone, neural tissue, and the lipoma (A, arrows). A shows the subarachnoid space (S) in a more normal position. B shows the subarachnoid space (S) and a meningocele (C) herniating into the lipoma.

zones of the dorsal roots. Thus, the raw, cleft surface of the neural plate lies medial to and outside the dural sac, (i.e., it is extradural). The arrangement of pia-arachnoid and of nerve roots in such lipomas is identical with that seen in myeloceles and myelomeningoceles. The lipoma inserts into the exposed dorsal "extradural" face of the neural plate and extends from there to the subcutaneous space (Fig. 5–15). Since the dorsal extradural surface of the neural plate is directly continuous with the central canal of the normal cord above, lipoma may also extend in continuity from the plate into the central canal of the cord, as in Figure 5–14. While the portion of lipoma within the central canal is certainly intramedullary, it is also extradural in the sense that it is not surrounded on all sides by dura. Rather, it is directly continuous with the extradural portion of the lipoma. This intramedullary component may increase in size as the child gains weight and may function as an expanding intramedullary tumor.[8, 14, 65] This may require a dorsal myelotomy and partial resection of the lipoma to preserve function in the surrounding neural tissue.

The junction of the lipoma and the spinal cord may be entirely within the spinal canal, may lie entirely outside the spinal canal, or may bridge the spina bifida to lie both inside and outside the spinal canal. When the spinal cord remains wholly within the spinal canal, the lipoma extends into the canal before entering into the cleft in the cord (Fig. 5–16). In these cases, the anatomic arrangement of the neural tissue is very similar to that of the myelocele, except that the raw dorsal surface of the neural plate is covered by fat, and the entire complex lies within the bifid spinal canal underneath an intact surface of skin. These lesions may be designated lipomyelocele.

When the cord herniates out of the canal, so the junction of fat and cord is at least partially outside the canal, the anatomic arrangement of the neural tissue is very similar to that of the myelomeningocele, except that the dorsal surface of the neural tissue is covered by fat and the entire complex is buried deep to intact skin. These lesions may be designated lipomyelomeningocele. In these cases,

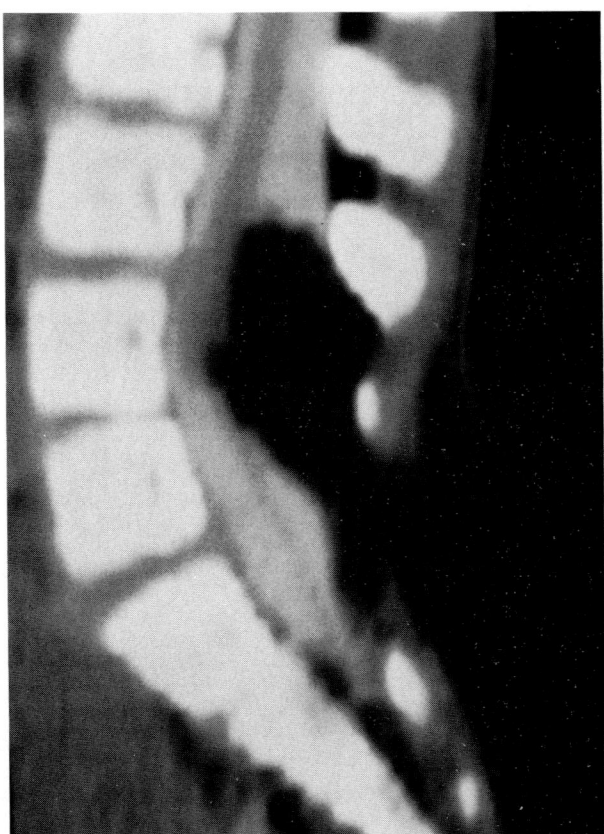

Figure 5–16. A re-formatted CT image of a water-soluble contrast-enhanced myelogram of lipomyelomeningocele. The lipoma extends into the canal under the first intact lamina, inserting into and pushing the spinal cord anteriorly.

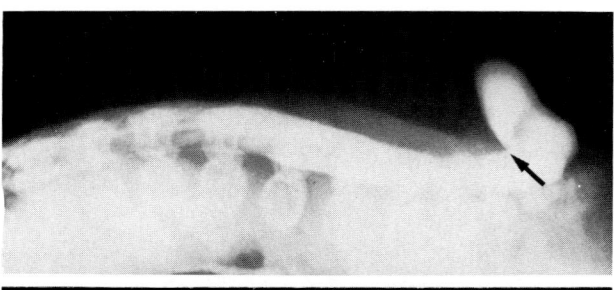
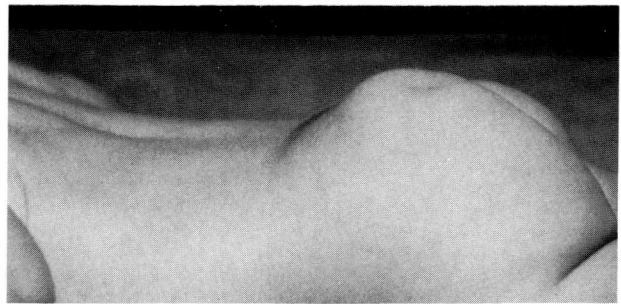

Figure 5–17. A myelogram of a child (below) with a lipomyelomeningocele shows the spinal cord angulating (arrow) under the last intact lamina, or fibrous band, and passing through the meningocele to the lipoma.

gross expansion of the subarachnoid space pushes the cord and the liponeural junction out of the canal into the sac (Fig. 5–17). The dura remains attached to the edges of the neural plate, so the lipoma itself remains extradural.

Typically, the neural plate rotates as it herniates out of the canal, so the dorsal surface faces posterolateral or lateral rather than directly posterior. The lipoma then lies dorsolateral or lateral to the neural tissue, while the sac bulges to the contralateral side (Fig. 5–15B). The left and right pairs of nerve roots become markedly different in length. The roots arising from the superficial side of the rotated spinal cord are long. The roots arising from the deep side of the rotated spinal cord are far shorter. These deep roots may be so short that they act to tether the spinal cord inferiorly.

The intradural lipomas and the lipomas with dural deficiency constitute 20 to 50 percent of all cases of occult spinal dysraphism. In these patients, computed tomography (CT) (Fig. 5–16) reveals the large, lucent subcutaneous mass of fat, the posterior spina bifida, insertion of the lucent lipoma into the dorsal surface of the cleft spinal cord, and any associated meningocele. The liponeural junction may be relatively smooth or stellate. A variably thick band of increased density is often observed at the liponeural junction and appears to represent fibrous tissue at the interface between neural tissue and fat. MRI necessarily demonstrates the same anatomic features (Fig. 5–18). The fat has high signal intensity on T1-weighted images and stands out distinctly from the low-signal CSF and intermediate signal neural tissue. In T2-weighted images, the signal intensity of fat decreases, while that of CSF increases, so the CSF may become as bright as or brighter than the fat. Currently, CT and MRI both display spinal lipomas satisfactorily.[69, 70, 82] MRI displays the sagittal plane more clearly than CT, whereas CT displays the axial plane more clearly than MRI.

Ultrasonography has become extremely useful in determining the structure of many of these congenital spinal lesions in infants. Because the immature bone allows ultrasound to penetrate and give excellent structural detail, tethering and the extent of the lesion can be determined (Fig. 5–19). The authors will now make a diagnosis and operate upon an infant solely on the basis of an ultrasound study. This is true not only for lipomas but also for tight filum terminale, dermal sinuses, and myelocystocele.

Dorsal Dermal Sinus

Clinically, dorsal dermal sinuses most frequently appear as pinpoint holes in the skin of the midline (Fig. 5–12).[1, 5, 17, 47] They occasionally lie just off the

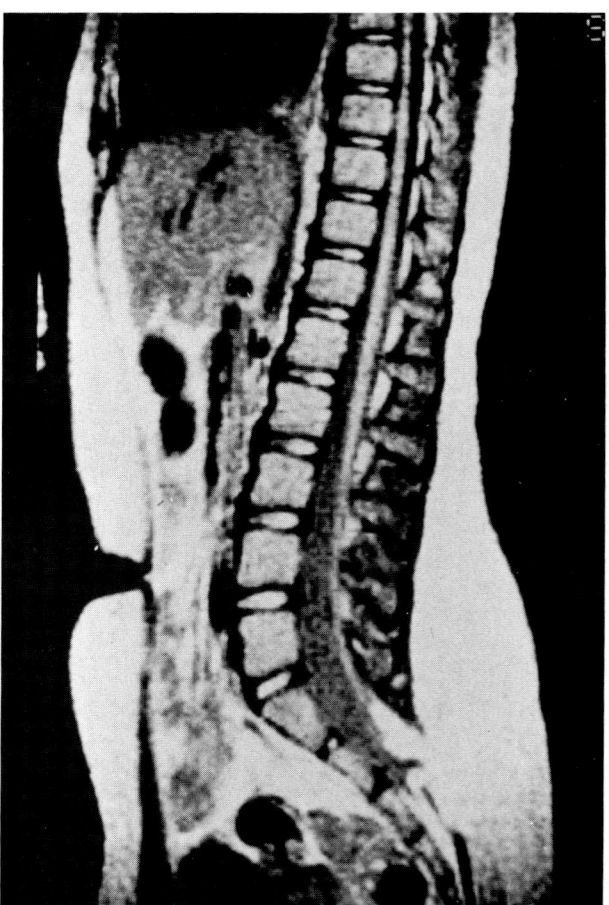

Figure 5–18. Magnetic resonance (MR) image of a lipoma passing into the spinal canal and attaching to the dorsal surface of the low-lying spinal cord. Note that, in this case, the spinal cord is tethered posteriorly, which is more typical.

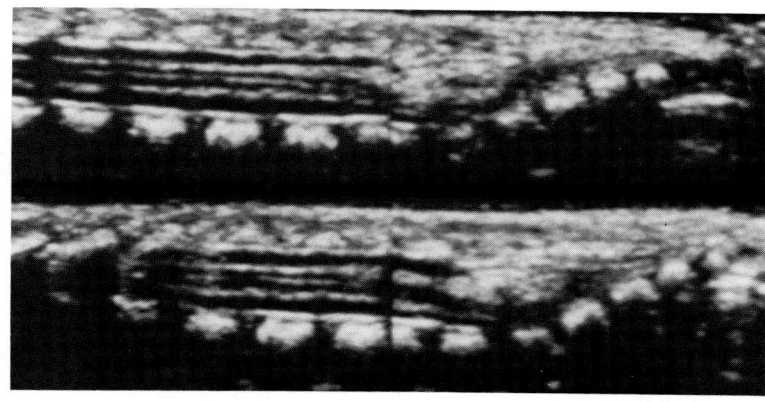

Figure 5–19. An ultrasound scan of an infant shows the low-lying spinal cord with its central echo fusing and passing under the echoic mass of the lipoma and the dermoid tumor.

midline and rarely are double. Small hemangiomas commonly surround the ostium. A tuft of short, sparse, wiry hairs may protrude from the ostium. In Wright's[99] collected series of 127 dermal sinuses, 57 percent were lumbosacral, and 24 percent were occipital. Sinuses at other sites are uncommon. Dermal sinuses frequently provide a path through which infection may ascend retrograde to the spinal canal. Such infection may lead to arachnoiditis, meningitis, and abscess.[15, 23, 54, 67, 77, 96]

Typically, the dermal sinus tract extends inward from the skin surface for a variable depth. It passes deeply through the subcutaneous layer and through the median raphe (or between bifid laminae) toward the dura. It may end at or before the dura. In most cases, the tract extends into the spinal canal deep to the dura (Fig. 5–20). A small midline sleeve of dura and arachnoid frequently marks the point at which the tract penetrates the dura. The tract may end in the subarachnoid space as an open tube through which CSF discharges. The dermal sinus may also end in a fibrous nodule situated among the roots of cauda equina.[52, 84] In up to 60 percent of cases, the tract incorporates or ends in a dermoid or epidermoid tumor (Fig. 5–21).[10, 31, 99] Approximately 30 percent of all spinal dermoid and epidermoid tumors are associated with dermal sinuses. The dermal sinus may cause tethering by a thick band of tissue attached to the conus medullaris or as a result of the scarring produced by chemical or bacterial meningitis.

On CT, dermal sinuses appear as dense linear tracts that extend inward from a skin dimple (the ostium) through the lucent subcutaneous tissue toward the dura. Occasionally, a thin lucent lumen can be observed within the tract. The intra-arachnoid course of the sinus is best displayed by water-soluble contrast-enhanced CT myelography[87] as a linear or tubular filling defect that ascends within the CSF toward the conus medullaris. Lucent masses along this course typically represent one or a string of dermoid or epidermoid tumors. MRI displays the extraspinal course of the dermal sinus as a low-signal tract that traverses the high-signal subcutaneous fat, toward the dura. MRI does not display readily the intradural course of the tract itself. The dermoid or epidermoid tumors have highly variable signal intensity on MRI and must be sought diligently with different pulse sequences to ascertain or rule out their presence.

Diastematomyelia

Clinically, most cases of diastematomyelia occur in females, 70 percent overall, up to 94 percent in

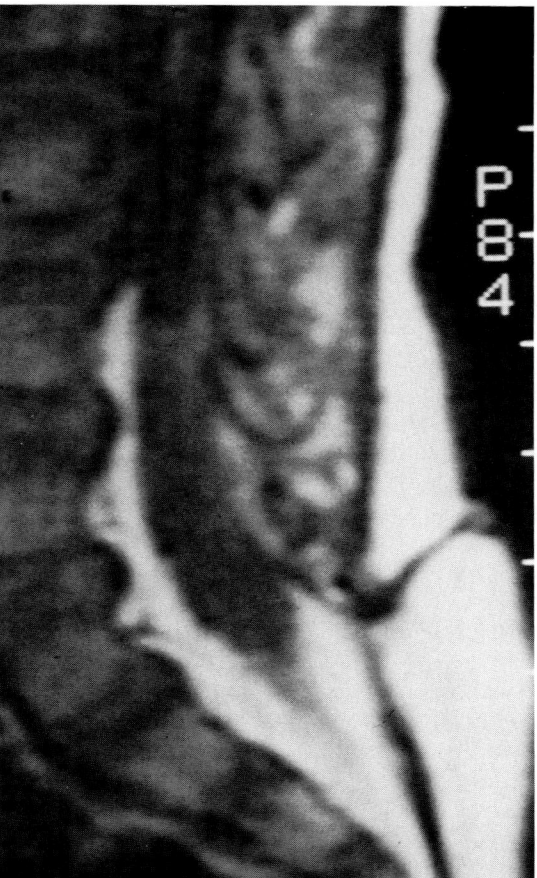

Figure 5–20. MR image showing a dermal sinus passing slightly caudally and then passing under a lamina before turning rostrally to attach to the conus medullaris.

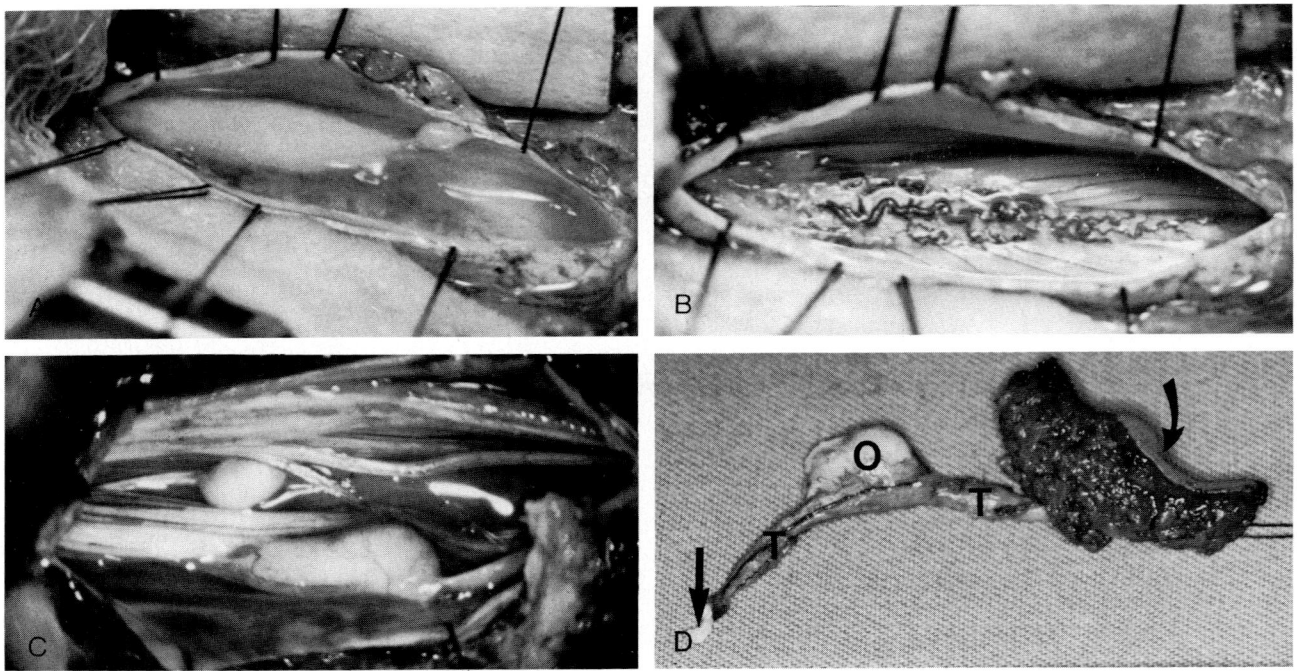

Figure 5–21. Operative photographs show a dermoid attached to the spinal cord (A), the same area after laser resection (B), and a patient with multiple dermoids (C). A specimen (D) shows skin dimple (curved arrow), tract (T), dermoid (O), and point of attachment to the conus medullaris (arrow).

some series.[19, 32, 55] Cutaneous nevi overlie the midline of the back, in some of the cases, usually near the site of the diastematomyelia. The most nearly characteristic cutaneous stigma is a large patch of long silky hairs (Fig. 5–12).[78]

The spinal canal is nearly always markedly abnormal in patients with diastematomyelia.[4, 40] Segmentation anomalies such as hemivertebrae, butterfly vertebrae, block vertebrae, and narrowed intervertebral disk spaces are present in approximately 85 percent of the cases. The sagittal dimension of the vertebral bodies is frequently decreased, and the interpediculate distance is characteristically widened at the level of the diastematomyelia. The laminae are abnormal in nearly all cases, with spina bifida, thickening of laminae, and fusion between laminae of adjacent segments. The combination of spina bifida and intersegmental fusion of laminae is present in 60 percent of cases and is highly suggestive of the diagnosis.

Scoliosis and kyphosis are present in 50 to 60 percent of cases of diastematomyelia and are directly related to the segmentation anomalies.[46] Whereas the kyphoscoliosis of myelomeningocele is typically neurogenic, the kyphoscoliosis of diastematomyelia is typically mechanical. The extent to which tethering of the spinal cord contributes to the scoliosis is unclear, and nearly 50 percent of patients with diastematomyelia also have hydromyelia. Such hydromyelia may contribute to the progression of the scoliosis.

In diastematomyelia, the conus medullaris is usually low in position. The two hemicords are each narrower than normal and nearly always (91 percent) reunite distally to re-form a single spinal cord below the cleft. In 30 percent of cases, the two hemicords are grossly asymmetric in size. When the hemicords are asymmetric, the cord above and below the cleft is usually asymmetrically smaller on the side of the smaller hemicord, and the smaller hemicord often lies ventral to the larger hemicord. Usually, each hemicord gives rise to the ipsilateral dorsal and ventral nerve roots. When there is asymmetry, one "hemicord" may give rise to three of the four roots, and the other only one root. Accessory nerve roots may also be present. The filum terminale is usually thickened, may itself tether the cord, and may itself require resection for release of tethering.[43, 66]

The meninges that surround the cord may also be cleft. The exact relationship of the arachnoid and dura to the hemicords is highly significant and defines two distinct forms of diastematomyelia that require two different approaches to treatment. In the majority of all cases of diastematomyelia (50 to 60 percent), the two hemicords are enveloped together in a single arachnoidal-dural sheath. In these cases, there is never a bone spur. No surgical intervention is required unless a thick filum terminale or adhesion is seen to tether the cord.

In the other 40 to 50 percent of cases, the meninges are also cleft, focally, so each hemicord is contained in its own arachnoidal-dural sheath (Fig. 5–22). The single cord above the cleft is contained in a single meningeal sheath that divides to surround each hemicord and that then reunites to a

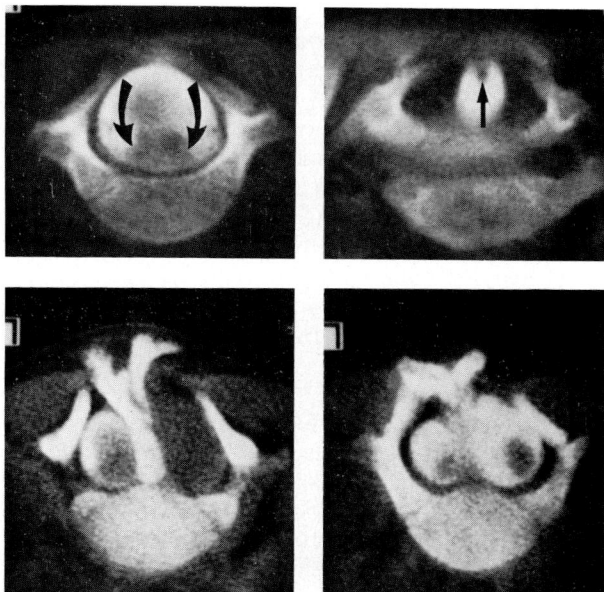

Figure 5–22. A water-soluble contrast-enhanced CT myelogram shows the bony spur dividing the canal and attached to the abnormal lamina. Each hemicord has its own canal. Note that distally the hemicords unite (curved arrows) and end in thickened filum terminale (arrow). Dorsally between the curved arrows is a Wilms's tumor, a rare additional lesion in congenital anomalies of the spine.

single sheath when the hemicords reunite to one cord below the cleft. In this group with cleft meninges, the cleft in the cord is always longer than the cleft in the meninges, often far longer, especially above the cleft. The medial walls of the two dural tubes form a double layered dural partition between the two hemicords. This is the so-called fibrous partition. The space between the two dural tubes (i.e., between the two medial layers of dura) may be called the interdural cleft.

In nearly all cases with cleft meninges, an osteo-cartilaginous spur forms in the interdural cleft between the two dural tubes.[72] Thus, this spur lies medial and external to the two dural tubes. The spur forms in cartilage from one or several ossification centers that mature with age, so that, depending on age, one may see no bone; several small fragments of bone separated by lucent cartilage; a nearly complete bone spur still separated from the vertebrae or laminae by lucent cartilage; or a complete septum of bone completely crossing the spinal canal. The lucent cartilage signifies the site at which the bone spur will fracture away during surgery. The spur itself may lie along the midline, dividing the canal into two symmetric hemicanals, or it may lie obliquely and asymmetrically. In 6 percent of cases, the spur projects posteriorly between bifid laminae. In approximately 5 to 6 percent of cases, double (rarely multiple) spurs are present near to or distant from each other.

In those patients with cleft meninges, the fibrous partition, bone spur, or both may tether the cord inferiorly. The bone spur typically lies at the caudal end of the cleft in the cord and appears to press against the medial surfaces of the two hemicords and the top of the reunited cord. In these patients, surgery is often required to resect the bone spur and the fibrous partition in order to release the spinal cord.

A note of caution: the epidural venous plexus (Fig. 5–23) surrounding the bony spur and deep to the two hemicords is usually substantial and should be controlled prior to removal of the spur, if possible. Once this space is decompressed and the spinal cord moves cephalad, bleeding can be difficult to control.

On CT, diastematomyelia with cleft meninges and bone spur is usually detected by virtue of the anomalous vertebrae and the spur itself. The two hemicords may be resolved separately.[93] The thickened filum terminale may be fully detectable owing to its lucency. However, in nearly all cases, the derangements in anatomy are better shown by water-soluble contrast-enhanced CT myelography.[88] That technique readily produces images of the individual hemicords and the nerve roots that arise from them and any occult pathologic conditions.

MRI readily displays the two hemicords, provided axial or coronal sections are obtained through

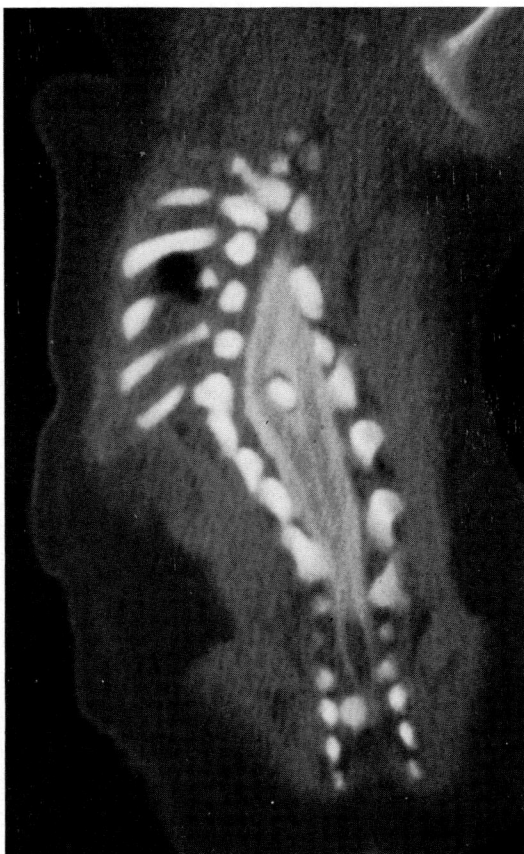

Figure 5–23. A direct coronal CT myelogram of a child with diastematomyelia, showing clearly the hemicords, bony spur, and distal fusion of the hemicords. Note also that the distal spinal cord ends in a lipoma. The dark ring around the bony spur is the epidural space, which usually contains a large venous plexus.

the cleft. Purely sagittal sections may not show each hemicord separately, leading to the misdiagnosis of a normal study. MRI displays concurrent hydromyelia more easily than does CT. When the diastematomyelia is accompanied by severe scoliosis, CT and MRI both may show the pathology only poorly. In such cases, standard myelography followed by CT appears to be most helpful (Fig. 5–23).

Tight Filum Terminale Syndrome

Patients with the tight filum terminale syndrome present with the clinical signs of tethered cord discussed earlier.[28, 53, 102] In this condition, by definition, (a) the spinal cord must be tethered, (b) the filum terminale must measure greater than 2 mm in diameter, and (c) no other cause for tethering can be present. The tip of the conus medullaris lies below L2 in 86 percent of these cases.[25] In 10 to 15 percent of cases, the spinal cord continues caudally, to attach to the distal thecal sac, without distinct termination. Filar fibrolipomas are present in 29 percent of cases (Fig. 5–24). Kyphoscoliosis is present in 14 percent of these cases and improves following section of the filum terminale, in one third of cases. In most cases, there is a midline defect in the arches of the lumbosacral spine, usually at L4, L5, S1, or all three. This suggests that normal spine radiographs almost exclude this diagnosis.

Both CT and MRI display the low-lying spinal cord, thick filum terminale, and the absence of other causes of spinal cord tethering. Filar lipomas appear as lucent or high-signal deposits within the filum terminale. The spina bifida appears as a focal defect in the union of the laminae. These findings are best demonstrated in the axial plane and may be missed if only sagittal MRI studies are performed.

The authors have found a high incidence of low-lying cords in newborns with anal stenosis or imperforate anus. The diagnosis can be made with ultrasound shortly after birth (Fig. 5–24).

Lipoma of the Filum Terminale

Persistence of caudal cells that differentiate toward fat could produce filar lipomas. Indeed, such lipomas are observed incidentally in 4 to 6 percent of normal adults and may be considered a normal variation, if they are not associated with spinal cord tethering or neurologic dysfunction.

Filar lipomas may involve the intradural portion of the filum terminale, the extradural portion, or both. Intradural lipomas tend to be fusiform in shape and taper down toward a point where the filum terminale pierces dura mater. They appear lucent on CT, have high-signal intensity on MRI, and are easily observed on good axial non–contrast-enhanced CT and MRI sections. Extradural lipomas of the filum terminale are far more diffuse, tend to merge with adjacent extradural fat, and are far more difficult to appreciate, even on good imaging studies.

Filar lipomas may be associated with lipomas of the distal half of conus medullaris—the portion of conus medullaris that is also formed by canalization and retrogressive differentiation. In some instances,

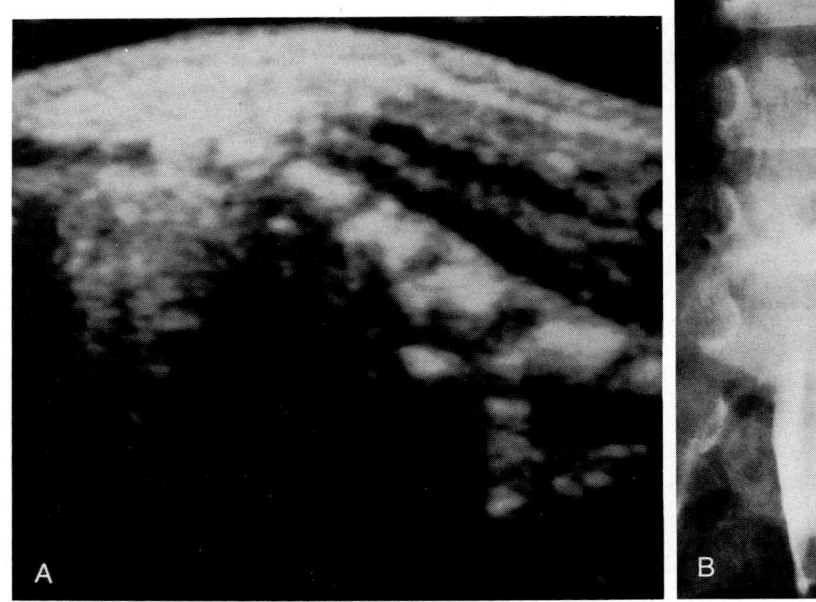
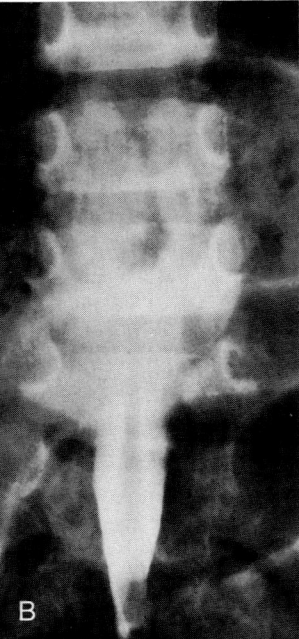
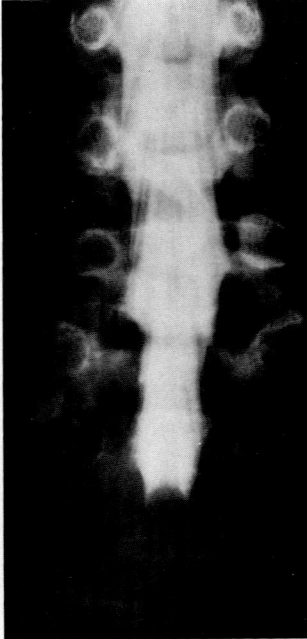

Figure 5–24. *A*, Ultrasound scan of the back of an infant who has an imperforate anus, showing a low-lying spinal cord with a thickened filum terminale. *B*, Myelograms of an older child show the thickened filum terminale ending in a lipoma.

accessory fila are present and may also exhibit lipomas.

Syndrome of Embryonic Deformation and Caudal Suppression

Children with the syndrome of caudal suppression (regression)[79] exhibit anomalies of the hind end of the trunk, including partial agenesis of the thoracolumbosacral spine, imperforate anus, malformed genitalia, bilateral renal dysplasia or aplasia, pulmonary hypoplasia, and (in the most severe deformities) extreme external rotation and fusion of the lower extremities (sirenomelia). There is a definite but incomplete association with diabetes mellitus: One percent of offspring of diabetic mothers have a form of this syndrome; 16 percent of patients with this syndrome have diabetic mothers (rarely diabetic fathers).[75, 76]

Isolated agenesis of the coccyx is an incidental finding in some patients. In patients with more extensive agenesis of the distal spine, the lowest vertebra present is T11 or T12 in one third of the patients, L1 to L4 in 40 percent of the patients, and L5 or below in 27 percent of the patients. The distal agenesis may be bilaterally symmetric or unilateral. Unilateral agenesis leads to marked pelvic tilt and scoliosis.

In these patients, the spinal canal narrows for a variable length above the last vertebra. Bone spurs and thickened dura may narrow the canal even further. Segmentation anomalies have been reported in 22 percent of these patients, and spina bifida in up to 33 percent of patients. The thecal sac tapers with the canal. The distalmost pair of root sleeves frequently extend downward vertically, side by side, simulating focal diastematomyelia. The distal cord may end rather abruptly and may be slightly bulbous at its end.

Patients with lumbosacral or sacral agenesis may have concurrent conditions such as tethered cords,[74] anterior sacral meningoceles, spinal lipomas and dermoid tumors, genitourinary anomalies, and anorectal stenoses. These concurrent malformations may result from constraints on the embryo at the time when these structures begin to form. Imaging studies readily display these bony anomalies and any associated tethered cord, lipoma, dermoid tumor, or anterior sacral meningocele.

Neurenteric Cysts

Neurenteric cysts are enteric-lined cysts that present within the spinal canal and exhibit a definite connection with the spinal cord, vertebrae, or both. They (1) may communicate around a hemivertebra or through a butterfly vertebra with an extraspinal component of cyst in the mesentery or mediastinum, (2) they may attach by a fibrous stalk to the vertebra, mesentery, or gut, or (3) they may do both.

The vertebral column usually exhibits a wide spinal canal with a widened interpediculate distance.[71] Spina bifida and segmentation anomalies of the bodies are common, but not invariable. In older patients, the vertebrae may be normal, aside from pressure erosion. Most cysts lie at the cervicothoracic junction or come into contact with the conus medullaris. The cyst usually lies ventral or ventrolateral to the spinal cord and may be deeply invaginated into the cord. CT and MRI display the cyst, the displaced cord, any bone abnormalities and any associated mediastinal or mesenteric lesion. Myelography typically displays a high-grade stenosis or a complete block of the flow of the contrast agent.

Anterior Meningocele

Although not a direct cause of tethering of the spinal cord, this lesion occasionally is associated with spinal lipomas, dermoid tumors, and thickened filum terminale. Familial cases have been reported.

Nearly all the children in our series have been girls with a history of chronic constipation. Many of these children have been followed for years and have had multiple gastrointestinal studies. Review of previous x-rays usually reveals the characteristic scimitar sacrum (Fig. 5–25). Myelography, CT, or MRI shows the extent of the meningocele and associated lesions.

SURGICAL MANAGEMENT

Myelomeningocele

These lesions are discussed in Chapter 4.

Lipomyelomeningocele and Lipomyelocele

Large series now document that spinal cord lipomas can be untethered successfully[16, 38] and that the intramedullary portion of the lipoma can be resected successfully, with nearly zero morbidity and no mortality.[60, 65] Further, the series prove that such operations lead to recovery of neurologic and urologic function in a significant number of patients with pre-existing deficits. In our study, for example, 40 percent of those with motor deficits and 12 percent of those with incontinence recovered normal function after effective operation.

Surgery is carried out with the child prone. Scalpels are used to incise the skin and the dura mater. All other dissection and all resection of lipoma are performed with a hand-held CO_2 laser (Sharplan No. 7033; Sharplan Industries, Tel Aviv, Israel) used at 10 watts, continuous mode, with beam focusing

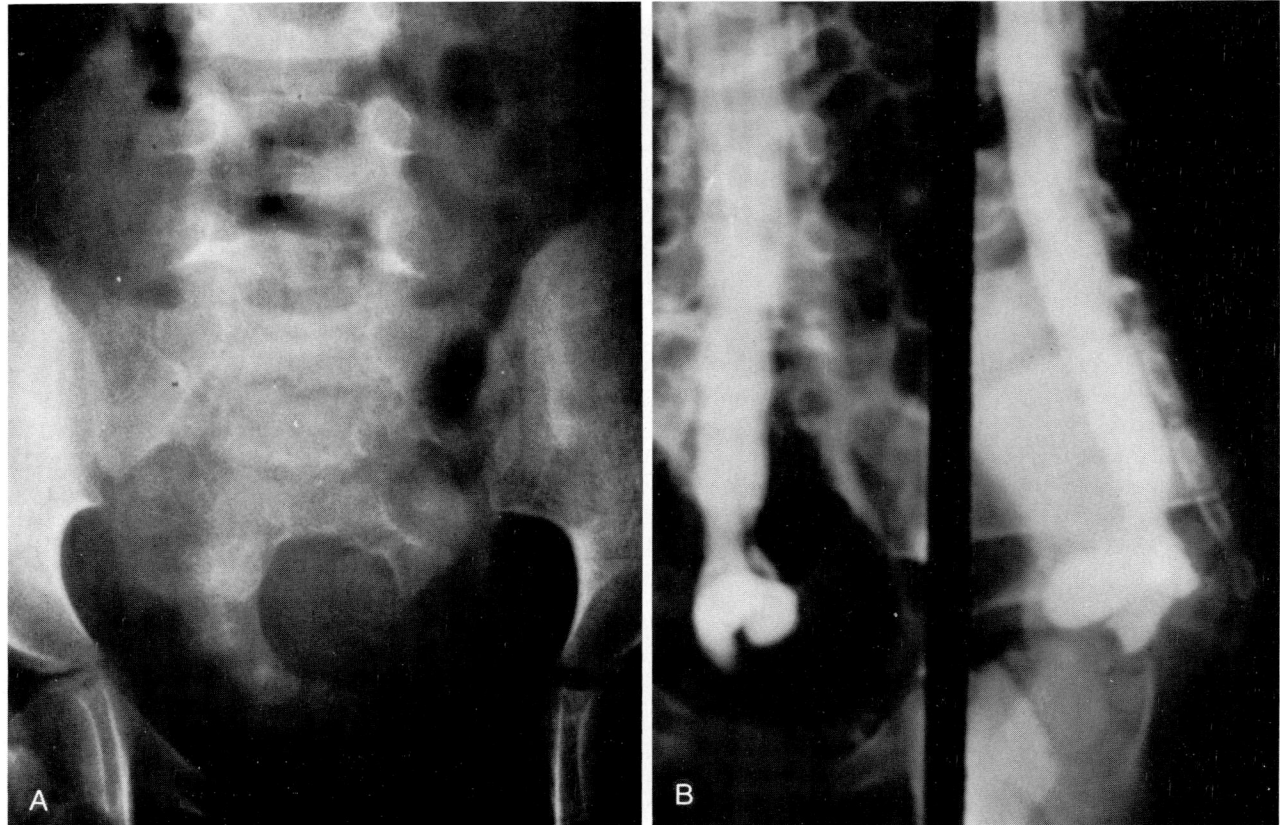

Figure 5–25. *A,* Spine x-ray film shows the scimitar sacrum. *B,* Myelography shows the opening and the extent of the meningocele. Note the low-lying spinal cord. The defects in the meningocele are a lipoma and a dermoid tumor.

for cutting and beam defocusing for vaporization. No attempt is made to resect the lipoma in toto (Fig. 5–26). Rather, lipoma is vaporized progressively until an interface between lipoma and neural tissue can be identified. Certainly, this operation can be done without the laser, but the laser has real advantages in removing the lipoma. The neural tube is then re-formed, when possible (Fig. 5–27), and the arachnoidal and dural tubes are reconstituted. Artificial dura mater is used, if necessary, to ensure that a slack dura and a capacious subarachnoid space surround the spinal cord. Then, the wound is closed in layers. Patients are maintained horizontally in bed, to reduce the incidence and the degree of the common, transient accumulations of cerebrospinal fluid in the subcutaneous pocket left by the lipoma resection.

In all patients, untethering of the spinal cord is the goal. In a few patients, the lipoma is resected, and the spinal cord is freed from lipoma. However, congenitally short nerve roots on one side may still anchor the spinal cord to the root sleeves. Such unilaterally short roots are encountered in three circumstances: (a) in patients with unilateral, partial sacral agenesis (on the side of agenesis), (b) in patients with conjoint neural foramina, and (c) in patients in whom the lipoma has rotated the cord 90 degrees, so that the left and right dorsal roots

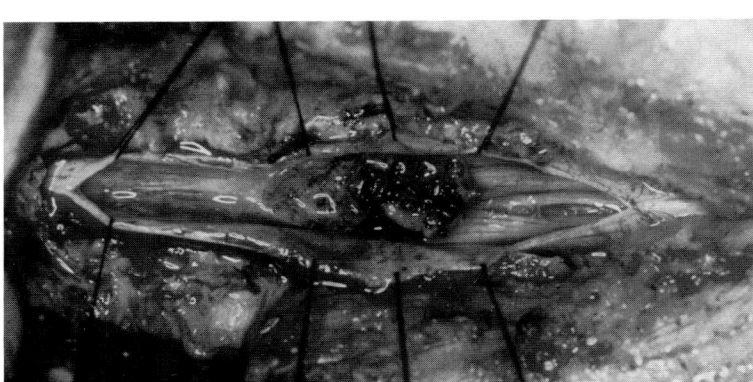

Figure 5–26. The conus medullaris after resection of a lipoma shows a layer of lipoma left over the neural tissue.

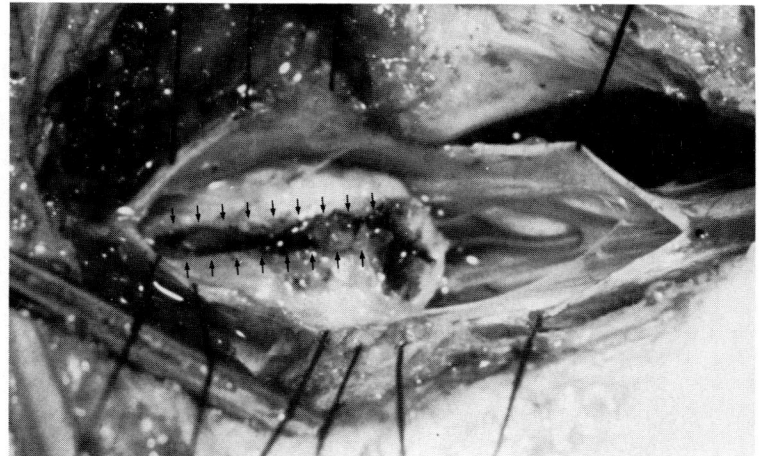

Figure 5–27. The conus medullaris after resection of the intramedullary component of a lipoma. The edges then can be approximated with pial-to-pial sutures (arrows).

lie anterior and posterior to each other in a (nearly) sagittal plane, rather than side by side in a coronal plane. In such patients, roots that are displaced and rotated anteriorly are invariably short, whereas those that come to lie posterior to the rotated spinal cord are unusually long. These circumstances can be anticipated in most patients by careful evaluation of plain roentgenograms, computed tomograms, and myelograms.

Terminal Myelocystocele

Figure 5–28 shows the typical myelocystocele in the intragluteal fold, and Figure 5–29 is an ultrasound scan demonstrating the two-compartment cyst. Surgery is performed with the patient in the prone position. The skin is incised in the midline, and the last intact neural arch above the spina bifida is exposed. If a fibrous band crosses the midline between the first (most cephalic) widely bifid laminae, this band is resected, and the next higher laminae are removed to expose the normal dura mater within the spinal canal and the posterior continuation of dura over the meningocele. The normal dura and arachnoid are opened, to visualize the spinal nerve roots. This incision is then carried over the meningocele, under direct vision, to expose the dilated spinal cord within the meningocele and to preserve the spinal nerve roots that arise from the cord and traverse the meningocele to re-enter the spinal canal.

At the caudal end of the meningocele, the pia-arachnoid is reflected from the "parietal" (arachnoid) wall of the meningocele onto the "visceral" (pial) wall of the spinal cord. The cord itself bulges caudal to the edge of the meningocele into the extra-arachnoid space, where it is covered by fat. Dissection through the fat exposes the terminal cyst. This is opened in the midline distal to the last spinal roots and is ependyma lined and directly continuous with the distal end of the central canal of the intra-arachnoid spinal cord (Fig. 5–30). The edges of the myelocystocele and the accompanying lipoma can be resected to the point just caudal to the arachnoid reflection, to preserve the third sacral

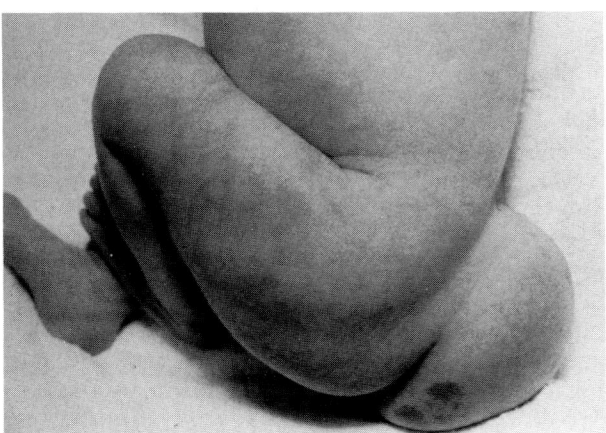

Figure 5–28. A typical skin-covered myelocystocele in the intragluteal fold of a child.

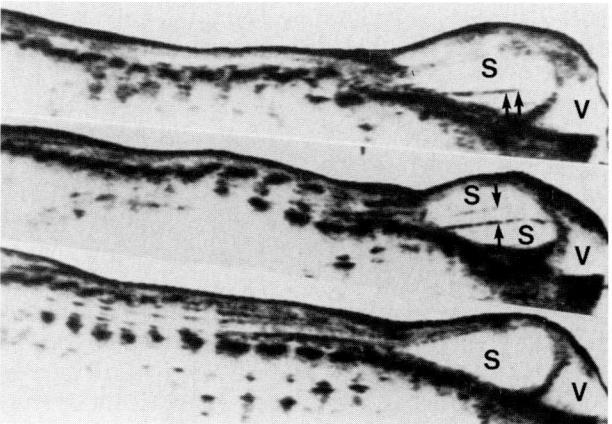

Figure 5–29. Ultrasound scans show the double cyst of the myelocystocele. Subarachnoid space (S) with the spinal cord (arrows) traversing it to join the distal dilated terminal ventricle (V).

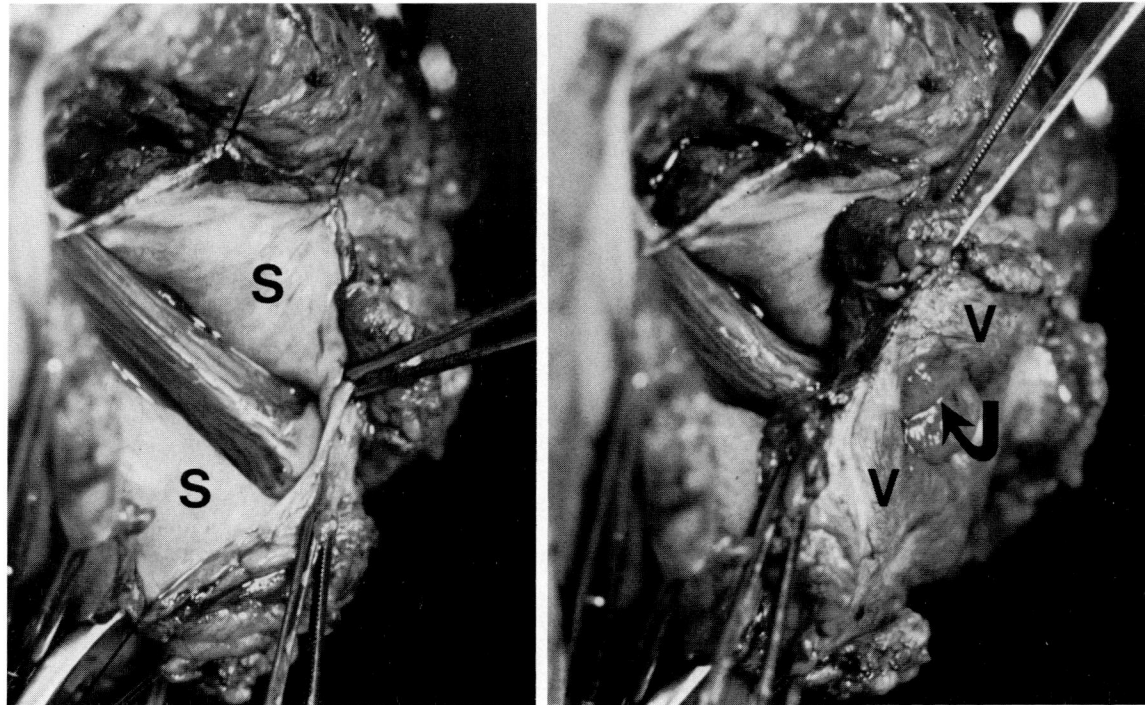

Figure 5–30. Operative pictures of a myelocystocele. *A* shows the proximal subarachnoid cyst (S). In *B*, the spinal cord traverses the cyst to attach to the distal cystic terminal ventricle (V), which contains the opening of the central canal (curved arrow).

nerve roots.[64] The edges of the cyst are then approximated to reconstitute a distal sac, and the abundant residual arachnoid and dura are used to reconstitute the meningeal tube and the spinal subarachnoid space. The midline incision is closed in layers.

SUMMARY

Armed with an understanding of the embryopathy and the consequent altered anatomy of the tethered spinal cord, the surgeon can plan the surgical procedure. Aided by ultrasonography, CT, and MRI, the position and the level of the lesion and its relation to functional tissue can be deduced. A basic surgical principle is essential in approaching the lesion: identify, and begin surgery at, the point where the anatomy is normal and work into the area of the lesion.

Prior to surgery, all patients should have a neurologic and a urologic evaluation. Preoperative muscle tests, electromyography, evoked potentials, and cystometrography add to the evaluation and make the determination of postoperative results more reliable.

The authors have found the CO_2 laser very useful for both dissection of the lesion and vaporization of tissues involved in the tethering process. Scalpels and sharp dissection are used only to incise the skin and the dura mater. Use of the CO_2 laser substantially reduces the time required for surgery and the intraoperative blood loss. This reduced blood loss is particularly important in infants because of their small blood volume. Use of the laser also reduces manipulation of tissue and, consequently, operative trauma.

Magnification, loupe or microscope, is an important adjunct to the laser. These recent improvements in operative technique and technology have allowed a more aggressive approach to these lesions.

The experience of watching patients who are not operated on deteriorate over time as well as the gratifying recovery often seen following surgery compels us to offer surgery to the asymptomatic child. Early intervention is effective prophylaxis against later, often irreparable, damage.

The time of onset and the rapidity of progression of the deficit cannot be predicted. The common experience of pediatric neurosurgeons confirms that the decline in function may be either insidious or precipitous. It is no longer tenable to advocate delayed or "cosmetic" surgery. Early, prophylactic intervention is now the standard of care, even in asymptomatic infants.

Release of the spinal cord from the tethering lesion is the aim of the surgical procedure. In the authors' experience, this is almost always possible. However, on occasion, the experience and judgment of the surgeon may cause the surgeon to stop short of that goal. To cause the very neurologic deficit you intend to prevent makes little sense.

Finally, when deterioration occurs in any child or adult who previously underwent surgery to untether the spinal cord, one must consider the spinal cord as having become retethered. These patients must be re-evaluated and, when the cause is determined, must undergo reoperation. To accept this deterioration as the natural course of the disease allows the patient to acquire preventable deficits. We have reoperated on 105 children because of retethering of the cord. Approximately half were children with previously repaired myelomeningoceles. The results of reoperation show that more than half will recover motor function, exhibit improvement in kyphoscoliosis, or both and that the others will remain stable. Unfortunately, if incontinence has developed, untethering the spinal cord will result in recovered function in only less than 15 percent of these children.

References

1. Amador LV, Hankinson J, Bigler JA: Congenital spinal dermal sinuses. J Pediatr 47:300, 1955.
2. Ammerman BJ, Henry JM, De Girolami U, et al: Intradural lipomas of the spinal cord: Clinicopathological correlation. J Neurosurg 44:331, 1976.
3. Anderson FM: Occult spinal dysraphism: Diagnosis and management. J Pediatr 73:163, 1968.
4. Arredondo F, Haughton VM, Hemmy DC, et al: The computed tomographic appearance of the spinal cord in diastematomyelia. Radiology 126:685, 1980.
5. Bailey IC: Dermoid tumors of the spinal cord. J Neurosurg 33:676, 1970.
6. Banta JV, Nichols O: Sacral agenesis. J Bone Joint Surg [Am] 51A:693, 1969.
7. Barson AJ: The vertebral level of termination of the spinal cord during normal and abnormal development. J Anat 106:489, 1970.
8. Bassett RC: The neurologic deficit associated with lipomas of the cauda equina. Ann Surg 131:108, 1950.
9. Berdon WE, Hochberg B, Baker DH, et al: The association of lumbosacral spine and genitourinary anomalies with imperforate anus. Am J Roentgenol 98:181, 1966.
10. Boldrey EB, Elvidge AR: Dermoid cysts of the vertebral canal. Ann Surg 110:273, 1939.
11. Breig A: Overstretching of and circumscribed pathological tension in the spinal cord. A basic cause of symptoms in cord disorders. J Biomech 3:7, 1970.
12. Bremer JL: Dorsal intestinal fistula, accessory neurenteric canal, diastematomyelia. Arch Pathol 54:132, 1952.
13. Bruce DA, Schut L: Spinal lipomas in infancy and childhood. Child's Brain 5:192, 1979.
14. Caram PC, Scarcella G, Carton CA: Intradural lipomas of the spinal cord, with particular emphasis on the "intramedullary" lipomas. J Neurosurg 14:28, 1957.
15. Cardell BS, Laurance B: Congenital dermal sinus associated with meningitis: Report of a fatal case. Br Med J 2:1558, 1951.
16. Chapman PH: Congenital intraspinal lipomas: Anatomic considerations and surgical treatment. Child's Brain 9:37, 1982.
17. Cheek WR, Laurent JP: Dermal sinus tracts. In: Chapman PH (ed): Concepts in Pediatric Neurosurgery, Vol. 6. Basel, S Karger, 1985, pp 63–75.
18. Choremis C, Economos D, Papadatos C, et al: Intraspinal epidermoid tumours (cholesteatomas) in patients treated for tuberculous meningitis. Lancet 2:437, 1956.
19. Dale AJD: Diastematomyelia. Arch Neurol 20:309, 1969.
20. Danforth CH: Artificial and hereditary suppression of sacral vertebrae in the fowl. Proc Soc Exp Biol Med 30:143, 1932.
21. Duhamel B: From the mermaid to anal imperforation: The syndrome of caudal regression. Arch Dis Child 36:152, 1961.
22. Ehni G, Love JG: Intraspinal lipomas: Report of cases, review of the literature, and clinical and pathologic study. Arch Neurol Psychiatry 53:1, 1945.
23. El-Gindi S, Fairburn B: Intramedullary spinal abscess as a complication of a congenital dermal sinus: Case report. J Neurosurg 30:494, 1969.
24. Emery JL, Lendon RG: The local cord lesion in neurospinal dysraphism (meningomyelocele). J Pathol 110:83, 1973.
25. Fitz CR, Harwood-Nash DC: The tethered conus. Am J Roentgenol Radium Ther Nucl Med 125:515, 1975.
26. Friede RL: Developmental Neuropathology. New York, Springer-Verlag, 1975, pp 166–271.
27. Frye FL, McFarland LZ, Enright JB: Sacrococcygeal agenesis in Swiss mice. Cornell Vet 54:487, 1964.
28. Garceau GJ: The filum terminale syndrome (the cord-traction syndrome). J Bone Joint Surg [Am] 35A:711, 1953.
29. Gardner WJ: Myelomeningocele, the result of rupture of the embryonic neural tube. Cleve Clin Q 27:88, 1960.
30. Gibson T, Norris W: Skin fragments removed by injection needles. Lancet 2:983, 1958.
31. Guidetti B, Gagliardi FM: Epidermoid and dermoid cysts: Clinical evaluation and late surgical results. J Neurosurg 47:12, 1977.
32. Guthkelch AN: Diastematomyelia with median septum. Brain 97:729, 1974.
33. Hamilton WJ, Boyd JD, Mossman HW: Human embryology. In: Hamilton WJ, Mossman HW (eds): Prenatal Development of Form and Function, 2nd ed. Baltimore, The Williams & Wilkins Co., 1952.
34. Heinz ER, Rosenbaum AE, Scarff TB, et al: Tethered spinal cord following meningomyelocele repair. Radiology 131:153, 1979.
35. Hendrick EB, Hoffman HJ, Humphreys RP: Tethered cord syndrome. In: McLaurin RL (ed): Myelomeningocele. New York, Grune & Stratton, 1977, pp 369–376.
36. Herren RY, Edwards JE: Diplomyelia (duplication of the spinal cord). Arch Pathol 30:1203, 1940.
37. Hoffman HJ, Hendrick EB, Humphreys RP: The tethered spinal cord: Its protean manifestations, diagnosis and surgical correction. Child's Brain 2:145, 1976.
38. Hoffman HJ, Taecholarn C, Hendrick EB, et al: Management of lipomyelomeningoceles. J Neurosurg 62:1, 1985.
39. Ignelzi RJ, Lehman RAW: Lumbosacral agenesis: Management and embryological implications. J Neurol Neurosurg Psychiatry 37:1273, 1974.
40. James CCM, Lassman LP: Diastematomyelia. Arch Dis Child 33:536, 1958.
41. James CCM, Lassman LP: Spinal dysraphism: An orthopaedic syndrome in children accompanying occult forms. Arch Dis Child 35:315, 1960.
42. James CCM, Lassman LP: Spinal dysraphism. The diagnosis and treatment of progressive lesions in spina bifida occulta. J Bone Joint Surg 44B:828, 1962.
43. James CCM, Lassman LP: Diastematomyelia and the tight filum terminale. J Neurol Sci 10:193, 1970.
44. Jones PH, Love JG: Tight filum terminale. Arch Surg 73:556, 1956.
45. Kallen B, Winberg J: Caudal mesoderm pattern of anomalies: From renal agenesis to sirenomelia. Teratology 9:99, 1974.
46. Keim HA, Greene AF: Diastematomyelia and scoliosis. J Bone Joint Surg [Am] 55A:1425, 1973.
47. Kooistra HP: Pilonidal sinuses occurring over the higher spinal segments with report of a case involving the spinal cord. Surgery 11:63, 1942.
48. Kunitomo K: The development and reduction of the tail and of the caudal end of the spinal cord. Contrib Embryol 8:161, 1918.
49. Lassman LP, James CCM: Lumbosacral lipomas: Critical

survey of 26 cases submitted to laminectomy. J Neurol Neurosurg Psychiatry 30:174, 1967.
50. Lemire RJ, Graham CB, Beckwith JB: Skin-covered sacrococcygeal masses in infants and children. J Pediatr 79:948, 1971.
51. Lemire RJ, Loeser JD, Leech RW, et al: Normal and Abnormal Development of the Human Nervous System. Hagerstown, MD, Harper & Row Publishers, Inc., 1975.
52. List CF: Intraspinal epidermoids, dermoids and dermal sinuses. Surg Gynecol Obstet 73:525, 1941.
53. Love JG, Daly DD, Harris LE: Tight filum terminale: Report of condition in three siblings. JAMA 176:31, 1961.
54. Matson DD, Jerva MJ: Recurrent meningitis associated with congenital lumbo-sacral dermal sinus tract. J Neurosurg 25:288, 1966.
55. Matson DD, Woods RP, Campbell JB, et al: Diastematomyelia (congenital clefts of the spinal cord): Diagnosis and surgical treatment. Pediatrics 6:98, 1950.
56. McAlister WH, Siegel JJ, Shackelford GD: A congenital iliac anomaly often associated with sacral lipoma and ipsilateral lower extremity weakness. Skeletal Radiol 3:161, 1978.
57. McLone DG: The subarachnoid space: A review. Child's Brain 6:113, 1980.
58. McLone DG: Embryonic deformation and caudal suppression. In: Marlin AE (ed): Concepts in Pediatric Neurosurgery. Basel, S Karger, 1987, pp 169–171.
59. McLone DG, Bondareff W: Developmental morphology of the subarachnoid space and contiguous structures in the mouse. Am J Anat 142:273, 1975.
60. McLone DG, Hayashida SF, Caldarelli M: Surgical resection of lipomyelomeningoceles in 18 asymptomatic infants. J Ped Neurosci 1:239, 1985.
61. McLone DG, Knepper PA: On the role of complex carbohydrates and neurulation. Pediatr Neurosc 12:2, 1986.
62. McLone DG, Mutluer S, Naidich TP: Lipomeningoceles of the conus medullaris. In: Raimondi AJ (ed): Concepts in Pediatric Neurosurgery, Vol. 3. Basel, S Karger, 1982.
63. McLone DG, Naidich TP: Spinal dysraphism: Experimental and clinical. In: Holtzman RNN, Stein BM (eds): The Tethered Cord. New York, Thieme-Stratton, 1985, pp 14–28.
64. McLone DG, Naidich TP: Terminal myelocystocele. Neurosurgery 16:36, 1985.
65. McLone DG, Naidich TP: Laser resection of fifty spinal lipomas. Neurosurgery 18:611, 1986.
66. Moes CAF, Hendrick EB: Diastematomyelia. J Pediatr 63:238, 1963.
67. Mount LA: Congenital dermal sinuses as a cause of meningitis, intraspinal abscess and intracranial abscess. JAMA 139:1263, 1949.
68. Naidich TP, McLone DG, Harwood-Nash DC: Spinal dysraphism. In: Newton TH, Potts DG (eds): Computed Tomography of the Spine and Spinal Cord. San Anselmo, CA, Clavadel Press, 1983.
69. Naidich TP, McLone DG, Mutluer S: A new understanding of dorsal dysraphism with lipoma (lipomyeloschisis): Radiologic evaluation and surgical correction. AJNR 4:103, 1983.
70. Naidich TP, McLone DG, Mutluer S, et al: Presurgical evaluation of lipomyelomeningoceles. Presented at the 19th Annual Meeting of the American Society of Neuroradiology, Chicago, Apr. 5–9, 1981. AJNR 3:93, 1982.
71. Neuhauser EBD, Harris GBC, Berrett A: Roentgenographic features of neurenteric cysts. Am J Roentgenol 79:235, 1958.
72. Neuhauser EBD, Wittenborg MH, Dehlinger K: Diastematomyelia: Transfixation of the cord or cauda equina with congenital anomalies of the spine. Radiology 54:659, 1950.
73. Osaka K, Matsumoto S, Tanimura T: Myeloschisis in early human embryos. Child's Brain 4:347, 1978.
74. Pang D, Hoffman HJ: Sacral agenesis with progressive neurological deficit. Neurosurgery 7:118, 1980.
75. Passarge E: Congenital malformations and maternal diabetes. Lancet 1:324, 1965.
76. Passarge E, Lenz W: Syndrome of caudal regression in infants of diabetic mothers: Observations of further cases. Pediatrics 37:672, 1966.
77. Perloff MM: Congenital dermal sinus complicated by meningitis: Report of a case. J Pediatr 44:73, 1954.
78. Perret G: Diagnosis and treatment of diastematomyelia. Surg Gynecol Obstet 105:69, 1957.
79. Price DL, Dooling EC, Richardson EP, Jr.: Caudal dysplasia (caudal regression syndrome). Arch Neurol 23:212, 1970.
80. Reigel DH: Tethered spinal cord. In: Humphreys RP (ed): Concepts in Pediatric Neurosurgery, Vol. 4. Basel, S Karger, 1983, pp 142–164.
81. Renshaw TS: Sacral agenesis: A classification and review of twenty-three cases. J Bone Joint Surg [Am] 60A:373, 1978.
82. Resjo IM, Harwood-Nash DC, Fitz CR, et al: Computed tomographic metrizamide myelography in spinal dysraphism in infants and children. J Comput Assist Tomogr 2:549, 1978.
83. Rogers HM, Long DM, Chou SN, et al: Lipomas of the spinal cord and cauda equina. J Neurosurg 34:349, 1971.
84. Sachs E, Jr., Horrax G: A cervical and a lumbar pilonidal sinus communicating with intraspinal dermoids: Report of 2 cases and review of the literature. J Neurosurg 6:97, 1949.
85. Sadler TW, Greenberg D, Coughlin P: Actin distribution patterns in the mouse neural tube during neurulation. Science 215:172, 1982.
86. Schut L, Pizzi FJ, Bruce DA: Occult spinal dysraphism. In: McLaurin RL (ed): Myelomeningocele. New York, Grune & Stratton, 1977, pp 349–368.
87. Scott G, Harwood-Nash DC, Hoffman HJ: Congenital thoracic dermal sinus: Diagnosis by computer-assisted metrizamide myelography. J Comput Assist Tomogr 4:675, 1980a.
88. Scotti G, Musgrave MA, Harwood-Nash DC, et al: Diastematomyelia in children: Metrizamide and CT metrizamide myelography. AJNR 1:403, 1980b.
89. Sensenig EC: The early development of the meninges of the spinal cord in human embryos. Contrib Embryol 34:147, 1951.
90. Storrs BB, Walker ML: Sacral dermal sinus—occult sacral masses discovered by routine ultrasound. In: Marlin AE (ed): Concepts in Pediatric Neurosurgery, Vol. 7. Basel, S Karger, 1987, pp 172–178.
91. Streeter GL: Factors involved in the formation of the filum terminale. Am J Anat 25:1, 1919.
92. Swanson HS, Barnett JC, Jr.: Intradural lipomas in children. Pediatrics 29:911, 1962.
93. Tadmor R, Davis KR, Roberson GH, et al: The diagnosis of diastematomyelia by computed tomography. Surg Neurol 8:434, 1977.
94. Van Gilder JC, Schwartz HG: Growth of dermoids from skin implants to the nervous system and surrounding spaces of the newborn rat. J Neurosurg 26:14, 1967.
95. Villarejo FJ, Blazquez MG, Gutierrez-Diaz JA: Intraspinal lipomas in children. Child's Brain 2:361, 1976.
96. Walker AE, Bucy PC: Congenital dermal sinuses: Source of spinal meningeal infection and subdural abscesses. Brain 57:401, 1934.
97. Walsh JW, Markesbery WR: Histological features of congenital lipomas of the lower spinal canal. J Neurosurg 52:564, 1980.
98. Warkany J, Wilson JG, Geiger JF: Myeloschisis and myelomeningocele produced experimentally in the rat. J Comp Neurol 109:34, 1958.
99. Wright RL: Congenital dermal sinuses. Prog Neurol Surg 4:175, 1971.
100. Yamada S, Schreider S, Ashwel S, et al: Pathophysiologic mechanisms in the tethered spinal cord syndrome. In: Holtzman RNN, Stein BM (eds): The Tethered Spinal Cord. New York, Thieme-Stratton, Inc., 1985, pp 29–40.
101. Yamada S, Zinke DE, Sanders D: Pathophysiology of tethered cord syndrome. J Neurosurg 54:494, 1981.
102. Yashon D, Beatty RA: Tethering of the conus medullaris within the sacrum. J Neurol Neurosurg Psychiatry 19:244, 1966.
103. Padget DH: Spina bifida and embryonic neuroschisis—a causal relationship; definition of postnatal confirmations of a bifid spine. Johns Hopkins Med J 128:233, 1968.

6
ENCEPHALOCELE, DERMOID SINUS, AND ARACHNOID CYST

Hector E. James, M.D.

ENCEPHALOCELES AND RELATED MALFORMATIONS

Encephaloceles are developmental anomalies that exhibit varying degrees of protrusion of the encephalon and its coverings through cranial midline closure defects. Congenital cranial closure defects and accompanying anomalies of the intracranial contents have significant pathologic variations and, therefore, varied clinical outcomes. A classification of the various cranial midline anomalies appears in Table 6–1.

Cranium bifidum (failure of cranial ossification, without herniation of the brain and the meninges) is associated with an abnormal outcome. A poor outcome is expected in the patient with a large encephalocele with associated hydrocephalus, because of the associated impaired maturation and migration of neuronal structures. Between these two extremes are cranial anomalies that show variations in anatomic pathology and clinical course.

Incidence

The incidence is reported to be as high as 1 in 5000 live births in areas of Southeast Asia[42, 44, 46] and as low as 1 in 10,000 live births in the Northern Continent.[11, 20, 29] Of all craniospinal malformations, 10 to 20 percent are encephaloceles.

The location of the encephalocele varies according to the geographic area in which the affected persons live. In Southeast Asia, encephaloceles are more commonly located in the anterior cranial vault;[42, 44, 46] in America and Europe, 70 percent are located in the posterior cranial vault.[11, 20, 29] The reason for this distribution is not known.

Pathology

The embryology and the etiology of these disorders are unclear. The pathogenesis has been compared with that of the myelomeningocele. The encephalocele represents a failure of the neural tube to fuse at the level of the anterior neuropore, on approximately the twenty-fifth day of gestation.[5, 23]

A classification of defects may be seen in Table 6–2. In occipital encephaloceles, there may be varying degrees of neuroectodermal displacements through the calvarial defect, at times containing primitive, disorganized glial elements with meninges, and no functional viability. Other displacements contain portions of one occipital lobe or both, with or without portions of the cerebellum and the fourth ventricle choroid plexus.[3, 24, 43] The bone defect may be confined to the occipital squamae or may involve the posterior arch of C1, and its size may vary. Large protrusions are commonly accompanied by small bony openings.[3] The base of the skull may be deformed in its entirety.[3] Hydrocephalus may not be present initially but may develop and become very symptomatic following repair of the defect.[24]

Sincipital encephaloceles may present with varying degrees of involvement of the frontal lobes, in the nasofrontal and frontoethmoidal types. The ethmoidal, sphenoethmoidal, and trans-sphenoidal types (Table 6–2) may have varying degrees of herniation of the hypothalamus and optic path-

Table 6–1. CRANIAL MIDLINE ANOMALIES

Cranium bifidum	Results from a failure of closure of the mesoderm in the midline cranium, without involvement of the meninges or the neuroectodermal derivatives. Radiologically, it is seen as a defect of the calvarium, occurring in various sizes.
Cranial meningocele	Produced by failure of mesodermal closure of the midline of the cranium, with herniation of the meninges through the cranial defect, without neural elements. For the most part, the brain is well formed and the outcome should be normal.
Encephalocele	Caused by failure of the anterior neuropore to fuse adequately during gestation. Consequently, there are varying degrees of protrusion of the encephalon, the meninges, and CSF through the cranium.
Encephalocystocele	In this type of encephalocele, there is herniation of the meninges, CSF, and the choroid plexus.
Encephalomeningocele	In this type of encephalocele, there is herniation of the meninges and the brain.

ways, with the clinical presentation being secondary to this involvement.[24]

Central nervous system (CNS) malformations of varying degrees have been noted in the presence of encephaloceles. Poor migration of neurones, heterotopias, displacement of the brainstem into the occipital encephaloceles, and changes in the commissures and the basal ganglia all may be seen.[3] In the Chiari type III anomaly, the presence of an occipital cervical encephalocele is noted to be accompanied with a hindbrain descended into the cervical canal and herniation of the cerebellum through the bone defect.[3]

Clinical Presentation

Cranial Vault Encephaloceles

These include the occipital, parietal, temporal, and frontonasal encephaloceles. Cranial vault encephaloceles are discovered usually at birth or with intrauterine imaging. Their size is extremely variable, and as a consequence, the smaller ones may not be detected by in utero sonography. These encephaloceles may present with or without skin covering; at times, a tenuous membrane covers the defect. They may be pedunculated or sessile; the stalk in the pedunculated ones may be vary narrow, despite the presence of a large external mass (Figs. 6–1 through 6–3). The size of the lesion does not allow an adequate assessment of the contents, and neural imaging is the way to determine the presence of an encephalocele or a meningocele as well as the extent of neural involvement.[19, 24] The lesions that are not skin covered exude varying amounts of cerebrospinal fluid (CSF).[24]

Encephaloceles of the Cranial Base

These may offer no evidence of their presence at birth. When they do manifest themselves, it may be in the form of obstruction of the airways (they are commonly thought to be nasal polyps or other masses[15, 24]) or in the form of meningitis resulting from communication between the airways and the subarachnoid spaces.[7] An intraorbital encephalocele may produce unilateral or bilateral exophthalmos.[6, 24]

Neurologic Assessment

Upon detecting the malformation at birth, the infant's neurologic examination is usually normal or may reflect increased flexor motor tone.[24] In severe occipital encephaloceles involving the brainstem, spells of apnea and bradycardia may be noted. The form of presentation that includes meningitis (due to communication between the airways and the subarachnoid space) usually occurs in later infancy or childhood.

Neural Imaging

Plain skull radiographs may readily document the location and extent of the bony defect in the vault encephaloceles but are less reliable for those located in the cranial base.[19] The smaller, rounded defects of the bone may be misinterpreted as being a dermoid cyst. Craniolacunia is very commonly seen in association with encephaloceles.[19] Associated anomalies of varying degrees of fusion, lack of fusion, or both of cervical vertebral elements are commonly seen with occipital encephaloceles. Frontonasal defects must be differentiated from those

Table 6–2. CLASSIFICATION OF ENCEPHALOCELES ACCORDING TO ANATOMIC LOCATION

Regional*	
Occipital	Nasopharyngeal
Parietal	Nasal
Frontal	

Topographic†
1. Cranial Vault Encephalocele
   a. Occipital
   b. Interfrontal
   c. Parietal
   d. Anterior and posterior fontanelle
   e. Temporal
2. Frontoethmoidal (Sincipital) Encephalocele
   a. Nasofrontal
   b. Nasoethmoidal
   c. Naso-orbital
3. Basal Encephalocele
   a. Transethmoidal
   b. Sphenoethmoidal
   c. Trans-sphenoidal
   d. Frontosphenoidal or spheno-orbital

*From Matson DD: Neurosurgery of Infancy and Childhood. Springfield, IL, Charles C Thomas, 1969.
†From Suwanwela C, Suwanwela N: A morphological classification of sincipital encephalomeningoceles. J Neurosurg 36:201, 1972.

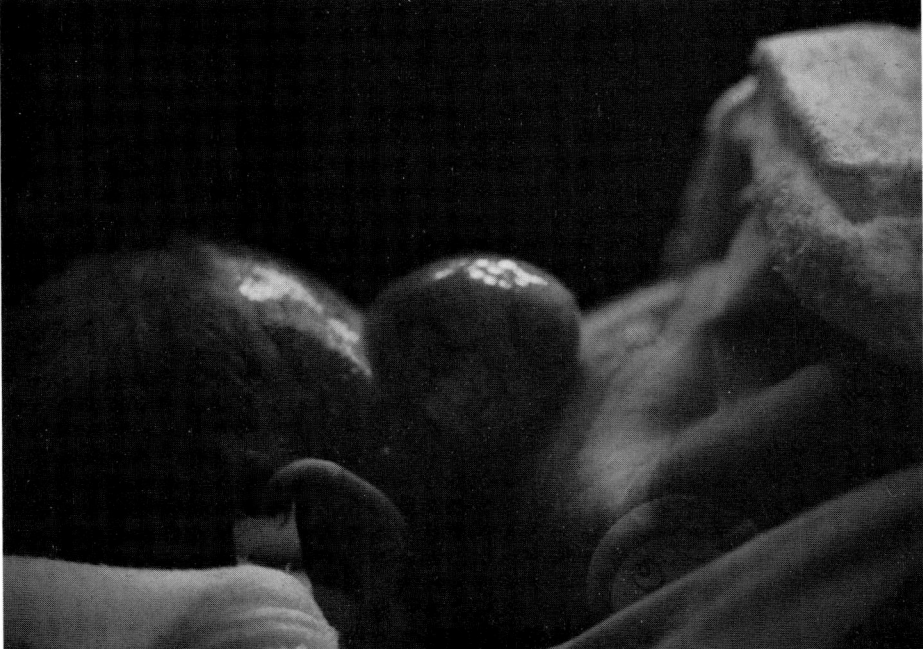

Figure 6–1. Occipital encephalocele. In this patient, the encephalocele contained only a thin gliotic membrane and CSF.

resulting from nasal gliomas.[19] With basal and frontoethmoidal encephaloceles, median cleft syndromes are commonly seen.[19] Hypertelorism may be present.

Computed tomography (CT) delineates the bony defects in encephaloceles with precise detail, and CT reconstruction allows for a better understanding of the abnormalities that at times are very complex in cranial base encephaloceles. This technique is superior to nuclear magnetic resonance imaging (NMRI) for abnormalities of the bone and is the study of choice for operative planning for corrective surgery. The author has found NMRI more useful for delineation of the contents of the encephaloceles and determining the type of neural structure in them. Thus, when faced with complex encephaloceles, the author routinely evaluates them with both CT and NMRI. However, NMRI is not a study that is readily performed in the infant who is not clinically stable and, thus, is in no situation to undergo the stress of transportation to the NMRI suite with life-support systems.

Cerebral angiography best demonstrates the presence of brain tissue in the encephalocele.[19] The pattern of vascularity and the vessels of origin may then permit the interpretation of the disordered

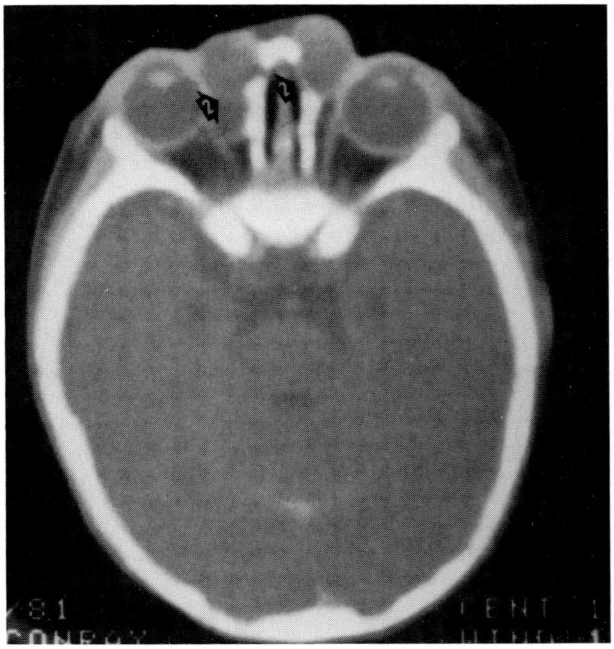

Figure 6–2. Nasal encephalocele with bilateral pedunculated orbital components (arrow no. 2).

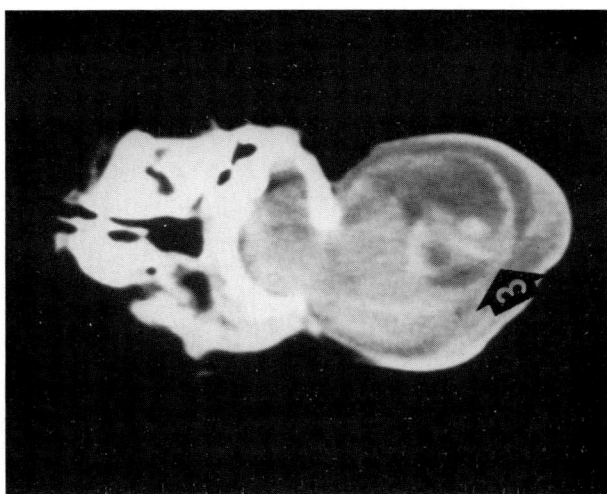

Figure 6–3. Encephalocystocele. Structure compatible with the ventricular system may be seen (arrow no. 3).

anatomy. Such vascular study may be of much assistance in complex occipital encephaloceles, since displacements of the basilar artery and its branches are not uncommon.[19] In these encephaloceles, the basilar artery may be hooked backward, which then leads to a sharp angulation of the posterior cerebral arteries so that they may then acquire their supratentorial course.[19] A situation of transposed brainstem, with the cerebellum in front of the basilar artery, may be diagnosed prior to operative intervention.[13]

CT and NMRI document the presence of associated anomalies of the CNS that are commonly seen in encephaloceles (see previous section on pathology). The presence or absence of hydrocephalus may be readily documented by these studies, and appropriate operative planning may then be performed.

In utero neural imaging is currently readily performed with high-resolution ultrasonography. These studies may document the presence of an abnormality early in gestation. Studies of the larger malformations may delineate the presence of neural elements in the sac. However, misinterpretation of encephalocele may lead to erroneous obstetric counseling. Discerning the presence of a cranial meningocele versus an encephalocele may not be easy. Since meningoceles are associated with normal outcomes, interrupting the pregnancy under these circumstances would not be appropriate. At times, in utero NMRI studies of the fetus may be of assistance, with the limiting factor being that fetal mobility may interfere with adequate neural imaging.

Therapy

The surgical treatment of midline cranial defects has to be considered on the basis of the pathologic condition. Cranium bifidum, a persistent large defect present well into childhood, does not require surgery. Patients with confirmed cranial meningoceles should have surgery early in life to minimize the risk of skin breakdown and secondary infection as well as for cosmetic correction. These interventions are not difficult, and the dura should be repaired to prevent infection and wound breakdown. No bone reconstruction is needed in most situations because once the protrusion is cared for, ossification of the defect will proceed over the months that follow.

Surgical correction should be considered in all encephaloceles unless death is imminent shortly after birth, or in the presence of severe associated anomalies. The rationale behind such decisions has been extensively discussed by other authors.[23, 24, 26] Even if the family is not going to assume care of the child, these defects should be removed to facilitate custodial and nursing care.[24] The open defects should be repaired immediately to minimize the risk of infection, in a way similar to the procedure for myelomeningocele.[23, 24, 26]

The basic operative principles are to repair the defects and, whenever possible, to preserve neural elements if they are not placing the closure of the defect at risk of dehiscence. The dura should be repaired to minimize the risks of CSF leakage and infection and to remove malformed or devitalized tissues.[23, 24, 26, 43] Repair of the bone defect need not be performed at this stage. In those situations in which the dural closure contains the defect, the ossification of the defect usually occurs in the months that follow. This is not the case when untreated progressive hydrocephalus is present, and the patient should be closely monitored for hydrocephalus in the postoperative period. When a large defect is present, closure of the scalp may be complex. Rotating cutaneous flaps may be needed.

In occipital encephaloceles, an elliptic, transverse incision is usually best. Circumferential dissection around the stalk of the lesion or the herniation permits identification of the dura, which should be carefully dissected for subsequent meticulous closure. In this region, the transverse sinuses and the torcular are the prime structures of concern, and they should be respected to avoid severe cerebrovascular congestion. Repair of parietal and temporal encephaloceles follows the same principles.

Anterior encephaloceles should be approached intracranially by bicoronal incision,[24] for several reasons. The first is to have an adequate exposure of all the pathology as well as the normal surrounding areas; this minimizes damage to normal structures during the dissection. The dura may then be readily reconstituted. If adequate amounts of dura exist, this approach gives the surgeon access to the surrounding normal pericranium, which is the ideal dural substitute. Another very important reason for the bicoronal approach is that it minimizes facial scars in an area that commonly is already distorted by the pathology. The extracranial approach may worsen the cosmetic result, and in the opinion of the author, the extracranial approach for anterior encephaloceles[43] should rarely, if ever, be employed.

Postoperative care should be that of close monitoring for hydrocephalus and for seizures. Seizures may be a consequence of cerebral maldevelopment and operative intervention and mandate aggressive medical control. Infection may manifest itself as local wound infection or meningitis, and appropriate steps should be taken when this is suspected.

Outcome

The outcome in infants with meningocele and cranium bifidum should be entirely normal, even in the case of meningocele with hydrocephalus. The outcome in patients with encephalocele is determined by a combination of factors: the extent of protrusion of the encephalon; the degree of perinatal damage from the mechanics of delivery; apnea spells; undetected seizures that lead to hypoventilation, hypoxemia, and acidosis; the presence or absence of hydrocephalus; and heterotopias and cerebral dysgenesis that may occur throughout the brain. These factors cannot be readily assessed in early life, and consequently, the prognosis given to the parents should always be qualified by the possibility of such conditions arising. Larger defects are more readily associated with developmental delay than are smaller ones, and ventral defects are more commonly associated with a better outcome than are occipital ones.[24] The combination of occipital encephalocele with hydrocephalus has a worse prognosis than that without hydrocephalus.[43] A much better outcome is expected in ventral defects unless there are associated complications. The majority of ventral defects have a normal outcome.[19, 24, 29]

Prevention

Encephaloceles are, for the most part, sporadic presentations, and therefore, their absolute prevention is infeasible. However, in the case of larger defects, intrauterine diagnosis can be made with routine high-resolution ultrasonography. Intrauterine sonography of the fetus also permits evaluation for associated anomalies, such as hydrocephalus. The limitations of the technique are obvious: At times, the ultrasonographer may not be able to ascertain whether the protruding mass is a cranial meningocele or an encephalocele, or a scalp or a cervical tumor. Diagnostic amniocentesis and measurement of amniotic alpha-fetoprotein levels may be of assistance only in those defects that have no cutaneous covering. When this occurs, there is a pathologic elevation of the level of alpha-fetoprotein; however, even in the presence of an encephalocele that has a cutaneous covering, the values may be normal. Therefore, caution is needed in interpreting these studies in the decision-making process and in considering interruption of the pregnancy.

DERMOID SINUSES

Intracranial dermoid sinuses are defined as developmental anomalies in which the end result is an abnormal communication between the dermis and the intracranial structures. The depth of communication is variable, involving subcutaneous tissues, bone, extradural or intradural spaces, or brain or cerebellum. Thus, intracranial dermoid sinuses may present clinically with varying degrees of drainage from their cutaneous openings; recurrent bouts of septic or aseptic meningitis; mass effect resulting from the cyst, brain abscess, or obstruction of the CSF pathways; and consequent hydrocephalus.

Incidence

Intracranial dermoid sinuses are less frequent than their counterparts in the lumbosacral region. In Matson's series[24] of 750 intracranial tumors in children, 12 were dermoid tumors with dermoid sinuses. Ten of these were in the posterior fossa. Cranial dermoid sinuses occur sporadically, with no known familial or genetic implication. Over 80 percent present before the age of four years.[14]

Pathology

Dermoid sinuses represent defects in the closure of the ectoderm that may be related to failures of closure of the anterior neuropore that are less severe than those leading to the encephaloceles previously discussed. They may occur toward the end of the fourth week of gestation.[24, 33, 38] The dermoid sinuses at times end blindly; on other occasions, they are accompanied by one or more dermoid or epidermoid tumors. In the former, the wall of the cyst is lined with dermis with hair follicles and sweat and sebaceous glands, and in the latter, the cyst wall is covered with stratified squamous epithelium.[38] The epidermoid tumors are believed to result from a failure of the ectoderm to close at a stage of gestation that is later than the stage that gives rise to dermoid tumors.

The involvement of the various intracranial structures relates to the stage of formation and the interrelationship of the mesodermal and neuroectodermal structures during their migration, in the closure of the midline. This is the reason that these defects are most common in the midline.[14, 24, 41]

Dermoid sinuses may contain more than one dermal tract,[41] may have more than one dermoid or epidermoid tumor on the tract,[41] and may present with concomitant brain or cerebellar abscesses because of recurrent infections.[41] Surrounding the wall of the tumor is usually a glial-fibrous vascular reactive capsule of varying degrees of thickness.[38, 41] The histology is benign, though there has been a case of a malignant change.[8]

Clinical Presentation

It is important to be aware that the clinical presentation may be varied. Dermoid sinuses often go unrecognized because of the feeling on the part of the parents of the child or the belief of the physician that only a minor cutaneous problem is present. The following sections describe the forms of presentation (Table 6–3).

Cutaneous Presentation. In this situation, one sees a small orifice with hairs in it, with or without a local small mass or hemangioma. There is intermittent drainage of a white, thick material from the

Table 6-3. CLINICAL PRESENTATION OF DERMOID SINUSES

Cutaneous presentation
Infectious presentation
Presentation with aseptic meningitis
Presentation with intracranial hypertension

sinus. At times, there may be inflammation of the surrounding tissues.[14, 24, 41] The sinus is most commonly located in the occipital region and less frequently in the parietal region, the frontal region, and the nasion and on the bridge of the nose (Fig. 6-4). Though most common in the midline, sinuses may occur off the midline, such as in the orbit, parapituitary areas, pontocerebellar recesses, cisterns, and lateral ventricles.[24, 34]

Presentation with Infection. Well recognized in the literature is the dermoid sinus that presents with bouts of meningitis, resulting from the communication of the dermis with the subarachnoid spaces.[14, 24, 38, 41] The most common etiologic organism is *Staphylococcus aureus*, although the etiologic role of other organisms has been well documented.[41] On examining the patient, the dermoid sinus may be noted, but in other situations, it is only detected after repeated infections of unexplained etiology.[14, 24, 41] On occasion, purulent material may be seen at the level of the dermoid sinuses.[24, 41] Brain abscesses may occur as a consequence of repeated infections and present a more acute and serious deterioration from intracranial hypertension or from seizures, fever, and prostration.[24, 41]

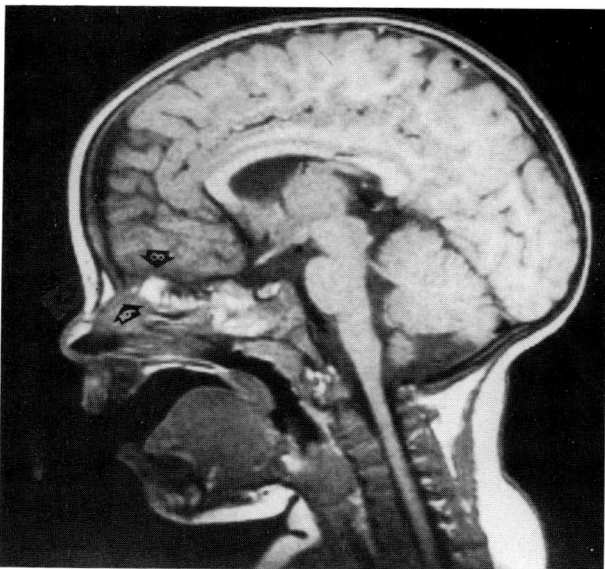

Figure 6-4. Magnetic resonance image of a one-year-old with a dermoid sinus on the bridge of the nose (arrow no. 4) and extending intracranially to the cribriform plate region. A dermoid tumor is seen in that location (arrow no. 8), making contact with the tract (arrow no. 6).

Presentation with Aseptic Meningitis. At times, the syndrome of meningitis seen in these patients may be mild and self-limiting.[33] The CSF exhibits pleocytosis; elevated protein levels; normal, or almost normal, glucose levels; and negative cultures.[33] These results are due to the passage of debris from the dermoid tumor into the CSF pathways, producing a chemical form of meningitis.[33] The diagnosis can be confirmed when cholesterol and squamous epithelial cells are noted in the CSF.[33]

Presentation with Intracranial Hypertension. Impairment of consciousness and neurologic deterioration with or without focal signs may be a consequence of the mass effect on local structures of the posterior fossa or supratentorial compartment.[14, 24, 41] The mass, as can occur with dermoid or epidermoid tumors of the fourth ventricle, may obstruct the CSF pathways and cause acute or subacute hydrocephalus. As previously noted, intracranial hypertension may also occur, not as much as from the tumor itself as from abscess formation.[14, 24, 41]

Neural Imaging

Intracranial dermoid sinuses and tumor may be seen on plain x-ray films as defects in the midline, or just off the midline, usually of small size, with sclerotic margins of the tracts in the bone.[19] However, on occasion, the opening of the bone may be so small that it may not be visible by any method of neural imaging and is found only upon surgical exploration.[24] The dermoid tumors may contain calcifications and, on occasion, teeth.[19]

Dermoid and epidermoid tumors contain fat and cholesterol, which may be readily visualized on CT and NMRI.[4, 31, 41] On CT scan, these tumors measure between -22 and $+26$ Hounsfield units.[4, 31, 41] The abscesses that may accompany these tumors may have measurements in Hounsfield units in the low twenties.[41] Following administration of contrast material, the tumor may have a thin rim of enhancement, whereas the abscess has a much larger and denser enhanced image. NMRI demonstrates the presence of fat and delineates the surrounding area well, except for the defect and the tract in the bone, which is more readily seen by CT, especially with the appropriate bone window.

Therapy

Upon recognizing a dermoid sinus, the appropriate studies should be performed, and radical surgical removal of the tract and any dermoid tumors is strongly recommended.[14, 24, 41] The objective is to prevent further growth of the mass, infections and abscess formation, and their complications. Surgical intervention needs to be performed with care and with the needed magnification to resect completely the tract and tumor and to minimize harm to the surrounding tissues.

According to the location of the tract and tumor, the surgery will require the necessary anatomic steps. Posterior fossa dermoid tumors of the midline may involve the torcular Herophili and the transverse, circular, and straight sinuses. Step-by-step dissection in these areas minimizes blood loss and prevents damage to the important venous-drainage structures.[14, 24, 41]

Patients with severe intracranial hypertension from severe hydrocephalus should be treated first for relief of the pressure from the hydrocephalus. Relief can be medically initiated with the early administration of furosemide, 1 mg/kg intravenously, followed by dexamethasone, 1 mg/kg. The patient should then undergo the immediate placement of a ventriculoperitoneal shunt or external ventricular drainage. After the patient's condition has improved as a result of the resolution of the changes secondary to hydrocephalus, the definitive operation for the dermoid sinus and tract should be performed.

In the presence of infection of the CSF pathways or abscess formation, external ventricular drainage is preferred over an internal CSF shunt for the treatment of hydrocephalus. Appropriate broad-spectrum antibiotic therapy should be promptly administered, especially when there exists significant neurologic impairment from distortion and mass effect from a posterior fossa abscess. Furosemide and dexamethasone, at a dose of 1 mg/kg each, should be given intravenously, and drainage of the abscess should follow immediately, leaving surgical treatment of the dermoid tumor and tract for a later date.[41]

During surgery, complete removal of the tumor wall and tract is necessary to avoid recurrence of the disease.[14, 24, 41] Appropriate care should be taken to avoid spilling the contents of the tumor into the CSF pathways. Aseptic meningitis may result from the passage of these contents into the CSF, and this complicates the postoperative management of the patient.[14] When aseptic meningitis occurs, therapy with dexamethasone may alleviate the symptoms.

Outcome

The outcome of this condition is directly related to the time of diagnosis, the success of the surgical removal, and the presence or absence of complications. Infections are of prime concern, as discussed earlier. The detection of the dermal sinuses before serious complications arise as well as surgical removal of the sinuses and associated tumors should result in an excellent outcome in most situations.[14, 24, 41]

CRANIAL ARACHNOID CYSTS

An arachnoid cyst is a pathologic condition in which an arachnoid-lined cavity fills with fluid similar to CSF, sometimes creating a disturbance in intracranial dynamics because of shift and displacement of surrounding structures and intracranial hypertension.

There are various types of CSF-containing cysts. Primary, or congenital, arachnoid cysts are maldevelopmental anomalies that are situated wholly within the arachnoid membrane, are lined by collagen and cells of the arachnoid, and contain clear CSF-like fluid.[32, 35-37, 39, 40] Secondary cysts may result from a variety of etiologies, such as trauma and infection. These cysts have, characteristically, something other than just arachnoid on their walls, including hemosiderin deposits, inflammatory cells, or glioependyma.[32, 40] Arachnoid diverticuli and pouches of the arachnoid are terms applied to cystlike malformations that rapidly communicate the CSF with the subarachnoid CSF, as documented by any contrast-enhanced study. Characteristically, the primary and secondary cysts previously defined do not freely communicate with the subarachnoid space.[32] The different types of cysts are summarized in Table 6–4.

This section addresses only the primary cranial arachnoid cysts.

Incidence

Intracranial arachnoid cysts occur as incidental findings in approximately 0.5 percent of autopsies and account for approximately 1 percent of intracranial space-occupying lesions.[25, 30] They are most

Table 6–4. CLASSIFICATION OF INTRACRANIAL CYSTS

Primary, or Congenital	These are maldevelopmental anomalies that are within the arachnoid membrane and are lined by collagen and cells of the arachnoid. They contain clear, CSF-like fluid and do not freely communicate with the subarachnoid CSF.
Secondary	These may result from a variety of insults, such as trauma or infection, and have something other than arachnoid on their walls (hemosiderin, inflammatory cells, or glioependyma). They do not freely communicate with the subarachnoid CSF.
Arachnoid Diverticuli	There are said to be intra-arachnoid CSF cavities that freely communicate with the subarachnoid CSF.

commonly sporadic presentations, but rarely they may present as more than one lesion or in siblings.[16] They affect males more frequently than females and most commonly present in the first two decades of life.[12, 39] In one series, two thirds of the girls were under one year of age.[19] Of importance is the fact that 9 of 17 girls had posterior fossa cysts.[19]

Pathology

Primary cysts probably arise as aberrations in the formation of the subarachnoid space. Initially, all CSF is contained within the ventricles, and there are no subarachnoid spaces. The future area of the subarachnoid space is a loose mesenchyme, and during fetal development, the ground substance of this mesenchyme undergoes a change.[27, 28] As the roof of the fourth ventricle becomes permeable, the pulsations of the CSF push the fluid into the subarachnoid space.[32, 40] Variations in the dispersal of the mesenchyme during this phase of development of the subarachnoid space could create areas of entrapment of CSF between the pia and the arachnoid, which have formed from the mesenchyme.[32]

Various theories have been put forward to explain the progressive expansion of the cysts and their mass effect.[19, 24, 32] Fluid could enter the wall of the cyst by an osmotic gradient, attracted by the higher oncotic pressure in the cyst, and then be retained in the cyst. Another theory describes a "ball-valve" mechanism in which CSF passively enters the cyst but is unable to leave. Another possible mechanism is that the wall of the cyst actively secretes CSF. The fluid is then unable to leave the cyst as quickly as it is produced. However, no theory has received uniform acceptance, and further research on this matter is necessary.[32]

In infants, arachnoid cysts are more commonly located in the posterior fossa. In older children, the supratentorial location is more frequent. Overall, the middle fossa is commonly said to be the most common location for primary cysts in children.[17, 24, 32] However, Harwood-Nash and Fitz[19] report that in 42 percent of patients in their series, the cysts were in the posterior fossa. The remainder were distributed as follows: middle fossa, 22 percent; cerebral convexity, 14 percent; suprasellar region, 12 percent; and posterior third ventricle, 10 percent. Posterior fossa arachnoid cysts have to be differentiated from the Dandy-Walker malformation and from a very large cisterna magna.

Clinical Presentation

The clinical presentation may be addressed from the standpoint of age of presentation as well as the region in which the cyst is located.

Intracranial arachnoid cysts detected in utero by

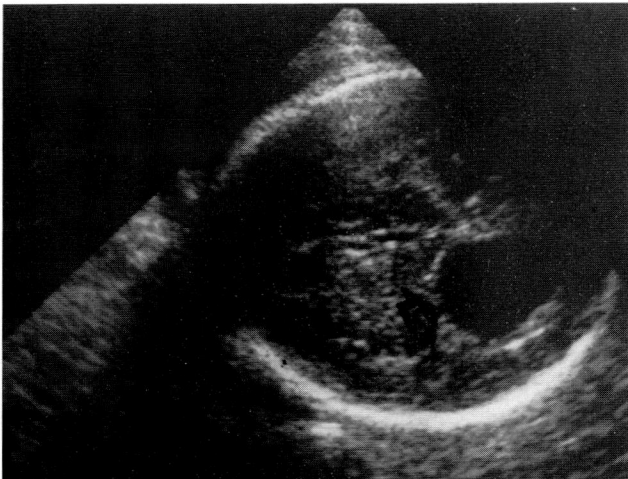

Figure 6–5. Intrauterine cranial ultrasound scan demonstrating a large, rounded, nonechogenic structure off the midline, in the substance of brain parenchyma (arrow no. 5). The remainder of the ventricular system appears normal.

obstetric ultrasonography are commonly misinterpreted as being hydrocephalus (Figs. 6–5 and 6–6). This may lead to erroneous counseling of the parents as well as to errors in intrauterine management. Additional information can be readily obtained by repeating the ultrasonography at a later date, before making a definitive diagnosis. If these studies are not satisfactory, further information may be gained with NMRI, using chloral hydrate to sedate the mother and, through her, the fetus.

Infants commonly present with increasing head size, fullness of the fontanelles, and, in more severe cases, frank signs of intracranial hypertension.[9, 10, 24] In older children, the signs and symptoms include

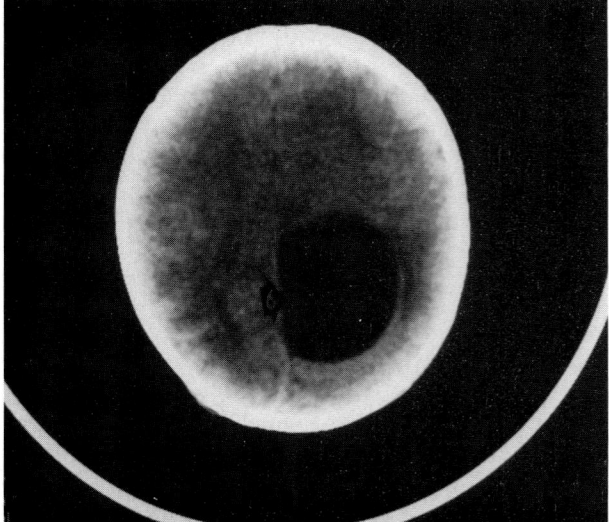

Figure 6–6. Cranial CT scan of the patient in Figure 6–5, at seven months of postuterine life, documenting the extent and location of the arachnoid cyst (arrow no. 6). The child subsequently underwent a cyst-peritoneum shunt.

increasing head size, headaches, seizures, and mental retardation.[9, 10, 24]

Presenting signs and symptoms vary according to the region involved. Posterior fossa cysts most commonly present with increased intracranial pressure from obstructive hydrocephalus.[9, 10, 24] In smaller children, asymmetry of the posterior fossa may be seen, or disproportion in size of the posterior cranium in reference to the anterior cranium may be noted.[9, 10, 24]

Children with supratentorial cysts may present with cranial asymmetry and macrocrania, with varying neurologic signs. In some patients, there may be no neurologic findings whatsoever, but others may present with motor and developmental delay, headaches, seizures, and hemiparesis.[1, 9, 10, 24, 30, 39] Suprasellar arachnoid cysts may create pressure on the optic pathways and then interfere with vision, and optic atrophy may be found.

Sudden, acute neurologic deterioration may occur as the result of three mechanisms: (1) worsening compliance due to mass effect and shifts, or decompensating obstructive hydrocephalus; (2) sudden rupture of the cyst that may occur following even minor head trauma, resulting in a sudden, subdural extra-arachnoid collection of CSF, with mass effect and displacement of structures;[45] and (3) sudden bleeding into the cyst, either spontaneous or induced by trauma.[45]

Neural Imaging

Plain skull radiographs may reveal evidence of intracranial hypertension, with split sutures and erosion of the cranium.[19, 24] With middle fossa arachnoid cysts, there may be rounding and outward bowing and thinning of the temporal squama and forward projection of the greater wing of the sphenoid.[39] Posterior fossa cysts may lead to elevation of the grooves of the transverse sinuses and torcular.[19]

The pathologic anatomy of the cyst and the distortion of the surrounding structures are readily demonstrated on CT. The cysts are usually large, rounded, clearly demarcated structures with the same density as CSF.[1, 19, 39] They are not enhanced following intravenous administration of contrast material.[1, 32] Variations in the CT images are present according to location, and this has been described in detail by Naidich and colleagues.[32] Cysts in the sylvian fissure are frequently trapezoidal or triangular, because of the mesial aspect of the cyst coming into contact with the limen of the insula.[32, 39] Anterior temporal cysts can extend into the orbit via the optic canal, causing local clinical findings.[22] Suprasellar cysts commonly expand in all directions. They may enlarge the sella turcica.[21]

NMRI also readily identifies the cysts because of the CSF-like signal that is obtained from them. NMRI images help to differentiate cysts from brain tumors, as the latter cannot be enhanced with contrast material and are of low density on the CT scan.

Therapy

Arachnoid cysts accompanied by symptoms and mass effect should always receive operative treatment.[1, 24] That is because clinical deterioration may occur in an insidious fashion or, worse, in a sudden catastrophic event resulting from rupture of the cyst or sudden hemorrhage into the cyst.[45]

In many reports, operative therapy has consisted of craniotomy and excision of the cyst wall.[1, 24, 39] However, if neural imaging of the lesion leaves little doubt that one is dealing with an arachnoid cyst, the author agrees with others that the simplest procedure is that of arachnoid-cyst peritoneal shunting with a low-pressure shunt system.[2, 18] Craniotomy for the cyst commonly fails to drain permanently the cyst because of arachnoidal reaction and cyst recurrence and postoperative scar formation.[18, 39] A shunt procedure will then be needed.[18] It is the author's experience that the shunt procedure alone is an intervention that not only is less invasive to the child but also is accompanied by a reduction in cyst size and expansion of the surrounding brain parenchyma.[18]

Outcome

Unrecognized or untreated arachnoid cysts may be associated with a poor outcome resulting from behavior and intellectual problems or motor and developmental delay.[9, 10, 24] On the other hand, normal or superior intelligence may be seen, since usually no other associated cerebral anomaly is present.[30]

Clinical deterioration following cyst drainage may occur as a consequence of insidious unresolved hydrocephalus, which may be present despite successful drainage of the cyst.[18, 24] Therefore, these patients should be followed on an ongoing basis, even though they have received what is considered a successful cyst treatment.

References

1. Anderson FM, Segal D, Caton WL: Use of computerized tomography scanning in supratentorial arachnoid cysts. J Neurosurg 50:333, 1979.
2. Archer CR, Darwish H, Smith K, Jr.: Enlarged cisternae magnae and posterior fossa cysts simulating Dandy-Walker syndrome on computed tomography. Radiology 127:681, 1978.
3. Blackwood W, Corsellis JAN: Greenfield's Neuropathology. Chicago, Year Book Medical Publishers, 1976, pp 377–380.
4. Braun IF, Naidich TP, Leeds NE, et al: Dense intracranial epidermoid tumors. Radiology 122:717, 1977.

5. Campbell JB: Congenital anomalies of the neural axis. Am J Surg 75:231, 1948.
6. Chohan BS, Parmar IPS, Bhatia JN: Anterior orbital meningoencephalocele. Am J Ophthalmol 68:144, 1969.
7. Coty M, Verret S, Langelier R, et al: Intranasal meningoencephalocele with recurrent meningitis. Surg Neurol 12:49, 1979.
8. Davidson S, Small J: Malignant change in an intracranial dermoid. J Neurol Neurosurg Psychiatry 23:176, 1960.
9. Di Rocco C, Caldarelli M, DiTrapani G, et al: Infratentorial arachnoid cysts in children. Child's Brain 8:119, 1981.
10. Di Rocco C, DiTrapani G, Ianelli A: Arachnoid cyst of the IV ventricle and "arrested" hydrocephalus. Surg Neurol 12:467, 1979.
11. Engel R, Buchan GC: Occipital encephaloceles with and without visual evoked potentials. Arch Neurol 30:314, 1974.
12. Galassi E, Tognetti F, Gaist G, et al: CT scan and metrizamide CT cisternography in arachnoid cysts of the middle cranial fossa: Classification and pathophysiological aspects. Surg Neurol 17:363, 1982.
13. Gilmor RL, Kalsbeck JE, Goodman JM, et al: Angiographic assessment of occipital encephaloceles. Radiology 103:127, 1972.
14. Giuffre R, Curatolo P: Cranial dermal sinuses in childhood and adolescence. Neurochirurgia 21:72, 1978.
15. Griffith BH: Frontonasal tumors: Their diagnosis and management. Plast Reconstr Surg 57:692, 1976.
16. Handa J, Okomato K, Sato M: Arachnoid cyst of the middle cranial fossa: Report of bilateral cysts in siblings. Surg Neurol 16:127, 1981.
17. Harrison MJG: Cerebral arachnoid cysts in children. J Neurol Neurosurg Psychiatry 34:316, 1971.
18. Harsh GR, IV, Edwards MSB, Wilson CB: Intracranial arachnoid cysts in children. J Neurosurg 64:835, 1986.
19. Harwood-Nash DC, Fitz CR: Neuroradiology in Infants and Children. St. Louis, The CV Mosby Co., 1976.
20. Karch SB, Urich H: Occipital encephalocele: A morphological study. J Neurol Sci 15:89, 1972.
21. Krawchenko J, Collins GH: Pathology of an arachnoid cyst: Case report. J Neurosurg 50:224, 1979.
22. Krohel GB, Hepler RS: Arachnoidal cyst invading the orbit. Arch Ophthalmol 97:2342, 1979.
23. Luyendijk W: Intranasal encephaloceles: A survey of 8 neurosurgically treated cases. Psychiatr Neurol Neurochir 72:77, 1969.
24. Matson DD: Neurosurgery of Infancy and Childhood. Springfield, IL, Charles C Thomas, 1969.
25. Matsuda M, Hirai O, Munemitsu H, et al: Arachnoid cysts—report of two cases in the interhemispheric fissure and over the cerebral convexity. Neurol Med Chir (Tokyo) 22:71, 1982.
26. McLaurin RL: Parietal cephaloceles. Neurology 14:764, 1964.
27. McLone DG: The subarachnoid space: A review. Child's Brain 6:113, 1980.
28. McLone DG, Bondareff W: Developmental morphology of the subarachnoid space and contiguous structures in the mouse. Am J Anat 142:273, 1975.
29. Mealey J, Jr, Dzenitis AJ, Hockey AA: The prognosis of encephaloceles. J Neurosurg 32:209, 1970.
30. Meche FGA, van der Braakman R: Arachnoid cysts in the middle cranial fossa: Cause and treatment of progressive and non-progressive symptoms. J Neurol Neurosurg Psychiatry 46:1102, 1983.
31. Mikhael M, Mattar A: Intracranial pearly tumors. The roles of computed tomography, angiography, and pneumoencephalography. J Comput Assist Tomogr 2:421, 1978.
32. Naidich TP, McLone DG, Radkowski MA: Intracranial arachnoid cysts. Pediatr Neurosci 12:112, 1985–86.
33. Nakamura S, Wakamatsu K, Tsubokawa T, et al: Sacral epidermoid cyst communicating with the spinal CSF canal. Child's Brain 6:103, 1980.
34. Parnell B, Hendrick EB, Hoffman HJ, et al: Dermoid cysts of the anterior fontanelle. Neurosurgery 10:317, 1982.
35. Rengachary SS: Parasagittal arachnoid cyst: Case report. Neurosurgery 9:70, 1981.
36. Rengachary SS, Watanabe I: Ultrastructure and pathogenesis of intracranial arachnoid cysts. J Neuropathol Exp Neurol 40:61, 1981.
37. Rengachary SS, Watanabe I, Brackett CE: Pathogenesis of intracranial arachnoid cysts. Surg Neurol 9:139, 1978.
38. Rubinstein L: Tumors of the central nervous system. Washington DC, Armed Forces Institute of Pathology, 1972.
39. Sato K, Shimoji T, Yaguchi K, et al: Middle fossa arachnoid cyst: Clinical, neuroradiological, and surgical features. Child's Brain 10:301, 1983.
40. Schachenmayr W, Friede RL: Fine structure of arachnoid cysts. J Neuropathol Exp Neurol 38:434, 1979.
41. Schijman E, Monges J, Cragnaz R: Congenital dermal sinuses, dermoid and epidermoid cysts of the posterior fossa. Child's Nerv Syst 2:83, 1986.
42. Suwanwela C, Chaturaporn H: Fronto-ethmoidal encephalocele. J Neurosurg 25:172, 1966.
43. Suwanwela C, Suwanwela N: A morphological classification of sincipital encephalomeningoceles. J Neurosurg 36:201, 1972.
44. Tandon PN: Meningoencephaloceles. Acta Neurol Scand 46:369, 1970.
45. Tiberin P, Gruzskiewicz J: Chronic arachnoidal cysts of the middle cranial fossa and their relation to trauma. J Neurol Neurosurg Psychiatry 24:86, 1961.
46. Whatmore WJ: Sincipital encephalomeningoceles. Br J Surg 60:261, 1973.

7
CRANIOSYNOSTOSIS

John P. Laurent, M.D.
William R. Cheek, M.D.

Cranial sutures function as hinges for the calvarium, permitting bending during childbirth and expansion as the brain grows. The major sutures (metopic, sagittal, coronal, and lambdoidal) are frequently involved in premature sutural synostosis (Fig. 7–1). The minor sutures (e.g., squamosal) may fuse without the dramatic morphologic changes seen with premature synostosis of the major sutures.

Open cranial sutures permit expansion of the cranial vault to accommodate the rapidly enlarging infant brain. Since brain growth is almost complete by the age of two years, the sutures begin to fuse by the age of three years, with complete fusion occurring by six to eight years of age. The sutures, which are the primary growth sites of the calvarium, separate to permit brain growth and to prevent premature fusion. Premature fusion may occur, however, if fibrous dural bands originating at the base of the calvarium hinder brain growth in a specific direction.[38] Virchow suggested that cranial growth occurs opposite a prematurely synostosed suture, following the path of least resistance, resulting in a skull deformity specific for the suture involved.[40] On occasion, an infant presents at birth with a characteristic skull deformity that suggests an intrauterine cause of premature suture fusion.

Craniosynostosis may cause neurologic damage. Increased intracranial pressure has been documented in children with a single premature fusion.[19] Shillito and Matson[35] reported symptomatic increased intracranial pressure in 2.6 percent of 287 children with sagittal synostosis, further describing papilledema, increased irritability, and separation of other sutures in 41 percent of the children with multiple suture synostoses and in 13 percent of those with sagittal synostosis. These symptoms were absent in children with lambdoidal synostosis.[35] Mental capacity and visual changes are directly related to intracranial pressure. Changes in visual acuity are rare except in oxycephalic children. Binocular vision can be affected by hypertelorism and plagiocephaly. Neuropsychologic problems are more commonly seen in craniodysostoses related to Crouzon's and Apert's diseases.

Routine skull roentgenograms confirm a clinical suspicion of premature sutural synostosis, although clinical acumen most frequently leads to the determination of the suture involved. Electroencephalograms and contrast-enhanced computerized axial tomography (CAT) scans reveal other cerebral abnormalities, and CAT scans of the skull demonstrate prematurely synostosed sutures.[9, 10] Radioisotope bone scanning (technetium-99m, or ^{99m}Tc) confirms questionable synostotic areas.[12]

Early surgical treatment has been advocated for craniosynostosis.[3, 24] The surgical procedure for a child under one year of age is much less extensive than that for an older child but produces the same morphologic results.

Lannelongue in 1890 and Lane in 1892 described the first craniectomies for surgical treatment of craniosynostosis.[16, 17] Surgical techniques for craniosynostosis include resection of portions of the cranium; resection of bone, with replacement and realignment of the cranium; and fragmentation of the calvarium. In a child younger than six months of age, rapid reossification of craniectomy sites

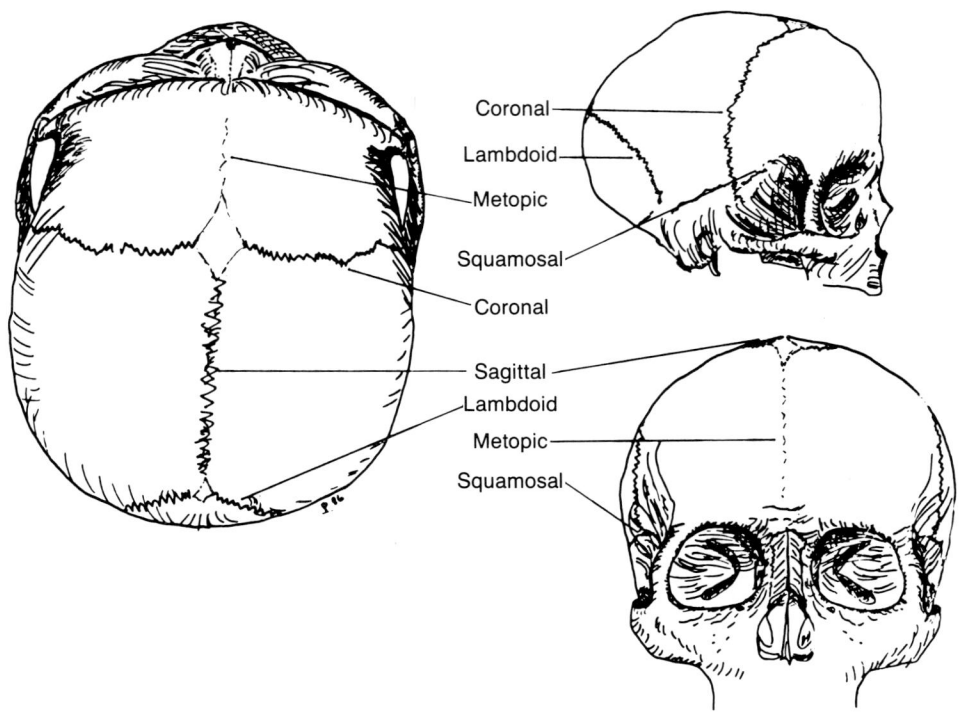

Figure 7–1. Diagram of major cranial sutures.

presents a major problem and may result in a recurrence of the sutural problems or in other defects. Inadequate reossification may require cranioplasty at a later date. The various methods developed to overcome postoperative reossification include the positioning of foreign material between bone edges,[4, 6-8, 36] the application of chemical solutions,[2, 21] and total craniectomy.[31] When reossification is incomplete, craniofacial reconstructive procedures may be considered.[18, 20, 32]

PREMATURE SAGITTAL SYNOSTOSIS

Premature sagittal synostosis accounts for 50 to 60 percent of all craniosynostoses. A male predominance has been noted, and some cases have been found to be of familial origin, suggesting a genetic aberration. Premature sagittal fusion produces a scaphocephalic appearance, with the skull elongated in the anteroposterior plane. Occipital and frontal bones typically expand posteriorly and anteriorly, respectively (Fig. 7–2), with diminution of the biparietal diameter. A prominent ridge is present, extending from the anterior to the posterior fontanelle. Depression of the sagittal suture at its midsection causes a saddle-shaped skull. Facial development is usually normal. There is no association of this condition with other clinical syndromes. Fusion of the sagittal suture appears to have no adverse effect on brain development. The degree of cosmetic abnormality varies, depending on when the premature closure occurred in utero. The most common cosmetic changes are apparent at birth, with both frontal and occipital bossing and a narrow head. Patients less severely affected may have a normal forehead, with the cranial vault pear-shaped from occipital expansion. Part of the suture may be synostosed with relatively little cosmetic effect.

Operative intervention is directed toward releasing the affected suture. The timing of surgery and the goal of achieving morphologic improvement assume major roles in the correction of premature sutural synostosis.

Surgical Procedures

Bilateral Parasagittal Craniectomies (Fig. 7–3). Matson[22] describes bilateral parasagittal craniectomies 1 cm in width, extending beyond both coronal and lambdoidal sutures, in children from eighteen months to three years of age. A single, midline scalp incision extending from in front of the anterior fontanelle to behind the lambda permitted access to the entire sagittal suture. In children younger than 18 months of age, all bony margins were covered with polyethylene film. Occasionally, the transverse craniectomies were connected at the posterior ends of the craniectomy sites. Suboptimal clinical response was seen in 33 percent of the children operated on in the manner just described. Restoration of a normal morphologic appearance was slow and often was not achieved in children over nine months of age.

Single Midline Sagittal Craniectomy (Fig. 7–4). Shillito[34] recommends a single midline sagittal cra-

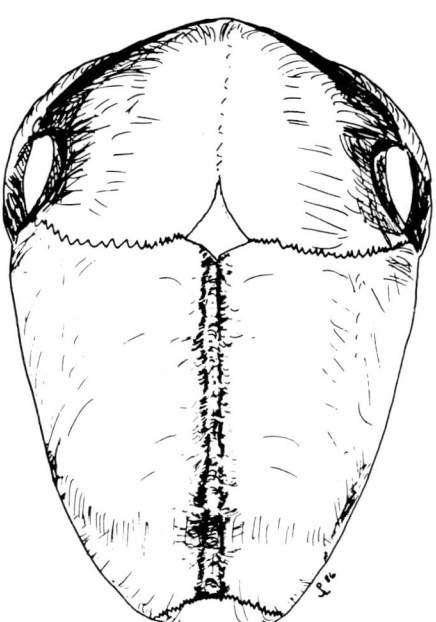

Figure 7–2. Premature sagittal synostosis.

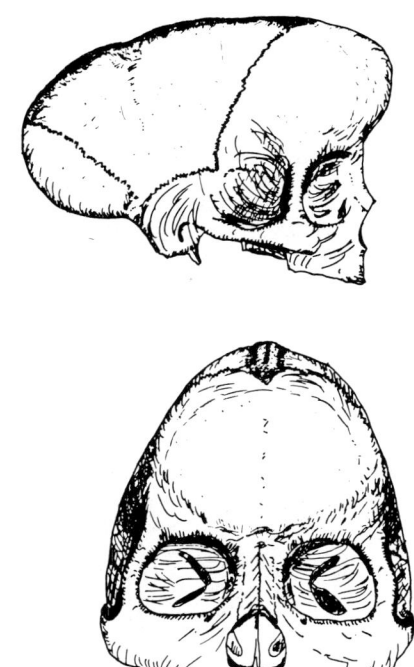

niectomy extending beyond the coronal and lambdoidal sutures, using the same scalp incision as that described by Matson, with the use of polyethylene film on bone edges.[22] Hoffman and colleagues[12] have performed this simple craniectomy in children during the first few months of life, using Silastic film, and report complete correction of the abnormal head shape by six months of age. Beyond these first few months, the use of Silastic film is probably not necessary, depending on the degree of bone maturation apparent during surgery. Restoration of normal vault contour is slow and variable.

A modification of the single midline sagittal craniectomy is used frequently at Texas Children's Hospital (Fig. 7–5). The craniectomy is wider and is done without Silastic interposition. Restoration of normal vault contour is faster and appears to be more reliable.

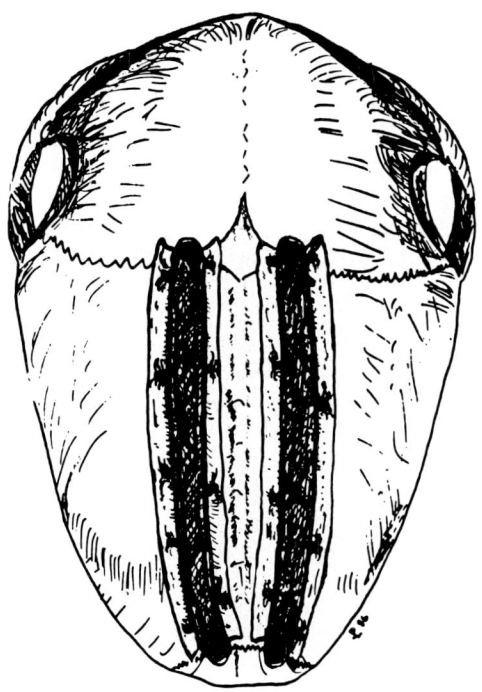

Figure 7–3. Bilateral midline sagittal craniectomy.

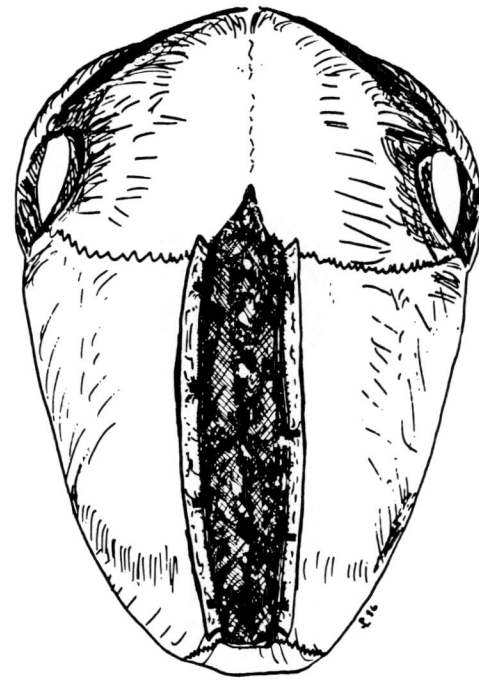

Figure 7–4. Single midline sagittal craniectomy.

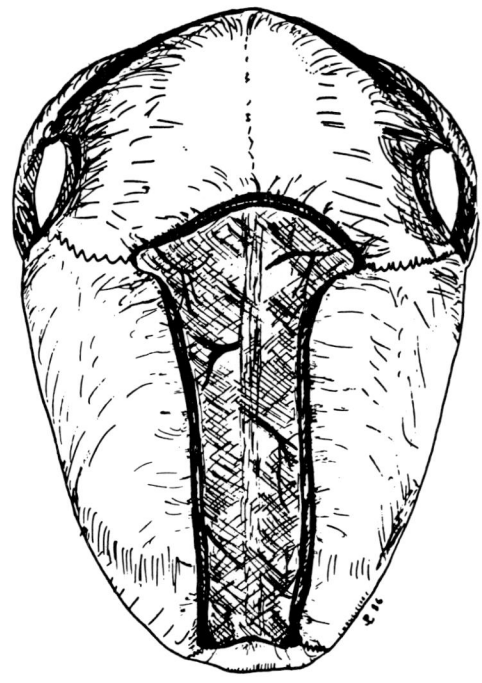

Figure 7–5. Single midline sagittal craniectomy without Silastic film interposition.

Modification of Single Midline Sagittal Craniectomy (Fig. 7–6). Venes and Sayers[39] modified the simple single midline sagittal craniectomy by adding the resection of the bony protuberances of the bregma and occiput. A portion of bone over the torcular was left intact. Normal skull contour became evident three to six weeks after surgery. The report made no mention of increased complications from this more extensive procedure.

"Clam Shell" Operation (Fig. 7–7). Stein and Schut[37] described an operative procedure to release the parietotemporal bone plates through a coronal incision. A wide sagittal craniectomy was extended laterally at the coronal and lambdoidal sutures to the squamosal sutures on both sides. The temporoparietal bone was mobilized from the dura by a greenstick fracture at its base. Optimal clinical results were seen in 96 percent of the children so treated when they were less than two months of age.

Vertex Craniectomy (Fig. 7–8). Epstein and associates[5] combined the operative procedure described by Stein and Schut with that of Venes and Sayers. The craniectomy was extended beyond the coronal and lambdoidal sutures, with a wide parasagittal craniectomy via a sagittal scalp incision preferred. The radical bone excision prevented bony re-fusion, without the need for Silastic implants. Blood loss during this operation was reported to have been considerable, and transfusion was begun at the time of the sagittal incision. The results in this study were excellent.

Modification of Vertex Craniectomy (Fig. 7–9). Olds and coworkers[29] modified the Epstein procedure by extending the craniectomy 2.5 cm down the coronal and lambdoidal suture lines. No interpositional material was used. The wide craniectomy prevented reunion of the bone edges. Widening of the biparietal diameter was usually apparent intraoperatively. Little morbidity was seen with this procedure.

The Pi (π) Procedure (Modification of Bilateral Parasagittal Craniectomies) (Figs. 7–10 through 7–12). Jane and colleagues[13] modified the bilateral parasagittal craniectomies of Matson through a co-

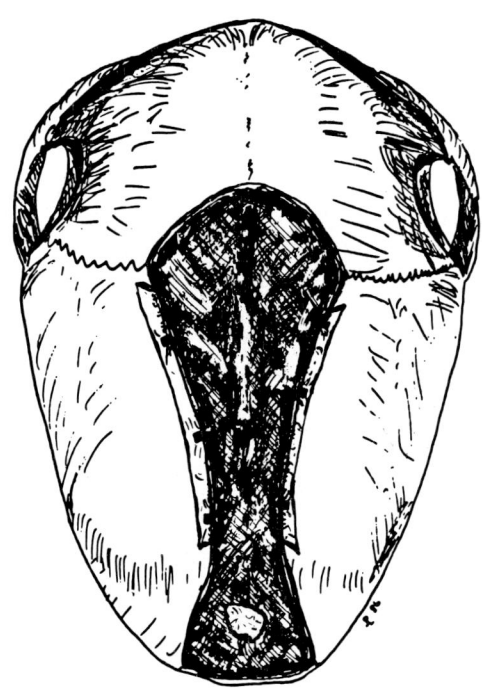

Figure 7–6. Modified single midline sagittal craniectomy.

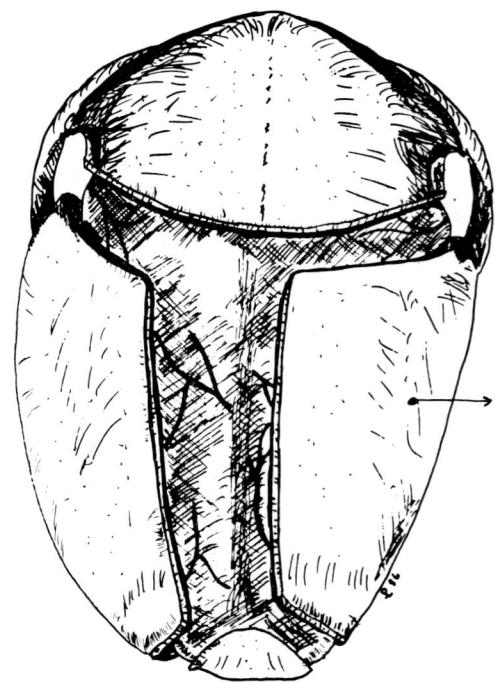

Figure 7–7. "Clam shell" craniectomy.

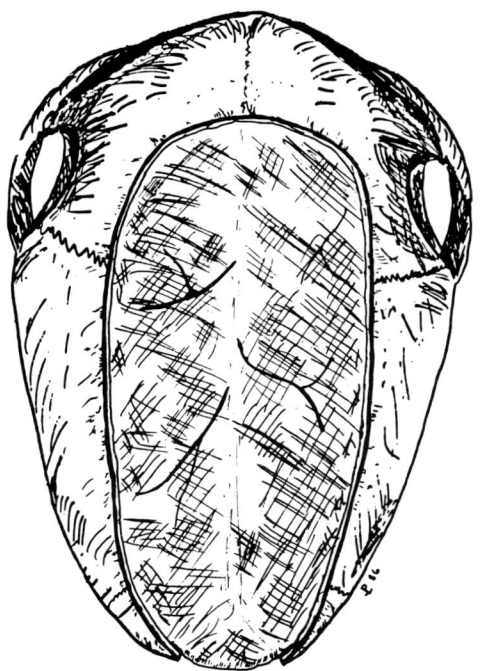

Figure 7–8. Vertex craniectomy.

ronal scalp incision, using bilateral parasagittal craniotomies with bilateral coronal craniectomies, extending as far as possible into the temporal region. Dura was separated from the frontal bone, coronal suture, and sagittal suture. The anteroposterior diameter of the vault was foreshortened via a stay suture through the frontal and parietal bones, and the reduced bone flap was replaced (Fig. 7–10). All the children so operated on were under eight months of age. In these patients, a normal appearance was achieved immediately after surgery. No postoperative cranial defect was present. Jane emphasized that the surgically induced changes in dura tension, especially in the coronal suture attachment, favored the normal calvarial growth that Moss advocated.[25, 26]

Vollmer and associates[41] modified the pi (π) procedure for variants of sagittal synostosis, describing alternative surgical methods to correct frontal bossing and prominent occipital bulging. In cases of frontal bossing, a major portion of the frontal bone was removed (Fig. 7–11), the anteroposterior diameter foreshortened, and bone replaced. With occipital prominence, a reverse pi (π) was employed (Fig. 7–12). Both Jane and Vollmer emphasize the lack of craniectomy defect as well as the immediate morphologic results and avoidance of synthetic materials. The effect on intracranial pressure was not mentioned in either description.

"Keyhole" Operation (Fig. 7–13). Albright[1] reported an operative procedure that incorporated both the Venes and Sayers technique and the pi (π) technique of Jane and associates. The children, who were less than six months of age at the time of surgery, attained normal head appearance by one to two years postoperatively. The children whose occiputs were not prominent underwent only sagittal and wedge craniectomies. Correction of the narrow biparietal diameter of sagittal synostosis was apparent immediately following surgery. None of

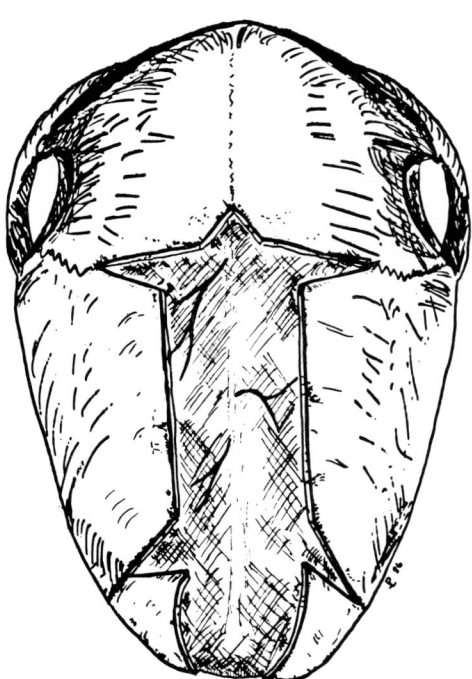

Figure 7–9. Modified vertex craniectomy.

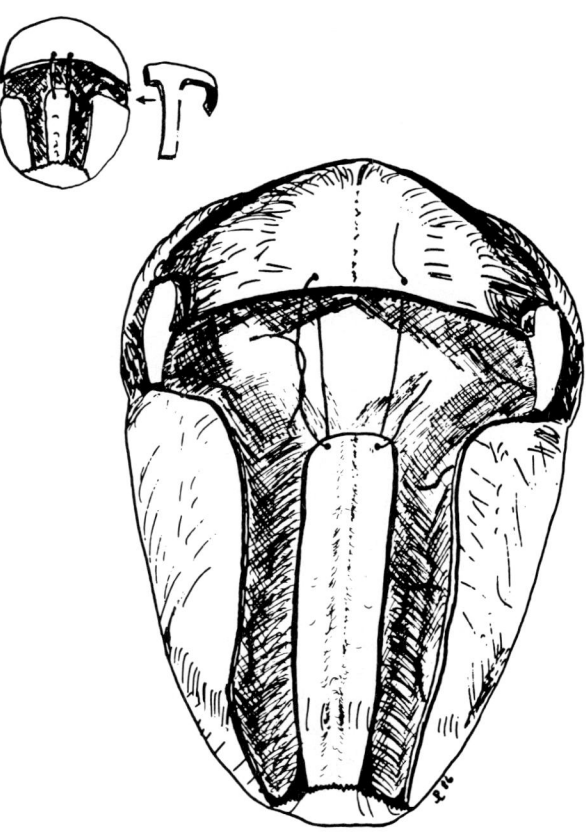

Figure 7–10. Pi (π) craniectomy.

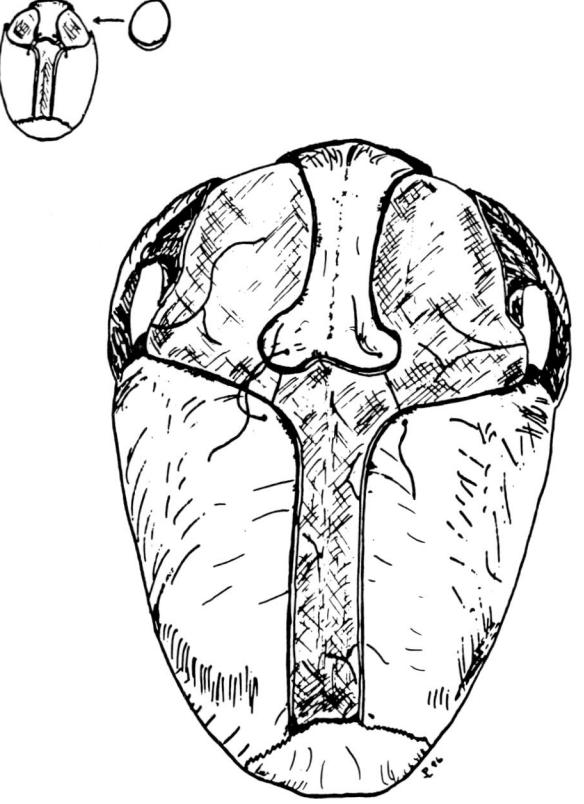

Figure 7–11. Modified pi (π) craniectomy for frontal prominence.

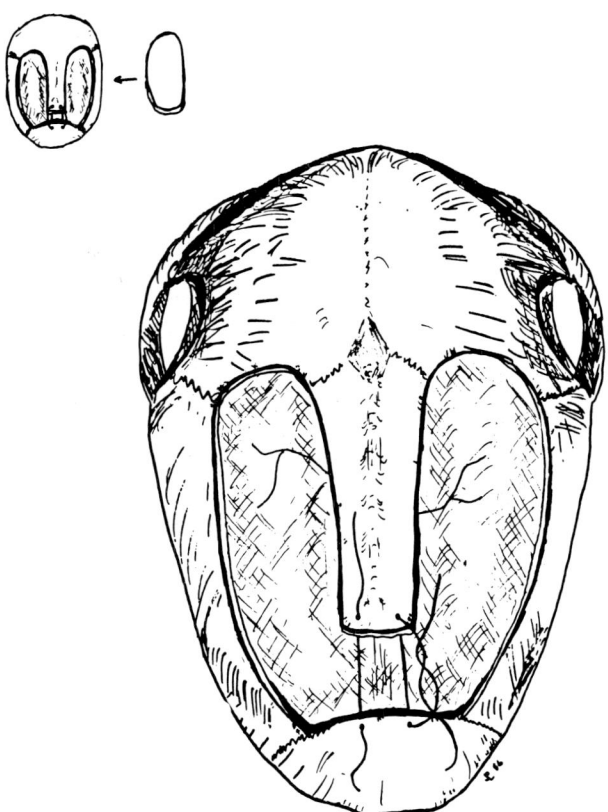

Figure 7–12. Modified pi (π) craniectomy for occipital prominence.

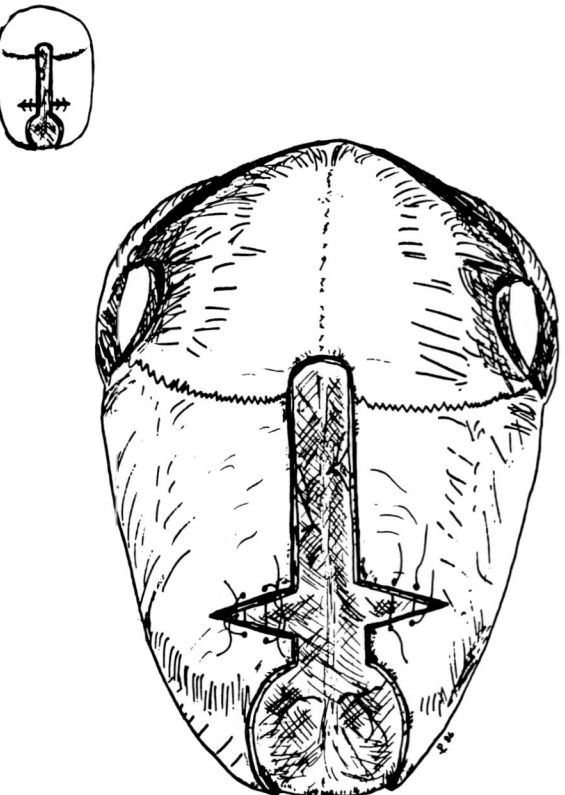

Figure 7–13. "Keyhole" craniectomy.

these children presented with severe frontal bossing.

Transposition with Frontal Bossing (Fig. 7–14). Marchac and Renier[18, 20] describe a procedure done on an older child with extensive frontal deformity. A posterior bicoronal skin incision exposed the occipital bones and the forehead. Transposition of four or five bony segments tilted backward and lowered the forehead, elevated the central cranial vault, permitted advancement of the occipital bone, and enlarged the transverse diameter. The procedure is especially useful in older children when other sutures are synostosed.

Vault Remodeling with Normal Forehead (Fig. 7–15). Rougerie and coworkers[32] report a technique for reconstruction of the cranial vault in children with sagittal synostosis and a normal forehead. Some modifications were made in the procedure for children under six months of age (i.e., the bony plates were left in place) (Fig. 7–15B). In older children, the bony plates were advanced, elevated, and maintained in position by bone wedges (Fig. 7–15A). The temporal bone was mobilized by a greenstick fracture at its base. Reossification of the craniectomy sites can occur rapidly in children less than six months of age, with resultant variability in correction of the deformity with this technique.

Discussion

Premature sagittal synostosis results in a progressive deformity of the skull. Surgical treatment

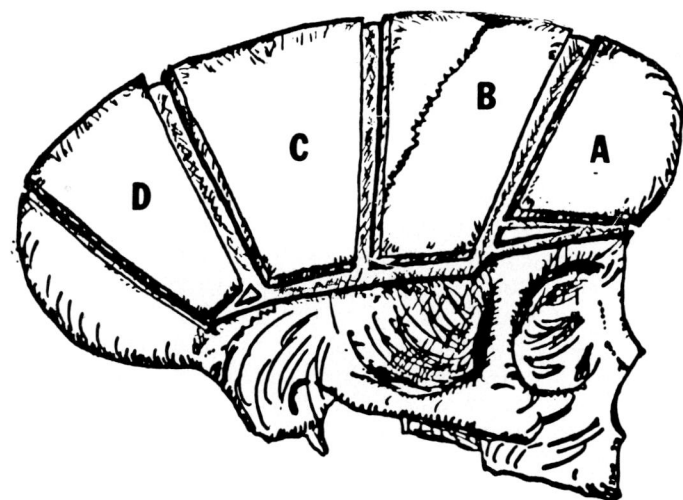

Figure 7–14. Transposition craniectomies.

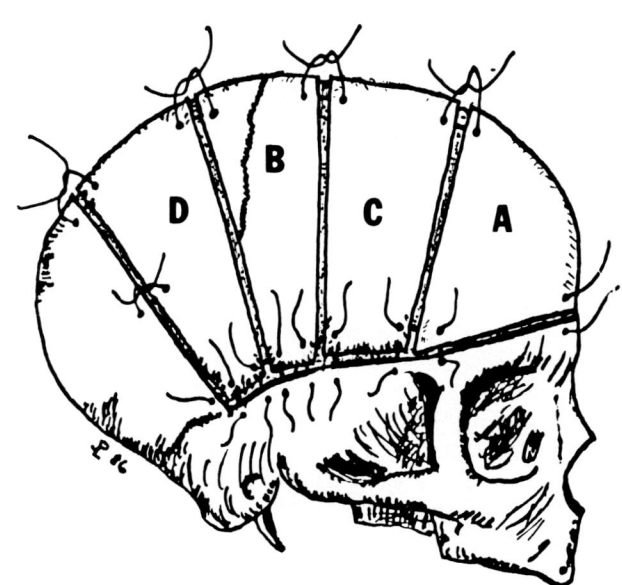

Figure 7–15. Vault remodeling with normal forehead.

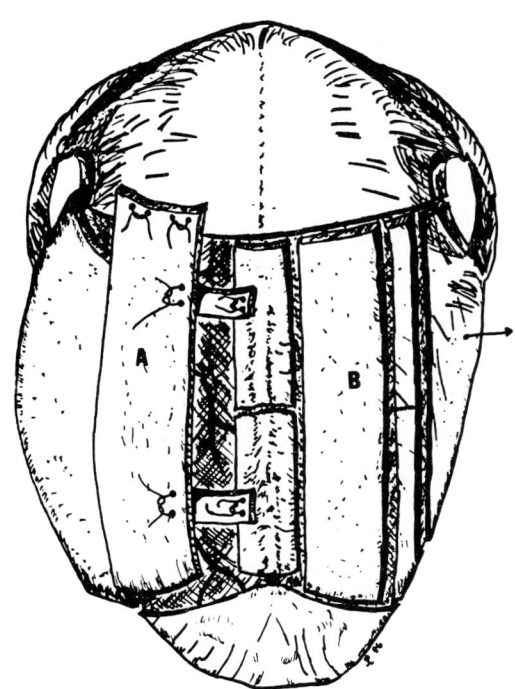

should correct the morphologic appearance without exposing the child to increased risks. In many surgical procedures, the morphologic changes are immediate (Figs. 7–7 and 7–9 through 7–15A), while other procedures facilitate progressive improvement in the child's appearance (Figs. 7–3 through 7–6 and 7–8). The problems of frontal and occipital prominence have prompted the development of specific surgical techniques for the correction of these variants of premature sagittal synostosis (Figs. 7–6, 7–10 through 7–12, 7–14, and 7–15). Parents often become quite anxious about extensive craniectomies, fearing that subsequent minor head trauma may badly injure the child. Some procedures offer more protection for the cranium and may help allay some of these fears (Figs. 7–3, 7–4, and 7–10 through 7–15).

Surgical correction of premature synostosis done by 12 weeks of age ensures a more satisfactory morphologic change (Figs. 7–3 through 7–9 and 7–13). This schedule takes advantage of rapid brain growth and skull expansion, while reossification potential remains optimal, thus avoiding future cranioplasty. Although children older than six months of age may require a more extensive procedure (Figs. 7–10 through 7–12, 7–14, and 7–15) to obtain the same morphologic results, the problem of reossification is precluded.

Strip craniectomy, with or without interpositional material, is the procedure chosen by many pediatric neurosurgeons to treat premature sagittal synostosis (Figs. 7–3, 7–4, 7–6). The extension of the craniectomies either across or along other suture lines has been advocated (Figs. 7–7 through 7–13). Morcellation, total craniectomy, and circular craniotomy have been abandoned. Craniofacial techniques for premature sagittal synostosis have been described since 1972; these are extensive procedures and should be reserved for the older child.

Because better cosmetic results are achieved with simpler surgical techniques in a child less than 12 weeks of age, the problem of premature regrowth of bone has arisen and has been handled in a variety of ways. Various materials have been interposed between bone edges to delay regrowth. Silastic sheets (Figs. 7–3, 7–4, and 7–6) have replaced tantalum and polyethylene; some problems encountered with Silastic sheets include extrusion, infection, persistent cranial defect, and subgaleal fluid collection.[3, 14, 24] Methyl methacrylate interposition has been associated with skin erosion.[36]

Chemical retardant (Zenker's solution) applied to the bone edges has had adverse effects.[23, 30] Larger craniectomies obviate the need for foreign material but increase parental anxiety about subsequent minor head trauma. The authors have not seen injury problems with large craniectomies in the child less than 12 weeks of age; the patient could wear a protective helmet until reossification is complete.

Cosmetic results from the surgical correction of premature sagittal synostosis are improved when (1) the child is under 12 weeks of age, (2) the use of interpositional material is avoided by extending craniectomies wide to include sutures other than the sagittal, (3) more extensive craniofacial techniques are used in children over six months of age, and (4) the simplest appropriate surgical technique, taking the age of the child into account, reduces anesthesia and surgery time, blood loss, and temperature problems.

PREMATURE LAMBDOIDAL SYNOSTOSIS

Premature lambdoidal synostosis is rare. Fewer than 5 percent of children with craniosynostosis at Texas Children's Hospital had lambdoidal involvement. Premature fusion of this suture causes flattening of the back of the head on the involved side, with a prominent sutural ridge (Fig. 7–16). The ear

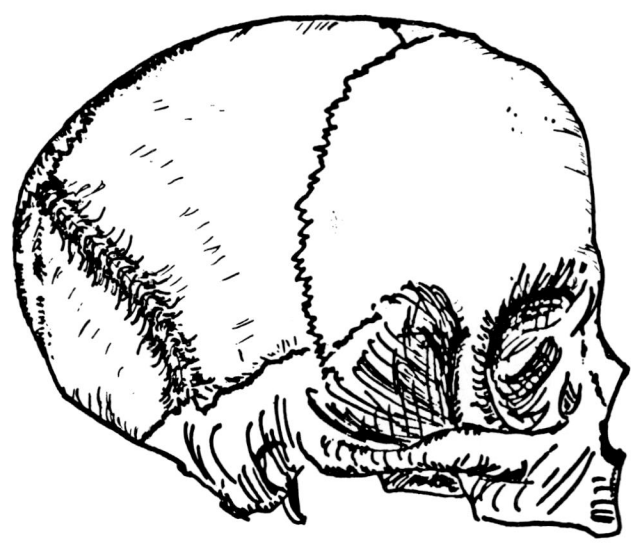

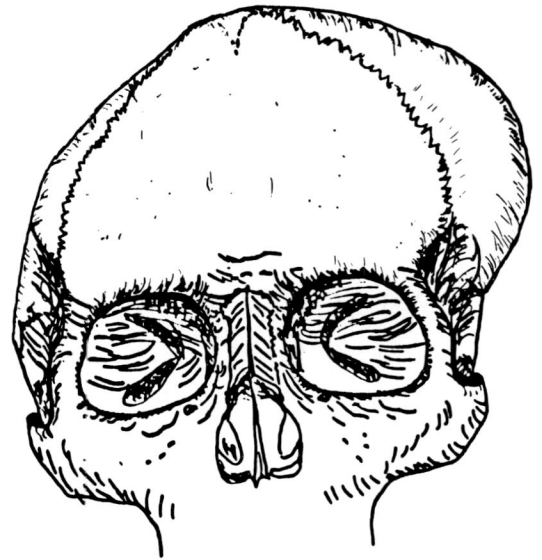

Figure 7–16. Premature lambdoidal synostosis.

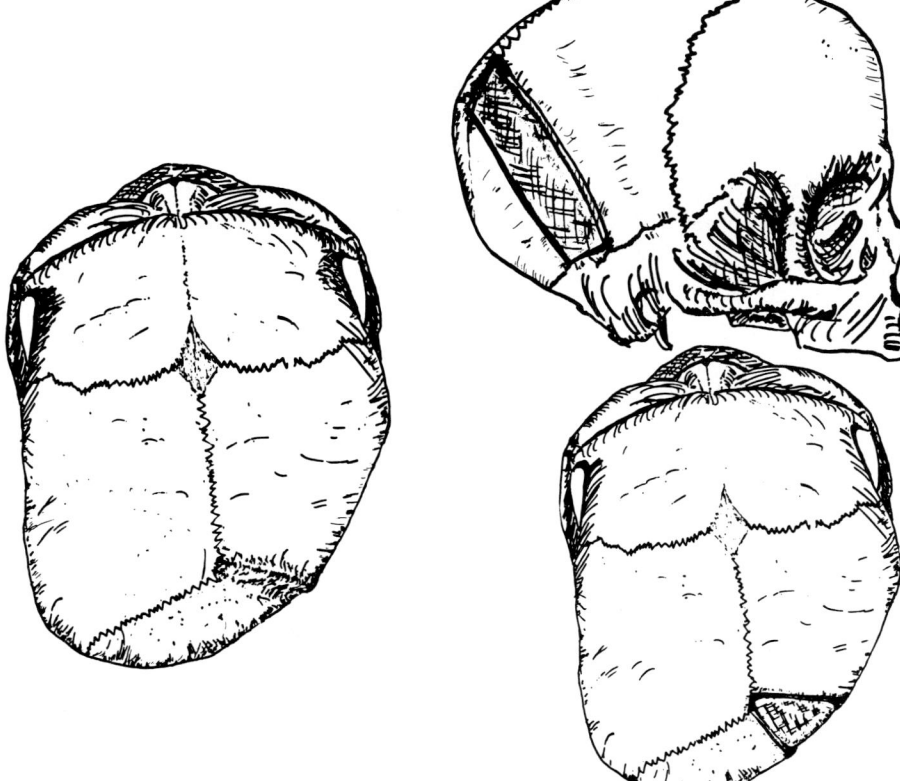

Figure 7–17. Simple linear craniectomy.

on the affected side will be more superiorly and anteriorly positioned. Partial lambdoidal synostosis may not cause severe flattening and, in females, may not require surgical correction.

Positional flattening of the occipital area must be differentiated from premature lambdoidal synostosis. Parental repositioning of the child's head during sleep often corrects the problem. A sclerotic margin at the edge of the suture seen on radiologic examination can confirm the diagnosis of synostosis.[11] Hoffman and colleagues[12] advocate bone scans to confirm the diagnosis, with no sclerotic activity evident when the suture is closed, and hyperactivity apparent when the suture is in the process of closing.[27]

Surgical Procedures

Simple linear craniectomy of the lambdoidal suture, from the sagittal suture to the asterion, gives good morphologic results in the child younger than 12 weeks (Fig. 7–17). In the older child, *split-thickness autologous calvarial transfers* give better results than does simple linear craniectomy (Fig. 7–18).

PREMATURE MULTIPLE SUTURAL SYNOSTOSES

Children with multiple premature sutural synostoses require early surgical release of all the major sutures. Hoffman and associates[12] reported that 7.6 percent of their patients with craniosynostoses had multiple sutures involved, predominantly sagittal and lambdoidal. Shillito and Matson[35] reported that 41 percent of children with multiple premature sutural synostoses showed clinical and radiologic evidence of increased intracranial pressure.

All the major sutures can be exposed by an ear-to-ear incision posterior to the coronal suture. In the child without hydrocephalus, a simple, wide, linear craniectomy of the involved sutures, without interpositional material, should be carried out as soon as the diagnosis of multiple premature sutural synostoses is made (Fig. 7–19).

Hydrocephalus complicates and accentuates premature sutural synostoses. Hydrocephalus and premature closure of all major sutures except the metopic (craniotelencephalic dysplasia) create severe forward frontal expansion (Figs. 7–20 and 7–21). Hydrocephalus and premature closure of all major sutures except the sagittal (kleeblattschädel, or cloverleaf skull) create a grotesque vertex expansion with wide bitemporal diameter (Figs. 7–22 and 7–23). In utero diagnosis of kleeblattschädel has been made with ultrasonography.[33] Those children with hydrocephalus and major premature sutural synostosis develop increased intracranial pressure, with concomitant neurologic results. Correction of the morphologic appearance by wide sutural craniectomies and treatment of the hydrocephalus may prevent institutionalization of these children. Rapid reossification is a problem, and, should the sutures

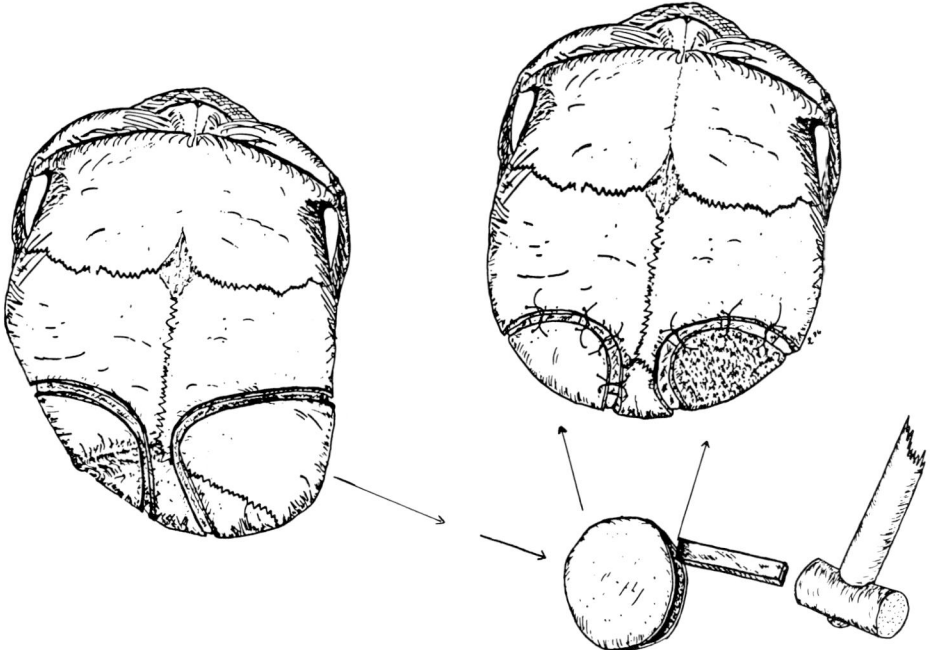

Figure 7–18. Split-thickness autologous calvarial transfer.

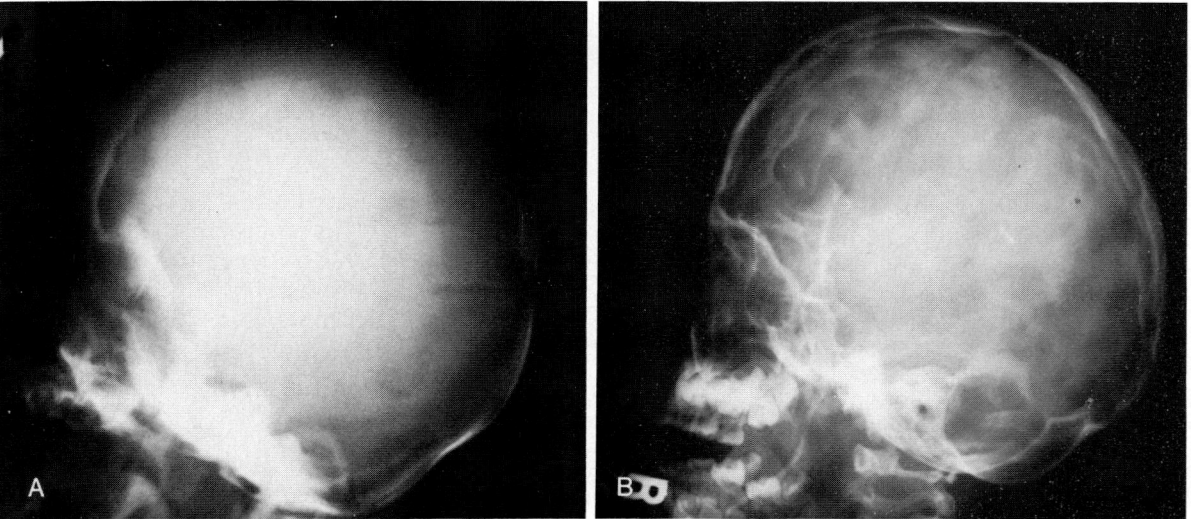

Figure 7–19. Roentgenograms of premature multiple sutural synostoses in a two-month-old (A) and recurrence of synostoses at three years of age (B).

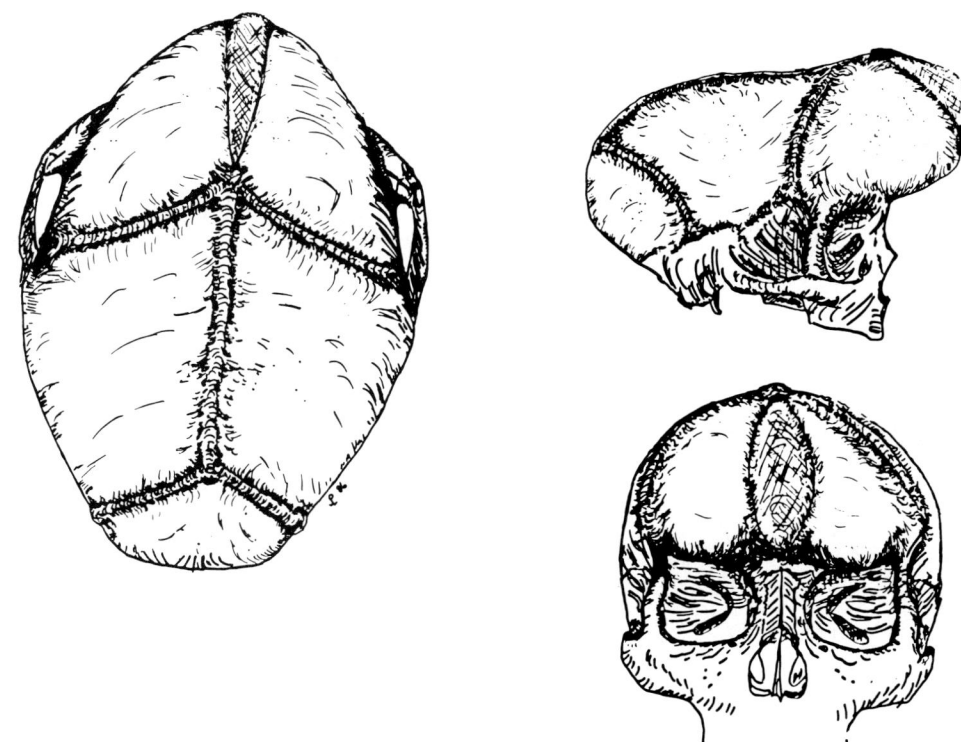

Figure 7–20. Craniotelencephalic dysplasia.

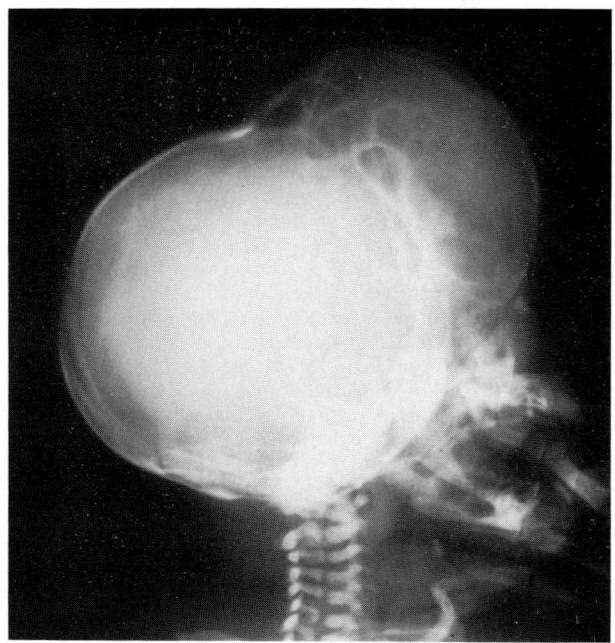

Figure 7–21. Roentgenogram of craniotelencephalic dysplasia.

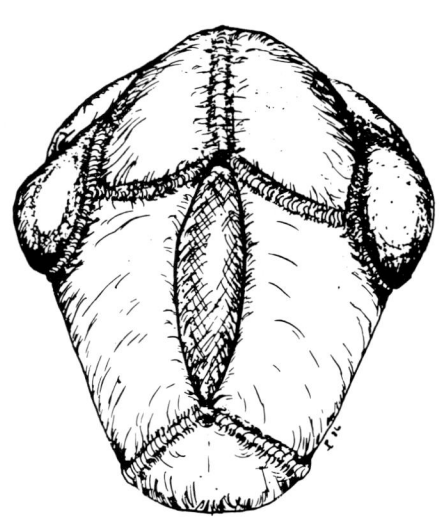
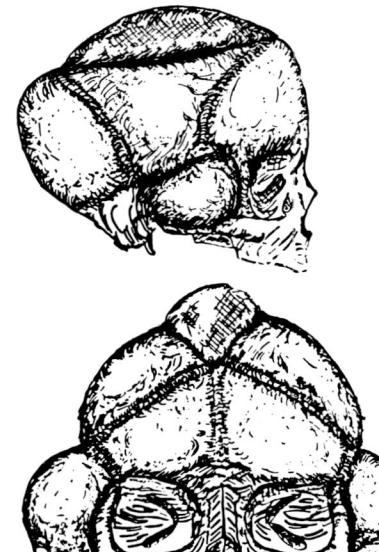

Figure 7–22. "Cloverleaf skull."

re-fuse, reoperation is necessary to prevent neurologic changes (Fig. 7–19).[28]

SUMMARY

The presence of sagittal, lambdoidal, and multiple sutural craniosynostoses causes typical morphologic changes to the calvarium. Compensatory brain growth along the path of least resistance is probably an epiphenomenon secondary to dural banding from the base of the skull occurring in utero. Release of the affected suture at an early age (less than 12 weeks) has been shown to yield favorable cosmetic results. In patients older than one year of age, surgical correction by linear craniectomies has little morphologic effect. Craniofacial techniques in children with delayed diagnosis of craniosynostosis (older than six months) have produced more favorable results. With the greater awareness of most clinicians of the various forms of craniosynostosis, early diagnosis is usually possible, and the simpler linear craniectomy is the procedure of choice.

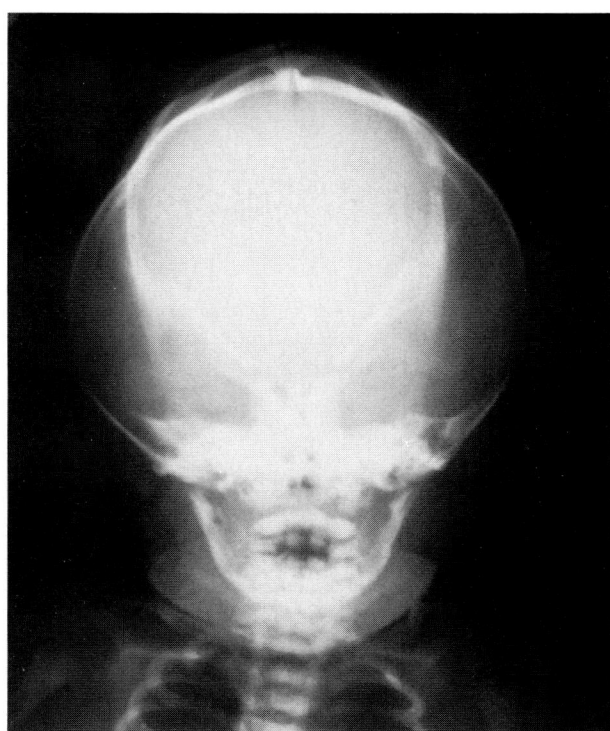

Figure 7–23. Roentgenogram of "cloverleaf skull."

References

1. Albright AL: Operative normalization of skull shape in sagittal synostosis. Neurosurgery 17:329, 1985.
2. Anderson FM: Treatment of coronal and metopic synostosis: 107 cases. Neurosurgery 8:143, 1981.
3. Anderson FM, Geiger L: Craniosynostosis: A survey of 204 cases. J Neurosurg 22:229–240, 1965.
4. Davis CH, Alexander E, Kelly DL: Treatment of craniosynostosis. J Neurosurg 30:630, 1969.
5. Epstein N, Epstein F, Newman G: Total vertex craniectomy for treatment of scaphocephaly. Child's Brain 9:309, 1982.
6. Fender FA: Device for isolation of bone edges in craniectomy for craniostenosis. J Neurosurg 16:347, 1979.
7. Foltz EL, Loeser JD: Craniosynostosis. J Neurosurg 43:48, 1975.
8. Fowler FO, Ingraham FD: A new method for applying polyethylene film to the skull in treatment of craniosynostosis. J Neurosurg 14:584, 1957.
9. Furuya Y, Edwards MSB, Alpers CE, et al: Computerized tomography of cranial sutures. Part 1. Comparison of suture anatomy in children and adults. J Neurosurg 61:53, 1984.
10. Furuya Y, Edwards MSB, Alpers CE, et al: Computerized tomography of cranial sutures. Part 2. Abnormalities of

sutures and skull deformity in craniosynostosis. J Neurosurg 61:59, 1984.
11. Hinton DR, Becker LE, Muakkassa KF, et al: Lambdoid synostosis. Part I: The lambdoid suture: Normal development and pathology of "synostosis." J Neurosurg 61:333, 1984.
12. Hoffman HJ, Hendrick EB, Munro IR: Craniosynostosis and craniofacial surgery. In: McLaurin RL (ed): Pediatric Neurosurgery. New York, Grune & Stratton, 1982, pp 121–156.
13. Jane JA, Edgeton MT, Futrell JW, et al: Immediate correction of sagittal synostosis. J Neurosurg 49:705, 1978.
14. Keener EB: Experimental observations on the use of rubber in treatment of craniosynostosis. J Neurosurg 15:642, 1958.
15. Kokick VG, Moffett BC, Cohen MM: The cloverleaf skull anomaly: An anatomic and histologic study of two specimens. Cleft Palate J 19:89, 1982.
16. Lane LC: Pioneer craniectomy for relief of the mental imbecility due to premature sutural closure and microcephalus. JAMA 18:29, 1892.
17. Lannelongue M: Craniectomy for microcephalus. Compta-Renda Academie de Sciena 110:1382, 1890.
18. Marchac D, Renier D: The forehead, treatment of craniofacial synostosis. Ann Chir Plast 24:121, 1979.
19. Marchac D, Renier D: Functional aspects of craniosynostosis. In: Marchac D, Renier D (eds): Craniofacial Surgery for Craniosynostosis. Boston, Little, Brown & Company, 1982, pp 9–16.
20. Marchac D, Renier D: Scaphocephaly. In: Marchac D, Renier D (eds): Craniofacial Surgery for Craniosynostosis. Boston, Little, Brown & Company, 1982, pp 88–92.
21. Marlin AE, Brown WE, Huntington HW, et al: Effect of dural application of Zenker's solution on the feline brain. Neurosurgery 6:45, 1980.
22. Matson DD: Craniosynostosis. In: Matson DD, Ingraham FD (eds): Neurosurgery of Infancy and Childhood. Springfield, IL, Charles C Thomas, 1969, pp 138–143.
23. McComb JG, Withers GJ, Davis RL: Cortical damage from Zenker's solution applied to the dura mater. Neurosurgery 8:68, 1981.
24. McLaurin RL, Matson DD: Importance of early surgical treatment of craniosynostosis. Review of 36 cases treated during the first six months of life. Pediatrics 10:637, 1952.
25. Moss ML: The pathogenesis of premature cranial synostosis in man. Acta Anat 37:351, 1959.
26. Moss ML: Functional anatomy of cranial synostosis. Child's Brain 1:22, 1975.
27. Muakkassa KF, Hoffman JH, Hinton DR, et al: Lambdoid synostosis. Part 2: Review of cases managed at The Hospital for Sick Children 1972–1982. J Neurosurg 61:340, 1984.
28. Norwood CW, Alexander E, David CH, et al: Recurrent and multiple suture closures after craniectomy for craniosynostosis. J Neurosurg 41:715, 1974.
29. Olds MV, Storrs B, Walker ML: Surgical treatment of sagittal synostosis. Neurosurgery 18:345, 1986.
30. Pawl RP, Sugar O: Zenker's solution in the surgical treatment of craniosynostosis. J Neurosurg 36:604, 1972.
31. Powiertowski H, Matlosz Z: Treatment of craniostenosis by a method of extensive resection of the vault of the skull. In: Proceedings of Third International Congress on Neurosurgery. Surg Excepta Med Internat Cong Series 110:834, 1965.
32. Rougerie J, Derome P, Anquez L: Craniostenosis and abnormal craniofacial deformities. Neurochirurgie 18:429, 1972.
33. Salvo AF: In utero diagnosis of kleeblattschädel. Prenat Diagn 1:141, 1981.
34. Shillito J: A new cranial suture appearing in the site of craniectomy for synostosis. Radiology 107:83, 1973.
35. Shillito J, Matson DD: Craniosynostosis: A review of 519 surgical patients. Pediatrics 41:829, 1968.
36. Simmons DR, Peyton WT: Premature closure of the cranial sutures. J Pediatr 31:528, 1947.
37. Stein C, Schut L: Management of scaphocephaly. Surg Neurol 7:153, 1977.
38. Venes JL, Burdi A: Proposed role of the orbitosphenoid in craniofacial dysostosis. In: Humphreys RP (ed): Concepts in Pediatric Neurosurgery, Vol. 5. New York, S Karger Publishing, 1985, pp 126–135.
39. Venes JL, Sayers MP: Sagittal synostectomy. J Neurosurg 44:390, 1976.
40. Virchow R: Uber den cretinismus, namentlich in franken und uber pathologische schadelformen. Verh Phys Med Ges Wurzburg 2:230, 1851.
41. Vollmer DG, Jane JA, Park TS, et al: Variants of sagittal synostosis: Strategies for surgical correction. J Neurosurg 61:557, 1984.

8
CRANIOFACIAL SURGERY

Harold J. Hoffman, M.D.
Corey Raffel, M.D., Ph.D.

The modern era of craniofacial surgery was ushered in by Paul Tessier in 1967, when he initially described his radical method for repairing the head and face in patients with craniofacial dysostosis.[34] Since then, the field of craniofacial surgery has rapidly expanded, so that many centers throughout the world are now performing corrective surgery on patients with disorders of the craniofacial skeleton.

In craniofacial dysostosis, there is deformity of the skull secondary to craniosynostosis in association with a deformity of the face. The deformities that occur with craniosynostosis have been recognized for centuries; the term oxycephaly was introduced in ancient Greece by Galen. The familial types of multiple suture synostoses were described in the early 1900's by Apert[2] and by Crouzon.[7]

Uncorrected craniofacial dysostosis results in severe abnormalities of skull shape, but other complications may also arise. Of male patients at the Royal Institute for the Blind in Copenhagen surveyed in 1913, one fifth (21 percent) had oxycephaly.[21] In a series of 171 patients with craniosynostosis, Bertelsen[4] reported that 26 had papilledema, 33 had optic atrophy, 85 had headaches, 39 had epilepsy, and 42 had below-normal intelligence. The lowered IQ frequently seen in patients with oxycephaly is now ascribed to raised intracranial pressure, hydrocephalus, or both (Fig. 8–1). The authors believe that early recognition of the problem and prompt surgical management can result in excellent cosmetic and intellectual results.

RATIONALE FOR EARLY SURGERY

Influenced by the rapidly growing brain of infancy, the skull increases in size by adding bone at the suture lines. The brain grows most dramatically during the first year of life, increasing from 335 gm to 925 gm (Fig. 8–2). By two years of age, most brain growth has occurred, and fibrous union of the sutures begins. The sutures are largely ossified by eight years of age. If a suture closes prematurely, irregular growth of the skull occurs, to make room for the growing brain. Compensatory growth occurs according to Virchow's law (i.e., parallel to the fused suture).

In order to take advantage of the skull-molding effects of the growing brain and to avoid the maximal defect that results if distorted skull growth continues through this period, the repair of craniofacial dysostosis is ideally undertaken during the first few weeks of life in patients presenting early. By removing the pathologic suture and allowing normal skull growth to occur under the influence of the growing brain, the best possible cosmetic results are achieved (Fig. 8–3). The authors have seen correction of the midface anomaly in brachycephaly and separation of the orbits in hypotelorism secondary to metopic synostosis under these circumstances. Furthermore, the early correction of a frontonasal encephalocele prevents this lesion from producing a progressive hypertelorism, as happens when therapy is delayed. Others have also stressed

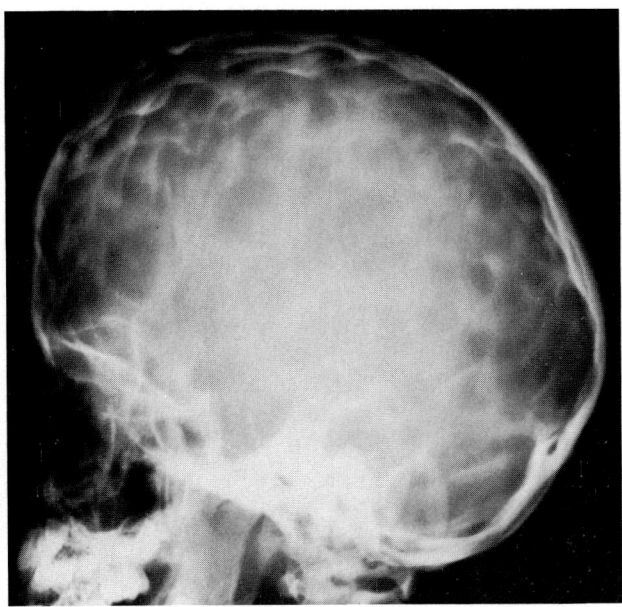

Figure 8–1. Lateral skull x-ray film of untreated older child with Crouzon's syndrome shows "beaten copper" skull secondary to multiple suture synostoses and raised intracranial pressure.

the improvement in cosmetic results obtained by early surgery.[29]

CRANIOFACIAL DYSMORPHISM

When calvarial synostosis is associated with abnormalities of the facial skeleton, the condition is termed craniofacial dysmorphism. In the past, these patients were socially ostracized and rarely were treated. This resulted in many patients with mental retardation secondary to hydrocephalus and with blindness secondary to raised intracranial pressure. These patients rarely married, and thus, the genetically determined craniofacial dysmorphic states were rare. The incidence is now increasing, as patients are receiving corrective surgery early in life, leading to an absence of sequelae and a pleasing cosmetic outcome.

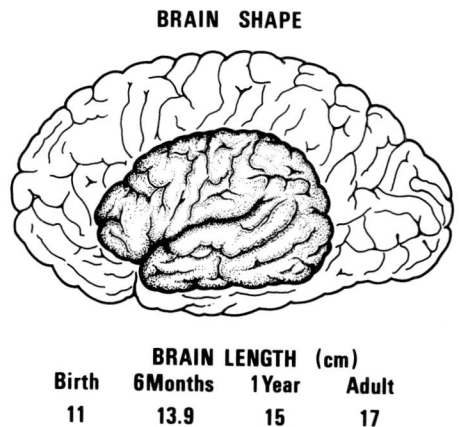

Figure 8–2. Diagrammatic depiction of change in brain size and shape with increasing age.

The most common of the craniofacial dysmorphic states is *Crouzon's syndrome*, characterized in its later stages by multiple suture synostoses, maxillary hypoplasia, and shallow orbits with proptosis.[7] The inheritance pattern is autosomal dominant; about two thirds of cases are familial, and one third sporadic.[3] Penetrance is either complete or extremely high. Mental deficiency occurs in about 10 percent of untreated patients and is usually associated with hydrocephalus. This figure is lower in patients treated with early corrective surgery.[19] The most common skull abnormality is brachycephaly, related to bilateral coronal synostosis with associated frontosphenoidal and frontoethmoidal closure. Frequently, other sutures are involved.

Apert's syndrome is also characterized by multiple suture synostoses and midface hypoplasia, associated with symmetric syndactyly of the hands and feet and, frequently, proptosis.[2] The facial anomalies may be asymmetric. The inheritance pattern is autosomal dominant, but most cases are sporadic. However, familial cases with almost complete penetrance have been reported.[5] The syndactyly usually involves the secondary third and fourth digits of the hands and feet. Progressive calcification and fusion of the bones of the hands, feet, and cervical spine occur with advancing age.[31] Mental retardation and hydrocephalus are more commonly seen in Apert's syndrome than in Crouzon's syndrome.

Pfeiffer's syndrome consists of craniosynostosis, broad thumbs and great toes, and variable partial soft-tissue syndactyly of the hands and feet. The inheritance pattern is autosomal dominant, with high penetrance and variable expression. Associated mental retardation and hydrocephalus are rare.

Saethre-Chotzen syndrome is characterized by craniosynostosis, low-set frontal hairline, facial asymmetry, ptosis, deviated nasal septum, and variable

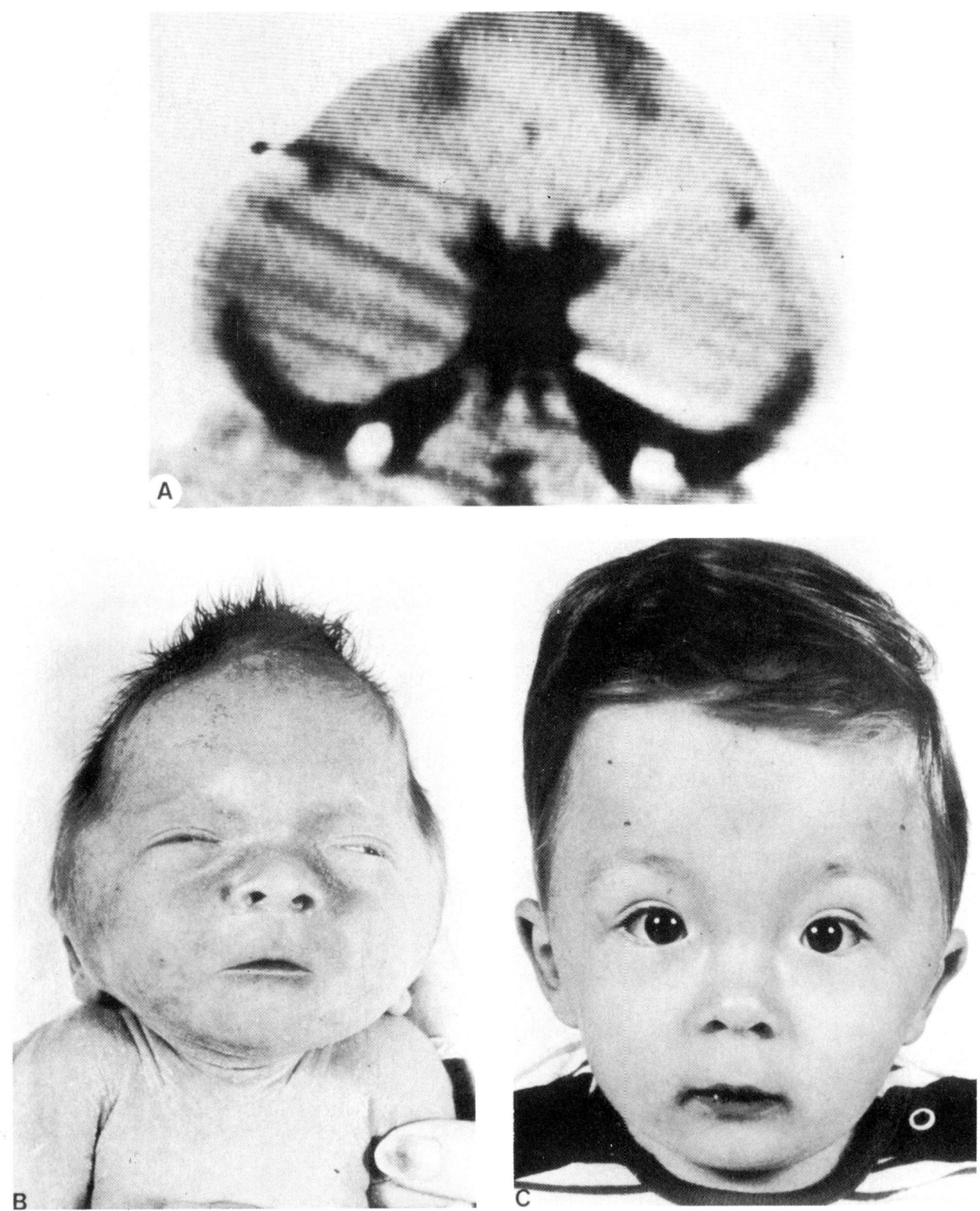

Figure 8–3. *A,* CT scan of neonate with characteristic trilobed skull of kleeblattschädel. *B,* Photograph of same infant. *C,* Same child at age two years, having undergone bilateral lateral canthal advancement and morcellation craniotomy at age two weeks. Not only does this child appear normal, but also he is functioning with a normal IQ.

Table 8–1. CONDITIONS ACCOMPANYING CLOVERLEAF SKULL MALFORMATION

Condition	Striking Features	Frequency of Cloverleaf Skull	Etiology
Monogenic Syndromes			
Apert's syndrome	Craniosynostosis, ocular proptosis, downslanting palpebral fissures, midface deficiency, symmetric syndactyly of all four limbs minimally involving digits 2–4, other anomalies	Rare	Autosomal dominant
Carpenter's syndrome	Craniosynostosis, mental deficiency, short stature, preaxial polysyndactyly of feet, brachydactyly, clinodactyly with variable syndactyly of hands, congenital heart defects, other anomalies	Rare	Autosomal recessive
Crouzon's syndrome	Craniosynostosis, ocular proptosis, midface deficiency	Probably uncommon; uncertain whether sporadic cloverleaf skull cases represent Crouzon's syndrome	Autosomal dominant
Pfeiffer's syndrome	Craniosynostosis, ocular proptosis, midface deficiency, broad thumbs and great toes, variable soft-tissue syndactyly of other digits, other anomalies	Common	Uncertain. All cases with cloverleaf skull are sporadic; Pfeiffer's syndrome without cloverleaf skull has autosomal dominant inheritance; may be etiologically heterogeneous
Thanatophoric dwarfism	Large skull; short limbs; short, thick limb bones; curved radii and fibulae; narrow thoracic cage	Common	Uncertain. Consanguinity and affected siblings have been reported, suggesting autosomal recessive inheritance; however, all cases without cloverleaf skull have been sporadic to date; may be etiologically heterogeneous
Environmentally Induced Syndromes			
Amniotic band syndrome	Ring constrictions and amputations of digits or limbs, variably distal syndactyly, facial clefts, encephalocele, other abnormalities	Rare	Amniotic bands
Iatrogenic malformation	Cloverleaf-shaped skull	Rare	Bilateral subtemporal decompression procedures in hydrocephalus
Unknown Genesis			
Isolated malformation	Cloverleaf-shaped skull	All cases	Uncertain. All cases sporadic to date
Various incompletely delineated syndromes with unique patterns	Cloverleaf-shaped skull with various anomalies such as bony ankylosis of limbs, unilateral anophthalmia, patent ductus arteriosus, Meckel's diverticulum, polydactyly, micropenis, cryptorchidism, other anomalies	?	Uncertain. Etiologically heterogeneous but poorly delineated group of disorders to date

(With permission from Cohen MM: Genetic perspectives on craniosynostosis and syndromes with craniosynostosis. J Neurosurg 47:886–898, 1977.)

brachydactyly and partial soft-tissue syndactyly, especially of the second and third fingers. The inheritance pattern is autosomal dominant, with high penetrance and variable expression. Hydrocephalus and mental retardation are rare.

Carpenter's syndrome includes craniosynostosis, preaxial polysyndactyly of the feet, brachydactyly, clinodactyly and variable soft-tissue syndactyly of the hands, short stature, and obesity. The inheritance pattern is autosomal recessive. One third of patients have an associated congenital heart defect. Mental deficiency is common and is not clearly related to hydrocephalus.

Kleeblattschädel, or *cloverleaf skull syndrome*, is a rare form of craniofacial dysostosis resulting in a characteristic trilobar skull configuration.[19] This deformity can be seen in association with either Crouzon's syndrome or Apert's syndrome. In the past, the condition was largely regarded as a curiosity, and the patients were frequently institutionalized.[6, 28] Modern craniofacial surgery carried out early in infancy can restore these patients to a normal appearance and normal intellectual function (Fig. 8–3).[26, 38, 42]

Numerous other genetically determined syndromes that include craniosynostosis as a feature have been described and are referred to in Table 8–1.[5]

CLINICAL EVALUATION

Clinical evaluation of the child with suspected synostosis is the most reliable guideline to establishing the diagnosis. The common combinations of suture fusion cause characteristic changes in head shape. The presence of synostosis can be confirmed by plain skull x-ray films. Radionuclide bone scanning after intravenous injection of technetium-99m (^{99m}Tc) methylene diphosphonate demonstrates decreased uptake along the closed suture, a useful study in questionable cases. Currently, computed tomography (CT) scanning is the examination of choice for evaluating patients with suspected synostosis. Not only are characteristic changes seen at the site of synostosis and in the shape of the skull, but also algorithms for three-dimensional reconstruction of the skull are available as an aid to planning surgical repair of the deformity.[12, 15, 24]

CORONAL SYNOSTOSIS

Coronal synostosis is the second most common single-suture synostosis, accounting for about 18 percent of cases at the Hospital for Sick Children.[16] Bilateral coronal synostosis is a common finding in patients with the inherited craniofacial dysmorphic syndromes listed in Tables 8–1 and 8–2. In these syndromes, premature closure of the frontoethmoidal and frontosphenoidal sutures is associated with the bilateral coronal synostosis.[33] This combination of multiple suture synostoses is tantamount to closure of a ring around the anterior end of the skull (Fig. 8–4). This results in severe limitation of anterior cranial fossa growth, with compensatory skull growth in the middle fossa. The anterior extent of the temporal lobes may actually be in front of the frontal lobes. Because growth of the midface is determined by growth of the floor of the anterior fossa to which it is attached, midface hypoplasia is a frequently associated anomaly in the craniofacial dysmorphic states (Fig. 8–5). The inhibited growth of the anterior cranial fossa and midface lead to shallow orbits and to progressive proptosis.

Patients with unilateral coronal synostosis present with a characteristic appearance (Figs. 8–6 and 8–7). The forehead on the involved side is flattened or concave; the contralateral forehead bulges out. The eye on the involved side is higher than its counterpart. The ipsilateral cheek is flattened, and the nose deviates away from the stenotic suture.

If both coronal sutures have closed prematurely, the forehead above both eyes is flattened. The anterior fossae are foreshortened, and the midface becomes progressively hypoplastic. The orbits are small, and progressive proptosis frequently occurs.

Surgical Repair

Early in infancy, the procedure of lateral canthal advancement[18] adequately deals with both unilateral and bilateral coronal synostoses. This procedure begins with a frontal craniotomy. An osteotomy through the floor of the anterior fossa, just behind the supraorbital margin, frees the supraorbital margin from adjacent structures. The pterion and sphenoid wing extending to the superior orbital fissure are removed. The lateral extent of the supraorbital margin is then advanced to a normal position and is secured in this position with a strut of bone that is fastened to the Silastic-edged parietal bone posteriorly. Thus, the open, artificial basal skull suture is continuous with the artificial coronal suture. The growing frontal lobe is then allowed to move the forehead and the attached face into a normal position (Figs. 8–8 and 8–9).

If unilateral coronal synostosis is treated with a lateral canthal advancement before six months of age, a perfectly normal appearance results. However, in the patient older than six months of age, the forehead can be restored to a normal appearance, but the nose tends to remain deviated away from the side of the closed suture.

In the case of craniofacial dysostosis with involvement only of the coronal sutures, the procedure of bilateral lateral canthal advancement done early in infancy allows for normal cranial and facial growth in more than 50 percent of the patients (Fig. 8–10).

After six months of age, brain growth slows down, and more radical procedures become necessary.

In 1979, Marchac and Renier described their technique of "floating forehead" as a method of treating the older infant with craniofacial dysostosis.[23] In this procedure, the entire supraorbital region is removed as a single supraorbital bar. The supraorbital bar is then fixed to the face only at the root of the nose and at the malar bones. They feel that this technique allows the growing brain to continue to push the forehead forward.

Although the floating forehead technique is an excellent technique in the older infant, it cannot be done before the metopic suture has fused sufficiently to allow removal of the entire supraorbital region as a single bar. Frequently, in the young neonate, the metopic suture is widely split and does not allow for this technique. In such situations, the procedure of lateral canthal advancement is preferable.[18]

In the older child with craniofacial dysmorphism who has not had an adequate repair in infancy, a radical craniofacial repair must be undertaken, as

Table 8-2. SYNDROMES WITH CRANIOSYNOSTOSIS

Syndrome	Striking Features	Frequency of Craniosynostosis	Etiology
Chromosomal Syndrome			
5p+ syndrome	Variable CNS anomalies, dolichocephaly, craniosynostosis, mental deficiency, respiratory difficulties, renal or ureteral malformations, short first toes, phenotype not completely delineated at present	?	Trisomy for most of the short arm of chromosome 5
7p− syndrome	Craniosynostosis and variable anomalies; phenotype not completely delineated at present	Apparently common	Deletion of short arm of chromosome 7
13q− syndrome	Microcephaly, lobar holoprosencephaly, trigonocephaly, craniosynostosis, mental deficiency, microphthalmia, iris coloboma, retinoblastoma, malformed ears, micrognathia, hypoplastic thumbs, imperforate anus, hypospadias, cryptorchidism, congenital heart defects	8/44	Deletion of long arm of chromosome 13
Monogenic Syndromes			
Apert's syndrome	Craniosynostosis, proptosis, downslanting palpebral fissures, strabismus, ocular hypertelorism, midface deficiency, highly arched palate, complete symmetric syndactyly of hands and feet minimally involving digits 2–4	Almost all cases	Autosomal dominant
Armendares syndrome	Craniosynostosis, microcephaly, retinitis pigmentosa, ptosis of the eyelids, malformed ears, micrognathia, highly arched palate, clinodactyly, simian creases, short stature	Apparently common	Probably autosomal or X-linked recessive
Baller-Gerold syndrome	Craniosynostosis, radial aplasia, absent or hypoplastic carpal bones and preaxial digits	Apparently common	Probably autosomal recessive
Berant's syndrome	Craniosynostosis involving sagittal suture, radioulnar synostosis	Apparently common	Probably autosomal dominant
Carpenter's syndrome	Craniosynostosis, mental deficiency, preaxial polysyndactyly of the feet, variable soft-tissue syndactyly with brachymesophalangy of the hands, displacement of patellae, genua valga, congenital heart defects, short stature, obesity	All reported cases	Autosomal recessive
Christian's syndrome I	Craniosynostosis, microcephaly, ocular hypertelorism, down-slanting palpebral fissures, cleft palate, arthrogryposis	Apparently common	Autosomal recessive
Christian's syndrome II	Craniosynostosis involving metopic suture, ocular hypertelorism, epicanthal folds, down-slanting palpebral fissures, C2–3 fusion, hemivertebrae, anomalous ears, clinodactyly, simian creases, foot abduction, imperforate anus, short stature	Apparently common	X-linked semidominant
Craniofacial dyssynostosis	Craniosynostosis involving lambdoidal and posterior sagittal suture and variably the coronal suture, prominent forehead, ocular hypertelorism, frequent Spanish ancestry	All known cases	? Autosomal recessive
Crouzon's syndrome	Craniosynostosis, shallow orbits with proptosis, strabismus, midface deficiency	Almost all cases	Autosomal dominant
Elejalde's syndrome	Craniosynostosis, swollen face, epicanthic folds, ocular hypertelorism, hypoplastic nose, malformed ears, redundant neck tissue, gigantism at birth, short limbs, polydactyly, omphalocele, lung hypoplasia, cystic renal dysplasia, sponge kidney, redundant connective tissue in skin and many viscera, proliferation of perivascular nerve fibers	Apparently common	Autosomal recessive
FG syndrome	Variable growth problems, disproportionately large head circumference, mental deficiency, congenital hypotonia, high narrow palate, imperforate anus, sacral dimple, partial 2–3 syndactyly of feet, and various other findings including craniosynostosis and frontal bossing	Apparently uncommon	X-linked
Frontonasal dysplasia	Ocular hypertelorism, cranium bifidum occultum, widow's peak, broad nasal root, flat nasal tip or bifid nose, notching or colobomas of nostrils, and median cleft lip in variable combinations; occurrence of many low-frequency anomalies including craniosynostosis	Uncommon	Etiologically heterogeneous, probably representing many poorly delineated entities; some cases are consistent with autosomal-dominant inheritance
Gorlin-Chaudhry-Moss syndrome	Craniosynostosis, midface deficiency, hypertrichosis, down-slanting palpebral fissures, upper eyelid colobomas, patent ductus arteriosus, hypoplastic labia majora	Apparently common	Probably autosomal recessive

Table continued on following page

Table 8–2. SYNDROMES WITH CRANIOSYNOSTOSIS *Continued*

Syndrome	Striking Features	Frequency of Craniosynostosis	Etiology
Monogenic Syndromes *Continued*			
Hootnick-Holmes syndrome	Frontal bossing, dolichocephaly, craniosynostosis involving sagittal suture, ocular hypertelorism, strabismus, preaxial and postaxial polysyndactyly of hands, preaxial polysyndactyly of feet	?	Probably autosomal dominant
Lowry's syndrome	Craniosynostosis, prominent eyes, strabismus, highly arched or cleft palate, fibular aplasia, talipes equinovarus, simian creases	Apparently common	Probably autosomal recessive
Pfeiffer's syndrome	Craniosynostosis, proptosis, strabismus, ocular hypertelorism, down-slanting palpebral fissures, midface deficiency, broad thumbs and great toes, mild cutaneous syndactyly of fingers and toes (variable)	All known cases	Autosomal dominant
Saethre-Chotzen syndrome	Craniosynostosis, facial asymmetry, low-set frontal hairline, ptosis of the eyelids, deviated nasal septum, variable brachydactyly and cutaneous syndactyly especially of the second and third fingers, normal thumbs and great toes	All known cases	Autosomal dominant
Summitt's syndrome	Craniosynostosis, strabismus, variable symmetrical syndactyly of hands and feet from partial to complete with clinodactyly, normal-sized thumbs and great toes, genua valga, obesity	Apparently common	Probably autosomal recessive
Washington's syndrome I	Craniosynostosis involving the sagittal suture, short fourth and fifth metacarpals	Apparently common	Probably autosomal recessive
Washington's syndrome II	Craniosynostosis, midface hypoplasia, lack of extension of the distal interphalangeal joints	Apparently common	Probably autosomal recessive
Weiss's syndrome	Craniosynostosis, medially deviated great toes, altered tarsal morphogenesis, mild syndactyly, wide variability of craniofacial involvement	Apparently common	Autosomal recessive
Teratogenically Induced Syndromes			
Aminopterin syndrome	Craniosynostosis, hypoplasia of cranial and facial bones, low-set ears, cleft palate, micrognathia, hypodactyly of feet, mild syndactyly of hands	Apparently common	Aminopterin or methotrexate during pregnancy
Sporadic, Incompletely Delineated Syndromes			
Andersen-Pindborg syndrome	Craniofacial dysostosis, ectodermal dysplasia, short stature	?	?
Antley-Bixler syndrome	Trapezoidocephaly, deformed ears and nose, elongated hands and feet, radiohumeral synostosis, digit contractures	?	?
Fairbanks's syndrome	Craniosynostosis, proptosis, short stature, brachydactyly, failure of tooth eruption	?	? (two sporadic cases known)
Hall's syndrome	Craniosynostosis and Turner-like phenotype	?	?
Hermann's syndrome I	Craniosynostosis, mental deficiency, hypoplastic supraorbital ridges, bitemporal flattening, ocular hypertelorism, ear anomalies, micrognathia, partial soft-tissue syndactyly of fingers 2–4, absent toes	?	?
Hermann's syndrome II	Craniosynostosis, microbrachycephaly, mental deficiency, anomalous ears, cleft lip and palate, symmetric limb reduction defects with absent fingers 4 and 5, short forearms, valgus positioning of the hands, ankylosis at knees, and varus positioning of feet	?	?
Idaho syndrome I	Craniosynostosis, scaphocephaly, strabismus, mental deficiency, congenital heart defect, umbilical hernia, complete anterior dislocation of tibia and fibula, talipes equinovarus, camptodactyly of fingers 2–5, deviation of fingers to ulnar side, proximally placed thumbs	?	?
Idaho syndrome II	Craniosynostosis, scaphocephaly, mental deficiency, down-slanting palpebral fissures, beaked nose, micrognathia, small low-set posteriorly angulated ears, preauricular tags, long neck, sloping shoulders, narrow thorax, pectus carinatum, winging of scapulae, cubitus valgus	?	?
Pederson's syndrome	Craniosynostosis, exostoses of the skull, premature exfoliation of deciduous teeth, linear verrucous nevi of neck, scaly patches on hands	?	?

Table 8-2. SYNDROMES WITH CRANIOSYNOSTOSIS Continued

Syndrome	Striking Features	Frequency of Craniosynostosis	Etiology
Teratogenically Induced Syndromes Continued			
Sakati's syndrome	Craniosynostosis, disproportionately small face, anomalous ears, patches of alopecia with atrophic skin, short limbs, polysyndactyly of feet, polydactyly of hands, congenital heart defect	?	?
Waardenburg's craniosynostosis syndrome	Craniosynostosis, hydrophthalmos, down-slanting palpebral fissures, cleft palate, micrognathia, low-set ears, malposed clavicles, contractures at elbows and knees, soft-tissue syndactyly of fingers 2-4, absent distal phalanx of thumb with absent nail, double nail with bifid terminal phalanx on second fingers, clinodactyly of fingers 4 and 5, hammertoes, ambiguous external genitalia, patent ductus arteriosus	?	?
Wisconsin syndrome	Craniosynostosis, mental deficiency, up-slanting palpebral fissures, microtia, short fourth metatarsals	?	? (two sporadic cases known)

(With permission from Cohen MM: Genetic perspectives on craniosynostosis and syndromes with craniosynostosis. J Neurosurg 47:886–898, 1977.)

described by Tessier.[36] The procedure begins with a tracheotomy. If there is some degree of hydrocephalus, it is useful to insert a lumbar drain to allow escape of cerebrospinal fluid (CSF). When the patient has an indwelling diversionary CSF shunt, this is not necessary. Mannitol, 20 percent in a dose of 2 gm/kg, is given to provide adequate brain shrinkage. Blood and fluid loss are carefully monitored during the procedure, with adequate replacement being carried out.

A bicoronal scalp incision, well behind the coronal suture and extending down to the ears bilaterally, is used. The periosteum is incised and carried down into the orbits with the scalp flap. The lacrimal sac is identified and dissected free from the orbital wall. Then, the periosteum is elevated from the lateral orbital wall, inferior orbital rim, and the zygoma.

The entire frontal bone, back to the coronal suture, is removed in one segment. The inferior frontal osteotomy is then extended horizontally to include the temporal bone and is continued in a step-by-step fashion inferiorly, toward the base of the skull. This outlines a posterior slot in the temporal bone, which guides the subsequent advancement of the supraorbital margin and allows maintenance of bony contact.

Horizontally, the osteotomy extends into the lateral orbital wall, then continues through the orbital roof and across the nasion. Once this is done bilaterally, it is possible to remove the supraorbital bar in one piece.

At this point, one has an excellent view of the dura along the floor of the anterior fossa, and thus, any dural leaks incurred during the removal of bone can be easily repaired. Frequently, with craniofacial dysostosis, there are numerous stalactites of bone protruding up from the floor of the anterior fossa, and many of these patients have undergone previous attempts at surgical correction as well. Consequently, dural lacerations are common during craniofacial repair. It is absolutely imperative that all these dural tears be adequately sealed, to avoid postoperative rhinorrhea, which is a dreaded complication.

The maxilla is advanced with a Lefort 3 osteotomy. The root of the nose is sectioned horizontally into the medial orbital wall; the osteotomy is then continued along the medial wall behind the lacrimal sac to the inner third of the orbital floor. The lateral wall of the orbit is split in a sagittal plane, and the osteotomy is continued into the orbital floor. The osteotomy is then extended to the malar bone, and the maxilla is advanced and fixed in position by interdental wiring. Consequently, the patient must be old enough to have primary dentition. If there are any abnormalities of the nasal structure, a rhinoplasty can be done. The advancement of the forehead can be as much as 20 to 30 mm in these children, and consequently, bone grafts (split skull) must be taken to fill in the defects created by the advancement. The frontal bone flap is then replaced (Figs. 8–11 and 8–12).

Since this procedure allows free communication between cranial cavity, face, and mouth, there is very significant risk of infection. Prophylactic antibiotics are used, and the wound is profusely irrigated with Betadine solution (10 percent povidone-iodine; manufactured by Purdue, Frederide Co., 123 Sunrise Avenue, Toronto, Canada).

TRIGONOCEPHALY

Premature fusion of the metopic suture gives rise to the deformity of trigonocephaly. With premature closure of the metopic suture in utero, a marked narrowing of the forehead occurs, as if the frontotemporal area had been pinched in. When examined from above, the forehead appears wedge-shaped, with a vertical keel along the midline of the forehead (Fig. 8–13). The lateral corners of the eyebrow tend

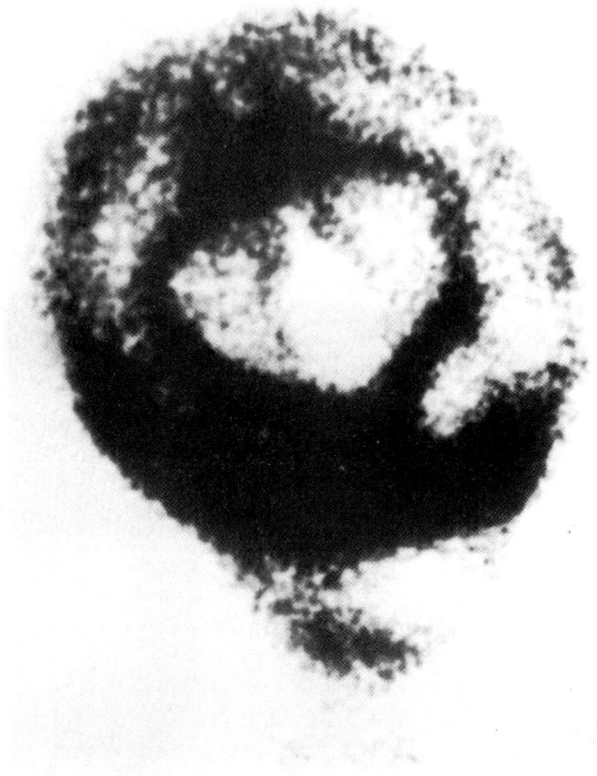

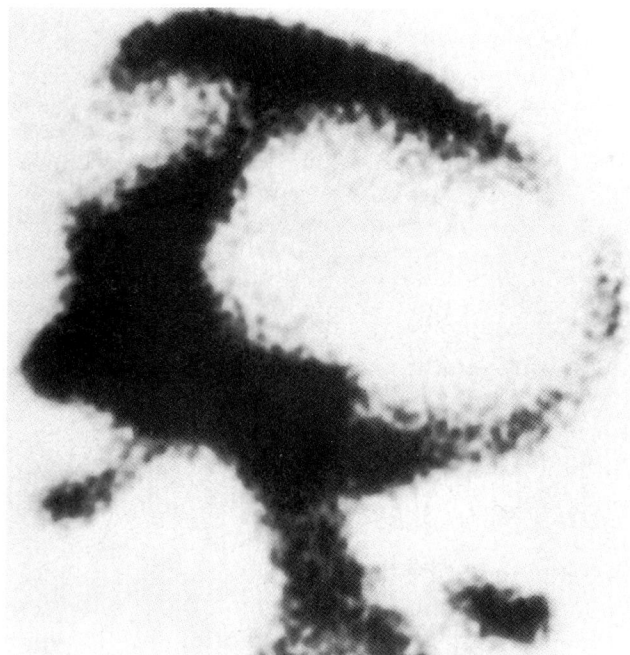

Figure 8–4. Bone scan of the skull of an infant with Crouzon's syndrome, showing increased activity in coronal, frontosphenoidal, and frontoethmoidal sutures, which form a ring around the anterior half of the skull. (With permission from Hoffman HJ: Craniofacial anomalies. *In* Wilson CB, Hoff JT [eds.]: Current Surgical Management of Neurologic Disease. New York, Churchill Livingstone, 1980.)

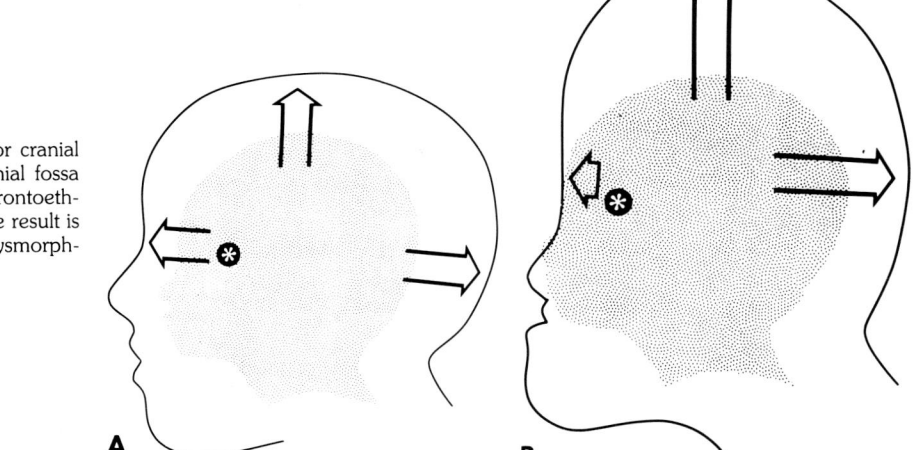

Figure 8–5. *A*, Normal growth of anterior cranial fossa. *B*, Lack of growth of anterior cranial fossa because of premature fusion of coronal, frontoethmoidal, and frontosphenoidal sutures. The result is characteristic deformity of craniofacial dysmorphism.

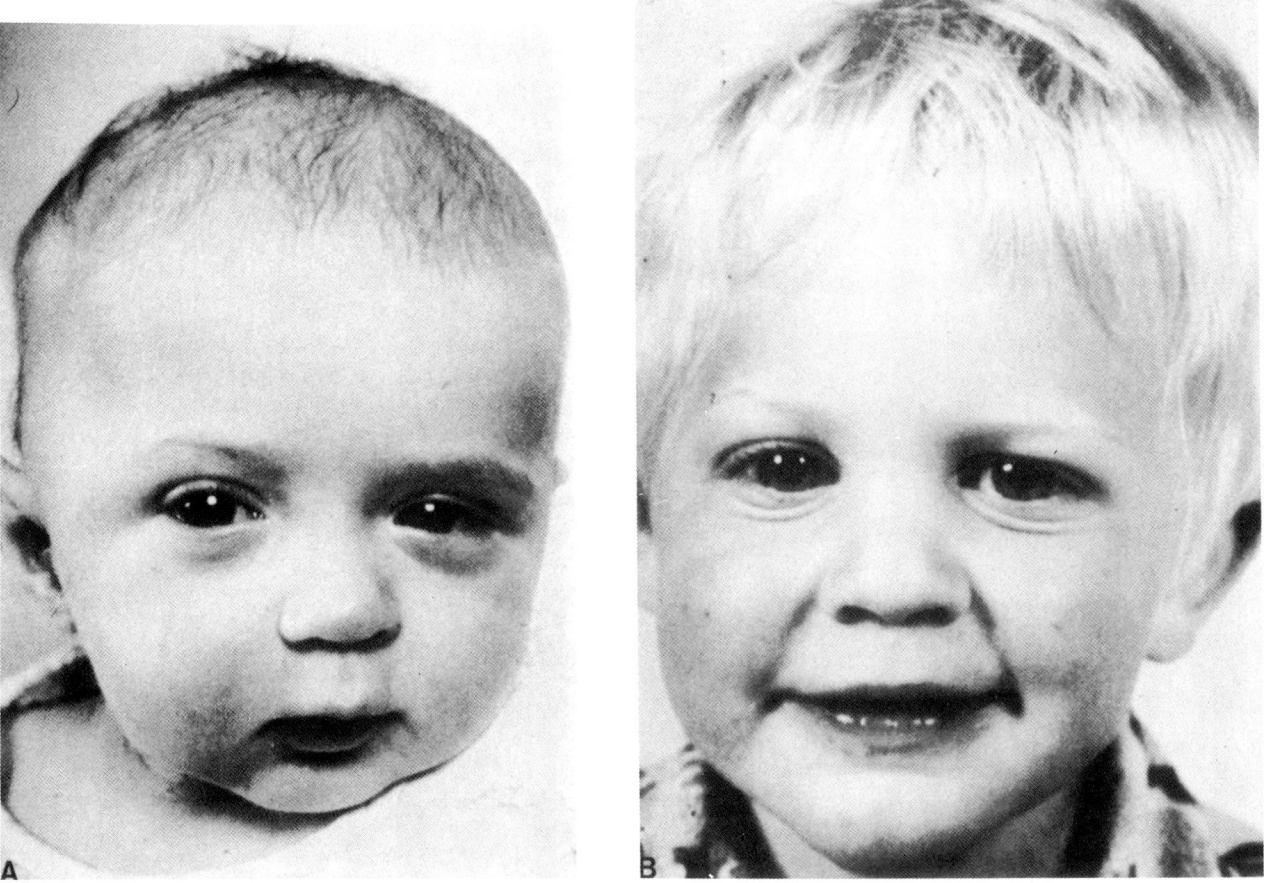

Figure 8–6. *A*, Infant with unilateral coronal synostosis, showing characteristic facies. Note higher eye on right, deviation of nose to left, and concavity of forehead above right eye. *B*, Same child at age four years, having undergone right lateral canthal advancement at age four weeks. Note complete correction of deformity.

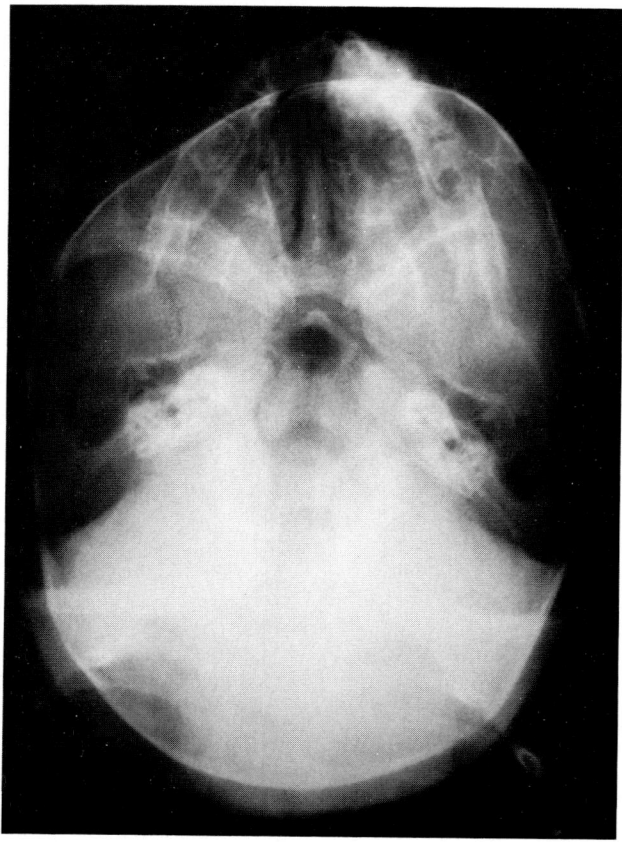

Figure 8–7. Basal skull view of child with unilateral coronal synostosis, showing flattening of ipsilateral forehead and thickening of ipsilateral pterion.

Figure 8–8. Diagrammatic depiction of operation of lateral canthal advancement from frontal view (A) and from superior view (B).

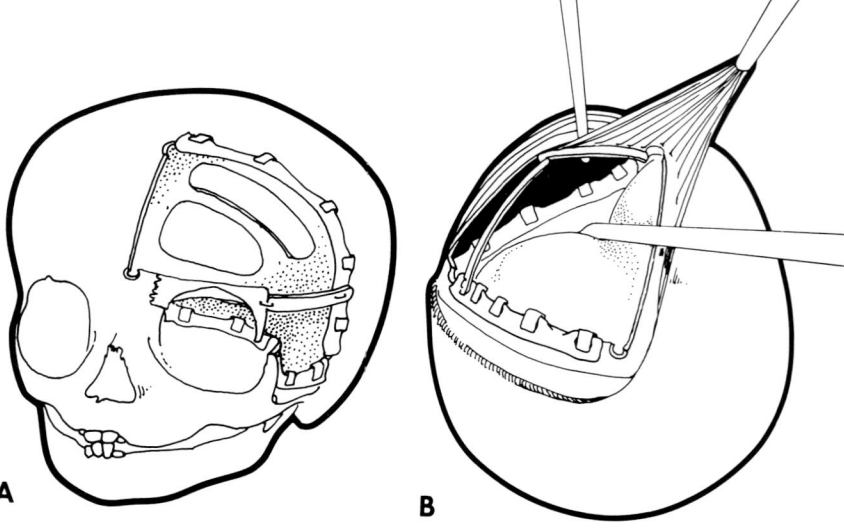

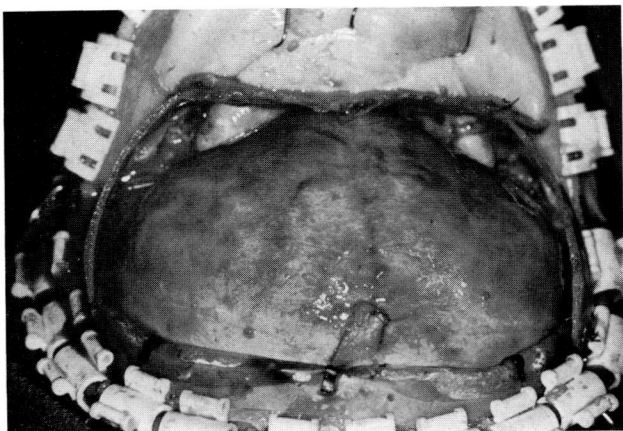

Figure 8–9. Operative view of procedure of bilateral canthal advancement in infant with Crouzon's syndrome.

to be elevated. Measurement of the distance between the medial canthi reveals hypotelorism.[8] In the most severe cases, the lateral supraorbital ridge is deficient. When the suture closes after birth, but before its usual closure time at two years of age, the abnormality is not as dramatic. Usually, there is only ridging of the metopic suture in its posterior portion; the forehead itself appears normal. As there is no cosmetic deformity, this type of synostosis requires no treatment, although surgical intervention has been recommended by some.[10] In the authors' experience, the milder forms of metopic synostosis are frequently familial.

In the past, the incidence of metopic synostosis has been reported as quite low. However, at the Hospital for Sick Children, metopic synostosis accounts for about 16 percent of cases of craniosynostosis.[16] There is a male predominance in most series.[9]

Trigonocephaly may be associated with underlying cerebral anomalies, the most common of which is holoprosencephaly.[27] The association of median cleft lip with metopic synostosis strongly suggests underlying holoprosencephaly, but the absence of the cleft does not rule out its occurrence.[9] In light of the possibility of underlying cerebral pathology, many series suggest the occurrence of decreased intelligence in some of these patients. Anderson and colleagues[1] report a 33 percent incidence of developmental delay. In the authors' experience, patients with uncomplicated trigonocephaly that is repaired early have normal intelligence; others report a similar experience.[9]

Although trigonocephaly was first described in 1862, surgical management was initially mentioned by Matson in 1960.[25]

Surgical Repair

The entire frontal bone is removed from just above the supraorbital margin to just in front of the coronal suture. The frontal bone is then fragmented, and these separate fragments are loosely applied to the dura and held there by the preserved sheet of frontal periosteum. Following this procedure, the forehead achieves a normal contour almost immediately, and with the passage of time, the orbits

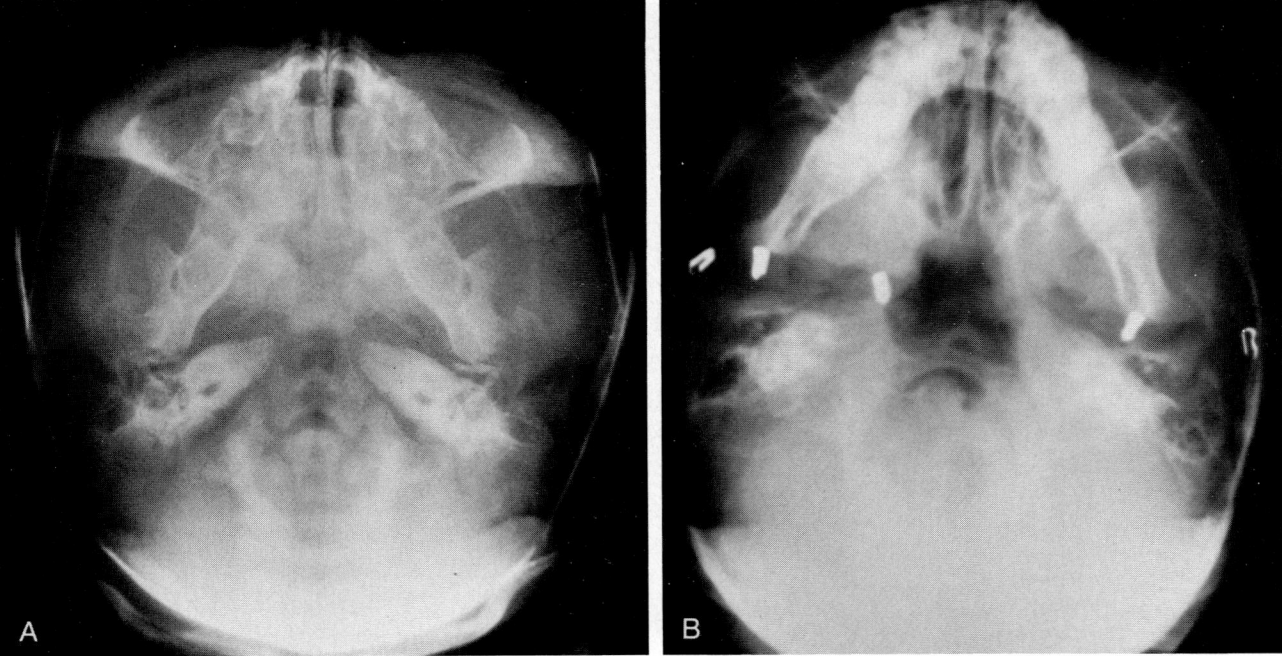

Figure 8–10. A, Basal skull view of neonate with Crouzon's syndrome, showing short anterior cranial fossa. B, Basal skull view of same patient as in A at age five years. Patient had bilateral lateral canthal advancement at age two weeks and now has normal anterior cranial fossa.

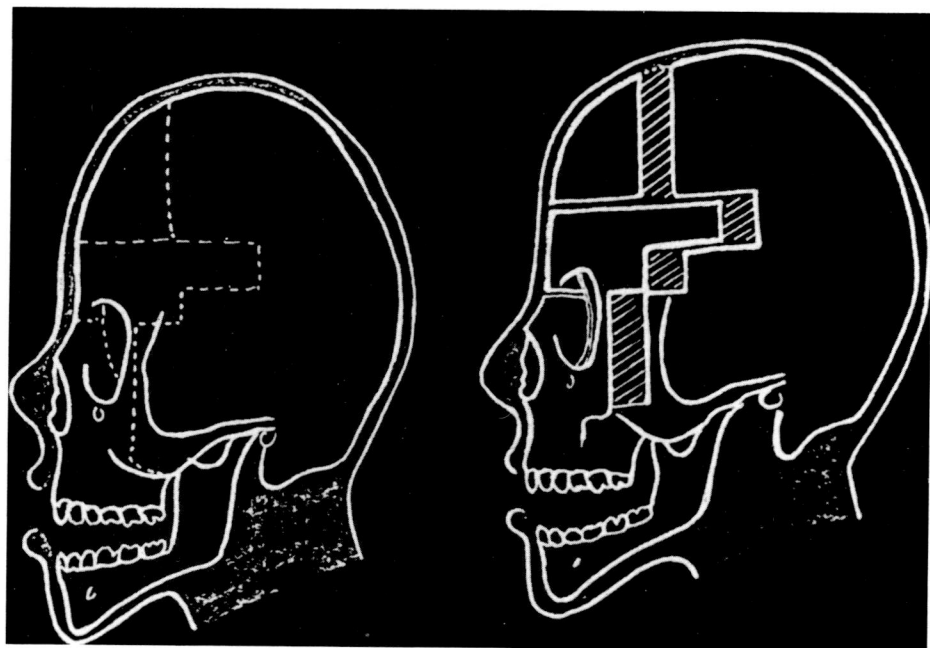

Figure 8–11. Operative diagram of technique of advancement of forehead and face in older patient with craniofacial dysmorphism.

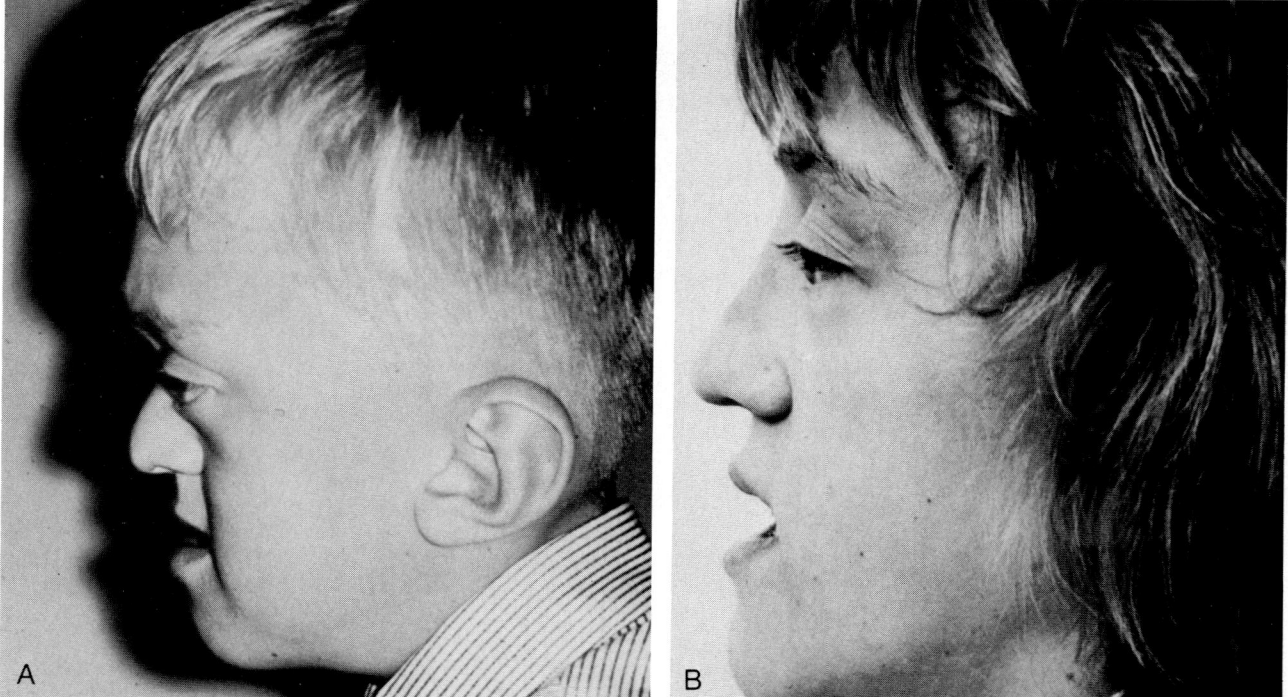

Figure 8–12. A, Photograph of child with Crouzon's syndrome. B, Photograph of same child as in A after Tessier-type repair.

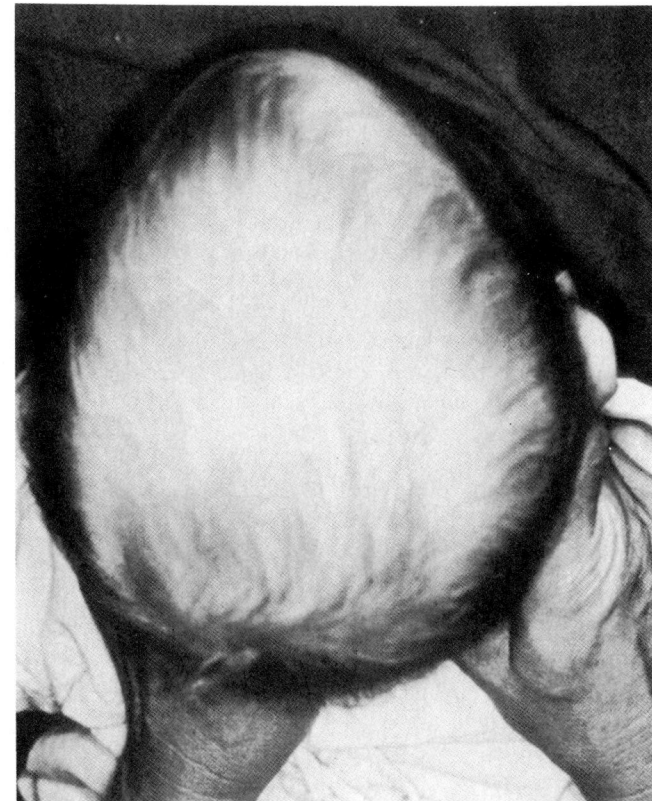

Figure 8–13. Photograph of infant with trigonocephaly.

move out into normal position and have a normal radiologic appearance.

In the severe forms of trigonocephaly, in which the forehead is markedly "depressed" above the orbits, a bilateral lateral canthal advancement is of value. This procedure is also used when trigonocephaly occurs in conjunction with bilateral coronal synostosis.

MULTIPLE SUTURE SYNOSTOSES

Multiple suture synostoses unassociated with craniofacial dysmorphism account for 7.6 percent of cases of craniosynostosis in the authors' series.[16] The head shape varies according to the sutures involved. A not infrequent combination is that of synostosis of the sagittal and both lambdoidal sutures (Fig. 8–14). Marked frontal bossing, ridging over the sagittal suture, and a very narrow head from posterior to the coronal suture are the result. Occasionally, patients with Crouzon's syndrome initially present in this fashion, and only at a later stage do the coronal sutures fuse.

Surgical Repair

In the past, multiple suture synostoses were frequently treated in several stages. With the modern techniques of pediatric neuroanesthesia, it is possible to open all sutures simultaneously. The head is supported by a special head rest applied to the cheeks and suboccipital region. A *meisterschnitt* incision is used so that the scalp can be reflected both anteriorly and posteriorly. Thus, it is possible to perform multiple linear craniectomies and, if necessary, a bilateral lateral canthal advancement, all at the same time.

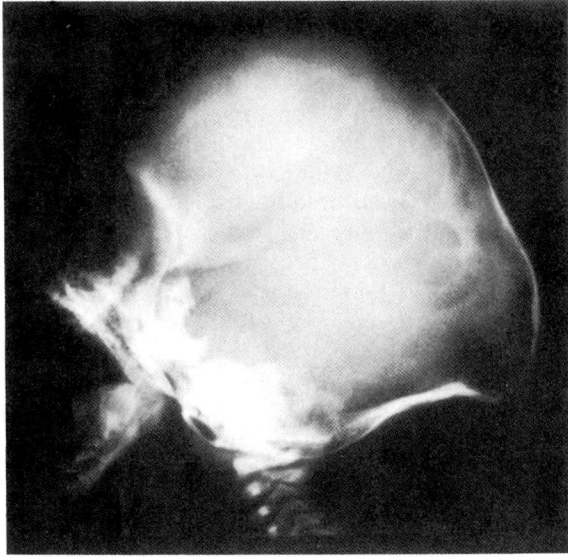

Figure 8–14. Lateral skull x-ray film of infant with Crouzon's syndrome who presented with closure of lambdoid and sagittal sutures.

HYPERTELORISM

Hypertelorism is a rare abnormality consisting of an increased distance between the eyes, occurring in 1 person in 60,000. Normally, during embryonic development, the eyes initially separate from the diencephalon as diverticula and migrate to a lateral position on the head as in lower animals. As the face matures, the eyes rotate forward, reducing the orbital angle from 180 degrees to 71 degrees by birth, and to 68 degrees by maturity. Therefore, hypertelorism may result not only from failure of this forward migration but also from its obstruction by congenital malformations such as encephaloceles.

In the median cleft face syndrome,[11] hypertelorism occurs in conjunction with one or more facial malformations, which include a V-shaped frontal hairline (widow's peak), cranium bifidum occultum, median cleft nose, and cleft lip and palate. Hypertelorism can also occur in association with the craniofacial dysmorphic states. Occasionally, hypertelorism is seen as a completely isolated event. In such instances, brain development and intellect are always normal.

Tessier[35] described hypertelorism according to the measured distance between the anterior lacrimal crests, as seen on skull x-ray films. This distance was called the intraorbital distance (IOD). The normal IOD ranges from 18.5 to 29.5 mm in women and from 19.6 to 30.7 mm in men. In first-degree hypertelorism, the IOD is between 30 and 34 mm; in second-degree hypertelorism, it is between 34 and 40 mm; and in third-degree cases, it is greater than 40 mm.

Early attempts at treating hypertelorism consisted only of altering soft-tissue structure. In 1966, Schmid[32] described his experience with shifting the bony medial walls of the orbit. In 1967, Tessier and associates[37] described the now classic procedure for moving both orbits medially, resulting in total correction of hypertelorism.

Unlike most cranial anomalies, hypertelorism is best corrected in the older child or the adult. However, when it coexists with a frontonasal encephalocele, repair should be done early in childhood.

Sincipital encephaloceles are divided into (1) nasofrontal lesions, which pass between nasal and frontal bone and produce a rounded, skin-covered mass in the midline of the root of the nose; (2) nasoethmoidal encephaloceles, which pass between ethmoidal, frontal, and nasal bones and appear on the side of the nose; and (3) naso-orbital encephaloceles, which pass between ethmoidal, frontal, and lacrimal bones into the anterior medial part of the orbit.[40]

The sincipital encephaloceles are associated with hypertelorism presumably produced by the protrusion of brain and meninges, which prevents the orbits from moving together during development. Furthermore, as the brain grows and if the encephalocele is not repaired, the continued pulsation of the encephalocele moves the orbits further apart.

The basal encephaloceles are associated with a split crista galli, and the encephalocele passes between the two halves of the crista galli into the nasal cavity, with no external evidence of the encephalocele.[40]

Surgical Repair

Early in infancy, sincipital encephaloceles can be easily repaired, and this may result in obviating the need for repair of the associated hypertelorism.

If hypertelorism persists or is present without an associated encephalocele, repair can be delayed.

Definitive repair of hypertelorism requires a bifrontal craniotomy, leaving a bar of bone 2.5 cm in height above the supraorbital margins. The floor of the anterior fossa is exposed back to and including the crista galli. The termination of the sagittal sinus at the foramen cecum must be divided, and the dura must be elevated off the crista galli. Where there is a frontonasal encephalocele, the crista galli is typically split, and the dural protrusion descends through this split. In such situations, the dura must be transected at the level of the crista galli and repaired. Through the coronal scalp incision, osteotomies can be made that free the anterior one third of the bony orbit from the skull and facial bones. Then, a carefully estimated central nasofrontal segment of bone is removed. A transverse bar of bone, 1.5 cm in height, is left intact just above the orbits, and this allows for correct horizontal and anteroposterior positioning of the orbits. The bony orbits are approximated to within a distance of 20 to 25 mm, depending on the age of the patient. Bone grafts consisting of split ribs taken from the patient are wired into the lateral orbital walls, and the frontal bone flap is replaced. A bilateral medial canthopexy is done, and the nose is rebuilt from a bone graft. If necessary, excessive skin of the nose is removed (Figs. 8–15 through 8–17).

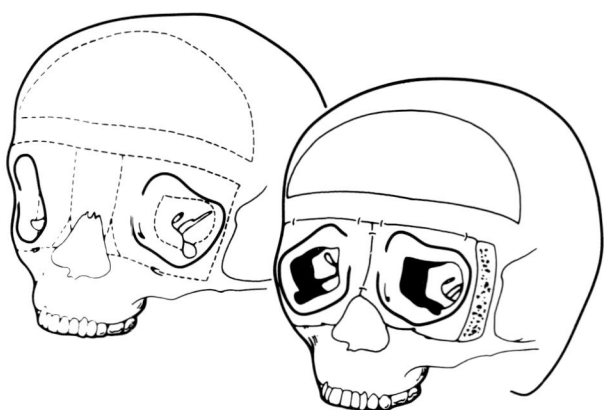

Figure 8–15. Diagrammatic depiction of repair of hypertelorism.

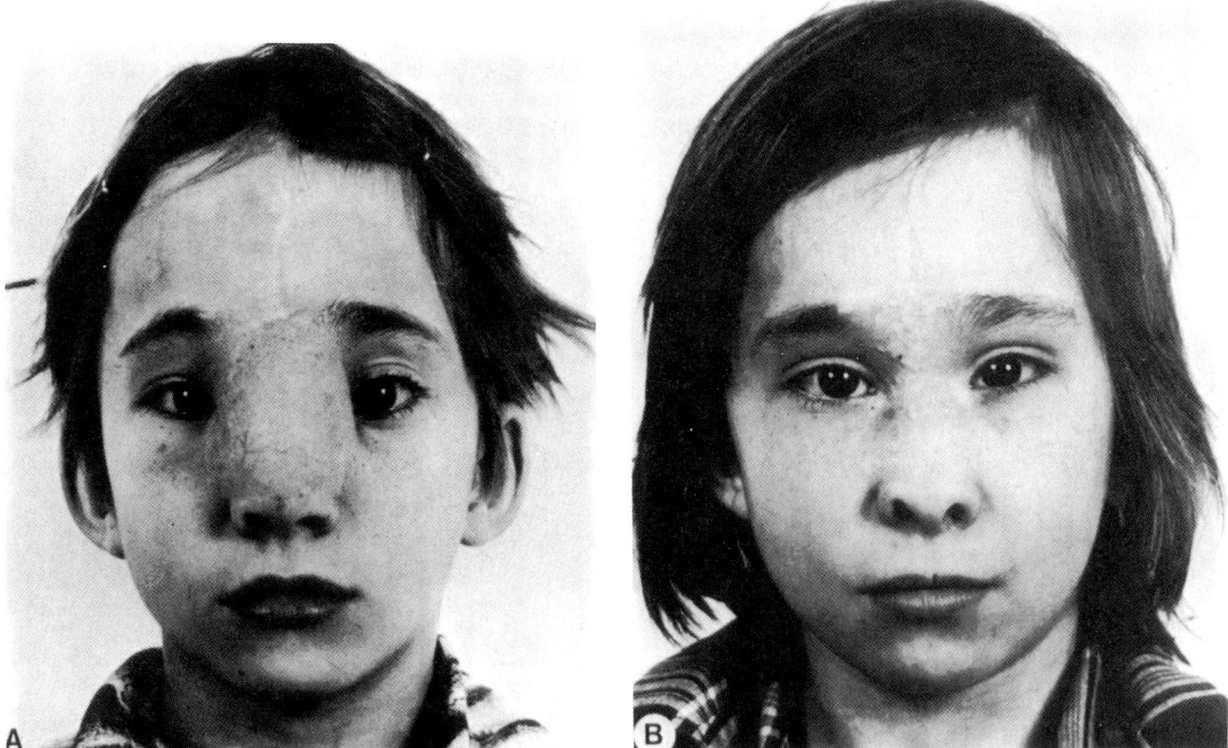

Figure 8–16. *A*, Child with frontonasal encephalocele and hypertelorism. *B*, Same child after repair.

Figure 8–17. *A*, Infant with median cleft and hypertelorism. *B*, Same patient after repair of hypertelorism.

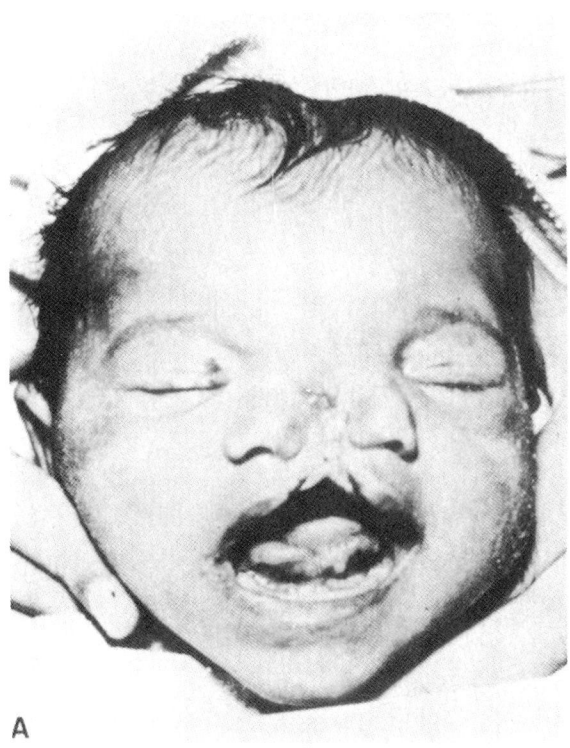
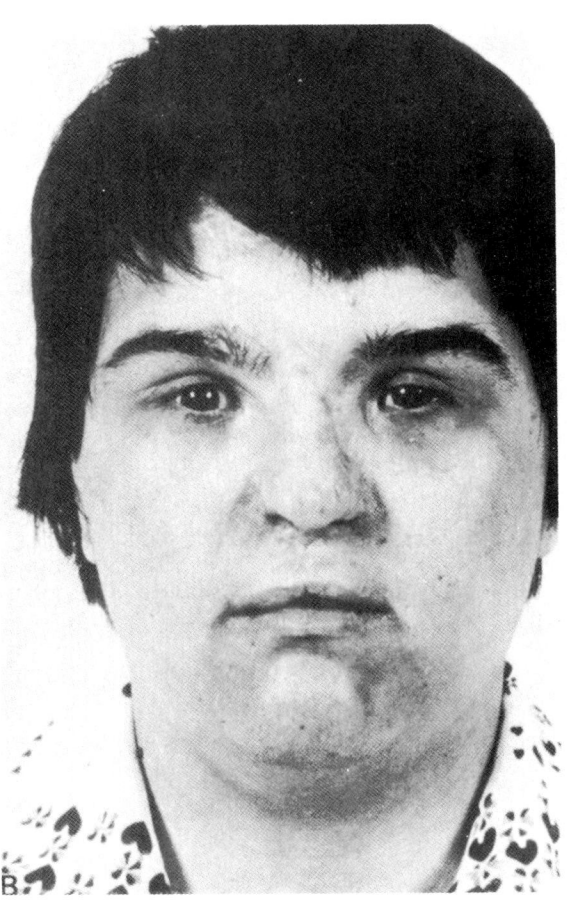

Because of the bony anomalies in the midline in these patients, tears in the dura and sagittal sinus can sometimes occur, leading to excessive blood loss and, even, air embolism. Failure to repair these dural tears may result in postoperative CSF leaks through the floor of the anterior cranial fossa, with the consequent risk of meningitis. Should a CSF leak develop postoperatively, it can be readily dealt with by external lumbar drainage or, rarely, by an indwelling lumboperitoneal shunt.

At the end of the procedure, visual acuity must be checked, since excessive traction on the optic nerve, distortion of the globe, and retinal detachment following hemorrhage behind the globe all are potential complications that become manifest by loss of visual acuity.

FIBROUS DYSPLASIA

Fibrous dysplasia is a disease of focal abnormal bone development of unknown etiology, in which cellular fibro-osseous tissue replaces normal bone in one or more locations. The abnormal lesions tend to expand during childhood and stabilize after puberty, although stabilization is not invariable.[13] The disease may be monostotic (limited to one bone) or polyostotic (present in two or more bones) or may be associated with endocrine hyperfunction and pigmented skin lesions (Albright's syndrome). Cranial involvement occurs in 50 percent of polyostotic cases and 10 to 27 percent of monostotic cases.[14, 22, 41] In the skull, the lesions tend to spread across sutures, but in the case of simple lesions, they are still classified as monostotic. Most commonly involved are the frontal, sphenoidal, and facial bones. Lesions are more frequent in the base of the skull than in the calvarium.

Gross enlargement of the involved bone is characteristic of fibrous dysplasia (Fig. 8-18). The abnormal masses of tissue may be gritty and yellowish gray. Histologic examination reveals fibroblasts, collagen, scattered islands of cartilage, occasional giant cells, and woven bone. An ample blood supply is typical. Malignant transformation of fibrous dysplasia has been reported but is rare in cranial lesions.[23]

Radiographically, large lesions are seen as cystic or sclerotic masses expanding the bone. The affected areas may have a "ground-glass" appearance. In the skull, increased density of the base, thickening of the occiput, obliteration of the paranasal and nasal sinuses, and displacement of the orbit are typical findings.[22]

Children with fibrous dysplasia usually come to neurosurgical attention because of cranial nerve compression (most often optic or auditory) and craniofacial deformity.

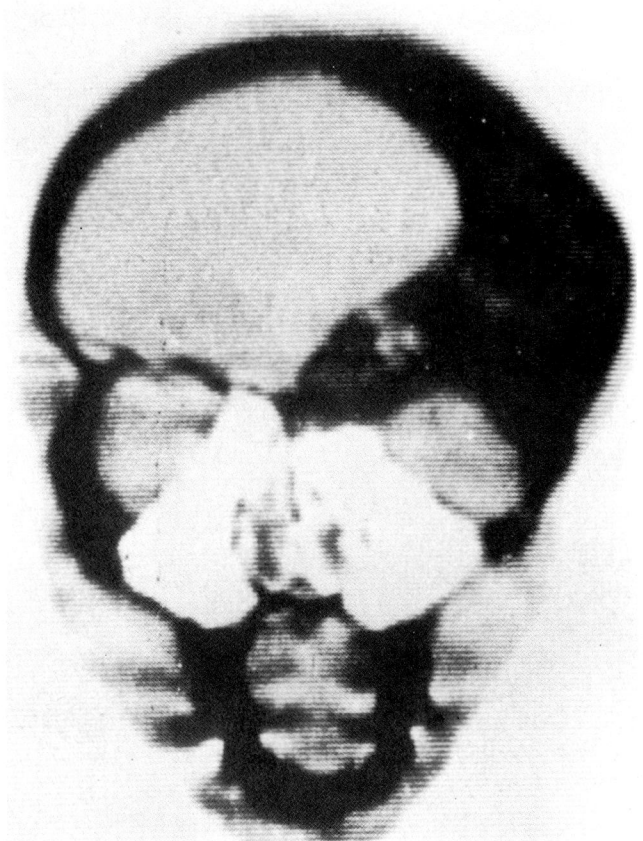

Figure 8-18. CT scan showing involvement of frontal and sphenoidal bone by fibrous dysplasia.

Surgical Repair

Surgical management of fibrous dysplasia has three goals: (1) decompression of affected neural elements, (2) removal of all the abnormal bone, and (3) achievement of a pleasing cosmetic result.

An attempt to remove all of the involved bone is necessary, as the lesion may recur and grow if a portion of dysplastic bone is left in place.

To achieve an adequate cosmetic result, the authors use split-thickness skull grafts to fill in the surgical bony defect. These grafts are harvested from calvarial bone not involved in the disease process. They can then be cut and molded to achieve an adequate facial appearance.

NEUROFIBROMATOSIS

In neurofibromatosis, there may be absence of the sphenoid wing. This allows contact between temporal lobe and the soft-tissues of the orbit, leading characteristically to a pulsating exophthalmos (Fig. 8–19).[20]

In this disorder, not only is there absence of the lesser and greater wings of the sphenoid bone, but the dura is deficient. In carrying out a repair, it is necessary to separate temporal lobe from the orbital soft tissues and to carry out a duraplasty. Once this is done, the sphenoid wing is reconstructed from split skull.

In Von Recklinghausen's disease, one can have neurofibromas arising in the three divisions of the fifth cranial nerve, with severe distortion of facial features, resulting in the "elephant man" syndrome. It is possible to resect facial tissues and remove the neurofibromas, which typically extend into middle cranial fossa. The face can then be rebuilt with bone grafts and appropriate soft-tissue flaps, allowing restoration of a reasonably normal appearance (Fig. 8–20).

CRANIOMETAPHYSEAL DYSPLASIA

Craniometaphyseal dysplasia was initially described by Pyle in 1931.[30] In this condition, there is failure of resorption of the secondary spongiosa, which produces increased thickening and density of the cranial base, cranial vault, facial bone, and mandible and leads to obliteration of the paranasal sinuses as well as the mastoid air cells. The laying down of this thick bone produces progressive hypertelorism with marked broadening of the root of the nose (Fig. 8–21). This produces a severe cosmetic deformity, which can in certain selected cases be treated with craniofacial surgery. The techniques are similar to those of treatment of hypertelorism. However, the skull is extremely thick and very hard, and high-speed drills and saws are necessary to carry out the procedure in craniometaphyseal dysplasia.

NEOPLASMS

The craniofacial surgery team are uniquely equipped to deal with tumors in the skull base, particularly when such tumors distort the patient's appearance.

Following surgical resection of such tumors, large, irregular bony defects may be created. The resection of dura beneath the involved bone may be necessary. Dural defects are repaired with cadaver freeze-dried dura. Bony defects in the base of the skull can then be reconstructed from split-thickness skull grafts (Fig. 8–22).

HYDROCEPHALUS

In the poorly treated hydrocephalic patient with a markedly enlarged calvarium, the calvarium can be reduced to a relatively normal size, utilizing the existing skull for the reconstruction of the newer small calvarium (Fig. 8–23).

CONCLUSIONS

Craniofacial anomalies have become a focus of attention in recent years. Reasonable treatment is being provided at last to patients with these disorders. In the past, such patients were objects of ridicule and frequently were housed in circuses and amusement parks to be gawked at by idle crowds. Modern surgical techniques have made it possible

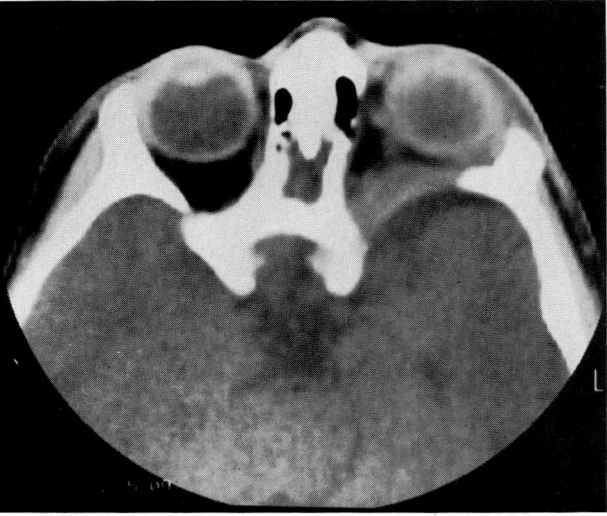

Figure 8–19. CT scan of a child with neurofibromatosis and unilateral agenesis of sphenoid wing.

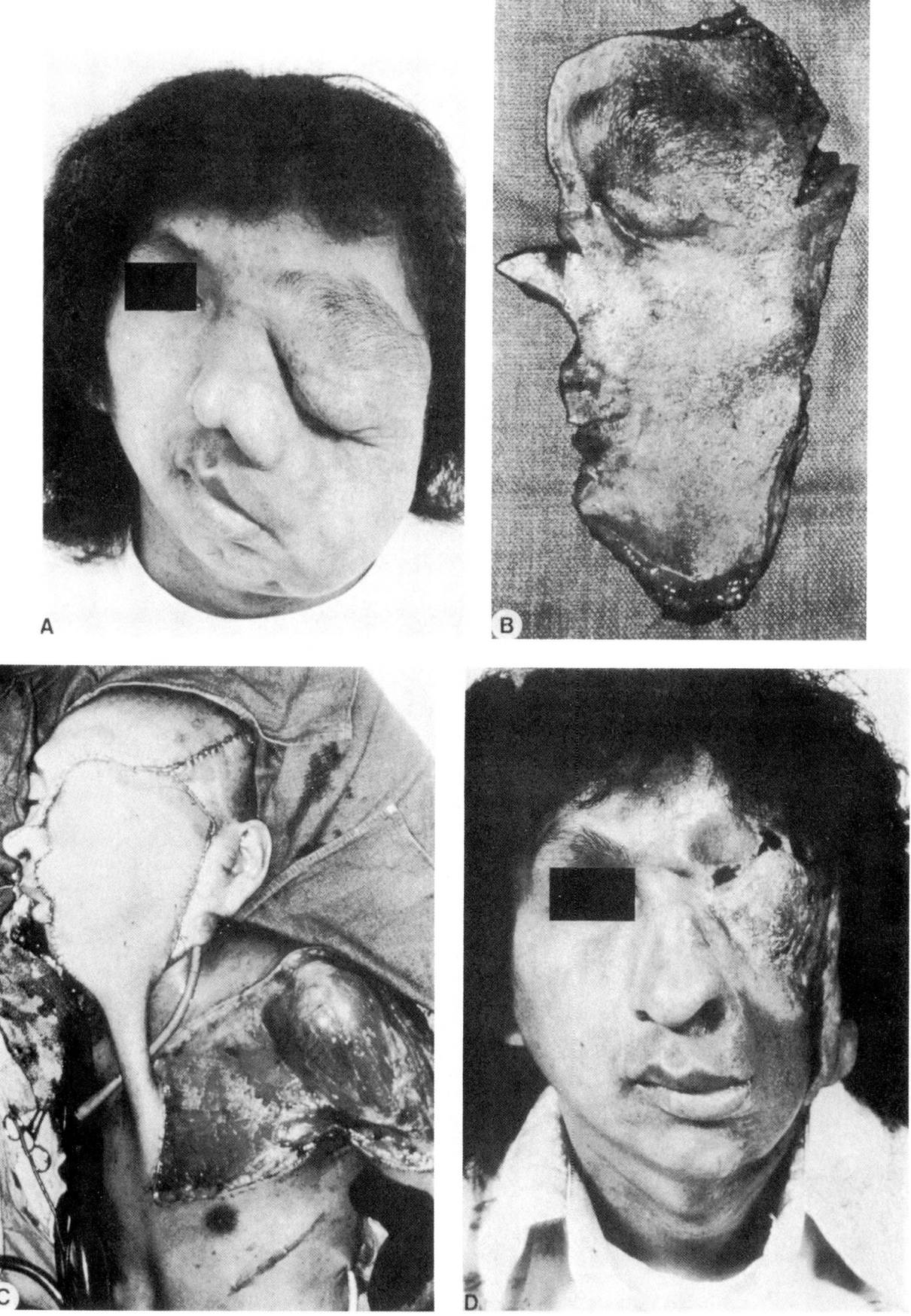

Figure 8–20. *A,* Young man with "elephant man" appearance due to facial neurofibromata. *B,* Surgical specimen at the time of repair. *C,* Repair by pedicle flap. *D,* Final appearance.

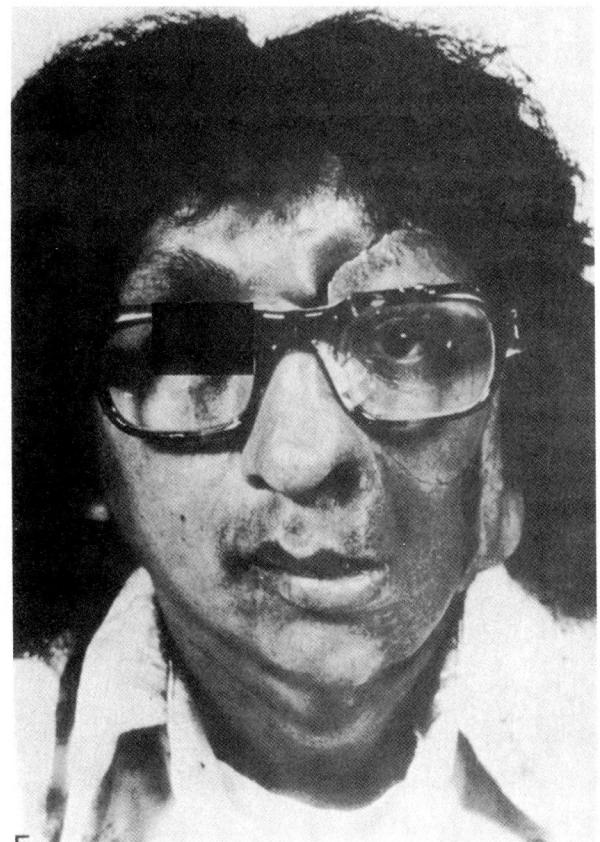

Figure 8–20 Continued. E, Final appearance with prosthesis.

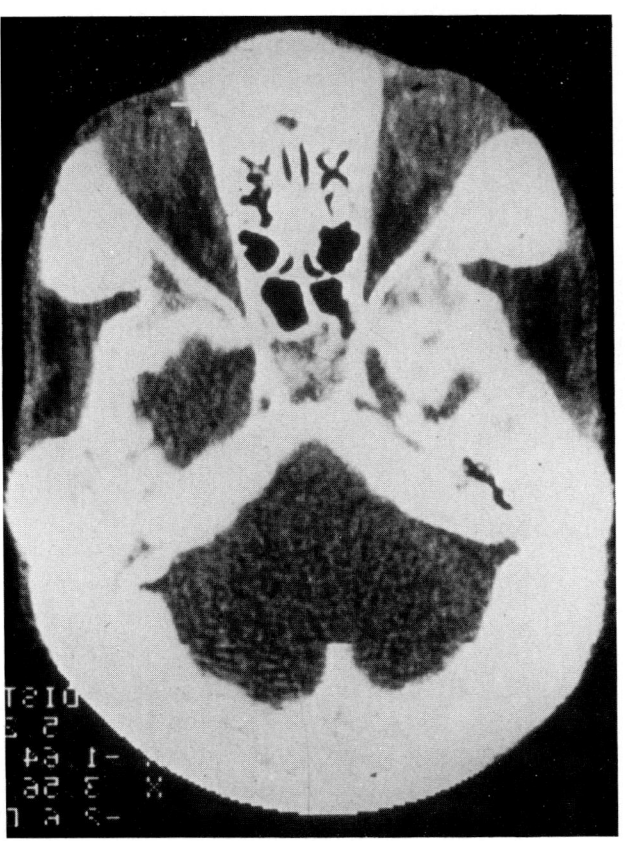

Figure 8–21. CT scan of a patient with craniometaphyseal dysplasia.

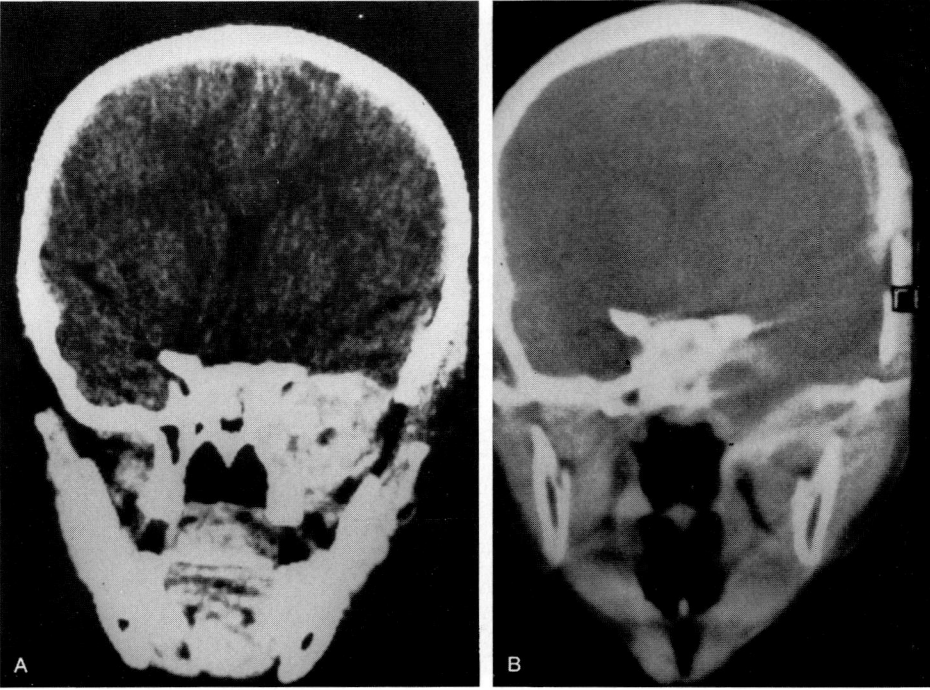

Figure 8–22. *A*, CT scan of a patient with benign osteoblastoma of the skull filling the left middle cranial fossa. *B*, CT scan of the same patient as in *A* after resection of the tumor and reconstruction of the middle cranial fossa.

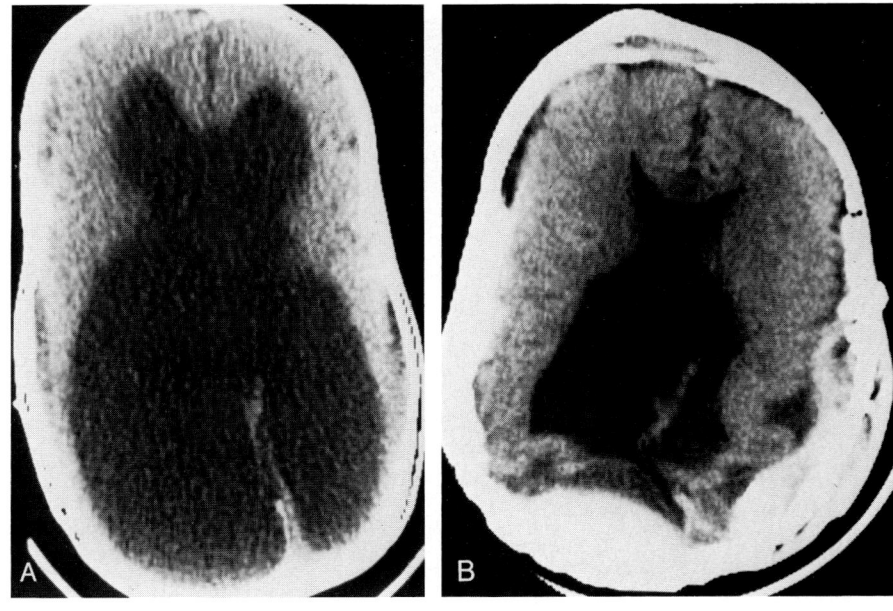

Figure 8–23. *A*, CT scan of a child with gross hydrocephalus. *B*, CT scan of the same child as in *A* after reduction cranioplasty.

for these patients to achieve a normal appearance and to lead a normal life.

References

1. Anderson FM, Gwinn JL, Todd JC: Trigonocephaly: Identity and surgical treatment. J Neurosurg 19:723, 1962.
2. Apert E: De l'Acrocephalosyndactylie. Bull Meme Soc Med Hop Paris 23:1310, 1906.
3. Atkinson FRB: Hereditary cranio-facial dysostosis, or Crouzon's disease. Med Press Circular 195:118, 1937.
4. Bertelsen TI: The premature synostosis of the cranial sutures. Acta Ophthalmol (Suppl)63:97, 1958.
5. Cohen MM: Genetic perspectives on craniosynostosis and syndromes with craniosynostosis. J Neurosurg 47:886, 1977.
6. Comings DE: The kleeblattschädel syndrome—a grotesque form of hydrocephalus. J Pediatr 67:126, 1965.
7. Crouzon O: Dystose cranio-faciale hereditaire. Bull Meme Soc Med Hop Paris 33:545, 1912.
8. Currarino G, Silverman F: Orbital hypotelorism, arhinencephaly, and trigonocephaly. Radiology 74:206, 1960.
9. David DJ, Poswillo DE, Simpson DA: The Craniosynostoses: Causes, History and Management. New York, Springer-Verlag, 1982, p 134.
10. Delashaw JB, Persing JA, Park TS, et al: Surgical approaches for the correction of metopic synostosis. Neurosurgery 19:228, 1986.
11. DeMyer W: The median cleft face syndrome. Differential diagnosis of cranium bifidum occultum, hypertelorism, and median cleft nose, lip, and palate. Neurology 17:961, 1967.
12. Furuya Y, Edwards MSB, Alpers CE, et al: Computerized tomography of cranial sutures. Part 2: Abnormalities of sutures and skull deformity in craniosynostosis. J Neurosurg 61:59, 1984.
13. Grabias SL, Campbell CJ: Fibrous dysplasia. Orthop Clin North Am 8:771, 1977.
14. Harris WH, Dudley HR, Jr., Barry RJ: The natural history of fibrous dysplasia: An orthopedic pathological and roentgenographic study. J Bone Joint Surg 44A:207, 1962.
15. Hemmy DC, David DJ, Herman GT: Three-dimensional reconstruction of craniofacial deformity using computed tomography. Neurosurgery 13:534, 1983.
16. Hoffman HJ: Congenital malformations of the spine and skull. In: Goldsmith HS (ed): Practice of Surgery. New York, Harper & Row, 1980.
17. Hoffman HJ, Hendrick EB: Early neurosurgical repair in craniofacial dysmorphism. J Neurosurg 51:796, 1979.
18. Hoffman HJ, Mohr G: Lateral canthal advancement of the supra-orbital margin. A new corrective technique in the treatment of coronal synostosis. J Neurosurg 45:376, 1976.
19. Holtermuller K, Wiedemann HR: Kleeblatschädel syndrome. Med Monatsschr 14:439, 1960.
20. Hunt JC, Pugh DG: Skeletal lesions in neurofibromatosis. Radiology 76:1, 1961.
21. Larsen H: Die Schadeldeformat mit Augensymptomen. Klin Monatsbl Augenkeilkd 51:145, 1913.
22. Leeds N, Seaman WB: Fibrous dysplasia of the skull and its differential diagnosis. Radiology 78:570, 1962.
23. Marchac D, Renier D: Le front flattant, traitement precoce de faciocraniostenoses. Ann Chir Plast 24:121, 1979.
24. Marsh JL, Schwartz HG: The surgical correction of coronal and metopic craniosynostosis. J Neurosurg 59:245, 1983.
25. Matson DD: Surgical treatment of congenital anomalies of the coronal and metopic sutures. J Neurosurg 17:413, 1960.
26. Muller PJ, Hoffman HJ: Cloverleaf skull syndrome. Case report. J Neurosurg 43:86, 1975.
27. Osaka K, Matsumoto S: Holoprosencephaly in neurosurgical practice. J Neurosurg 48:787, 1978.
28. Partington MW, Gonzales-Crussi F, Khakee SG, et al: Cloverleaf skull and thanatophoric dwarfism. Report of four cases, two in the same sibship. Arch Dis Child 46:656, 1971.
29. Persing J, Babler W, Winn HR, et al: Age as a critical factor in the success of surgical correction of craniosynostosis. J Neurosurg 54:601, 1981.
30. Pyle E: Case of unusual bone development. J Bone Joint Surg 13:874, 1931.
31. Schauerte EW, St-Aubin PM: Progressive synosteosis in Apert's syndrome (acrocephalosyndactyly), with a description of roentgenographic changes in the feet. Am J Roentgenol 97:67, 1966.
32. Schmid E: Surgical management of hypertelorism. In: Longacre JJ (ed): Craniofacial Anomalies, Pathogenesis and Repair. Philadelphia, J.B. Lippincott Co., 1965, pp 155–161.
33. Seeger JF, Gabrielson TO: Premature closure of the frontosphenoidal suture in synostosis of the coronal suture. Radiology 101:631, 1971.
34. Tessier P: Osteotomies totales de la face, syndrome de Crouzon, syndrome d'Apert, oxycephalies, scaphocephalies, turricephalies. Ann Chir Plast 12:273, 1967.
35. Tessier P: Experiences in the treatment of orbital hypertelorism. Plast Reconstr Surg 53:1, 1974.
36. Tessier P: Relationship of craniostenoses to craniofacial dysostoses and to faciostenosis. Plast Reconstr Surg 48:224, 1971.
37. Tessier P, Guiot G, Rougerie J, et al: Osteotomies cranio-naso-orbito-faciales. Hypertelorisme. Ann Chir Plast 12:103, 1967.
38. Turner PT, Reynolds AF: Generous craniectomy for kleeblattschädel anomaly. Neurosurgery 6:555, 1980.
39. Ventureyra ECG, DaSilva VF: Reduction cranioplasty for neglected hydrocephalus. Surg Neurol 15:236, 1981.
40. Vincken PH, Bruyn GW: Handbook of Clinical Neurology, Vol. 30: Part I, Congenital Malformations of the Brain and Skull. Amsterdam, Elsevier, North-Holland, 1977, pp 219–225.
41. Windholz F: Cranial manifestations of fibrous dysplasia of bone. Their relation to leontiasis ossea and to simple bone cysts of the vault. Am J Roentgenol 58:51, 1947.
42. Zuleta A, Basauri L: Cloverleaf skull syndrome. Child's Brain 11:418, 1984.

9
ANOMALIES OF THE CRANIOCERVICAL JUNCTION

Steven L. Wald, M.D.
Robert L. McLaurin, M.D.

Anomalies of the craniocervical junction have been a source of confusion to the clinician since the first description of deformity of the skull base by Ackermann in 1790.[68] The extent of involvement of bony, neural, or meningeal elements, the relationship to clinical symptomatology, and the pattern of association with other skeletal or neural structures are diverse and complicated. Multiple classification schemes have been proposed, based on presumed etiology, functional presentation, radiologic findings, and dynamic pathophysiology. A basic understanding of the embryologic development of this region is required and assists in the understanding and classification of the various bony anomalies of the craniocervical junction.[50]

EMBRYOLOGY

The basicranium, or skull base, is defined as the bony structure that surrounds the foramen magnum. These structures include the basisphenoid and occipital bone (Fig. 9-1). The occipital bone can be subdivided into basioccipital (or basal portion), exoccipital, and squamosal sections. The basioccipital bone will become the clivus, while the paired exoccipital bones that develop on either side of the foramen magnum eventually become its lateral boundaries as well as the hypoglossal canals and the occipital condyles. The squamosal portion of the occipital bone develops from supraoccipital and interparietal centers. These two centers are fused at birth, while fusion between the other centers occurs postnatally. Ossification between the sphenoid and basioccipital bone begins at age 12, with closure completed between 16 and 20 years of age.[77] Growth and development of the skull base is dependent on several factors, including lengthening of the midbrain and brainstem, enlargement of the overlying cerebral hemispheres, and maturation of facial structures. The presence of synchondroses allows progression from the relatively flat basicranium of the newborn to the markedly curved structure of the adult.

The basicranium develops by a process of membrane formation, chondrification, and ossification. Cartilage, which is formed from condensations of mesenchymal cells during the fifth to sixth week of intrauterine life, undergoes ossification from centers that appear in the cartilage during the sixth to eighth week of intrauterine life. The occipital bone below the nuchal line develops by the same process of endochondral ossification. The occipital squama, however, develops by a process of membranous ossification that entails a stage of mesenchymal differentiation to a prebone stage but does not involve a cartilaginous phase.

The atlas is formed by the fusion of the caudal half of the last occipital sclerotome and the cranial and caudal halves of the first cervical sclerotome. The first cervical sclerotome also gives rise to the odontoid process. The tip of the odontoid is prob-

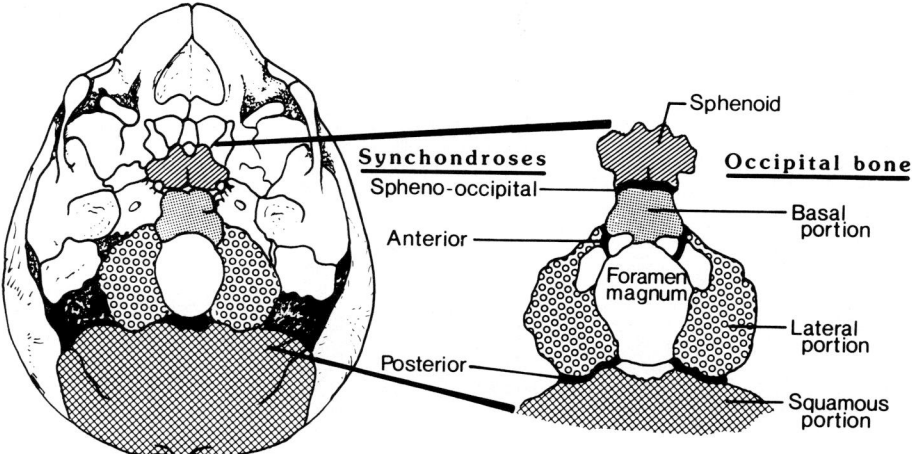

Figure 9–1. Diagrammatic representation of the neonatal basicranium. The sphenoid and representative parts of the occipital bone are shaded with heavy black lines, demonstrating the synchondroses.

ably derived from the most caudal occipital sclerotome, although disagreement on this point persists.

RADIOLOGIC ANATOMY AND MEASUREMENTS

Multiple roentgenologic methods and measurements have been advised for evaluation of the craniocervical junction. While each is valuable for determining certain aspects of anatomic relationships, differences in technique, lack of specificity, dependence on facial structures, and variance during flexion or extension require that multiple views and positions be obtained. Standard views may suggest an abnormality in the craniovertebral region, but tomography is often required to clarify pathologic relationships and is particularly valuable for demonstrating normal and pathologic sutures and synchondroses.

Standard radiologic measurements include the basilar angle, Bull's angle,[8] Chamberlain's line,[14] McGregor's line,[57] the diagastric line of Fischgold and Metzger,[29] the bimastoid line,[29] the height index,[43] and the anteroposterior dimension of the foramen magnum.[59] The basilar angle is drawn from the nasion to the tuberculum sella to the anterior lip of the foramen magnum (Fig. 9–2). This angle should not exceed 140 degrees. Chamberlain's line extends from the posterior aspect of the hard palate to the posterior rim of the foramen magnum (Fig. 9–3). McGregor's line joins the posterior end of the hard palate to the lowest point of the occipital bone. The digastric line joins the digastric notches. The bimastoid line connects the mastoid tips and should be within 2 mm of the odontoid tip. Klaus's height index is determined by drawing a line from the tuberculum sella to the internal occipital protuberance and measuring the distance from this line to the tip of the odontoid. The normal anteroposterior diameter of the foramen magnum, as described by

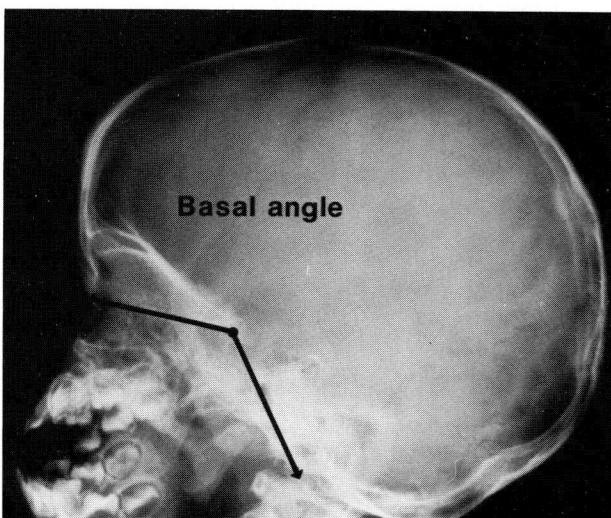

Figure 9–2. The basal angle. This angle should normally not exceed 140 degrees.

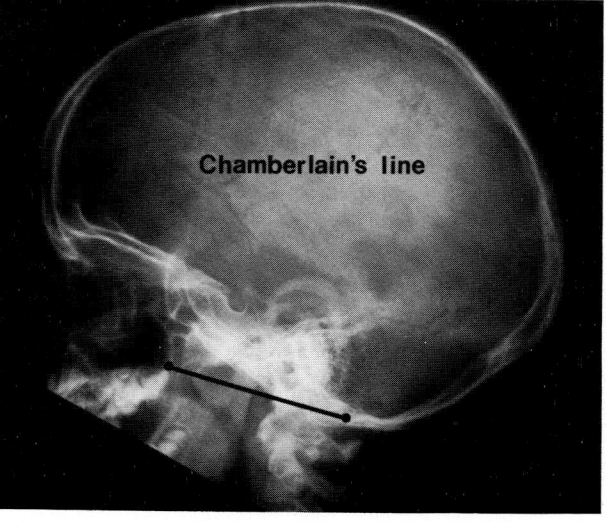

Figure 9–3. Chamberlain's line. Basilar impression is suggested when the tip of the odontoid is 5 mm or more above this line.

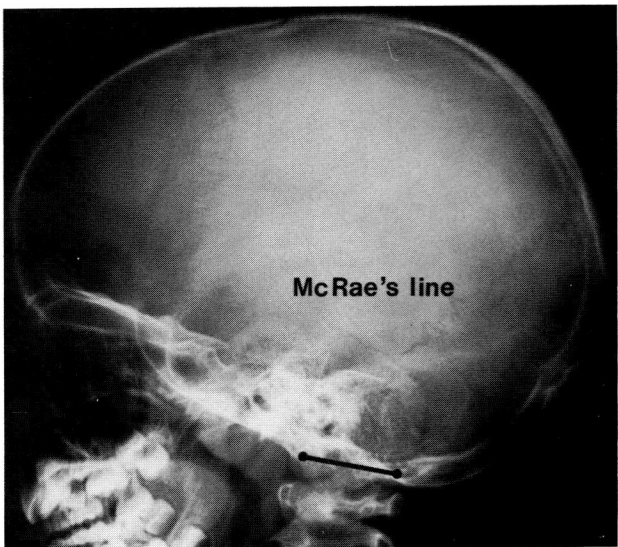

Figure 9–4. McRae's line determines the anteroposterior boundaries of the foramen magnum and should not be less than 18 mm.

McRae and Barnum, should exceed 19 mm (Fig. 9–4).[59]

Myelography is required to clarify the relationships of bony abnormalities to neural structures. Supine myelography is considered a necessary part of the procedure by some authors.[90] Dynamic testing during myelography is useful in planning surgical therapy. Vertebral angiography has been utilized, although its usefulness is questioned.[4] Computerized tomography (CT) is widely employed to visualize the anatomy of the posterior fossa, foramen magnum, and upper cervical spine.[66] Combined with myelography, CT provides valuable information about the relationships of bony structures to the nervous system. Sagittal and parasagittal reconstruction adds further information, providing the neurosurgeon with a multidimensional appreciation of these relationships. The high incidence of artifact encountered with CT of the lower posterior fossa and craniocervical junction limits, on occasion, the value of this study. Nuclear magnetic resonance imaging (NMRI) has been utilized recently to evaluate these complex relationships at the craniocervical junction.[5] In addition to producing artifact-free images, NMRI is able to demonstrate anatomy in multiple planes. The superior definition of neural structures makes NMRI a valuable adjunct in the understanding and diagnosis of anomalies in this area.

ANOMALIES OF THE CRANIOCERVICAL JUNCTION

As shown in Tables 9–1 through 9–3, numerous bony abnormalities have been reported in the area of the craniocervical junction. Many of these anomalies are found in combination with other skeletal dysplasias, and combinations of anomalies involving the cranial base and cervical spine are common. Furthermore, many of these abnormalities are asymptomatic and are called to attention only during incidental radiographic procedures. The discussion of the various craniocervical anomalies will concentrate on those lesions with symptomatic manifestations and their surgical management.

MALFORMATIONS OF THE BASIOCCIPUT AND THE FORAMEN MAGNUM

Basilar Impression

In 1844, Rokitansky described indentation of the skull base by the cervical spine.[68] In 1855, Berg and Retzius provided a more detailed report of this abnormality.[3] Basilar impression and platybasia are terms often used synonymously, although they represent different processes. Platybasia implies an abnormal basilar angle of greater than 140 degrees, such that the basiocciput, or clivus, assumes a more horizontal course with respect to the axis of the spine. This is of primary interest to anatomists and anthropologists but has little use in clinical medicine.

Basilar impression, or invagination, represents the upward displacement of the margins of the foramen magnum into the posterior fossa. The elevation is most prominent medially, such that the rim of the foramen magnum curves upward, while the lateral parts of the posterior fossa angle downward.[90] There is reduction of volume in the posterior fossa and an irregular contour to the foramen magnum. The clivus is reduced in length.[75] The cerebellar tonsils may be situated below the rim of the foramen magnum, as in the Arnold-Chiari deformity. However, the abnormal tonsillar herniation is not necessarily representative of a true Arnold-Chiari malformation, as the cervical roots pass in the usual rostral-caudal direction, and associated brainstem and cerebellar anomalies are not present.

Etiology

The causes of basilar impression can be divided into primary, or congenital, and secondary, or acquired (Table 9–1). Although considerable areas of overlap exist, and combinations of abnormalities are common, primary causes represent a true congenital malformation. Secondary basilar impression, however, is associated with a disease process leading to structural change of the skull base. Acquired basilar impression is relatively rare, being found in only 3 to 8 percent of all cases.[75] Paget's disease is the most frequently mentioned secondary cause, although it is uncommon in children.[72] Disordered calcium and phosphorus metabolism is infrequently

Table 9-1. MALFORMATIONS OF THE BASIOCCIPUT AND THE FORAMEN MAGNUM

Basilar Impression[37, 60, 68, 76]
  Primary or Congenital
    Familial[8, 49]
    Down's syndrome[63]
    Achondroplasia[54, 80, 88]
    Mucopolysaccharidosis
    Arnold-Chiari malformation[19, 20, 31]
    Cleidocranial dysplasia[42, 56]
    Osteogenesis imperfecta[38, 56, 68, 73]
  Secondary or Acquired
    Osteomalacia[8, 13, 39]
    Paget's disease[9, 27, 83]
    Fibrous dysplasia[43]
    Rickets[39]
    Hypothyroidism[26]
    Hyperparathyroidism[8, 51]
    Neoplastic process[22]
    Infectious process[10]
    Birth trauma[2]
    Trauma
Basioccipital clefts[41, 46, 53, 75, 85]
Hypoplasia of the clivus[21]
Occipital condylar hyperplasia[22, 45, 78]
Third occipital condyle[53, 61, 78]
Occipital vertebra[53, 61]
Paracondylar process[75, 78]
Basilar processes[17, 75, 78]
Bone masses on the anterior rim of the foramen magnum[17, 75]
Persistent mendosal suture
Premature closure of the occipital synchondrosis[15, 45]

reported as a cause of basilar impression.[39] Traumatic basilar impression is extremely rare, although trauma is a frequent precipitating event.[68] The higher-than-expected frequency of birth trauma found in adults with basilar impression led Battersby and Williams[2] to hypothesize that an abnormal or difficult labor might contribute to or be responsible for some examples of basilar impression resulting from disruption of normal growth and development of the basicranium.

While many instances of presumed congenital etiology can be found in the literature, the paucity of clinical reports in infants and younger children is striking. Gardner[32] and Lindgren[51] felt that the invagination could be explained by the transition from a recumbent posture to an upright stature. The weight of the relatively heavy skull and brain presumably exerts more pressure than the craniocervical junction can support. While the disease is congenital, the bony abnormality is developmental. In addition, constant radiographic landmarks required for measurements are obscured in the infant by incomplete ossification and calcification of the chondrocranium and cervical spine.

Congenital causes of basilar impression are represented by a group of diseases characterized by both biochemical and structural bony abnormalities of a genetic origin. The inheritance pattern of achondroplasia is autosomal dominant. Inadequate endochondral bone formation leads to retardation of growth of the skull base. The clivus is shortened and assumes a more vertical orientation. The posterior fossa is deformed, although recent studies indicate that its volume is preserved by a compensatory elevation of the tentorium.[71] The odontoid is high, although Pierre-Kahn found true basilar impression in only one of ten patients.[71] The atlas lies in close proximity to the occiput. Atlanto-occipital assimilation has not been reported, although fibrous fusion between the posterior arch and the occiput is implied and may account for the radiographic appearance of basilar impression.[16] Significant deformation and stenosis of the foramen magnum is characteristic and may be symptomatic (Fig. 9–5).[54, 71, 88]

Down's syndrome also involves the skull base and the foramen magnum. In reviewing this topic, Michejda suggested multiple factors that might be responsible or might play a role in the abnormal development of the basiocciput.[63] Delayed fusion of basal synchondroses coupled with endocrine factors and abnormal mucopolysaccharide metabolism are areas requiring further research.

Basilar impression is a well-recognized although rare complication in patients with osteogenesis imperfecta. Pozo and colleagues[73] noted that all cases reported in the literature had the mild form of the disease, defined as osteogenesis imperfecta tarda. He further suggested that the differences in occurrence might be due to aberrations in the collagen DNA sequence.

Associated Conditions

Herniation of the cerebellar tonsils has often been reported with basilar impression.[19, 20, 31, 81] While these two entities are seen in association and as isolated malformations, supporting a primary congenital etiology, tonsillar herniation has also been described in secondary basilar impression (Fig. 9–6).[27]

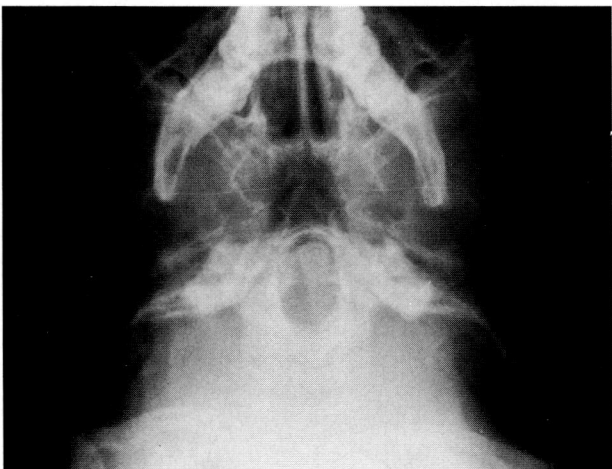

Figure 9–5. An abnormally shaped foramen magnum is identified in a child with achondroplasia. Spasticity, gait problems, and urinary incontinence prompted posterior decompression. The results were excellent.

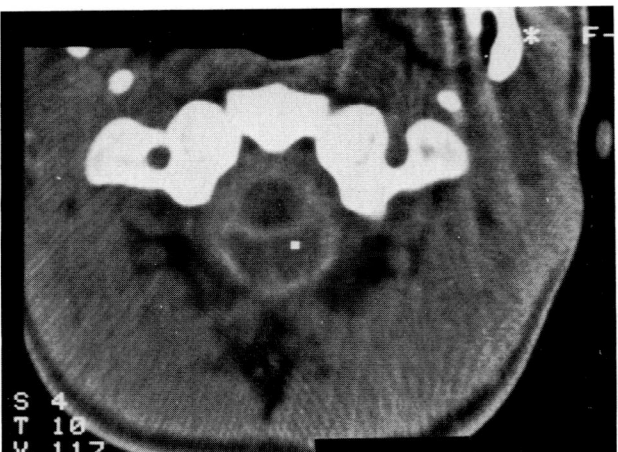

Figure 9–6. Tonsillar herniation is demonstrated by CT myelography (white box on the left cerebellar tonsil) in a child with a mucopolysaccharidosis, Maroteaux-Lamy syndrome.

Although less frequent, an association of basilar impression and syringomyelia is reported.[36, 58, 72] Hertel and associates[36] noted that one third of 81 cases of syringomyelia had basilar impression, although age was not considered. It is always difficult to determine whether the syrinx is primary or secondary, as symptoms may be related to either lesion. Several additional intrinsic neural anomalies have been reported, including familial aqueductal stenosis.[74]

Other skeletal malformations have been reported in association with basilar impression.[75] Associated anomalies include a high-arched palate, polydactyly and syndactyly, pes cavus, iris heterochromia, Sprengel's deformity, scoliosis, torticollis, and skull abnormalities.

Symptoms

Basilar impression is a radiologically detected abnormality. As such, it may be associated with clinical symptoms, although Burrows[10] found that only 45 percent of patients manifested appropriate signs and symptoms. In infants, developmental abnormalities in the region of the craniocervical junction are often accompanied by hydrocephalus, whereas in the symptomatic adult or adolescent, ventricular dilatation is much less frequent. The onset of symptoms is insidious and usually progressive.[28] Diffuse, bilateral headache and occipital pain, often precipitated by head movement, are the most common symptoms. The pain is often most severe in the morning and may be unilateral, resembling occipital neuralgia. Weakness of one or both legs or arms, paresthesias, and dysesthesias are less frequently reported. Symptoms and signs referable to cranial nerve dysfunction include diplopia, facial pain, dysphagia, and hearing disturbances. Symptoms attributed to disruption of the vertebrobasilar circulation are drop attacks, transient paralysis, and amaurosis fugax.[82] The concept of a vascular etiology as responsible for neurologic symptoms is supported by a high incidence of vascular changes in association with craniocervical junction abnormalities.[4, 40]

Signs

A characteristic physical feature, although infrequently noted, is a stocky, short neck with restriction of passive movements of the head. Facial asymmetry may accompany this finding.

Neurologic signs can be grouped into those causing disturbances of the cerebellum, of the pyramidal tracts, and of the cranial nerves. Rarely do these signs occur in isolation. Nystagmus is the most common sign of basilar impression but is nonspecific. Movement of the eyes may be in any direction and is reported to be supravestibular in origin.[75] Ataxia and dysmetria are less frequently found.

Paraparesis with hyper-reflexia and extensor plantar responses are the hallmark of pyramidal tract involvement. Upper extremity paresis rarely occurs as the only or predominant sign. Sensory changes are usually not striking, although pain of a sharp, shooting nature may be elicited (Lhermitte's sign). Bladder disturbance is rare.

Hypoglossal paresis may be the only neurologic sign.[75] Accessory nerve palsy is probably more common than its reported frequency. Vocal cord paresis and dysarthria point to the vagus or its branches. Facial paresis and trigeminal involvement have been reported.[1, 69]

Radiographic Investigation

A complete skull series and cervical spine survey are always indicated. Careful determination of relationships of structures to constructed lines is required and often leads to the diagnosis as well as suggesting the need for tomography. The odontoid tip should not be greater than 5 mm above Chamberlain's line or 7 mm above McGregor's line.[37] The normal distance of the digastric line is 10 mm and is reduced in the presence of invagination. The digastric line is the upper limit in position of the odontoid tip.[22] Klaus's height index should not be less than 30 mm. McRae's line, the anteroposterior diameter of the foramen magnum, should be greater than 19 mm.

Additional Investigation

EEG abnormalities have been reported in 45 percent of 50 patients.[75] CSF studies are nonspecific, with elevations in protein levels observed in a substantial number of patients.

Differential Diagnosis

Basilar impression must be differentiated from other lesions of the posterior fossa and foramen magnum. Tumors of the brainstem, cerebellum, and fourth ventricle rarely produce the characteristic bone changes and are often associated with hydrocephalus, which is not common in uncomplicated basilar impression. McRae[61] has presented 68 patients, noting their referring diagnosis at the time of admission. These include multiple sclerosis, cervical fracture or dislocation, degenerative spinal disease, spinocerebellar degenerative disease, and hysteria. To this can be added myelitis, amyotrophic lateral sclerosis, and variants of bulbar and pseudobulbar palsy.

Treatment

In the presence of significant and particularly progressive signs and symptoms, treatment is directed to providing adequate space. While conservative measures, including head and neck immobilization, may offer temporary relief, surgical decompression is eventually required.

Standard neurosurgical treatment has consisted of occipital craniectomy, including excision of the posterior rim of the foramen magnum and bilateral cervical decompressive laminectomy. Although rare, the surgeon must be aware of the possibility of respiratory dysfunction that can occur with flexion of the neck.[7, 44, 65] A preoperative trial of flexion in addition to measurement of resting blood gases and determination of respiratory function is suggested. The dura is opened, and arachnoid adhesions, if present, are lysed. The dura is left open, or preferably, a graft is employed. Prior to 1960, the operative mortality rate was as high as 36 percent, but recent operative experience indicates a mortality rate of 5 percent.[24, 70] Nearly two thirds of patients either show improvement or demonstrate cessation of their progressive disease.[23]

Menezes and coworkers[62] have formulated a physiologic approach to the cervicomedullary region, based on the mechanism of compression and the ability to achieve reduction at the craniocervical junction. Myelography and pluridirectional tomography demonstrated the direction of compression and dictated the surgical approach. Patients with anterior compression underwent resection of the offending structure (i.e., odontoid, clivus, or atlas), by a transoral approach.[34] Instability required posterior or posterolateral fusion. Dorsal impingement on neural structures was treated by suboccipital craniectomy and cervical decompression. All patients showed improvement or recovered, and morbidity was minimal.

Basioccipital Clefts

Retention of sclerotomal segmentation results in complete or partial clefts or fissures in the basiociput. They are best visualized using a modified Waters' projection and tomography. The clefts are similar to the normal synchondroses, being smooth, often paired, and 3–5 mm in depth.[41] They may be associated with additional fetal malformations or may be entirely asymptomatic.

Occipital Condylar Hypoplasia

Hypoplasia of the occipital condyles is most commonly asymptomatic. Because of the relatively elevated position of the atlas, the foramen magnum may be compromised, producing neurologic dysfunction. Roentgenograms demonstrate the odontoid to be high in relation to Chamberlain's and McGregor's lines. Anteroposterior tomography reveals elevation of the dens above the digastric line and allows for an estimation of the height of the occipital condyles. Occipital condylar hypoplasia has been described in Morquio's disease, spondyloepiphyseal dysplasia, and Conradi's syndrome.[22, 33, 39, 86]

Third Occipital Condyle, Occipital Vertebra, and Occipitalization of the Atlas

Anomalous bony formations around the foramen magnum may be difficult to classify because of their diversity. A third condyle is located in the midline above the anterior arch of the atlas but is separated from the atlas. While it may be a type of occipital vertebra, it should not be misdiagnosed as an occipitalized atlas.[53] Often, the lateral condyles are hypoplastic, the atlas is high, and the clivus is short. The condyle is usually asymptomatic, but it may restrict head and neck movements.

Differentiation between an occipital vertebra and an occipitalized atlas is often difficult. McRae has reviewed and established criteria for differentiating these lesions.[61] The lack of a foramen for the passage of the vertebral artery or suboccipital nerve supports a diagnosis of occipital vertebra. Both lesions are usually asymptomatic.

Paracondylar Process

This accessory bony structure extends from the paracondylar surface of the occipital bone towards the transverse process of the atlas. In its pure form it is asymptomatic, but it is usually found in conjunction with other anomalies of the craniocervical region. The epitransverse process of the atlas is its mirror image projecting from the transverse process of the atlas toward the occiput.

Premature Closure of the Occipital Synchondroses

As development of the chondrocranium proceeds, sutures between the two exoccipital centers and the basioccipital bone anteriorly (anterior synchondrosis) and the supraoccipital bone posteriorly (innominate synchondrosis) can be seen.

They are easily visualized at one year of age and persist until nearly four years of age. Premature synostosis of these sutures has been documented by Kruyff.[45] Anterior synostosis results in improper migration and formation of the occipital condyles and asymmetry of the foramen magnum. Of the eight infants reported by Kruyff, all were neurologically intact, although he speculated that problems might develop as the children grew. Careful observation was suggested.

CONGENITAL SKULL DYSPLASIAS

The skeletal dysplasias are a diverse group of inherited disorders (Table 9–2). Many of these disorders are characterized by prominent changes in the calvarium, and others produced pronounced thickening or sclerosis of the skull base and the foramen magnum.

Osteopetrosis is a rare disorder characterized by dense, compact, homogeneous bone. Encroachment of the skull base foramina may result in cranial nerve deficits, especially affecting the optic nerve.[48, 87] Surgical decompression of the optic nerves may be required to preserve vision. The need for decompression of other cranial nerves of the skull base has not been reported.

Pyknodysostosis combines the features of cleidocranial dysostosis and osteopetrosis.[25] The disease is characterized by multiple long-bone fractures and a thickened skull base.

Engelmann-Camurati disease involves sclerotic enlargement of the diaphyseal portion of the long bones and thickening of the skull base.[79] Blindness associated with optic atrophy and deafness have been reported.

Van Buchem and colleagues[84] have described in detail seven patients with tremendous thickening and sclerosis of the skull and osteosclerosis of the diaphyseal portions of the long bones. Disturbances of vision, abnormalities of the optic fundi, deafness, and facial palsies were encountered.

Pyle's disease is also characterized by skull base sclerosis and multiple cranial nerve palsies.[64]

ABNORMALITIES OF THE FIRST CERVICAL SCLEROTOME

Occipitalization of the Atlas

The incidence of assimilation of the atlas to the foramen magnum has been variously reported as between 0.08 and 3 percent of the general population (Table 9–3).[11] Fusion of the atlas to the occiput is most commonly anterior and results in flexion and extension at the atlantoaxial joint rather than

Table 9–2. CONGENITAL SKULL DYSPLASIAS

Osteopetrosis (Albers-Schönberg disease)[48, 87, 89]
Pyknodysosteogenesis[25]
Progressive diaphyseal dysplasia (Engelmann-Camurati disease)[79, 87]
Van Buchem's disease[84]
Endemic fluorosis
Craniometaphyseal dysplasia (Pyle's disease)[12, 64]
Achondroplasia[54, 80, 88]

at the atlanto-occipital level. The area of fusion becomes the effective foramen magnum. The odontoid often is high because of the assimilation and is situated at the point of movement in flexion or extension. McRae[61] found that all patients were symptomatic if the anteroposterior diameter from the odontoid to the posterior margin of the effective foramen magnum was less than 19 mm. Symptoms are localized to disturbances of the medulla and upper cervical spine, with torticollis, weakness, pain, ataxia, and numbness being frequently encountered.[6, 35] Stress at the atlantoaxial joint may produce dislocation if ligamentous laxity is present. Fusion of C2 to C1 and degrees of Klippel-Feil syndrome are commonly associated with atlantic assimilation.[7] Although basilar impression has been a frequent accompanying abnormality, it is not an absolute association. Likewise, basilar impression does not cause assimilation of the atlas.[4, 11, 27, 70, 82]

Atlanto-occipital fusion is usually a congenital abnormality resulting from failure of segmentation. Rarely, it may be secondary to a neoplastic or infectious process.

Surgical treatment consists of decompression of the foramen magnum by either odontoidectomy or suboccipital craniectomy and removal of the posterior arch of the atlas. Atlantoaxial dislocation requires bony fusion.

Dysplasia and Dysraphism

Most of the defects or anomalies in this category are asymptomatic and require differentiation from other conditions, such as trauma, that may produce neurologic deficit. A spicule of bone extending from

Table 9–3. ABNORMALITIES OF THE FIRST CERVICAL SCLEROTOME AND ATLAS

Fusion
  Assimilation or occipitalization of the atlas[6, 7, 11, 35, 52, 60, 61, 67, 81]
  Atlantoaxial fusion
Dysplasia
  Malformations of the transverse processes
  Ponticulus lateralis[61]
  Ponticulus posticus[61]
  Epitransverse process[78]
  Malformations of the lateral masses
  Hypoplasia of C1:[30, 83] Turner's syndrome
Dysraphism[47, 61]
  Anterior arch defects[35, 75]
  Posterior arch defects[18, 70]

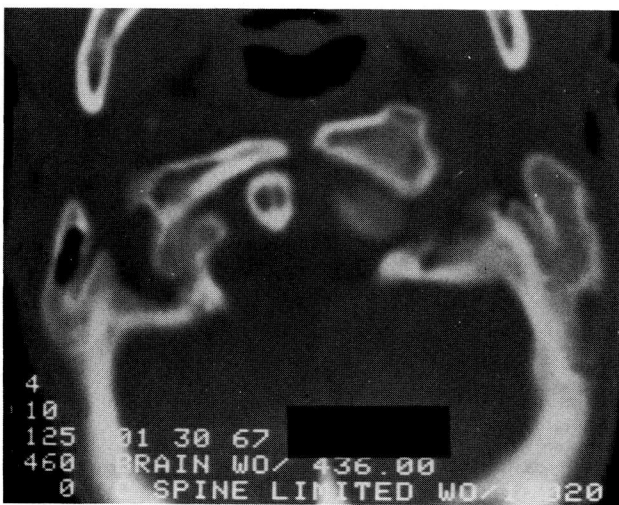

Figure 9–7. CT scan of the craniocervical junction demonstrates anterior spina bifida of C1. The patient is slightly rotated.

the lateral edge of the superior facet of the atlas to the transverse process represents a ponticulus lateralis. This bony bridge extends over the posterolateral margin of the foramen transversarium. If the spicule passes over the posterior margin, it is labeled a ponticulus posticus.

Anterior or posterior defects in the atlas or axis (spina bifida occulta) are rare. McRae[61] found isolated posterior rachischisis in 2 percent of asymptomatic persons and only one case of isolated anterior rachischisis, although the authors have recently seen a 14-year-old with asymptomatic C1 anterior spina bifida (Fig. 9–7). Isolated cases have been described with unilateral absence of the posterior arch.[55]

ABNORMALITIES OF THE DENS

Congenital abnormalities of the odontoid process do not properly fall into a consideration of anomalies of the craniocervical junction. However, they are sufficiently frequent and significant to justify a very brief description. The odontoid bone may be completely absent, separated from the body of the axis, partially developed, or represented by a bony process extending downward from the occipital bone. Regardless of the precise configuration of the defect, there may be instability between the axis and the atlas, leading to subluxation at the junction during normal flexion and extension movements. Treatment by fusion of the two vertebral segments is essential to preventing this abnormal movement and may be accomplished by external immobilization in some children.

References

1. Bares L: Basilar impression and the so-called associated anomalies. Eur Neurol 13:92, 1975.
2. Battersby RD, Williams B: Birth injury: A possible contributory factor in the aetiology of primary basilar impression. J Neurol Neurosurg Psychiatry 45:879, 1982.
3. Berg FT, Retzius A: Fasc 1, Museum Anatomicium Holmiensae, Stockholm. Quoted by Spillane JD, 1957.
4. Bernini FP, Elefante R, Smaltino F, et al: Angiographic study on the vertebral artery in cases of deformities of the occipitocervical joint. Am J Roentgenol 107:526, 1969.
5. Bewermeyer H, Dreesbach HA, Hunermann B, et al: MR imaging of familial basilar impression. J Comput Assist Tomogr 8:953, 1984.
6. Bezi I: Assimilation of the atlas and compression of the medulla. Arch Pathol 12:333, 1931.
7. Bharucha EP, Dastur HM: Craniovertebral anomalies. Brain 87:469, 1964.
8. Bull JWD, Nixon WLB, Pratt RTC: The radiological criteria and familial occurrence of primary basilar impression. Brain 78:229, 1955.
9. Bull JWD, Nixon WLB, Pratt RTC, et al: Paget's disease of the skull and secondary basilar impression. Brain 82:10, 1959.
10. Burrows EH: Clinical relevance of radiological abnormalities of the craniovertebral junction. Br J Radiol 54:195, 1981.
11. Burwood RJ, Watt I: Assimilation of the atlas and basilar impression: A review of 1,500 skull and cervical spine radiographs. Clin Radiol 25:327, 1974.
12. Caffey J: Pediatric X-Ray Diagnosis, 5th ed. Chicago, Year Book, 1967.
13. Chakrabarti AK, Johnson SC, Samantray SK, et al: Osteomalacia, myelopathy, and basilar impression. J Neurol Sci 23:227, 1974.
14. Chamberlain WE: Basilar impression (platybasia). Yale J Biol Med 11:487, 1939.
15. Coin CG, Malkasian DR: Foramen magnum. In: Newton TH, Potts DG (eds): Radiology of the Skull and Brain, Vol 1. St. Louis, CV Mosby Co, 1971, pp 275–286.
16. Crawford DB, Ensor RE, Dorst JP: The chondrocranium in achondroplasia. In: Bosma JF (ed): Development of the Basicranium. Washington, DC, Dept. HEW Publication No. NIH 76–989, 1976, pp 301–318.
17. Custis DL, Verbrugghen A: Basilar impression resembling cerebellar tumor. Arch Neurol Psychiatry 52:412, 1944.
18. Dalinka MK, Rosenbaum AE, Van Houten F: Congenital absence of the posterior arch of the atlas. Radiology 103:581, 1972.
19. DeBarros MC, Farias W, Ataide L, et al: Basilar impression and Arnold-Chiari malformation. J Neurol Neurosurg Psychiatry 31:596, 1968.
20. DeBarros MC, DaSilva WF, DeAzevedo HC, et al: Disturbances of sexual potency in patients with basilar impression and Arnold-Chiari malformation. J Neurol Neurosurg Psychiatry 38:598, 1975.
21. DeChiro G, Anderson WB: The clivus. Clin Radiol 16:211, 1965.
22. Dolan KD: Cervicobasilar relationships. Radiol Clin North Am 15:155, 1977.
23. Driesen W, Oldenkott P, Ross V, et al: Results of surgical treatment of basilar impression. Acta Neurochir 15:83, 1966.
24. Driesen W: Craniospinal malformations as a particular example of pathogenetic significance of biomechanical factors. In: Modern Aspects of Neurosurgery, Procedures, German Society for Neurosurgery, Vol 3. Dusseldorf, Nov. 14–17, 1971.
25. Dusenberry JF, Kane JJ: Pyknodysostosis. Am J Roentgenol 99:717, 1967.
26. Engel MD, Bronstein IP, Brodie AG, et al: A roentgenographic cephalometric appraisal of the untreated and treated hypothyroidism. Am J Dis Child 61:1193, 1941.
27. Epstein BS, Epstein JA: The association of cerebellar tonsillar herniation with basilar impression incident to Paget's disease. Am J Roentgenol 107:535, 1969.
28. Erickson TC, Paul LW, Suckle HM: Clinical observations on basilar impression of the skull. Trans Am Neurol Assoc 75:180, 1950.
29. Fischgold H, Metzger J: Etude radiotomographique de l'impression basilare. Rev Rhumat 19:261, 1952.

30. Fromm GH, Pitner SE: Large progressive quadriparesis due to odontoid agenesis. Arch Neurol 9:291, 1963.
31. Gardner WJ, Goodall RJ: The surgical treatment of Arnold-Chiari malformation in adults. J Neurosurg 7:199, 1950.
32. Gardner WJ: Anomalies of the craniovertebral junction. In: Youmans JR (ed): Neurological Surgery, Vol 1. Philadelphia, WB Saunders Co, 1973, pp 628–643.
33. Gilles RH, Bina M, Sotrel A: Infantile atlanto-occipital instability. The potential danger of extreme extension. Am J Dis Child 133:30, 1979.
34. Greenberg AD, Scoville WB, Davey LM: Transoral decompression of the atlantoaxial dislocation due to odontoid hypoplasia. Report of two cases. J Neurosurg 28:266, 1968.
35. Hadley LA: Atlanto-occipital fusion, ossiculum terminale, and occipital vertebra as related to basilar impression with neurological symptoms. Am J Roentgenol 59:511, 1948.
36. Hertel G, Naddmi M, Kunze J: A statistical comparative study of the basilar impression in syringomyelia. Eur Neurol 11:363, 1974.
37. Hinck VC, Hopkins CE, Savara BS: Diagnostic criteria of basilar impression. Radiology 76:572, 1961.
38. Hurwitz LJ, McSwiney RR: Basilar impression and osteogenesis imperfecta in a family. Brain 83:138, 1960.
39. Hurwitz LJ, Shepard WH: Basilar impression and disordered metabolism of bone. Brain 89:223, 1966.
40. Janeway R, Toole JF, Leinbach LB, et al: Vertebral artery obstruction with basilar impression. Arch Neurol 15:211, 1966.
41. Johnson GF, Israel H: Basioccipital clefts. Radiology 133:101, 1979.
42. Keats T: Cleidocranial dysostosis: Some atypical roentgen manifestations. Am J Roentgenol 100:71, 1967.
43. Klaus E: Die basilare Impression. Leipzig, S Hirzel, 1969.
44. Krieger AJ, Rosomoff HL, Kuperman AS, et al: Occult respiratory dysfunction in a craniovertebral anomaly. J Neurosurg 31:15, 1969.
45. Kruyff E: Occipital dysplasia in infancy. Radiology 85:501, 1965.
46. Kruyff E: Transverse cleft in the basi-occiput. Acta Radiol 6:41, 1967.
47. Lawrence WS, Anderson WD: Rare developmental abnormality of atlas. Radiology 28:55, 1937.
48. Lehman RAW, Reves JD, Wilson WB, et al: Neurological complications of infantile osteopetrosis. Ann Neurol 2:378, 1977.
49. Lehman RAW, Stears JC, Wesenberg RL, et al: Familial osteosclerosis with abnormalities of the nervous system and meninges. J Pediatr 90:49, 1977.
50. Lemire RJ, Loeser JD, Leech RW, et al: Skull. In: Lemire RJ (ed): Normal and Abnormal Development of the Human Nervous System. Hagerstown, Harper & Row, 1975, pp 289–309.
51. Lindgren E: Roentgenologic views on basilar impression. Acta Radiol (Stockh) 22:297, 1941.
52. List CF: Developmental anomalies of the craniovertebral border. In: Kahn EA, Bassett RC, Schneider RC, et al (eds): Correlative Neurosurgery. Springfield, Charles C Thomas, 1955, pp 335–362.
53. Lombardi G: The occipital vertebra. Am J Roentgenol 86:260, 1961.
54. Luyendijk W, Matricali B, Thomeer RTWM: Basilar impression in an achondroplastic dwarf: Causative role in tetraparesis. Acta Neurochir 41:243, 1978.
55. MacAlister A: Notes on development and variations of the atlas. J Anat Physiol 27:519, 1892.
56. Maroteaux P: Bone Diseases of Children. Philadelphia, JB Lippincott Co, 1979, pp 158–161.
57. McGregor M: The significance of certain measurements of the skull in the diagnosis of basilar impression. Br J Radiol 21:171, 1948.
58. McRae DL: Bony abnormalities in the region of the foramen magnum. Correlation of anatomic and neurologic findings. Acta Radiol 40:335, 1953.
59. McRae DL, Barnum AS: Occipitalization of the atlas. Am J Roentgenol 70:23, 1953.
60. McRae DL: Bony abnormalities at the craniospinal junction. In: Ojemann RG (ed): Clinical Neurosurgery, Vol 16. Baltimore, Williams & Wilkins, 1969, pp 356–375.
61. McRae DL: Craniovertebral junction. In: Newton TH, Potts DG (eds): Radiology of the Skull and Brain, Vol 1. St. Louis, CV Mosby Co, 1971, pp 260–286.
62. Menezes AH, VanGilder JC, Graf CJ, et al: Craniocervical abnormalities. A comprehensive surgical approach. J Neurosurg 53:444, 1980.
63. Michejda M, Menolascino FJ: Skull base abnormalities in Down's syndrome. Ment Retard 131:24, 1975.
64. Mori PA, Holt JF: Cranial manifestations of familial metaphysical dysplasia. Radiology 66:335, 1956.
65. Mullan S, Raimondi A: Respiratory hazards of the surgical treatment of the Arnold-Chiari malformation. J Neurosurg 19:675–678, 1962.
66. Murtagh FR: Visualization of basilar invagination by computerized tomography. Arch Neurol 36:659, 1979.
67. Nicholson JT, Sherk HH: Anomalies of the occipitocervical articulation. J Bone Joint Surg 50A:295, 1968.
68. O'Connell JEA, Turner JWA: Basilar impression of the skull. Brain 73:405, 1950.
69. Paradis RW, Sax DS: Familial basilar impression. Neurology 22:554, 1972.
70. Peyton WT, Peterson HO: Congenital deformities in the region of the foramen magnum: Basilar impression. Radiology 38:131, 1942.
71. Pierre-Kahn A, Hirsch JF, Renier D, et al: Hydrocephalus and achondroplasia. Child's Brain 7:205, 1980.
72. Poppel MH, Jacobsen HG, Duff BK, et al: Basilar impression and platybasia in Paget's disease. Radiology 61:639, 1953.
73. Pozo JL, Crockard HA, Ransford AO: Basilar impression in osteogenesis imperfecta. A report of three cases in one family. J Bone Joint Surg 66B:233, 1984.
74. Sajid MH, Copple PJ: Familial aqueductal stenosis and basilar impression. Neurology 18:260, 1968.
75. Schmidt H, Sartor K, Heckl RW: Bone malformation of the craniocervical region. In: Vinken PJ, Bruyn GW (eds): Handbook of Clinical Neurology, Vol. 32, pt. 1. Amsterdam, Elsevier, North Holland, 1978, pp 1–83.
76. Scoville WB, Sherman IJ: Platybasia. Ann Surg 133:496, 1951.
77. Shapiro R, Robinson F: Embryogenesis of the human occipital bone. Am J Roentgenol 126:1063, 1976.
78. Shapiro R, Robinson F: Anomalies of the craniovertebral border. Am J Roentgenol 127:281, 1976.
79. Singleton EB, Thomas JR, Worthington WW, et al: Progressive diaphyseal dysplasia (Engelmann's disease). Radiology 67:233, 1956.
80. Spillane JD: Three cases of achondroplasia with neurological complications. J Neurol Neurosurg Psychiatry 15:246, 1952.
81. Spillane JD, Pallis C, Jones AM: Developmental abnormalities in the region of the foramen magnum. Brain 80:11, 1957.
82. Taylor AR, Chakravorty BC: Clinical syndromes associated with basilar impression. Arch Neurol 10:475, 1964.
83. Tishler J, Martel W: Dislocation of the atlas in mongolism. Radiology 84:904, 1965.
84. Van Buchem FSP, Hadders HN, Hansen JF, et al: Hyperostosis corticalis generalisata. Am J Med 33:387, 1962.
85. Wackenheim A: Roentgen Diagnosis of the Craniovertebral Region. Berlin, Springer-Verlag, 1974.
86. White AA, Panjabi MM: The clinical biomechanics of the occipitoatlantoaxial complex. Orthop Clin North Am 9:867, 1978.
87. Winchester PH, Grossman H: Congenital skull dysplasias. In: Newton TH, Pitts DG (eds): Radiology of the Skull and Brain, Vol 2. St. Louis, CV Mosby Co, 1971, pp 653–661.
88. Yamada H, Nakamura S, Tajima M, et al: Neurologic manifestations of pediatric achondroplasia. J Neurosurg 54:49, 1981.
89. Yarington C, Sprinkle P: Facial palsy in osteopetrosis: Relief by endotemporal decompression. JAMA 202:549, 1967.
90. Zingesser LH: Radiologic aspects of anomalies of the upper cervical spine and craniocervical junction. In: Wilkins RH (ed): Clinical Neurosurgery, Vol 20. Baltimore, Williams & Wilkins, 1973, pp 220–231.

10
MEDICAL ETHICS: THE RESOLUTION OF MORAL DILEMMAS IN THE MANAGEMENT OF CHILDREN WITH SEVERE CONGENITAL ANOMALIES

Anthony E. Gallo, Jr., M.D.

HISTORY

Medical ethics has been an integral part of the practice of medicine in the Western world since the earliest historical recordings. The hippocratic oath (500 B.C.?) codified the moral behavior and ethical stance of physicians for the next 2500 years. This has been attested to by the graduation ceremonies of medical schools throughout the Western world, where, as a part of the ceremony, the graduates swore to the oath of Hippocrates. Many schools continue this tradition to this day, though a number of schools now recite the Declaration of Geneva or similar modern updates of the oath of Hippocrates.[8]

The principles espoused through the ages have included (1) a regard for one's teachers and, even, a concern for their well-being, (2) a dedication to the well-being of one's patients and, even, a positive role in protecting them from harm and injustice, (3) the utmost respect for life, including an unwillingness to participate in an act leading to the death of the patient, (4) a respect for the person of the patient regardless of his station, and (5) holding of the physician-patient relationship in strict confidentiality.

The increasing complexity of medicine, the development of multiple health care systems, and the development of a huge, largely federally funded research establishment have, in recent decades, resulted in the proliferation of reports, statements, and guidelines designed to legitimize the behavior of various parts of the medical profession. These documents have been generated from bodies as diverse as the American Medical Association, the American Nursing Association, the American Hospital Association,[1] and, most recently, the American Association of Neurological Surgeons (AANS), which published "The American Association of Neurological Surgeons Code of Ethics" in the AANS yearbook for 1986.[2] It is interesting to note that the ethical concerns of the medical profession are reflected not only in the wide variety of documents that have been created in recent times but also in the size of these documents. The oath of Hippocrates contains ten sentences detailing the relationship of physicians to their teachers and their patients. This is to be contrasted with the AANS Code of Ethics, which contains 27 sentences, subdivided into seven sections, that deal with the ethics of (1) the neurologic surgeon, (2) the physician-physician relationship, (3) the relationship of the physician with the patient and with the patient's family, (4) the physician and the legal profession, (5) the relationship of the neurologic surgeon with the government, (6) the relationship of the physician with the insurance compensation and reimbursement agencies, and (7) the physician's relationship with the community and concern with world affairs.

One can readily see from this brief historical survey of codes of ethics that their increasing complexity is related to the resolution of modern moral dilemmas (including the care of severe congenital anomalies) that came into existence only after World War II.

TECHNOLOGY

It is interesting to note the influence of technology on our values and on the way we resolve moral dilemmas. This is no better demonstrated than in the changing selection criteria used in the treatment of myelodysplasia. The absence of aseptic technique, antibiotic therapy, and endotracheal anesthesia limited surgical repair of myelomeningoceles to occasional anecdotal reports consisting largely of sac ligation.[20]

The twentieth century heralded new attempts at the repair of these lesions, with surgery restricted mostly to the repair of the epithelialized sac in surviving children with little evidence of hydrocephalus or paralysis.[15]

The development of antibiotic therapy and cerebrospinal fluid shunting techniques made surgical therapy realistically available to a large number of infants who previously could not be considered for treatment on purely technical grounds. With the advent of these new skills came a Pandora's box of ethical problems. Now for the first time, the question "Who should survive?" was not to be answered by the limits of surgical skills alone. In the first half of the sixties, the advantages of early closure and a multidisciplinary approach to the longitudinal care of children with myelodysplasia took hold and spread rapidly from a small base in Sheffield, England, to multiple centers around the North American continent. The monumental paper of Sharrard and colleagues[25] kindled both altruism and surgical imagination around the world. This was reinforced by the conviction, energy, and zeal of Sharrard, who championed the early repair of myelomeningoceles in all but the most severely afflicted children.

This movement was not to silence all other voices, however, as others cautioned and argued for a more selective approach. Matson[19] argued for early surgical therapy in the infant with good lower extremity function and for more expectant but supportive care for the infant with total paralysis of the lower extremities. This would permit a delayed repair in early childhood for those who survived. He stressed the need to consider all the factors that contribute to the child's well-being, including intellectual impairment and the physical and emotional support systems available to the child. It was clear to Matson that the responsibility of the neurosurgeon was to serve as an *advocate for the patient*.[19]

In 1971, a dramatic shift occurred in the treatment of myelodysplasia. In a highly controversial paper reviewing the experience with 524 patients, Lorber[18] suggested that selection criteria be much stricter in the treatment of myelodysplasia. His justification sprang from the documentation of poorer results in the more severely afflicted children. The guidelines were quite specific, with recommendations that those children with severe hydrocephalus, significant associated anomalies, kyphosis, and extensive paralysis remain untreated.[18] This therapeutic philosophy became widespread in many centers treating myelodysplasia.

In recent years, increasing experience has significantly modified this trend, as further observations substantiate that many untreated infants do not die and that many infants with severe hydrocephalus that is treated early can be intellectually normal. The ethical dilemmas of the early seventies were beautifully reviewed by Freeman in an extensive article entitled "To Treat or Not To Treat: Ethical Dilemmas of Treating the Infant with a Myelomeningocele."[9] The worrisome conclusion inevitably drawn from the publications of this period was that technology was advancing at such a rapid rate that selection criteria were virtually invalidated at the same time that the criteria were being disseminated throughout the medical community.

Advancements in urologic care (particularly intermittent catheterization techniques), pediatric and neonatal intensive care units, central nervous system imaging, and the treatment of kyphoscoliosis (to name but a few areas) continue to improve the prognosis in the surgical treatment of myelodysplasia, to the point where fewer and fewer children are left untreated, if for no other reason than the uncertainty about prognosis.[12]

GENERAL SUBSTRATES OF ETHICAL CONFLICT

The Society

The populations of the United States and Canada are nonhomogeneous and are becoming more so with extensive immigration. In addition, both countries, because of their great land masses, have multiple, relatively isolated minisocieties with their own special value systems. Whether or not to offer surgical therapy to a newborn infant with a severe congenital deformity remains a significant ethical and legal controversy in the United States;[23] however, it would not have been an issue in ancient Greece and still is not an issue in many parts of the world today. This discrepancy increases the probability of conflict, as physicians unwittingly bring to the physician-patient relationship a value system different from that of their patient.

There is no doubt that societal values have their most forceful impact on treatment decisions in areas of medical uncertainty. This was elegantly demonstrated by Nancy K. Rhoden, associate professor of law at Ohio State University, when she studied the treatment strategies used in the management of extremely premature infants in Sweden versus those in Great Britain versus those in the United States. Her comments are equally applicable to the management of myelodysplasia and other severe congenital anomalies:

> The ethical tensions inherent in all Baby Doe treatment conditions are compounded by medical uncertainty. Physicians both here and abroad have adopted various strategies. Swedish doctors tend to withhold treatment from the beginning from infants for whom statistical data suggest a grim prognosis. The British are more likely to initiate treatment but withdraw it if the infant appears likely to die or suffer severe brain damage. The trend in the U.S. is to start treating any baby who is potentially viable and continue until it is virtually certain that the infant will die. The "least worst" strategy is an individualized one: starting treatment, gathering data, and then reassessing the decision.[24]

What the cultural factors are that account for these differences remain conjecture, but it is clear, as others have noted, that U.S. physicians are exposed to nonmedical social pressures that are minimal or unknown in other Western societies. For instance, physicians are becoming increasingly aware of the potential legal liability of treating the infant who subsequently is found to be significantly impaired. This is probably felt most acutely in obstetrics and neurologic surgery. In contrast, malpractice suits are rare in Great Britain and have little influence in medical decision making in Sweden, where a no-fault compensation system for medical accidents currently exists.[24]

More recently, treatment decisions have been greatly influenced by the policies of government agencies. The Department of Health and Human Services' (DHHS) recent regulations concerning nontreatment of infants exerted considerable force on medical decision makers when coupled with their fear of being reported to child abuse agencies and with the possibility of withdrawal of financial support to the treating institution. There is little doubt that the legal interests and fears of both hospitals and physicians are factors in the treatment decisions in the management of severely compromised infants.[10, 24, 26] The roles of government and the law in the regulation of treatment decisions remain uncertain,[23] but the 9 June 1986 decision of the Supreme Court of the United States, vacating the aforementioned regulations of DHHS, criticized the role of the federal government in intervening in private and sensitive treatment decisions.[3] Such action gives new hope for preserving the hippocratic tradition.

Economic Factors

There is a sparsity of literature dealing with the influence of economic factors on medical ethics and, more particularly, on therapeutic choices in the treatment of severely compromised neonates.[10, 13, 24, 27]

The literature that does exist tends to focus on successful cost containment, the decreasing use of hospitals, shortening of the hospital stay, and other easily measurable parameters of medical health financing.[5, 13] Logic would dictate that the allocation of scarce resources and specialized methods of remuneration such as diagnosis-related groups (DRG) have an impact on treatment strategies. In spite of the fact that conclusions of some writers are rather guarded as to what specific effects economic factors have on treatment decisions, recent personal experiences and the experiences of many of the author's colleagues across the United States argue that economic factors are having a significant effect on treatment choices and, even, on the traditional role of the physician as patient advocate.[24, 27]

The utilization review committee, now present in virtually all major hospitals, clearly has such an influence. A typical example is the distribution of countless letters to physicians across the land, denying Medicare or Medicaid hospital payments for the last few days of hospitalization of the patient because, in the judgment of the utilization review committee, the hospitalization was unnecessarily prolonged. Even more common is the committee determination that hospitalization was *not* indicated.[22] In fact, this is the most common action taken by the hospital utilization review committee in the author's own institution. As a corollary, it should be noted that this institution has been exceedingly successful in reducing the average hospital stay of its patients (from 12.4 days in 1966 to 5.6 days in 1987), as has generally been the case across the nation. There is overwhelming evidence that such systems have a profound influence on the allocation of scarce resources, namely money, but it is equally clear that there is both an ethical and a medical price. The exhaustion, pain, and sense of neglect of a new mother unwillingly discharged on the first postpartum day, with little children at home, will never be reflected in the mortality and morbidity statistics of an obstetric service but remain vivid in the author's mind.[16]

The establishment of DRGs as a system of prospective payment is rapidly expanding. They are already applied to Medicare patients and are being studied by major third-party carriers. Such a system, by its fundamental design, has profound ethical implications for the practice of medicine. First, the advocacy role of the physician must, of necessity, change as he or she shifts from the position of providing the patient with the very best that medical science can offer regardless of the cost to the position of caring for the "diagnosis" within the financial constraints placed on the physician's "institution."[7]

Such a system also creates pressure for the physician both from the hospital administration and from his peer group, if his method of practice consistently results in cost overruns that are not easily justified (and thus funded) by such obvious medical factors as severity of disease, in-hospital complications, and a medically expensive subgroup (such as the indigent, chronic alcoholic, and the aged).

An increasing concern among thoughtful observers of the medical scene is the expanding role of health maintenance organizations (HMOs), in which the physician is the employee of the HMO and benefits financially by decreasing the utilization of hospitals and expensive technology. The potential risk of a significant change in ethical framework from that of patient advocate to that of institutional advocate is obvious. What remains unclear is whether there is a net social benefit to the reallocation of financial resources in such a fashion.[7] There is little question that the principles of patient-centered beneficence (physicians' choices are always directed toward patient benefit) can frequently be in conflict with the social ethical principle of full beneficence (the most good for the most people). In like manner, it can easily be seen how the principle of patient autonomy (the patient's right to self-determination) can clash with the principle of social justice (equal access to health care for all). It is difficult in these rapidly changing times, when one is both a member of society and a physician, to sort out these ethical conflicts as they relate to our individual patients. At least with regard to DRGs, Veatch has given some thoughtful commentary:

> To allocate resources ethically under DRGs, we need an expanded medical ethic. Appealing to traditional patient-centered principles such as individual beneficence and autonomy will not be sufficient. We also need to take into account the social principles of full beneficence and justice. If marginal benefits must be eliminated, clinicians should *not* participate in deciding who should get less care but *should remain committed to their patient's interest.*[27] [Italics mine.]

It would certainly seem reasonable that the role of patient advocate, wedded to an intelligent application of scientific principles, will guide medicine through the changing economic realities, as it guides us through the gray areas of surgical care in severe myelodyplasia.

Competence

More ethical controversy is centered around the issue of competence and informed consent than any other single issue in the care of the newborn. Obviously, the newborn is not competent, and therefore, one must look to the parents or the legal guardian to represent the best interests of the infant in getting an informed consent for surgical therapy.

In the intensely emotional arena of myelodysplasia treatment, when the expected "perfect" child is born not only imperfect but permanently disabled, it becomes difficult to determine what constitutes competence. There is a very constricted time frame for action. The large surgical defect in the spine requires early repair, preferably in the first 24 hours. Parents have little time to digest the large volume of totally unfamiliar medical information that is showered upon them. There is no time for them to acclimate themselves to the intensely emotionally charged atmosphere of the hospital and, particularly, the pediatric intensive care unit, when they are advised that the child will be at least partially paralyzed in the lower extremities and will require bracing, that the child will be incontinent of urine and feces, and that the probabilities are exceedingly high that the child will develop hydrocephalus and will require a ventriculoperitoneal shunt.[9, 10, 12] One can readily appreciate the conflict and anxiety that must arise in young parents.

Under these circumstances, it is not unreasonable to be concerned about the ability of the parents to safeguard the present and enhance the future of the newborn child. The management of the newborn with severe congenital anomalies of necessity raises alarming questions, such as whose future is to be enhanced, the parents, their families, or the newborn? This is particularly so in the severely compromised infant, who can be expected to achieve only limited goals at a significant economic and emotional price.

While ethicists continue to argue over what constitutes competence sufficient to give informed consent, experienced physicians uniformly recognize that competence, in any truly intellectual sense, cannot be achieved under such circumstances and that the emotional content and urgency of the situation does not permit the giving of a truly informed consent.* It is uncertain whether this problem will ever be resolved, whether the concept of a "valid consent" can be developed ethically and legally to resolve this moral dilemma. In the absence

---

*References 6, 9, 10, 12, 21, 23, 24

of new guidelines or another authority, physicians will continue to work with parents, informing them and guiding them to decisions that serve the best interests of the newborn child.

Autonomy

Patient autonomy (the right of self-determination) is often viewed as being in direct conflict with medical paternalism (the obligation of the physician to make decisions in the best interest of the patient). In the pediatric neurosurgical population and in the treatment of most children, the responsibility for treatment decisions and, therefore, patient autonomy is transferred from the patient to the parent. If the child is of sufficient age and intelligence to participate, ethicists and physicians alike would insist that he or she do so. In the vast majority of circumstances, patient autonomy and paternalism do not clash. Certainly, almost no one takes issue with the view that the autonomous state is a desirable state or that the patient (or the parents) should whenever possible assume the responsibility for therapeutic consent. In fact, the conflict centers around the *role* of medical paternalism, and the polar positions of "paternalism is good and necessary" versus "paternalism is evil, since it robs patients of their autonomy." However, recent thoughtful observers of the scene are less and less willing to participate in the argument, as insight into the dynamics of the physician-nurse-patient relationship tempers theoretical positions. If one recognizes that patient autonomy is not a steady state, that it is compromised by stress, unfamiliarity, illness, the needs of other members of the family, and the dependent position associated with the terror of illness, then the appropriate role of medical paternalism becomes clearer.[4, 14] Therefore, it becomes the responsibility of treating physicians to recognize when it is necessary to assume a paternalistic role in making treatment decisions for the patient in order to *restore* patient autonomy. Paternalism certainly is not a constant feature of the interaction between physicians and patients. In the autonomously well patient (Haavi Morreim would say "in the reflectively competent patient"[21]), paternalism plays no role. Certainly, in counseling parents concerning a largely elective procedure, for example sagittal craniectomy and the treatment of sagittal synostosis, interaction between the parents and the physician involves no decision making for the family by the physician, but rather a simple description of the procedure, associated expectations, complications, and available alternatives. The absence of paternalism in such a relationship is based on the elective nature of the treatment, which is evidenced by the fact that the refusal of surgery would not have a high probability of interfering with the ability of the patient to function appropriately in his or her environment and that surgery could be deferred for a significant period of time, measured at least in weeks, if not permanently.

Paternalism enters as a strong factor in the relationship when patients require decisions either wholly or in part, either actively or passively, to be made for them so that their best interests are protected and that they have a good chance, as a result of treatment, to achieve the autonomous state. The most commonly cited and simplistic expression of appropriate medical paternalism is the giving of blood to infants over the objection of, and contrary to the religious beliefs of, the parents. In this circumstance, when surgery is essential, most surgeons will do everything within the limits of their surgical skill to avoid transfusing the infant and yet deliver necessary surgical treatment (e.g., repair of a large myelomeningocele). However, if the well-being and survival of the child are at stake, blood is ordered and is administered, usually under the authority of a court order. This highly paternalistic behavior might easily be viewed as compromising the autonomy of the parents. It might more appropriately be perceived as preserving and potentiating the autonomy of the child in circumstances in which family members, through no fault of their own, are incapable of protecting the best interests of the child as perceived by the larger society in which they reside. Rarely does paternalism result in making a decision for the patient against the wishes of the parents. It usually represents making a decision in the patient's best interest, when the parents are incapable of doing so by virtue of the effects of the disease and the environment on their ability to function as an autonomous people.[9, 12, 14, 27]

Physician paternalism is essential when advising parents as to appropriate therapy in severely compromised newborn children. In such situations, the physician must make recommendations in the best interest of the child, including both short-term and long-term considerations. Although the family as a unit participates in the doctor-family-nurse-patient relationship, the impact of such a birth on the emotional resources of the parents is so profound as to make decision making for the child a necessary part of the attending physician's responsibility. Such an interaction transpires even when both parents and physician are *unaware* of it. An example is the child with myelomeningocele born to a young inexperienced couple. Such a family, counseled as to the probabilities of hydrocephalus, incontinence, paraparesis, the necessity and complications of shunting, Arnold-Chiari malformation, syringomyelia, and tethered cord, cannot begin to comprehend the significance of these issues and almost invariably accepts the recommendations of the attending physician, as evidenced by the very high compliance rate in the treatment of infants with myelodysplasia regardless of whether the recommendation is to operate or to withhold all therapy.[9, 10, 12]

The role of nurses in family counseling, particularly in the management of the severely compromised newborn, is paramount. Nurses clearly have the broadest view of the social and emotional dynamics. Their counseling should always strive to restore family autonomy and, in contrast to the physician's role, is virtually never paternalistic.[11]

Another widely held position among physicians is their responsibility to preserve life. Many hold this as a basic tenet. Others are confounded by the uncertainty of the situation and, therefore, recommend therapy. A few, though holding neither of the aforementioned positions, feel that to always treat is, at least, safe and defensible. Certainly, the sanctity of life is such a widely held belief in the Judeo-Christian world that it is not difficult to see its influence in fostering paternalism, particularly in the care of the nonautonomous newborn infant.[26]

The Surrogate Role

The practice of pediatrics, particularly pediatric neurosurgery of the severely compromised infant, is complicated by the surrogate responsibility of parents who frequently must make life or death decisions regarding the treatment of the child. The surrogate role abounds with ethical conflict, as does most surrogate responsibility, since it requires the parent to predict what decision the infant would make, were he or she autonomous and competent. It borders on absurdity to believe that one can project oneself into such a position. This role is substantially different from the other responsibilities of parenthood in that the order of magnitude of the decision is unique in the experience of the parent. Since the appearance of the child is markedly different from the preconceived hopes and aspirations of the parents, the associated grieving and acute remorse is often viewed as influencing the reflective competence of the parents. Under these circumstances, the parents find it difficult to get a clear view of the standards that should be used to guide decisions as to medical therapy.

Finally, there is the balancing of rights. Conflict inevitably arises when either the family or the physician is attempting to make a balanced judgment in regard to family rights versus the newborn infant's rights.

Concerns about the influence of a badly compromised infant on siblings, the immense long-term emotional and financial costs, and the value placed on the body image of wholeness all influence parents in carrying out the surrogate role and create an ethical dilemma that is not easily resolved. A realization of this only further emphasizes the responsibility of the physician to serve as a patient advocate.

Prognosis

Uncertainty regarding prognosis remains and is, in many ways, an ever-increasing source of ethical conflict. Occasionally, this is the result of mixed signals given to the parents during the early hours after birth, when the opinions of family, nursing service, neonatologist, and pediatric neurosurgeon are perceived by confused parents as being at variance (which may well be the case). The improvements in the treatment of myelodysplasia have been so rapid over the past two decades as to change dramatically selection criteria, so that now few patients are refused therapy. Improvements in neonatology have resulted in the survival of premature infants with birth weights of 500 gm, when only a few years ago the chances of survival of the 900-gm infant were marginal. This information is disseminated slowly in the medical community and even more slowly in the folklore of the society. In spite of these improvements, for many of these infants, prognosis is difficult and is further complicated by the short track record of the medical profession in the treatment of many of these conditions. In 1972, Freeman noted that uncertainty drove him to almost invariably treat infants with myelodysplasia.[9] Today, uncertainty continues to influence treatment decisions, not only for these children but for all infants in the great gray area of uncertain prognosis.

After 24 centuries, the ethical counsel reflected in these words from the oath of Hippocrates still serves well: "Whatever houses I may visit, I will come for the benefit of the sick, remaining free of all intentional injustice."[8]

References

1. A Perspective on Teaching Medical Ethics. Report of the Committee on Ethics. American Heart Association, 1978, pp 64–101.
2. American Association of Neurological Surgeons Code of Ethics: Yearbook 1986, The American Association of Neurological Surgeons, p. 11.
3. Bowen vs. American Hospital Association. 54LW4579 (1986).
4. Cassell EJ: The Function of Medicine. Restoring autonomy to the patient. Hastings Cent Rep, December 1977, pp 16–19.
5. Center for Health Affairs, Case Approach to DRG Assignment: A Guide for Physicians. Cleveland, Greater Cleveland Hospital Association, 1984.
6. Childress JF: Who Should Decide? Paternalism in Health Care. New York, Oxford University Press, 1982.
7. Dolenc CA, Dougherty CJ: DRGs: The counterrevolution in financing health care. Hastings Cent Rep 15:19, 1985.
8. Edelstein L: The Hippocratic Oath: Text, Translation and Interpretation. In: Bulletin of the History of Medicine, Supplement 1. Baltimore, Johns Hopkins Press, 1943, p 3.
9. Freeman JM: To treat or not to treat: Ethical dilemmas of treating the infant with a myelomeningocele. Clin Neurosurg 20:134, 1973.
10. Frohock FM: Special Care, Medical Decisions at the Beginning of Life. Chicago, Univ. of Chicago Pr., 1986.
11. Gadow S: A model for ethical decision making. Oncol Nurs Forum 7:44, 1980.
12. Gallo A: Spina bifida: The state of the art of medical management. Hastings Cent Rep, February 1984, pp 10–13.
13. Homan S: DRG's: Forcing physicians into a business role? Hosp Physician, Vol. 20, 1984.
14. Ingelfinger J: Arrogance. N Engl J Med 303:1507, 1980.
15. Ingram FD, Swan H: Spina bifida and cranium bifidum. I: A

survey of five hundred and forty-six cases. N Engl J Med 228:559, 1943.
16. Kinzer DM: "Board Management." Oral presentation, Medical Staff Leadership Conference. Sisters of Providence. Scottsdale, AZ, April 17, 1986.
17. Kinzer DM: Ten testing questions: Five years later. Health Prog, December 1985, pp 36–40.
18. Lorber J: Results of treatment of myelomeningocele. An analysis of 524 unselected cases with special references to special selection for treatment. Dev Med Child Neurol 13:279, 1971. For a critique of the Lorber guideline, see Veatch RM: The Technical Criteria Fallacy. Hastings Cent Rep 7:15, 1977.
19. Matson DD: Neurosurgery of Infancy and Childhood, 2nd ed. Springfield, IL, Charles C Thomas, 1969.
20. Moore JE: Spina bifida with a report of 385 cases treated by excision. Surg Gynecol Obstet 1:137, 1905.
21. Morreim H: Three concepts of patient competence. Theor Med 4:232, 1983.
22. Personal communication: Utilization Review Committee. Portland, OR, University Hospital, Oregon Health Sciences University, 1987.
23. Porter KD: Treatment of the handicapped—an emerging controversy. Cases in Medical Ethics, The University Case Presentations Series, Vol. 1, 1986, pp 14–15.
24. Rhoden N: Treating Baby Doe: The ethics of uncertainty. Hastings Cent Rep 16:34, 1986.
25. Sharrard WJW, Zachary RB, Lorber J, et al: A controlled trial of immediate and delayed closure of spina bifida cystica. Arch Dis Child 38:18, 1963.
26. Smith WB: Judeo-Christian teaching on euthanasia. NY Med Q 6:181, 1986.
27. Veatch RM: DRG's and the ethical reallocation of resources. Hastings Cent Rep 16:32, 1986.

II Hydrocephalus and Intracranial Hypertension

11

CEREBROSPINAL FLUID FORMATION AND ABSORPTION

J. Gordon McComb, M.D.

Under normal physiologic conditions, most of the cerebrospinal fluid (CSF) is secreted by the choroid plexus and flows through the ventricular system to emerge from the fourth ventricle. The CSF then traverses the subarachnoid spaces (SAS), to drain from the central nervous system (CNS) through unidirectional open channels, as a result of a hydrostatic pressure difference. This chapter reviews the clinical and experimental evidence for these conclusions as well as the physiologic alterations that occur in hydrocephalus.

CHOROID PLEXUS

The choroid plexus, the major source of CSF, is found in the lateral ventricles; the third ventricle, including the suprapineal recess; and the fourth ventricle, with an extension of this tissue out the lateral foramina of Luschka into the cerebellopontine angles. In humans, most of the choroid plexus resides in the lateral ventricles and is attached to the medial ventricular wall, where branches of the anterior and posterior choroidal arteries provide the vascular input. The remainder of the choroid plexus hangs from the roof of the third and fourth ventricles and is supplied by branches of the medial posterior choroidal and posterior inferior cerebellar arteries, respectively. The choroidal veins drain mainly into the internal cerebral veins, which are part of the deep venous, or galenic, system.

During development, the choroid plexus forms lobules, which become fronds covered with villi. Each villus is lined with a single layer of cuboidal epithelium, which is a modified ependyma covering a stromal core derived from a layer of pia. Microvilli and a few cilia cover the apical, or ventricular, surface of these epithelial cells, while on the basal side, lateral infoldings interdigitate with neighboring cells. Tight junctions are present at the apical sides of the cells. The cells lay on a basement membrane, beneath which is a stromal space containing collagen, fibroblast, and nerve fibers. A capillary, with the endothelium of the fenestrated type and devoid of tight junctions, is at the center of each villus (Fig. 11–1). A blood-CSF barrier results from the presence of tight junctions at the apical end of the choroid epithelium, rather than at the capillary endothelium of the villus (Fig. 11–2A).[13] This is in contradistinction to the capillaries of the parenchyma, in which the tight junctions between the endothelial cells constitute the blood-brain barrier (Figs. 11–2B and 11–3). The blood-CSF-brain barrier complex is completed by the presence of tight junctions in the outer layers of the arachnoid membrane (Fig. 11–2C).[71] Together, these barriers help mitigate changes in the chemical composition of the CSF, thereby improving the stability and consistency that are essential to normal brain function (Fig. 11–2D).

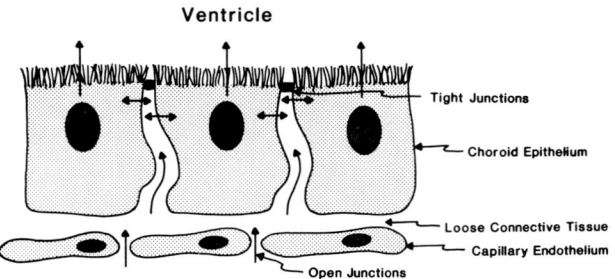

Figure 11–1. Diagrammatic representation of the choroid plexus. The capillary endothelium is of the attenuated fenestrated type, which allows an ultrafiltrate of plasma to reach the basal side of the epithelial cells. Tight junctions at the apical, or ventricular, side of the epithelial cells restrict molecular movement and constitute the blood-CSF barrier.

FORMATION OF CEREBROSPINAL FLUID

Formation Sites

It is generally agreed that most of the CSF is formed within the ventricular system. The possible sites of origin include the choroid plexus, the ependyma, and the rest of the parenchyma. A method has not been developed to separate the function of the ependyma from that of the remainder of the parenchyma. Thus, the role of the ependyma in the mass formation of CSF is not known, although from morphologic considerations, its contribution is most probably insignificant. The choroidal epithelium, however, has histologic features characteristic of epithelia specialized for transcellular transport of solutes and solvents.[21, 25] The discussion that follows is limited to mass secretion of CSF.

Results from isolated choroid plexus preparations would indicate that 80 percent or more of CSF production is from this source alone.[68, 106] Perfusion of the portion of the ventricular system devoid of choroid plexus has demonstrated that 30 to 60 percent of CSF is produced from a nonchoroidal source.[65, 75] This may explain the failure of choroid plexectomy in the clinical setting to control adequately progressive hydrocephalus.[65] It may be added that this surgical procedure removes the choroid plexus only from the lateral ventricles and not from the third or fourth ventricle. The contribution of the remaining intact choroid plexus to the formation of CSF is not clear. Whether or not the remaining choroid plexus can compensate for the portion that was removed is not known.

The various groupings of evidence showing the extracellular space (ECS) to be approximately 15 percent of the brain volume have been summarized by Welch.[108] The established presence of a substantial amount of ECS, the lack of ependymal resistance to free exchange between the extracellular fluid (ECF) and the CSF, and the similar composition of ECF and CSF have a direct bearing on the possibility that the parenchyma may be the main source of nonchoroidal CSF formation.[13, 14, 78, 108] It appears that usually about 80 to 90 percent of CSF secretion is derived from the choroid plexus, with the remaining portion most probably originating from the parenchyma. The obvious candidate for the parenchymal source is the capillary endothelium, as its

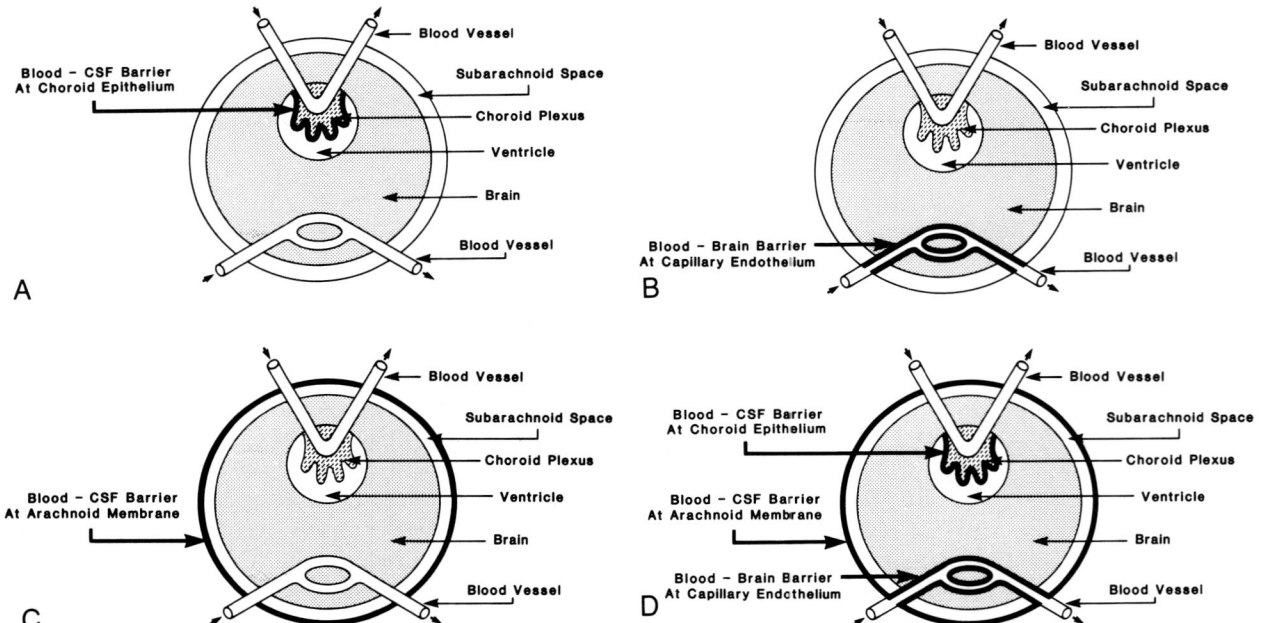

Figure 11–2. Diagrammatic representation of the central nervous system. A, Blood-CSF barrier at the choroid epithelium. B, Blood-brain barrier at the capillary endothelium. C, Blood-CSF barrier at the arachnoid membrane. D, It is the three barriers depicted in A, B, and C that provide the specialized environment of the central nervous system.

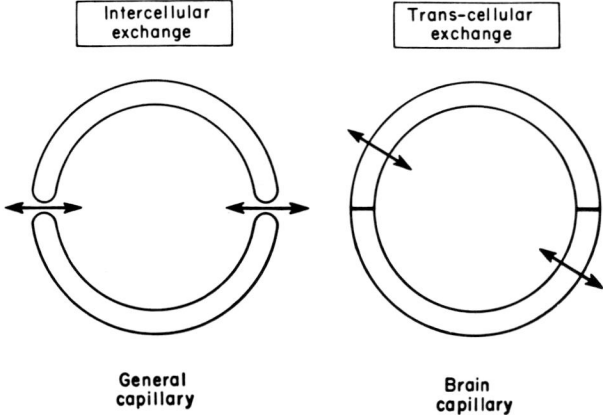

Figure 11–3. Diagrammatic representation of the differences between the general and brain capillaries. General capillaries allow all small molecules to diffuse through clefts between adjacent endothelial cells (i.e., extracellular). In contrast, brain capillaries permit exchanges only through the cells (i.e., transcellular). (With permission from Oldendorf WH: Blood-brain barrier. In, Bito LZ, Davson HM, Fenstermacher JD [eds.]: The Ocular and Cerebrospinal Fluids. New York, Academic Press, 1977.)

high content of mitochondria could provide the metabolic energy required for such a function.[73]

Mechanisms of Formation

The first step in the formation of CSF is the passage of an ultrafiltrate of plasma through the section of the choroidal capillary endothelium that does not have tight junctions, by hydrostatic pressure, into the surrounding connective tissue stroma beneath the epithelium of the villi. The ultrafiltrate is subsequently transformed into a secretion (namely, CSF) by an active metabolic process within the choroidal epithelium, via a mechanism that is largely speculative (Fig. 11–4).[21, 108] Using the information available, Wright[113] and Segal and Pollay[90] have constructed a model based on the "standing gradient" hypothesis of Diamond and Bossert,[23] which assumes that local osmotic forces within the cell are responsible for the movement of water.

Sodium-potassium-adenosine triphosphatase (Na-K-ATPase) pumps sodium into the basal side of the cell, with water entering by the osmotic gradient created. Chloride may be coupled with the sodium or may enter the cell separately.[113] Carbonic anhydrase catalyzes the formation of bicarbonate inside the cell, with the hydrogen ion being fed back to the sodium pump as a counter ion with potassium.[57, 114] In a manner analogous to that involving the basal side of the epithelium, Na-K-ATPase located in the microvilli on the apical surface extrudes sodium into the ventricle, followed by osmotically drawn water. Since the cells do not swell or shrink, the sum of the two processes must be in balance.[89] That water readily equilibrates in this process is indicated by the negligible difference in the osmolalities of plasma, plasma ultrafiltrate, and CSF.[49]

Formation Rate

The earliest method of estimating the rate of CSF formation entailed simply measuring the amount of fluid drained per unit of time or removing a known volume of CSF and noting the time required for the original pressure to be restored. The validity of the results obtained in this way can be criticized because it is necessary to assume that neither formation nor absorption rates are changed by alterations in pressure. In spite of this objection, the volumes obtained by these methods are remarkably close to those determined by the more precise ventriculocisternal or ventriculolumbar perfusion techniques introduced by Heisey, Pappenheimer, and associates.[42, 74] Although this method is employed extensively in animals, its clinical use had been very limited because the procedure is invasive. The experimental protocol requires the infusion of artificial CSF containing a nondiffusible reference material, which moves only by bulk flow (such as radioiodinated serum albumin, RISA), into the ventricles while removing artificial CSF diluted with the newly formed CSF from the cisterna magna or lumbar SAS at a constant low pressure. By quantitating the volumes of fluid going into and coming out of the system and

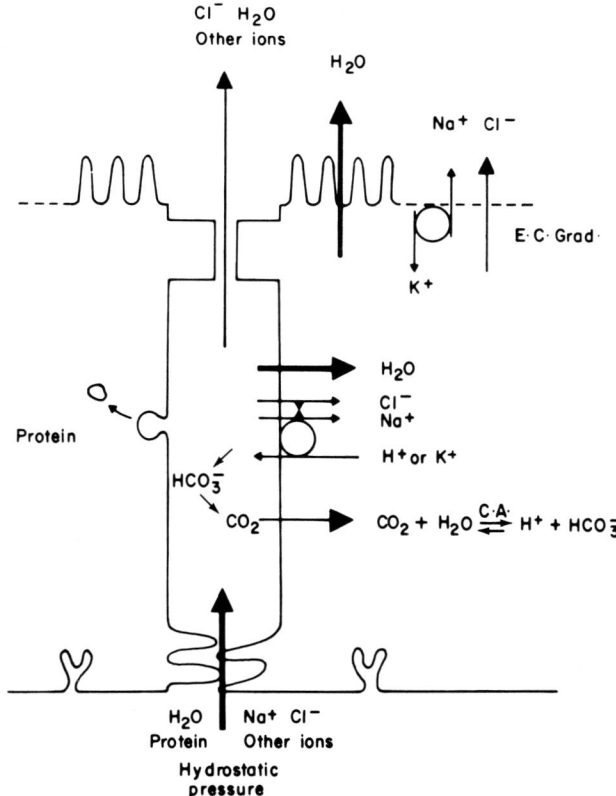

Figure 11–4. Diagrammatic summary of CSF secretion by the choroid plexus. The direction and the location of the metabolic pumps are speculative, although their presence is documented. An ultrafiltrate of plasma enters the basal side of the cell, where it is modified by metabolic processes to produce a secretion at the apical, or ventricular, side. (With permission from Segal MB, Pollay M: The secretion of cerebrospinal fluid. Exp Eye Res 25:127, 1977.)

measuring the difference in the concentration of the reference marker in the two fluids, it is possible to evaluate the rate of CSF formation and absorption. Clinical studies have indicated a CSF formation rate of about 20 ml/hr or 500 ml/day.[18, 54, 82] Since the total volume of CSF in the ventricles and SAS in the adult averages approximately 150 ml, a threefold turnover of CSF occurs daily.

Alterations in Formation Rate

Under normal physiologic conditions, CSF formation can be considered independent of pressure.[18, 42, 82] The process is pressure-responsive, but the effect of pressure is insignificant until the intraventricular pressure becomes markedly elevated. Such elevated intraventricular pressure diminishes the cerebral perfusion pressure[105] and probably interferes with the first step in CSF production, by reducing the quantity of ultrafiltrate from the choroidal capillary.[108] The effect of temperature on CSF production in patients is not known and probably has little relevance, except in marked hypothermia. Acute serum hyperosmolality in animal experiments has been claimed to reduce CSF formation, whereas acute serum hypo-osmolality is said to increase the rate.[44, 96] Little doubt exists that a decrease in serum osmolality increases the observed CSF volume flow, secondary to movement of ECF within the parenchyma, but as none of the studies has dealt with an isolated choroid plexus preparation, no statement can be made regarding whether or not changes in serum osmolality, in and of themselves, alter CSF formation. No data exist on the effect of a change in serum osmolality, be it acute or chronic, on CSF production in the clinical setting.

It has long been suspected that oversecretion of CSF occurs in cases of choroid plexus papilloma.[59] Unequivocal evidence for this has been documented by ventriculolumbar infusion studies, on several occasions.[26, 67] Evidence for overproduction of CSF in the absence of a choroid plexus papilloma does not at present exist. The clinical observation of what appears to be a temporary reduction in CSF production associated with ventriculitis is supported by two experimental studies.[11, 19] Through its presumed action on cyclic adenosine monophosphate (cAMP), cholera toxin has been reported to double the flow of CSF,[28] a finding that has not been confirmed by another investigation.[45]

Drugs that reduce CSF formation do so by interfering with the entire cellular metabolic process or the specific transport mechanisms. Dinitrophenol, an uncoupler of oxidative phosphorylation, is an example of a drug that acts on the former process, while cardiac glycosides, furosemide, and acetazolamide (Diamox) are examples of drugs that act on the latter. It is not clear whether glucocorticoids alter CSF formation, since some investigations show no change[58, 99] with their use, while others report a diminished CSF production rate.[85, 104] Furosemide decreases CSF formation by what appears to be interference with chloride transport rather than by any direct effect on carbonic anhydrase.[60] Acetazolamide decreases CSF production by interfering with the function of carbonic anhydrase and appears to diminish significantly CSF formation in humans, both acutely and chronically.[18, 82] Rapid intravenous injection of acetazolamide can also cause a transient elevation in intracranial pressure (ICP), consequent to the release of tissue carbon dioxide, with a resultant increase in cerebral blood volume and cerebral blood flow. This could be hazardous in a patient with a marked elevation in ICP. As Fishman[32] has observed, ICP is far more dependent upon cerebral hemodynamics than is the rate of CSF formation. Cutler and associates[18] have noted that as a result of the nature of the formation curve versus the absorption curve, reduction of normal CSF production by one third would cause the ICP to decrease by only 15 mm H_2O, or 1 torr. This helps explain why acetazolamide and other agents that reduce CSF formation have not proved to be particularly useful in the control of hydrocephalus. The first report of CSF formation and absorption in humans studied by the ventriculolumbar perfusion technique was that of Rubin and colleagues,[82] who concluded that future studies into the pathogenesis of hydrocephalus should be focused on CSF absorption and not on CSF formation.

ABSORPTION OF CEREBROSPINAL FLUID

The absorption of CSF and its constituents depends upon bulk flow, in addition to passive or facilitated diffusion and active transport of specific solutes. This section will deal exclusively with bulk flow, the forces involved, and where it does occur.

Absorptive Forces

That the rate of CSF absorption is pressure-dependent and relatively linear over a fairly wide physiologic range has been well established.[5, 18, 42, 48, 69, 82] The resistance to flow appears to diminish at higher than normal physiologic pressures[22, 56] and may be related to the opening of channels not available at lower pressures.

Weed[102] proposed an incremental colloid osmotic force, in addition to hydrostatic force, which would by necessity require the presence of a semipermeable membrane between the CSF and its site of absorption. Subsequent physiologic studies have shown that a colloid osmotic force does not exist; instead, Weed's prior observations are explained by particulate matter or an increase in viscosity occluding the absorptive sites, which slows bulk flow.[22, 77, 109] Studies have shown that the presence of pinocytotic vesicles in the arachnoid endothelial cells lining the venous sinuses is influenced by pressure.[2, 37] However, the process may not be metabolically dependent, as the absorption process is reported to be unaltered by the death of the animal.[76, 112] Thus, the only proven force responsible for CSF absorption is that of a hydrostatic gradient.

The Arachnoid Villus

The arachnoid villus would seem to be ideally situated to drain CSF from the SAS into the major dural sinuses, as it consists of a cell cluster that projects from the SAS into the lacunae laterales adjacent to these venous structures. Electron microscopic studies have shown that the villi are covered by a layer of endothelium with tight junctions that are continuous with the inner surface of the venous sinuses.[1, 91] The villi that are grossly visible, termed "arachnoid granulations," or "pacchionian bodies," are functionally similar to the villi that are not.[101] Key and Retzius[50] and Weed[100] firmly established that these structures drain CSF. Welch and Friedman,[109] using a flux chamber containing a section of monkey superior sagittal sinus (SSS) with arachnoid villi, found unidirectional flow from the SSS to the venous sinuses when a critical opening pressure was exceeded.

A point of controversy regarding the structure of the arachnoid villus is the existence of open channels connecting the arachnoid side with the venous side, for the presence or absence of such channels would mean a basic physiologic difference in the manner in which CSF and its constituents drain. The open villus model would be solely pressure-responsive and would allow for passive escape of macromolecules. On the other hand, a villus covered by an endothelial membrane with continuous tight-junctions would add the factors of osmosis and filtration, and macromolecules would require an active transport process to cross this barrier. The various anatomic studies are fairly evenly divided between these two possibilities. The discrepancy in findings may relate wholly or in part to the manner in which the villus is prepared for histologic study. A zero pressure gradient between the arachnoid and the venous sides of the villus during fixation would allow for its collapse, and as a result, open channels would not be apparent. This explanation is supported by a recent study.[52]

Another possible mechanism that could bridge the gap between the open-channel and the closed-channel theories of CSF drainage has been proposed by Tripathi.[98] He reported the presence of a dynamic transendothelial vacuolization process that temporarily creates an open channel through the villus endothelium, during which time CSF and its constituents could flow from the SAS to the blood.[97] The effect of pressure on this mechanism was not investigated.

Attempts have been made to determine the size of the passageways in the arachnoid villus[110] and also to see if they are responsive to pressure. They were found not to be pressure-responsive.[46] The size of the passageways in the arachnoid villus is only pertinent if this site is virtually the exclusive location for bulk egress of CSF into the blood stream. If a significant fraction of CSF and its constituents drains elsewhere, the size of the channels in the arachnoid villus is less relevant.

The Lymphatic System

Until recently, the fact that CSF might drain at sites other than the arachnoid villus, under normal physiologic conditions, has been given scant consideration. If an alternative route is postulated, it is usually associated with the hydrocephalic brain.

Weed's work[100] firmly established the arachnoid villus as a major site for bulk CSF outflow. It is rarely mentioned, though, that Weed acknowledged that some of his injected solutions drained into the mucosa of the paranasal sinuses, nasal mucosa, cranial nerve root sheaths, and cervical lymph nodes; he thought that these routes were accessory. The idea that a portion of CSF could and did drain via the lymphatics was gradually relegated to obscurity, and for more than a generation now, standard texts and teachings have limited CSF drainage solely to the arachnoid villus.

The concept of CSF drainage via the lymphatic system has been given additional support by a number of recent laboratory investigations that indicate that a significant quantity of CSF, and under certain circumstances even the majority, can drain via the lymphatic channels.* Substances with different molecular weights that are infused into the lateral ventricles can be found in the same concentrations in the deep cervical lymph, indicating that the process of transport is by way of bulk flow.[7] Additional studies have shown that elevations in intraventricular pressure increase the volume of CSF directed into the lymphatic pathways.[55, 62]

At the present time, no studies show the extent to which lymphatic drainage of CSF exists in humans, but some support for this concept comes from the clinical observation that, occasionally, parents of children with CSF diverting shunts report nasal congestion and periorbital or facial swelling when their child's shunt becomes obstructed.

The Brain

A question debated for some time is whether or not CSF can be absorbed by the brain. Penetra-

---

*References 7–10, 29, 30, 36, 55, 62, 63, 93

tion of substances into the periventricular region in the hydrocephalic animal has been well documented.[47, 111] With the advent of computerized tomographic (CT) scanning, periventricular hypodensity may be noted in the presence of hydrocephalus and has been shown to be the result of CSF migrating into the area surrounding the ventricles, as a result of increased intraventricular pressure.[43] Nuclear magnetic resonance imaging (NMRI) has demonstrated this as well. However, CSF in the parenchyma, indicative of migration, does not necessarily equate with absorption. Bulk flow of CSF is usually measured via the clearance of various reference macromolecules, such as albumin, which by necessity would have to enter the lumen of the blood vessel and be removed by the systemic circulation. It has been shown that cerebral capillaries have a very low permeability to albumin and that most of any given quantity of albumin injected into the brain can be recovered from the lymph and CSF, with very little being lost to the blood.[8] Zervas and coworkers[116] have found that horseradish peroxidase (HRP), which has nearly the same molecular weight as albumin, can penetrate to the basal lamina of the capillary endothelium but not beyond. In addition to the impermeability of the capillaries to the various reference markers, clearance of which is the measure of CSF absorption, Welch[108] has pointed out that, as absorption occurs in response to a pressure drop, it would require a higher pressure outside the lumen of the capillary than inside, which obviously would lead to its collapse and would preclude absorption. The ECS in the brain (about 15 percent of brain volume) readily allows fluid flow in the parenchyma. This flow of fluid within the parenchyma is present under normal physiologic conditions,[80] and its velocity and direction are responsive to changes in hydrostatic[79] and osmotic pressure gradients.[80] Macromolecules injected into the CSF of the ventricles or SAS have been observed to penetrate readily the ECF of the parenchyma, and vice versa.[14, 16, 116] Thus, evidence supports the contention that the brain, rather than absorbing CSF, is acting as a conduit for fluid to move from the ventricles to the SAS or into the prelymphatic channels of the blood vessels.

The Blood Vessels

As was noted in the discussion on absorption of CSF by the brain, there is no evidence to support CSF being absorbed by the capillary endothelium. However, this does not preclude net water changes when disequilibrium in the blood-brain osmotic gradient occurs, as there is no barrier in this regard. Casley-Smith and associates[16] found that carbon black injected into the parenchyma could be later traced to the SAS, the walls of the cerebral blood vessels, the adventitia of the internal carotid artery outside the cranium, and the cervical lymph nodes.

The findings of Bradbury and colleagues[8] are at variance with the observation that macromolecules travel extracranially in the adventitia of the major cerebral blood vessels, for in their study, labeled albumin injected into the brain stopped abruptly when the blood vessels exited the SAS. It is their contention that the parenchymal vessels provide a passageway for macromolecules to reach the SAS, where absorption into the lymphatic system occurs from the cranial nerve root sleeves, particularly those sleeves surrounding the olfactory nerve roots.

The Nerve Root Sleeves

Schwalbe[88] first postulated drainage of CSF into the nasal submucosa, a finding that has subsequently been confirmed on many occasions.* Yoffey and Drinker[115] noted that the best injections of the nasal lymphatics were made by placing tracers in the cranial SAS. The nasal submucosa has a dense network of lymphatic channels that subsequently drain into the deep cervical lymph nodes.[12, 31, 50, 88, 100, 115] The pathway of CSF into the nasal submucosa is via the extension of the SAS that surrounds each olfactory filament as it passes through the lamina cribrosa and can be blocked if the continuity of the space is disrupted.[9, 34] The pia-arachnoid layer progressively thins and blends into a perineural sheath as the olfactory filament passes through the cribriform plate. This perineural sheath becomes but a single cell layer in the submucosa. The perineural space between the filament and the sheath is reported to be in continuity with the SAS.[12, 115] A point of uncertainty has been whether or not open channels connect the perineural spaces (and, thus, the SAS) with the ECS of the submucosa. The presence or absence of open channels would mean a basic physiologic difference in the manner in which CSF and its constituents drain, just as with the arachnoid villus. A recent electron microscopic study indicates that an endothelial membrane with tight junctions is not present, thus allowing for the passive escape of macromolecules via bulk fluid flow on a pressure-responsive basis alone (Fig. 11–5).[32] Two additional studies found that the SAS surrounding the optic nerve divided into numerous tortuous channels to form an "arachnoid trabecular meshwork" containing "microcanals" that allow for ferritin to pass through and reach the posterior intraorbital connective tissue. At the sclera, a barrier was present that prevented tracer entrance into the choroidal interstitium. Once again, the passageways were open and similar to those found in the olfactory region.[30, 93]

A physiologic study looking at drainage from the spinal nerve roots indicates that the same physiologic processes operative at the cranial nerves occur in the spinal nerves as well.[64] CSF drainage from

---
*References 12, 24, 31, 50, 87, 100, 115

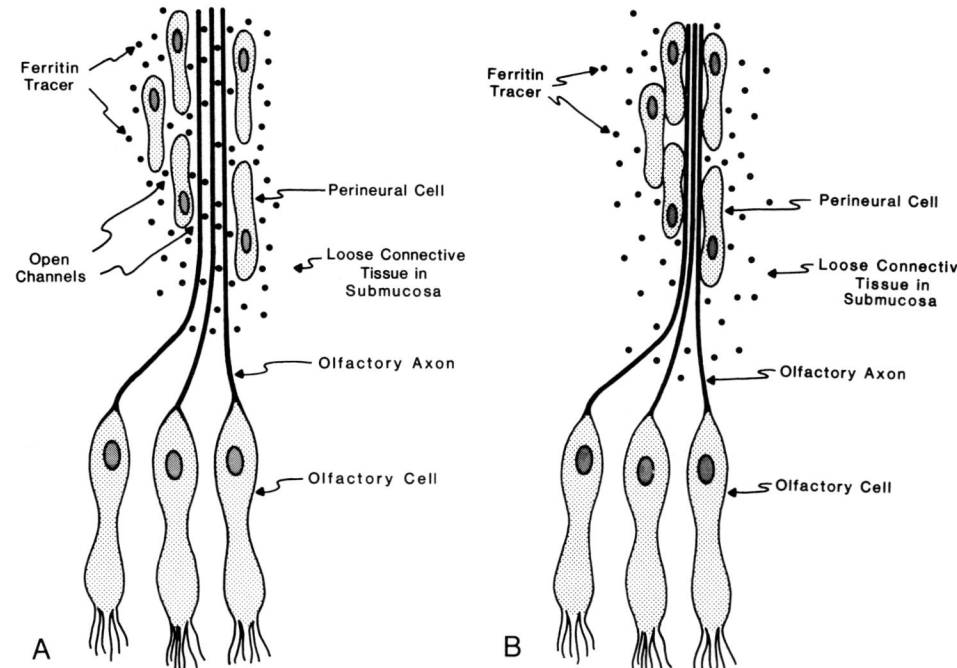

Figure 11–5. Schematic representation of the passage of macromolecules from the perineural space into the submucosal connective tissue. A, Positive hydrostatic gradient from the perineural space allows for passive drainage of cerebrospinal fluid and macromolecules. B, It is speculated that a negative hydrostatic gradient from the SAS to the nasal submucosa collapses the perineural space and acts as a one-way valve, preventing reflux into the SAS. (With permission from Erlich SS, McComb JG, Hyman MS, Weiss MH: Ultrastructural morphology of the olfactory pathway for cerebrospinal fluid drainage in the rabbit. J Neurosurg 64:466, 1986.)

the spinal nerve root sleeves has yet to be studied from a morphologic standpoint, but so far, evidence favors an open channel passageway similar to that found for the optic and olfactory nerves.

The Subarachnoid Space

Experiments document CSF drainage from the SAS surrounding the cranial and spinal nerves, with entry into the lymphatic system, but the question of fluid egress from the membrane itself remains. Dandy and Blackfan[20] contended that CSF absorption was a diffuse process from the SAS, with the arachnoid villi accounting for only a small percentage of the fluid drained. Weed[101] found that under normal physiologic conditions, the arachnoid membrane acted as a barrier but could be readily broached with cellular damage. Bowsher[6] injected radioisotope-labeled protein into the SAS of cats and found an uptake at the arachnoid villi, around the blood vessels both on the surface and within the cortex, and along the cranial and spinal nerve root sheaths but no penetration through the arachnoid membrane, thus confirming the work of Weed.

Electron microscopic studies by Nabeshima and associates[71] have shown several layers of arachnoid cells between the SAS and dura; the cells in the outer portion of these layers exhibit tight junctions, with occlusion of the intercellular clefts serving as an effective barrier to large molecules (i.e., they function as the blood-CSF barrier in this location) (Fig. 11–2C). Butler[15] has noted that, contrary to the findings at normal pressure, the arachnoid barrier layer is disrupted at higher pressures, and HRP can penetrate through the arachnoid membrane to reach the ECS of the dura mater and dural lymphatic channels. Normally, it does not seem as if that much, if any, CSF drains through the arachnoid membrane, whereas at unphysiologically high pressures, disruption of this barrier may allow for significant bulk flow.

ALTERATION OF CSF PHYSIOLOGY IN HYDROCEPHALUS

The observation that several laboratory animals and several infants have arachnoid villi but no arachnoid granulations was cited by Dandy and Blackfan[20] as an argument against these structures having an important role in CSF absorption. Subsequent investigations have shown that the arachnoid villi and granulations are anatomically and functionally the same, the only difference being that the arachnoid villi are not visible to the unaided eye.[17,101] If the arachnoid villi constitute the major site of CSF absorption, their numbers and individual structures should have some bearing on the development of hydrocephalus. That the number and size of arachnoid granulations increase with age need not have any implications, as there does not appear to be any relationship between the visibility of villi and their ability to absorb CSF. Few investigators have studied the villus in hydrocephalus. Those who have done so have mainly concentrated on the villi associated with the SSS, since the greatest concentration of these structures per volume of dural sinus exists in this region.[17,35,109] Lesser concentrations of villi are present along all the other major sinuses, some of the major cerebral veins, and veins associated with the cranial and spinal nerves.[17, 50, 61, 92, 110]

Gilles and Davidson[35] examined only the SSS region for arachnoid villi at autopsy in an infant and a child, each with communicating hydrocephalus. In one case, no villi were present, and in the other, only a few displastic villi were found. In a more thorough postmortem study, Gutierrez and colleagues[39] examined the superior sagittal, straight, and lateral sinuses of two children, searching for arachnoid villi. No villi were found in one child who had communicating hydrocephalus, and only two small patches containing a few villi were found in the second child, who did not have hydrocephalus. In spite of the near or complete lack of observed villi, CSF was being absorbed somewhere, albeit inadequately in three of the four patients. Obviously, CSF could have been absorbed via villi elsewhere, at sites not studied, or at locations without villi.

In the clinical setting, spontaneous subarachnoid hemorrhage can lead to hydrocephalus.[33] Experimental studies of the arachnoid villi following the introduction of blood into the SAS have shown a variable degree of villus distention and trapping of the red blood cells (RBCs) within.[1, 27] That RBCs can fill the villus, following entry of blood into the SAS, and can be associated with hydrocephalus does not necessarily imply that the villus is the sole or major site of CSF absorption, as the RBCs could affect all routes of drainage that have been previously considered. The same argument also holds true for those instances of hydrocephalus associated with elevated levels of protein in the CSF.[32]

The pressure relationships between the SSS and the SAS have been of some interest, since CSF drainage occurs in response to a hydrostatic difference and the greatest concentration of arachnoid villi are in this location. Under normal conditions, the pressure in the SAS is higher than that in the SSS, an observation made by Weed and Hughson[103] and confirmed on a number of occasions since. In a study of kaolin-induced hydrocephalus in dogs, Shulman and associates[95] found that the substantial pressure gradient present before hydrocephalus was induced was virtually absent after. Studies of hydrocephalus in humans have shown that the mean pressure in the SSS is often equal to or higher than that in the SAS.[72, 94] These observations indicate that little or no CSF absorption could be taking place in this region. CSF could certainly drain via the villi in different areas where a hydrostatic gradient still remained or at locations other than the villus.

Experimental attempts to produce hydrocephalus by occlusion of the SSS,[3] torcular,[38] or vein of Galen[20, 41] have not been successful. Ventricular enlargement has not been reported following acute thrombosis of the dural sinuses in humans.[83] Although hydrocephalus cannot be produced with venous obstruction intracranially, it appears to be possible to cause hydrocephalus with extracranial venous obstruction. Following ligation of all the major cephalic veins in the neck, Bering and Salibi[4] noted moderate ventricular dilatation. The clinical reports of hydrocephalus associated with impairment of venous drainage have revealed that obstructions are invariably extracranial.[40, 81] One explanation could be that intracranial venous obstruction may not be sufficient to raise significantly the venous pressure throughout the intracranial venous bed. This is supported by Schlesinger,[86] who found that venous flow can be bidirectional because no valves are present and that the deep and superficial venous systems communicate with one another. Another theory is that the hydrocephalus did not result primarily from the impairment of cephalic venous drainage but rather from obstruction of the cervical lymphatic system.

With the single exception of CSF overproduction by a choroid plexus papilloma, hydrocephalus results from impaired CSF absorption.[5, 53, 54, 84] Production of CSF is only slightly pressure-responsive[108] and does diminish noticeably until cerebral perfusion pressure is markedly reduced.[105] Production of CSF in hydrocephalus is either normal or near normal.[5, 51, 53, 54] In compensated hydrocephalus, the rate of absorption must equal the rate of formation (approximately 500 ml/day). In the noncompensated form, only a small fraction of the total amount secreted is retained; thus, the overwhelming majority of CSF output is still absorbed. As CSF formation is relatively constant, the change in resistance to absorption determines CSF pressure and whether or not the hydrocephalus is progressive.

Impairment of CSF absorption in communicating hydrocephalus could occur at some or all of the following sites: the arachnoid villus, the lymphatic channels associated with the cranial and spinal nerves, lymphatic channels in the adventitia of the cerebral vessels, and the arachnoid membrane. If CSF outflow from the ventricles is blocked (noncommunicating hydrocephalus), fluid flow could still take place via the blood vessel adventitia and ECS of the cortical mantle to reach the SAS on the brain surface. Assuming a complete ventricular blockage, which is not always the case,[66, 83] additional ways for CSF to exit the ventricles would be via the dilated spinal cord central canal[70, 107] and through a fistulous opening created by a rupture of the ventricular system into the SAS, at the lamina terminalis or the suprapineal recess.[63]

References

1. Alksne JF, Lovings ET: The role of the arachnoid villus in the removal of red blood cells from the subarachnoid space. An electron microscope study in the dog. J Neurosurg 36:192, 1972.

2. Alksne JF, White LE, Jr.: Electron-microscope study of the effect of increased intracranial pressure on the arachnoid villus. J Neurosurg 22:481, 1965.
3. Beck DJK, Russell DS: Experiments on thrombosis of the superior longitudinal sinus. J Neurosurg 3:337, 1946.
4. Bering EA, Jr., Salibi B: Production of hydrocephalus by increased cephalic-venous pressure. Arch Neurol Psychiatry 81:693, 1959.
5. Bering EA, Jr., Sato O: Hydrocephalus: Changes in formation and absorption of cerebrospinal fluid within the cerebral ventricles. J Neurosurg 20:1050, 1963.
6. Bowsher D: Pathways of absorption of protein from the cerebrospinal fluid: An autoradiographic study in the cat. Anat Rec 128:23, 1957.
7. Bradbury MWB, Cole DF: The role of the lymphatic system in drainage of cerebrospinal fluid and aqueous humour. J Physiol (Lond) 299:353, 1980.
8. Bradbury MWB, Cserr HF, Westrop RJ: Drainage of cerebral interstitial fluid into deep cervical lymph of the rabbit. Am J Physiol 240:F329, 1981.
9. Bradbury MWB, Westrop RJ: Factors influencing exit of substances from cerebrospinal fluid into deep cervical lymph of the rabbit. J Physiol (Lond) 339:519, 1983.
10. Bradbury MWB, Westrop RJ: Lymphatics and the drainage of cerebrospinal fluid. In: Shapiro K, Marmarou A, Portnoy H (eds): Hydrocephalus. New York, Raven Press, 1984, pp 69–82.
11. Breeze RE, McComb JG, Hyman S, et al: Cerebrospinal fluid formation in acute ventriculitis. Presented at the American Association of Neurological Surgeons, Pediatric Section. Pittsburgh, PA, December 2–4, 1986.
12. Brierley JB, Field EJ: The connections of the spinal subarachnoid space with the lymphatic system. J Anat 82:153, 1948.
13. Brightman MW: The intracerebral movement of proteins injected into blood and cerebrospinal fluid of mice. Prog Brain Res 29:19, 1968.
14. Brightman MW, Reese TS: Junctions between intimately opposed cell membranes in the vertebrate brain. J Cell Biol 40:648, 1969.
15. Butler A: Correlated physiologic and structural studies of CSF absorption. In: Shapiro K, Marmarou A, Portnoy H (eds): Hydrocephalus. New York, Raven Press, 1984, pp 41–58.
16. Casley-Smith JR, Földi-Börsök E, Földi M: The prelymphatic pathways of the brain as revealed by cervical lymphatic obstruction and the passage of particles. Br J Exp Pathol 57:179, 1976.
17. Clark WEL: On the Pacchionian bodies. J Anat 55:40, 1920.
18. Cutler RWP, Page L, Galicich J, et al: Formation and absorption of cerebrospinal fluid in man. Brain 91:707, 1968.
19. Dacey RG, Welsh JE, Scheld WM, et al: Alterations of cerebrospinal fluid outflow resistance in experimental bacterial meningitis. Ann Neurol 4:173, 1978 (abstract).
20. Dandy WE, Blackfan KD: Internal hydrocephalus. An experimental, clinical and pathological study. Am J Dis Child 8:406, 1914.
21. Davson H: Physiology of the Cerebrospinal Fluid. London, Churchill, 1967.
22. Davson H, Hollingsworth G, Segal MB: The mechanism of drainage of the cerebrospinal fluid. Brain 93:665, 1970.
23. Diamond JM, Bossert WH: Standing-gradient osmotic flow. A mechanism for coupling of water and solute transport in epithelia. J Gen Physiol 50:2061, 1967.
24. DiChiro G, Stein SC, Harrington T: Spontaneous cerebrospinal fluid rhinorrhea in normal dogs. Radioisotope studies of an alternative pathway of CSF drainage. J Neuropathol Exp Neurol 31:447, 1972.
25. Dohrmann GJ: The choroid plexus in experimental hydrocephalus. A light and electron microscopic study in normal, hydrocephalic, and shunted hydrocephalic dogs. J Neurosurg 34:56, 1971.
26. Eisenberg HM, McComb JG, Lorenzo AV: Cerebrospinal fluid overproduction and hydrocephalus associated with choroid plexus papilloma. J Neurosurg 40:381, 1974.
27. Ellington E, Margolis G: Block of arachnoid villus by subarachnoid hemorrhage. J Neurosurg 30:651, 1969.
28. Epstein MH, Feldman AM, Brusilow SW: Cerebrospinal fluid production: Stimulation by cholera toxin. Science 196:1012, 1977.
29. Erlich SS, McComb JG, Hyman S, et al: Ultrastructural morphology of the olfactory pathway for CSF drainage in the rabbit. J Neurosurg 64:466, 1986.
30. Erlich SS, McComb JG, Hyman S, et al: Ultrastructure of the rabbit orbital pathway for cerebrospinal fluid drainage. Exp Eye Res (in press).
31. Faber FW: The nasal mucosa and the subarachnoid space. Am J Anat 62:121, 1937.
32. Fishman RA: Cerebrospinal Fluid in Diseases of the Nervous System. Philadelphia, W.B. Saunders Co., 1980.
33. Foltz EL, Ward AA, Jr.: Communicating hydrocephalus from subarachnoid bleeding. J Neurosurg 13:546, 1956.
34. Galkin WS: Uber die bedentung der 'nasenbahn' fur arbfluss aus subarachnoidalraum. Z Gesamte Exp Med 72:65, 1930.
35. Gilles FH, Davidson RI: Communicating hydrocephalus associated with deficient dysplastic parasagittal arachnoidal granulations. J Neurosurg 35:421, 1971.
36. Gomez DG, Fenstermacher JD, Manzo RP, et al: Cerebrospinal fluid absorption in the rabbit: Olfactory pathways. Acta Otolaryngol 100:429, 1985.
37. Gomez DG, Potts DG, Deonarine V, et al: Effects of pressure gradient changes on the morphology of arachnoid villi and granulations of the monkey. Lab Invest 28:648, 1973.
38. Guthrie TC, Dunbar HS, Karpell B: Ventricular size and chronic increased intracranial venous pressure in the dog. J Neurosurg 33:407, 1970.
39. Gutierrez Y, Friede RL, Kaliney WJ: Agenesis of arachnoid granulations and its relationship to communicating hydrocephalus. J Neurosurg 43:553, 1975.
40. Haar FL, Miller CA: Hydrocephalus resulting from superior vena cava thrombosis in an infant. J Neurosurg 42:597, 1975.
41. Hammock MK, Milhorat TH, Earl K, et al: Vein of Galen ligation in the primate. Angiographic, gross and light microscopic evaluation. J Neurosurg 34:77, 1971.
42. Heisey SR, Held D, Pappenheimer JR: Bulk flow and diffusion in the cerebrospinal fluid system of the goat. Am J Physiol 203:775, 1962.
43. Hiratsuka H, Tabata H, Tsurouka S, et al: Evaluation of periventricular hypodensity in experimental hydrocephalus by metrizamide CT ventriculography. J Neurosurg 56:235, 1982.
44. Hochwald GM, Wald A, Malhan C: The sink action of cerebrospinal fluid volume flow. Effect on brain water content. Arch Neurol 33:339, 1976.
45. Hyman S, McComb JG, Megerdichian L, et al: Blood-CSF barrier alteration following intraventricular administration of cholera toxin. Brain Res 419:104, 1987.
46. James AE, Jr., McComb JG, Christian J, et al: The effect of cerebrospinal fluid pressure on the size of the drainage pathways. Neurology 26:659, 1976.
47. James AE, Jr., Strecker EP, Sperber E, et al: An alternative pathway of cerebrospinal fluid absorption in communicating hydrocephalus. Transependymal movement. Radiology 111:143, 1974.
48. Katzman R, Hussey F: A simple constant-infusion manometric test for measurement of CSF absorption. I. Rationale and method. Neurology 20:534, 1970.
49. Katzman R, Pappius HM: Brain Electrolytes and Fluid Metabolism. Baltimore, Williams & Wilkins, 1973, p 419.
50. Key EAH, Retzius MG: Studien in der Anatomie des Nervensystems und des Bindegewebes. Stockholm, Samson and Walin, 1875.
51. Levin VA, Milhorat TH, Fenstermacher JD, et al: Physiological studies on the development of obstructive hydrocephalus in the monkey. Neurology 21:238, 1971.
52. Levine JE, Povlishock JT, Becker DP: The morphological correlates of primate cerebrospinal fluid absorption. Brain Res 241:31, 1982.

53. Lorenzo AV, Bresnan MJ, Barlow CF: Cerebrospinal fluid absorption deficit in normal pressure hydrocephalus. Arch Neurol 30:387, 1974.
54. Lorenzo AV, Page LK, Watters GV: Relationship between cerebrospinal fluid formation, absorption and pressure in human hydrocephalus. Brain 93:679, 1970.
55. Love JA, Leslie RA: The effects of raised ICP on lymph flow in the cervical lymphatic trunks in cats. J Neurosurg 60:577, 1984.
56. Mann JD, Butler AB, Johnson RN, et al: Clearance of macromolecular and particulate substances from the cerebrospinal fluid system of the rat. J Neurosurg 50:343, 1979.
57. Maren TH: Bicarbonate formation in cerebrospinal fluid: Role in sodium transport and pH regulation. Am J Physiol 222:885, 1972.
58. Martins AN, Ramirez A, Solomon LS, et al: The effect of dexamethasone on the rate of formation of cerebrospinal fluid in the monkey. J Neurosurg 41:550, 1974.
59. Matson DD, Crofton FDL: Papillomas of the choroid plexus in childhood. J Neurosurg 17:1002, 1960.
60. McCarthy KD, Reed DJ: The effect of acetazolamide and furosemide on cerebrospinal fluid production and choroid plexus carbonic anhydrase activity. J Pharmacol Exp Ther 189:194, 1974.
61. McComb JG, Davson H, Hollingsworth JR: Attempted separation of blood-brain and blood–cerebrospinal fluid barriers in the rabbit. Exp Eye Res 25:333, 1977.
62. McComb JG, Davson H, Hyman S, et al: Cerebrospinal fluid drainage as influenced by ventricular pressure in the rabbit. J Neurosurg 56:709, 1982.
63. McComb JG, Hyman S, Weiss MH: Lymphatic drainage of cerebrospinal fluid in the cat. In: Shapiro K, Marmarou A, Portnoy H (eds): Hydrocephalus. New York, Raven Press, 1984, pp 83–98.
64. McComb JG, Hyman S, Weiss MH: Contribution of the spinal compartment to cerebrospinal fluid drainage. Presented at the American Association of Neurological Surgeons, Pediatric Section. Salt Lake City, Utah, December 11–13, 1984.
65. Milhorat TH: Hydrocephalus and the Cerebrospinal Fluid. Baltimore, Williams & Wilkins, 1972.
66. Milhorat TH, Hammock MK, Chandra RS: The subarachnoid space in congenital obstructive hydrocephalus. Part 2: Microscopic findings. J Neurosurg 35:7, 1971.
67. Milhorat TH, Hammock MK, Davis DA, et al: Choroid plexus papilloma. I. Proof of cerebrospinal fluid overproduction. Child's Brain 2:273, 1976.
68. Miner LC, Reed DJ: Composition of fluid obtained from choroid plexus tissue isolated in a chamber *in situ*. J Physiol (Lond) 227:127, 1972.
69. Mortensen OA, Weed LH: Absorption of isotonic fluids from the subarachnoid space. Am J Physiol 108:458, 1934.
70. Murthy VS, Deshpande DH: The central canal of the filum terminale in communicating hydrocephalus. J Neurosurg 53:528, 1980.
71. Nabeshima S, Reese TS, Landis DMD, et al: Junctions in the meninges and marginal glia. J Comp Neurol 164:127, 1975.
72. Norrell H, Wilson C, Howieson J, et al: Venous factors in infantile hydrocephalus. J Neurosurg 31:561, 1969.
73. Oldendorf WH, Cornford ME, Brown WJ: The large apparent work capability of the blood-brain barrier: A study of the mitochondrial content of capillary endothelial cells in brain and other tissues of the rat. Ann Neurol 1:409, 1977.
74. Pappenheimer JR, Heisey SR, Jordan EF, et al: Perfusion of the cerebral ventricular system in unanesthetized goats. Am J Physiol 203:763, 1962.
75. Pollay M, Curl F: Secretion of cerebrospinal fluid by the ventricular ependyma of the rabbit. Am J Physiol 213:1031, 1967.
76. Potts DG, Deonarine V, Welton W: Perfusion studies of the cerebrospinal fluid absorptive pathways in the dog. Radiology 104:321, 1972.
77. Prockop LD, Schanker LS, Brodie BB: Passage of lipid-insoluble substance from the cerebrospinal fluid to blood. J Pharmacol Exper Ther 135:266, 1962.
78. Rall DP: Transport through the ependymal linings. Prog Brain Res 29:159, 1968.
79. Reulen HJ, Tsuyumu M, Tack A, et al: Clearance of edema fluid into cerebrospinal fluid. A mechanism for the resolution of vasogenic brain edema. J Neurosurg 48:754, 1978.
80. Rosenberg GA, Kyner WT, Estrada E: Bulk flow of brain interstitial fluid under normal and hyperosmolar conditions. Am J Physiol 238:F42, 1980.
81. Rosman NP, Shands KN: Hydrocephalus caused by increased intracranial venous pressure: A clinicopathologic study. Ann Neurol 3:445, 1978.
82. Rubin RC, Henderson ES, Ommaya AK, et al: The production of cerebrospinal fluid in man and its modification by acetazolamide. J Neurosurg 25:430, 1966.
83. Russell DS: Observations on the Pathology of Hydrocephalus. Medical Research Council Special Report Series No. 265. London, His Majesty's Stationery Office, 1949.
84. Sahar A, Hochwald GM, Sadik AR, et al: Cerebrospinal fluid absorption in animals with experimental obstructive hydrocephalus. Arch Neurol 21:638, 1969.
85. Sato O: The effect of dexamethasone on cerebrospinal fluid production rate in the dog. Brain Nerve 19:485, 1967.
86. Schlesinger B: The venous drainage of the brain, with special reference to the Galenic system. Brain 62:274, 1939.
87. Schurr PH, McLaurin RL, Ingraham FD: Experimental studies on the circulation of the cerebrospinal fluid, and methods of producing communicating hydrocephalus in the dog. J Neurosurg 10:515, 1953.
88. Schwalbe G: Der Arachnoidalraum ein Lymphraum und sein Zusammenhang mit den Perichoriodalraum. Zentralbl Med Wiss 7:465, 1869.
89. Segal MB, Burgess AMC: A combined physiological and morphological study of the secretory process in the rabbit choroid plexus. J Cell Sci 14:339, 1974.
90. Segal MB, Pollay M: The secretion of cerebrospinal fluid. Exp Eye Res 25:127, 1977.
91. Shabo AL, Maxwell DS: The morphology of the arachnoid villi: A light and electron microscopic study in the monkey. J Neurosurg 29:451, 1968.
92. Shantaveerappa TR, Bourne GH: Arachnoid villi in the optic nerve of man and monkey. Exp Eye Res 3:31, 1964.
93. Shen JY, Kelly DE, Hyman S, et al: Intraorbital cerebrospinal fluid outflow and the posterior uveal compartment of the hamster eye. Cell Tissue Res 240:77, 1985.
94. Shulman K, Ransohoff J: Sagittal sinus venous pressure in hydrocephalus. J Neurosurg 23:169, 1965.
95. Shulman K, Yarnell P, Ransohoff J: Dural sinus pressure in normal and hydrocephalic dogs. Arch Neurol 10:575, 1964.
96. Stern J, Hochwald GM, Wald A, et al: Visualization of brain interstitial fluid movement during osmotic disequilibrium. Exp Eye Res 25:475, 1977.
97. Tripathi BJ, Tripathi RC: Vacuolar transcellular channels as a drainage pathway for cerebrospinal fluid. J Physiol (Lond) 239:195, 1974.
98. Tripathi RC: Ultrastructure of the arachnoid matter in relation to outflow of cerebrospinal fluid. A new concept. Lancet 2:8, 1973.
99. Vela AR, Carey ME, Thompson BM: Further data on the acute effect of intravenous steroids on canine CSF secretion and absorption. J Neurosurg 50:477, 1979.
100. Weed LH: Studies on cerebrospinal fluid. No. III. The pathways of escape from the subarachnoid spaces, with particular reference to the arachnoid villi. J Med Res 31:51, 1914.
101. Weed LH: The absorption of cerebrospinal fluid into the venous system. Am J Anat 31:191, 1923.
102. Weed LH: Forces concerned in the absorption of the cerebrospinal fluid. Am J Physiol 114:40, 1935.
103. Weed LH, Hughson W: Intracranial venous pressure and

cerebrospinal fluid pressure as affected by the intravenous injection of solutions of various concentrations. Am J Physiol 58:101, 1921.
104. Weiss MH, Nulsen FE: The effect of glucocorticoids on CSF flow in dogs. J Neurosurg 32:452, 1970.
105. Weiss MH, Wertman N: Modulation of CSF production by alterations in cerebral perfusion pressure. Arch Neurol 35:527, 1978.
106. Welch K: Secretion of cerebrospinal fluid by the choroid plexus of the rabbit. Am J Physiol 205:617, 1963.
107. Welch K: Selected topics relating to hydrocephalus. Exp Eye Res 25:345, 1977.
108. Welch K: The principles of physiology of the cerebrospinal fluid in relation to hydrocephalus, including normal pressure hydrocephalus. In: Friedlander WJ (ed): Current Reviews. Advances in Neurology, Vol 13. New York, Raven Press, 1975, pp 247–332.
109. Welch K, Friedman V: The cerebrospinal fluid valves. Brain 83:454, 1960.
110. Welch K, Pollay M: Perfusion of particles through arachnoid villi of the monkey. Am J Physiol 201:651, 1961.
111. Wislocki GB, Putnam TJ: Absorption from the ventricles in experimentally produced internal hydrocephalus. Am J Anat 29:313, 1921.
112. Wolfson LI, Katzman R: Infusion manometric test in experimental subarachnoid hemorrhage in cats. Neurology 22:856, 1972.
113. Wright EM: Active transport of iodide and other anions across the choroid plexus. J Physiol (Lond) 240:535, 1974.
114. Wright EM, Wiedner G, Rumrich G: Fluid secretion by the frog choroid plexus. Exp Eye Res 25:149, 1977.
115. Yoffey JM, Drinker CK: Some observations on the lymphatics of the nasal mucous membrane in the cat and monkey. J Anat 74:45, 1939.
116. Zervas NT, Liszczak TM, Mayberg MR, et al: Cerebrospinal fluid may nourish cerebral vessels through pathways in the adventitia that may be analogous to systemic vasa vasorum. J Neurosurg 56:475, 1982.

12
CIRCULATION OF THE CEREBROSPINAL FLUID

Thomas H. Milhorat, M.D.

Although the discovery of the cerebrospinal fluid (CSF) can be attributed to Cotugno (1764), who proved against all galenic authority that a watery fluid and not a vapor was present within the cerebral ventricles, the circulatory nature of this unique body fluid was scarcely recognized until the beginning of the twentieth century. Long regarded as little more than a "cushion for the brain," the cerebrospinal fluid is in fact a dynamic medium whose flowing character and biologic functions justify its description as the "third circulation."[11, 32] Among its many roles, the CSF serves as a modified lymphatic system for the brain and spinal cord, as a closely regulated internal milieu for nervous tissue, and as a vehicle for the intracerebral transport of neurochemicals.[32, 33]

ANATOMY OF THE CSF SYSTEM

Nature saw fit to provide nervous tissue, which generates and conducts electrical impulses, with a highly specialized environment that is sheltered from the blood and is watery in composition and chemically precise. To isolate this environment, the system was surrounded by a unique vascular membrane (the blood-brain barrier), and to contain the fluid within it, a series of interconnecting channels was arranged that surround, support, and protect the nervous elements. The internal fluid of the system, or CSF, is maintained as a protein-poor product of the plasma and is the ideal milieu for the proper functioning of nerve cells.[32, 33] The CSF system of humans and other higher vertebrates consists of two separate but continuous compartments: (1) the interstitial space, which surrounds the individual cellular elements, and (2) the macroscopic CSF cavities, which encircle the brain and spinal cord. These internal and external spaces are in direct anatomic continuity so that it is appropriate to regard the ventriculospinal pathways as expanded lacunae of brain interspaces.[32, 42]

Interstitial Space

The interspaces of the brain and spinal cord, in contrast to those in other organs of the body, are comparatively narrow channels that are separated from the vascular compartment by a highly impermeable capillary membrane (Fig. 12–1). This membrane constitutes the structural basis of the blood-brain barrier and consists of a double layer of cells, formed by a specialized capillary endothelium, and a circumferential investment of astrocytes. In most areas of the brain, the cells of the capillary endothelium are joined by pentalaminar tight junctions (zonulae occludentae) that are capable of restricting the intercellular movement of molecules having a diameter of 2 nm or more.[2, 18, 48]

Beyond the blood-brain barrier, the extracellular spaces of the brain and spinal cord form a maze of interconnecting and patent channels that are anatomically continuous with the macroscopic cavities in which CSF accumulates. As Brightman[4-6] has demonstrated, when proteins such as ferritin and

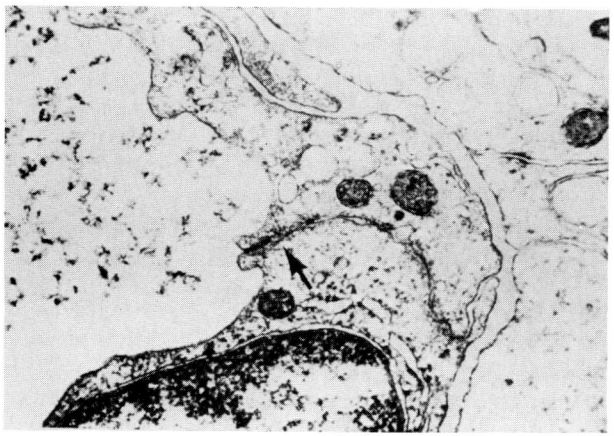

Figure 12-1. Electron micrograph of a cerebral capillary of a rat, showing intercellular tight junction (arrow) between two adjacent endothelial cells. This feature, plus a system of specialized heterolytic vesicles within the endothelial cell cytoplasm, constitutes the morphologic basis of the blood-brain barrier. Note that the lumen *(left)* of the capillary is filled with horseradish peroxidase, which is prohibited from moving extravascularly by a highly impermeable vascular membrane. Beyond the cerebral capillary *(right)* is a series of interconnecting perivascular and intercellular spaces (the extracellular compartment) that have widths of 10 to 200 nm and are anatomically continuous with adjacent CSF spaces ($\times$ 10,500).

Macroscopic Cavities

The macroscopic CSF cavities consist of the three cerebral ventricles, the aqueduct of Sylvius, the fourth (cerebellar) ventricle, the central canal of the spinal cord, and the subarachnoid space (Fig. 12-2). Each cavity is continuous with the next through one or more well-defined openings, and the system terminates at the level of the dural sinuses where expansions of the subarachnoid space, the arachnoid villi, protrude into the venous circulation.

The lining of the macroscopic cavities is formed by a single layer of cells that functions as a semipermeable membrane. Within the ventricles and central canal of the spinal cord, the surface is lined by a ciliated, low columnar epithelium (the ependyma) that lacks tight junctions, except for a specialized segment covering the choroid plexuses. The cisterns and sulci of the subarachnoid space are bounded by an "open" epithelium that is formed inwardly by the pia and outwardly by a loose investment of arachnoid cells containing tight junctions.

NORMAL CSF CIRCULATION

There are two mechanisms by which the CSF is elaborated: (1) secretion by the choroid plexuses and (2) "lymphatic-like" drainage of the brain extracellular fluid.[32, 33, 42] Although the exact contributions from choroidal and extrachoroidal sites remain to be determined, the latter are probably significant, since the maximum reduction in the rate of CSF formation that can be achieved by choroid plexectomy is only 40 percent.[29, 45]

horseradish peroxidase are injected into CSF, these large markers move with relative ease between ependymal and pial cells to distribute widely throughout the brain extracellular space. Ventricular perfusion studies, employing a variety of substances including inulin, sulfate, and dextran, have shown a similar distribution.[25, 26, 47] From these and other data, the extracellular channels of the brain and spinal cord have been estimated to have an average width of about 15 nm.[32, 42]

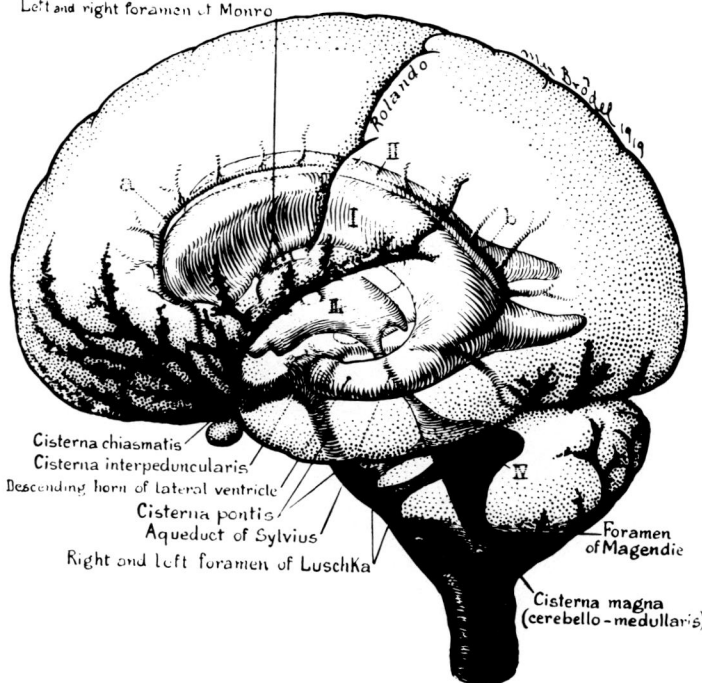

Figure 12-2. The macroscopic CSF spaces. (From Dandy WE: The brain. *In* Lewis D [ed.]: Practice of Surgery, vol. 12. Hagerstown, WF Prior, 1932.)

Minor Pathways of Flow

Early investigators, including Cushing,[10] Weed,[53] and Flexner,[19] favored the view that there is a steady bulk flow of brain extracellular fluid (ECF) from the perivascular spaces into the perineuronal spaces, and subsequently into the CSF. In contrast, a number of later investigators argued that the CSF cavities do not receive accessions of fluid from the brain interspaces and that the ECF is neither formed nor circulated in the conventional sense but serves primarily as a medium for diffusional exchange between the blood and the brain or between the CSF and the brain. This latter point of view has been especially emphasized during the past three decades by the work and writings of Davson.[12, 14]

Renewed interest in the proposal that there is a "lymphaticlike" drainage of brain ECF into the CSF cavities is attributable to many new pieces of information. These include evidence that (1) a substantial fraction of the CSF is formed at extrachoroidal sites,[29, 46, 50, 52] (2) the sodium exchange kinetics of the brain parenchyma can be correlated with the rate of CSF formation,[45] (3) regional variations in the composition of fluid within the cerebral ventricles, cisterna magna, and subarachnoid space cannot be accounted for by the secretory activity of the choroid plexuses,[30] and (4) some and perhaps many substances are cleared from the brain into the CSF by net transport.[7, 32] Final proof that the CSF is formed in part by the lymphaticlike drainage of ECF across the ependymal and pial surfaces will depend upon evidence of a true bulk flow of fluid within the interspaces of the brain and spinal cord. Although this question is obviously difficult to study, it has been addressed in several interesting ways. In 1974, Cserr and Ostrach[9] noted that when dextran blue 2000 is injected into the caudate nucleus of the rat, the dye is rapidly transported, predominantly along extracellular channels, to the globus pallidus, internal capsule, stria terminalis, and junction of the lateral and third ventricles. Since the molecular size of this marker is too large for it to move appreciably by diffusion, this finding provided the first solid suggestion of a bulk circulation within the brain interspaces.[32] Subsequently, Cserr and coworkers[8] refined these studies and examined the distribution of intracerebrally injected anionic isoenzymes of horseradish peroxidase (HRP). These experiments were much more convincing and provided substantive evidence that the interstitial fluid (ISF) of the brain flows from the narrow intercellular clefts of the neuropil, along extracellular pathways between fiber tracts and through perivascular and periventricular spaces, to drain ultimately into the ventricles and subarachnoid space and, possibly, into fenestrated capillaries lining these cavities.[8]

Recently, additional proof of bulk flow within the brain interspaces has been provided by studies on cerebral edema following injury or "physiologic opening" of the blood-brain barrier.[42] In a startling series of experiments utilizing quantitative autoradiography (QAR) to examine the freeze-lesion model of Klatzo and colleagues,[22-24] Blasberg and coworkers[1] demonstrated that when radioactive carbon–labeled (^{14}C) sucrose and radioactive indium–labeled (^{111}In) transferrin are injected into the blood simultaneously, these solutes cross injured or otherwise permeable cerebral capillaries to enter the brain extracellular space. From this point, the tracers move rapidly, and at identical rates, into the adjacent CSF cavities (Fig. 12–3). This pattern of movement, by molecules of greatly different sizes and diffusion coefficients, can occur only by bulk flow and excludes, for practical purposes, diffusion as a significant means for the transport of interstitial fluid in brain edema.[42] Whether normal ECF moves in a similar fashion awaits final confirmation, but the evidence to date seems overwhelming.[32, 35, 42]

Taken together, the foregoing data support the view that the ECF of the brain is formed continuously across the cerebral endothelium as a protein-poor "lymph"[32] that flows in bulk toward the adjacent CSF cavities (Fig. 12–4). Since the interspaces of the brain and spinal cord communicate freely with the surrounding CSF cavities, a steady, net addition of new fluid probably occurs at all points along the ventriculosubarachnoid pathway until the major sites of CSF absorption are reached.[30] The fact that, in different regions of the nervous system, the chemical compositions of the ECF and CSF are probably similar[30] provides further support for this view.

Major Pathways of Flow

On the basis of extensive data concerning the migration of dyes, radioisotopes, and other tracers injected into the macroscopic CSF cavities, it is now firmly established that the CSF flows in bulk from the sites of its origin to sites of absorption (Fig. 12–5).[30] The fluid that is formed in the lateral ventricles passes out through the paired interventricular foramina of Monro to reach the third ventricle. This fluid then flows caudally through the aqueduct of Sylvius and the fourth ventricle, from which point it passes into the subarachnoid space by three exits: through the paired lateral foramina of Luschka (which direct the fluid around the brainstem into the cerebellopontine angle and prepontine cisterns) and through the midline foramen of Magendie (which directs fluid through the vallecula into the cisterna magna). In addition, a small volume of fluid may exit through the central canal of the spinal cord.[17] From the cisterna magna, CSF then flows in several directions: superiorly, into the subarachnoid space investing the cerebellar hemispheres; caudally, into the spinal subarachnoid space; and cephalad, into the premedullary, prepontine, and cerebellopontine cisterns.

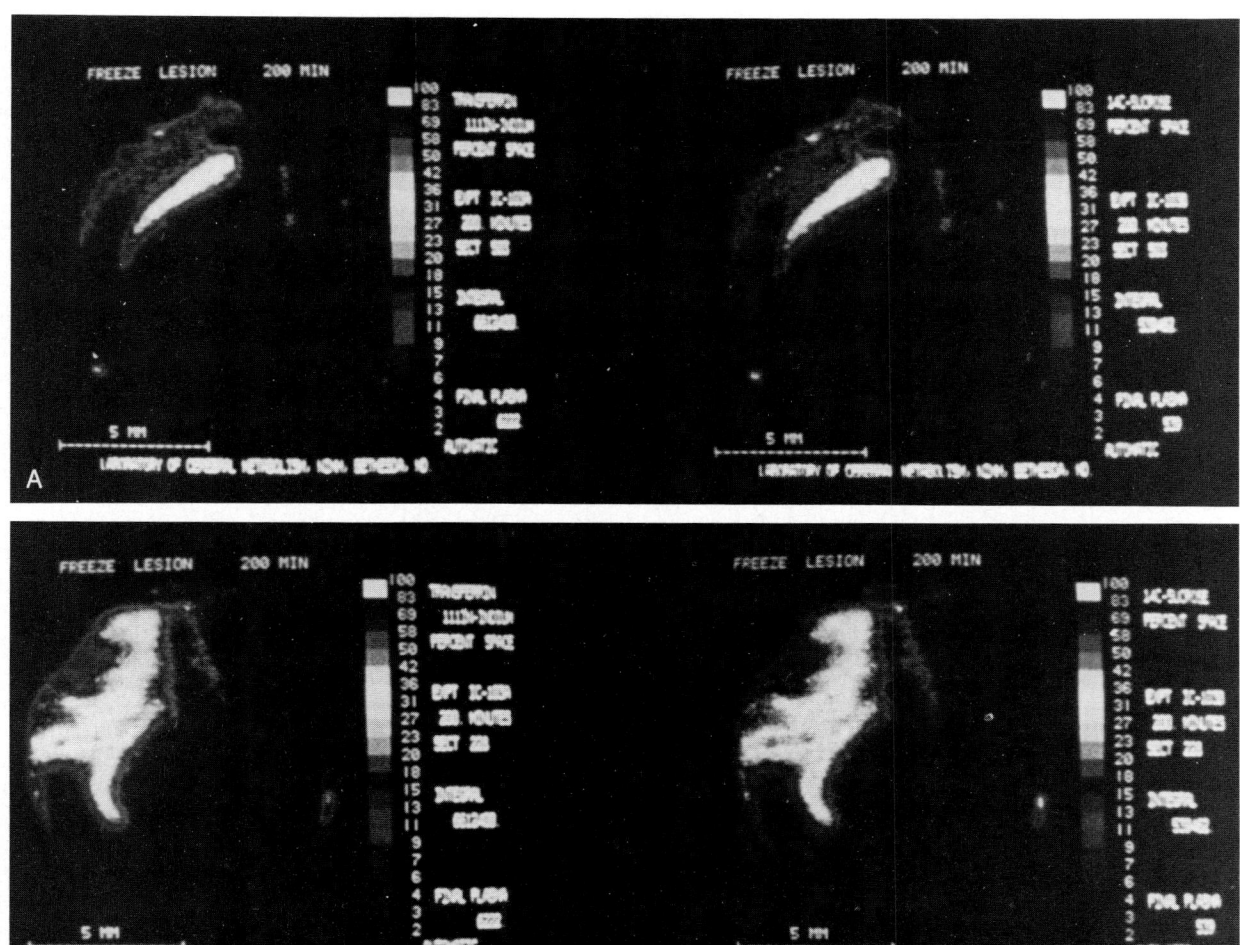

Figure 12–3. Quantitative autoradiography (QAR) study of brain interstitial fluid movement, utilizing freeze-lesion model and double-marker technique. In this experiment, carbon-14–labeled sucrose and indium-111–labeled transferrin were administered simultaneously by the intravascular route at various times following cerebral freeze lesion. A, Twenty minutes after injection of double marker, reconstructed images of sucrose activity (left) and transferrin activity (right) are identical. B, Four hours after injection of double marker, reconstructed images of sucrose activity (left) and transferrin activity (right) are identical. Note that tracers have moved rapidly and at equal rates to fill ipsilateral lateral ventricle. This pattern of movement, by molecules of greatly different molecular size and diffusion coefficients, can occur only by bulk flow and excludes, for practical purposes, diffusion as a significant means for transport of interstitial brain edema.

From the basilar cisterns, the bulk flow of CSF continues cephalad along two major routes: (1) a ventral route through the interpeduncular cistern, from which the fluid passes, mainly through the sylvian fissure and prechiasmatic cisterns, to the subarachnoid space investing the lateral and frontal aspects of the cerebral hemispheres, and (2) a dorsomedial route through the ambient cisterns and cisterna venae magnae cerebri, from which fluid passes to the subarachnoid space investing the medial and posterior aspects of the cerebral hemispheres. In the spinal subarachnoid space, the bulk flow of fluid appears to follow a downward route behind the cord (posterior to the dentate ligaments) to the lumbar theca and then upward in front of the cord to the basilar cisterns.[17] The circulation of the CSF within the macroscopic cavities terminates at the level of the dural sinuses, where absorption takes place across the arachnoid villi. A limited absorption of CSF may also occur proximal to the arachnoid villi, across fenestrated capillaries lining the ventriculosubarachnoid pathways and through perineural lymphatics investing the spinal and cranial nerves.[8, 30, 34] The manner in which fluid circulates within the CSF cavities has been a controversial subject. For many years, it was thought that no true circulatory current existed and that CSF traveled by simple ebb-and-flow movements resulting from the arterial pulse as modified by such factors as respiration, body position, and coughing.[20, 49] However, with the advent of isotope cisternography, the existence of a characteristic pattern of flow

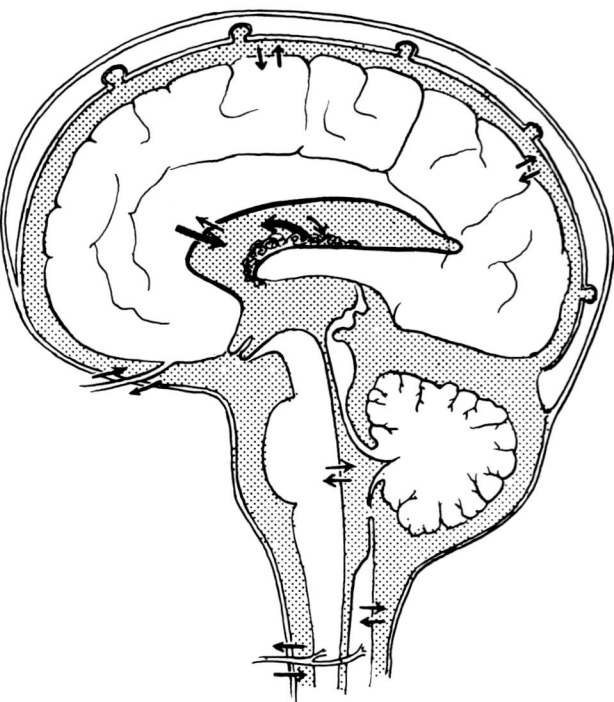

Figure 12–4. Lesser pathways of CSF bulk flow. (With permission from Milhorat TH: Hydrocephalus and the Cerebrospinal Fluid. Baltimore, Williams & Wilkins, 1972.)

toward the cerebral convexities was soon established (Fig. 12–6). DiChiro has shown that the position of the body and the physical activity of the patient do not affect the pattern of spreading[15, 16] and that although an ebb-and-flow component is

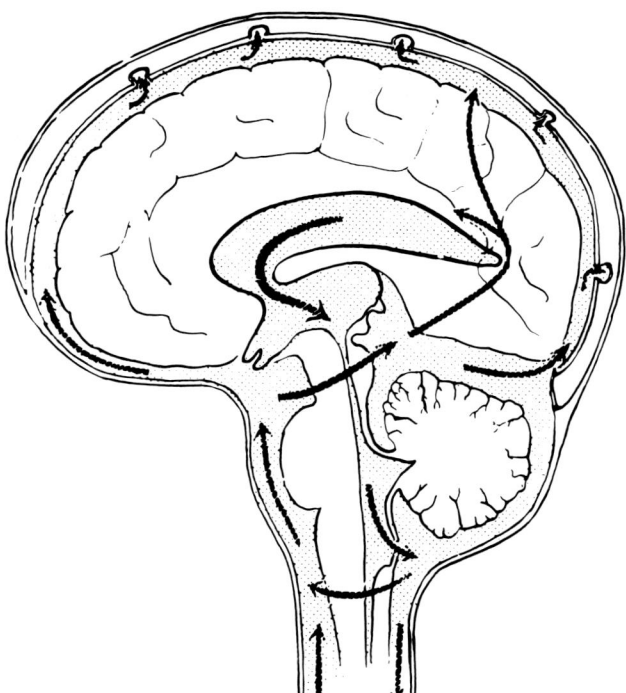

Figure 12–5. Major pathways of CSF bulk flow. (With permission from Milhorat TH: Hydrocephalus and the Cerebrospinal Fluid. Baltimore, Williams & Wilkins, 1972.)

probably present, the CSF moves in a true circulatory current.[17]

Whereas the exact mechanism by which the CSF is propelled along its circulatory route is incompletely understood, the following factors are probably involved to some extent: (1) the continuous outpouring of newly formed CSF, (2) the ciliary action of the ventricular ependyma, (3) the ventricular pulsations, representing the combined effects of respiratory variations and the pulsations emanating from the choroid plexuses and cerebral arteries, and (4) the pressure gradient across the arachnoid villi.[30] Of these, the last factor is probably the most important. As Shulman and colleagues[51] have shown, the mean CSF pressure in humans (150 mm H_2O) is considerably higher than the pressure in the superior sagittal sinus (90 mm H_2O). This differential is required to promote drainage and absorption across the arachnoid villi and, doubtless, contributes to the cephalad movement of the CSF.[30] Bradley[3] has emphasized that the dural sinuses also exercise a "suction-pump" action. This phenomenon, which depends upon the high velocity of central blood flow through the fixed diameter of the sinuses, and the low intraluminal pressure that develops at the circumference of the sinus wall where the arachnoid villi enter, may explain how the circulation of the CSF continues through a wide range of postural pressures.[30]

It is probable that in certain areas of the CSF system, the circulation stagnates. A notable example of this is in the lumbosacral cul-de-sac, where intrathecal drugs, blood, and purulent material may be retained for prolonged intervals.[30] In discussing neoplasms that seed along the CSF pathways, Zulch[54] pointed out that the locations of metastatic tumor implants often coincide with areas where the circulation "sludges down." Thus, the frequent spread of pinealomas to the anterior recess of the third ventricle, and of medulloblastomas to the cauda equina, may indicate areas of circulatory stagnation.

CSF CIRCULATION IN HYDROCEPHALUS

Obstruction of the CSF pathways, regardless of its cause, leads inevitably to an altered pattern of CSF circulation. Although these patterns vary according to the location and completeness of the block, there is, in almost every case, an attempt by the body to establish compensatory pathways of absorption.

Communicating Hydrocephalus

When lesions obstruct the subarachnoid space, there is a free flow of fluid out of the ventricles up

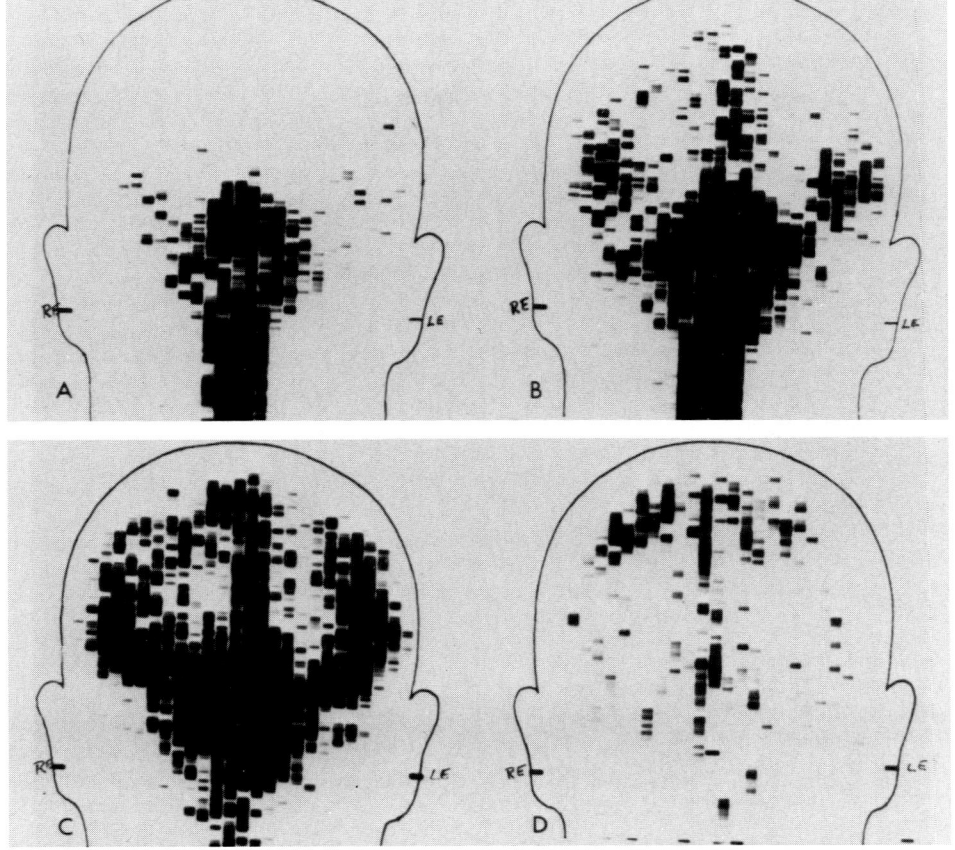

Figure 12–6. RISA cisternogram in a normal human. A, At one hour; B, at three hours; C, at six hours; D, at 24 hours. (With permission from DiChiro G: Movement of the cerebrospinal fluid in human beings. Nature [London] 204:209, 1964.)

to the level of the block. However, since the circulatory flow beyond this point is impeded, there is a net accumulation of fluid within the trapped chambers, and the forward circulation of the CSF is slowed or even totally arrested. As a consequence of the continuous ventricular pulsations, fluid proximal to the block undergoes "mixing." This "mixing effect" is important and accounts for the fact that when tracers are injected into the lumbar theca, they tend to disperse throughout the obstructed system and will usually migrate upward into the lateral ventricles. In patients undergoing isotope cisternography, retrograde filling of the ventricular system is a characteristic sign of communicating hydrocephalus (Fig. 12–7).

Noncommunicating Hydrocephalus

In cases of noncommunicating hydrocephalus, the cerebral ventricles are separated from the subarachnoid space, and the fluid proximal to the block is subjected to the "mixing" forces previously cited. Distal to the block, the flow of fluid may or may not be altered. In some cases, the subarachnoid fluid flows normally toward the cerebral convexities. This can occur even when the ventricular obstruction is comparatively complete (e.g., aqueductal stenosis) and indicates that the circulation of fluid in the subarachnoid space is not entirely dependent upon pulsations emanating from the choroid plexuses or upon the flow of fluid out of the cerebral ventricles.[30] However, in most cases, both the convexity subarachnoid space and the basilar cisterns are mechanically obstructed by the enlarged ventricular system (Fig. 12–8).[43, 44] This phenomenon probably contributes to the frequent failure of internal shunts, such as third ventriculostomy or ventriculocisternostomy (Torkildsen's shunt), in the treatment of noncommunicating hydrocephalus.[30]

Compensatory Pathways of Flow

A constant finding in hydrocephalus of any type is a greatly increased permeability of the surfaces lining the obstructed system. When dyes or radioisotopes are injected into the CSF, the tracers can be demonstrated to migrate rapidly and in increased amounts into structures such as the septum pellucidum, the choroid plexuses, the periventricular zone of the brain, and the leptomeninges proximal to the block (Fig. 12–9).[36, 37] In humans, the easy penetrability of the periventricular boundaries in hydrocephalus was first shown convincingly in patients undergoing isotope ventriculography.[41] Under these conditions, a "double density" pattern was often seen consisting of (1) a dense inner area

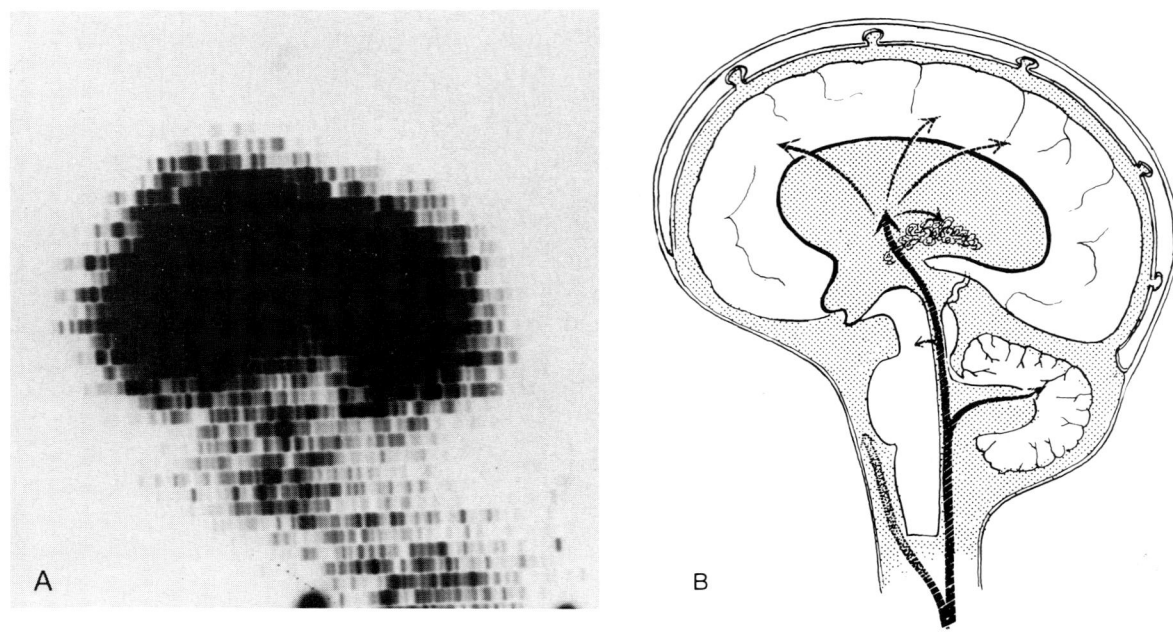

Figure 12–7. Retrograde circulation of CSF in communicating hydrocephalus. *A,* RISA cisternogram of a patient with hydrocephalus secondary to subarachnoid hemorrhage. Twenty-four hour scan shows reflux of radiotracer into the lateral ventricles and nonfilling of the basilar cisterns and subarachnoid space. The halo, or "double-density" pattern, around the lateral ventricles represents migration of the tracer into the periventricular tissue. *B,* Diagram of CSF circulation in communicating hydrocephalus. (With permission from Milhorat TH: Hydrocephalus and the Cerebrospinal Fluid. Baltimore, Williams & Wilkins, 1972.)

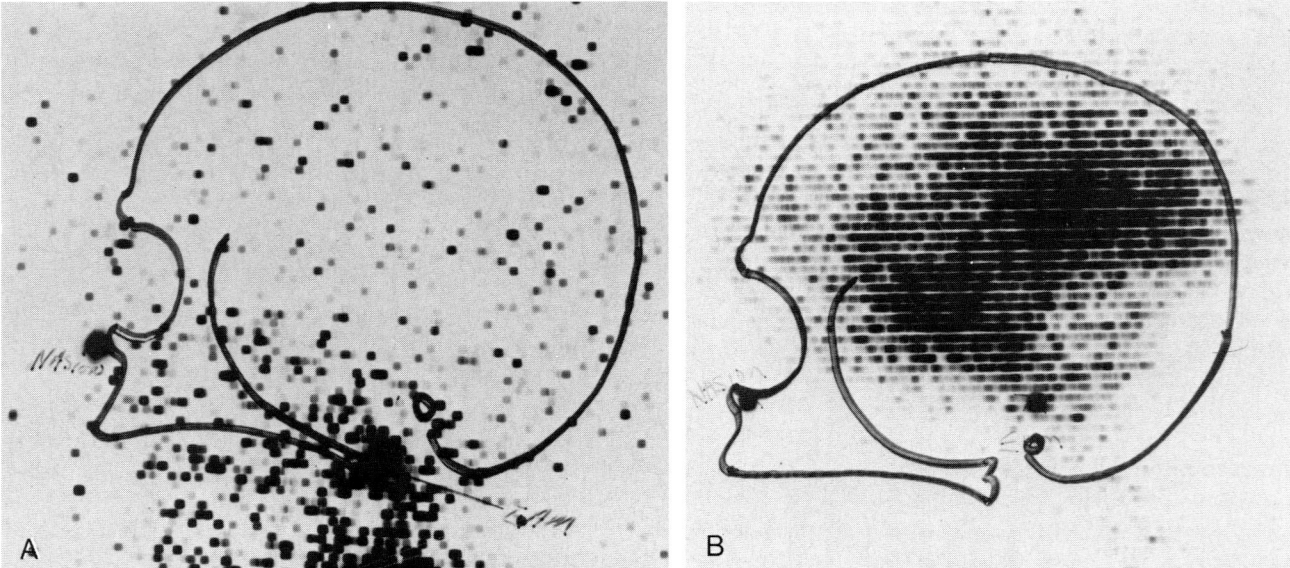

Figure 12–8. Flow of subarachnoid fluid in noncommunicating hydrocephalus. *A,* RISA cisternogram in a patient with congenital aqueductal stenosis and massive ventricular enlargement. On 48-hour scan, little or no tracer has passed above the level of the cisterna magna. *B,* RISA scan of same patient at 48 hours, following ventricular shunt. The convexity subarachnoid space has re-expanded. (With permission from Milhorat TH: Hydrocephalus and the Cerebrospinal Fluid. Baltimore, Williams & Wilkins, 1972.)

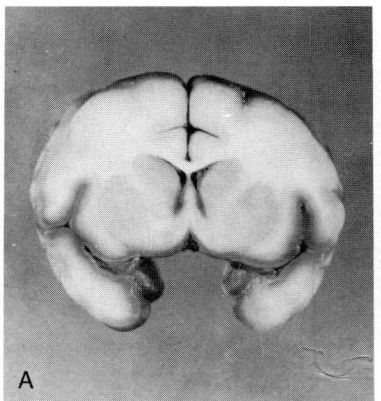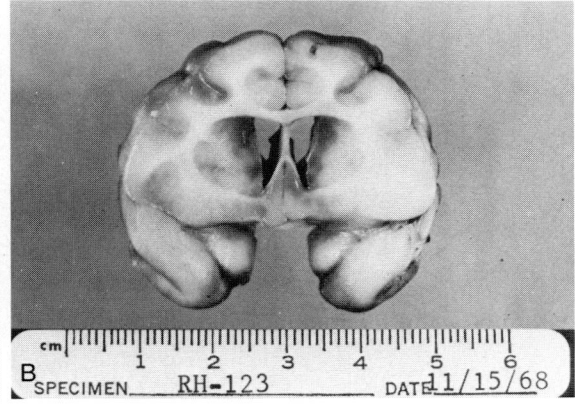

Figure 12-9. Increased permeability of ventricular surface in experimental hydrocephalus. A, Distribution of intraventricularly injected phenolsulfonphtalein (PSP) in a normal rhesus monkey. After 45 minutes, the dye has migrated across the ependyma to a depth of 1 to 2 mm. B, Distribution of intraventricularly injected PSP in a rhesus monkey with obstruction of the fourth ventricle (inflatable balloon). After 45 minutes, the dye has migrated deeply into the periventricular gray and white matter. (With permission from Milhorat TH, Clark RG: Some observations on the circulation of phenolsulfonphthalein in cerebrospinal fluid: Normal flow and flow in hydrocephalus. J Neurosurg 35:522, 1970.)

of uptake corresponding to the presence of the radiotracer in the cerebral ventricles and (2) a less dense outer area of uptake corresponding to the presence of the radiotracer in the brain surrounding the ventricles (Fig. 12–7). With the advent of computed tomography (CT) and nuclear magnetic resonance imaging (NMRI), the presence of periventricular white matter edema can now be graphically demonstrated without the use of special tracers (Fig. 12–10). This finding is often useful in distinguishing examples of normal pressure hydrocephalus and cerebral atrophy.[34]

The fate of fluid once it has entered the cerebral parenchyma is not known. There is growing evidence that much of this fluid is probably absorbed across the fenestrated capillaries lining the ventriculosubarachnoid pathways.[8, 30, 35] Levin and associates[27] have reported an apparent increase in cerebral capillary permeability in experimental hydrocephalus, and McLone[28] has presented evidence that when lanthanum colloid is injected into the lateral ventricles of hydrocephalic mice, the tracer moves transcerebrally by extracellular routes to enter cerebral vessels in the subarachnoid space. However, before transependymal absorption can be accepted unequivocally as a major compensatory mechanism in hydrocephalus, it is obvious that more work needs to be done.[34, 35]

Despite the foregoing uncertainties, it is evident that a major adjustment in the dynamics and circulation of the CSF must take place in almost every case of chronic hydrocephalus. Were this not to occur, then in patients with complete blocks, the ventricles would be forced to enlarge by several hundred cubic centimeters a day. In this regard, it is appropriate to point out that Hammock and colleagues[21] have shown that in cases of "complete" ventricular obstruction, radioisotopes invariably bypass the block, albeit at a delayed rate. This suggests that a considerable volume of fluid may actually circulate along normal pathways. Overall, it is probable that within any obstructed CSF system, fluid flows along the route or routes of least structural resistance. This probably explains the phenomenon

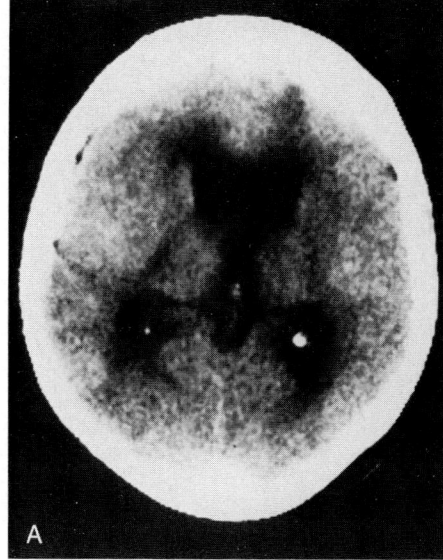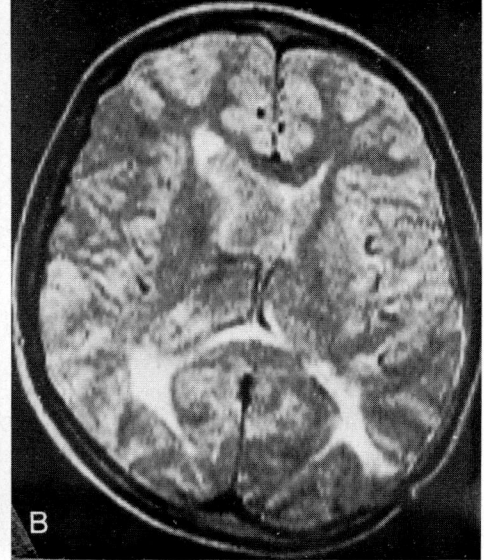

Figure 12-10. Periventricular edema associated with hydrocephalus. A, CT scan of a patient with acute hydrocephalus ten days after subarachnoid hemorrhage. B, Nuclear magnetic resonance image of patient with malfunctioning ventriculoperitoneal shunt, demonstrating asymmetric ventricular enlargement (greater on side opposite shunt).

of periventricular edema as well as the development of ventricular diverticula and hydromyelia in certain types of hydrocephalus.

References

1. Blasberg RG, Gasendam J, Patlak CS, et al: Quantitative autoradiographic studies of brain edema and a comparison of multi-isotope autoradiographic techniques. In: Cervos-Navarro J, Ferszt R (eds): Brain Edema. New York, Raven Press, 1980, pp 225–269.
2. Bodenheimer TS, Brightman MW: A blood-brain barrier to peroxidase in capillaries surrounded by perivascular spaces. Am J Anat 122:244, 1968.
3. Bradley KC: Cerebrospinal fluid pressure. J Neurol Neurosurg Psychiatry 33:387, 1970.
4. Brightman MW: The distribution within the brain of ferritin injected into cerebrospinal fluid compartments. 1. Ependymal distribution. J Cell Biol 26:99, 1965.
5. Brightman MW: The distribution within the brain of ferritin injected into cerebrospinal fluid compartments. 2. Parenchymal distribution. Am J Anat 117:193, 1965.
6. Brightman MW: The intracerebral movement of proteins injected into blood and cerebrospinal fluid of mice. Prog Brain Res 29:19, 1968.
7. Cserr HF: Physiology of the choroid plexus. Physiol Rev 51:273, 1971.
8. Cserr HF, Cooper DN, Milhorat TH: Flow of cerebral interstitial fluid as indicated by removal of extracellular markers from rat caudate nucleus. In: Bito LZ, Davson H, Fenstermacher JD (eds): The Ocular and Cerebrospinal Fluids. Exp Eye Res 25:461, 1977.
9. Cserr HF, Ostrach LH: Bulk flow of interstitial fluid following intracranial injection of Blue Dextran 2000. Exp Neurol 45:50, 1974.
10. Cushing H: Studies on the cerebrospinal fluid. 1. Introduction. J Med Res 26:1, 1914.
11. Cushing H: The Third Circulation. London, Oxford University Press, 1926.
12. Davson H: The blood–cerebrospinal fluid and blood-brain barriers. Ergeb Physiol 52:20, 1963.
13. Davson H: Physiology of the Cerebrospinal Fluid. London, Churchill, 1967.
14. Davson H: The cerebrospinal fluid. In: Lajtha A (ed): Handbook of Neurochemistry, Vol 2. New York, Plenum Press, 1969, pp 23–48.
15. DiChiro G: Movement of the cerebrospinal fluid in human beings. Nature (Lond) 204:209, 1964.
16. DiChiro G: New radiographic and isotopic procedures in neurological diagnosis. JAMA 188:524, 1964.
17. DiChiro G: Observations on the circulation of the cerebrospinal fluid. Acta Radiol (Diagn) (Stockh) 5:988, 1966.
18. Fenstermacher JD, Johnson JA: Filtration and reflection coefficients of the rabbit blood-brain barrier. Am J Physiol 211:341, 1966.
19. Flexner LB: Some problems of the origin, circulation and absorption of the cerebrospinal fluid. Q Rev Biol 8:397, 1933.
20. Grundy HF: Circulation of cerebrospinal fluid in the spinal region of the cat. J Physiol (Lond) 163:457, 1962.
21. Hammock MK, Milhorat TH, Davis DA: Isotope cisternography and ventriculography in the diagnosis of hydrocephalus. Dev Med Child Neurol 16:58, 1974.
22. Klatzo I: Presidential address: Neuropathological aspects of brain edema. J Neuropathol Exp Neurol 26:1, 1967.
23. Klatzo I, Miquel J, Ostenasek R: The application of fluorescein-labeled serum proteins (FLSP) to the study of vascular permeability in the brain. Acta Neuropathol 2:144, 1962.
24. Klatzo I, Wisniewski H, Steinwall O, et al: Dynamics of brain edema. In: Klatzo I, Feitelberger F (eds): Brain Edema. New York, Springer-Verlag, 1967, pp 554–563.
25. Levin VA, Fenstermacher JD: Cortical ECS and diffusion profiles in the cat, dog and monkey perfused through the subarachnoid space. Fed Proc 28:578, 1969 (abstract).
26. Levin VA, Fenstermacher JD, Patlak CS: Sucrose and inulin space measurements of cerebral cortex in four mammalian species. Am J Physiol 219:1528, 1970.
27. Levin VA, Milhorat TH, Fenstermacher JD, et al: Physiological studies on the development of obstructive hydrocephalus in the monkey. Neurology (Minn) 21:238, 1971.
28. McLone DG: Development of brain extracellular space in hydrocephalus (Hy-3) mice. J Neurol Neurosurg Psychiatry 36:155, 1972.
29. Milhorat TH: Choroid plexus and cerebrospinal fluid production. Science 166:1514, 1969.
30. Milhorat TH: Hydrocephalus and the Cerebrospinal Fluid. Baltimore, Williams & Wilkins, 1972.
31. Milhorat TH: Failure of choroid plexectomy as treatment for hydrocephalus. Surg Gynecol Obstet 139:505, 1974.
32. Milhorat TH: The third circulation revisited. J Neurosurg 42:628, 1975.
33. Milhorat TH: Structure and function of the choroid plexus and other sites of cerebrospinal fluid formation. Int Rev Cytol 47:225, 1976.
34. Milhorat TH: Circulation of the cerebrospinal fluid. In: McLaurin RL (ed): Pediatric Neurosurgery. Surgery of the Developing Nervous System. New York, Grune and Stratton, 1982, pp 171–182.
35. Milhorat TH: Interstitial compartment of brain in hydrocephalus. In: Shapiro K, Marmarou A, Portnoy H (eds): Hydrocephalus. New York, Raven Press, 1984, pp 99–108.
36. Milhorat TH, Clark RG: Some observations on the circulation of phenolsulfonphthalein in cerebrospinal fluid. Normal flow and flow in hydrocephalus. J Neurosurg 35:522, 1970.
37. Milhorat TH, Clark RG, Hammock MK, et al: Structural, ultrastructural, and permeability changes in the ependyma and surrounding brain favoring equilibration in progressive hydrocephalus. Arch Neurol (Chicago) 22:397, 1970.
38. Milhorat TH, Davis DA, Hammock MK: Localization of ouabain-sensitive Na-K-ATPase in frog, rabbit, and rat choroid plexus. Brain Res 99:170, 1975.
39. Milhorat TH, Davis DA, Hammock MK: Experimental intracerebral movement of electron microscopic tracers of various molecular sizes. J Neurosurg 42:315, 1975.
40. Milhorat TH, Davis DA, Lloyd BJ: Two morphologically distinct blood-brain barriers preventing the entry of cytochrome c into the cerebrospinal fluid. Science 180:76, 1973.
41. Milhorat TH, Hammock MK: Isotope ventriculography. Interpretation of ventricular size and configuration in hydrocephalus. Arch Neurol (Chicago) 25:1, 1971.
42. Milhorat TH, Hammock MK: Cerebrospinal fluid as a reflection of the internal milieu of the brain. In: Wood JH (ed): Neurobiology of Cerebrospinal Fluid 2. New York, Plenum Pub. Corp., 1983, pp 1–23.
43. Milhorat TH, Hammock MK, Chandra RS: The subarachnoid space in congenital obstructive hydrocephalus. Part II. Microscopic findings. J Neurosurg 35:7, 1971.
44. Milhorat TH, Hammock MK, DiChiro G: The subarachnoid space in congenital obstructive hydrocephalus. Part I. Cisternographic findings. J Neurosurg 35:1, 1971.
45. Milhorat TH, Hammock MK, Fenstermacher JD, et al: Cerebrospinal fluid production by the choroid plexus and brain. Science 173:330, 1971.
46. Pollay M, Curl F: Secretion of cerebrospinal fluid by the ventricular ependyma of the rabbit. Am J Physiol 213:1031, 1967.
47. Rall DP, Oppelt WW, Patlak CS: Extracellular space of brain as determined by diffusion of inulin from the ventricular system. Life Sci 1:43, 1962.
48. Reese TS, Karnovsky MJ: Fine structural localization of a blood-brain barrier to exogenous peroxidase. J Cell Biol 34:207, 1967.
49. Sachs E, Wilkins H, Sams CF: Studies on cerebrospinal

circulation by a new method. Arch Neurol Psychiatry 23:130, 1930.
50. Sato O, Bering EA: Extraventricular formation of cerebrospinal fluid. Brain Nerve (Tokyo) 19:883, 1967.
51. Shulman K, Yarnell P, Ransohoff J: Dural sinus pressure in normal and hydrocephalic dogs. Arch Neurol 10:575, 1964.
52. Sonnenberg H, Soloman S, Frazier DT: Sodium and chloride movement into the central canal of the spinal cord. Proc Soc Exp Biol Med 124:1316, 1967.
53. Weed LH: Studies on the cerebrospinal fluid. The dual source of cerebral spinal fluid. J Med Res 26:93–113, 1914.
54. Zulch KJ: *In*: Olevacrona H, Tonnis W (eds): Handbucher Neurochirugie, Vol. 3. Berlin, Springer-Verlag, 1956.

13
HYDROCEPHALUS: ETIOLOGY, PATHOLOGIC EFFECTS, DIAGNOSIS, AND NATURAL HISTORY

David C. McCullough, M.D.

> Hydrocephalus is not a disease. It is a pathological condition with many variations, but it is always characterized by an increase in the amount of cerebrospinal fluid which is or has been under increased pressure. It may be found at any period of life...
>
> DONALD D. MATSON[60]

Matson's concise definition of hydrocephalus scarcely requires elaboration. However, it would be accurate to append that hydrocephalus is a condition caused by a discrepancy between the production and the absorption of cerebrospinal fluid (CSF), so that the cerebral ventricles dilate. The condition arises from three basic disease processes: (1) congenital anomalies, (2) neoplasms, and (3) inflammatory conditions (Table 13–1). It should be appreciated that hydrocephalus may be congenital or acquired. Thus, it can occur prenatally or at any time during life.

Hydrocephalus usually results from obstruction of CSF flow, but as Matson also stated, this is not an "all or none" phenomenon. Therefore, its presentation varies according to age of onset, degree of blockage of CSF flow, rate of accumulation of ventricular fluid, etiology, and associated intracranial pathology.

Twentieth-century discoveries in pathophysiology nurtured the understanding of clinical hydrocephalus, yielding vastly improved diagnostic techniques. The latter have fundamentally influenced the control of hydrocephalus; however, prevention and cure remain elusive objectives.

BRIEF HISTORICAL NOTE

Recognition of this condition dates from at least the hippocratic era.[68] Early writings on "the dropsy of the brain" reflect imprecise understanding of the location of the fluid. In some accounts, hydrocephalus seems to have been confused with subdural effusions. Galenic teaching perpetuated this confusion for several centuries, probably institutionalizing the phrase "water on the brain," which prevails to this day. During the sixteenth century, Vesalius first accurately concluded that the pathologic accumulation of fluid was within the cerebral ventricles.[94]

With refinements in the knowledge regarding cerebral and ventricular anatomy and the concept of CSF circulation came increasingly valid interpretation of the pathology of hydrocephalus. Eighteenth- and nineteenth-century investigators began to specify sites and causes of obstruction of CSF pathways. Morgagni[70] and others sequentially described acquired adult-onset hydrocephalus, post-meningitic varieties, and congenital and neoplastic types.[63, 68]

Methodic elucidation of CSF circulation originated during the nineteenth century. Magendie[58] has been credited with the concept of an active bulk flow process. The pathways were meticulously detailed in the anatomic treatises of Key and Retzius.[49] Although the intracacies of the CSF circulation are still incompletely understood, contemporary clinical thinking on the diagnosis and management of hydrocephalus owes much to twentieth-century physiologists, pathologists, neurosurgeons, and radiologists. Weed,[97] Dandy and Blackfan,[17] Bering,[5] Davson,[19] Milhorat,[67] Pappenheimer and colleagues,[74] Cutler and coworkers,[15] and many others have contributed basic data to undergird clinical thinking. Russell[82] added systematic pathologic descriptions, which continue to sustain diagnostic and therapeutic efforts.

Dandy's initial neurosurgical approaches were firmly supported by laboratory experiments and his sagacious radiologic innovations. Diagnostic capability advanced dramatically after he introduced pneumoventriculography in 1918.[16] However, nearly six decades were to pass before the appearance of safer, noninvasive techniques such as computerized tomography (CT) and, more recently, cranial ultrasonography and nuclear magnetic resonance imaging (NMRI). These have virtually eliminated a number of sophisticated, although cumbersome, testing methods that characterized diagnosis and evaluation of hydrocephalic patients prior to 1974. Current facilities for the diagnosis of hydrocephalus in utero have engendered the real prospect of the fetus as a neurosurgical patient.[4, 13]

CLASSIFICATION AND ETIOLOGY

Terms and Definitions

Terminology becomes confusing at times, even to the initiated, and definitions demand greater precision. Some terms should be eliminated. When therapy was more diverse (and air studies in vogue), clinicians frequently spoke of noncommunicating and communicating hydrocephalus. The former presumes a blockage of CSF pathways at or proximal to the outlet foramina of the fourth ventricle. With the latter, the obstruction is located in the basal subarachnoid cisterns, subarachnoid sulci (convexities), or arachnoid villi. The designations internal and external hydrocephalus had similar meanings, respectively, although some clinicians clearly confused external hydrocephalus with subdural hygromas. Therefore, it seems appropriate to eliminate the terms internal and external hydrocephalus from current usage. Since most hydrocephalus results from obstruction, the terms obstructive and nonobstructive should also be de-emphasized.

Concerning the two labels noncommunicating and communicating, present diagnostic testing, for practical purposes, only implies these conditions. Although they are still useful categories, it is proper to classify the disorder in a patient with respect to (1) site of the blockage, (2) probable or precise etiology, and (3) state of progression.

The additional consideration in the classification scheme is the dynamic status of the disorder. Is it progressive or nonprogressive (active or arrested)? All persons with large ventricles do not have hydrocephalus. Furthermore, progressive ventriculomegaly may not signify a CSF absorptive deficit. For example, a patient incurring a localized or diffuse cerebral insult or a progressive dementing degenerative disorder may show a subtly increasing ventriculomegaly (usually with cortical atrophy) over a prolonged interval. This is often called hydrocephalus ex vacuo, an unfortunate term indicating neither previous nor ongoing obstruction of CSF circulation.

On the other hand, compensation may occur in the hydrocephalic condition, usually resulting in stable ventriculomegaly. The labels nonprogressive, compensated, or arrested hydrocephalus are often used interchangeably. They imply that the patient previously experienced a CSF absorptive deficit (block), but then production and absorption became balanced. There is no increasing (progressive) ventriculomegaly, escalating functional impairment, or continuing cerebral injury. This clinical determination is difficult to make and is always subject to revision with future evidence. From the foregoing, the definitions of spontaneous or therapeutically (surgically) compensated hydrocephalus should be obvious.

The meaning of "acute" hydrocephalus is also largely self-explanatory, denoting the abruptness of onset of dramatic clinical symptoms with increased intracranial pressure. Furthermore, it alludes to the brief time interval of symptomatic progression when a known cause can be assigned.

Etiologic-Anatomic Classification

Table 13-1 provides a simple categorization of etiology, assuming that in rare instances, the hydrocephalic condition can be caused purely by overproduction of CSF. Table 13-2 expands the diagnostic categories, including the sites and the causes of obstruction. Table 13-3 illustrates the author's experience with the congenital and the acquired forms. Any of the three diseases processes—congenital malformation, neoplasms, and inflammatory conditions—may produce hydrocephalus of the

Table 13–1. SIMPLIFIED ETIOLOGIC CLASSIFICATION OF HYDROCEPHALUS

Obstruction of CSF Pathways
Congenital malformations
Neoplasms
Inflammatory conditions
Infectious
Chemical
Overproduction of CSF
Neoplastic (choroid plexus papilloma)

noncommunicating or communicating variety. However, hydrocephalus originating from congenital and neoplastic causes tends to be noncommunicating, and that caused by infections or subarachnoid or intraventricular hemorrhage tends to be communicating.

Common Sites and Causes of Anatomic Obstruction

Noncommunicating hydrocephalus may be highly focal. This is exemplified by a neoplasm, such as an ependymoma or astrocytoma, that obstructs a temporal or frontal ventricular horn. Indeed, a conceptual tour through the CSF pathways from lateral ventricles to the arachnoid villi discloses astonishing numbers and types of lesions that may produce hydrocephalus. These include the possibilities of unilateral hydrocephalus from congenital atresia of a foramen of Monro and bilateral hydrocephalus from a colloid cyst of the anterior third ventricle. Bilateral ventriculomegaly also occurs with neoplastic obstruction of the third ventricle (e.g., ependymoma, astrocytoma, suprasellar craniopharyngioma), various congenital or neoplastic obstructions of the aqueduct (e.g., arteriovenous anomalies of the vein of Galen, pineal neoplasms), and anomalies or tumors distorting the fourth ventricle.

Continuing this figurative tour through the cisterns, the diagnostician encounters acute inflammatory processes and chronic adhesive leptomeningeal obstructions from hemorrhage and bacterial, fungal, and, possibly, viral meningitis. Occasionally, neoplastic meningeal infiltration with leukemia or carcinomatosis produces communicating hydrocephalus. At the terminus of the pathway, maldevelopment of arachnoid villi[32] or engorgement of those structures with blood and particulate matter may produce an absorptive deficit.[26, 43]

Congenital Hydrocephalus—Causes

Common Malformation Syndromes

Congenital hydrocephalus is associated with a number of recognized malformation syndromes (Table 13–4).[88] The various aqueductal anomalies—forking, narrowing, septum, gliosis—are among the leading hydrocephalic birth defects.[82] The X-linked hereditary form is unusual (affecting only two brothers in the author's 380 cases; Table 13–3).[6, 44] Two other types, spina bifida cystica with Chiari II anomaly and the Dandy-Walker syndrome, merit amplification.

A strong association between myelodysplasia and congenital hydrocephalus pertains almost exclusively to patients with myelomeningocele (spina bifida cystica). A well-documented 80 to 90 percent

Table 13–3. CAUSES OF PROGRESSIVE HYDROCEPHALUS IN 380 PEDIATRIC PATIENTS*

	No. Overt at Birth	No. Not Overt	Total	Percentage
Congenital				
With spina bifida	37	45	82	21.6
Other (aqueductal atresia, Dandy-Walker malformation, developmental cyst, encephalocele, simple communicating type, Crouzon's disease, AVM)	44	50	94	24.7
Tumor	1	1	2	0.5
Acquired				
Posthemorrhagic				
Premature	—	—	59	15.5
Full term	—	—	3	0.8
Traumatic	—	—	5	1.3
Postmeningitic				
Infectious	—	—	15	4.0
Other	—	—	5	1.3
Late-onset aqueductal atresia	—	—	4	1.1
Tumor or Colloid Cyst	—	—	111	29.2
TOTAL			380	100

*Author's personal series, excluding cases with spontaneous compensation.

Table 13–2. ANATOMIC-ETIOLOGIC CLASSIFICATION OF HYDROCEPHALUS

Noncommunicating	Communicating
Congenital	**Congenital**
Aqueductal obstruction	Arnold-Chiari malformation
Atresia of foramen of Monro	Dandy-Walker malformation
Arnold-Chiari malformation	Leptomeningeal inflammation
Dandy-Walker malformation	Incompetent arachnoid villi
Neoplasms	Encephalocele
Benign intracranial cysts	Benign cysts
Skull base anomalies	**Neoplastic**
Neoplastic	**Inflammatory**
Inflammatory	Infectious meningitis
Infectious ventriculitis	Subarachnoid hemorrhage (spontaneous, traumatic, surgical)
Intraventricular hemorrhage	
Chemical ventriculitis	Chemical arachnoiditis

Table 13–4. CONGENITAL HYDROCEPHALUS—ASSOCIATION WITH MALFORMATION SYNDROMES*

Frequent Occurrence of Hydrocephalus
 X-linked recessive hydrocephalus
 Familial type of Dandy-Walker malformation
 Spina bifida cystica
 Albers-Schönberg disease (severe osteopetrosis)

Occasional Occurrence of Hydrocephalus
 Achondroplasia
 Acrodysostosis
 Apert's disease
 Basal cell nevus
 Hurler's disease
 Incontinentia pigmenti
 Linear sebaceous nevus sequence
 Meckel-Gruber syndrome
 Oral-facial-digital syndrome
 Osteogenesis imperfecta
 Riley-Day syndrome
 Thanatophoric dwarfism
 Triploidy†
 Trisomy 13†
 Trisomy 18†

*Adapted from Smith DW: Recognizable Patterns of Human Malformation, 3rd ed. (Vol. 7 in the series Major Problems in Clinical Pediatrics). Philadelphia, W. B. Saunders Co., 1982.
†Chromosomal anomalies.

incidence of congenital ventriculomegaly in patients with myelomeningocele is appreciated by neurosurgeons.[54] The majority of newborns (55 percent of the author's cases; Table 13–3) paradoxically have normal or small head circumferences. Progressive ventriculomegaly and increased intracranial pressure characteristically develop after myelomeningocele repair. This may result from the elimination of the myelomeningocele sac as a CSF reservoir, or a pressure cushion, that nullifies CSF pulsations.[53] The sites of obstruction vary, depending somewhat on whether there is complicating infection of CSF pathways. All myelomeningocele patients have some expression of the Arnold-Chiari malformation. Thus, trapping at or near the foramen magnum plays an important role. Radiographic experience suggests that the aqueduct is completely obstructed in at least 50 percent of patients.[64] Conversely, the examination of brains removed at autopsy has uniformly shown some degree of aqueductal patency.[27]

The Dandy-Walker malformation, consisting of dysgenetic cerebellar vermis and cystic dilation of the fourth ventricle, occurs as a familial anomaly but more commonly is sporadic. Numerous associated cerebral and systemic birth defects have been described in affected patients. Midline defects, particularly agenesis of the corpus callosum, are common. The hydrocephalus has been attributed to prenatal obstruction of fourth ventricular outlet foramina. However, communication between ventricles and subarachnoid spaces has often been demonstrated clinically. Therefore, the etiology is in doubt but is probably complex.[76] Hydrocephalus may be expressed only at the fourth ventricle, or the entire system may be dilated. Macrocephaly does not always appear at birth. In fact, in some cases, symptoms are delayed beyond adolescence. Differences in clinical expression relate to the severity of the hydrocephalus, the integrity of the adjacent brainstem, and the magnitude of associated anomalies. Ventricular disconnection resulting from intermittent or persistent mechanical compression of the aqueduct may be associated with discrepancy in intercompartmental pressures.[75]

Table 13–5 depicts other structural and developmental anomalies frequently found with congenital hydrocephalus.

Viruses and Congenital Hydrocephalus

Substantial laboratory and some clinical evidence suggests that many of the patients with idiopathic congenital hydrocephalus were victims of intrauterine viral infections. The list of viruses capable of producing aqueductal atresia or communicating varieties of hydrocephalus comprises at least 20 agents.[64] Cytomegalovirus (CMV) infections, mumps, rubella, varicella, Asian influenza, and others have been recognized as causatic factors in human hydrocephalus.[7, 18, 67]

Linked to the issue of viral hydrocephalus is the mechanistic theory of the cause of aqueductal stenosis or atresia. While true inflammatory ependymal and subependymal conditions may strike the narrow aqueduct, Williams[102] and others have hypothesized that aqueductal occlusion often represents a mechanical consequence of more distal obstruction. The sequence has been induced by intracerebral or surface inoculations in experimental animals. Progressive ventriculomegaly with caudal displacement of the hindrain allows midbrain compression and, hence, aqueductal narrowing.

Parasites

Toxoplasma has long been recognized as a serious pathogen that produces congenital hydrocephalus.[55] The infestation was found to be an etiologic factor in 39 percent of 38 pediatric patients with hydrocephalus in a recent study from Yugoslavia[59] but could be documented in only 0.5 percent of the

Table 13–5. CONGENITAL HYDROCEPHALUS—SOME ASSOCIATED STRUCTURAL AND DEVELOPMENTAL ANOMALIES

Agenesis of corpus callosum
Arteriovenous malformation (AVM)
Craniofacial dysostosis (Crouzon's disease, Apert's disease)
Dandy-Walker malformation
Developmental cysts (arachnoid, ependymal)
Encephalocele, cranial meningocele
Holoprosencephaly
Lissencephaly
Midline (central) cysts
Myelomeningocele (Chiari II anomaly)
Neoplasms

author's cases. The parasite is often recovered from CSF in affected newborn infants with pleocytosis, indicating persistent infestation, with a low-grade inflammatory response.

Intracranial Tumors

In the author's series, the incidence of neoplasm among patients with overt congenital hydrocephalus was only 1.2 percent. The potential variety of lesions is extensive, prominently including medulloblastoma, teratoma, astrocytoma, and craniopharyngioma.

Choroid plexus papilloma, a rare cerebral neoplasm, has recently been proved to secrete excessive volumes of CSF.[14, 25, 69] Thus, the associated hydrocephalus can be a consequence of pure overproduction of CSF. However, many patients exhibit obstruction of CSF flow, resulting from the inflammatory effects of intermittent tumoral hemorrhage and proteinaceous CSF.

Developmental Cysts

The etiology of arachnoid (interarachnoid) cysts and the less common ependymal cysts is not always evident.[65] Some may be true malformations, whereas others may stem from inflammatory events in the CSF pathways after infection or hemorrhage.[78, 89] Ependymal cysts have been interpreted as complications of aberrant rests of ependymal cells in subarachnoid locations or pockets of ependymal expansion occurring after blockage of CSF compartments.[2, 65] Macrocrania in congenital cases results directly from expanded cysts or from secondary hydrocephalus.

Toxic and Nutritional Factors

Other etiologic factors have been implicated in a number of human cases, and various teratogens have been employed to produce animal models of hydrocephalus (Table 13–6).[46] Suggested but unconvincing risk factors in humans are race, ethnicity, maternal age, parity, and socioeconomic conditions.

Acquired Hydrocephalus—Causes

Inflammatory Conditions

Chemical Irritants. Prominent among all causes of human hydrocephalus is chronic adhesive arachnoiditis or ventriculitis secondary to subarachnoid or intraventricular hemorrhage.[56] The possibility of spontaneous or traumatic intracranial hemorrhage is, of course, a lifelong threat. Intrauterine or parturitional hemorrhage may account for occasional cases of "congenital" hydrocephalus as well.[99]

The incidence of germinal plate hemorrhage in premature babies approaches 30 to 40 percent. Incipient obstruction of CSF pathways may result from hemorrhagic engorgement of arachnoid villi.[43] Progressive hydrocephalus from adhesive arachnoiditis or ventriculitis is a frequent sequel. Fifteen percent of the author's cases of juvenile hydrocephalus were premature infants with this condition (Table 13–3).

Table 13–6. CONGENITAL HYDROCEPHALUS—ASSOCIATED TOXIC AND NUTRITIONAL FACTORS*

Azo dyes
Bromolysergic acid
Folic acid deficiency
Hypervitaminosis A
Irradiation
Lysergic acid diethylamide (LSD)
Mescaline
Triamcinolone acetonide
Vitamin A deficiency
Vitamin B_{12} deficiency

*From laboratory and clinical investigations.

The clinician should also be sensitive to the possibility of posthemorrhagic hydrocephalus from tumors, bacterial meningitis, closed head injury, and intracranial surgery.

Other threatening chemical irritants include the cholesterol-laden fluid discharged from craniopharyngiomas or dermoid tumors and injected substances such as preservatives for intrathecal and intraventricular antibiotics. Experimental hydrocephalus has been produced with numerous substances such as lampblack, kaolin, paraffin, and silicone oils.

Infections. Although little is established regarding the influence of postnatally acquired viral leptomeningitis in the etiology of hydrocephalus, bacterial, fungal, and parasitic infections are recognized offenders. Acute, self-limited hydrocephalus is probably more common than the late form, which develops with chronic adhesive arachnoiditis.[8]

Approximately 1 percent of survivors of bacterial meningitis go on to develop progressive hydrocephalus.[23] Newborns are at greater risk than older children. Intraventricular obstruction and aqueductal and fourth ventricular outlet obstruction occur at all ages, but neonates are especially susceptible to noncommunicating hydrocephalus. Infections with gram-negative organisms (e.g., *Escherichia coli*) at early ages are especially offensive. Common bacterial agents associated with adhesive arachnoidal fibrosis and communicating hydrocephalus are *Haemophilus influenzae*, *Mycobacterium tuberculosis*, *Streptococcus pneumoniae*, and Group B streptococci.

Acquired postnatal cysticercosis is an important but rare antecedent of pediatric hydrocephalus in endemic regions. The racemose form is implicated in both the intraventricular and the cisternal varieties.[52] Single cysts may obstruct narrow internal channels, or grapelike clusters of cysts may incite inflammatory responses in the basal cisterns. Occasionally, the parenchymal form produces internal obstruction of narrow CSF channels. This type usually provokes only mild inflammatory reactions in distal pathways. For both forms, the time of latency until the emergence of hydrocephalus may be years or decades.

Tumors

Neoplasms at diverse intracranial loci may incite hydrocephalus. The predisposition to neoplasms originating in the posterior fossa in infants and children increases the proportion of such patients presenting with ventriculomegaly. In the author's series, 54 percent of intracranial tumors in children were accompanied by hydrocephalus. They represent 29 percent of diagnosed cases with the condition (Table 13–3). Choroidal tumors may become symptomatic at any age. Hydrocephalus in conjunction with neurofibromatosis is often, but not always, of neoplastic origin.

Other Causes

Acquired leptomeningeal cysts and posterior fossa subdural, epidural, and cerebellar hemorrhages occasionally contribute.[32] Idiopathic aqueductal atresia presenting in late childhood or adolescence may have no apparent connection with inflammatory or neoplastic events (Table 13–3). The same applies to membranous obstruction of the fourth ventricle.[3]

Venous Obstruction

Occlusion of multiple cerebral veins, jugular veins, or a major sinus has been proposed as an etiologic factor in hydrocephalus. The concept remains theoretical and unsubstantiated.[68] The author has witnessed a single convincing case of bilateral transverse sinus thrombosis with severe, self-limited noncommunicating hydrocephalus. The latter appeared to be secondary to extreme swelling of the cerebellum. Recently, Friedman and Mickle[30] postulated venous outflow obstruction as the mechanism of ventriculomegaly in achondroplasia.

The term "otitic" hydrocephalus,[93] meaning ventriculomegaly from lateral sinus thrombophlebitis with otitis media, has largely passed from the vocabulary. True progressive hydrocephalus emanating from sagittal sinus thrombosis is a chimeric, albeit appealing, construction. Although hydrocephalus does result from arteriovenous shunts involving the posterior venous circulation, the ventriculomegaly associated with thrombosis is probably an atrophic process following an interlude of intense cerebral edema.

INCIDENCE AND EPIDEMIOLOGY

Because congenital hydrocephalus is often occult at birth (Table 13–3), statistics from surveys of congenital malformations are suspect. Adding the fact that the condition may be acquired throughout life, authoritative data on incidence is just not available.

Having first impeached the sources, it can be stated that the incidence of congenital hydrocephalus without spina bifida has been variously estimated as 1.2 to 15 cases per 10,000 births.[9, 10, 12, 68] These figures include cases detected at autopsy from studies covering stillborn infants and live-born infants and from other studies covering only live-born infants. Data from the Birth Defects Monitoring Program in the United States between 1975 and 1982 show a slowly increasing incidence, from 3.9 to 5.5 cases per 10,000 births.[9, 10] A similar but stable number of cases of spina bifida was detected over the same period. Considering the expected proportion of hydrocephalic patients with spina bifida, approximately 7 to 9 cases of congenital hydrocephalus per 10,000 births may have been detected.

Contrary to the subtle trend of increase in the United States, Lorber and Ward[57] recently revealed a decline in hydrocephalic births (without spina bifida) from 4.8 to 3.1 per 10,000 births in England and Wales between 1974 and 1983. Considering the multiple risk factors for acquired conditions, the incidence must exceed 0.15 percent, the figure reported from the Collaborative Perinatal Project in the United States.[12]

PATHOLOGIC EFFECTS OF HYDROCEPHALUS

Many published sources review the primary lesions causing CSF absorptive defects. The reader is referred to monographs by Russell[82] and Milhorat[67] and standard neuropathology texts for detailed descriptions of aqueductal-periaqueductal and other anomalies and acquired leptomeningeal fibrosis. Several chapters in this volume also discuss major anomalies and tumors.

Secondary pathologic effects of hydrocephalus potentially augment the rates of cerebral injury, functional deficit, and eventual mortality. In the context of pre-existing cerebral malformation or insult, the injury superimposed by hydrocephalus on the developing, myelinating brain may be severe.

Gross distention of the cerebral ventricles proceeds sequentially downward toward obstructed segments. Ependymal disruption is initiated at the angles of the lateral ventricles.[67] This may progress to extensive denudation of ventricular surfaces. The interhemispheric commissures become stretched, and the septum pellucidum ruptures. Eventually, deformed cortical gyri atrophy. Pseudopolymicrogyria may be a consequence of this process. Choroidal structures atrophy and fibrose in long-standing cases.[82]

Spontaneous ventriculostomy is a clinically recognized[47] and pathologically verified[82] entity in certain congenital cases. Ballooning of ventricular chambers and recesses leads to pooling of CSF in cisterns or subdural spaces after ventricular rupture. Arachnoid and ependymal cysts can originate from ruptured or ballooned ventricular diverticula.[2, 82]

Classic pathoanatomic signs of incisural and transforaminal herniation are obvious gross secondary effects of hydrocephalus in autopsy specimens. Cerebellar, mesencephalic, and pontine signs of upward herniation also occur with posterior fossa pathologic conditions.

Speculative concerns of many clinicians find answers from gross and micropathologic study of secondary blocks. These questions relate to sequential mechanisms of CSF obstruction in noncommunicating and communicating hydrocephalus. It appears to be established that aqueductal atresia can result from mechanical effects of ventricular expansion after obliteration of subarachnoid spaces.[27, 102] Furthermore, Milhorat and coworkers[67] have shown that distal subarachnoid spaces become physically compressed in patients with noncommunicating hydrocephalus. They found no evidence of deficient initial development of cortical subarachnoid spaces. Whether or not the frequently observed subarachnoid fibrosis can be purely a consequence of ventricular expansion is an unanswered question.

Examination of the effects of acute and chronic hydrocephalus on brain parenchyma with light and electron microscopy discloses a sequential pathologic process. Limited human material and many experimental studies document a pattern of subependymal edema, gliosis, myelin degradation, and reduction of the microvasculature.[33, 100, 101, 104] Lipid and protein fractions of deep white matter quantitatively decline.[28] Microcysts and macrocysts may appear. Some authors have described a regenerative process in chronic experimental hydrocephalus, consisting of ependymal recovery and subependymal gliosis.

Although the fate of axons in this process is less well understood, cortical neurons seem to escape injury. Using quantitation of DNA fractions as an index, Rubin and colleagues[80] reported excellent cellular preservation, a condition anticipated by earlier investigators. These observations sustain the argument for reversibility of brain injury in hydrocephalus.[79]

CLINICAL PRESENTATION

The symptoms and signs of hydrocephalus are age related. Additional determinants are the primary causes of the condition, associated malformations or cerebral insults, severity of obstruction of CSF flow, and the intracranial pressure. Contemporary diagnostic approaches (especially cranial ultrasonography) have convinced clinicians that rapidly progressive ventriculomegaly, in the early stages, occurs without classic signs or cranial enlargement.[42, 50, 96]

Infantile Hydrocephalus

Head Size, Growth Rate, and Associated Symptoms

The diagnosis may be obvious in newborns with macrocrania and other typical symptoms such as irritability, lethargy, vomiting, and poor feeding. Pediatricians are usually alert to the rate of cranial expansion. In the absence of obvious signs of increased intracranial pressure, serial circumferential head measurements provide adequate guides to the detection of macrocrania.[61] Maximum occipitofrontal circumference compared with standard curves for full-term or premature babies should be recorded at four- to eight-week intervals during the first year of life. Variations from standard may eventually be accompanied by behavioral and neurologic signs of progressive hydrocephalus.

Discrepancies between head and chest circumferences may suggest pathology. Normally, heads measure about 1 cm larger than chests until late in the first year, when the relationship reverses. Comparison of head measurements with weight and length measurements may be helpful in children of large size or with family histories of large heads, when signs of increased intracranial pressure are absent (Fig. 13–1).

In premature and nutritionally deprived infants,[20] spurts of head growth may in fact be accompanied by some evidence of increased intracranial pressure, which often provokes additional diagnostic studies.

Another source of confusion is the tendency of the premature cranium to mold in a scaphocephalic fashion. The ellipsoidal head has a greater average circumference than does the spheroidal head of comparable volume. This is also the reason for occasional confusion between macrocrania and the scaphocephaly of sagittal craniosynostosis, which is rarely associated with untreated hydrocephalus.[55]

Examination—Neurologic Signs

Bulging of the anterior fontanelle (Fig. 13–2) is typical of infantile hydrocephalus. Estimation of intracranial tension involves fontanelle palpation in both reclining and relaxed sitting positions. Normally, intracranial pressure is negative in the latter situation, although moderate respiratory congestion may produce slight fontanelle bulging. Welch[98] has described a quantitative procedure for estimating intracranial pressure at cribside. This requires measurement of the vertical distance between the bregma and a central venous point (clavicle), at the point where the fontanelle flattens or sinks when the infant is slowly lifted from a horizontal to a vertical

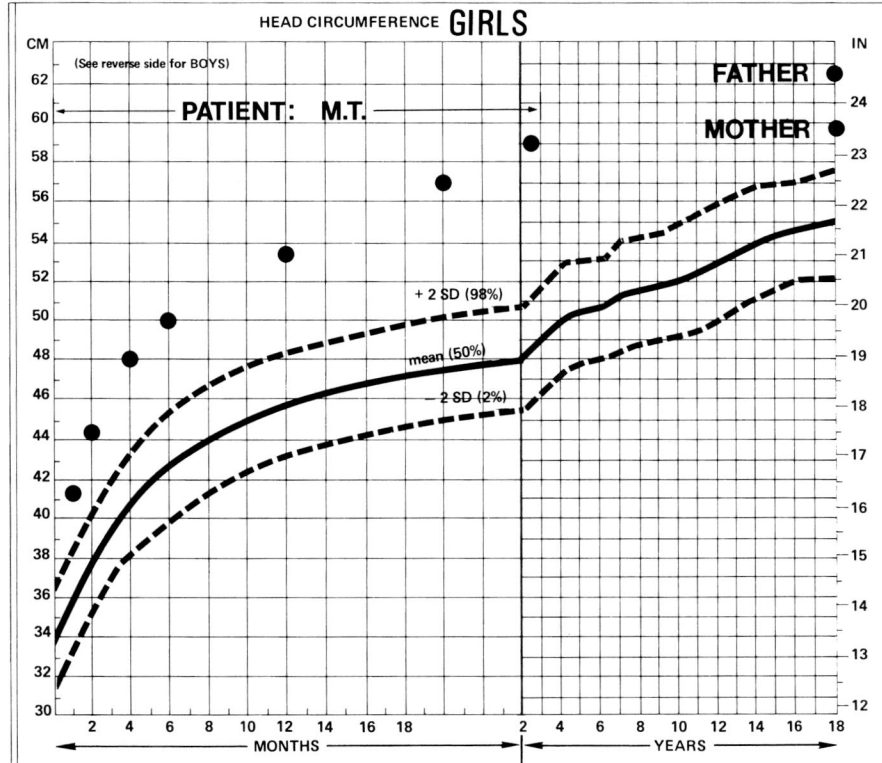

Figure 13–1. Head circumference plot of macrocephalic infant, also showing measurements of father and mother. Benign familial macrocephaly.

position. The normal measurement is 3 to 5 cm. The author has found this maneuver to be practical and its accuracy to be consistent.

Widened cranial sutures may be detected by palpation. The "cracked pot" sound on cranial percussion may be a reliable early indicator of increased pressure for the experienced observer. Head shape per se can provide clues to specific pathologic conditions (e.g., prominent posterior fossa is a clue to cysts in that region, and asymmetry can indicate unilateral ventriculomegaly).

Increased collateral venous drainage often leads to scalp vein dilation, especially in infants with the Arnold-Chiari malformation in which dural venous sinuses are aberrant.[72] Auscultation over the head may disclose augmented physiologic cranial bruits, under conditions of elevated intracranial pressure. An extremely loud murmur suggests the possibility of an arteriovenous malformation (AVM) of the vein of Galen, especially if cervical carotid arteries and jugular veins are prominent.

The sunset sign of forced downward deviation of the eyes is a neurologic sign nearly unique to hydrocephalus (Fig. 13–2). It appears to be most common with aqueductal occlusion or pathology, in juxtaposition to the mesencephalic tectum. A similar phenomenon may be observed transiently in normal infants with position changes or rapid changes in room lighting. A sustained instance of the sunset sign may be preceded by impaired ocular convergence and upward gaze, which can be detected in attentive infants, using appropriate visual stimuli.

A more tentative case can be made for other ocular findings. The deficient visual tracking characteristic of many infants with progressive hydrocephalus may be caused by oculomotor or gaze palsies. Internal strabismus is one example. Visual tracking disorders could also signify cortical blind-

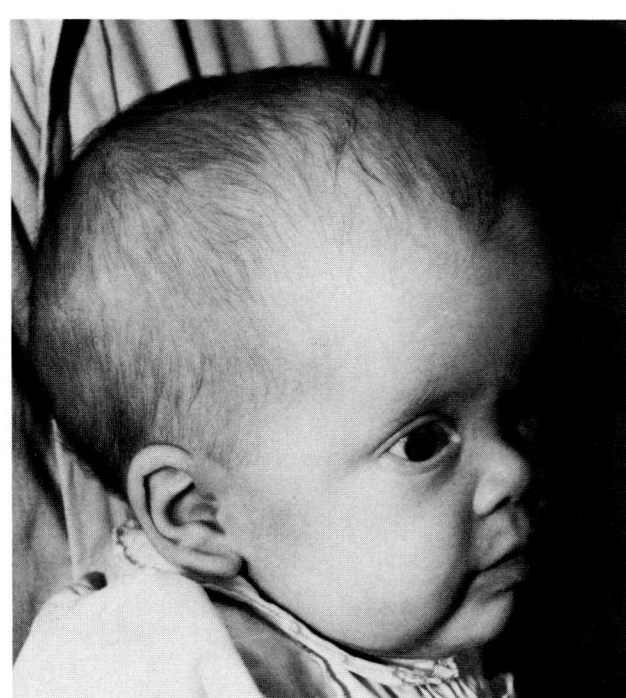

Figure 13–2. Hydrocephalic three-month-old infant.

ness. The lateral ventricles of the infant expand most prominently in the parieto-occipital dimension, thereby stretching the optic radiations and compressing the occipital lobes. This perhaps results in lack of appreciation of visual stimuli and may persist in some measure as the explanation of abnormal visual association and visual-motor performance in older, treated patients with hydrocephalus.

Papilledema is only occasionally observed in infantile hydrocephalus. Retinal hemorrhages of the discrete subhyaloid variety suggest an alternative diagnosis of subdural hematoma.

Poor head control is observed frequently in infants with macrocrania and in hydrocephalic infants. It can signify motor retardation but often reflects difficulty in mobilizing the large head. Forcible head retraction may be seen.

Pediatricians frequently attribute episodes of apnea and bradycardia in premature and neurologically impaired infants to progressive hydrocephalus. Although apneic bouts, poor feeding and swallowing, and failure to thrive occasionally appear in infants with posterior fossa anomalies and tumors, episodic apnea and bradycardia rarely complicate other types of progressive hydrocephalus. They cannot be routinely ascribed to bouts of increased intracranial pressure.[62]

Hydrocephalus per se does not often lead to early neurologic signs other than developmental delay. The existence of frank signs may reflect a primary pathologic condition such as perinatal asphyxia, intracranial hemorrhage, meningoencephalitis, and major cerebral malformation or tumor. However, there are a few helpful indicators that point to the possibility of infantile hydrocephalus. These include hypertonicity of the lower extremities, decreased active leg motion, ankle clonus, and poor placing and positive-support reflexes. Retarded ambulation is a typical consequence. Presumedly because of the long, circuitous course of the corticospinal fibers supplying the lower extremities over and around the distended lateral ventricles, these tracts are damaged by stretching before the inferolateral fibers to the arms become involved.[105]

Although hemiparesis, nystagmus, or obvious ataxia strongly imply associated intracranial pathology, some clinicians have interpreted infantile hypotonia as a direct consequence of hydrocephalus.[36]

Cranial transillumination has declined in importance in the present era of noninvasive, sophisticated imaging. Its performance requires a totally dark room and a shielded cupping device to inhibit stray light. Occasionally, it helps disclose large fluid collections such as porencephalic, Dandy-Walker, and arachnoid cysts.

Differential Diagnosis in the Infant

Hydrocephalus accounts for the majority of cases of pathologic macrocrania. However, many children referred because of large head size or rapid head growth are found to have benign conditions. The single most common referral to a pediatric neurosurgeon is a developmentally normal infant with a flat fontanelle and a large head. Many have parents and ancestors with large heads.[1] Such individuals with constitutional or familial macrocrania do not require immediate CT or sonography. Others with benign macrocrania include large children (some may have gigantism) and dwarves. Some of the latter are found to be achondroplastic dwarves with increased intracranial pressure.

Table 13–7 lists most of the conditions with macrocrania that can be initially mistaken for hydrocephalus.[21] The important ones that may require urgent intervention are lead encephalopathy, primary mass effect from intracranial tumor, and subdural effusions or hematomas. CT scans readily distinguish among them. Serious metabolic disorders with macrocrania are rare and usually untreatable (Fig. 13–3). Convulsions may occur in hydrocephalus but far more frequently point to subdural hematomas. Scaphocephaly with craniosynostosis should be obvious to neurosurgeons.

Hydranencephaly, a disorder characterized by extensive prenatal cerebral destruction, may or may not present with macrocrania. If there is abnormal growth of the head, a hydrocephalic component must be assumed. Poor feeding, suppressed activity, hypothermia, and deficient visual and reflex performances are typical findings. The etiology is probably diverse, but vascular infarction (porencephaly) represents a common cause. Historically, clinicians have struggled to differentiate this malformation from extreme neonatal hydrocephalus (Fig. 13–4).[24, 90]

Hydrocephalus in Older Children

Except for similarities occurring at intermediate ages from 18 months to 3 years, the clinical presentation of hydrocephalus in childhood differs from

Table 13–7. MACROCRANIA*

Hydrocephalus	Megalencephaly
Subdural fluid	Benign
Hygroma	Familial or constitutional
Hematoma	scaphocephaly
Effusion	Pathologic
Brain edema	Gigantism
Toxic (e.g., lead	Dwarfism
encephalopathy)	Neurocutaneous syndrome
Endocrine (e.g., hypopara-	Aminoaciduria
thyroidism galactosemia)	Leukodystrophy (e.g.,
Thickened skull	Alexander's disease)
Anemia (e.g., thalassemia)	Lysozymal disorders (e.g.,
Cranioskeletal dysplasia	metachromatic
(e.g., osteopetrosis,	leukodystrophy,
Russell's dwarf)	mucopolysaccharidosis)

*Adapted from DeMyer W: Megalencephaly in children. Neurology (Minn) 22:634, 1972.

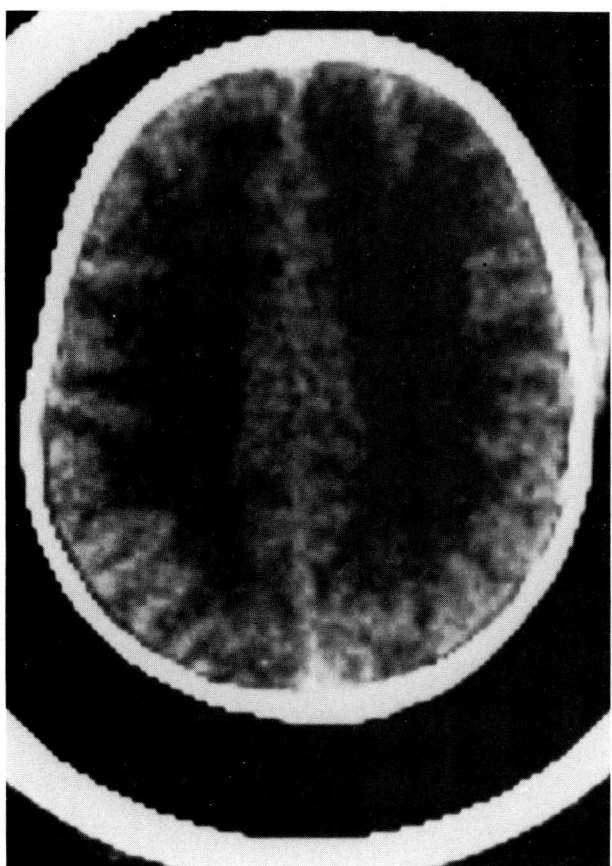

Figure 13–3. Example of a CT scan in a megalencephalic infant with prominent low-density lesions in centrum semiovale. No ventriculomegaly (Alexander's disease).

that in newborns and infants. Frequently, the child in question has abnormal head measurements, but the rate and extent of growth only subtly deviate from normal.

Acute Presentation

In hydrocephalus of acute onset, cranial expansion is more limited at older ages. Severe headaches, protracted vomiting, oculomotor symptoms, and unconsciousness may supervene. Although not a symptom in the majority of patients, convulsions are more frequent at older ages. Papilledema is not unusual in older children. Signs of uncal herniation have been observed in rapidly progressive cases.

Chronic Hydrocephalus

In the more common slowly progressive or chronic variety of hydrocephalus, episodic headaches, early morning vomiting, deteriorating gait, and declining school performance promote consideration of hydrocephalus. Delayed onset of independent walking may be part of the history. Personality changes often occur. If the cause is a tumor, symptoms of intracranial hypertension almost invariably antedate cerebellar and brainstem signs.

Diabetes insipidus suggests specific tumor involvement of the pituitary stalk or hypothalamus rather than hydrocephalus per se. Conversely, precocious puberty may be a specific effect of hydrocephalus, observed in cases with late onset or as a delayed symptom after early successful therapy.

Examination in chronic cases may or may not disclose macrocrania. Eye signs can include sixth nerve palsy, deficient ocular convergence, and limited upward gaze as well as papilledema or optic atrophy. Neurologic examination often reveals fine motor performance deficit, increased tendon reflexes, spasticity, and gait disturbance. Ataxia, lower cranial nerve palsies, or hemiparesis specifically argues for primary hindbrain anomalies or tumors. The physician should also carefully examine the integument for signs of a neurocutaneous disease.

So-called "normal pressure" hydrocephalus has been described in children and adolescents.[34, 38] The symptomatic triad described by Hakim and Adams,[37] consisting of dementia, gait apraxia, and urinary incontinence, is a rare but recognized aspect of juvenile hydrocephalus.

In chronic hydrocephalus, psychologic testing reveals discrepancies between verbal and performance intelligence quotient (IQ), with impairment of spatial perception and visual-motor function.[36, 51]

Antenatal Presentation

For practical purposes, hydrocephalus is asymptomatic in the fetus, unless there is intrauterine demise. Although polyhydramnios has been incriminated as a harbinger of neonatal hydrocephalus, its disclosure is far from specific and is often absent. Most fetal cases are discovered when prenatal ultrasonography is performed for assessment of fetal age or for screening for spina bifida and genetic conditions. With the extensive use of prenatal ultrasonography, hydrocephalus is being diagnosed in the fetus[39] quite as often as in the newborn infant, in some clinics. Recent reports show that fetal hydrocephalus frequently accompanies other birth defects that do not readily lend themselves to early disclosure.[103] Furthermore, fetal hydrocephalus is not infrequently a transient phenomenon (Fig. 13–5).

DIAGNOSTIC STRATEGY AND TESTS

It is not difficult to establish a diagnosis of hydrocephalus in this modern era of accurate and safe neuroradiologic imaging. Clinical judgment involves the timing of diagnostic testing and a systematic approach for characterizing the disorder. In all cases, the diagnostician attempts to ascertain the

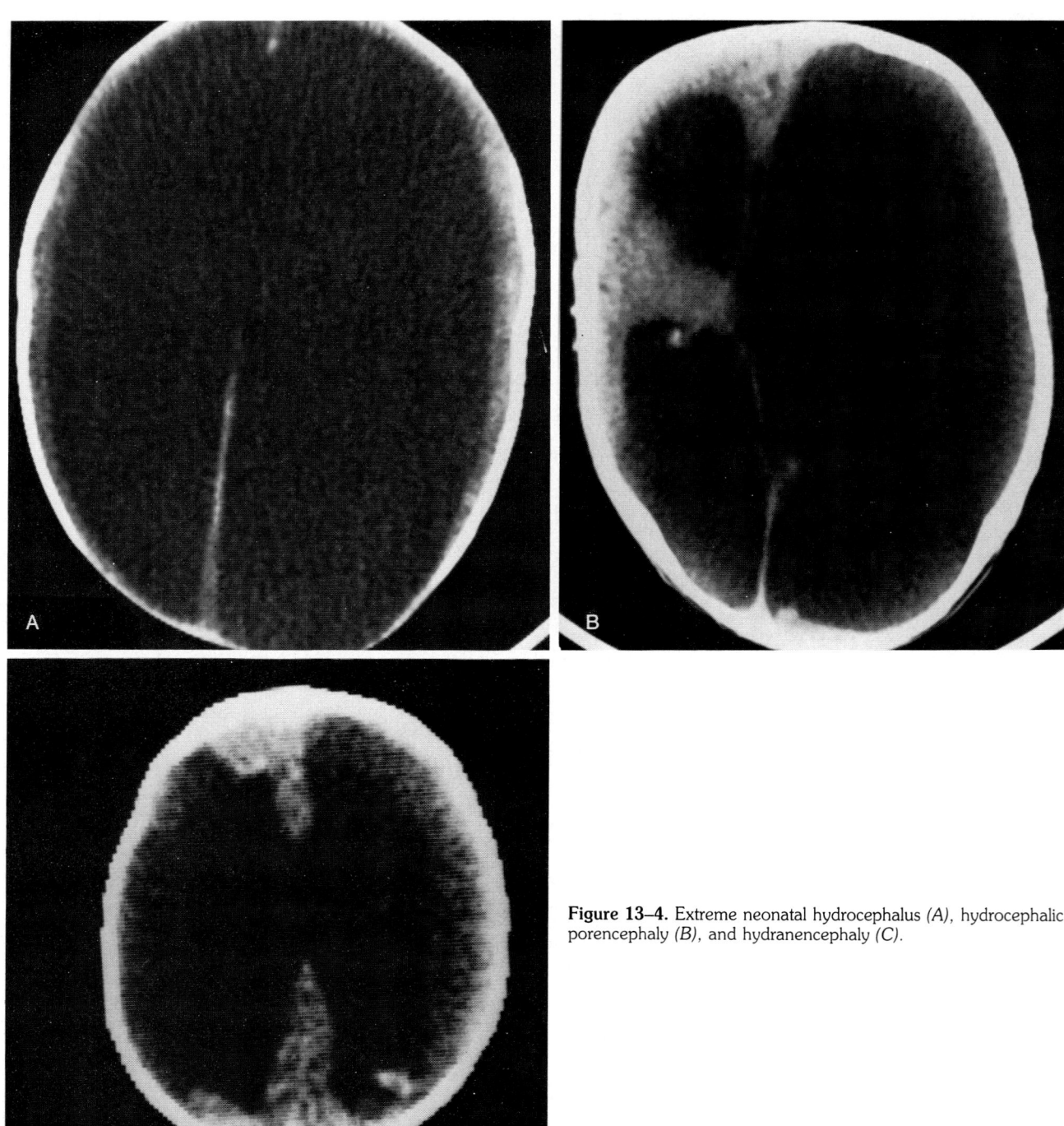

Figure 13–4. Extreme neonatal hydrocephalus (A), hydrocephalic porencephaly (B), and hydranencephaly (C).

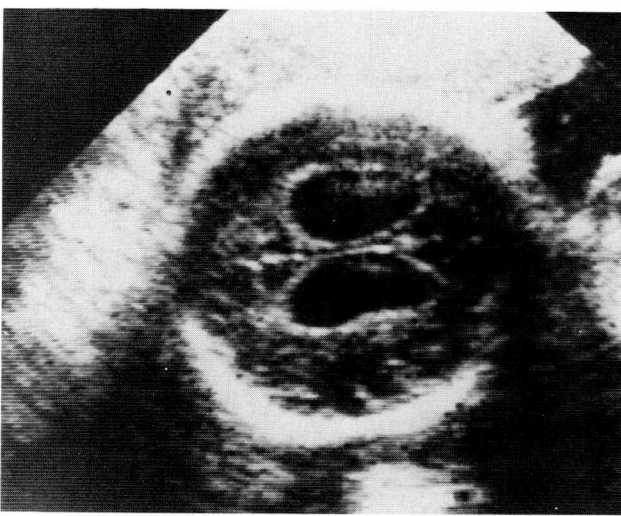

Figure 13–5. Prenatal ultrasonogram at 28 weeks, showing fetal ventriculomegaly. Cranial ultrasonography at birth and CT scan at one year were normal. (With permission from Michejda M, McCullough, DC, Bacher J, Queenan JD: Investigational approaches in fetal neurosurgery. In Humphreys R [ed.]: Concepts in Pediatric Neurosurgery, vol. 4. Basel, S. Karger, 1983, p. 45.)

site of impairment of CSF circulation, assign an etiology, and produce an assessment of the severity of the condition. Is it progressive or static? The delineation of the site of block and the judgment concerning progression may have important therapeutic implications.

Certain diagnostic procedures provide anatomic information related to the existence of hydrocephalus: the probable cause and the site of block. Others contribute pathophysiologic data that influence therapeutic decisions. Some of the imaging techniques provide both types of information. Table 13–8 lists diagnostic and prognostic procedures.

Table 13–8. HYDROCEPHALUS—LABORATORY DIAGNOSTIC PROCEDURES

Neuroimaging Procedures	Auxiliary Procedures
Primary diagnostic	*Diagnostic*
CT	CSF culture, cell count, protein
Cranial ultrasonography	level determination
NMRI	*Prognostic-Pathophysiologic*
Supplementary	Intracranial pressure monitoring
Radionuclide scanning	Ventricular perfusion
Contrast scanning	Ventricular or lumbar infusion
Arteriography	Pressure-volume indices
	Biochemical analyses
	Neurotransmitter levels
	Lipid–fatty acid ratios
	Lactate-pyruvate ratios
	Cyclic nucleotide levels
	Myelin basic proteins
	Cerebral blood flow
	Psychologic testing
	Visual evoked responses

Clinical Laboratory Diagnosis

Imaging Techniques

For clinical purposes, the three imaging techniques, CT scanning, cranial ultrasonography, and NMRI invariably reveal hydrocephalus if it exists in suspected cases. Not infrequently, they disclose unexpected or occult cases.

CT. CT represents the standard tool.[71] In evaluating infants and children with macrocrania, the method has the advantage of delineating widespread intracranial pathology. It is more accurate than sonography for depicting cerebral mantle thickness, cortical surfaces, subarachnoid spaces, and subdural hematomas or hygromas. It also provides suggestive evidence of the sites of block (Figs. 13–6 and 13–7). Contrast-enhanced scanning complements the imaging of intracranial tumors (Fig. 13–8) and provides suggestive if not confirmative evidence of arteriovenous malformations. CT may suggest a rapidly progressive process or the possibility of alternative absorptive pathways, exemplified by periventricular low densities (Fig. 13–8). Calcifications in tumors or periventricular inflammatory processes such as cytomegalovirus inclusion disease or toxoplasmosis are readily discerned (Fig. 13–9). Serial CT assists decision making in both untreated and treated patients under follow-up.

Cranial Ultrasonography. Cranial ultrasonography has advanced impressively in the past decade. The equipment is portable, and therefore, cranial ultrasonography is ideal for screening and follow-up of premature babies in neonatal nurseries (Fig. 13–10). The method accurately detects intracranial hemorrhages but is currently less reliable for vascular malformations, surface hematomas, neoplasms, and posterior fossa anomalies. As the anterior fontanelle (ultrasonic "window") closes, the usefulness of ultrasonography declines and then subsides.

NMRI. NMRI is apparently safe and allows the patient to avoid radiation exposure. To date, experience attributes a high degree of accuracy to this modality in detecting hydrocephalus and almost all types of intracranial lesions. NMRI reliably generates coronal, sagittal (Fig. 13–11), and parasagittal detailed images, with fewer manipulations than with CT. Useful information on CSF flow appears to be attainable. If NMRI becomes widely available and economical, it will become the first choice as a screening and anatomic monitoring technique for hydrocephalus in patients of all ages.

Other Techniques. Ventriculography has been relegated to a minor role with the emergence of CT, NMRI, and sonography. Pneumography is virtually defunct. Positive contrast-enhanced ventriculography and cisternography persist in some clinics, for confirmation of ventricular loculations[45] and dynamic studies of the communications between intracranial cysts.[65]

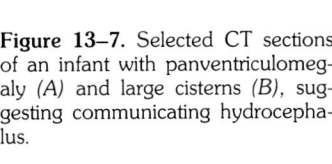

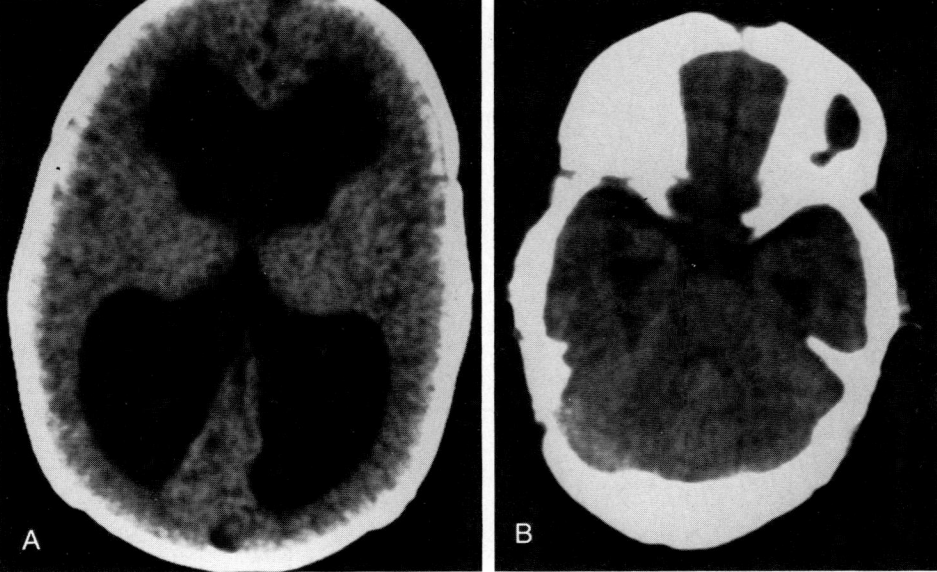

Figure 13–6. Selected CT sections of an infant with triventriculomegaly *(A)* and a small fourth ventricle *(B)*, which suggests noncommunicating hydrocephalus (aqueductal atresia).

Figure 13–7. Selected CT sections of an infant with panventriculomegaly *(A)* and large cisterns *(B)*, suggesting communicating hydrocephalus.

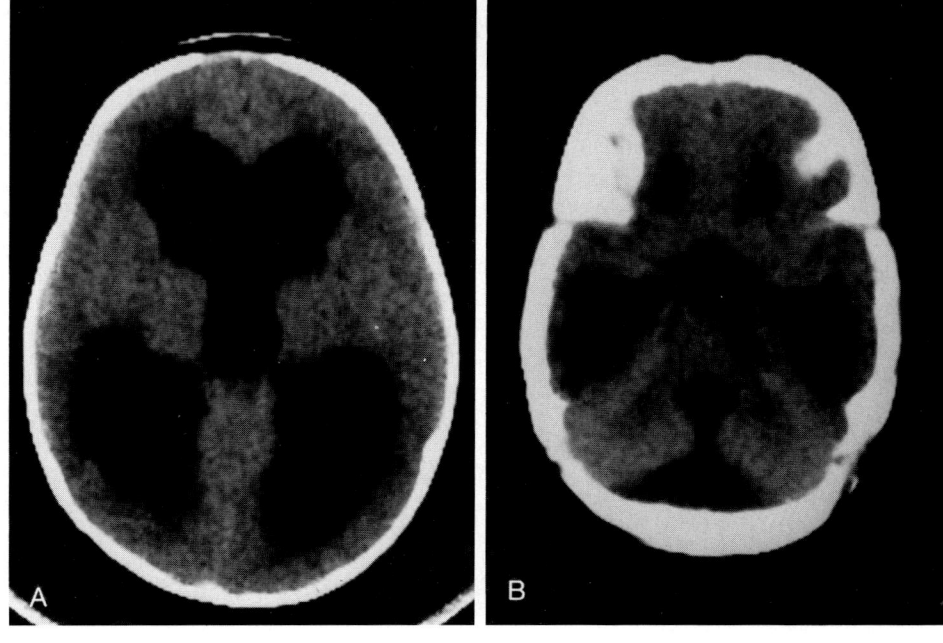

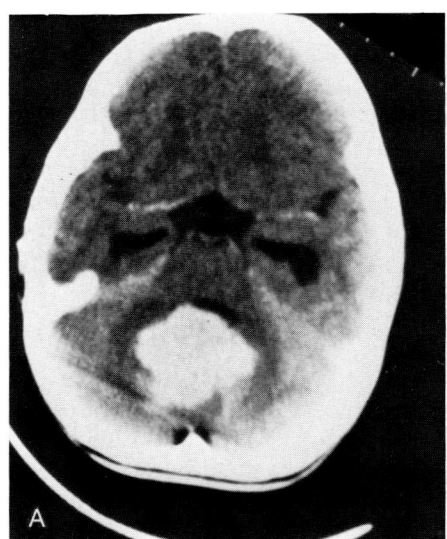
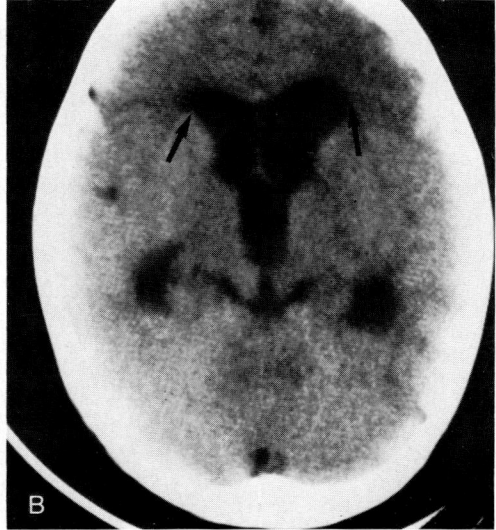

Figure 13–8. Contrast-enhanced CT sections depicting cerebellar medulloblastoma *(A)* and low densities adjacent to the anterior horns *(B, arrows)*.

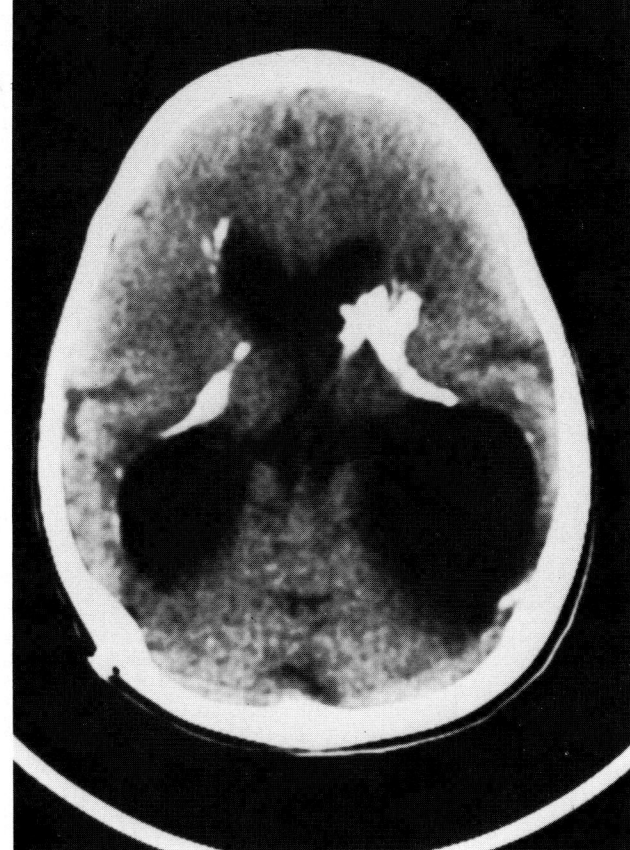

Figure 13–9. Periventricular calcifications with ventriculomegaly in toxoplasmosis.

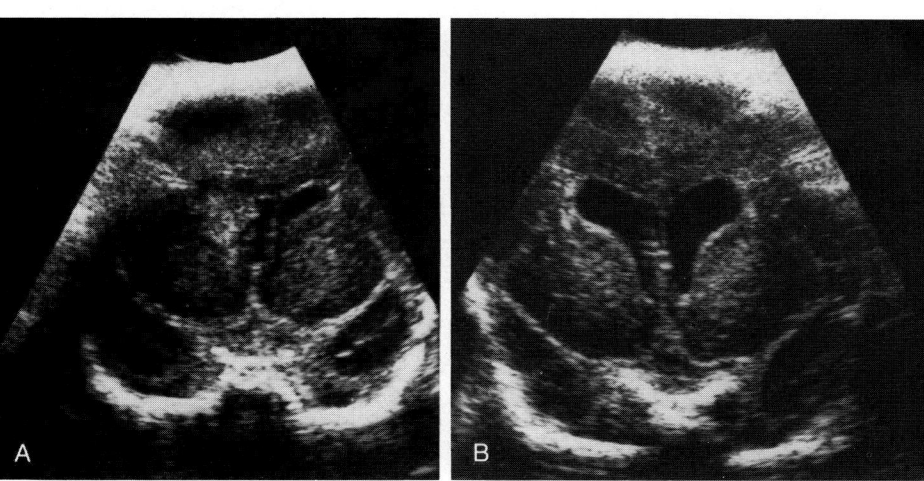

Figure 13–10. Cranial sonograms in a 1200-gm, premature infant. Early right ventricular hemorrhage (A); later scan shows ventriculomegaly (B).

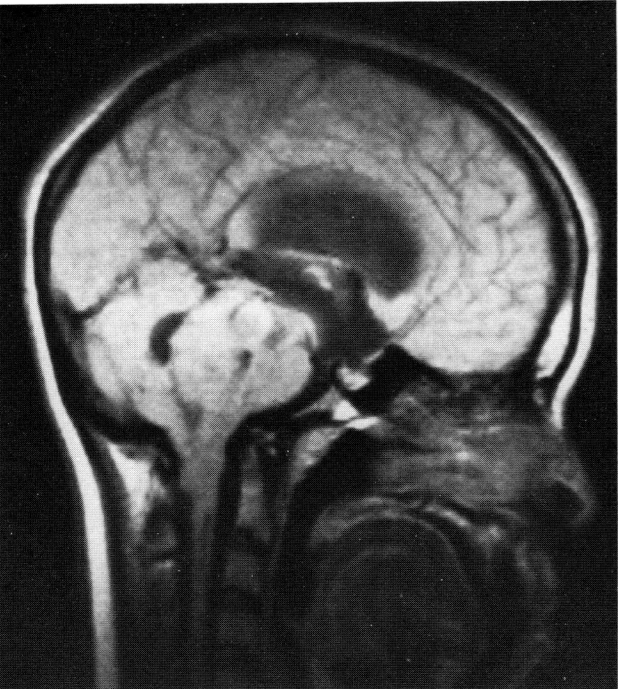

Figure 13–11. Sagittal magnetic resonance section in hydrocephalic adolescent with ependymoma.

Cerebral arteriography has no place in screening for hydrocephalus but remains essential for examining vascular malformations (Fig. 13–12) and in preoperative planning for some tumors. Arteriography has been used to differentiate hydranencephaly, which shows absence rather than displacement of major cerebral vessels.[24]

Tests for Prognostic Data

After the disclosure of hydrocephalus, the neurosurgeon may need information regarding therapeutic indications, timing, and approach. Anatomic data from imaging usually satisfactorily suggests the cause and probable site of obstruction when used in conjunction with a history and an examination. Rational decisions about therapy are often forthcoming from single scans. However, especially in postinfectious, posthemorrhagic, chronic, or unexpected cases of hydrocephalus, additional information is important to proper therapy selection and timing. Most of the appropriate procedures are invasive.

CSF Analysis. Knowledge of ventricular fluid cell count and bacteriologic culture results is essential when there is the slightest suspicion of ongoing infection. The character of the CSF with respect to blood and protein levels influences treatment decisions in posthemorrhagic cases. CSF glucose levels are often low in such cases, indicating ongoing aseptic ventriculitis when cultures are negative.

Certain biochemical tests of CSF have also been suggested for determining progressive hydrocehalus. Theoretically, they reflect cerebral injury. These tests include CSF fat stains;[11] lipid,[73] biogenic amine,[40] and myelin basic protein[91] levels; lactate-pyruvate ratios;[77] and cyclic nucleotide determinations.[81] They should be considered investigational procedures.

Radionuclide Studies. Before CT, radionuclide cisternography and ventriculography were fashionable for screening and for developing prognostic information in pediatric hydrocephalus.[66] Some clinicians still utilize cisternography in attempts to judge the progressive nature of suspected cases of chronic, "normal pressure" hydrocephalus. In the author's experience, adequate therapeutic judgments derive from serial neurologic and neuropsychologic examinations and from CT.

Intracranial Pressure Monitoring. Similar questions regarding the severity or progressiveness of hydrocephalus have been approached with ventriculostomy or intrathecal cannulation for continuous monitoring. Most of the data have research connotations, but there are important implications concerning pathophysiology. Briefly, the detection of prolonged pressure waves,[22] frequent short-term waves,[92] augmented pulsatile indices,[29] and abnor-

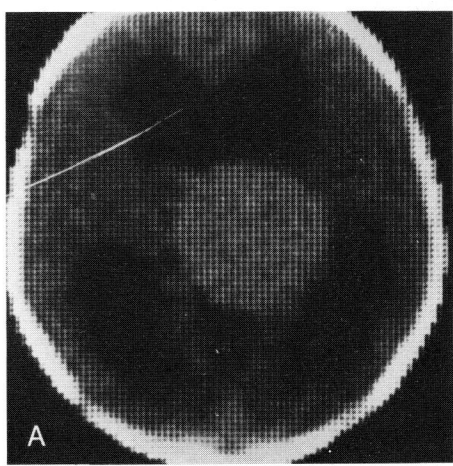
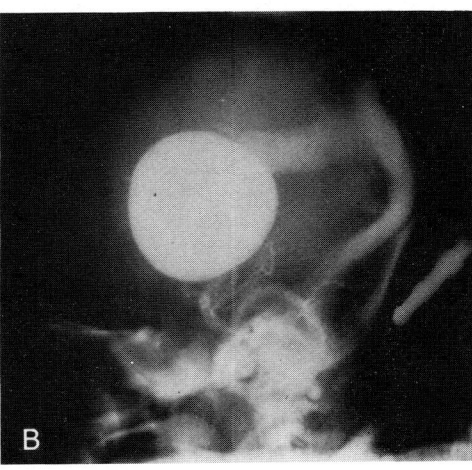

Figure 13–12. Hydrocephalic four-month-old infant with arteriovenous anomaly of vein of Galen. A, CT scan; B, angiogram.

mal volume-pressure responses with small bolus injections[86] implies low compliance and sparse absorptive reserve. Prognostically, it may be inferred that the patient has progressive hydrocephalus, which requires intervention. Shapiro and colleagues[86] recently documented that infants with hydrocephalus actually have increased volume buffering capacity. However, most candidates for these tests are older children with chronic communicating hydrocephalus or, conversely, a compensated condition.

In some instances, neonates and infants are reliably monitored with external transducers over the fontanelle.[95] There are many limitations to this practice, not the least being rapid progression of ventriculomegaly[50] with low intracranial pressure and unimpressive waves.[62]

Perfusion and Infusion Studies. Much physiologic enlightenment has resulted from elegant clinical research using the Pappenheimer perfusion technique[74] in humans. Clinical applications with these and the less sophisticated CSF infusion methods[48, 87] have no primary diagnostic importance. Useful CSF production and absorption data[15] emerged in the 1970's, but conflicting results have prohibited standardization and clinical acceptance. Alternative, qualitative findings from imaging techniques have supplanted these earlier quantitative tests for answering clinical questions about progression.

Psychologic and Neuropsychologic Tests. Serial developmental evaluations contribute to diagnosis in suspected or confirmed hydrocephalus of infancy. They can be recommended for prognostic purposes in untreated or mildly progressive cases in which intervention has been deferred. In concert with intracranial imaging from CT or sonography, psychologic testing facilitates prognostication to some degree. Similarly, serial psychologic or neuropsychologic monitoring may discern trends that are useful in categorizing older children and adolescents with either chronic progressive or compensated hydrocephalus.

Cerebral Blood Flow. Several investigators have provided interesting data with inhalation or intravascular radionuclide regional blood flow methods.[35] Most of the studies have been performed in adults with chronic hydrocephalus.[83] The results argue for a global ischemic state that improves after therapy. These tests are research tools.

Process of Evaluation

Newborns and Infants

The infant with macrocrania who exhibits normal development, has an estimated normal intracranial pressure, and has forebears with large heads should be followed serially by a neurosurgeon or a competent pediatrician. If neurologic, intracranial pressure, or development signs emerge, a CT scan (or NMR image) suffices to exclude hydrocephalus. Infants with so-called "benign familial macrocrania"[1] frequently exhibit increased extraventricular CSF spaces, which may be difficult to differentiate from small subdural hygromas (Fig. 13–13). In the author's experience, this is a self-limited condition. If mild ventriculomegaly is detected, serial sonography may be used while the fontanelle is open. If the ventricles are markedly enlarged, treatment is appropriately recommended after proximate cause is determined.

Newborns with large heads and CT-diagnosed hydrocephalus should have ventricular fluid sampled prior to therapy. Many have surprisingly xanthochromic or bloody fluid. Lingering ventriculitis must be excluded after recent leptomeningeal infection. CSF cell count, protein level measurement, and culture are recommended. Torch (*T*oxoplasma, *r*ubella, *c*ytomegalovirus, and *h*erpes simple virus) titers of ventricular fluid and serum may be performed but are seldom helpful. When periventricular calcifications are apparent, *Toxoplasma* or cytomegalovirus (CMV) is often encountered. Examination for chorioretinitis is warranted.

Premature Babies. In the premature infant with documented ventriculomegaly, exclusion of the possibility of active ventriculitis is required, and some consideration of the hemorrhagic character of the fluid is necessary. Scans should be surveyed for persistent intraventricular blood and the possibility

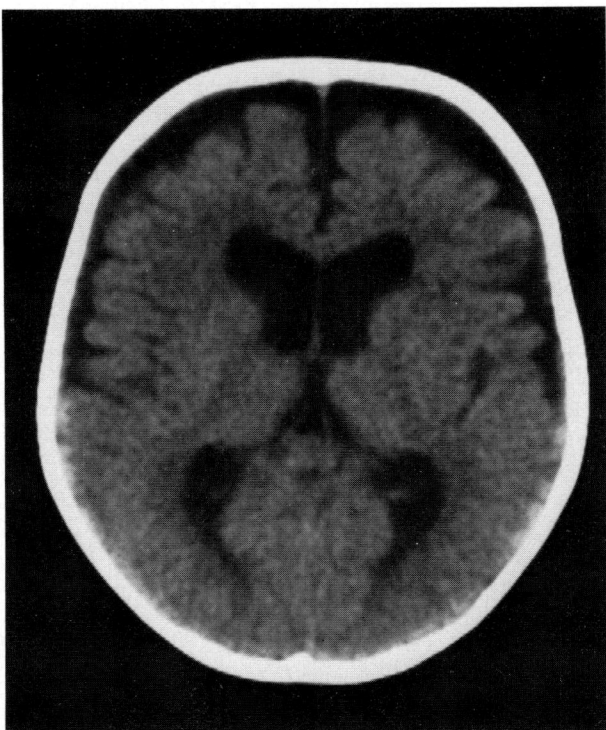

Figure 13–13. CT section of an infant with mild ventriculomegaly and frontal extracerebral fluid collections.

of septations.[24, 85] Serial sonography will settle questions of progression, when therapy is delayed.

Signs of Increased Pressure. An infant or child presenting with signs and symptoms of increased intracranial pressure and a large head requires a CT or an NMRI scan. The proper scan survey for signs of a mass lesion should include intravenous injection of contrast material. Disclosure of a mass dictates arteriography in certain cases, especially if a galenic system anomaly appears probable. A Dandy-Walker cyst with panventriculomegaly (Fig. 13-14) should be studied for aqueductal patency if only a single cavity shunt is contemplated.[76]

Dysraphic Conditions. Regardless of head size, a newborn with myelomeningocele or encephalocele should have an intracranial imaging procedure. Serial studies may be required, since ventriculomegaly can be subtly progressive. If hydrocehalus is diagnosed after repair of the primary anomaly or beyond the first few hours of life, preoperative CSF sampling is advisable to exclude ventriculitis.

Older Children

Older children presenting with hydrocephalus require careful evaluation for neoplasm. If tumor is excluded, and signs of increased intracranial pressure cannot be found, baseline and serial neuropsychologic testing, office follow-up, and periodic CT usually help in prognostication. When subtle intellectual deterioration, decline in school performance, and gait disturbances appear, it is often in the context of a past history of slow development and mental retardation. Here, the issue of more invasive testing often arises. Intracranial pressure monitoring or radionuclide flow studies may occasionally be useful. Intracranial cysts may be studied with radionuclide or positive-contrast cisternography, but these tests have declined in importance with recent changes in therapeutic approach.[41]

Fetal Macrocrania, Hydrocephalus, and Dysraphism

After disclosure of these gestational conditions with prenatal ultrasonography, sequential sonographic studies are recommended. Careful serial examinations should aim to disclose progression or regression of the hydrocephalus and associated central nervous system or systemic anomalies.[103]

NATURAL HISTORY

Prior to the acceptance of modern neurosurgical treatment of juvenile hydrocephalus, a number of studies traced the course of the untreated disorder. The absence of recent reports on this subject offers some testimony to therapeutic success.

These accounts described patients whose conditions had disparate etiologies. Primary etiology and associated neuropathologic conditions should influence outcome. This consideration notwithstanding, a fairly uniform pattern of mortality and morbidity emerged in reported series from several Western countries.[106]

Laurence and Coates[51] provided the most exhaustive analysis, including 182 referral patients who were "selected," at least to a degree that excluded the mildest and the most severe cases. Survival projections for this group pointed to a 20 percent chance of an infant patient reaching adulthood. Two thirds of the deaths had occurred before the age of 18 months. The deaths were attributed primarily to cardiorespiratory failure from hydrocephalus. Some patients died of pulmonary complica-

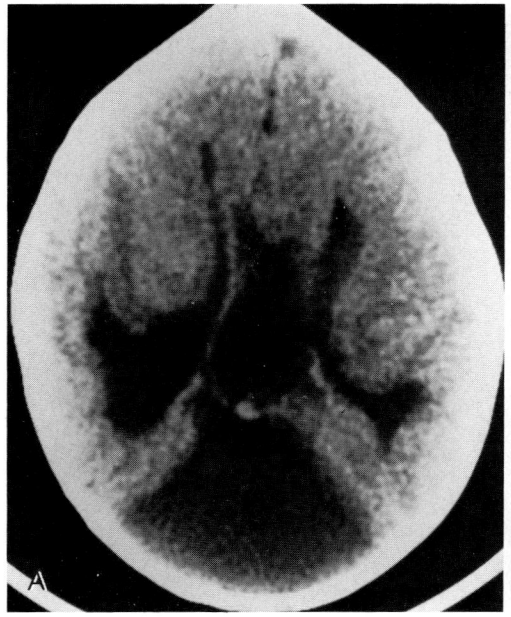 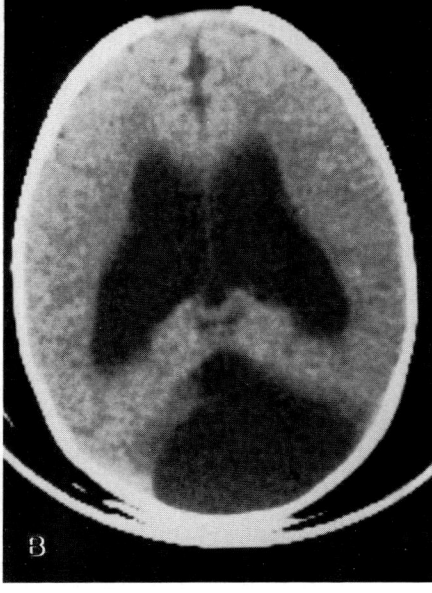

Figure 13-14. Dandy-Walker syndrome with agenesis of corpus callosum and small lateral ventricles (A). B, A second patient with panventriculomegaly.

tions or, in the few reported spina bifida patients, meningitis. Other patients died after lumbar punctures or air studies.

Survivors in the series by Laurence and Coates and in a smaller kindred from Sweden[36] were thought to have arrested hydrocephalus according to criteria of that era.[84] Laurence and Coates opined that the condition stabilized between nine months and two years of age. Exacerbations were recognized.

A pattern of handicap including physical, neurologic, visual, and intellectual impairment prevailed in the majority of survivors of untreated hydrocephalus. None of these factors was related to head size or thickness of the remaining cortical mantle. Dysplastic body builds (girdle obesity) and precocious puberty were often recognized. A total of 60 to 70 percent of patients had slight to extreme degrees (19 percent) of motor deficit. Ataxia was a major problem. Visual disorders typical of this population were divergent squints and, to a much lesser extent, blindness with optic atrophy.

Intellectual impairment characterized roughly 62 percent of surviving children. Surprising accounts of normal intellect described some children with remarkably large heads and thin pallium. However, 25 percent were completely ineducable. Spatial perception and reasoning ability were especially deficient. About 25 percent demonstrated the peculiar, vacant loquaciousness that has been labeled the "chatterbox" or "cocktail party" syndrome. Finally, spiraling downhill courses or incidents of sudden death were recognized among children thought to have compensated hydrocephalus.

References

1. Alvarez LA, Maytal J, Shinnar S: Idiopathic hydrocephalus: Natural history and relationship to benign familial macrocephaly. Pediatrics 77:901, 1986.
2. Alvord EC: The pathology of hydrocephalus. In: Fields WS, Desmond MM (eds): Disorders of the Developing Nervous System. Springfield, IL, Charles C Thomas, 1961, pp 343–419.
3. Amacher AL, Page LK: Hydrocephalus due to membranous obstruction of the fourth ventricle. J Neurosurg 35:672, 1971.
4. Bannister CM: Fetal neurosurgery—a new challenge on the horizon. Dev Med Child Neurol 26:827, 1984.
5. Bering EA, Jr.: Circulation of the cerebrospinal fluid. Demonstration of the choroid plexuses as the generator of the force for flow of fluid and ventricular enlargement. J Neurosurg 19:405, 1962.
6. Bickers DS, Adams RD: Hereditary stenosis of the aqueduct of Sylvius as a cause of congenital hydrocephalus. Brain 72:246, 1949.
7. Bray PF: Mumps—a cause of hydrocephalus? Pediatrics 49:446, 1972.
8. Centeno RS, Winter J, Bentson JR, et al: CT evaluation of Haemophilus influenzae meningitis with clinical and pathological correlation. Comput Radiol 7:243, 1983.
9. Centers for Disease Control, Annual Summary 1980: Reported morbidity and mortality in the United States. Morbidity Mortality Weekly Rep 29:106, 1981.
10. Centers for Disease Control, Annual Summary 1983: Reported morbidity and mortality in the United States. Morbidity Mortality Weekly Rep 32:85, 1984.
11. Chester DC, Emery JL, Penny SR: Fat-laden macrophages in cerebrospinal fluid as an indication of brain damage in children. J Clin Pathol 24:753, 1971.
12. Chung CS, Myrianthopoulos NC: Factors affecting risks of congenital malformations. I. Epidemiological analysis. In: Bergsma D (ed): Birth Defects Original Article Series, Vol. XI, No. 10, Miami, Symposia Specialists. The National Foundation–March of Dimes, 1975, p 11.
13. Clewell WH, Johnson ML, Meier PR, et al: A surgical approach to the treatment of fetal hydrocephalus. N Engl J Med 306:1320, 1982.
14. Cutler RWP, Murray JE, Moody RA: Overproduction of cerebrospinal fluid in communicating hydrocephalus. Neurology (Minn) 23:1, 1973.
15. Cutler RWP, Page L, Galicich J: Formation and absorption of cerebrospinal fluid in man. Brain 91:707, 1968.
16. Dandy WE: Ventriculostomy following the injection of air into the cerebral ventricles. Ann Surg 68:5, 1918.
17. Dandy WE, Blackfan KD: Internal hydrocephalus. An experimental clinical and pathological study. Am J Dis Child 8:406, 1914.
18. Davis LE: Communicating hydrocephalus in newborn hamsters and cats following vaccinia virus infection. J Neurosurg 54:767, 1981.
19. Davson H: Physiology of the Cerebrospinal Fluid. London, Churchill, 1967.
20. DeLevie M, Nogrady M: Rapid brain growth upon restoration of adequate nutrition causing false radiologic evidence of increased intracranial pressure. J Pediatr 76:523, 1970.
21. DeMyer W: Megalencephaly in children. Neurology (Minn) 22:634, 1972.
22. DiRocco C, McLone DG, Shimoji T, et al: Continuous intraventricular cerebrospinal fluid pressure recording in hydrocephalic children during wakefulness and sleep. J Neurosurg 42:683, 1975.
23. Dodge PR, Swartz MN: Bacterial meningitis—a review of selected aspects II. Special neurological problems, postmeningitic complications and clinicopathological correlations. N Engl J Med 272:954, 1965.
24. Dublin AB, French BN: Diagnostic image evaluation of hydranencephaly and pictorially similar entities with emphasis on computed tomography. Radiology 137:81, 1980.
25. Eisenberg HM, McComb JG, Lorenzo AV: Cerebrospinal fluid overproduction and hydrocephalus associated with choroid plexus papilloma. J Neurosurg 40:381, 1974.
26. Ellington E, Margolis G: Block of arachnoid villus by subarachnoid hemorrhage. J Neurosurg 30:651, 1969.
27. Emery JL: Deformity of the aqueduct of Sylvius in children with hydrocephalus and myelomeningocele. Dev Med Child Neurol 16:40, 1974.
28. Fishman RA, Greer M: Experimental obstructive hydrocephalus. Changes in the cerebrum. Arch Neurol 8:156, 1963.
29. Foltz EL, Aine C: Diagnosis of hydrocephalus by CSF pulse-wave analysis: A clinical study. Surg Neurol 15:283, 1981.
30. Friedman WA, Mickle JP: Hydrocephalus in achondroplasia: A possible mechanism. Neurosurgery 7:150, 1980.
31. Gilles FH, Davidson RI: Communicating hydrocephalus associated with deficient dysplastic parasagittal arachnoid granulations. J Neurosurg 35:421, 1971.
32. Gilles FH, Shillito J: Infantile hydrocephalus: Retrocerebellar subdural hematoma. J Pediatr 76:529, 1970.
33. Gonzalez-Darder J, Barbera J, Cerda-Nicolas M, et al: Sequential morphological changes in kaolin-induced hydrocephalus. J Neurosurg 61:918, 1984.
34. Gordon N: Normal pressure hydrocephalus and arrested hydrocephalus. Dev Med Child Neurol 19:540, 1977.
35. Greitz T: Effect of brain distention on cerebral circulation. Lancet 1:863, 1969.
36. Hagberg B, Sjorgen I: The chronic brain syndrome of infantile hydrocephalus. A follow-up study of 63 spontaneously arrested cases. Am J Dis Child 112:189, 1966.

37. Hakim S, Adams RD: The special clinical problem of symptomatic hydrocephalus with normal cerebrospinal fluid pressure. Observations on cerebrospinal fluid hydrodynamics. J Neurol Sci 2:307, 1965.
38. Hammock MK, Milhorat TH, Baron IS: Normal pressure hydrocephalus in patients with myelomeningocele. Dev Med Child Neurol 18:55, 1976.
39. Hanigan WC, Gibson J, Kleopoulos NJ, et al: Medical imaging of fetal ventriculomegaly. J Neurosurg 64:575, 1986.
40. Hansson O: Hydrocephalus and 5-hydroxy indoleacetic acid in the CSF. Dev Med Child Neurol 12:101, 1970.
41. Harsh GR, IV, Edwards MSB, Wilson CB: Intracranial arachnoid cysts in children. J Neurosurg 64:835, 1986.
42. Hill A, Volpe JJ: Normal pressure hydrocephalus in the newborn. Pediatrics 68:623, 1981.
43. Hill A, Shackelford GD, Volpe JJ: A potential mechanism of pathogenesis for early posthemorrhagic hydrocephalus in the premature newborn. Pediatrics 73:19, 1984.
44. Holmes LB, Nash A, Zu Rhein GM, et al: X-linked aqueductal stenosis: Clinical and neuropathological findings in two families. Pediatrics 51:697, 1973.
45. Kalsbeck JE, DeSousa AL, Kleiman MB, et al: Compartmentalization of the cerebral ventricles as a sequel of neonatal meningitis. J Neurosurg 52:547, 1980.
46. Kalter H: Teratology of the Central Nervous System. Chicago, University of Chicago, 1968.
47. Kapila A, Naidich TP: Spontaneous lateral ventriculocisternostomy documented by metrizamide CT ventriculography. Case report. J Neurosurg 54:101, 1981.
48. Katzman R, Hussey F: A simple constant infusion manometric test for measurement of cerebrospinal fluid absorption. I. Rationale and method. Neurology (Minn) 20:534, 1970.
49. Key EAH, Retzius G: Studien in der Anatomie des Nervensystems und des Bindegewebes. Stockholm, Samson and Wallin, 1875.
50. Korobkin R: The relationship between head circumference and the development of communicating hydrocephalus in infants following intraventricular hemorrhage. Pediatrics 56:74, 1975.
51. Laurence KM, Coates S: The natural history of hydrocephalus. Detailed analysis of 182 unoperated cases. Arch Dis Child 37:345, 1962.
52. Leblanc R, Knowles KF, Melanson D, et al: Neurocysticercosis: Surgical and medical management with praziquantel. Neurosurgery 18:419, 1986.
53. Linder M, Nichols J, Sklar FH: Effect of meningomyelocele closure on the intracranial pulse pressure. Child's Brain 11:176, 1984.
54. Lorber J: Systematic ventriculographic studies in infants born with meningomyelocele and encephalocele. The incidence and development of hydrocephalus. Arch Dis Child 36:381, 1961.
55. Lorber J, Bassi U: The etiology of neonatal hydrocephalus (excluding cases with spina bifida). Dev Med Child Neurol 7:289, 1965.
56. Lorber J, Bhat US: Posthemorrhagic hydrocephalus. Diagnosis, differential diagnosis, treatment and long-term results. Arch Dis Child 49:751, 1974.
57. Lorber J, Ward AM: Spina bifida—a vanishing nightmare? Arch Dis Child 60:1086, 1985.
58. Magendie F: Memoire sur le liquide qui se trouve le crane et le pine de l'homme et des animaux. J Physiol Exp Pathol 5:27, 1825.
59. Martinovic J, Sibalic D, Djordjevic M: Frequency of toxoplasmosis in the appearance of congenital hydrocephalus. J Neurosurg 56:830, 1982.
60. Matson DD: Neurosurgery of Infancy and Childhood. Springfield, IL, Charles C Thomas, 1969, p 199.
61. McCullough DC: Large and growing heads. Pediatr Portfolio 3:1, 1974.
62. McCullough DC: A critical evaluation of continuous intracranial pressure monitoring in pediatric hydrocephalus. Child's Brain 6:225, 1980.
63. McCullough DC: A history of the treatment of hydrocephalus. Fetal Ther 1:38, 1986.
64. McCullough DC: Unpublished data.
65. McCullough DC, Harbert JC, Manz HJ: Large arachnoid cysts at the cranial base. Neurosurgery 6:76, 1980.
66. McCullough DC, Harbert JC, Miale A, et al: Radioisotope cisternography in the evaluation of hydrocephalus of infancy and childhood. Radiology 102:645, 1972.
67. Milhorat TH: Hydrocephalus and the Cerebrospinal Fluid. Baltimore, Williams & Wilkins, 1972.
68. Milhorat TH: Hydrocephalus: Historical notes, etiology and clinical diagnosis. In: McLaurin RL (ed): Pediatric Neurosurgery. New York, Grune and Stratton, 1984, pp 197–210.
69. Milhorat TH, Hammock MK, Davis DA, et al: Choroid plexus papilloma. I. Proof of cerebrospinal fluid overproduction. Child's Brain 2:273, 1977.
70. Morgagni CB: The Seats and Causes of Disease Investigated by Anatomy. London, Millar and Cadell, 1761.
71. Naidich TP, Epstein F, Lin JP, et al: Evaluation of pediatric hydrocephalus by computed tomography. Radiology 119:337, 1976.
72. Norrell H, Wilson C, Howieson J, et al: Venous factors in infantile hydrocephalus. J Neurosurg 31:561, 1969.
73. Onodera Y, Ito H: Fatty acid in cerebrospinal fluid of congenital hydrocephalus. Child's Brain 3:101, 1977.
74. Pappenheimer JR, Heisey SR, Jordan EF: Perfusion of the ventricular system in anesthetized goats. Am J Physiol 203:763, 1962.
75. Raimondi AJ, Samuelson G, Yarzagaray L, et al: Atresia of the foramina of Luschka and Magendie: The Dandy Walker cyst. J Neurosurg 31:202, 1969.
76. Raimondi AJ, Sato K, Shimoji T: The Dandy-Walker Syndrome. Basel, S Karger, 1984.
77. Raisis JE, Kindt GW, McGillicuddy JE, et al: Cerebrospinal fluid lactate and lactate/pyruvate ratios in hydrocephalus. J Neurosurg 44:337, 1976.
78. Rengachary SS, Watanabe I, Brackett CE: Pathogenesis of arachnoid cysts. Surg Neurol 9:139, 1978.
79. Rowlatt U: The microscopic effects of ventricular dilation without increase in head size. J Neurosurg 48:957, 1978.
80. Rubin RC, Hochwald G, Liwnicz B, et al: The effect of severe hydrocephalus on the size and number of brain cells. Dev Med Child Neurol 14:117, 1972.
81. Rudman D, O'Brien MS, McKinney AS, et al: Observations on cyclic nucleotide concentrations in human cerebrospinal fluid. J Clin Endocrinol Metab 42:1088, 1976.
82. Russell DS: Observations on the Pathology of Hydrocephalus. Medical Research Council Special Report Series, No. 265, London, Her Majesty's Stationery Office, 1949.
83. Salmon JH, Timperman AL: Cerebral blood flow in posttraumatic encephalopathy. The effect of ventriculoatrial shunt. Neurology (Minn) 21:34, 1971.
84. Schick RW, Matson DD: What is arrested hydrocephalus? J Pediatr 58:791, 1961.
85. Scotti G, Musgrave MA, Fitz CR, et al: The isolated fourth ventricle in children: CT and clinical review of 16 cases. AJNR 1:419, 1980.
86. Shapiro K, Fried A, Marmarou A: Biomechanical and hydrodynamic characterization of the hydrocephalic infant. J Neurosurg 63:69, 1985.
87. Sklar FH, Beyer CW, Ramanthan M, et al: Servo-controlled lumbar infusions: A clinical tool for the determination of CSF dynamics as a function of pressure. Neurosurgery 3:170, 1978.
88. Smith DW: Recognizable Patterns of Human Malformation, 3rd ed. (Vol. 7 in the series Major Problems in Clinical Pediatrics). Philadelphia, W. B. Saunders Co., 1982, p 617.
89. Starkman SP, Brown TC, Linnell EA: Cerebral arachnoid cysts. J Neuropathol Exp Neurol 17:484, 1958.
90. Sutton LN, Bruce DA, Schut L: Hydranencephaly versus

maximal hydrocephalus: An important clinical distinction. Neurosurgery 6:35, 1980.
91. Sutton LN, Wood JH, Brooks BR, et al: Cerebrospinal fluid myelin basic protein in hydrocephalus. J Neurosurg 59:467, 1983.
92. Symon L, Dorsch NWC: Use of long-term intracranial pressure measurement to assess hydrocephalic patients prior to shunt surgery. J Neurosurg 42:259, 1975.
93. Symonds C: Otitic hydrocephalus. Neurology (Minn) 6:681, 1956.
94. Vesalius A: Opera Omnia Anatomica et Chirgica Cura Hermanni Boehaave et Bernhardi Siegfried Albini, Vol. 1. Leyden, Apud Joannem du Vivie, Ludguni Batavorum, 1725.
95. Vidyasagar D, Raju TNK, Chiang J: Clinical significance of monitoring anterior fontanelle pressure in sick neonates and infants. Pediatrics 62:996, 1978.
96. Volpe JJ, Pasternak JF, Allan WC: Ventricular dilation preceding rapid head growth following neonatal intracranial hemorrhage. Am J Dis Child 131:1212, 1977.
97. Weed LH: Certain anatomical and physiological aspects of the meninges and cerebrospinal fluid. Brain 58:383, 1935.
98. Welch K: The emergence of hydrocephalus after ventricular hemorrhage and the estimation of intracranial pressure in infants. Am J Dis Child 131:1203, 1977.
99. Welch K, Strand R: The contribution of trauma at birth to the problem of hydrocephalus. Z Kinderchir 37:124, 1982.
100. Weller RO, Shulman K: Infantile hydrocephalus: Clinical, histological, and ultrastructural study of brain damage. J Neurosurg 36:255, 1972.
101. Weller RO, Wisniewski H: Histological and ultrastructural changes with experimental hydrocephalus in adult rabbits. Brain 92:819, 1969.
102. Williams B: Is aqueduct stenosis a result of hydrocephalus? Brain 96:399, 1973.
103. Williamson RA, Schauberger CW, Varner MW, et al: Heterogenicity of prenatal onset hydrocephalus: Management and counseling implications. Am J Med Genet 17:497, 1984.
104. Wozniak M, McLone DG, Raimondi AJ: Micro- and macrovascular changes as the direct cause of parenchymal destruction in congenital murine hydrocephalus. J Neurosurg 43:535, 1973.
105. Yakovlev PI: Paraplegias of hydrocephalics. A clinical note and interpretation. Am J Ment Defic 51:561, 1947.
106. Yashon D, Jane JA, Sugar O: The course of severe untreated infantile hydrocephalus. Prognostic significance of the cerebral mantle. J Neurosurg 23:509, 1965.

14
TREATMENT OF HYDROCEPHALUS

Harold L. Rekate, M.D.

Hydrocephalus is not an "all or none" phenomenon. Although overproduction of cerebrospinal fluid (CSF) may account for hydrocephalus in a small number of choroid plexus papillomas, hydrocephalus in the overwhelming majority of cases is due to an obstruction of CSF flow between its point of production within the ventricular system and its normal point of absorption in the superior sagittal sinus. This obstruction of CSF outflow may be *complete,* as that in aqueductal stenosis, or quite *partial,* as that following subarachnoid hemorrhage. When the obstruction is incomplete, the elevation in intracranial pressure (ICP) and the degree of ventriculomegaly may be very mild before a new steady state is established. Nonetheless, the latter condition is hydrocephalus, but often no therapy is indicated. An important aspect of hydrocephalus management is to determine initially whether the patient indeed requires treatment.

PATIENT SELECTION

If there were no risks accompanying the performance of a shunting procedure, it would be recommended for all patients with the slightest degree of moderate ventriculomegaly. However, shunting is not innocuous, and it is not clear whether ventriculomegaly results in a decrease in cognitive ability. Therefore, each child must be assessed individually, balancing the risks of shunting versus the risks of untreated hydrocephalus. A theoretical representation of the risks of shunting and the risks of hydrocephalus not treated with a shunt as a function of the depth of the cerebral mantle (thickness of the brain) can be seen in Figure 14–1.[76]

The risks involved in performing a shunt procedure are low and are independent of ventricular size, except when the ventricles are extremely small. Improved techniques and instruments and supplies have greatly reduced the risks accompanying a shunt, but the possibility of shunt infection or malfunction is always present. Shunt infection is the most serious threat to life and intellectual function. It has been shown that when hydrocephalus is associated with the Arnold-Chiari malformation,

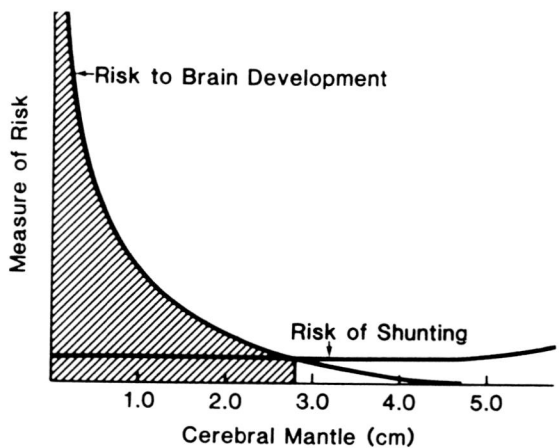

Figure 14–1. Theoretical representation of risk-benefit ratio of shunting versus ventriculomegaly. (With permission from Rekate HL: "To Shunt or Not To Shunt." Clin Neurosurg 32:593, 1985.)

shunt infection in the first six months of life can lead to intellectual downgrading.[42, 49, 50]

When considering the risks of hydrocephalus to the developing brain, there is much conflicting information. Certain patients tolerate ventriculomegaly better than others. A portion of this information is anecdotal, such as the intriguing discussion in *Science*, "Is the brain really necessary?" in which the computerized tomographic (CT) scan of a graduate student in mathematics is presented showing a cerebral mantle of less than 1 cm.[38] Other patients attain a low level of intellectual functioning despite early aggressive and effective control of their hydrocephalus.

In trying to arrive at a rationale for patient selection, one of the most difficult tasks is to discern differences between the effects caused by the hydrocephalus itself, and the underlying damage to neural function resulting from the cause of the hydrocephalus. The best information regarding the degree of hydrocephalus needed to cause intellectual downgrading was derived from the work of Young and colleagues.[93] Previous attempts to correlate outcome with severity of hydrocephalus with or without treatment had been unsuccessful.[2, 19, 37] Young and associates were able to correlate outcome with depth of the cerebral mantle following treatment. In their study, patients who had no associated central nervous system anomalies or perinatal asphyxia, but whose cerebral mantle remained less than 2.0 cm at the foramen of Monro, reached an intelligence quotient (IQ) as measured on the Wechsler intelligence Scale for Children (WISC) or the Stanford-Binet test of no better than 80. The IQ distribution became normal when the 2.8 cm level was reached. There did not seem to be an advantage in having a normal (i.e., 5 cm) cerebral mantle. This study also showed the time dependency of the treatment of hydrocephalus. After five months, the child with hydrocephalus was less likely to attain the stated goal of 3.5 cm than was the child treated earlier. The decision "to shunt or not to shunt" in infantile hydrocephalus should be made by five months of age.

From the above discussion and Figure 14–1, it is possible to make rational decisions regarding who is and who is not likely to benefit from a shunt. The neurosurgeon's goal for the infant with hydrocephalus should be to attain a 3.5 cm cerebral mantle by five months of age. The 3.5 cm mantle is chosen because the risk of shunting is not increased between 2.8 cm and 3.5 cm, and this higher number provides some added safety to the child. It does not seem to matter how this 3.5 cm mantle is obtained (shunting, nonsurgical measures, or close observation).

The one modifying factor is the neurologic and developmental status of the child. Although one cannot correlate results from the Denver Developmental screening test (DDST) easily with later IQ, it is clear that poor performance on this test is likely to be associated with delayed intellectual development. Accurate measurement by formal psychologic testing cannot be performed prior to age three.[21] Because there is a minimum of data on very young children, it is difficult to determine whether the prognosis for a child (who will probably be delayed intellectually) can be improved by shunting. It has been the author's policy to shunt developmentally delayed children with ventriculomegaly of nearly any degree to assure both himself and the family that all that could be done has been done.

Figure 14–2 represents the author's approach to the evaluation of the child who presents in infancy with enlarged ventricles and evidence of hydrocephalus. According to this format, only one child who had obtained a cerebral mantle of 3.5 cm by five months subsequently needed shunting. All children with or without shunting should be followed for the first two years with CT scans at 12 and 24 months.

NONSURGICAL TREATMENT

Once an objective measurement of cerebral mantle is defined as a treatment goal, alternative methods of obtaining those goals can be assessed. The wrapping of the infant's distensible head with a compressive dressing was evaluated by Epstein and colleagues,[15] and in certain patients, it was effective in reversing progressive hydrocephalus. The theory underlying head wrapping was that in cases of moderate infantile hydrocephalus, the infant cranium could enlarge at relatively low pressures. Head wrapping led to a closed intracranial cavity, as if the skull were fully formed and therefore not distensible. Higher pressures could then be generated, with a concomitant increase in CSF absorption and stabilization of ventricular size.[15]

Other mechanical measures have been advocated to prevent the need for shunting or to prevent shunt dependency. The use of an on-off valve with the shunt in infants has been advocated to prevent shunt dependency. In the child with hydrocephalus, a shunt is placed with an on-off valve, and the shunt is opened to flow for only a short period of time each day. This technique may allow stabilization of head circumference and ventricular size and will avoid shunt dependency in certain cases.[16]

MANAGEMENT OF HYDROCEPHALUS SECONDARY TO NEONATAL INTRAVENTRICULAR HEMORRHAGE

In the special case of premature infants with hydrocephalus secondary to neonatal intraventricular hemorrhage, a number of nonsurgical meas-

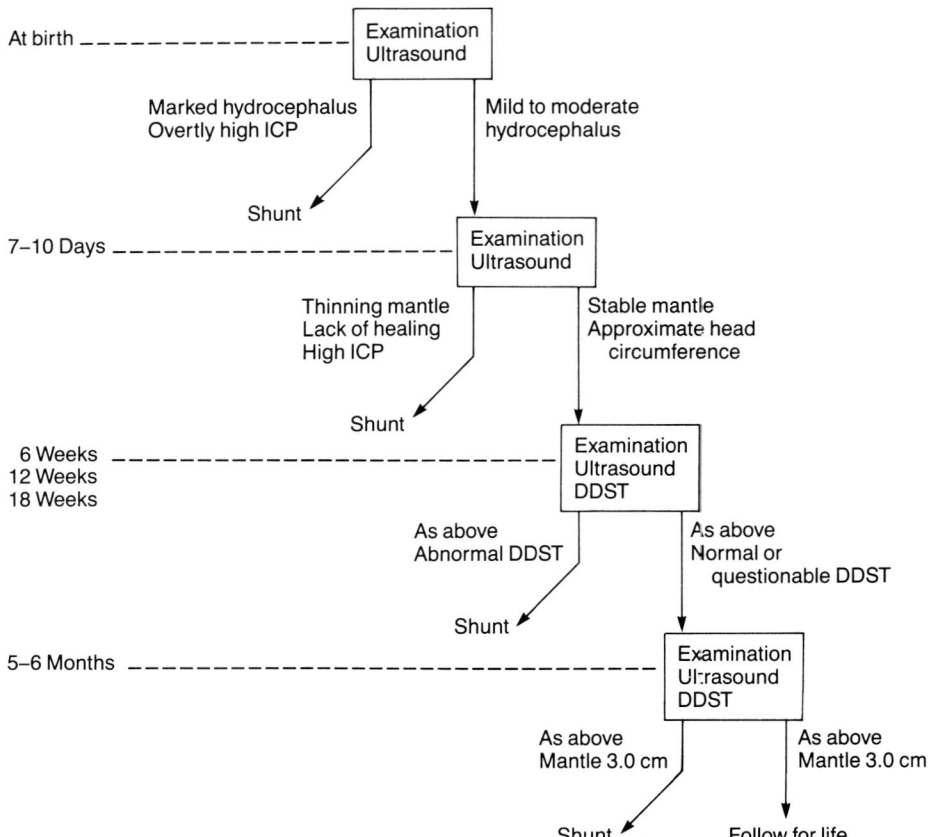

Figure 14–2. Algorithm for making treatment decisions in neonatal hydrocephalus. (Modified from Rekate HL: To Shunt or Not to Shunt." Clin Neurosurg 32:605, 1985. Reprinted with permission.)

ures have been employed that stabilize or improve ventricular size in critically low birthweight children. Various children subsequently need shunts, but some never require permanent shunts. For example, the use of intermittent lumbar punctures decreases ICP and helps clear the CSF of toxic chemicals with the dissolution of the intraventricular hemorrhage.[3, 23] This procedure has been used in many premature neonates and has proved to be effective in preventing the need for shunting in some children. There are reports of resolution of hydrocephalus with this form of treatment alone, and there is one report of the resolution of progressive hydrocephalus after only one spinal tap.[3] However, this form of treatment does present some technical difficulties. To obtain adequate volumes of CSF to affect the intraventricular pressure and volume is often technically difficult. It requires prolonged periods of time with the spinal needle in place. These taps are usually done with the patient in an upright position, and for the time of the tap, the infants are not in a closed Isolette. This is difficult in children on a respirator or on high concentrations of oxygen. The amount of handling needed to perform such taps may be dangerous to these infants of fragile health and could conceivably lead to an increased risk of further intraventricular hemorrhage. Although in some children, intermittent spinal taps are effective in controlling hydrocephalus, great care must be used in selecting patients and in performing these procedures.

Intermittent ventricular punctures serve a function similar to that of intermittent lumbar punctures. They can be performed in a shorter period of time and are more effective in removing large volumes of cerebrospinal fluid. The risk with ventricular puncture in untreated hydrocephalus is the production of large porencephalic cysts ("needle porencephaly"). Because of this risk, the procedure has been abandoned as a prolonged temporizing measure.[81] The use of external ventricular drainage has a number of advantages in that large volumes of CSF can be removed under controlled circumstances. Except for the time of placement, the child may remain in the Isolette while CSF is withdrawn, and it can be used as an access to the ventricles for the purposes of removing toxic chemicals from the CSF by irrigation. The usefulness of external ventricular drainage is limited by the risk of infection, by highly viscous CSF, and by the propensity of the ventricular catheter to become encased in the blood clot. When employing this or any technique in which relatively large volumes of CSF are removed from small infants, the neurosurgeon or pediatrician must be constantly aware of the loss of volumes of CSF that are quite large relative to the circulating blood volume and contain ions and blood elements.[56] CSF should be replaced intravenously, cubic centimeter for cubic centimeter, with a fluid containing salt and electrolytes. Assessments of hemoglobin and albumin levels in peripheral blood should be performed routinely several times per week.

Manwaring and colleagues[41] have developed a technique called pulsed lumbar cisternostomy to manage children with hydrocephalus secondary to neonatal intraventricular hemorrhage. Using a Touhy needle, polyethylene (PE) tubing is introduced into the spinal subarachnoid space. Then, the PE tubing is connected to a special pump that applies a "to and fro" pulsation to the fluid in the tubing. Finally, a drainage bag is used, the height of which determines the pressure and flow characteristics of the system. The pulsations in the system effectively prevent blockage of the lumbar catheter and allow prolonged (weeks) treatment of the infants. The technique works well as a temporizing measure and prevents the need for shunting in some infants.

Several authors have advocated the use of a subcutaneous reservoir attached to a ventricular catheter. This technique allows the removal of large volumes of CSF on an intermittent basis. Because it is a closed system, it has a lower infection risk than does external ventricular drainage. As in other techniques mentioned in this section, ventricular size is assessed frequently using ultrasonography, by the amount of CSF withdrawn and the frequency of its withdrawal (modified as needed). Using this technique, Marlin and colleagues reported that less than half the infants required eventual internal shunting. Some patients had subsequent stabilization of ventricular size, and a few died of other causes related to prematurity.[43, 48]

One very exciting area of investigation involves the intraventricular installation of agents that dissolve the intraventricular clot without damaging the brain or causing further bleeding. Pang and colleagues at the University of Pittsburgh have tested the efficiency of injecting urokinase intraventricularly, in a canine model of intraventricular hemorrhage.[62-64] Urokinase was successful in accelerating clot lysis and preventing posthemorrhagic hydrocephalus, without any demonstrable effect on central nervous system tissue. A clinical trial in humans has been proposed by the researchers.[64] Kaufman,[35] in his comment on this work, points out that the newly available tissue plasminogen activator (Genentech, San Francisco, CA) may be superior to urokinase in this regard.

USE OF DRUGS TO CONTROL HYDROCEPHALUS

Many drugs that affect ICP and production of CSF have been used to treat hydrocephalus, with varying degrees of success. These drugs generally are categorized into two groups: (1) osmotic diuretics and (2) drugs that decrease CSF production at the choroid plexus level. Mannitol and urea, when administered intravenously, decrease ICP by removal of brain extracellular fluid, using an osmotic gradient with plasma. Since these drugs must be given intravenously, their use in the chronic management of hydrocephalus was not practical. Isosorbide is a dehydric alcohol derived from sorbitol that has been shown to lower effectively ICP in both laboratory animals and humans. The drug is effective when administered orally in doses of 2 to 3 gm per kg. However, the lowering of ICP is not associated with decreases in ventricular volume, since its mechanical function is to decrease brain extracellular fluid. Lorber[39] reported gratifying results when using isosorbide in a large number of patients with myelomeningoceles, stating that the use of this drug obviated the need for shunting in such children. Other authors have not been able to demonstrate avoidance of the need to perform shunting, resulting from the use of this drug.[27] Isosorbide is not available in the United States for the treatment of hydrocephalus.

Approximately 50 percent of CSF is produced by the choroid plexus in an energy-requiring process that is dependent on the enzyme carbonic anhydrase. The remainder of CSF production occurs as a result of bulk flow of CSF from brain extracellular fluid.[55] Acetazolamide, a potent inhibitor of carbonic anhydrase, has been shown to decrease CSF production by 49 percent in rabbits[65] and 16 to 66 percent in humans.[80] Several early reports of the use of acetazolamide showed the drug to be effective in up to one half of infnts in whom it was tried.[80, 84] In one trial of 32 infants with myelomeningoceles, no effect could be seen with the drug.[51] Acetazolamide has proved to be effective as a temporizing measure in patients with transient CSF absorption defects and in patients with borderline shunt function.

In a very recent study involving premature neonates with progressive hydrocephalus secondary to neonatal intraventricular hemorrhage, the combination of acetazolamide and furosemide was shown to be effective in preventing the need for shunting.[87] Furosemide is a diuretic that acts at the loop of Henle. The mechanism of decrease in ICP with this drug is unclear, but its action seems to be to decrease brain extracellular fluid. This combination seems a logical approach to the management of infantile hydrocephalus, but in the author's experience the treatment seems to involve the risk of severe dehydration of these fragile children. A multicentered study of this form of treatment seems indicated.

SURGICAL TREATMENT OF HYDROCEPHALUS

The modern era of the surgical treatment of hydrocephalus begins with the development of valve mechanisms for use in shunt systems.[61] For an excellent historical perspective on earlier management techniques in hydrocephalus, the reader is directed to the fine review article by Pudenz.[69] Only a brief view will be presented here. Whether shunts went from the ventricular or lumbar subarachnoid space to a variety of absorbing reservoirs, prior to the advent of valve-regulated shunting, they were largely unsuccessful for technical reasons. The lack of valves led to reflux of blood and coagulation, which resulted in blockage. Rapid overdrainage of massively enlarged ventricles led to fatal subdural hematomas. Finally, the materials available for implantation at that time characteristically excited an intense inflammatory response, which resulted in obstruction of the shunt systems. The lumboureteral shunt was the most effective form of treatment available prior to the early 1950's.[45] As originally conceived by Heile in 1927, the renal pelvis was sutured to the dura arachnoid.[69] Later, Matson[45] performed a nephrectomy and inserted a piece of polyethylene tubing from the spinal subarachnoid space to the ureter. While mostly successful, a few patients experienced a profound hyponatremic dehydration resulting from CSF loss through the bladder.

In 1918, Dandy introduced the choroid plexectomy for the treatment of hydrocephalus, based on experiments performed by Blackfan and himself, which defined the choroid plexus as the site of CSF production.[7] Early experiences with this technique resulted in a high rate of operative mortality. Later, this procedure was attempted using an endoscope, with equivocal results.[70,83] However, the procedure has been abandoned for the most part. It is now known that the choroid plexus is responsible for only one half of CSF production, and the beneficial results of choroid plexectomy were usually of only temporary benefit. Further, Milhorat[53,54] has been able to demonstrate normal rates of CSF production five years after choroid plexectomy.

Procedures that bypassed the site of obstruction of CSF pathways were successful in a limited way, and some are employed today in very specific situations. The earliest of these techniques involved such fenestration of the ventricular system into the subarachnoid space, either at open surgery or using a ventriculoscopic technique.[8] Contemporary authors report encouraging results, using stereotactic techniques to create holes from the third ventricle to the cortical subarachnoid space. Sayers and Kosnick[82] emphasized the need to demonstrate open subarachnoid pathways and intact absorptive mechanisms in order properly to select patients.

Ventriculocisternostomy, or the creation of a bypass channel between the lateral ventricle and the cisterna magna, was originally described by Torkildsen[90] and has been shown to be an effective procedure in patients with secondary obstructive hydrocephalus (e.g., from tumors). Enthusiasm for this procedure was dampened by the finding that it was not applicable in infantile hydrocephalus, presumably because of the lack of development of adequate absorptive mechanisms.[44]

Treatment of Hydrocephalus by Valve-Regulated Shunts

A great majority of children with hydrocephalus are managed by valve-regulated shunting systems. All these systems have common biologic and mechanical components, which will be discussed. All commercially available shunting systems are capable of managing hydrocephalus in most children.[13] While some prejudices in the reader will be unavoidable from the following discussion, the author does not intend to advocate the use of one product over another. As experience with the idiosyncrasies of the individual systems is gained, the neurosurgeon becomes comfortable with one system and, except in very specific circumstances, should abandon it only with great trepidation.

The first component of the shunting system is the proximal catheter. This plastic tube of multiple designs is placed within the CSF pathways proximal to the site of obstruction of CSF. Most commonly, this means the placement of a catheter in the lateral ventricle. There is general agreement that it is technically advantageous to place the ventricular catheter anterior to the foramen of Monro in order to avoid the likelihood of having the holes in the catheter become occluded by the choroid plexus.[57,58] There are two acceptable approaches to proper ventricular catheter placement. These are (1) the insertion of the ventricular catheter in the anterior horn of the lateral ventricle, by a parieto-occipital placement, and (2) the more direct approach through the frontal lobe at the area of the coronal sutures. Both procedures normally result in proper placement of the ventricular catheter in the frontal horn, anterior to the foramen of Monro.

When using the anterior approach, the hole in the skull is made 3 cm lateral to the sagittal suture and just anterior or posterior to the coronal suture (Fig. 14–3). The catheter is directed perpendicular to the skull, aiming generally at the inner canthus of the ipsilateral eye unless the ventricular antomy is distorted. In patients with small ventricles, particularly when replacing a ventricular catheter in a chronically shunted ventricle, it is often advantageous to drape the face (which is in a brow-up position), using sterile, transparent plastic so that these landmarks can be observed during the passage of the ventricular catheter. A tripod-shaped device has recently been introduced to make this pass easier.[22] Conceptually, the device is logical, but the author has no experience with it.

The anterior placement has an advantage in that the pass is a shorter distance through the brain and does not traverse elegant areas of the brain. It is also more likely to lead to ventricular catheter placement in the proper position anterior to the choroid

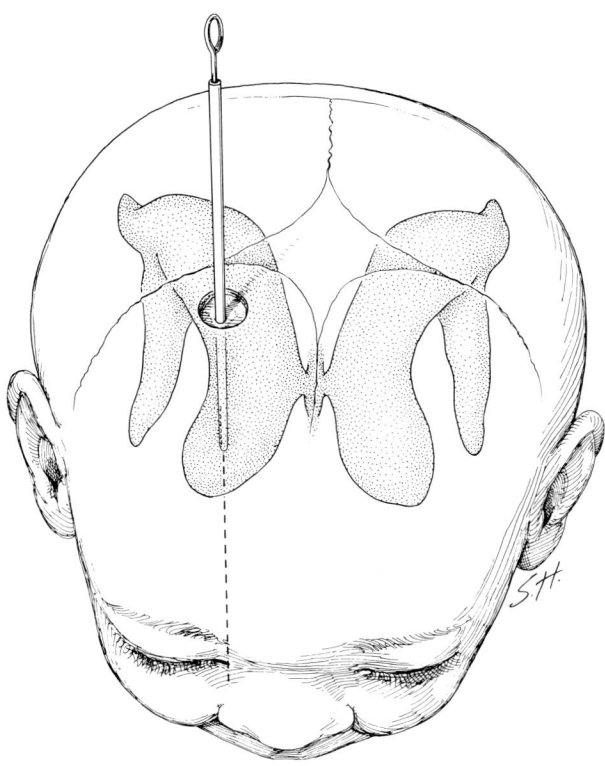

Figure 14–3. Anterior placement of ventricular catheter. (Courtesy of Barrow Neurological Institute.)

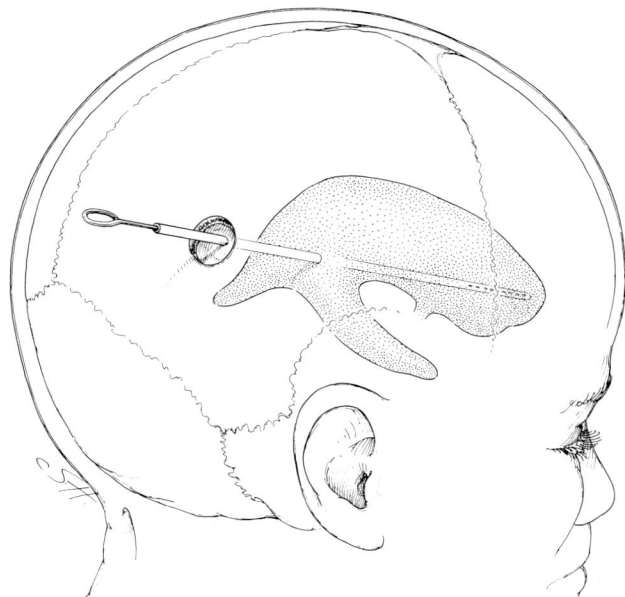

Figure 14–4. Posterior placement of ventricular catheter. (Courtesy of Barrow Neurological Institute.)

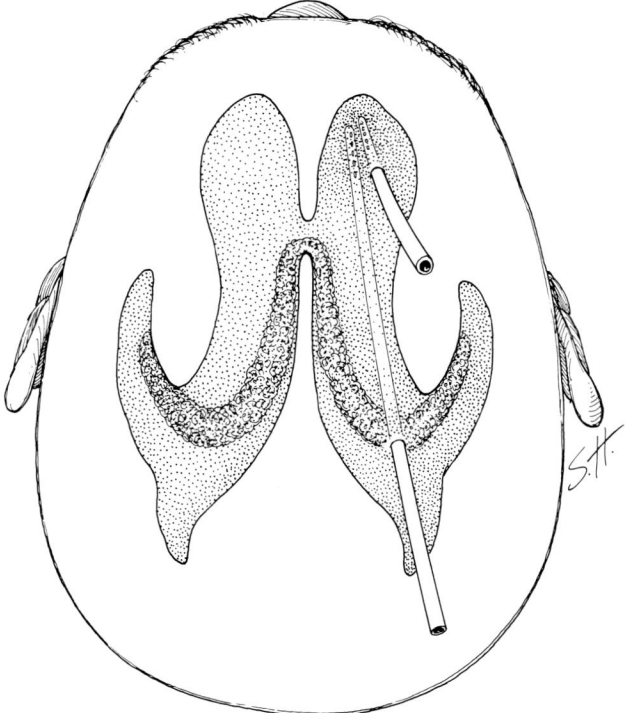

Figure 14–5. Relationship of ventricular catheters to foramen of Monro and choroid plexus. (Courtesy of Barrow Neurological Institute.)

plexus. The disadvantage of the anterior placement relates to the distance the catheter must travel subgaleally. If this placement is used in infants, as the infant grows the external catheter under the scalp is fixed at each point by the dense adherence of scalp to periosteum. As the head grows, a minimal amount of sliding or no sliding of this catheter is permitted, and a slowly applied distracting force is applied to the catheter end, which frequently leads to disconnection or breakage of the catheter at points of stress. When used in the child older than two years of age or in adults, the rate of head growth is rarely fast enough to result in such problems.

Landmarks for the posterior approach to ventricular cannulation vary somewhat with the neurosurgeon and the purpose for which this approach was chosen. Positioning of patients and landmarks for the placement of ventricular catheters are strictly followed (Fig. 14–4). The patient is placed in a lateral decubitus position, with the hole 3 cm above and 3 cm behind the tip of the ear.[58] The catheter is aimed parallel to the sagittal suture in the direction of the ipsilateral eye. The length of the catheter should be approximately 1 cm longer than the distance from the hole to the coronal suture. The advantage of this placement is that the catheter runs along the long axis of the ventricle, yielding a longer segment of the ventricular catheter containing drainage holes within the ventricular system itself (Fig. 14–5). It also has the advantage of a shorter subgaleal distance for the external tubing and, therefore, a smaller chance of disconnection. The disadvantage of this placement is the potential for harm to more elegant areas of the brain, particularly the visual cortex. In infants, there is a selective dilation of the occipital horns of the lateral ventricles when the thickness of the brain in that location is less than 1 cm (Fig. 14–6). Ventricular

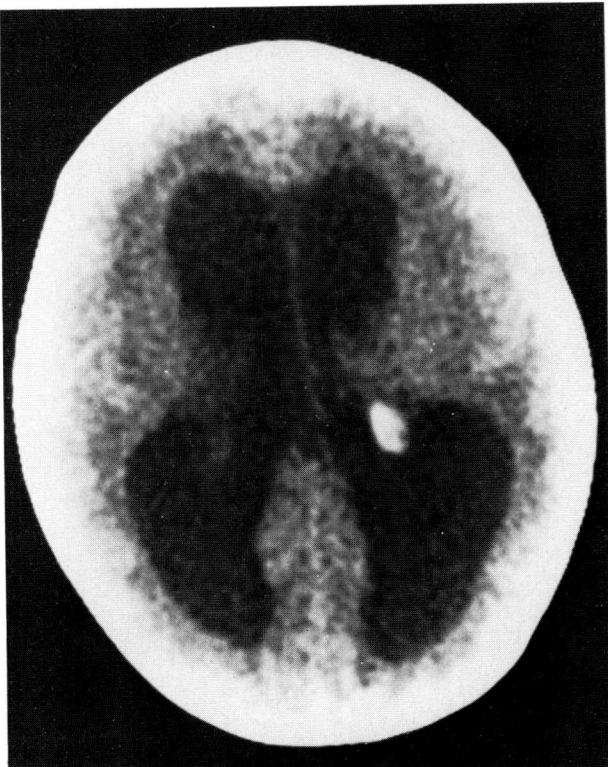

Figure 14–6. Computed tomographic scan of infant with hydrocephalus, showing selective dilatation of occipital horns.

catheter placement in the high parietal region traverses very little cortex.

After the ventricular catheter has been placed and free flow of CSF is ensured, anteroposterior and lateral x-ray films should be obtained to verify that the shunt catheter tip is in the correct location. A reservoir attached to the ventricular catheter is strongly recommended. Whether the neurosurgeon uses a separate reservoir (e.g., Rickham's reservoir) or one that is incorporated into the valve system is a matter of personal preference. The reservoir should allow the sampling of ventricular CSF and the measurement of intraventricular pressure.

In patients who have communicating hydrocephalus or, as Ransohoff and colleagues[73] have described, extraventricular obstructive hydrocephalus, the lumbar theca can be an excellent site of placement for the proximal catheter. The major advantage of this form of treatment is that it trends to maintain the integrity of the CSF pathways (e.g., it will not lead to secondary obstruction of the aqueduct of Sylvius). Also, it does not lead to collapse of the ventricular wall around the catheter tip, resulting in obstruction. Although classically performed using a limited laminectomy and subarachnoid placement under direct vision, it is now possible to perform this procedure percutaneously, using a Touhy needle.[30, 86] Reports of scoliosis and nerve root deficits in growing children have tended to result in a less frequent use of this technique.[36] The ability to perform lumboperitoneal shunts without the need to do a laminectomy in children over two years of age and the use of less irritating implantable (Silastic) materials make this procedure more attractive.

Testing the patency of lumboperitoneal shunts is difficult. If one attempts actually to follow the path of a radionuclide or radiopaque tracer through the shunt system, equivocal results are often obtained. If one remembers that in order for CSF to be absorbed by natural pathways it must ascend to the level of the sagittal sinus and that no absorption of CSF occurs at the level of the spinal subarachnoid space, a simple test of lumboperitoneal shunt patency can be derived. Radionuclide or radiopaque tracer introduced into the spinal subarachnoid space can be absorbed in one of two ways, either by normal absorptive pathways or via the shunt catheter. The peritoneal surface absorbs CSF quickly, but in the patient with partial obstruction of CSF pathways, CSF is slowly absorbed into the blood stream, for clearance through the kidneys. If the shunt is patent, the tracer will be detectable in the bladder within one hour and could not have arrived there by natural pathways.

The Distal Catheter

In shunt systems, the distal catheter is a plastic tube that can be simply open on the end, can have a distal slit valve that adds a resistance element (to be discussed under valve systems), or can have holes in the sides to give multiple sites for release of CSF into the distal receptacle. The superiority of one form of tube over another has not been demonstrated. There remains some controversy as to the optimal receptacle for placement of the distal catheter. Since the development of Silastic materials, which do not usually incite walling off by the omentum, the peritoneal cavity has become the preferred site of distal catheters both for ventricular and lumbar shunt systems.[4, 92]

The Peritoneal Cavity. The peritoneum is an extremely efficient site of absorption of both fluids and drugs and, in many ways, is the ideal receptacle for the distal catheter of a shunt system. Attempts to use the peritoneum as a receptacle in the treatment of hydrocephalus date from Ferguson, who in 1898 attempted to link the lumbar theca with the peritoneum, using a silver wire.[10] Early ventriculoperitoneal (VP) shunts without valves led to overly rapid ventricular decompression, subdural hematoma, and death. The development of pressure-activated valve systems made the peritoneum a feasible receptacle for CSF diversion. However, valve-regulated VP shunts were unreliable because of a high incidence of distal obstruction resulting from the inflammatory response that they incited. Suprahepatic or intrapelvic placement was advocated, but peritoneal placement was considered only a temporizing measure awaiting a permanent vascular placement.

With the development of Silastic tubing in 1968, the reliability of VP shunts increased greatly.[4, 92] VP shunts have two compelling advantages over vascular shunts and, at present, should be considered the receptacle of choice for shunts in children. The performance of all shunts is associated with a risk of infection, with published incidences of 2 to 20 percent per procedure.[85, 91] If a patient with a ventriculoatrial (VA) shunt develops an infection, there exists a potential for the life-threatening complications of septic endocarditis, septic pulmonary emboli, and immune complex glomerulonephritis. Conversely, infection in peritoneal shunts usually presents with distal obstruction from the local inflammatory process or may present as localized or generalized peritonitis, conditions that are rarely life-threatening.[79] The second major advantage of VP shunting has to do with the growth of the infant. VA shunts, to be reliable and safe, must be placed well proximal to the tricuspid valve and must extend at least into the large superior vena cava (usually at the level of the fourth thoracic vertebra).[57, 58] As the child grows, the distal catheter tends to pull out of this desired placement, and when it pulls into the jugular vein, the venous flow is often not great enough to prevent obstruction due to fibrosis at the end of the catheter. To maintain a working VA shunt usually requires several elective revisions with time. When the peritoneum is chosen, a nearly unlimited length of tubing can be placed within the peritoneal cavity that can uncoil as the child grows normally, resulting in fewer revisions during childhood. Figure 14–7 demonstrates the techniques available for the placement of the peritoneal catheter.

Occasionally, a child is found who will not tolerate peritoneal shunting, and an atrial or other distal receptacle will be required. There are three potential causes of this problem. The most common cause is unrecognized indolent infection of the shunt system. These cryptic infections may be due to anaerobic diphtheroids, the identification of which requires special culturing techniques and prolonged incubation times.[78] The second cause is the chemical content of the CSF being very irritating to the peritoneal surface, such as following intraventricular hemorrhage or with extremely high protein levels seen in intraventricular tumors. Finally, some patients have a peritoneal surface that will not absorb CSF.

The Venous System. With the development of adequate valve systems, the right atrium became the preferred site of distal CSF diversion. Shunts inserted into the atrium were more reliable, and as long as they stayed radiologically between T-7 and T-4, they remained patent, for the most part.[57] Atrial shunts are a low-pressure system relative to intra-abdominal pressures, and because of the much shorter distance from the ventricle to the right atrium when the shunt is in the erect position, the effects of siphoning are minimized.

Maintaining VA shunts is often extremely difficult because of the limited number of points of access to the vascular tree. The first VA shunt placed into the right jugular vein, usually via the common facial vein, led to a direct path to the atrium, with little difficulty. However, when this access point was not available, much difficulty in cannulating the right atrium was often encountered. Left jugular or subclavian cannulation tended to result in the tube tending to go into the right subclavian vein. Likewise, right subclavian cannulation would result in the tubing tending to be directed to the left subclavian vein.

The difficulties of atrial cannulation could often be overcome by using fluoroscopy and Seldinger's guide wires. Certain patients underwent right atrial cannulation by open thoracotomy, after multiple previous venous placements made cannulation difficult. Kaufman[34] developed a technique for placing right atrial catheters, using a transfemoral venous Seldinger technique. The catheter was passed through the right atrium into a vein in the neck, allowing the surgeon to palpate the wire in the neck, to prepare the area, and to cut down on the length of the guide wire. The atrial catheter was placed over the guide wire and was drawn into the atrium. There it was disconnected with a quick tug, to remain in the proper position in the atrium, and then was connected to the rest of the shunt system in the neck (Fig. 14–8).[34]

Other Sites of Distal Catheter Placement. Many sites for distal placement of shunt systems have been tried, with varying success. Most are used extremely rarely in contemporary practice. The use of the *stomach* and the *fallopian tube* has probably been abandoned altogether. The *gallbladder* continues to be used by various neurosurgeons when the difficulty in performing atrial shunts or the futility of performing peritoneal shunts justifies the risk of potential infection of the system.

The *pleural cavity* has been advocated for the treatment of hydrocephalus and does adequately absorb CSF in numerous patients.[52, 72] The length of time that the pleura retains its absorptive capacity varies from individual to individual. There have been cases in which the pleural cavity ceased to be an absorptive surface, and the patient presented with severe respiratory compromise, with hydrothorax.

The *ureter* as a site of distal catheter placement is of special interest from a historical perspective. In 1925, Heile reported suturing of the renal pelvis to the lumbar subarachnoid space.[69] Matson,[45] who developed both lumbar and ventricular ureteral shunts, connected the CSF pathway to the ureter, using polyethylene tubing after performing a nephrectomy. As late as 1956, Matson considered ureterostomy to be the most reliable form of treatment for hydrocephalus. This procedure involved unique problems. CSF was released into the bladder and was irrevocably lost from the circulation. In

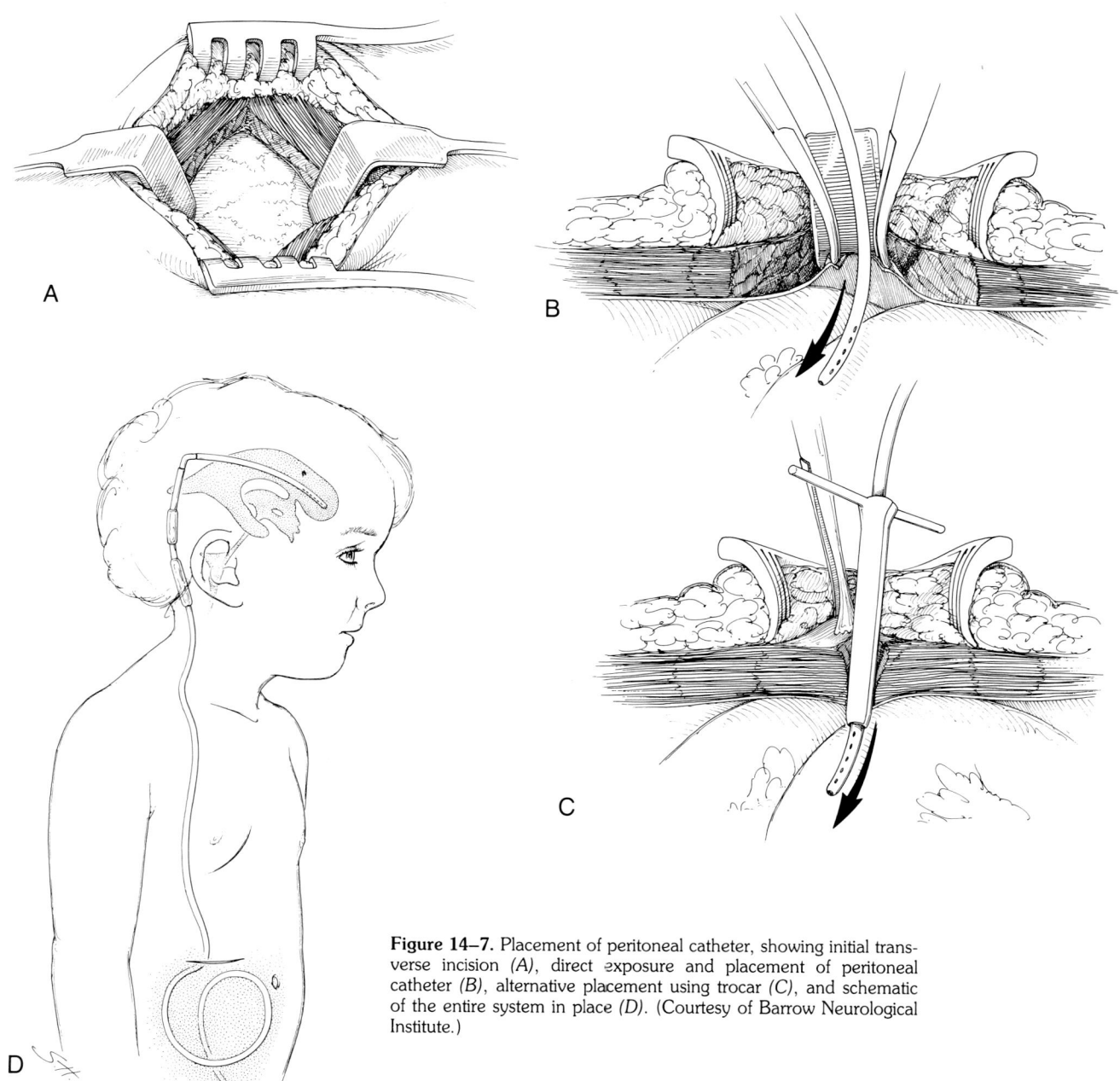

Figure 14–7. Placement of peritoneal catheter, showing initial transverse incision (A), direct exposure and placement of peritoneal catheter (B), alternative placement using trocar (C), and schematic of the entire system in place (D). (Courtesy of Barrow Neurological Institute.)

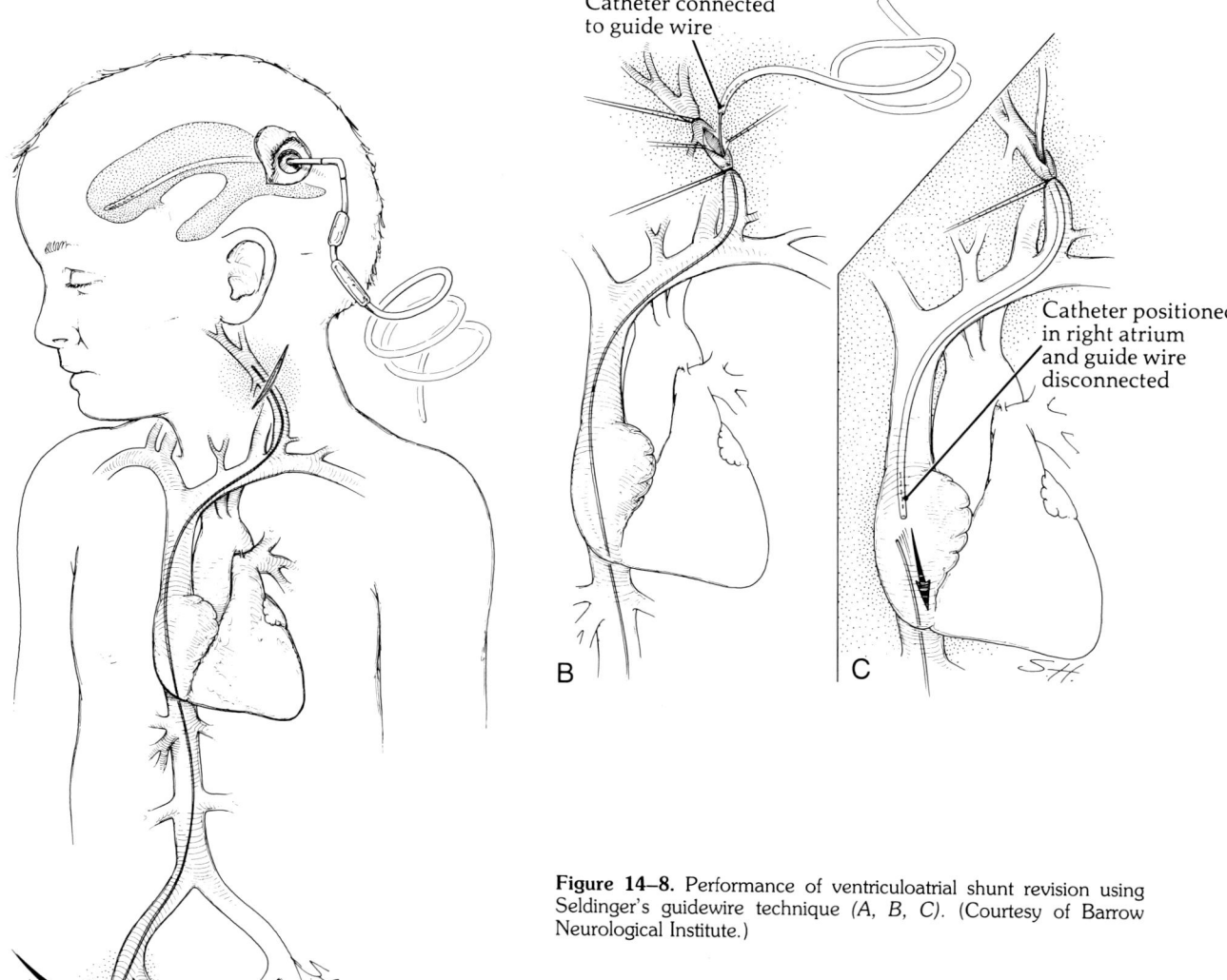

Figure 14–8. Performance of ventriculoatrial shunt revision using Seldinger's guidewire technique (A, B, C). (Courtesy of Barrow Neurological Institute.)

certain instances in small children, this resulted in profound hyponatremic dehydration. It was also essential to prove that the ureterovesical junction was a competent valve that would prevent retrograde passage of urine and bacteria to the shunt system. Recently, ureterostomy has been modified by Smith and colleagues[88] to preserve the kidney. They perform a ureteroureterostomy in which both kidneys drain into one ureter, with the tubing being placed in the other ureter. This is an effective procedure in patients in whom it is difficult or unwise to place the catheter in the atrium or peritoneum, such as patients with chronic fungal meningitis or active neoplastic meningeal seeding.

THE VALVE SYSTEM

While a few authors advocate the use of shunts without valves in the specific case of posthemorrhagic hydrocephalus in premature infants, it was the development of the valve-regulated shunting systems that led to the expectation of successful treatment of hydrocephalus in the vast majority of patients.[61] There are many different valve designs marketed by nearly as many manufacturers, but they all share important characteristics. The most important shared characteristic is that all valve systems marketed within the United States have been proved to control successfully hydrocephalus. This point is extremely important. The dogmatic stances taken by neurosurgeons that one system is always the best or that another does not adequately treat hydrocephalus are not justified by the available statistical information. Certain valve characteristics of opening or closing pressure or of valve resistance may or may not be more desirable in one or another clinical setting. The decision as to which valve system one should use depends to a great extent on the individual experiences of the neurosurgeon

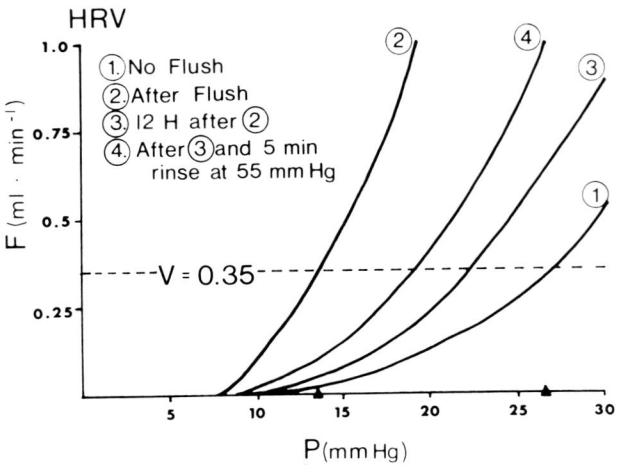

Figure 14–9. Pressure-flow characteristics of high-resistance shunts (i.e., slit valves).

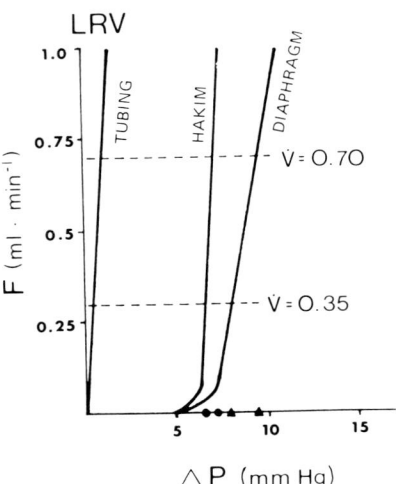

Figure 14–10. Pressure-flow characteristics of low-resistance shunts (i.e., Hakim's and diaphragm valves).

who does the implantation and who will perform the patient follow-up.

The other characteristic that all valves currently share is that they represent a fixed preset resistance that is dependent on the differential pressure between the CSF compartment and the distal receptacle flow, as determined solely by the valve characteristics and this differential pressure. There is no valve that is a controller based on flow. Further, minimal information is available relative to the rate

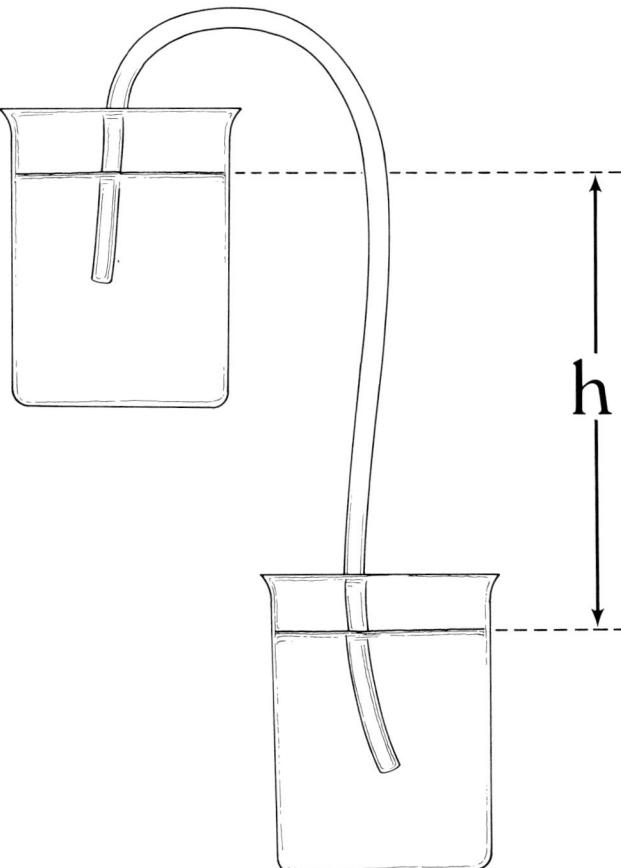

Figure 14–11. Representation of the concept of siphoning as it relates to CSF shunts. When a column of water is in an enclosed space, the hydrostatic pressure driving fluid flow is dependent only on the distances between the upper and lower reservoirs and not on the course that the fluid takes. In this equation, the driving pressure equals height times the mass of CSF times the acceleration of gravity ($P = mhg$). (Courtesy of Barrow Neurological Institute.)

of flow through shunts over a 24-hour period. Some evidence exists that there may be prolonged periods during the day when there is actually no or extremely little flow through shunt systems as well as other times when flow is extremely rapid.[89]

This resistance element in the shunt can be extremely simple (such as the inherent resistances to flow in a small-lumen tube or a distal slit-valve) or very complicated. Portnoy[66, 68] has divided all shunt systems, according to their resistance to flow characteristics, into two categories, which he terms "high-pressure" shunts and "low-pressure" shunts. By high-pressure (high-resistance) shunts, he means that as the differential pressure across the valve decreases, the rate of flow becomes slower and slower (Fig. 14–9). These valves are mostly of the slit-valve type (Holter, Holter-Hausner, distal slit valve). The low-pressure (low-resistance) valve shows a very low resistance to flow until the closing pressure of the valve is reached, at which time it stops flow abruptly (Fig. 14–10). All diaphragm valves (Pudenz, Pudenz-Shulte, LPV) are in this category, as well as the spring-loaded ball in a cup (Hakim).[66, 68] Both high-pressure and low-pressure shunt valves respond to differential pressures across the valve's resistance element and, therefore, are subject to the effects of siphoning. Siphoning occurs when the height of fluid at one end of a closed system is greater than that at the other end; therefore, gravity causes a pressure differential that would not be seen with the patient in a recumbent-position (Fig. 14–11). This phenomenon can lead to ICPs in shunted patients that are markedly negative with respect to atmospheric pressure and possibly can collapse the ventricular system.[59, 60] In patients who are symptomatic from low ICP, the use of a valve system containing an anti-siphon device often reverses the symptoms.[32] For mechanical reasons, Portnoy and associates recommend that anti-siphon devices be used only with low-pressure shunt systems.[67]

MANAGEMENT OF COMPARTMENTALIZED HYDROCEPHALUS

Often, neurosurgeons dealing with a large hydrocephalic population are confronted by shunt surgery complicated by the presence of CSF compartments that may or may not be drained by a ventricular shunting procedure. Managing these conditions is controversial. Each form of compartmentalization will be discussed separately.

The Dandy-Walker Malformation

The Dandy-Walker malformation is a term used to describe several abnormalities of brain development that have posterior fossa cysts, hypoplasia of the cerebellar vermis, and hydrocephalus in common.[9, 29] The condition is associated with multiple other anomalies including agenesis of the corpus callosum, cleft palate, eye abnormalities, and subnormal intelligence in a significant percentage.[29, 49] That this syndrome is not uniform pathologically is emphasized by the work of Entzian and colleagues,[11] who demonstrated two pathologically distinct cysts: one lined simply with ependyma and presenting after the perinatal period, and one that they thought represented a porencephaly of the cerebellar vermis presenting at or near delivery.

Therapy for this condition remains very controversial. Direct surgical attack, as advocated by Matson, has been abandoned by contemporary authors as dangerous and futile.[5, 29, 33, 46, 71] Carmel and colleagues[5] point to the fact that free communication between the supratentorial ventricular system and the cyst can usually be demonstrated. They advocate the shunting of lateral ventricles only. However, they do emphasize the potential change in the comunicating nature of the cyst-ventricle relationship and recommend combined shunting of the cyst and the ventricle when free communication cannot be demonstrated.[5] In Hirsch's series of 25 patients treated primarily by shunting, 12 had ventriculoperitoneal shunts, and 13 had cyst-peritoneum shunts. One of his patients with a ventricular shunt subsequently required incorporation of the cyst into the system.[29]

From the previous discussion, it follows that in the majority of cases, the ventricles communicate with the cyst of the posterior fossa; therefore, shunting of either compartment is usually successful. Raimondi and coworkers[71] and Carmel and associates[5] point out that even though communication can be shown early in the course, it does not necessarily prove that communication will remain throughout life. If mono-compartment shunting is selected, diligence must be maintained, or late deterioration will result from late ventricular isolation. Shunting of the lateral ventricles has resulted in upward herniation and prolonged apneic spells in a few patients.[71] In James's series, all six patients who were initially treated by only shunting the lateral ventricles subsequently required posterior fossa shunting.[33]

Because the incidence of late noncommunication between the supratentorial and the infratentorial compartments is difficult to discern and because of the theoretical benefit of ensuring that a pressure gradient does not exist across the tentorial ring, the author suggests that ventricular catheters be placed into the lateral ventricle and the posterior fossa cyst and that the tubing be spliced together proximal to the valve. On one occasion, in attempting to perform such a procedure, the two leaves of the dura were found to be separated in multiple areas by a venous sinus of the entire posterior fossa. It was not possible to place a posterior fossa shunt. In this case, simply shunting the ventricle produced an excellent clinical outcome.

The Isolated Fourth Ventricle

Since the advent of CT scanning, the area of the posterior fossa can be easily visualized. Unexpectedly, dilatation of the fourth ventricle in chronically shunted patients (difficult to diagnose before CT scanning) is being recognized with increasing frequency. Foltz and Shurtleff[20] recognized early the possibility that communicating hydrocephalus could be converted to aqueductal stenosis if the distending force (i.e., hydrocephalus) was removed by shunting, particularly with an inflammatory condition such as infection or hemorrhage. Isolation of the fourth ventricle occurs under these circumstances. The sequence is described in Figure 14–12. Foltz and associates[18, 20] apparently recognized this condition in the era preceding CT scanning and treated it by performing a Torkildsen shunt with a lateral ventricle shunt. In this situation, the original level of obstruction is at the basal meninges, theoretically creating a block to CSF passage between the spinal subarachnoid space (SSAS) and the cortical subarachnoid space (CSAS). Alternatively, the blockage may occur at the level of the outlet foramina of the fourth ventricle. After shunting, the pressure distending the aqueduct of Sylvius is removed. The aqueduct, which has the form of a collapsable tube, then chronically assumes its collapsed position, with the walls abutting. Chronic opposition of these ependymally lined surfaces can lead to a scar that will eventually cause permanent stenosis of the aqueduct. During this time, CSF is still being produced within the fourth ventricle, which contains choroid plexus. Now that the aqueduct is closed, the CSF cannot be removed by flow through the shunt and is still obstructed from its normal absorption pathways, either by obstruction of the outlet foramina of the fourth ventricle or by a block of flow at the area of the basal cisterns. Pressure increases in the fourth ventricle are followed by distention of this compartment.

Signs and symptoms related to fourth ventricular or double compartment hydrocephalus have been reported to include headache, ataxia, coma, cranial nerve palsies, anorexia, and vomiting.[6, 18, 25, 26, 40] In the course of routine surveillance of shunted hydrocephalic patients, dilatation of the fourth ventricle is occasionally found in patients without overt symptoms referable to posterior fossa mass lesions. In some of these, isolated fourth ventricular hydrocephalus leads to behavioral disturbances, short attention span, and deterioration in school performance. Such signs are difficult to interpret but dramatic improvement in behavior and school performance may result from treating this condition.

It should be pointed out that the etiology of the hydrocephalus or subsequent complications of treatment play a significant role in the pathogenesis of the isolated fourth ventricle. The majority of patients reported to have this condition have had postmeningitic hydrocephalus or have suffered from multiple shunt infections.[6, 18, 26, 40] This condition seems to be frequently associated with fungal meningitis.[18, 25] This condition can also be encountered in patients whose hydrocephalus is a result of tumorous obstruction of CSF outflow, which in

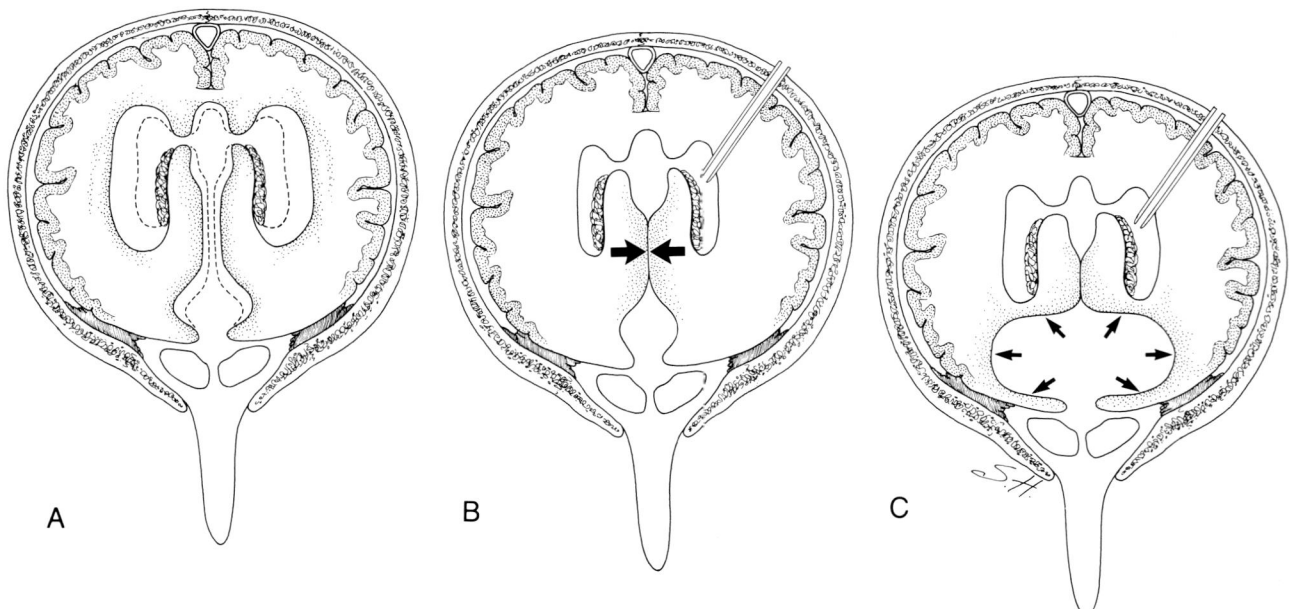

Figure 14–12. Representation of the pathophysiology of the isolated fourth ventricle (A) and panventricular hydrocephalus with dilatation of the aqueduct of Sylvius and blockage of the basal cisterns (B). The shunting of the lateral ventricles leads to collapse of the aqueduct of Sylvius, which, with time, becomes irreversible (C). Since CSF is still being produced within the fourth ventricle and cannot be drained from above or below, progressive dilatation of the fourth ventricle occurs. (Courtesy of Barrow Neurological Institute.)

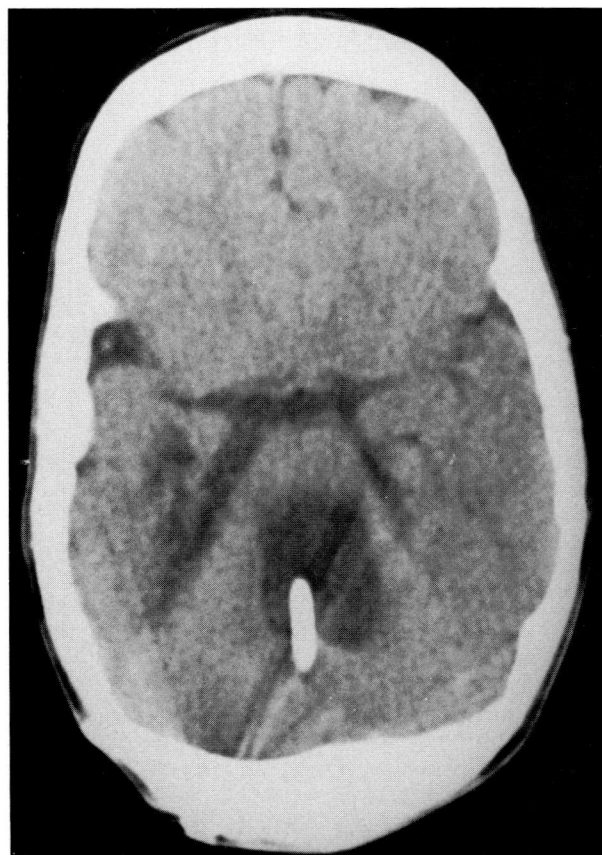

Figure 14–13. CT scan of the placement of a catheter in the fourth ventricle.

the author's experience includes one case of CSF seeding from medulloblastoma and one case of CSF obstruction at multiple sites in neurofibromatosis and which also includes a case of subependymoma, with blockage of the outlet foramina of the fourth ventricle.[1]

The treatment of this condition is controversial and often difficult. Foltz and Shortleff[20] seem to advocate a direct surgical attack on the site of obstruction if it can be determined that this obstruction has a veil-like quality. Most authors recommend cannulating the cystlike fourth ventricle, usually creating a splice into the existing shunt system.[6, 25, 26, 40] Cannulation of the fourth ventricle may be difficult, requiring multiple passes. Estimating the required length of the ventricular catheter may also be difficult. For this reason, the author recommends placing the ventricular catheter under CT scan control. In the author's experience, it is best to trephine the posterior fossa, to incorporate the shunting system into the existing shunt in the operating room, and to close the incisions not directly over the trephine. The patient is then transported to the CT scanner, where the length and the trajectory of the ventricular catheter can be accurately assessed (Fig. 14–13). Then, the wound is copiously irrigated with antibiotic solution and is closed. This allows accurate placement with minimum CT scan time and gives access to operating room equipment (for hemostasis) for the major portion of the operative procedure.

Cannulation of the fourth ventricle is not without risk. The author has had two patients who had cannulation of a fourth ventricular cyst, in whom the catheter was found to be in an appropriate location postoperatively. These patients were asymptomatic at the time. Days to weeks later, one patient returned with a fifth nerve palsy, and the other had a seventh nerve palsy with some ataxia. Follow-up CT scans showed that as the fourth ventricle returned to normal size, the ventricular catheter came to lie on the floor of the fourth ventricle, in the area of the appropriate cranial nerve nuclei (Fig. 14–14). Use of CT scan control may minimize the possibility of this complication.

If the site of obstruction is from the spinal subarachnoid space to the cortical subarachnoid space rather than involving the outlet foramina of the fourth ventricle, the risks and difficulties just described can be obviated by using a lumboperitoneal shunt. Before performing such a procedure, it is essential to prove that the fourth ventricle is in communication with the lumbar theca. This is best accomplished by injecting iodinated contrast material into the lumbar thecal sac and tipping the head down to roll the dye into the posterior fossa. If the fourth ventricle fills with contrast material, the patient is a candidate for the much easier and safer percutaneous lumboperitoneal shunt.[86]

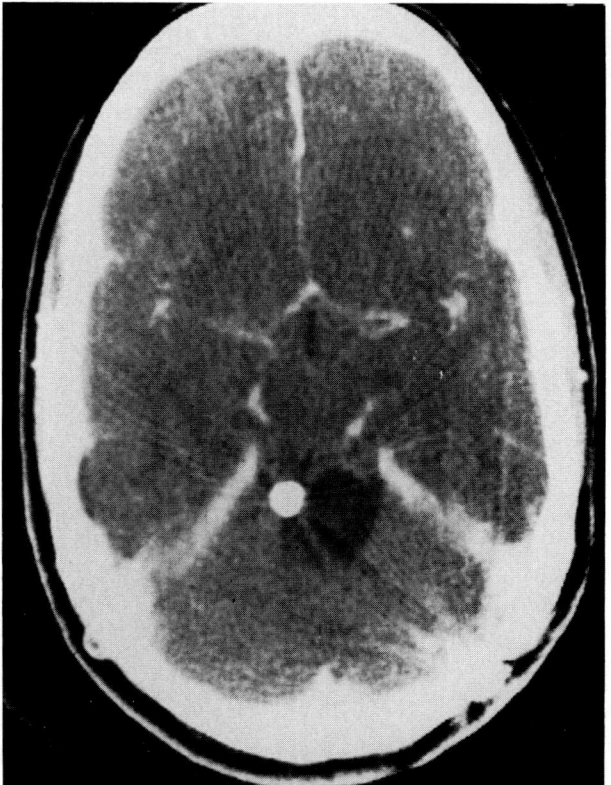

Figure 14–14. Catheter in the fourth ventricle. As the fourth ventricle became smaller, it came to lie within the brainstem, at the area of the cerebellar peduncle.

Supratentorial CSF Cysts

Intraventricular and other supratentorial cysts represent a broad spectrum of disease, and for the most part, their diagnosis and management lie outside this discussion. However, if they are seen in the context of hydrocephalus or as a complication of its treatment, two options are available to the neurosurgeon: (1) direct attack, with removal or fenestration into the ventricle, *or* (2) cannulation of the cystic structure and incorporation of the new ventricular shunt into the pre-existing shunt system. These cysts can be developmental, or they can result from the lifting off of ependymal surface from the ventricular wall, occurring in infection, as described by McLone and coworkers.[47]

When cysts that contain CSF are found in chronically shunted patients and there is no evidence of enhancement on CT scans, these lesions can usually be managed best by placing a ventricular cannula within the cyst and incorporating the cyst into the existing shunt system. It is often necessary to outline the cyst anatomically by injecting metrizamide (Amipaque, Winthrop-Breon Laboratories, New York) into the ventricular system. This procedure usually shows the extent of the lesion and guides cannulation (Fig. 14–15).

Occasionally, these cysts have firm capsules that tend to resist cannulation. The ventricular catheters may actually bounce off the cyst wall and fail to drain the cyst (Fig. 14–16). In this situation or in cases in which the actual diagnosis of the cyst is unknown, a direct surgical approach to the cyst is warranted. Figure 14–16 shows a large cyst, probably arising from the area of the quadrigeminal

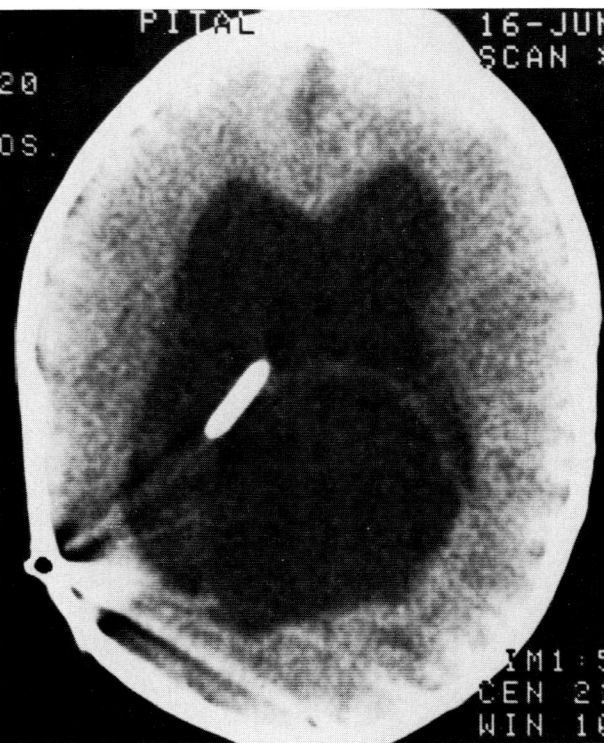

Figure 14–16. Demonstration of the placement of a ventricular catheter that failed to enter a large cyst of the quadrigeminal plate.

cistern, in a child with hydrocephalus secondary to the Arnold-Chiari malformation. The cyst is outlined by injecting metrizamide into the catheter that has been used to cannulate the cyst. This catheter bounced off the wall of the cyst and is present in the ventricular system. The patient was treated with a transcallosal approach to the cyst, with exploration and placement of the shunt tubing in the cyst under direct vision.

WHO CAN DO WITHOUT A SHUNT?

A discussion of the treatment of a disease process must always contain an evaluation of when such treatment may be discontinued. In a child or adult who is shunt-dependent, treatment must be continued throughout the life of the patient. Neurosurgical assessment of the child or adult to document the physical integrity of the shunt system should be performed at least once a year. The continuing higher cognitive functioning of the patient and the patient's neurologic functioning also should be assessed on at least a yearly basis. If a change occurs, the patient should be reassessed with CT scanning or nuclear magnetic resonance imaging (NMRI) to determine ventricular size. Known shunt-dependent patients must have shunts repaired even if they do not have overt evidence of increased ICP. Within this category are shunts found to be discon-

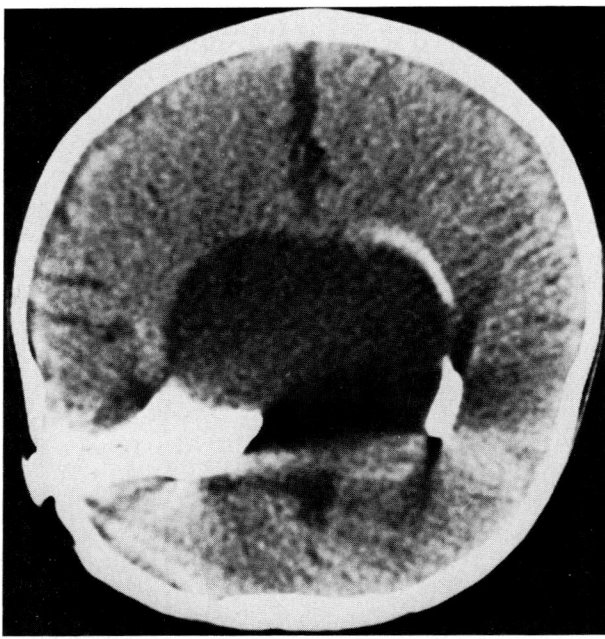

Figure 14–15. Injection of metrizamide through a shunt system outlines a cyst of the quadrigeminal cistern in a child with Arnold-Chiari malformation.

nected or to be too short in the abdomen or jugular vein on x-ray film. The essential part of this discussion is who is and who is not dependent on shunting for life. An alternative way of stating this is who can do without a shunt?

The presence of a shunt, to some extent, creates a dependence on the shunt system. Flow of CSF is preferentially directed into the shunt system rather than through the partially obstructed and intrinsically higher resistance natural pathways for CSF absorption. Abnormally low intraventricular pressures intrinsic to nearly all shunt systems in the erect position may lead to collapse of the ventricular system, to the extent that the walls of the ventricles may collapse completely. When this occurs at the level of the aqueduct of Sylvius, a secondary aqueductal stenosis may occur that converts communicating (extraventricular obstructive) hydrocephalus to noncommunicating (intraventricular obstructive) hydrocephalus.[20] Especially in the face of an inflammatory response, this process may be irreversible, and all chance for shunt independence is lost.

Hydrocephalus is "arrested" when the natural pathways of CSF absorption have been re-established, ICP has returned to normal, and ventricular volume has stabilized. This term implies that the patient is not being harmed by the process and would not be helped by the repair of a shunt or the placement of a new shunt. Hydrocephalus is "compensated" when ventricles have ceased to enlarge, and there are no overt signs of increased ICP. This term implies that, in subtle ways, the patient is being harmed by the condition and that intellectual, psychologic, or motor function would somehow be improved by the placement of a shunt.[12] Making this distinction is frequently very difficult, but it is essential to the proper management of patients with hydrocephalus.[13] Views on this subject range from that of Foltz[17] and Hemmer,[28] "Once a shunt—always a shunt," to that of Holtzer and DeLange,[31] who believe that shunt independence can be obtained in all forms of hydrocephalus.

Some guidelines are useful in making treatment decisions. While this discussion is not intended to lead to decisions to remove shunts, neurosurgeons are frequently faced with patients whose shunts are not working or with pediatric patients who have shunts that are barely functioning and who do not show signs of increased ICP. VA shunts have been pulled into the jugular vein above the T-4 level. VP shunts have become disconnected or have been pulled up along the anterior chest wall. In these situations, the shunts either are not functioning or will soon be nonfunctioning, and decisions as to whether or not to fix the shunt must be made. The first decision to be made is: "Is this shunt functioning?" If on CT scan or NMR image, the ventricles are normal-sized or smaller than normal, the shunt is performing well.[12, 13] Hydrocephalus becomes arrested or compensated only when the ventricles are at least normal-sized and usually when they are larger than normal. Disconnected shunts may continue to function through fibrous tracks around the shunt. For the most part, a tenuously functioning shunt should be repaired.

If the ventricles are larger than normal, the shunt may not be adequate, and the next decision depends on the level of functioning of the patient. If there are any signs or symptoms of increased ICP such as morning headaches, the shunt should be repaired. If there are any signs of decreases in higher cognitive functioning, the shunt should be repaired. Frequently, these problems are subtle and difficult to assess. Formal neuropsychologic evaluation may be necessary. A decrease in attention span or an increase in temper may indicate that the hydrocephalus is compensated rather than arrested. When there are emotional difficulties or poor school performance, it may be impossible to discern whether it is due to the hydrocephalus. Therefore, it may be necessary to re-establish the shunt to ensure the possible benefit from its functioning. "When in doubt, shunt."

The final step in determining whether it is essential to re-establish a shunt that may be malfunctioning is to determine the etiology of the hydrocephalus. Patients with noncommunicating hydrocephalus are extremely unlikely to have arrested hydrocephalus unless alternative pathways of CSF absorption are formed. Therefore, patients with aqueductal stenosis should be considered shunt-dependent for life.

With very few exceptions, children born with myelomeningoceles have the Arnold-Chiari malformation. In this anomaly, the posterior fossa is extremely small, and most of the medulla oblongata lies in the cervical canal and not in the posterior fossa. Syringomyelia is common in these children, and it seems that compensation for hydrocephalus occurs at the expense of dilatation of the central canal of the spinal cord. In this condition, syringomyelia can lead to weakness of shoulder and hand musculature as well as progressive scoliosis without overt signs of increased ICP.[24]

In a review of the concept of shunt independence from Case Western Reserve University in Cleveland, Ohio, four patients who had documented nonfunctioning shunts and spina bifida exhibited arrested hydrocephalus between 24 hours and five years after the shunt had been proved nonfunctional or had been removed for infection. Two of these patients died, and two suffered severe motor and intellectual downgrading. These patients were apparently asymptomatic prior to the arrested hydrocephalus.[77] Reigel[74] presented a series of patients, the majority of whom had the Arnold-Chiari malformation, with massive ventriculomegaly and no overt signs of increased ICP. Shunt repair led to rapid reconstitution of cerebral mantle and improvement in intellectual performance.[74] Deterioration from hydrocephalus in the Arnold-Chiari malformation may be insidious, and generally, once children receive shunts for hydrocephalus with the Arnold-Chiari malformation, they should be considered shunt-dependent for life.

Communicating hydrocephalus resulting from obstruction of CSF flow between the spinal subarachnoid space through the cortical subarachnoid space to the sagittal sinus is not an "all of none" phenomenon, and when the cause (infection or hemorrhage) resolves, the increased resistance to CSF flow often resolves as well. It is in these patients that nonsurgical measures are often successful in preventing the need for shunting in the first place. It is also these patients who have the potential to develop shunt independence. In the Case Western Reserve University study, 50 percent of children with documented communicating hydrocephalus who were tested for shunt independence were found to have the capacity to be shunt-independent. This represented 25 percent of cases in the series with this etiology. Long-term assessment of intellectual and neurologic performance failed to show any evidence of potential for late deterioration. In children with documented (by a form of dye study) communicating hydrocephalus, shunt independence is a realistic and valuable goal. If they have mild ventricular enlargement, stable intellectual functioning, and no new severe emotional disturbances, continued observation without shunt repair is indicated.[77]

SUMMARY: GOALS IN THE TREATMENT OF HYDROCEPHALUS

While each child who presents to the neurosurgeon must be assessed as an individual, based on the previous discussion, it is possible to define a series of goals, some obvious and some subtle, that should link the treatment plans of most if not all patients, including to

1. Decrease intracranial pressure to at least safe, if not to normal, values.
2. Increase the volume of brain tissue (at least 3.5 cm of cortical mantle) to maximize the child's potential for intellectual, emotional, and motor development.
3. Minimize the frequency and the severity of crises of ICP.
4. Minimize the likelihood of complications of treatment.
5. Maintain the integrity of CSF pathways, to prevent ventricular coaptation and maximize the potential for life without shunt dependency.

Of these goals, the first two are met by most, if not all, shunt systems that are currently available. Failures are probably due to lack of careful follow-up of shunt function. Children who have been treated with or without shunting should be followed at least at three-month intervals for the first year, with examinations including head circumference measurements and ventricular size determinations (ultrasonography, CT, or NMRI) when indicated, to make certain the shunt performs as intended.

Goals no. 3 and no. 4 are outside the scope of this chapter and will be dealt with elsewhere in this volume.

Goal no. 5 is the most controversial, and several authors claim that collapsed or coapted ventricles should be an acceptable goal of shunting. In growing children, all shunt systems currently existing have been associated with the "slit-ventricle syndrome" or proximal shunt failure from ventricular collapse. Several authors hve been successful in treating this condition by simply increasing valve resistance, while others have advocated subtemporal decompression.[14] In the series by Hyde-Rowan and colleagues,[32] the use of high-resistance valves with an anti-siphon device has been shown to be effective in re-expanding previously collapsed ventricles, in preventing ventricular coaptation, and in treating the symptomatic slit-ventricle syndrome (small ventricles on CT, intermittent severe headaches lasting 10 to 90 minutes, and extreme slowness of valve refill).

To avoid these complications, which frequently interfere with the lives of shunt-dependent children, requires some hardware development, in the form of a variable-resistance or a variable-flow valve. This is the technologic challenge remaining in the treatment of hydrocephalus.[75]

References

1. Azzarelli B, Rekate HL, Roessmann NW: Subependymoma: A case report with ultrastructural study. Acta Neuropathol 40:297, 1977.
2. Badell-Ribera A, Shulman K, Paddock N: The relationship of non-progressive hydrocephalus to intellectual functioning in children with spina bifida cystica. Pediatrics 37:787, 1960.
3. Blumenthal I, MacMillan M, Costalos C: Lumbar puncture in transient hydrocephalus: Letter to the Editor. Lancet 1:756, 1976.
4. Braley S: The silicones as subdural engineering materials. Ann NY Acad Sci 146:148, 1968.
5. Carmel PW, Antunes JL, Hilal SK, et al: Dandy-Walker syndrome: Clinico-pathological features and re-evaluation of modes of treatment. Surg Neurol 8:132, 1977.
6. Collada M, Kott J, Kline DG: Documentation of fourth ventricle entrapment by metrizamide ventriculography with CT scanning: Report of two cases. J Neurosurg 55:838, 1981.
7. Dandy WE: Extirpation of the choroid plexus of the lateral ventricle in communicating hydrocephalus. Ann Surg 68:569, 1918.
8. Dandy WE: Diagnosis and treatment of strictures of aqueduct of Sylvius (causing hydrocephalus). Arch Surg 51:1, 1945.
9. Dandy WE, Blackfan KD: Internal hydrocephalus. An experimental, clinical and pathological study. Am J Dis Child 8:406, 1914.
10. Davidson RI: Peritoneal bypass in the treatment of hydrocephalus: Historical review and abdominal complications. J Neurol Neurosurg Psychiatry 39:640, 1976.
11. Entzian W, Szepan B, Wappenschmidt J, et al: The so-called Dandy-Walker syndrome: Comments on morphologic, di-

agnostic and therapeutic problems. Monogr Neural Sci 8:215, 1982.
12. Epstein F: Diagnosis and management of arrested hydrocephalus. Monogr Neural Sci 8:105, 1982.
13. Epstein FJ: How to keep shunts functioning, or "The Impossible Dream." Clin Neurosurg 32:608, 1985.
14. Epstein FJ, Fleischer AS, Hochwald GM, et al: Subtemporal craniectomy for recurrent shunt obstruction secondary to small ventricles. J Neurosurg 41:29, 1974.
15. Epstein F, Hochwald G, Ransohoff J: Neonatal hydrocephalus treated by compressive head wrapping. Lancet 1:634, 1973.
16. Epstein FJ, Hochwald GM, Wald A: Avoidance of shunt dependency in hydrocephalus. Dev Med Child Neurol 17:71, 1975.
17. Foltz E: The first seven years of a hydrocephalus project. In: Shulman K (ed): Workshop in Hydrocephalus. Philadelphia, University of Pennsylvania, 1965, pp 79–14.
18. Foltz EL, DeFeo DR: Double compartment hydrocephalus—a new clinical entity. Neurosurgery 7:551, 1980.
19. Foltz EL, Shurtleff DB: Five-year comparative study of hydrocephalus in children with and without operation (113) cases. J Neurosurg 20:1064, 1963.
20. Foltz EL, Shurtleff DB: Conversion of communicating hydrocephalus to stenosis or occlusion of the aqueduct during ventricular shunt. J Neurosurg 24:520, 1966.
21. Garrity L, Servos A: Comparison of measures of adaptive behavior in pre-school children. J Consult Clin Psychol 46:228, 1978.
22. Ghajar JB: A guide for ventricular catheter placement: Technical note. J Neurosurg 63:985, 1985.
23. Goldstein GW, Chaplin ER, Maitland J: Transient hydrocephalus in premature infants: Treatment by lumbar punctures. Lancet 1:512, 1976.
24. Hall P, Lindseth R, Campbell R, et al: Scoliosis and hydrocephalus in myelocele patients: The effects of ventricular shunting. J Neurosurg 50:174, 1979.
25. Harrison HR, Reynolds AF: Trapped fourth ventricle in coccidioidal meningitis. Surg Neurol 17:197, 1982.
26. Hawkins JC, Hoffman HJ, Humphreys RP: Isolated fourth ventricle as a complication of ventricular shunting: Report of three cases. J Neurosurg 49:910, 1978.
27. Hayden PW, Foltz EL, Shurtleff DB: Effect of an oral osmotic agent on ventricular fluid pressure of hydrocephalic children. Pediatrics 41:955, 1968.
28. Hemmer R: Can a shunt be removed? Monogr Neural Sci 8:227, 1982.
29. Hirsch JF, Kahn AP, Renier D, et al: The Dandy-Walker malformation: A review of 40 cases. J Neurosurg 61:515, 1984.
30. Hoffman HJ, Hendrick EB, Humphreys RP: New lumboperitoneal shunt for communicating hydrocephalus. J Neurosurg 44:258, 1976.
31. Holtzer GJ, De Lange SA: Shunt-independent arrest of hydrocephalus. J Neurosurg 39:698, 1973.
32. Hyde-Rowan MD, Rekate HL, Nulsen FE: Reexpansion of previously collapsed ventricles: The slit ventricle syndrome. J Neurosurg 56:536, 1982.
33. James HE, Kaiser G, Schut L, et al: Problems of diagnosis and treatment in the Dandy-Walker syndrome. Child's Brain 5:24, 1979.
34. Kaufman B: Revision of ventriculoatrial shunt by transfemoral cannulation of neck veins. Presented at The Pediatric Section, AANS Meeting, Cleveland, Ohio, Dec. 1977.
35. Kaufman HH: Comments on lysis of intraventricular blood clot with urokinase in a canine model. Part 3. Effects of intraventricular urokinase on clot lysis and posthemorrhagic hydrocephalus. Neurosurgery 19:572, 1986.
36. Kushner J, Alexander E, Davis CH, et al: Kyphoscoliosis following lumbar subarachnoid shunts. J Neurosurg 34:783, 1971.
37. Laurence KM: Neurological and intellectual sequelae of hydrocephalus. Arch Neurol 20:73, 1974.
38. Lewin R: Is your brain really necessary? Science 210:1232, 1980.
39. Lorber J: Isosorbide in the medical treatment of infantile hydrocephalus. J Neurosurg 39:702, 1973.
40. Lourie H, Shende MC, Krawchenko J, et al: Trapped fourth ventricle: A report of two unusual cases. Neurosurgery 7:279, 1980.
41. Manwaring KH, Pittman HW, Tarby TJ, et al: New techniques in the investigation and management of post-hemorrhagic hydrocephalus. BNI Q 1:24, 1985.
42. Mapstone TB, Rekate HL, Nulsen FE, et al: The relationship of CSF shunting and IQ in children with myelomeningocele: Retrospective analysis. Child's Brain 11:112, 1984.
43. Marlin AE: Protection of the cortical mantle in premature infants with posthemorrhagic hydrocephalus. Neurosurgery 7:464, 1980.
44. Matson DD: The treatment of hydrocephalus. Surg Clin North Am 34:1021, 1954.
45. Matson DD: Current treatment of infantile hydrocephalus. N Engl J Med 255:933, 1956.
46. Matson DD: Prenatal obstruction of the fourth ventricle. Am J Roentgenol 76:499, 1956.
47. McLone DA, Killian M, Yogeb R: Ventriculitis: Of mice and men. In: Raimondi A (ed): Concepts in Pediatric Neurosurgery, Vol. 2. New York, S Karger, 1982, p 112.
48. McComb JG, Ramos AD, Platzker AC, et al: Management of hydrocephalus secondary to intraventricular hemorrhage in the preterm infant with a subcutaneous ventricular catheter reservoir. Neurosurgery 13:295, 1983.
49. McLone DG: Effect of complications on intellectual function in 173 children with myelomeningocele. Child's Brain 5:A561, 1979.
50. McLone DG, Czyzewski D, Raimondi AJ, et al: Central nervous system infections as a limiting factor in the intelligence of children with myelomeningocele. Pediatrics 70:338, 1982.
51. Mealey J, Barket DT: Failure of oral acetazolamide to avert hydrocephalus in infants with myelomeningocele. J Pediatr 72:257, 1968.
52. Milhorat TH: Hydrocephalus and the Cerebrospinal Fluid. Baltimore, Williams & Wilkins, 1972, p 237.
53. Milhorat TH: Failure of choroid plexectomy as treatment for hydrocephalus. Surg Gynecol Obstet 139:505, 1974.
54. Milhorat TH, Hammock MK, Chien T, et al: Normal rate of cerebrospinal fluid production five years after bilateral choroid plexectomy. J Neurosurg 44:735, 1976.
55. Milhorat TH, Hammock MK, Fenstermacher JD, et al: Cerebrospinal fluid production by the choroid plexus and brain. Science 173:330, 1971.
56. Mori K, Raimondi AJ: An analysis of external ventricular drainage as a treatment for infected shunts. Child's Brain 1:243, 1975.
57. Nulsen FE, Becker DP: Control of hydrocephalus by valve-regulated shunt: Infections and their prevention. Clin Neurosurg 14:256, 1967.
58. Nulsen FE, Becker DP: Control of hydrocephalus by valve-regulated shunt. J Neurosurg 26:361, 1967.
59. Nulsen FE, Rekate HL: Results of treatment for hydrocephalus as a guide to future management. In Pediatric Neurosurgery: Surgery of the Developing Nervous System. New York, Grune & Stratton, 1982, pp 239–241.
60. Nulsen FE, Rekate HL, Leung A, et al: Telemetry intracranial pressure monitoring in children. In: Paraicz E (ed): ICP in Infancy and Childhood (Monographs in Paediatrics, Vol. 15). Basel, S Karger, 1982, pp 17–21.
61. Nulsen FE, Spitz EB: Treatment of hydrocephalus by direct shunt from ventricles to jugular vein. Surg Form 2:399, 1952.
62. Pang D, Sclabassi RR, Horton JA: Lysis of intraventricular blood clot with urokinase in a canine model. Part 1. Canine intraventricular blood cast model. Neurosurgery 19:540, 1986.
63. Pang D, Sclabassi R, Horton JA: Lysis of intraventricular blood clot with urokinase in a canine model. Part 2. In vivo safety study of intraventricular urokinase. Neurosurgery 19:547, 1986.
64. Pang D, Sclabassi R, Horton JA: Lysis of intraventricular blood clot with urokinase in a canine model. Part 3. Effects

of intraventricular urokinase on clot lysis and posthemorrhagic hydrocephalus. Neurosurgery 19:553, 1986.
65. Pollay M, Davson H: The passage of certain substances out of the cerebrospinal fluid. Brain 86:137, 1963.
66. Portnoy HD: Treatment of hydrocephalus. In: Pediatric Neurosurgery: Surgery of the Developing Nervous System. New York, Grune & Stratton, 1982, pp 229–241.
67. Portnoy HD, Schulte RR, Fox JL, et al: Antisiphon and reversible occlusion valves for shunting in hydrocephalus and preventing post shunt subdural hematomas. J Neurosurg 38:729, 1973.
68. Portnoy HD, Tripp L, Croissant PD: Hydrodynamics of shunt valves. Child's Brain 2:242, 1976.
69. Pudenz RH: The surgical treatment of hydrocephalus: An historical review. Surg Neurol 15:15, 1981.
70. Putnam TJ: Results of treatment of hydrocephalus by endoscopic coagulation of the choroid plexus. Arch Pediatr 52:676, 1935.
71. Raimondi AJ, Samuelson G, Yarzagaray L, et al: Atresia of the foramina of Luschka and Magendie: The Dandy-Walker cyst. J Neurosurg 31:202, 1969.
72. Ransohoff J: Ventriculopleural anastomosis in treatment of midline obstructional neoplasms. J Neurosurg 11:295, 1954.
73. Ransohoff J, Shulman K, Fishman RA: Hydrocephalus. J Pediatr 56:399, 1960.
74. Reigel D: Changes in the subdural space following cerebral spinal fluid shunts. In: Raimondi AJ (ed): Concepts in Pediatric Neurosurgery, Vol. 3. New York, S Karger, 1983, p 145.
75. Rekate HL: Closed loop control of intracranial pressure. Ann Biomed Eng 8:515, 1980.
76. Rekate HL: To shunt or not to shunt: Hydrocephalus and dysraphism. Clin Neurosurg 32:593, 1985.
77. Rekate HL, Nulsen FE, Mack HL, et al: Establishing the diagnosis of shunt independence. Monogr Neural Sci 8:223, 1982.
78. Rekate HL, Ruch T, Nulsen FE: Diphtheroid infections of cerebrospinal fluid shunts: The changing pattern of shunt infection in Cleveland. J Neurosurg 52:553, 1980.
79. Rekate HL, Yonas H, White RJ, et al: The acute abdomen in patients with ventriculoperitoneal shunts. Surg Neurol 11:442, 1979.
80. Rubin RC, Henderson ES, Ommaya AK, et al: The production of cerebrospinal fluid in man and its modification by acetazolamide. J Neurosurg 25:430, 1966.
81. Salmon JH: Puncture porencephaly: Pathogenesis and prevention. Am J Dis Child 114:72, 1967.
82. Sayers MP, Kosnick EJ: Percutaneous third ventriculostomy: Experience and technique. Child's Brain 2:24, 1976.
83. Scarff JE: The treatment of non-obstructive (communicating) hydrocephalus by endoscopic cauterization of the choroid plexuses. J Neurosurg 33:1, 1970.
84. Schain RJ: Carbonic anhydrase inhibitors in chronic infantile hydrocephalus. Am J Dis Child 117:621, 1969.
85. Schoenbaum SC, Gardner P, Shullito J: Infections of cerebrospinal fluid shunts: Epidemiology, clinical manifestations, and therapy. J Infect Dis 131:543, 1975.
86. Selman WR, Spetzler RF, Wilson CB, et al: Percutaneous lumboperitoneal shunt: Review of 130 cases. Neurosurgery 6:255, 1980.
87. Shinner S, Gammon K, Bergman EW, et al: Management of hydrocephalus in infancy: Use of acetazolamide and furosemide to avoid cerebrospinal fluid shunts. J Pediatr 107:31, 1985.
88. Smith JA, Lee RE, Middleton RG: Ventriculoureteral shunt for hydrocephalus without nephrectomy. J Urol 123:224, 1980.
89. Stein SC, Apfel S: A non-invasive approach to quantitative measurement of flow through CSF shunts. Technical note. J Neurosurg 54:556, 1981.
90. Torkildsen A: A new palliative operation in cases of inoperable occlusion of the sylvian aqueduct. Acta Chir Scand 82:117, 1939.
91. Venes JL: Control of shunt infection: Report of 150 consecutive cases. J Neurosurg 45:311, 1976.
92. Weiss SR, Raskind R: Twenty-two cases of hydrocephalus treated with a Silastic ventriculoperitoneal shunt. Int Surg 51:13, 1969.
93. Young HF, Nulsen FE, Weiss MH, et al: The relationship of intelligence and cerebral mantle in treated infantile hydrocephalus. J Pediatr 52:38, 1973.

15
VENTRICULAR SHUNTS: COMPLICATIONS AND RESULTS

Robert L. McLaurin, M.D.

COMPLICATIONS

The history of the evolution of ventricular shunting for hydrocephalus in largely a history of efforts to prevent or treat the complications of shunting. Until such time as pharmacologic control of cerebrospinal fluid (CSF) production is achieved, the treatment of hydrocephalus will necessarily rely mainly on the establishment of artificial conduits for the venting of CSF from the ventricular system. Such devices have been fraught with mechanical and biologic complications. This chapter attempts to summarize these untoward occurrences.

Complications Common to All Types of Shunts

Malfunction

The most common complication of a ventricular shunt, regardless of the terminus, is mechanical malfunction of the shunt system. Malfunction may be the result of either obstruction or disconnection of the component parts of a shunt system. Obstruction may occur at the proximal (ventricular) end, within the pumping device or valve, or at the distal end.

There have been several reviews of the complications occurring in sizable series of shunts. The largest series reported to date is that of Forrest and Cooper,[11] which included 455 cases of ventriculoatrial (VA) shunts in which 520 revisions were performed. Complications involving the proximal catheter were the most frequent, and this has been true in nearly all reported series.

Malfunction at the proximal end of the shunt may be due to disconnection, with separation of the ventricular catheter from the rest of the shunt system. This complication has become less frequent in recent years, as a result of the use of a one-piece ventricular catheter reservoir. Prior to utilization of this particular device, it was not uncommon for ventricular catheters to become disconnected and to lie free within the ventricle. There has been no report to indicate that a free catheter within the ventricle causes any harm. However, it may be noted that it is not possible to cure ventricular or shunt infections in the presence of a free-floating ventricular catheter (Fig. 15–1).

A second cause of malfunction at the ventricular end is blockage of the ventricular catheter by choroid plexus and glial tissue growing into the lumen of the ventricular catheter (Fig. 15–2). This complication can be minimized by proper placement of the ventricular catheter; the tip of the catheter should be placed sufficiently far anteriorly in the lateral ventricle so that it is beyond the anterior extent of the choroid plexus. Ideally, the tip of the ventricular catheter, therefore, should be anterior to the foramen of Monro.

A third cause of proximal shunt failure is the catheter tip becoming embedded in the periventricular ependymal and neural tissue. This may occur from improper placement of the catheter initially or from collapse of the ventricle as a result

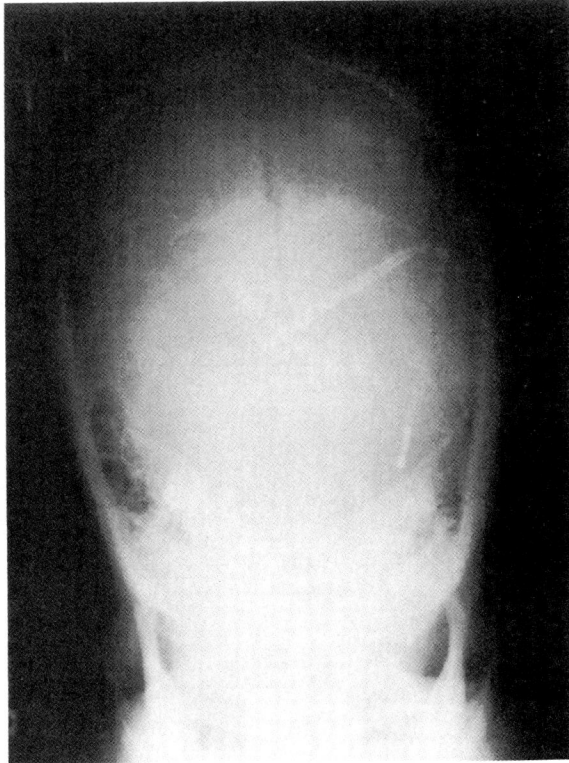

Figure 15–1. A free-floating catheter within the shunted ventricular system. It was essential to remove the catheter in order to cure the shunt infection.

of decompression. Intermittent obstruction in the "slit-ventricle" syndrome (see following) may precede permanent blockage of an embedded catheter tip.

Malfunctions involving the valve and pumping device have been quite few in nearly all reported series. Incompetence of a valve may allow retro-

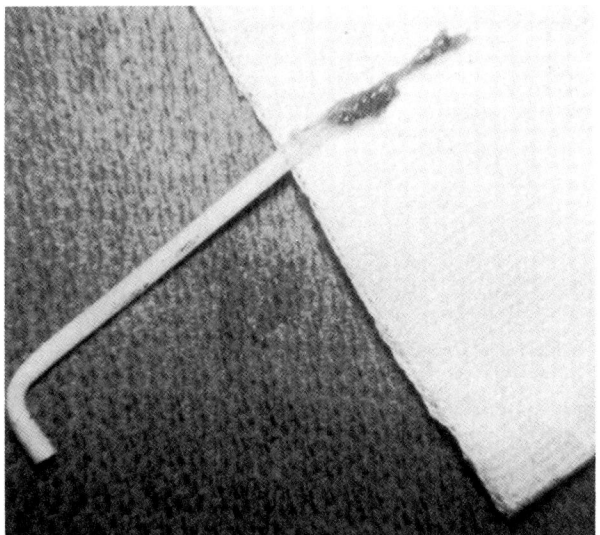

Figure 15–2. Ventricular catheter removed because of malfunction. Adherent choroid plexus had grown through multiple openings and had obstructed the catheter lumen.

grade blood flow, with clotting and occlusion in a vascular shunt. It is fortunate that such valve incompetence is quite rare and generally can be detected prior to insertion of the valve by meticulous testing at the time of surgery. The hazard of retrograde incompetence is considerably less in the presence of peritoneal shunting than it was previously, when vascular shunts were used more commonly.

Although there has been concern generally about the effect of the high protein content of the CSF on valve function, it is noteworthy that no definite relationship has been substantiated. This writer has seen several instances of CSF protein levels in excess of 1000 mg% with no apparent effect on the functional integrity of the shunt system.

Malfunction relating to the distal part of the shunt also may be attributed to disconnection, to migration, or to blockage at the distal end. Obstruction at the distal end within the vascular system or the peritoneal cavity is considered in more detail in subsequent sections of this chapter. Disconnection may occur at the site of attachment of the distal catheter to the lower end of the pumping device or at the site of a more distal connection. Raimondi and colleagues[30] have advocated the use of a one-piece shunt and reported the complications occurring in 357 patients have peritoneal shunts. Of these, 161 had a one-piece shunt and 196 a three-piece shunt. The complications were fewer in those with the one-piece shunt, and this difference was partially attributable to the lack of problems caused by disconnection. Distal shunt tubing can migrate from the peritoneal cavity or vascular compartment, and the direction of migration is generally toward the ventricular end of the shunt system (Fig. 15–3).

Several diagnostic procedures have been advocated to determine the functional status of a shunt system. Evans and associates[9] describe the use of valvography employing a water-soluble contrast medium instilled directly into the shunt system. With this method, patency of the distal end of the shunt could be seen directly on injection, and reflux into the ventricular system also could be visualized. The authors noted that no instances of false-positive valvograms were encountered, but occasional false-negative results were obtained. A similar type of shuntogram has been described,[31] using radionuclides injected directly into the shunt system and followed by scintillation scanning in its passage distally in the shunt system.

Infection

Infection constitutes the second most frequent type of shunt complication. Two types of shunt infection can be delineated. The first is an infection occurring primarily on the external surface of the shunt, involving the subcutaneous soft tissues. This may appear as an acute sepsis shortly after the insertion of a shunt system, accompanied by inflammation at the site of insertion and evidence of

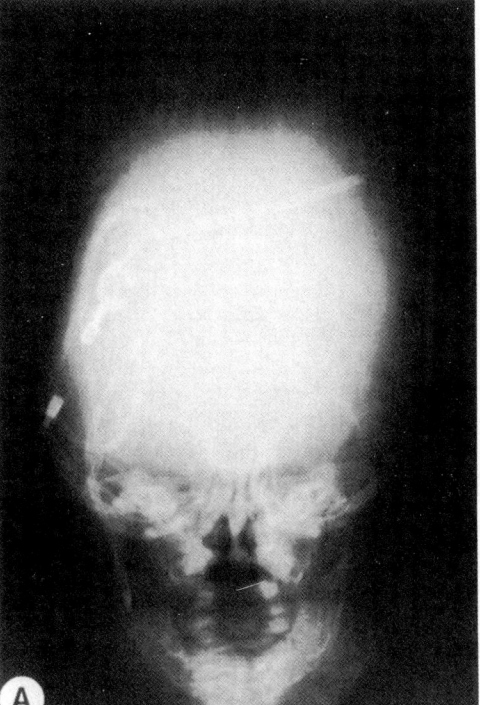
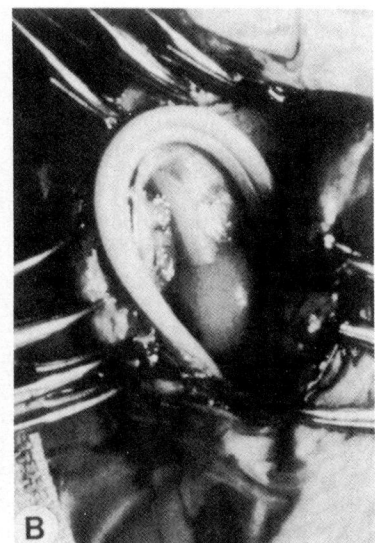

Figure 15-3. *A*, X-ray appearance of a peritoneal catheter that has migrated and become coiled beneath the scalp. *B*, Operative appearance of coiled shunt.

infection spreading along the entire length of the shunt, detectable as a reddened, hyperthermic streak along the course of the subcutaneous shunt tubing. The patient shows the usual systemic signs of acute infection.

A delayed form of the external infection may occur as a result of necrosis of the skin overlying the shunting device. This complication may be prevented by the use of low-profile reservoirs and pumping devices and by the proper placement of the shunt apparatus. The ventricular insertion and the pumping device should be sufficiently posterior so that the device is not directly at the site of maximum prominence and pressure when the infant's head is lying on that side. Excessive weight of the enlarged head and the delicate attenuated skin of the hydrocephalic scalp likewise contribute to such a problem. Embedding the rigid metallic portion of a shunting device in the outer skull table may be useful in preventing pressure against the overlying scalp, which may lead to decubitus ulceration.

The second principal type of infection is one that is primarily within the shunt system. Since it is usually the result of a less virulent organism, this type of infection generally is not associated with evidence of acute inflammation. The infection is one of the CSF, but usually there is no acute inflammation of the ventricular system. The most frequent organism accounting for this type of indolent infection is *Staphylococcus epidermidis.*

Although infection may occur in either vascular or peritoneal shunts, there appears to be a greater incidence in vascular shunts, and additionally the consequences of infection are greater in this type of shunt system. Little and coworkers,[22] in an attempt to compare the complications occurring in peritoneal and vascular shunts, noted that infection was a much greater problem in the latter group. The comparison included 37 patients in each group, and infection occurred in 15 vascular shunts and in only four peritoneal shunts. Keucher and Mealey,[20] in a more recent effort to compare the two principal types of shunts, found no significant difference between vascular and peritoneal shunts in relation to the case infection rate or the operative infection rate. However, there were significant differences in other respects. Vascular shunts led to septicemia and bacteremia with renal damage, endocarditis, and septic emboli. Peritoneal shunt infections led only to malfunction of the distal catheter. Moreover, the continuous presence of the catheter within the blood stream in vascular shunts led to its repeated exposure to transient bacteremias. For this reason, the authors concluded that infections in peritoneal shunts were more closely related to the time of shunt surgery, whereas infection in vascular shunts might occur at any subsequent time, as a result of bacteremia. The infection rate was 7 percent in both vascular and peritoneal shunts.

A specific complication of low-grade shunt infection is shunt nephritis. This has occurred primarily in the course of vascular shunt infection, although it has been reported to occur also in the presence of an indolent peritoneal shunt infection. The renal lesion results from glomerular deposition of immune complexes composed of antigen derived from the infecting organism, antibody, and complement

Table 15–1. ANTIBIOTICS FOR CSF SHUNT INFECTIONS—RECOMMENDATIONS FOR EMPIRIC THERAPY*

Organism	Intrashunt	Systemic
Staphylococcus epidermidis	Vancomycin	Rifampin plus trimethoprim/sulfamethoxazole (oral) or Vancomycin (IV)
Staphylococcus aureus	Same	Same
Enterococci	Vancomycin plus gentamicin	Vancomycin
Other streptococci		
Penicillin MIC ≤0.1	Gentamicin	Penicillin G (IV)
Penicillin MIC ≥0.2	Same as enterococcus	
Aerobic gram-negative rods	Gentamicin	Cefotaxime
Diphtheroids	Vancomycin	Vancomycin
		Trimethoprim/sulfamethoxazole (oral is susceptible)

*These recommendations are intended as starting recommendations based on culture results. Susceptibility testing might indicate changes in therapy, especially for streptococci, aerobic gram-negative organisms, and diphtheroids.

components. The result is a nephritis characterized by proteinuria and hematuria. Shunt nephritis is a rare but serious complication that fortunately responds favorably to the elimination of infection, indicating that the renal changes are generally reversible.[40]

The treatment of shunt infection has been the subject of differences of opinion over several years. The concept of removal of a foreign body in the presence of infection has been an accepted principle of management of infections in all parts of the body, and this principle has been followed in the management of shunt infections by removal of the shunting device, followed by appropriate antibiotic therapy. However, it has been demonstrated that in many instances, shunt infection can be cured without removal of the foreign body, by administration of a high concentration of antibiotics to the CSF compartment.

Experience has indicated that infection of vascular shunts can be successfully treated without removal of the shunts in about 75 percent of cases.[12] The treatment consists of intensive intraventricular and systemic antibiotics, based on bactericidal concentrations of the appropriate antibiotics and employment of frequent monitoring of the CSF levels. It must be recalled that since no immune mechanisms, leukocytes or antibodies, are present in the CSF in low-grade shunt infections, it is necessary to achieve bactericidal, rather than inhibitory, titers. Table 15–1 shows the recommended antibiotics for CSF shunt infections, and Table 15–2 lists the suggested dosages.

Peritoneal shunt infections present a unique problem, since the peritoneum has a strong tendency to wall off infection, resulting in loculated cystic pools around the terminus of infected peritoneal catheters. For this reason, it is usually necessary to remove the peritoneal portion of the shunt. If an attempt is to be made to preserve the remaining part of the shunt, as can be successfully done in about 90 percent of patients, the peritoneal catheter may be externalized and later replaced with a fresh catheter, after sterilization of the proximal portion of the shunt.[23]

Prevention of shunt infection is, of course, preferable to treatment, and several specific factors should be noted. Venes[39] has emphasized the importance of skin preparation for the shunting procedure and, by utilizing this meticulous skin preparation, was able to reduce the incidence of shunt infection to 7 percent. It should also be noted that the same type of skin preparation is necessary when tapping of the ventricular system or the shunt is performed, to prevent introduction of skin organisms by that procedure. Nulsen and Becker[25] have emphasized the higher incidence of shunt infection when the distal end of a vascular shunt is below the level of the seventh dorsal vertebra. This relationship, however, has not been borne out by other observers.

Finally, the use of prophylactic antibiotics at the

Table 15–2. DOSAGES OF RECOMMENDED ANTIBACTERIAL DRUGS*

Antibiotic	Route	Children	Newborns	Expected Peak Serum Levels	Expected Trough CSF Levels
Vancomycin	Intravenous	15 mg/kg/8 hr	15 mg/kg/12 hr	20–40 μg/ml	
Gentamicin		2.5 mg/kg/8 hr	2.5 mg/kg/12 hr	5–10 μg/ml	
Cefotaxime		30 mg/kg/4 hr	50 mg/kg/12 hr	70–100 μg/ml	
Rifampin	Oral	10 mg/kg/12 hr		Sulfamethoxazole 75–150 μg/ml	
Trimethoprim/sulfamethoxazole		5 mg/kg/8 hr			
Vancomycin	Intrashunt	20 mg daily	10 mg daily		10 μg/ml
Gentamicin		8 mg daily	8 mg daily		4 μg/ml

*Drug dosages should be modified according to measured serum and CSF levels.

time of insertion or revision of a shunt has been advocated by some individuals and questioned by others. In general, though, the trend has been toward the use of prophylactic antibiotics, and in the author's experience, such a regimen has reduced the incidence of infection to less than 5 percent. However, it is recognized that other factors, such as the use of computerized tomography (CT) scanning or ultrasonography rather than ventriculography, also may have contributed to this reduced rate of infection.

Overdrainage

The third most frequent category of shunt complications includes those resulting from overdrainage of CSF from the intracranial cavity. Three such complications are described.

Slit-Ventricle Syndrome. This complication, though recognized for nearly two decades, has defied agreement concerning diagnosis, pathophysiology, and treatment. Clinically, it is characterized by intermittent episodes resembling shunt malfunction, with symptoms including headache, vomiting, lethargy, and occasionally extraocular disturbances. However, the CT scan, instead of revealing ventriculomegaly, demonstrates very small slit-like ventricles (Fig. 15–4). One explanation for this syndrome is based on a concept that the ventricles collapse around the ventricular catheter, causing temporary blockage until there is sufficient ventricular dilatation to allow drainage and consequent relief of symptoms. The overdrainage of CSF is thought to

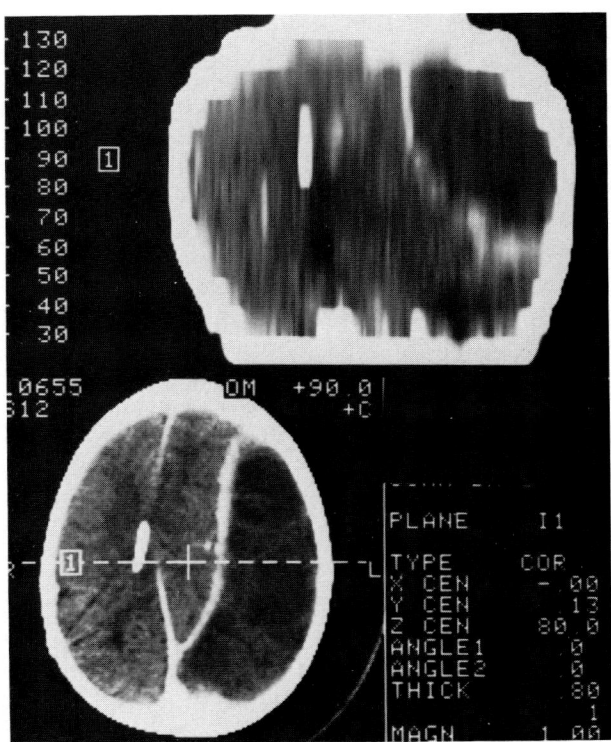

Figure 15–5. Axial and reconstructed coronal CT scans of a nine-year-old girl, showing chronic subdural hematoma with enhancing inner membrane that followed ventriculoperitoneal shunting.

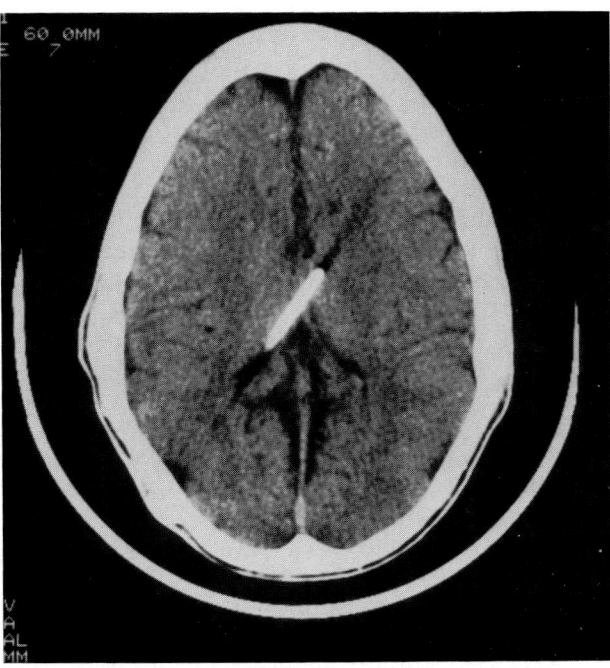

Figure 15–4. A 16-year-old boy with intermittent episodes of headache, vomiting, and ataxia, whose shunt had been placed seven years earlier (i.e., slit-ventricle syndrome). The symptoms were relieved by insertion of an anti-siphon device.

be due to the siphoning effect of a peritoneal catheter, as the syndrome occurs principally in children who have assumed the upright posture.

The treatment of this complication has stimulated a diversity of recommendations. Portnoy and colleagues[29] described a device that prevents flow through a shunt when a negative pressure of 100 to 200 mm H$_2$O is exerted at the outlet of the device. This, in effect, counteracts the siphoning action of the hydrostatic pressure of a fluid column between the head and the abdominal cavity. Epstein and associates[8] advocated subtemporal craniectomy to decompress intracranial contents and allow ventricular dilatation. Salmon[33] advised upgrading the valve resistance. The author's experience has indicated that inserting an anti-siphon device and upgrading the valve resistance simultaneously relieves the symptoms of the slit-ventricle syndrome in most instances, although it is not necessarily accompanied by visible change in the ventricular size, as seen on CT scan.

Subdural Accumulations. Subdural hematomas and effusions have been a recognized complication of successful shunting of hydrocephalic patients, but it is significant that this complication only rarely exhibits clinical manifestations. Unilateral subdural accumulations may cause focal neurologic deficit resulting from shift of the intracranial structures (Fig. 15–5). More often, however, bilateral and rather symmetric effusions may be present without clinical evidence. The existence of such accumulations has become increasingly apparent since the advent of CT scanning. It appears likely that subdural effusions are frequently a manifestation of the existence of a craniocephalic disproportion and that no specific treatment is necessary in most instances.

Craniosynostosis. Craniosynostosis has been reported as a complication of shunting. Anderson[2] reported three such instances, two of which occurred in patients with associated myelomeningocele, and the third in a patient treated for aqueductal stenosis. In addition to premature closure of the sutures, there was a marked increase in the thickness of the skull bones. The author recommended that low-pressure valves not be used because of this particular complication. It should be noted that while this complication may have some cosmetic effect, there has been no definite indication that it restricts brain growth in the treated hydrocephalic patient.

A rare complication of shunting has been described by Hoffman and Tucker[18] as "cephalocranial disproportion," in which there occurred cerebellar and brainstem herniation into the upper spinal canal. Six of the eight reported cases had communicating hydrocephalus treated by lumboperitoneal shunts. The symptoms included signs of lower brainstem dysfunction, and myelography and air study demonstrated tonsillar herniation. Posterior fossa decompression was carried out, with significant improvement in all patients. The authors speculate that the basic problem is that secondary craniosynostosis results from overshunting of the patients. Further normal growth of the brain then leads to a cephalocranial disproportion, and this in turn leads to herniation downward as the brain volume exceeds the available space.

Seizures

An increased incidence of seizures has been recognized in shunted patients. One of the first indications of potential seizure disorder following shunting was reported by Laws and Niedermeyer,[21] who noted that 15 of 18 patients with shunts had electroencephalogram (EEG) abnormalities. Lateralization of the abnormality was to the right hemisphere in 11 patients. In a comparative group of infants with hydrocephalus and no shunting, there was a high incidence of normal traces and no significant lateralization. The matter was pursued further by Graebner and Celesia,[14] who also compared a group of shunted hydrocephalic patients with a nonshunted group. There was a higher incidence of abnormal records in the shunted group and focal paroxysmal discharges were seen much more frequently in the shunted patients. In addition, there was an incidence of clinical seizures in 48 percent of the shunted group and 20 percent of the nonshunted group. Ines and Markand[19] later evaluated a large series of hydrocephalic patients for EEG abnormalities and seizures; in 65 patients with right-sided shunts, there were 22 patients with grand mal seizures and 6 patients with other minor seizures. The authors noted that the majority of seizures began within four years after placement of the shunt.

Another recent report was that of Varfis and associates,[38] who noted that 19 of 29 shunted hydrocephalic patients developed an epileptogenic focus and that during a follow-up period of four years, 17 of the 19 patients experienced clinical seizures. By observing serial EEGs, it was found that the irritative abnormalities occurred usually during the second year after surgery and that a slow wave pattern usually preceded the occurrence of the irritative abnormality. It was further noted that myelomeningocele patients had the lowest incidence of epilepsy, while the highest incidence occurred in paients with hydrocephalus resulting from cerebral hemorrhage. The authors also concluded that the younger the patient at the time of surgery, the greater the chance of developing an epileptogenic scar.

It must be concluded that the incidence of EEG abnormality and seizure activity is sufficiently high after shunting to indicate some routine evaluation of this potential complication. Routine use of anticonvulsant therapy is probably not necessary, except in the high-risk groups (e.g., cerebral hemorrhage, porencephalic cyst), but serial observation of EEGs during the first few years after shunting is indicated so that anticonvulsant therapy can be used if an irritative focus occurs.

Complications Unique to Vascular Shunts

The complications that are unique to ventriculovascular shunts fall into two principal groups, cardiac and pulmonary. Although the incidence of such complications is difficult to determine, their severity has led to preference, in most instances, for the use of peritoneal shunting.

The following cardiac complications have been reported: (1) mural thrombosis occurring in the right atrium or extending into the atrium from the superior or inferior vena cava; (2) bacterial endocarditis; (3) cardiac arrhythmias, which have been attributed to irritation by the distal catheter; (4) cardiac tamponade resulting from perforation of the right atrium by the distal shunt catheter; and (5) detachment of distal shunt tubing remaining in the heart, or embolization to the pulmonary arteries.

Emery and Hilton[7] reported the necropsy findings on 15 patients with vascular shunts. In every instance, the catheter entering the heart was surrounded by fibrinous material extending for various distances into the auricle. Attached to the end of the fibrinous collar were masses of fibrinous clot. On one occasion, the tricuspid valve was obstructed by such a clot. In 6 of the 15 cases, the wall of the right atrium contained vegetation that was probably the result of trauma.

The existence of clots within the atrium may not produce any specific manifestations until emboli occur in the pulmonary vascular system. Therefore, the first indication of the existence of such a problem may be either a malfunction of the distal end of the shunt or irreversible secondary changes resulting from pulmonary hypertension. The presence of a detached catheter lying within the cardiac chambers may be correctable by retrieval, under radiographic control, through the inferior venous drainage system (Fig. 15–6).[36]

Obstruction of the venous system above the heart is another vascular complication that only rarely proceeds to a symptomatic state. Obstruction of the superior vena cava has occurred infrequently but results in the characteristic evidence of blockage of the venous drainage from the head and neck. It may be noted that the distal shunt catheter introduced into the jugular vein may become misdirected into the subclavian vein rather than progressing toward the atrium. Again, it is possible in many instances to redirect the catheter under radiographic control, by manipulation performed via the inferior venous system.[36]

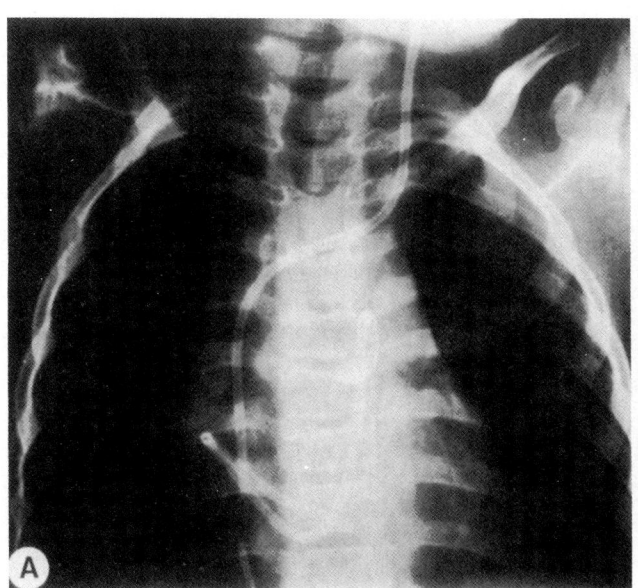
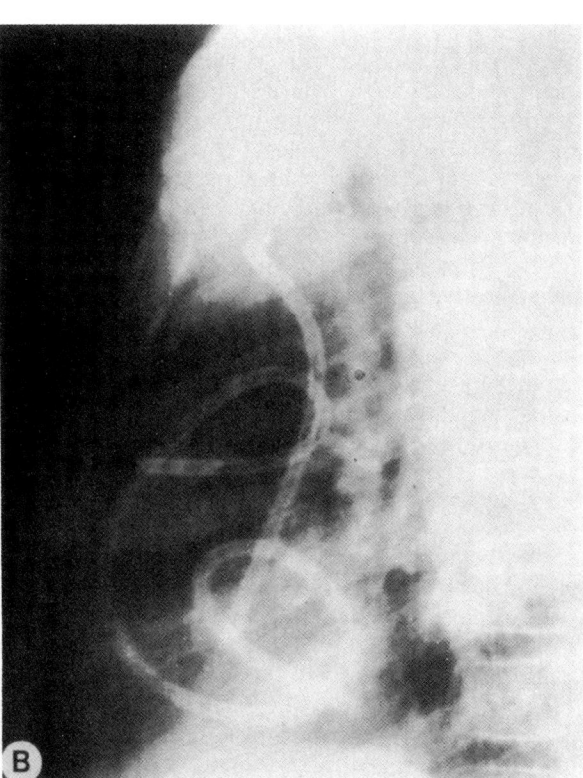
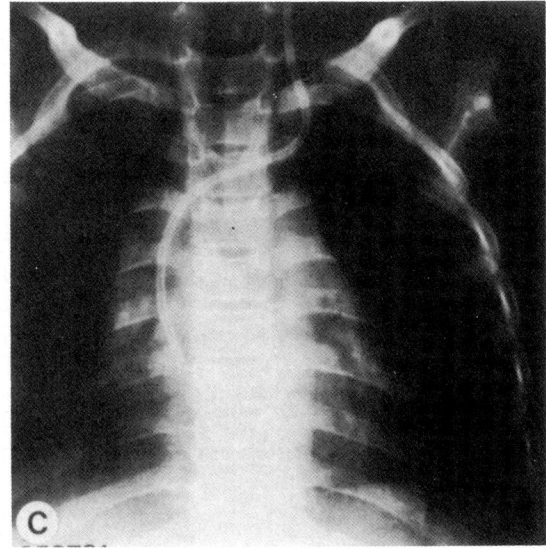

Figure 15–6. *A*, Left ventriculoatrial (VA) shunt in proper position. Embolized right VA shunt is coiled in the heart, with the distal end in the main pulmonary artery. *B*, Lateral view of same. *C*, Following removal of embolized shunt tubing by transvenous retrieval.

The most consistent vascular complication consists of emboli in the pulmonary system. Emery and Hilton[7] found pulmonary emboli in all but 1 of 15 patients studied at necropsy. The emboli varied markedly in size but in the majority of instances had completely occupied and obstructed small arteries. In many instances, there was no edema or cellular infiltration of the vessel walls around the embolized vessel. Friedman and coworkers,[13] in reviewing the pulmonary vascular histology in 65 patients who had died following ventriculojugular shunting, found that approximately half of the patients had pulmonary vascular lesions. They noted that the age of the patient, composition of the tubing, location of the distal tubing, and nature of coexisting disease did not seem to influence the incidence of pulmonary thromboembolism. This is at some variance with the opinion of Nugent and colleagues,[24] who concluded that infection played a major role in the occurrence of thrombosis in their patients. They reported that most of the patients who had thromboembolic phenomena were myelomeningocele patients and had experienced repeated septicemia. Emery and Hilton[7] also noted mycotic aneurysms, periarteritis, and intimal degeneration in several of their patients.

The signs of pulmonary thromboembolism are the result of pulmonary hypertension. This includes accentuation of the second heart sound and disappearance of physiologic "splitting" of the second heart sound. The most serious consequence of pulmonary hypertension is the development of right heart failure (cor pulmonale). Although this is a rare complication of vascular shunting, it appears to represent an end state that is irreversible.

Complications Unique to Peritoneal Shunts

Intra-abdominal complications of peritoneal shunts include (1) inguinal hernia, hydrocele, or both; (2) ascites and cyst formation; (3) intestinal volvulus and obstruction; (4) perforation of a viscus or to the outside; and (5) spread of neoplasm or infection to the peritoneal cavity. An extensive review of intra-abdominal complications was made by Davidson[4] in 1976, which included a very complete bibliography up to that time.

A frequent complication of peritoneal shunts is the occurrence of inguinal hernia. Grosfeld and associates[15] noted an incidence of 16.8 percent in a series of 185 peritoneal shunts. All the patients underwent hernia repair, and bilateral hernias or patent processus vaginalis occurred in 75 percent. The authors attribute this high incidence to the fact that in most instances, shunting is performed while the processus vaginalis is still patent. The superimposed CSF in the peritoneal cavity then converts itself into a clinical hernia. Prompt surgical treatment of the inguinal hernia is recommended, and bilateral exploration seems advisable. A less common complication has been described by Scherzer.[34]

Abdominal cysts and ascites have been discussed by several authors. Fischer and Schillito,[10] on the basis of the character of the cyst wall, speculate that infection from previous abdominal procedures contributes to the occurrence of a cyst. Parry and coworkers,[28] on the other hand, describe cysts that were formed solely by intestinal serosal surfaces but no fibrous cyst wall. Although most authors believe that the occurrence of an abdominal cyst precludes re-establishment of a functioning shunt, Parry and associates[28] report instances of subsequent use of the peritoneal cavity with no sign of cyst recurrence or shunt malfunction. Two series of abdominal pseudocysts have recently been reviewed. In one series of 26 patients, infection was found in 16 (62 percent),[16] while in the other series of eight patients, there was infection in all patients.[6] Therefore, it seems reasonable to conclude that when a pseudocyst is demonstrated, it must be assumed to be due to shunt infection and should be treated accordingly (Fig. 15–7). Treatment includes removal of the peritoneal catheter. If infection is demonstrated and eradicated, the peritoneal catheter can usually be reinserted into the abdomen; if malfunction then occurs, a vascular shunt is indicated.

Surprisingly, the occurrence of intestinal volvulus and obstruction has been a rare complication. Sakoda and colleagues[32] reported the first such case in 1971, in which a single adhesive band was found in the region of the tubing, about which the volvulus had occurred.

Perforation may occur into the bowel, bladder, or vagina. Grosfeld and associates[15] reported seven instances of perforation of a viscus in 185 cases. In 1975, Schulhof and coworkers[35] reviewed the literature concerning bowel perforation and found descriptions of only 12 patients. In almost all instances, the shunt had continued to function despite the perforation. Only two of the 12 patients had evidence of peritonitis, although six patients had ventriculitis from gram-negative bacilli. Gros-

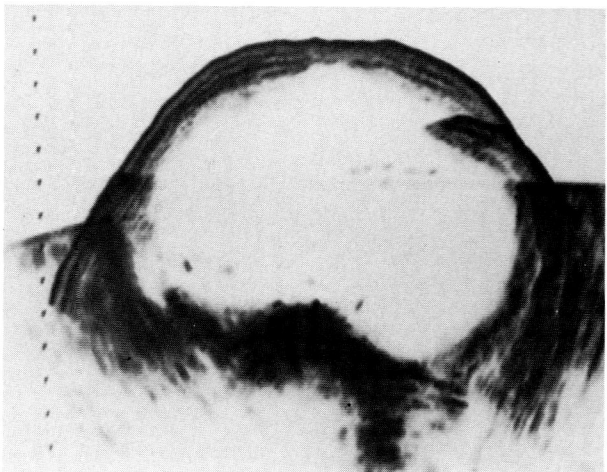

Figure 15–7. Peritoneal pseudocyst as seen by ultrasonography. This was associated with a shunt infection.

feld and associates[15] noted that four of the five patients with colon perforation were asymptomatic and were treated conservatively without femoral laparotomy or attempts at colon repair, and all survived.

Perforation of the vagina had been reported in several instances, and umbilical perforation and fistulae have also been noted.[3]

The peritoneal shunt also may act as a conduit for the spread of neoplasm when the shunt is performed as a part of the management of intracranial tumors. Hoffman and colleagues[17] have reported an incidence of approximately 10 percent of peritoneal metastases when shunting is performed in the presence of medulloblastoma. As a result of this experience, the authors have recommended the use of a Millipore filter encased in the shunt system.[17]

Comparison of Vascular and Peritoneal Shunt Complications

In recent years, there has been a definite trend toward peritoneal rather than vascular shunting. The principal reason for this has been that while the incidences of complications in the two groups may not differ significantly, the severity and consequences of the complications have been greater in the vascular shunts. A recent review by Keucher and Mealey[20] analyzed the relative incidence of complications in the two types of shunt. The series included 119 patients who had initial vascular shunts and 72 with initial peritoneal shunts. Children who survived until five years of age with uninfected vascular shunts required an average of 1.46 revisions, whereas those with uninfected peritoneal shunts averaged 1.02 revisions. Distal obstructions and prophylactic lengthening accounted for more than half of the revisions in vascular shunts. Proximal revisions were more common in peritoneal systems, while distal revisions were more common in vascular systems. Twice as many children with peritoneal shunts did not need revision as did those with vascular shunts. The authors also noted that although the infection rate was the same in vascular and peritoneal shunts, the consequences of infection were much more serious in the vascular systems. Therefore, it was concluded that peritoneal shunts required fewer revisions and the patients suffered from fewer and less serious complications. On the basis of this review and the experience of other observers, it seems reasonable to conclude that at present, peritoneal shunts should be used, if possible, whenever shunting is necessary in the treatment of hydrocephalus.

RESULTS OF TREATMENT

The results of treated hydrocephalus have been the subject of numerous reviews during the past one and a half decades, since the advent of shunting has allowed sufficient numbers to be observed over an adequate follow-up period. These reviews may be considered from the standpoints of mortality rate and intellectual development.

Mortality rate is related more to associated anomalies or diseases than to the effects of hydrocephalus. Because of the broad spectrum of associated problems, it is difficult to obtain sound figures concerning mortality. Keucher and Mealey,[20] reviewing 228 children with non-neoplastic hydrocephalus, followed for at least seven years, found a mortality rate of 19 percent for those treated with vascular shunts and 11 percent for those treated with peritoneal shunts. More recently, Amacher and Wellington[2] have reported a five-year survival rate of 93.8 percent in infantile hydrocephalus, ranging from 71 percent in patients with myelomeningoceles to 100 percent in those with post-traumatic hydrocephalus. It must be concluded that the overall mortality rate from the hydrocephalic process itself is very low.

It is equally as difficult to establish with accuracy any predictive or prospective criteria on the intellectual development of patients with infantile hydrocephalus. One of the initial efforts was made by Young and coworkers,[41] who attempted to relate intelligence to the thickness of the cerebral mantle. They analyzed 147 treated hydrocephalic patients older than three years of age. The cortical mantle was determined by bubble ventriculography. The authors concluded that in patients with pure hydrocephalus, a cerebral mantle thicker than 2.8 cm after shunting was consistent with normal development. With a cerebral mantle thinner than 2.8 cm, mental retardation was virtually ensured. It should be recognized that the cortical mantle is not that which is found before shunting, as this has no predictive value. However, the final attained mantle thickness must be the consequence of shunting before six months of age.

Nulsen and Rekate[26] later reported a follow-up carried out over a longer period that included patients in the earlier study. The results indicated that patients with mantles thinner than 2 cm were either just educable or uneducable. Patients with cerebral mantles between 2 and 3 cm exhibited IQs below 100; however, patients with mantles thicker than 3 cm had normal IQs. The implication is that successful intellectual development does not depend on shunting ventricles to a normal size, reflected by a mantle of 5 to 6 cm. The failure to achieve a mantle consistent with normal development appeared to be related to delay in shunting during infancy. Therefore, it is suggested that as hydrocephalus progresses, irreversible damage does not occur until a critical point is reached, and thereafter the damage results in poor development performance.

A more recent study based on CT scans was reported by Oberbauer.[27] A computer program based on the different densities of CSF and brain was designed, and the results expressed as brain-ventricle index (BVI). The normal BVI is 35 to 40. Hydrocephalic children ranged from 0.5 to 12.5. In the patients with initial BVIs of less than 1.5, there was little chance of normal development. However, above that level, there was poor relationship. Follow-up BVIs showed a better relationship.

Dennis and associates[5] have also reviewed in detail a series of 78 children between 5 and 15 years of age who were shunted within the first year after diagnosis of hydrocephalus. They noted that there had been uneven cognitive development reported previously, so that some studies have shown patients' language to be lacking in substantive content.[37] Other studies have shown a selective loss of visual or perceptual motor skills. These authors found that the particular etiology of hydrocephalus affected the pattern of intelligence. Children with aqueduct stenosis demonstrated lower levels of nonverbal intelligence in relation to their verbal cognitive skills than those with postnatal etiologies. It was also noted in this study that the type or number of shunts performed did not affect intelligence. It was concluded that the cognitive defects were not related to hydrocephalus but rather to other developmental brain anomalies.

To summarize the data available concerning results of treatment, it may be said that the cause of hydrocephalus, the duration of the condition prior to treatment, and the associated brain abnormalities are of greater prognostic significance than the initial ventricular size and the initial thickness of the cortical mantle.

References

1. Amacher AL, Wellington J: Infantile hydrocephalus: Long-term results of surgical therapy. Child's Brain 11:217, 1984.
2. Anderson H: Craniosynostosis as a complication after operation for hydrocephalus. Acta Paediatr Scand 55:192, 1966.
3. Antunes ACM, Riberio TR: Spontaneous umbilication fistula from ventriculoperitoneal shunt drainage. J Neurosurg 43:481, 1975.
4. Davidson RI: Peritoneal bypass in the treatment of hydrocephalus. Historical review and abdominal complications. J Neurol Neurosurg Psychiatr 39:640, 1976.
5. Dennis M, Fitz CR, Netley CT, et al: The intelligence of hydrocephalic children. Arch Neurol 38:607, 1981.
6. Egelhoff J, Babcock DS, McLaurin RL: Cerebrospinal fluid pseudocysts: Sonographic appearance and clinical management. Pediatr Neurosci 12:80, 1985–86.
7. Emery JL, Hilton HB: Lung and heart complications of the treatment of hydrocephalus by ventriculoauriculostomy. Surgery 50:309, 1966.
8. Epstein FJ, Fleischer AS, Hochwald GM, et al: Subtemporal craniectomy for recurrent shunt obstruction secondary to small ventricles. J Neurosurg 41:29, 1974.
9. Evans RC, Thomas MD, Williams LA: Shunt blockage in hydrocephalic children: The use of the valvogram. Clin Radiol 27:489, 1976.
10. Fischer EG, Shillito J, Jr.: Large abdominal cysts: A complication of peritoneal shunts. J Neurosurg 31:441, 1969.
11. Forrest DM, Cooper DGW: Complications of ventriculoatrial shunts. A review of 455 cases. J Neurosurg 29:506, 1968.
12. Frame PT, McLaurin RL: Treatment of CSF shunt infections with intrashunt plus oral antibiotic therapy. J Neurosurg 60:354, 1984.
13. Friedman S, Zita-Gozum C, Chatten J: Pulmonary vascular changes complicating ventriculovascular shunting for hydrocephalus. J Pediatr 64:305, 1964.
14. Graebner RW, Celesia GG: EEG findings in hydrocephalus and their relation to shunting procedures. Electroencephologr Clin Neurophysiol 35:517, 1973.
15. Grosfeld JL, Cooney DR, Smith J, et al: Intra-abdominal complications following ventriculoperitoneal shunt procedures. Pediatrics 54:791, 1974.
16. Hahn YS, Engelhard H, McLone DG: Abdominal CSF pseudocyst: Clinical features and surgical management. Pediatr Neurosci 12:75, 1985–86.
17. Hoffman NJ, Hendrick EB, Humphreys RP: Metastasis via ventriculoperitoneal shunt in patients with medulloblastoma. J Neurosurg 44:562, 1976.
18. Hoffman HJ, Tucker HJ: Cephalocranial disproportion. A complication of the treatment of hydrocephalus in children. Child's Brain 2:167, 1976.
19. Ines DF, Markand ON: Epileptic seizures and abnormal electroencephalographic findings in hydrocephalus and their relation to the shunting procedures. Electroencephalogr Clin Neurophysiol 42:761, 1977.
20. Keucher TR, Mealey J: Long-term results after ventriculoatrial and ventriculoperitoneal shunting for infantile hydrocephalus. J Neurosurg 50:179, 1979.
21. Laws ER, Jr., Niedermeyer E: EEG findings in hydrocephalic patients with shunt procedures. Electroencephalogr Clin Neurophysiol 29:325, 1970.
22. Little JR, Rhoton AL, Jr., Mellinger JF: Comparison of ventriculoperitoneal and ventriculoatrial shunts for hydrocephalus in children. Mayo Clin Proc 47:396, 1972.
23. McLaurin RL, Frame PT: The role of shunt externalization in the management of shunt infection. In Chapman PH (ed): Concepts in Pediatric Neurosurgery, Vol. 6. Basel, S Karger, 1985, pp 133–146.
24. Nugent GR, Lucas R, Judy M, et al: Thrombo-embolic complications of ventriculoatrial shunts. Angiocardiographic and pathologic correlations. J Neurosurg 24:34, 1966.
25. Nulsen FE, Becker DP: Control of hydrocephalus by valve-regulated shunt. J Neurosurg 26:362, 1967.
26. Nulsen FE, Rekate HL: Results of treatment for hydrocephalus as a guide to future management. In: Pediatric Neurosurgery. New York, Grune & Stratton, 1982, pp 229–241.
27. Oberbauer RW: The significance of morphological details for developmental outcome in infantile hydrocephalus. Child's Nerv Syst 1:329, 1985.
28. Parry SW, Schumacher JF, Llewellyn RC: Abdominal pseudocysts and ascites formation after ventriculoperitoneal shunt procedures. Report of four cases. J Neurosurg 43:476, 1975.
29. Portnoy HD, Schulte RR, Fox JL, et al: Anti-siphon and reversible occlusion valves for shunting in hydrocephalus and preventing postshunt subdural hematomas. J Neurosurg 38:729, 1973.
30. Raimondi AJ, Robinson JS, Kuwamura K: Complications of ventriculoperitoneal shunting and a critical comparison of the three-piece and one-piece systems. Child's Brain 3:321, 1977.
31. Rudd TG, Shurtleff DB, Loeser JD, et al: Radionuclide assessment of cerebrospinal fluid shunt function in children. J Nucl Med 14:683, 1973.
32. Sakoda TH, Maxwell JA, Brackett CE, Jr.: Intestinal volvulus secondary to a ventriculoperitoneal shunt. Case report. J Neurosurg 35:95, 1971.
33. Salmon JH: The collapsed ventricle: Management and prevention. Surg Neurol 9:349, 1978.
34. Scherzer AL: Hydrocele following placement of a ventriculoperitoneal shunt. J Pediatr 86:811, 1975.
35. Schulhof LA, Worth RM, Kalsbeck JE: Bowel perforation due

to peritoneal shunt. A report of seven cases and a review of the literature. Surg Neurol 3:265, 1975.
36. Schwartz DC, McSweeney WJ: Intravascular manipulation of ventriculoatrial shunt catheters. *In*: McLaurin R (ed): Myelomeningocele. Proceedings of a Multidisciplinary Symposium. New York, Grune & Stratton, 1976.
37. Tew B, Laurence KM: The clinical and psychological characteristics of children with the "cocktail party" syndrome. Z Kinderchir 28:360, 1979.
38. Varfis G, Berney J, Beaumanoir A: Electro-clinical follow-up of shunted hydrocephalic children. Child's Brain 3:129, 1977.
39. Venes JL: Control of shunt infection. Report of 150 consecutive cases. J Neurosurg 45:311, 1976.
40. Wald SL, McLaurin RL: Shunt-associated glomerulonephritis. Neurosurgery 3:146, 1978.
41. Young HF, Nulsen FE, Weiss MH, et al: The relationship of intelligence and cerebral mantle in treated infantile hydrocephalus (IQ potential in hydrocephalic children). Pediatrics 52:38, 1973.

16
ACQUIRED PROBLEMS OF THE NEWBORN

Charles C. Duncan, M.D.
Laura R. Ment, M.D.
Eileen Ogle, P.A.-C.

Although the development of sophisticated perinatal care has brought steady improvement in the mortality rates among small and critically ill infants, the incidence of major neurodevelopmental abnormalities in this population of patients has remained essentially unchanged over the past decade.[31, 59] Ten to 20 percent of the survivors of newborn special care have been reported to experience serious neurodevelopmental handicaps including seizures, developmental delay, and motoric problems.[55, 60, 75, 78] Therefore, increasing attention has been paid both to the early identification of affected infants, such as those with parenchymal involvement in intraventricular hemorrhage, cerebral infarction, and bacterial meningitis, who are believed to be at risk for later neurodevelopmental handicaps, and to understanding the pathophysiology of these insults.

Many of the perinatal cerebral insults to be discussed in this chapter are thought to be secondary to alterations in cerebral blood flow (CBF).[30, 53] CBF is believed to be largely independent of autonomic stimuli and to be controlled by local metabolic needs.[3, 18] In addition, CBF is believed to be constant over a wide range of blood pressures, a phenomenon known as "autoregulation."[35] However, when blood pressure becomes too low, CBF falls, and infarction may ensue.[51] Similarly, a rapid increase in blood pressure may markedly increase CBF, causing hemorrhage into damaged tissues.[53] Finally, hypoxia, hypercapnia (hypercarbia), and acidosis may all override autoregulation to produce increases in CBF.[3]

INTRAVENTRICULAR HEMORRHAGE

Intraventricular hemorrhage (IVH), or hemorrhage into the germinal matrix tissues with possible rupture into the ventricular system and parenchymal involvement of the developing cerebrum, remains a common problem in preterm neonates. Although Bejar and colleagues[6] noted a very high incidence of germinal matrix hemorrhage and intraventricular hemorrhage (GMH/IVH) on the first postnatal day and an overall incidence of almost 90 percent among infants whose gestational age was less than 34 weeks, most other investigators have reported an incidence of 40 to 50 percent in similar populations.[19, 25, 64, 76, 84] GMH/IVH has been noted within the first postnatal hour, and a substantial number of hemorrhages occur by the sixth postnatal hour.[63] Perlman and Volpe have reported that approximately 50 percent of all infants with hemorrhage were found to have this lesion on the first postnatal day; only a small percentage have hemorrhage after the fourth or fifth postnatal day.[63, 80]

Utilizing either computed tomography (CT) scanning techniques or, more commonly, cranial ultrasonography (Fig. 16–1), GMH/IVH is descriptively graded based on both the location of the hemorrhage and the ventricular size.[66] Grade I hemorrhage is germinal matrix hemorrhage only; grade II is hemorrhage into the ventricular system without ventricular distention. Grade III describes hemorrhage filling and dilating the ventricular system, and grade IV includes all of those hemorrhages with a parenchymal component. The most common site for parenchymal involvement in hemorrhage is the frontal region, with many hemorrhages occurring bilaterally. Less commonly, the caudate nuclei and occipital periventricular white matter are involved. In 10 to 20 percent of infants, progression of hemorrhage is documented. Infants with the earliest onset of hemorrhage appear to have the greatest chance for progression of hemorrhage and the highest mortality rate.[63]

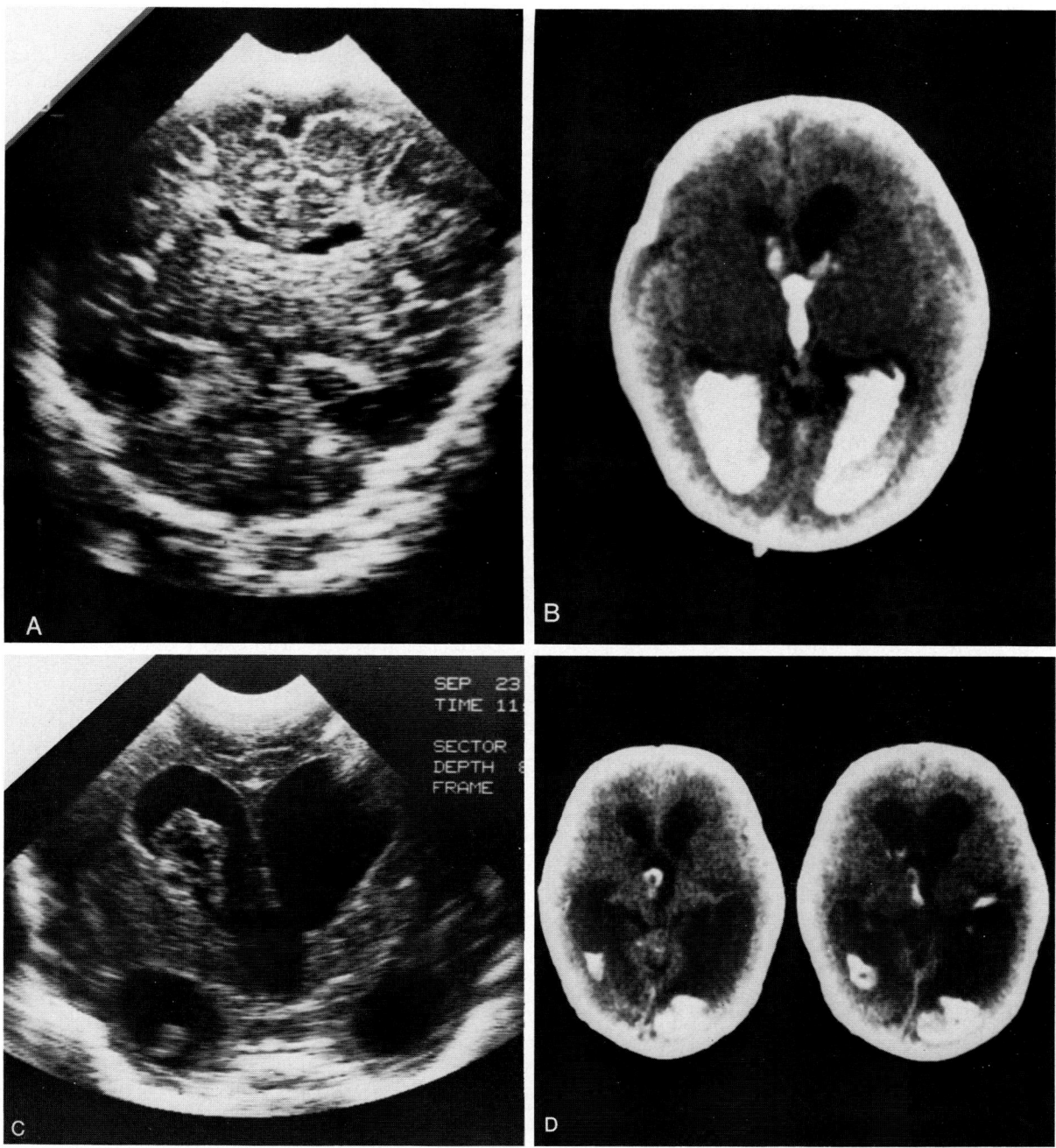

Figure 16–1. CT scans and cranial ultrasonograms of a preterm neonate with severe perinatal asphyxia and seizures beginning on the first postnatal day. *A*, Cranial ultrasonogram performed on the first postnatal day demonstrated no evidence of germinal matrix or intraventricular hemorrhage. *B*, CT scan performed on the second postnatal day demonstrated a grade IV intraventricular hemorrhage with blood in the left occipital parenchyma and dilated ventricular spaces. *C*, Cranial ultrasonogram performed on the tenth postnatal day because of somnolence and increasing occipitofrontal head circumference demonstrated enlargement of the ventricular system. *D*, CT scan performed on the same day confirmed these findings. A spinal tap performed shortly thereafter demonstrated an opening pressure of 220 mm Hg, consistent with posthemorrhagic hydrocephalus.

Numerous studies have correlated IVH with events such as hypercapnia, volume expansion, seizures, and pneumothorax, all of which are known to alter CBF.[19, 25, 37, 63, 76, 80] Increases in the CBF index have been reported in infants who had hypercapnia and volume expansion with subsequent IVH.[13, 69] Similarly, others have noted an increased CBF velocity in neonates with seizures before the development of IVH. Of equal concern, and perhaps more important for the neurodevelopmental outcome of these tiny patients, is the observation of markedly diminished CBF after GMH/IVH.[53-57, 86, 89]

Studies of clinically relevant animal models have demonstrated that acute hypercapnia, acute hypertension, and hemorrhagic hypotension followed by volume re-expansion may lead to alterations in CBF and neuropathologic lesions similar to those caused by GMH/IVH.[29, 30, 66, 68] Experimental data appear to demonstrate that IVH may be the result of alterations in CBF to a previously damaged germinal matrix capillary bed.[66, 68]

Infants with GMH/IVH are known to have a higher incidence of neonatal seizures than occurs in infants without hemorrhage.[63, 76] In addition, those with IVH may develop posthemorrhagic hydrocephalus.[1, 40, 65, 76] The mortality rate is clearly higher in groups of infants with hemorrhage, as compared with normal neonates matched for birth weight, gestational age, or both.[63, 76, 84] Finally, although very low birth weight preterm infants have long been noted to have lower developmental quotients than those of their full-term siblings, and the long-term neurodevelopmental outcome in infants with lower grades of hemorrhage compared with those of their nonhemorrhage peers remains unclear, most observers would agree that those with the most severe grade of IVH with parenchymal involvement have a high incidence of neurodevelopmental handicaps.[75, 78, 84]

POSTHEMORRHAGIC HYDROCEPHALUS

The posthemorrhagic hydrocephalus (PHH) that infants with IVH develop must be carefully defined as the combination of ventriculomegaly diagnosed either by CT or echoencephalography and increased intracranial pressure (ICP).[65, 85] It is generally believed to be secondary to obliterative posterior fossa arachnoiditis that is evoked by the presence of red blood cells and cellular debris following hemorrhage. Occasionally, acute PHH is attributed to a noncommunicating hydrocephalus at the level of the aqueduct; this has also been attributed to the accumulation of red blood cells and cellular debris along that area.[38, 48, 50]

The incidence of PHH is reported to vary from 25 to 74 percent in low birth weight infants with IVH, and the problem has been noted to occur with greater frequency in those infants with more severe degrees of hemorrhage.[1, 76] In addition, despite the grade of the hemorrhage, infants of relatively younger gestational ages seem to be at lower risk for PHH.[63, 76, 84] Low ICP ventriculomegaly is relatively common in very low birth weight infants with and without GMH/IVH.[9, 32] However, patients with true PHH classically present with a rapidly increasing occipitofrontal head circumference, apnea, lethargy, and vomiting, and the diagnosis is generally made on the triad of dilated ventricular system and increased intracranial pressure of greater than 120 to 140 mm H_2O in addition to the altered clinical state. With the routine use of serial head ultrasonography, lumbar punctures, and serial clinical examinations in infants with IVH, PHH is diagnosed early. Although neurologic damage may have already occurred at the time of the initial insult, it is important that treatment be instituted promptly in order to prevent further damage to the periventricular white matter by the PHH itself.[32, 65]

The treatment of PHH has included mechanical, pharmacologic, and surgical intervention.* The aim of management is to control the resultant increase in ICP and ventricular size by medical modalities, in an attempt to avoid surgical shunting procedures and long-term shunt dependence. Certainly, all infants with noncommunicating PHH require ventricular shunting procedures. The treatment of those infants with communicating PHH remains varied.

Although prophylactic daily lumbar punctures are known not to prevent the development of PHH, careful daily or twice daily lumbar punctures may be utilized to treat the major clinical symptoms of PHH (i.e., lethargy, apnea, and poor feeding), all of which may be attributed to the increased intracranial pressure, until the chemical arachnoiditis may spontaneously resolve.

Serial lumbar punctures remove excessive cerebrospinal fluid (CSF) and, thereby, reduce ICP and decrease ventricular size. There is very little risk to the patient when it is performed properly. Electrolyte disturbances may occur as a result of the fluid removal, hyponatremia being the most frequent. One case of osteomyelitis at the procedure site has also been reported. Infants undergoing this treatment may require lumbar punctures one to three times daily or less frequently, depending upon the rate of excessive CSF accumulation, as indicated by the ventricular size on head ultrasonography, lumbar puncture opening pressure, and the clinical examination.

Acetazolamide and furosemide (Lasix) as combined therapy is reported to decrease CSF production by as much as 50 percent, thus reducing CSF

---

*References 9, 32, 33, 38, 40, 45, 58-60

volume, CSF pressure, and ventricular size.[59] The administration of these medications is outlined by Shinnar and colleagues,[85] who reported a 50 percent success rate with the use of acetazolamide in dosages up to 100 mg/kg/day and furosemide (Lasix), 1 mg/kg/day. Acetazolamide can cause lethargy, tachypnea, diarrhea, electrolyte imbalance, and metabolic acidosis. To counteract the side effects of the metabolic acidosis, alkylating agents such as Bicitra, Polycitra, and sodium bicarbonate (NaHCO$_3$) are administered concurrently.

Serial head ultrasound scans should be performed throughout the duration of treatment as well as occipitofrontal circumference measurements and neurologic examinations. Either of the treatments, lumbar puncture or acetazolamide and furosemide, is considered successful if there is stabilization or diminution of ventricular size, normalization of head growth, and stabilization of the results of physical examination. In the event that one treatment modality does not achieve these results, that treatment should be discontinued, and an alternative treatment sought. This includes infants who cannot undergo serial lumbar punctures because of mechanical restraints that preclude positioning for the procedure or who develop localized inflammation at the procedure site, and infants receiving acetazolamide and furosemide (Lasix) who develop side effects from the medications that cannot be controlled by dosage adjustments. Alternatives would include switching from one type of medical management to the other, or a shunting procedure.

The duration of treatment for infants receiving either therapy is dependent upon the severity of the initial insult and the rate of progression of the PHH. Therefore, the length of treatment must be individualized for each infant, with a projected range up to six weeks for infants receiving lumbar punctures and six months for infants receiving acetazolamide and furosemide. The frequency of serial lumbar punctures depends on the infant's clinical examination, ventricular size, and pressure measurements. Infants receiving acetazolamide and furosemide whose PHH is successfully managed without side effects may be discharged from the hospital on medication, and then followed weekly with head ultrasonography, serum electrolyte determinations, and occipitofrontal circumference measurements. When stabilization of the ventricular size and the other previously mentioned determinations of health occurs, the medication may be slowly tapered.

Although draining ventriculostomy with either open or closed systems has been utilized by some for the treatment of PHH, this technique is associated with a high degree of infection and is not recommended at this time. Whatever the mode of therapy chosen for the treatment of PHH, the ventricular size, neurologic examination, and occipitofrontal head circumference must be carefully monitored. If the ventricular size and occipitofrontal circumference appear to be increasing despite vigorous therapeutic intervention, then ventriculoperitoneal shunting may be warranted.[25, 77, 82]

PERINATAL CEREBRAL INFARCTION

Perinatal cerebral infarction, or stroke, may be defined as a severe disorganization or even complete disruption of the gray and white matter architecture caused by embolic, thrombotic, or ischemic events.[2, 4, 12, 38] Stroke with discrete areas of cystic infarction is more commonly noted in full-term than in preterm infants, in whom many small cystic lesions may be found throughout both the cerebral hemispheres and brainstem structures.[21-24, 26, 73, 74] Although Barmada and associates[5] reported a 5.4 percent incidence of cerebral infarction in a large series of neonates who came to post-mortem studies, examination of the literature reveals only scattered reports of infants surviving well-documented neonatal cerebral infarction. However, with the increasing survival of many high-risk neonates and the ready availability of diagnostic imaging techniques to define intracranial anatomy, this diagnosis is suggested more often than previously noted.[46, 55, 62]

Larroche[48] observed that infarcts in early fetal life result in cortical neuronal loss and architectural changes resembling polymicrogyria. Strokes later in gestation are characterized by cavitary changes, or porencephalies, and appear similar to well-defined adult cerebral infarctions. In neonates with stroke caused by perinatal events, cortical necrosis, basal ganglia changes, and hemorrhage into gray and subcortical white matter structures may be apparent. Both subarachnoid and intraventricular hemorrhage may be noted as well. Although neonatal cerebral infarcts are reported to be caused by embolic events related to cyanotic congenital heart disease, thrombotic events associated with polycythemia, trauma, or meningitis, and hemorrhagic events secondary to vascular malformations and congenital tumors, it appears that perinatal asphyxia, with its attendant hypoxia and hypotension, is the most commonly determined reason for stroke in most recent series.[3, 10, 11, 67, 81, 87, 92]

Perinatal asphyxia in experimental animals results in both bradycardia and hypotension.[87] Tracer studies reveal loss of normal blood-brain barrier integrity, pressure-passive CBF, and edema in parasagittal cerebral regions.[53] Edema formation may, in turn, result in further diminution of CBF. The relative roles of hypoxia, hypotension, and edema in the production of cerebral damage remain to be clarified.[41-43, 67] Newborn infants with perinatal asphyxia are frequently noted to have experienced episodes of fetal bradycardia. At delivery, they may be profoundly hypotensive and may require vigorous resuscitation, and later they may continue to demonstrate systemic evidence of ischemia-induced problems as well as persistent heart rate and blood pressure changes. Sankaran and associates[81] used jugular venous plethysmography to demonstrate prolonged depression of CBF in asphyxiated full-term patients. Lou and coworkers[51, 52] reported the loss of cerebrovascular autoregulation in asphyxiated preterm neonates, with respiratory distress and marked increases in CBF in the presence of seizures and apnea. As in animal tracer studies, full-term asphyxiated infants have been reported to have abnormal technetium-99m brain scans,[90] suggesting a disruption of the normal neonatal blood-brain barrier, and CT studies have shown a diffuse pattern of low density throughout the cerebral hemispheres. Follow-up CT scans demonstrate ventriculomegaly and cortical and central atrophy as well as porencephalies in many infants.[26, 32]

Though stroke has been reported only rarely in preterm neonates, Lou and colleagues[53, 54] have hypothesized that hypoxic-ischemic lesions and IVH are often found in the same patient, and Volpe and Pasternak[90] have used positron emission tomography in preterm infants with IVH and stroke to document this occurrence. Preterm neonates may readily lose cerebrovascular autoregulation in re-

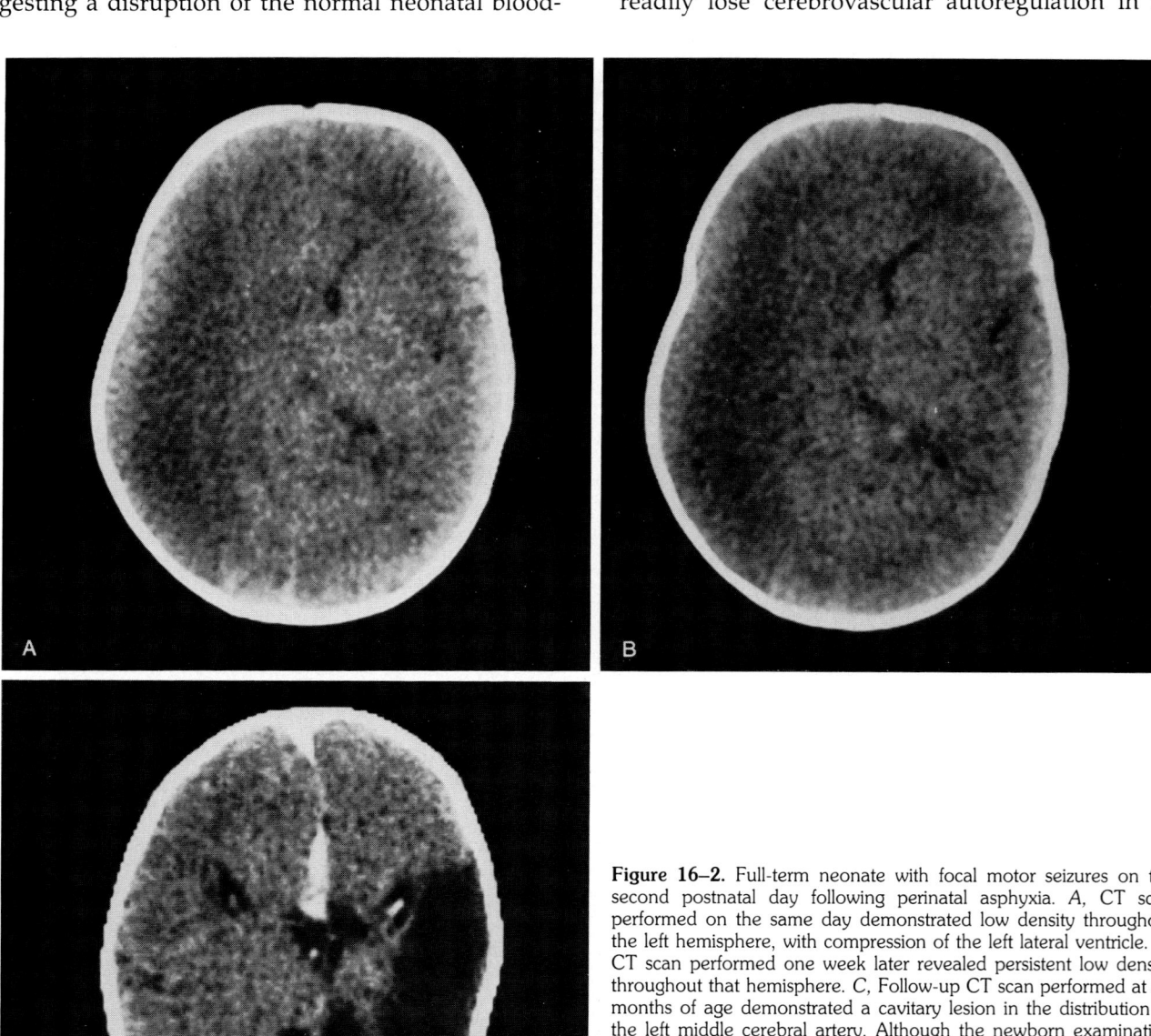

Figure 16–2. Full-term neonate with focal motor seizures on the second postnatal day following perinatal asphyxia. A, CT scan performed on the same day demonstrated low density throughout the left hemisphere, with compression of the left lateral ventricle. B, CT scan performed one week later revealed persistent low density throughout that hemisphere. C, Follow-up CT scan performed at six months of age demonstrated a cavitary lesion in the distribution of the left middle cerebral artery. Although the newborn examination was nonfocal, the patient demonstrated a right spastic hemiparesis and developmental delay at six months of age.

sponse to a perinatal hypotensive insult, resulting in pressure-passive CBF. Hypercapnia and hypoxia, apnea, seizures, and volume manipulations may elevate CBF episodically, which may in turn result in hemorrhage into infarcted germinal matrix tissues. Fitzhardinge and coworkers[25] studied 67 preterm infants with perinatal asphyxia, apnea, or both. Initial CT studies demonstrated hypodensities in all; only 4 of the 56 scans repeated at six months of corrected age (i.e., age from the maternal due date) were believed to be normal (Fig. 16–2). Ventricular dilatation and cortical atrophy were most commonly present. The neuropathologic study of Barmada[5] indicates that stroke in preterm patients is most frequently manifested by multiple, small infarcts. When these infarcts are found in the region of periventricular white matter, thought to be a watershed zone for the developing brain, periventricular leukomalacia may develop, and the clinical correlates of spastic diplegia may be found.[2, 4, 16]

Like preterm neonates with IVH, infants with both subarachnoid hemorrhage and hemorrhagic infarction with an intraventricular component may be at risk for the development of PHH. In addition to repeated neurologic examinations, both occipitofrontal head circumference measurements and determinations of ventricular size by echoencephalography should be carefully followed. In addition, in those infants with parenchymal hemorrhage, the rare diagnoses of congenital tumors, especially medulloblastoma and choroid plexus papillomas, and vascular malformations must be considered and excluded by neuroradiologic investigations.

NEONATAL BACTERIAL MENINGITIS

Despite improvement in mortality rates, the survivors of neonatal bacterial meningitis continue to experience a significant incidence of neurologic sequelae, including seizures, hydrocephalus, and developmental delay.* *Escherichia coli* and group B streptococcus (GBS) represent the two major causative organisms of neonatal meningitis. Cerebral angiographic studies on acutely ill infants have demonstrated arteritis, thrombosis, thrombophlebitis, and vascular narrowing, and neuropathologic studies on infants who have died of neonatal bacterial meningitis have reported arachnoiditis, vasculitis, encephalomalacia, and focal areas of infarction.[7, 8, 28]

Infants with bacterial meningitis commonly experience increased ICP, and this may be attributable to the sequelae of the prominent vasculitis that these patients experience as well as to a communicating hydrocephalus that is secondary to the arachnoiditis they suffer. Vasculitis, with involvement of both arterial and venous pathways, is an early and almost constant concomitant of neonatal meningitis, and the edema, regions of cerebral infarction, and periventricular cystic changes all arise in part from vasculitic processes. Cerebral infarction has been reported to occur in almost 30 percent of the patients in neuropathologic studies and has been found in infants who have died within the first week of illness.[8, 28] Although the neuropathologic data have emphasized the presence of multiple cortical and subcortical areas of infarction, usually of venous origin, cerebral infarction has been described in arterial distributions as well. These arterial distribution strokes have been attributed to inflammation of the adventitia and involvement of the vasa vasorum of the large vessels entering the brain at the base of the skull. Vasoconstriction and luminal narrowing of the major cerebral arteries ensue.

References

1. Allan WC, Holt PJ, Sawyer LR, et al: Ventricular dilatation after neonatal periventricular-intraventricular hemorrhage. Natural history and therapeutic implications. Am J Dis Child 136:589, 1982.
2. Armstrong D, Norman MG: Periventricular leucomalacia in neonates. Complications and sequelae. Arch Dis Child 49:367, 1974.
3. Ashwal S, Dale PS, Longo LD: Regional cerebral blood flow: Studies in the fetal lamb during hypoxia, hypercapnia, acidosis, and hypotension. Pediatr Res 18:1309, 1984.
4. Banker BQ, Larroche JC: Periventricular leukomalacia of infancy. A form of neonatal anoxic encephalopathy. Arch Neurol 7:386, 1962.
5. Barmada MA, Moossy J, Shuman RM: Cerebral infarcts with arterial occlusion in neonates. Ann Neurol 6:45, 1979.
6. Bejar R, Curbelo V, Coen RW, et al: Diagnosis and follow-up of intraventricular and intracerebral hemorrhages by ultrasound studies of infant's brain through the fontanelles and sutures. Pediatrics 66:661, 1980.
7. Bell WE, McCormick WF: Neonatal meningitis. In: Bell WE, McCormick WF (eds): Neurologic Infections in Children. Philadelphia, W.B. Saunders Co., 1981, pp 105–133.
8. Berman PH, Banker BQ: Neonatal menigitis: A clinical pathological study of 29 cases. Pediatrics 38:6, 1966.
9. Boynton BR, Boynton CA, Merritt TA, et al: Ventricular peritoneal shunts in low birth weight infants with intracranial hemorrhage: Neurodevelopmental outcome. Neurosurgery 18:141, 1981.
10. Brann AW, Jr., Myers RE: Central nervous system findings in the newborn monkey following severe in utero partial asphyxia. Neurology 25:327, 1975.
11. Cavazzuti M, Duffy TE: Regulation of local cerebral blood flow in normal and hypoxic newborn dogs. Ann Neurol 11:247, 1982.
12. Chin KC, Fitzhardinge PM: Sequelae of early-onset group B hemolytic streptococcal neonatal meningitis. J Pediatr 106:819, 1985.
13. Chiswick ML, Johnson M, Woodhall C, et al: Protective effect of vitamin E (DL-alpha-tocopherol) against intraventricular haemorrhage in premature babies. Br Med J 287:81, 1983.
14. Cooke RWI, Rolfe P, Howat P: Apparent cerebral blood-flow in newborns with respiratory disease. Dev Med Child Neurol 21:154, 1979.
15. Cussen LJ, Ryan GB: Hemorrhagic cerebral necrosis in neonatal infants with enterobacterial meningitis. J Pediatr 71:771, 1967.

16. DeReuck J, Chattha AS, Richardson EP: Pathogenesis and evolution of periventricular leukomalacia in infancy. Arch Neurol 27:229, 1972.
17. Donn SM, Roloff DW, Goldstein GW: Prevention of intraventricular haemorrhage in preterm infants by phenobarbitone: A controlled trial. Lancet 2:215, 1981.
18. Duffy TE, Cavazzuti M, Cruz NF, et al: Local cerebral glucose metabolism in newborn dogs: Effects of hypoxia and halothane anesthesia. Ann Neurol 11:233, 1982.
19. Dykes FD, Lazzara A, Ahmann P, et al: Intraventricular hemorrhage: A prospective evaluation of etiopathogenesis. Pediatrics 66:42, 1980.
20. Edwards MS, Rench MA, Haffar AAM, et al: Long-term sequelae of group B streptococal meningitis in infants. J Pediatr 106:717, 1985.
21. Ergander U, Eriksson M, Zetterstrom R: Severe neonatal asphyxia: Incidence and prediction of outcome in the Stockholm area. Acta Paediatr Scand 72:321, 1983.
22. Feldman GB, Freiman JA: Prophylactic Ceasarean section at term? New Engl J Med 312:1264, 1985.
23. Fenichel GM: Hypoxic-ischemic encephalography in the newborn. Arch Neurol 40:261, 1983.
24. Finer NN, Robertson CN, Richards RT, et al: Hypoxic-ischemic encephalopathy in term neonates: Perinatal factors and outcome. J Pediatr 98:112, 1981.
25. Fitzhardinge PM, Flodmark O, Fitz CR, et al: The prognostic value of computed tomography of the brain in asphyxiated premature infants. J Pediatr 100:476, 1982.
26. Fitzhardinge PM, Flodmark O, Fitz CR, et al: The prognostic value of computed tomography as an adjunct to assessment of the term infant with postasphyxia encephalopathy. J Pediatr 99:777, 1981.
27. Fitzhardinge PM, Kazemi M, Ramsay M, et al: Long-term sequelae of neonatal meningitis. Dev Med Child Neurol 16:3, 1974.
28. Friede RL: Cerebral infarcts complicating neonatal leptomeningitis. Acta Neuropathol (Berl) 23:245, 1973.
29. Goddard J, Lewis RM, Alcala H, et al: Intraventricular hemorrhage—an animal model. Biol Neonate 37:39, 1980.
30. Goddard-Finegold J: Periventricular, intraventricular hemorrhages in the premature newborn. Arch Neurol 41:766, 1984.
31. Hack M, Fanaroff AA, Merkatz IR: The low-birth-weight infants—evolution of a changing outlook. N Engl J Med 301:1162, 1979.
32. Hahn YS, McLone DG, Raimondi AJ, et al: Surgical outcome of preterm newborns with severe periventricular-intraventricular hemorrhage and posthemorrhagic hydrocephalus. In Humphreys RP (ed): Concepts in Pediatric Neurosurgery, Vol. 4. Basel, S Karger, 1983, pp 66–80.
33. Harbaugh RE, Saunders RL, Edwards WH: External ventricular drainage for control of post hemorrhagic hydrocephalus in premature infants. J Neurosurg 55:766, 1981.
34. Haslam RHA, Allen JR, Dorsen MM, et al: The sequelae of Group B B-hemolytic streptococcal meningitis in early infancy. J Dis Child 131:845, 1977.
35. Hernandez MJ, Brennan RW, Bowman GS: Autoregulation of cerebral blood flow in the newborn dog. Brain Res 184:202, 1980.
36. Hill A, Martin DJ, Daneman A, et al: Focal ischemic cerebral injury in the newborn: Diagnosis by ultrasound and correlation with computed tomographic scan. Pediatrics 71:790, 1983.
37. Hill A, Perlman MB, Volpe JJ: Relationship of pneumothorax to occurrence of intraventricular hemorrhage in the premature newborn. Pediatrics 69:144, 1982.
38. Hill A, Shackelford GD, Volpe JJ: A potential mechanism of pathogenesis for early posthemorrhagic hydrocephalus in the premature newborn. Pediatrics 73:19, 1984.
39. Hill A, Volpe JJ: Seizures, hypoxic-ischemic brain injury and intraventricular hemorrhage in the newborn. Ann Neurol 10:109, 1981.
40. James HE, Bejar R, Merritt A, et al: Management of hydrocephalus secondary to intracranial hemorrhage in the high-risk newborn. Neurosurgery 14:612, 1984.
41. Kennedy C, Grave GD, Jehle JW: Effects of hyperoxia on the cerebral circulation of the newborn puppy. Pediatr Res 5:659, 1971.
42. Kjellner I, Karlsson K, Olsson T, et al: Cerebral reactions during intrauterine asphyxia in the sheep. I. Circulation and oxygen consumption in the fetal brain. Pediatr Res 8:50, 1974.
43. Koehler RC, Jones MD, Traystman RJ: Cerebral circulatory response to carbon monoxide and hypoxic hypoxia in the lamb. Am J Physiol 243:H27, 1982.
44. Kontos HA, Wei EP, Raper AJ, et al: Role of tissue hypoxia in local regulation of cerebral microcirculation. Am J Physiol 234:H582, 1978.
45. Kreuser KL, Tarby TJ, Kovnar E, et al: Serial lumbar punctures for at least temporary amelioration of neonatal posthemorrhagic hydrocephalus. Pediatrics 75:719, 1985.
46. Lacey DJ: Inability to verify parasagittal cerebral injury as a neuropathologic entity in the asphyxiated term neonate. Pediatr Neurol 1:100, 1985.
47. Laptook A, Stonestreet BS, Oh W: The effects of different rates of plasmanate infusions upon brain blood flow after asphyxia and hypotension in newborn piglets. J Pediatr 100:791, 1982.
48. Larroche JC: Post-haemorrhagic hydrocephalus in infancy. Anatomical study. Biol Neonate 20:287, 1972.
49. Levene MI, Starte DR: A longitudinal study of posthaemorrhagic ventricular diltation in the newborn. Arch Dis Child 56:905, 1981.
50. Lorber J, Bhat US: Posthaemorrhagic hydrocephalus: Diagnosis, differential diagnosis, treatment, and long-term results. Arch Dis Child 49:751, 1974.
51. Lou HC, Lassen NA, Friis-Hansen B: Low cerebral blood flow in hypotensive neonatal distress. Acta Neurol Scand 56:343, 1977.
52. Lou HC, Lassen NA, Friis-Hansen B: Impaired autoregulation of cerebral blood flow in the distressed newborn infant. J Pediatr 94:118, 1979.
53. Lou HC, Lassen NA, Tweed WA, et al: Pressure passive cerebral blood flow and breakdown of the blood-brain barrier in experimental fetal asphyxia. Acta Paediatr Scand 68:57, 1979.
54. Lou HC, Skov H, Pedersen H: Low cerebral blood flow: A risk factor in the neonate. J Pediatr 95:606, 1979.
55. Mannino FL, Trauner DA: Stroke in neonates. J Pediatr 102:605, 1983.
56. Mantovani JF, Pasternak JF, Mathew OP, et al: Failure of daily lumbar punctures to prevent the development of hydrocephalus following intraventricular hemorrhage. J Pediatr 97:278, 1980.
57. McCarthy KD, Reed DJ: The effect of acetazolamide and furosemide on cerebrospinal fluid production and choroid plexus carbonic anhydrase activity. J Pharmacol Exper Ther 189:194, 1974.
58. McComb JG, Ramos AD, Platzker AC, et al: Management of hydrocephalus secondary to intraventricular hemorrhage in the preterm infant with a subcutaneous ventricular catheter reservoir. Neurosurgery 13:295, 1983.
59. McCormick MC: The contribution of low birth weight to infant mortality and childhood morbidity. N Engl J Med 312:82, 1985.
60. McCracken GH, Mize SG: A controlled study of intrathecal antibiotic therapy in gram-negative enteric meningitis of infancy. J Pediatr 89:66, 1976.
61. McCracken GH, Threlkeild N, Mize S, et al: Moxalactam therapy for neonatal meningitis due to gram-negative enteric bacilli. JAMA 252:1427, 1984.
62. Ment LR, Duncan CC, Ehrenkranz RA: Perinatal cerebral infarction. Ann Neurol 16:559, 1984.
63. Ment LR, Duncan CC, Ehrenkranz RA, et al: Intraventricular hemorrhage in the preterm neonate: Timing and cerebral blood flow changes. J Pediatr 104:419, 1984.
64. Ment LR, Duncan CC, Ehrenkranz RA, et al: Randomized indomethacin trial for prevention of intraventricular hemorrhage in very low birth weight infants. J Pediatr 107:937, 1985.

65. Ment LR, Duncan CC, Scott DT, et al: Posthemorrhagic hydrocephalus. J Neurosurg 60:343, 1984.
66. Ment LR, Stewart WB, Duncan CC: Beagle puppy model of intraventricular hemorrhage: Ethamsylate studies. Prostaglandins 27:245, 1984.
67. Ment LR, Stewart WB, Duncan CC, et al: Beagle puppy model of perinatal cerebral infarction: Acute changes in cerebral blood flow and metabolism during hemorrhagic hypotension. J Neurosurg 63:441, 1985.
68. Ment LR, Stewart WB, Scott DT, et al: Beagle puppy model of intraventricular hemorrhage: Randomized indomethacin prevention trial. Neurology 33:179, 1983.
69. Milligan DWA: Failure of autoregulation and intraventricular haemorrhage in preterm infants. Lancet 1:896, 1980.
70. Morgan MEI, Benson JWT, Cooke RWI: Ethamsylate reduces the incidence of periventricular hemorrhage in very low birth weight babies. Lancet 2:830, 1981.
71. Morgan MEI, Massey RF, Cooke RWI: Does phenobarbitone prevent periventricular hemorrhage in very-low-birth-weight babies? A controlled trial. Pediatrics 70:186, 1982.
72. Myers RE: Two patterns of perinatal brain damage and their conditions of occurrence. Am J Obstet Gynecol 112:246, 1972.
73. Nelson KB, Broman SH: Perinatal risk factors in children with serious motor and mental handicaps. Ann Neurol 2:371, 1977.
74. Nelson KB, Ellenberg JH: Obstetric complications as risk factors for cerebral palsy or seizure disorders. JAMA 251:1843, 1984.
75. Palmer P, Dubowitz LMS, Levene MI, et al: Developmental and neurological progress of preterm infants with intraventricular haemorrhage and ventricular dilatation. Arch Dis Child 57:748, 1982.
76. Papile LA, Burstein J, Burstein R, et al: Incidence and evolution of the subependymal and intraventricular hemorrhage: A study of infants with birth weights less than 1,500 gm. J Pediatr 92:529, 1978.
77. Papile LA, Burstein J, Burstein R, et al: Posthemorrhagic hydrocephalus in low-birth-weight infants: Treatment by serial lumbar punctures. J Pediatr 97:273, 1980.
78. Papile LA, Munsick-Bruno G, Schaefer A: Relationship of cerebral intraventricular hemorrhage and early childhood neurologic handicaps. J Pediatr 103:273, 1983.
79. Perlman JM, Goodman S, Kreusser KL, et al: Reduction in intraventricular hemorrhage by elimination of fluctuating cerebral blood-flow velocity in preterm infants with respiratory distress syndrome. N Engl J Med 312:1353, 1985.
80. Perlman JM, Volpe JJ: Cerebral blood flow velocity in relation to intraventricular hemorrhage in the premature newborn infant. J Pediatr 100:956, 1982.
81. Sankaran K, Peters K, Finer N: Estimated cerebral blood flow in term infants with hypoxic-ischemic encephalopathy. Pediatr Res 15:1415, 1981.
82. Scarff TB, Anderson DE, Anderson CL, et al: Complication of ventriculo-peritoneal shunts in premature infants. In: Humphreys RP (ed): Concepts in Pediatric Neurosurgery, Vol. 4. Basel, S Karger, 1983, pp 81–89.
83. Shankaran S, Cepeda EE, Hagan N, et al: Antenatal phenobarbital for the prevention of neonatal intracerebral hemorrhage. Am J Obstet Gynecol 154:53, 1986.
84. Shankaran S, Slovis TL, Bedard MP, et al: Sonographic classification of intracranial hemorrhage. A prognostic indicator of mortality, morbidity, and short-term neurologic outcome. J Pediatr 100:469, 1982.
85. Shinnar S, Gammon K, Bergman EW, et al: Management of hydrocephalus in infancy: Use of acetazolamide and furosemide to avoid cerebrospinal fluid shunts. J Pediatr 107:31, 1985.
86. Skov H, Lou H, Pederson H: Perinatal brain ischaemia: Impact at four years of age. Dev Med Child Neurol 26:353, 1984.
87. Snyder RD, Stovring J, Cushing AH: Cerebral infarction in childhood bacterial meningitis. J Neurol Neurosurg Psychiatry 44:581, 1981.
88. Vannucci RC, Duffy TE: Cerebral metabolism in newborn dogs during reversible asphyxia. Ann Neurol 1:528, 1977.
89. Volpe JJ, Herscovitch P, Perlman JM, et al: Positron emission tomography in the newborn: Extensive impairment of regional cerebral blood flow with intraventricular hemorrhage and hemorrhagic intracerebral involvement. Pediatrics 72:589, 1983.
90. Volpe JJ, Pasternak JF: Parasagittal cerebral injury in neonatal hypoxic-ischemic encephalopathy: Clinical and neuroradiologic features. J Pediatr 91:472, 1977.
91. Wolfe LS: The role of prostaglandins in the central nervous system. Ann Rev Physiol 41:669, 1979.
92. Young RSK, Hernandez MJ, Yagel SK: Selective reduction of blood flow to white matter during hypotension in newborn dogs: A possible mechanism of periventricular leukomalacia. Ann Neurol 12:445, 1982.

17
MECHANISMS OF INTRACRANIAL HYPERTENSION IN CHILDREN

Kenneth Shapiro, M.D.
Anthony Marmarou, Ph.D.

"The control of intracranial pressure is perhaps the principal task in the neurosurgical care of infants."[20] This statement may be extended to patients with a wider range of ages, encountered in pediatric neurosurgery, because many of the medical and surgical diseases encountered in children are accompanied by intracranial hypertension. Widely differing conditions, including congenital lesions, neoplasms, metabolic and infectious syndromes, and trauma, require evaluation and treatment for elevated intracranial pressure. Because intracranial hypertension frequently accompanies disease processes in children, an understanding of the mechanisms leading to intracranial hypertension is of paramount importance to the neurosurgeon.

The neurosurgeon involved in the care of children must be cautious in applying to children the concepts of intracranial hypertension derived from experience with adults. Although many of the clinical manifestations of intracranial hypertension are similar in both age groups, distinct differences exist. Children may harbor an intracranial mass for some time without overt signs of intracranial hypertension, only to deteriorate rapidly and dramatically to an unsalvageable state. Often, intracranial masses may be accompanied by phenomena not encountered in adults, such as failure to reach developmental milestones or rapid increase in head circumference. Unique properties of the immature brain and its container affect the brain's response to changes in intracranial pressure. The following discussion addresses the mechanisms that lead to raised intracranial pressure and integrates these mechanisms with the properties of the immature nervous system.

NORMAL INTRACRANIAL PRESSURE

The upper limit of normal intracranial pressure (ICP) in adults and older children is usually given as 15 mmHg. Transient changes resulting from coughing, sneezing, or straining often produce pressures exceeding 30 to 50 mmHg, but ICP returns rapidly to baseline levels. Efforts to measure ICP in younger children and infants by spinal puncture using manometers can be criticized because of the poor cooperation from the child and the displacement of fluid into the manometric measuring device. Given these practical difficulties, published norms for children range from 3 to 7.4 mmHg, and for infants from 1.5 to 5.9 mmHg.[10, 12, 20] Using visual estimates of fontanelle configuration, Welch[20] reported a normal ICP of 3 to 4 mmHg in patients from the first hours of life to seven months of age.

By applying a noninvasive applanation transducer to the fontanelle, Salmon and colleagues[12] reported that the normal ICP of infancy is approximately 8 mmHg.

All reported values for the ICP of younger children are lower than those reported for adults but are probably reasonable approximations of the actual level of ICP. A teleologic explanation might account for this relatively low normal ICP in children. In adults, the ability to perfuse the brain effectively depends on the maintenance of an adequate cerebral perfusion pressure (CPP). Usually, a CPP greater than 50 mmHg is needed to maintain adequate cerebral perfusion in adults.[3] The critical CPP of the immature brain has not been determined. Since the mean arterial blood pressure of infants and children is considerably lower than that of adults, a lower normal ICP may be a mechanism for maintaining adequate cerebral perfusion of the brain in younger children.

Measurements of ICP using low-volume displacement, electric transducers to interface with the CSF pathways yield considerably more information than an absolute pressure that exceeds atmospheric pressure by 4 to 8 mmHg. A strip chart recorder can be used to display the pulsatile ICP wave form, which can be divided into three major components (Fig. 17–1). The *baseline*, or diastolic, level is commonly referred to as the ICP, while the rhythmic components are associated with *cardiac* and *respiratory* activity. In order to describe completely ICP, one should specify the magnitude of the baseline, or

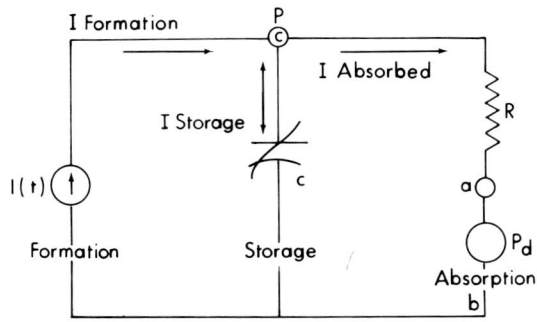

Figure 17–2. The CSF system was depicted by an equivalent electric circuit that distributed the CSF parameters among three fundamental mechanisms: formation, represented by a constant-current generator; storage, represented by a nonlinear capacitance (C); and absorption, represented by a resistance element (R). The venous outflow site (dural sinus) was represented by a constant pressure source P_d. The system equations were derived from this configuration.

"steady state," level and the amplitude and periodicity of the pulsatile components. Although some workers report ICP as a mean pressure, paralleling the convention used in systemic blood pressure, this has not been universally adopted. Many eliminate the pulsatile components and specify diastolic pressure as the ICP.

Steady State Dynamics

In the condition of physiologic equilibrium, both the baseline ICP and the amplitude of the pulsatile components of ICP remain constant. This implies that the net intracranial volume is also in a state of dynamic equilibrium, or a steady state. If volume is removed or added to the system, the net seepage of fluid into or out of the cerebrospinal fluid spaces will be in a direction that returns pressure to its steady state level. Since this dynamic equilibrium occurs in a system with continuous changes of volume produced by the heartbeat and CSF formation, it is logical to ask what the factors are that govern volume interchange in the steady state, and how these changes affect baseline ICP.

These questions were addressed by using a mathematical model of the cerebrospinal fluid system that subdivided the physical mechanisms into three major categories: (1) mechanisms associated with CSF formation, (2) mechanisms for volume storage, or compliance, and (3) mechanisms dealing with fluid absorption (Fig. 17–2).[6] Conceptually, the formation of CSF was depicted as a fluid pump that continuously introduces fluid into the CSF spaces of the neural axis. The rate of formation of fluid (I_f) was considered constant and independent of the pressure head seen by the pump mechanism, in accordance with observations that the rate of CSF formation is minimally, if at all, affected by changes in the ICP.

According to this model, the newly formed fluid enters a compliant storage space, which can expand

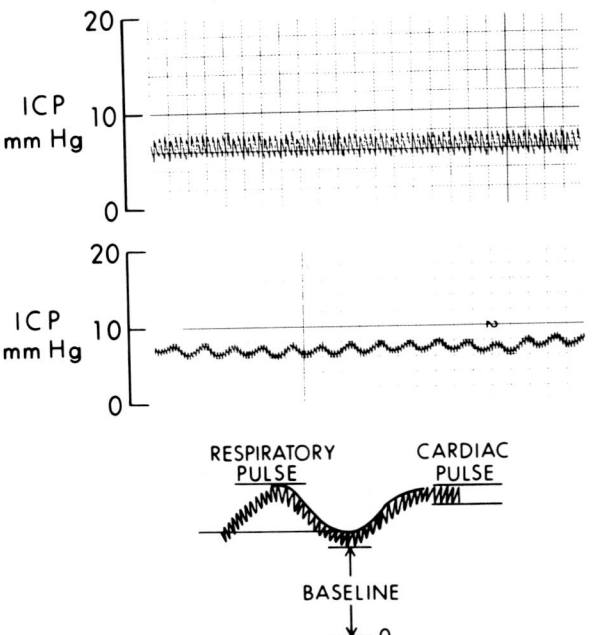

Figure 17–1. The intracranial pressure (ICP) wave form consists of respiratory and cardiac variations superimposed upon a steady-state level that is usually above atmospheric pressure. The upper panel displays the ICP at fast chart speed to accentuate the cardiac pulsations. Specification of ICP should include a measure of both baseline level and amplitude of pulsatile components.

to accommodate the added volume, or proceeds via outflow pathways and is absorbed across the arachnoid villi into the dural venous sinuses. The compliance mechanism was represented by an element (C), which decreased its contractibility with increasing volume, much like the resistance offered by a rubber balloon at maximum inflation. Both the resistance of the CSF channels leading to the arachnoid villi and the resistance of the villi to fluid flow were combined into a single resistance element (R_o). This component represented the total resistance to the outflow of CSF, which, under normal conditions, was considered to remain fixed and independent of ICP. The final element of this model is the dural sinus pressure (P_d). Fluid crossing the arachnoid villi must overcome the P_d, so the exit pressure of CSF is determined by P_d.

From this conceptual framework, a theory was developed to describe the interaction of the formation, storage, and absorption elements in the steady state. First, both pressure and volume are in equilibrium, and there can be no net increase or decrease in the total volume of the CSF spaces. The CSF formed must pass through the absorptive elements, so that no net fluid is stored and the total volume within the CSF spaces remains constant.

Since all fluid formed passes through the resistive element (R_o), a pressure gradient will be developed across the absorptive element that is equal to the product of fluid flow (I_f) and the fluid resistance (R_o). The greater the magnitude of flow or resistance, the greater the pressure gradient ($I_f \times R_o$). As long as a condition of equilibrium is imposed upon the system, the pressure of the CSF spaces must be of sufficient magnitude to force continuously all newly formed fluid through the arachnoid villi and overcome the exit pressure. This requires that the CSF pressure (ICP) be equal to the sum of the pressure gradient developed by the absorptive element ($I_f \times R_o$) and the exit pressure. Thus, ICP = ($I_f \times R_o$) + P_d.[1]

Thus, the steady state ICP is proportional to three parameters: the rate of CSF formation, the resistance to CSF absorption, and the dural sinus pressure. When these parameters remain constant, the ICP level remains unchanged, and the compliance element does not participate actively.

How is this dynamic equilibrium altered in cases of raised ICP? According to the model, a sustained elevation of pressure can develop with an increase in CSF formation, an increase in outflow resistance, or an increase in the venous pressure at the site of fluid absorption. Computer studies show that the contribution of the product of outflow resistance and the formation rate ($I_f \times R_o$) is approximately 10 percent of the total ICP.[9] The remainder is attributed to the magnitude of the dural sinus pressure (P_d). With this distribution, the outflow resistance would have to increase markedly in order to effect a significant rise in the ICP. However, elevations of sagittal sinus pressure caused by venous sinus obstruction would be transmitted directly to the CSF system, resulting in an increase in resting ICP. Since the increase in P_d equals the change in ICP, the gradient across the arachnoid villi is not altered, CSF absorption remains constant, and the equilibrium shift to a higher ICP level is sustained. This concept is supported by the work of Johnston,[3] who demonstrated normal CSF resistance in the presence of raised ICP induced by venous obstruction, and by observations in children with anomalous venous return.[18] In both conditions, there is no net storage of CSF volume and presumably no change in the compliant element. When the latter two events occur, neural axis dynamics are no longer in a steady state, and new concepts must be invoked.

Non–Steady State Dynamics

As implied in the preceding paragraph, steady state pressure dynamics cannot be transposed directly to pathologic conditions. In contrast with the physiologic steady state in which net volume storage does not occur, pathologic states are often associated with net changes in volume within the neural axis. In order to understand the interaction between pressure and volume changes, additional concepts and parameters are required.

The cornerstone for analyzing these volume-pressure interactions is the Munro-Kellie doctrine. This states that, after fontanelle and suture closure, the container of the neural axis forms a rigid box with the craniospinal, intradural volume being *nearly* constant. Since the components of neural axis volume (i.e., neural parenchyma, CSF, and blood) are essentially incompressible, any change in one of these components must be accompanied by reciprocal changes in one or both of the others in order to preserve the constancy of neural axis volume. When an additional component is introduced, such as a hematoma, the same principle applies. Exchanges of volume must also be analyzed in terms of rate because changing properties of tissue may allow volume exchanges to occur over time that may not be possible acutely. In children with open fontanelles or unfused sutures, the container is not rigid, thereby modifying the Munro-Kellie hypothesis.

The interaction between the three components of neural axis volume depends on the ease of egress and the amount of each component that is available for exchange with the other components. The largest constituent of neural axis volume is the brain, comprising approximately 80 percent of total volume. The brain can respond to volume added to the neural axis by undergoing compression, dislocation, or shift. The effectiveness of the brain as a buffer to added volume depends on the rate at which the volume is added. As an example, a slowly growing brain tumor is more likely to cause compression and deformation than a rapidly enlarging epidural hematoma, which will shift the brain through the tentorial hiatus. The ability of the brain to adapt itself to masses also depends upon the viscoelastic properties of the brain. Theoretically, cerebral edema might alter the elasticity of the brain, rendering it less capable of accommodating volume added to the neural axis.

The second component of neural axis volume is the CSF, constituting approximately 10 per cent of total neural axis volume. Since CSF absorption can increase with increasing pressure gradients across the arachnoid villi,[21] significant compensatory reserves are available for volume exchange. Approximately 30 to 70 percent of total compensatory reserves for volume exchange or buffering occur through the mechanism of increased absorption or displacement of CSF into the spinal subarachnoid spaces.[5, 7] Since the capacity to increase CSF absorption is not infinite, the rapidity of volume interchange required to preserve the relative constancy of total neural axis volume is important.

The final component of intracranial volume is blood, which normally constitutes the remaining 8 to 10 percent of total neural axis volume. Since most of the blood is contained on the venous or capacitance side of the vasculature, many view the cerebrovascular volume as the mechanism for the rapid interchange of volume. Although attractive, this mechanism has not been well documented. This mechanism must play some role in young children, as evidenced by the scalp veins supplied via the emissary system that characteristically become engorged in children with intracranial hypertension and must represent a mechanism to dissipate ICP.

The elastic properties of the components within the "closed box" also determine the changes in ICP induced by volume. Many inanimate containers have "ideal" elastic properties, including a coefficient of deformation that does not vary with time and is constant for all degrees of expansion of that container. In such an "ideal" container pressure varies directly with volume so that a pressure-volume relationship can be described that is linear, with the compliance, or rate of volume-pressure change ($\Delta V/\Delta P$), being constant. However, the containers of the neural axis and neural parenchyma do not have ideal elastic properties. This results in a nonlinear relationship between ICP and volume added to the neural axis. For equal volume increments, the $\Delta V/\Delta P$ ratio, or compliance, decreases as pressure increases. This was first demonstrated in 1953 by Ryder and coworkers,[11] who described the general form of the curve as hyperbolic.

The relationship between neural axis volume and ICP is hyperbolic, or exponential, up to an ICP of 50 mmHg (Fig. 17–3A). When pressure exceeds 50 mmHg, the curve tends to flatten as the arterial blood pressure is approached. Thus, over the entire range of ICP, the pressure volume curve may be described by a sigmoid-shaped curve. The pressure-volume relationship is measured by rapidly inserting known volumes of fluid into the CSF pathways and recording the magnitude of ICP change. Compliance, according to physical definition, is given by the ratio of volume and pressure changes ($\Delta V/\Delta P$), which is graphically equivalent to the slope of the pressure volume curve. Elastance, the reciprocal of compliance, can be extracted from the pressure-volume curve or can be computed by similar bolus techniques. Since the slope of this curve reflects the ability of the neural axis to accommodate or buffer additional increments of volume, steeper curves identify settings that have limited compensatory reserves. However, since compliance changes with

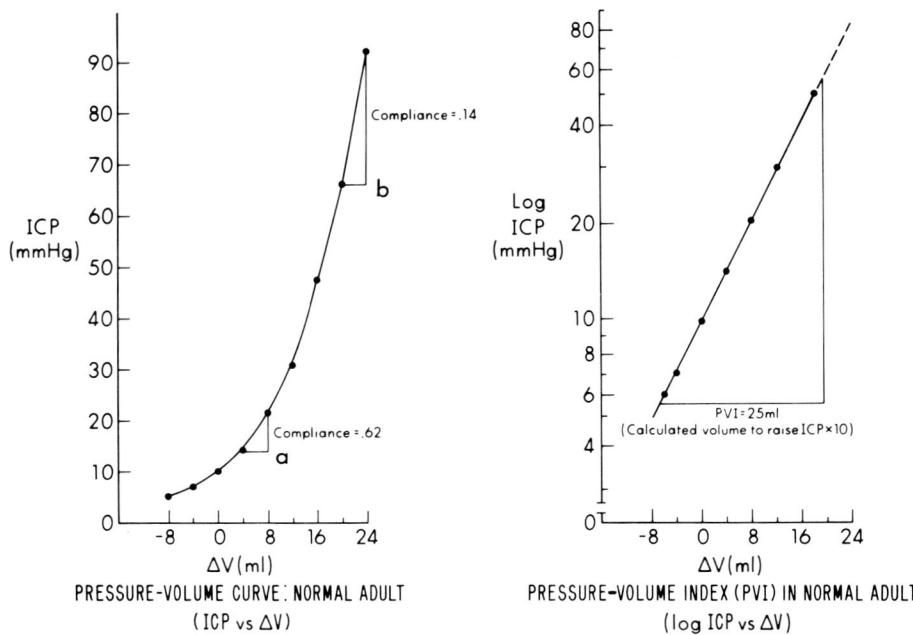

Figure 17–3. Neural axis pressure-volume curve obtained by measuring the immediate cerebrospinal fluid pressure response to successive bolus injections ($+\Delta V$) or withdrawals ($-\Delta V$) of CSF in a normal adult. Compliance ($\Delta V/\Delta P$) is measured at two points on this curve: at point a compliance is greater than at point b. The differences in compliance at these points are a normal function of CSF pressure. B, The same pressure-volume curve has been transformed to a linear function by plotting the response of CSF pressure on a logarithmic scale. Only two points are needed to define this linear function. The pressure volume index (PVI) is the calculated volume (ml) needed to raise CSF pressure by a factor of 10.

pressure, the authors have found little use for these numerical determinations of compliance.

When pressure-volume data is plotted on a logarithmic pressure axis against volume, the exponential curve is transformed into a straight line (Fig. 17–3B). The slope of this straight line transformation is the pressure volume index (PVI) and is the calculated volume (ml) needed to raise ICP by a factor of 10.[7] A *steep* exponential curve is associated with a *reduced* buffering capacity and is characterized by a low PVI. An exponential curve with a more gradual increase in slope describes a *more* compliant system and is characterized by a higher PVI.

In adult humans, the normal PVI is approximately 25 ml. This level of PVI can be expressed in more physical terms and indicates that 25 ml of fluid must be added to the CSF compartment in order to raise baseline ICP by a factor of 10.[17] The PVI is directly proportional to the available buffering capacity. A 50 percent reduction in PVI is equivalent to a 50 percent reduction in volume-buffering capacity at all points along the exponential portion of the pressure-volume curve.

In clinical settings, the PVI can be determined by adding a known volume (ΔV) to the CSF space at initial pressure (P_o) and recording the peak pressure (P_p) measured immediately after the bolus addition. Both pressures must be measured on the same relative portion of the respiratory and cardiac ICP pulse wave to avoid error. The PVI can be calculated using the formula $PVI = \Delta V/\log_{10}(P_p/P_o)$ (Fig. 17–4). In normal children ranging from infancy to 14 years of age, the authors have found that PVI varies in proportion to estimated neural axis volume.[17] Normal infants have PVIs below 10 ml, while the adult PVI of 25 ml is reached at around 14 years of age. These studies provide important reference data for assessing pressure-volume relationships in pathologic conditions. More important, the authors have found that the slope of a normal infant's or a young child's pressure-volume curve is greater than that of a normal teenager (Fig. 17–5). A 10 ml volume added to the neural axis of a teenager may produce modest elevations in ICP, but the same increment can be lethal in an infant.

The factors responsible for volume buffering represent the combined storage ability of both intracranial and spinal compartments. Most researchers agree that, theoretically, the venous capacitance

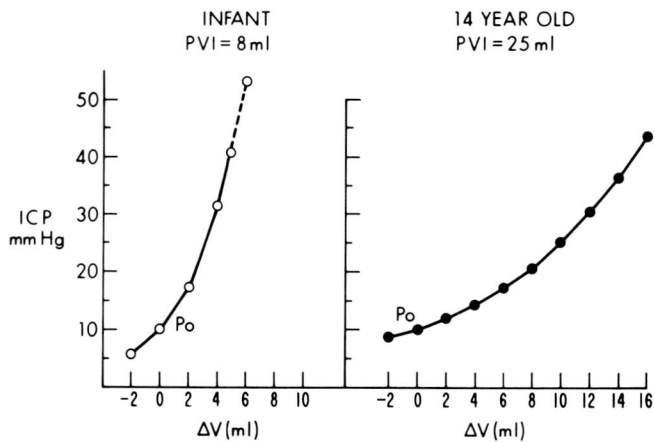

Figure 17–5. The pressure-volume curves shown were generated by injecting and withdrawing CSF from a normal infant *(left)* and a normal teenager *(right)*. The slope of the infant's pressure-volume curve is steeper than that of the teenager, resulting in less ability to buffer equal increments of volume.

system is at least partly responsible for volume buffering, so that as added volume accumulates within the neural axis, venous blood is expressed from these capacitance vessels. Additional buffering capacity may be gained by the relative ease of distending the spinal dural tube, at the expense of epidural venous blood volume. The authors have estimated that 48 percent of this "pool" of compensatory reserve is derived from the supratentorial compartment, 20 percent infratentorially, and 32 percent from the spinal canal.[8]

The expression of these non–steady state dynamics depends on many factors. Conceptually, the simplest situation exists when neural axis pressure-volume relationships describe a stable pressure-volume curve. As volume is added to this system, ICP rises along this curve, and the pressure response to each increment of added volume is predicted by this curve. This situation often fails to materialize in many clinical settings, for most disease processes are dynamic, with shift from one pressure-volume curve to another.[16] This dynamic shift may be caused by such factors as increases in cerebral blood volume and cerebral edema, exhausting the compensatory reserve that functions to preserve normal ICP. The authors have observed this shifting of pressure-volume curves without significant changes in ICP, in a variety of neurosurgical conditions and also as a response to treating these conditions (Fig. 17–6). Intuitively, this concept of varying pressure-volume curve as opposed to movement along a single curve is reasonable, for not only is there redistribution of volume, but also there are probably changes in the biomechanical properties of the brain in response to a variety of insults.

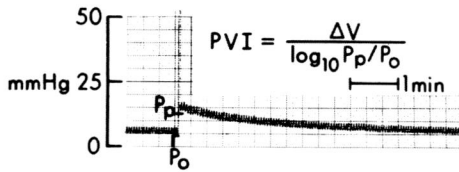

Figure 17–4. This strip chart recording shows the ICP response to a bolus injection of CSF into the cisterna magna of a child. Following injection, the baseline pressure P_o is immediately raised to P_p, the peak pressure response to the injection. Pressure then begins to return toward P_o as CSF is absorbed. The PVI can be calculated from the formula *(inset)*, using data derived from the bolus injection.

Younger Children

The conceptual model and analysis discussed in the preceding sections are based on the "rigid box"

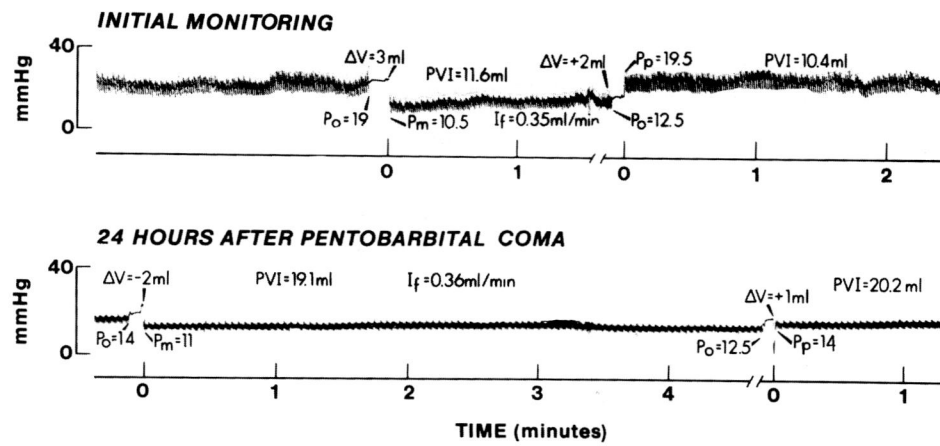

Figure 17–6. The strip chart recordings shown were obtained through a ventricular catheter placed in a child with severe closed head injury. The upper tracing shows that PVI was markedly reduced from the predicted normal value (23 ml) for this child and was manifested by dramatic elevations of intracranial pressure. The lower tracing shows a PVI determination performed after barbiturate coma was induced in this child. The increased PVI of 19 ml represents an improvement in the slope of this child's pressure-volume curve and was associated with normalization of intracranial pressure.

container of the neural axis implicit in the Munro-Kellie hypothesis. Weed[19] observed that this does not hold in infants because the skull has not acquired the rigid container property found in the adult. Clinicians caring for infants with hydrocephalus have repeatedly observed that infants with open sutures accommodate added intracranial volumes by skull expansion, often with little elevation in ICP. The response of the infant to osmotic dehydration that reduces total neural axis volume, as evidenced by a sunken fontanelle, is yet another exception to the Munro-Kellie hypothesis found in younger children.[19]

In the preceding section, the authors stated that the pressure-volume relationship in infants described curves similar to, but steeper than, those found in older children and in adults. At first glance, this evidence appears to contradict the work of Weed. However, our studies in infants were not carried to extreme ICP levels. With the rapid absorption of the added CSF, it is unlikely that the generation of a pressure-volume curve stretched the container of the brain in these infants, so the tensile properties of the sutures were probably not affected by these tests. These studies demonstrated that the smaller pressure-volume indices could be accounted for by the smaller size of these infants and that the open fontanelles and sutures did not enhance the ability to accommodate volume. However, laboratory studies show that, once the container of the brain has been altered in a way that simulates sutural *separation,* the pressure-volume index increases, which indicates that the storage of volume is facilitated.[15] When infants and younger children have increases in intracranial volume, they often experience a period of intracranial hypertension, which is partially dissipated as the head enlarges. Once the force at the cranial sutures has been overcome, the immature brain can accommodate volume more readily than the adult brain enclosed in its rigid skull. As the authors have shown in a variety of clinical situations, this unique property has important implications in the progression of certain disease processes.[13, 14, 16]

The preceding discussion of the factors responsible for steady state ICP and the mechanisms of its change form the foundation for analyzing ICP dynamics in clinical settings. Many of the principles previously detailed require modification when applied to the pediatric patient. In addition to the Monro-Kellie hypothesis, other basic concepts of ICP physiopathology may not be directly applicable to the immature nervous system. The notion of a critical cerebral perfusion pressure, well described in adults, has yet to be investigated in young children. The effect of raised ICP on the immature brain, with its high water content and changing myelin content, has not been systematically investigated. These issues, while beyond the scope of this chapter, may influence the response of the immature brain to raised ICP.

References

1. Davson H: Physiology of the Cerebrospinal Fluid. London, Churchill Livingstone, 1967, p 445.
2. Galford JE, McElahany JH: A viscoelastic study of the scalp, brain and dura. J Biomech 3:211, 1969.
3. Johnston I: Reduced CSF absorption syndrome. Reappraisal of benign intracranial hypertension and related conditions. Lancet 2:418, 1973.
4. Johnston IH, Rowan JO, Harper AM, et al: Raised intracranial pressure and cerebral blood flow. 1. Cisterna magna infusion in primates. J Neurol Neurosurg Psychiatry 35:285, 1972.
5. Lofgren J, Zwetnow NN: Cranial and spinal components of the cerebrospinal fluid pressure-volume curve. Acta Neurol Scand 49:575, 1973.
6. Marmarou A: A Theoretical and Experimental Evaluation of the Cerebrospinal Fluid System. Drexel University, Ph.D. thesis, 1973.
7. Marmarou A, Shulman K: Pressure-volume relationships—basic aspects. In: McLaurin RL (ed): Head Injuries. New York, Grune & Stratton, 1976, pp 233–236.
8. Marmarou A, Shulman K, LaMorgese J: Compartmental analysis of compliance and outflow resistance of the cerebrospinal fluid system. J Neurosurg 43:523, 1976.
9. Marmarou A, Shulman K, Rosende R: A nonlinear analysis of the cerebrospinal fluid system and intracranial pressure dynamics. J Neurosurg 48:332, 1978.
10. Munro D: Cerebrospinal fluid pressure in the newborn. JAMA 90:1688, 1928.

11. Ryder HW, Epsey FP, Kimbell FD, et al: The mechanism of the change in cerebrospinal fluid pressure following an induced change in the volume of the fluid space. J Lab Clin Med 41:428, 1953.
12. Salmon JH, Hajjar W, Bada HS: The fontogram: A noninvasive intracranial pressure monitor. Pediatrics 60:721, 1977.
13. Shapiro K, Fried A: Pressure-volume relationships in shunt-dependent childhood hydrocephalus: The zone of pressure instability in children with acute deterioration. J Neurosurg 64:390, 1986.
14. Shapiro K, Fried A, Marmarou A: Biomechanical and hydrodynamic characterization of the hydrocephalic infant. J Neurosurg 63:69, 1985.
15. Shapiro K, Fried A, Takei F, et al: Effect of the skull and dura on neural axis pressure-volume relationships and CSF hydrodynamics. J Neurosurg 63:76, 1985.
16. Shapiro K, Marmarou A: Clinical applications of the pressure-volume index in treatment of pediatric head injuries. J Neurosurg 56:819, 1982.
17. Shapiro K, Marmarou A, Shulman K: Characterization of clinical CSF dynamics and neural axis compliance using the pressure-volume index. I. The normal pressure-volume index. Ann Neurol 7:508, 1980.
18. Shapiro K, Shulman K: Facial nevi associated with anomalous venous return and hydrocephalus. J Neurosurg 45:20, 1976.
19. Weed LH: Some limitations of the Munro-Kellie hypothesis. Arch Surg 18:1049, 1929.
20. Welch K: The intracranial pressure in infants. J Neurosurg 52:693, 1980.
21. Welch K, Friedman V: The cerebrospinal fluid valves. Brain 83:454, 1961.

18
TREATMENT OF INTRACRANIAL HYPERTENSION

Derek A. Bruce, M.D.

In Chapter 17, the mechanisms that function to maintain a normal intracranial pressure–volume relationship were discussed. This chapter reviews the therapeutic means available to treat increased intracranial pressure (ICP). The fact that the pressure is altered suggests that some resetting of the homeostatic mechanisms or some dysfunction thereof has occurred. Increased ICP is not a disease but a symptom of some underlying pathologic process in the intracranial cavity. It is rare that events external to the cranium produce intracranial hypertension, although bilateral acute obstruction of the internal jugular veins can produce transient intracranial hypertension, as can prolonged CO_2 retention and severe systemic hypertension. The normal intracranial cavity is exposed to intermittently high pressures (e.g., in coughing, sneezing, and straining). As long as mechanisms such as vascular pressure autoregulation are functioning and the period of increased pressure is short, no ill effects from intracranial hypertension occur. The deleterious effects of increased ICP appear to be those of secondary brain ischemia and displacement and herniation of brain substance—cingulate, uncal, and tonsillar.[6] Thus, the ICP that produces deterioration of neurologic function varies, depending upon the course of the intracranial hypertension and the state of the various homeostatic mechanisms within the cranium. It appears that diffuse increases in ICP (hydrocephalus, pseudotumor cerebri) are better tolerated than focal lesions, since the latter are more likely to produce herniation syndromes.

There is no single therapy for intracranial hypertension, since elevated ICP is not a disease but merely a symptom of a variety of pathologic events that can occur within the cranium. Therapy must be directed toward correction of the underlying pathologic factors, if possible. The intracranial space contains blood, cerebrospinal fluid (CSF), brain, and any other pathologic lesion (e.g., hematoma, tumor) that may be added. An increase in any one compartment, if large enough or rapid enough, can lead to increased ICP. Correction of the increased ICP may be directed against a primary event, as in hydrocephalus, or designed to decrease some nonpathologic compartment in an effort simply to decrease overall volume, as in the use of mannitol to lower ICP in the face of a mass lesion. With the multiplicity of therapies available, selection of the best method of treatment of elevated ICP has to be based on an accurate diagnosis of the underlying pathology. This is important not only in selecting the most effective initial therapy but also in planning later therapy. Hyperventilation, for example, may be very effective in lowering the ICP following head trauma or in Reye's syndrome in the initial stages of disease. However, after several days, increased cerebral edema may be present or a hematoma may have formed, and now a different type of therapy will be required. The physician must not be restricted to the use of one or two modalities of therapy, since, in the patient with severe intracranial hypertension, a whole gamut of therapy from physiologic manipulation to surgical decompression may be necessary to prevent secondary brain ischemia resulting from intracranial hypertension.

When considering the causes of increased ICP, the following equation is helpful in visualizing the various compartments of the cranium:

$$V_{CSF} + V_{blood} + V_{brain} + V_{other} = V_{intracranial\ space}$$

Each of these compartments will be discussed separately, to examine what diseases affect each compartment and what methods are available for treatment (Table 18-1).

V_{OTHER}

Under this heading are all the lesions that add a new component to the intracranial space (e.g., tumor, abscess, hematoma). When one of these lesions is the cause of intracranial hypertension, the best therapy is surgical removal of the mass. This may be definitive therapy, and therefore, such a treatable cause of increased ICP must always be sought. The other various methods of treatment to be discussed below and shown in Table 18-1 may well be applicable, particularly when the added intracranial mass lesion is not readily removable or has been present for a long period and is associated with significant cerebral edema.

Surgery is the ideal therapy when the cause of increased intracranial volume is an increased V_{other}. Thus, such conditions as tumor, abscess, hemorrhage, giant aneurysms, and arteriovenous malformations (AVMs) all lend themselves to surgical removal and re-establishment of the normal intracranial volume. There are situations in which a mass lesion may be present (e.g., infection and metastatic disease), yet surgery may not be indicated. The intracranial hypertension must then be treated by some other method, such as corticosteroids, antibiotics, chemotherapy, or radiation. In patients with rapid neurologic deterioration secondary to a rapidly expanding mass lesion (e.g., epidural hematoma), there is a need to apply general therapy to lower ICP until a diagnosis is made. These therapies include head-up position, hyperventilation, and endotracheal intubation, *if done with full anesthetic precautions for rapid sequence induction and osmotic therapy.* The dangers of some increase in size of the hematoma are offset by reversal of any associated herniation and improvement in cerebral perfusion. The danger of the therapy comes in seeing an improvement in the patient's neurologic examination and then not continuing to make a definitive diagnosis of the underlying pathophysiology. If an expanding mass is present, the sequence of increased ICP and herniation will repeat itself. This is not "rebound" but a manifestation of the progressive nature of the primary lesion, which must be diagnosed and treated. When a difficult-to-approach mass lesion is present (e.g., deep hematoma secondary to ruptured AVM), ICP monitoring can be very useful in helping to decide whether immediate surgery is advisable or necessary. If the ICP is easily controlled below 20 torr and there are no signs of progressive herniation, the surgery can be postponed until the patient is in a more favorable condition for a complex operation and the brain swelling and increased ICP have subsided. The use of ICP monitoring can also be helpful when multiple lesions are present and surgery is deemed inadvisable or impossible (e.g., multiple abscesses or mycotic aneurysm). The knowledge of the level of ICP permits rational selection of therapy and allows the physician to measure the response to therapy, thereby helping to define when further therapy or a different type of therapy is necessary. It is the author's firm belief that severe intracranial hypertension associated with coma can be adequately treated only with the help of intracranial pressure monitoring.

Besides the role of surgery in the definitive removal of an intracranial mass lesion, there are two other situations in which surgical intervention may be helpful: the performance of internal and of external decompressions. Internal decompression is the surgical excision of a portion of the brain to decrease intracranial volume, at least temporarily. This is a technique that has little role in the treatment of children with brain disease. It has been particularly applicable to traumatic injuries in adults when relatively silent polar areas are involved with hemorrhagic contusion and edema. Because these lesions act as a focal mass, surgical removal of the frontal or temporal pole has been advocated. In adults, ICP monitoring can be used in a predictive fashion; that is, those with an ICP over 20 torr despite therapy require surgery, whereas those in whom the ICP remains below 20 torr are likely to recover without surgical intervention.[41] Whenever therapy involves the removal of potentially viable brain, the treatment must be questioned, and in children, this type of destructive surgery is rarely necessary or justifiable.

The final role of surgery is in the treatment of intracranial hypertension by external decompression. This, as the name implies, is the removal of portions of the cranium to enlarge the intracranial

Table 18-1. TREATMENTS AVAILABLE TO LOWER ICP OR IMPROVE INTRACRANIAL COMPLIANCE

Blood Volume	CSF	Brain Bulk
Head-up position	Acetazolamide	Steroids
Midline head position	Furosemide	Osmotic diuretics
Controlled intrathoracic pressure	Ethacrynic acid	Tubular diuretics
	CSF drainage	Barbiturates (?)
	Steroids	Controlled blood pressure
Decrease $PaCO_2$		
Barbiturates (?)		

volume. This type of therapy can be rationalized when an ultimately self-limiting process that does not produce primary brain damage is present, the ICP cannot be kept below 20 to 25 mmHg with intensive medical therapy, and the chances of recovery are good if secondary ischemia and herniation can be avoided. In trauma, the results have been discouraging, probably because the traumatically damaged brain does not fulfill these criteria. Hoffman has suggested a role for decompressive craniectomy in children with Reye's syndrome and has reported encouraging results. The role for this type of therapy is very limited, and careful judgment is required before such an operation is performed. The potential benefit of bifrontal craniectomy with opening of the dura is that transtentorial herniation is less likely to occur because the brain can now decompress anteriorly. Cerebral perfusion pressure also may be improved. In the author's experience, craniectomy in Reye's syndrome is rarely associated with a significant lowering of the ICP, and the beneficial results obtained are probably due to decreased tentorial herniation. Residual brain damage may be very severe (Fig. 18–1).

When the increase in intracranial volume is due to an increased V_{other}, the most satisfactory treatment is the surgical removal of the offending mass lesion, when possible. When this is impossible, other ancillary methods to decrease intracranial volume by removing CSF, brain, water, or blood may all be applicable. These treatments are discussed in the following.

V_{CSF}

Ventricular shunting or ventricular drainage is the treatment of choice when increased CSF is the cause of the increase in intracranial pressure in hydrocephalus. The treatment of hydrocephalus is discussed in Chapter 14 and will not be elaborated on here. However, other situations lend themselves to CSF drainage as an ancillary measure to control intracranial hypertension. These may be divided into acute and subacute cases. Many care units still use an intraventricular catheter to monitor the ICP, even when ventriculomegaly is not present. One of the advantages of this technique is that it gives access to the CSF, and removal of small amounts of CSF can terminate waves of ICP. The second theoretic reason for the use of CSF drainage is to create a gradient of pressure from the edematous brain to the ventricles, thereby encouraging movement of water from the brain into the ventricles and aiding in the resolution of cerebral edema.[10, 37] Practically, this does not seem to be effective as a continuous therapy, since when the ventricles are small, the removal of CSF leads to collapse of the ventricle around the catheter, loss of drainage capability, and frequently loss of ICP recording. In the patient with a swollen brain (i.e., small ventricles), therefore, although intermittent removal of small amounts of ventricular CSF may be an effective ancillary measure to maintain the ICP below 20 mmHg, it cannot be done continuously and is of limited value. The subacute instances in which CSF drainage may be effective are during the resolution of an episode of cerebral edema. There are a number of situations during which the ventricular size enlarges abnormally during the course of treatment for increased ICP. This is especially true following trauma in children but may occur during recovery from Reye's syndrome, meningitis, or subarachnoid or ventricular hemorrhage. In the child with severe closed-head injury, subarachnoid hemorrhage, and diffuse brain swelling, the ICP can usually be controlled in the first three to ten days, by a combination of position, hyperventilation, and medications. It is not uncommon that after a period of 24 to 48 hours of a stable, normal ICP, the pressure again rises between the third and fifteenth day. At this time, a repeat computerized tomographic (CT) scan will show enlarged subarachnoid spaces, especially frontally; ventricular dilation; or both (Fig. 18–2).[9] At this time, therapy to maintain a normal pressure is primarily removal of the excess CSF via lumbar or ventricular drainage. A permanent ventricular shunt usually is not necessary in these children, as this is a transient phase. The cause of the increased CSF is believed to be an increase in outflow resistance. This change from the swollen brain with little *extracerebral* CSF to excess CSF emphasizes that disturbances of the intracranial homeostatic mechanisms are dynamic events, and a constant review of the underlying pathology is required to govern the sensible choice of specific therapy. Changes in therapy based on changes in the underlying pathology are frequently necessary. The formation of CSF, which also contributes to intracranial pressure, can be decreased by a variety of drugs, and in children with acute hydrocephalus, ICP may be transiently controlled by the use of such medica-

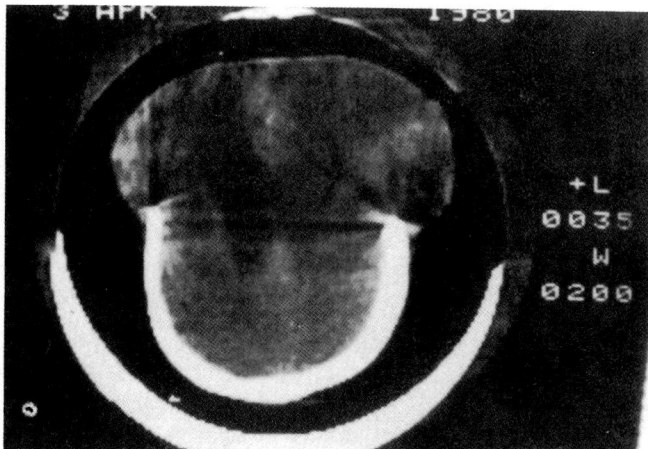

Figure 18–1. CT scan two weeks following decompressive craniotomy in a patient with Reye's syndrome. Note enlarged ventricular system and marked decreased density of both frontal lobes.

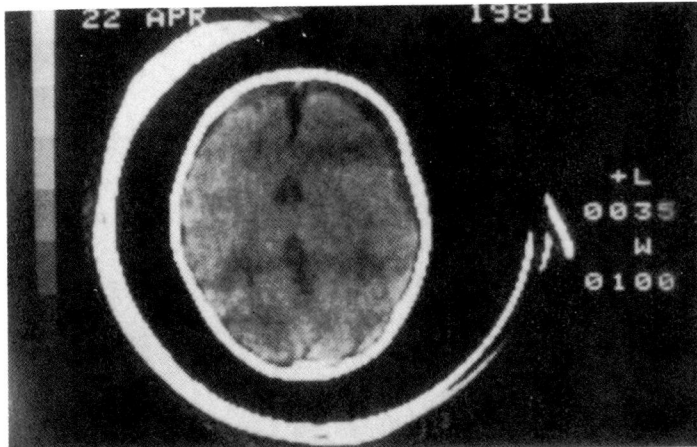

Figure 18–2. CT scan in a two-year-old with head trauma, taken two weeks following trauma. Note increased subarachnoid spaces over the frontal lobes.

tions. Acetazolamide (Diamox Sequel tablets; Lederle Laboratories, Pearl River, NY, 10965),[34] furosemide (Lasix; Hoechst-Roussel, Somerville, NJ 08876),[13] and corticosteroids[43] all may transiently decrease CSF production. There is good evidence[5] that the use of corticosteroids very rapidly decreases pressure waves and, ultimately, lowers the ICP in patients with posterior fossa tumors and hydrocephalus. Except in the sickest children, the author routinely uses steroids rather than ventricular drainage or shunting to treat posterior fossa lesions, especially those that are malignant, in an effort to avoid peritoneal metastases. Unfortunately, none of the methods of decreasing CSF production have been shown to have any long-term benefit in the treatment of intracranial hypertension, and all are associated with side effects. One other medication, isosorbide,[27] has been used chronically in the treatment of borderline hydrocephalus in childhood and seems to have some minor role to play.

Whether or not the increase in ICP is due to an increase in CSF, a variety of therapies that reduce the volume of CSF are available. These range from the use of drugs that decrease CSF formation to withdrawal and removal of CSF from the lumbar space or the ventricles, and they can help maintain a normal ICP.

V_{BLOOD}

Most of the intracranial blood volume is in the venous sinuses and pial blood vessels. Only quite small amounts, 5 ml/100 gm of gray matter and 3.5 ml/100 gm of white matter, are present within the brain parenchyma.[23] Theoretically the displacement of pial venous blood is one of the factors responsible for acute compensation for volume changes in the cranium. However, there is good evidence that intracerebral blood volume increases with increasing ICP,[17] and this is believed to be due to vasodilatation in response to lowered cerebral perfusion pressure (CPP), or pressure autoregulation. As the ICP is elevated, there is, in fact, a shift of blood volume from the pial vessels at the venous end of the system to the arterial end because of arterial dilatation. Two separate events may occur in response to elevation of ICP. The intracerebral blood volume may increase, whereas the total intracranial blood volume, at least in the early stages of increasing ICP, may decrease as blood is squeezed from the pial circulation to the sinuses. Thus, the net effect on the intracranial blood volume is not a simple one and remains to be completely clarified.

It is possible to have a primary increase in cerebral blood volume that can produce swelling of the brain, increased ICP, and, depending on the location of the blood, a change in the elastic properties of the brain itself. In this situation, the compliance in the cranium could be either increased or decreased, depending on whether the increased blood volume was in the pial circulation and, therefore, readily expressible into the venous sinuses or within the cerebral substance itself. Increased $PaCO_2$ leads to an increase in cerebral blood flow (CBF) and cerebral blood volume (CBV); increased ICP; and papilledema. Also, in the face of acute infarction, it can produce vasodilatation and acute hemorrhage, as a result of the increased CBF.[25]

Can an increase in CBV alone be adequate to raise the ICP, and if so, under what conditions? Carbon dioxide intoxication has already been mentioned. Raichle and colleagues[35] have demonstrated an increased CBV in patients with pseudotumor cerebri but concluded that the increase in CBV was insufficient to account for the increase in ICP. Cerebrovascular dilatation occurs following experimental head injury,[38] and there is a suggestion that this vasodilatation may be blocked by prostaglandin inhibitors.[42] Following certain types of head injury in children, acute swelling of the brain is seen. Bruce and associates[7] have suggested that in children the swelling is most probably due to increased intracranial blood volume. As yet, studies on regional cerebral blood volume (rCBV) have not conclusively proved that all the swelling is due to blood volume, although CT scan density measurements suggest that the increased brain bulk is not the result of edema but more probably of increased blood volume.[44] In the acute encephalopathy of Reye's syndrome, increased CBF is present, and this must also be accompanied by an increase in CBV. The author believes that there is adequate evidence that in many acute brain insults in childhood, increased blood volume is at least one factor contributing to the decrease in intracranial compliance and the increase in ICP.

The simplest way of decreasing intracranial blood volume is to place the patient in a 30-degree head-up tilt. This decreases the venous pressure in intracranial dural sinuses and permits collapse of the upper cervical extradural veins, thus allowing a decrease in ICP. Proper ventilator settings, if the patient is on mechanical ventilation, are important, since too long an inspiratory phase produces prolonged increased intrathoracic pressure—increased venous pressure reflecting back to the head with increased venous sinus pressure. Similarly, too high levels of positive end-expiratory pressure (PEEP) theoretically produce increases in central venous pressure that could also be reflected back to the intracranial space. In practice, the author has not found the use of PEEP to be associated with elevated ICP. The best explanation for this is that when large amounts of PEEP are required, there is usually markedly reduced pulmonary compliance and the intrapulmonary pressure is not transmitted directly to the central veins. Therefore, significant rises in central venous pressure do not occur. While lowering of systemic arterial pressure (SAP) might be expected to decrease intracranial blood volume, the reverse is true. This is so because the decrease in systemic arterial pressure produces a fall in CPP that results in vasodilatation at the arterial end of the tree. However, there is evidence that lowered SAP does have some beneficial effect in lowering brain compliance, and this is discussed in the following.[26]

The single most effective therapy to decrease rCBV is to reduce the arterial CO_2. This results in decreased vascular caliber and reduction of CBF and CBV.[24, 36] The response of the cerebral vessels to changes in $PaCO_2$ is preserved in most disease states until the point of impending brain death, and therefore, a good response to hyperventilation can usually be expected. Acutely, hyperventilation can almost always be performed adequately in the child, with the use of an oral airway, bag, and mask. While adult studies suggest that lowering the $PaCO_2$ below 20 torr has little further effect on CBF,[36] this does not appear to hold true for children. Clinically, the author has found that a favorable decrease in ICP occurs with lowering of the $PaCO_2$ from 20 to 17 torr. When severe hyperventilation to this degree is used, it is advisable to have a jugular venous bulb catheter in place to monitor the cerebrovenous arteriovenous difference (AVD) O_2 and the venous PaO_2, since a fall in cerebrovenous PaO_2 below 20 torr may be a sign of too large a decrease in CBF. The jugular bulb catheter can also be used to monitor the match between cerebral blood flow and metabolism.[40] It is unlikely that true cerebral ischemia can be produced by hyperventilation, since, because CBF decreases owing to decreased $PaCO_2$, the local increase in metabolites will produce vascular dilatation and prevent a severe decrease in CBF. Metabolic studies by MacMillan and Seisjö[28] showed no evidence of changes in energy charge potential until the CO_2 was decreased below 10 torr.

It seems probable that one of the beneficial effects of barbiturates on intracranial hypertension is due to vasoconstriction, with an acute decrease in CBV inside the brain. Whether this is a secondary effect of decreased metabolism or a prime effect on the cerebral vessels remains unclear. The barbiturates are discussed in greater detail below.

V_{BRAIN}

The final intracranial component that can expand is the brain tissue itself. The processes underlying expansion of the brain can be tumor, in which case the definitive therapy is to remove the lesion if possible; infection; or, most frequently, brain edema. Brain edema is an increase in the water content of the brain and occurs as a result of either disturbances of cellular function interfering with cell pumping mechanisms, disruption of the blood-brain barrier, or disturbances of transcapillary pressures, or in association with disturbance of CSF circulation or with hydrocephalus. The last has been discussed under CSF increases and will not be considered here. When brain edema is believed to be the pathologic process responsible for the increased ICP, therapeutic considerations have to be based on the location and cause of the cerebral edema. The approach to therapy can be divided into three phases: (1) decreasing the formation of the edema, (2) improving neuronal or axonal function in the presence of edema, and (3) increasing the rate of removal of the edema fluid.

The edema fluid may be intracellular—neurons, glial, or both; in the extracellular space; or occasionally between the lamellae of the myelin. While removal of fluid from the brain may not depend upon the location of the fluid, the effect of other drugs that influence edema is dependent upon the location of the edema fluid. When the excess water is intracellular, this is the result of some disturbance of cellular metabolism, usually interference with energy production (e.g., following anoxia or ischemia), and the edema is secondary to the cellular dysfunction. The ideal therapy in these instances is to correct the disordered cell function. At present few, if any, agents are available for this purpose. When anoxia or ischemia is of limited duration, re-establishment of oxygen delivery will correct the metabolic defect. Therefore, maintenance of adequate cerebral circulation and oxygen and glucose delivery are primary considerations in all types of cellular edema.

The most common type of edema requiring therapy is extracellular edema, so-called vasogenic, which occurs as a result of disturbances of the blood-brain barrier, or a combination of extra- and intracellular edema, as occurs in the later stages of infarction. At present, the way in which this type of extracellular edema influences cerebral function is unclear. There appear to be three major detrimental effects: (1) interference with local neuronal-axonal function (mechanism not yet known); (2) local expansion of the brain, with distortion and displacement of the brain leading to cerebral herniation, subfalcine, transtentorial, or cerebellar tonsillar herniation; and (3) diffuse increase in ICP, producing pressure waves, decreased CBF, and focal or global ischemia as a result of lowered CPP. Experimental studies on vasogenic edema have demonstrated that removal of the area of damaged blood-brain barrier can limit and stop the progressive accumulation of edema fluid.[1] While it is very rare to use resection of the brain as a treatment for brain edema, the removal of severely contused brain (e.g., temporal tip lobectomy) following trauma is occasionally performed to control the ICP, and this has the additionl benefit of removing the source of the edema fluid. The concept of removing the source of the edema is more pertinent when the edema source is not normal or damaged brain but a separate pathophysiologic lesion (e.g., brain tumor, abscess, and hematoma). Here, removal of the source stops edema formation. When large mass lesions are removed, the decompression of the brain may be followed by a period of increased swelling and edema, and therefore, other methods of therapy to control brain edema may have to be continued for several days following removal of mass lesions. The factors involved in edema formation are the state of the hydraulic conductance of the cerebral capillaries, the compliance of brain tissue, the intravascular hydrostatic pressure, the intravascular oncotic pressure, the cerebral tissue hydrostatic pressure, and the cerebral oncotic pressure. Although most of these factors cannot be manipulated, the systemic arterial pressure, the intravascular oncotic pressure, and possibly the hydraulic conductance of the capillaries can be affected. Experimental studies show that if the SAP is lowered sufficiently, little or no cerebral edema will occur following a cold lesion of the cortex.[2] In practice, the use of this information should lead at least to preventing cerebrovascular hypertension (age-appropriate) in children with brain edema. To lower the blood pressure below the normal mean can be safely performed only if both blood pressure and ICP are continuously monitored to ensure that adequate CPP is preserved. When there is severe brain edema with coma and difficult-to-control ICP, modest lowering of the SAP can occasionally be a useful ancillary measure. This is discussed again under barbiturates.

Increasing the intravascular osmolality, thus speeding removal of edema fluid, is probably the most widely used method of treating cerebral edema and intracranial hypertension. The three commonly used agents are urea, mannitol, and glycerol. Mannitol is the one most frequently used. The theory behind the use of these agents is that by increasing serum osmolality, fluid, mostly free water, will move from the brain tissue into the blood down an osmotic gradient. It has been demonstrated that the maximum water removal is from the normal brain rather than from the edematous brain.[32, 33] This remains a poorly explained phenomenon and cannot be the result of disturbances of the blood-brain barrier, since it has been shown that the barrier is intact in all but the area of edema formation. Urea has been shown to enter the brain through an intact barrier. This knowledge led to the theoretic concern that urea might leak into the brain and end up reversing the osmotic gradient, thus producing a rebound in ICP. There is little or no hard evidence that rebund is a clinically significant phenomenon, and urea has one advantage over the other drugs mentioned. It is a smaller molecule, and less volume has to be given to obtain the same osmotic effect. Over the past two or three years, the initial doses of both urea and mannitol have decreased from the more standard doses of 1 to 2 gm/kg to small doses of 0.25 to 0.5 gm/kg. The ideal mode of delivery is to give the smallest amount that will effectively lower the ICP. The complications associated with osmotic therapy are electrolyte imbalance, dehydration, and possibly renal failure. Repeat measurements of serum electrolytes and osmolality are necessary with repeated use of osmotic therapy. Fluid replacement is performed to preserve vascular volume, and the ideal situation is to preserve isovolemia with increased serum osmolality. With both urea and mannitol, as the serum osmolality rises about 320 to 330 mOsm, there is increasing concern for the effects on the renal tubules, and it is advised that another agent be used at this time. Gycerol has been used intravenously (IV) and by mouth (PO) to lower ICP and shows promise as a valuable agent for control of increased ICP. The most obvious benefit is that glycerol is not excreted via the kidneys but is metabolized in the body. Therefore, the concentration gradients in the renal tubules are not disturbed, and tubular failure has not been reported. Very high levels of serum osmolality can be obtained, over 400 mOsm, with apparent safety. This is a drug that is likely to see increasing use.

Hyperosmotic therapy should be valuable in lowering the ICP and reducing edema in both cellular and extracellular edema. The amount of water removed depends upon the tissue perfusion and the osmotic gradient, but also upon the site and the state of the brain water. Little is known about the state of brain water (i.e., bound or unbound). The major contraindication to the use of osmotic agents is the presence of hyperemia and an increased CBV. Hyperosmotic agents increase CBF[8] independently of their effect on ICP and, therefore, should be used with caution in the early treatment of head injuries or Reye's syndrome.

Dimethyl sulfoxide (DMSO) is again being investigated as an agent to reduce ICP. At present, there is no good information on the efficacy of the drug, the best methods of administration, the best dose, or complications. While there is an osmotic effect, this does not seem to be the prime mechanism whereby ICP is decreased. Studies are under way to investigate the usefulness of and complications associated with this drug. It is not recommended as an agent for intracranial hypertension control at the present time and is not available for general use.

In discussing the factors responsible for edema formation, alterations of blood-brain barrier and increased capillary hydraulic conductance were mentioned. In vasogenic edema, in particular, therapy to restore the integrity of the blod-brain barrier should be useful. Corticosteroids, especially methylprednisolone and dexamethasone, have been demonstrated to have a clinically beneficial effect on certain patients with cerebral edema. The best clinical responses are seen in patients with brain tumors or abscesses. A beneficial role of steroids in the outcome of patients with brain trauma or infarction remains unproved. The effect of corticosteroids is not clear. A simple decrease in tissue water content does not occur, yet clinical and experimental improvement in neurologic function, the electroencephalogram (EEG), and intracranial compliance all are seen early after administration.[19, 31] Crocker and coworkers[14] demonstrated that steroids appear to decrease the area and amount of blood-brain barrier leakage and may be beneficial by decreasing edema formation or by some direct membrane effect in the area of edema. Methylprednisolone has been shown to facilitate the release of oxygen from hemoglobin, and it is possible that some systemic effect facilitating substrate delivery to the brain underlies the beneficial actions of these drugs. Whatever the mechanism involved, corticosteroids have a firm place in the therapy of brain edema secondary to tumor or infection. In other lesions (e.g., trauma or infarction), the use of steroids is very much the decision of the individual physician. When used to control symptomatic cerebral edema, large doses are employed (1 mg/kg/day divided into four doses). Once the reason for the edema has resolved, the dosage is cut rapidly, and every effort is made to stop the steroids within the shortest possible time.

Work by Bourke[3] and with his coworkers[4] has shown that swelling of the glial cells accompanies trauma and hypoxia and that this swelling appears to be related to a chloride-mediated transport system within the glial cell membrane. These investigators have demonstrated that ethacrynic acid decreases this glial cell swelling and, in animal models, improves mortality statistics. They have also tested ethacrynic acid derivaties that have little or no diuretic effect but appear to be even more potent against the glial swelling. This field of research seems to hold promise for the development of a whole new group of specific agents with which to treat brain edema, particularly that associated with glial swelling.

Diuretic agents, such as furosemide and ethacrynic acid, also decrease CSF production and may lower ICP by removing water from the body or by effects on sodium pumping at the membrane. In children, furosemide is most effective in lowering ICP when there is evidence of fluid overload. When a rapid decrease in ICP is desired, a combination of a tubular diuretic plus a hyperosmolar agent may produce a better response than either drug alone. When tubular diuretics are employed to treat edema and ICP, a careful management of fluid status is necessary, with close monitoring of intake and output, electrolytes, and serum osmolarity.

The final group of drugs that have received clinical and experimental support as agents to control brain swelling, edema, and increased ICP are the barbiturates. Three barbiturates have been used: thiopental sodium, pentobarbital, and phenobarbital. The mechanism of action of these drugs is unknown. They do decrease CBF and cerebral metabolism, however. The decrease in CBF tends to limit formation of edema by lowering end-capillary pressure. The decrease in cerebral metabolism may permit the cells to tolerate a degree of ischemia or anoxia that would otherwise be detrimental. While experimental studies of focal ischemia, particularly, have shown some protective effect of barbiturates, this has yet to be demonstrated in the clinic. The use of barbiturate therapy, then, is mainly to lower the ICP. The use of high doses of barbiturates is a major undertaking and requires a pediatric intensive care unit. Of the three drugs, phenobarbital appears to have the fewest cardiovascular side effects but also appears to have the least effect on the EEG and, at present, appears to be less capable of controlling intracranial hypertension. Pentobarbital has been the most commonly used agent, but when levels above 3 mg% are obtained in children, hypotension is common. This drop in SAP is due to decreasing peripheral resistance, not to altered cardiac output, and can be controlled with fluid volume and dopamine, if necessary.

Significant dangers from hypotension and infection exist when barbiturates are administered, and their use should be restricted to areas where continuous supervision of therapy can be maintained. There seems to be a definite value in the use of barbiturates following head trauma in children and for Reye's syndrome. In both of these states, there is significant cerebral hyperemia, and it may be that the barbiturates have a maximum effect in those situations where flow is greater than metabolism. In patients with severe brain swelling after anoxia or ischemia, the author has not found the use of baributrates to lead to an improved outcome.[35] While it has proved possible to control the ICP, no patient recovered beyond the vegetative state. However, in those patients who did not develop intracranial hypertension, 30 percent recovered to a moderately disabled or better state.

PSEUDOTUMOR CEREBRI

This term is used to describe the appearance of signs and symptoms of intracranial hypertension in the absence of either hydrocephalus or an identifiable mass lesion. The syndrome is most common in prepubertal overweight children, boys and girls, but can be seen at any age throughout childhood. The presentation is of headache, often relatively nonspecific, and on examination of the child, papilledema is found. There can be sixth nerve palsies and visual loss as the syndrome progresses. Thus, the alternative name for the syndrome, benign intracranial hypertension, is a misnomer. In younger children, the headache may be a very minor complaint, and the only evidence of a problem is the finding of papilledema, or the realization that visual loss is present. The earliest visual manifestation of the chronic papilledema is enlargement of the blind spot, which is rarely complained of by the child. If left untreated, the chronic intracranial hypertension can produce chronic papilledema, resulting in optic atrophy. Up to 10 percent of patients with this syndrome have been reported to have permanent visual loss.[21] Disturbance of consciousness does not occur, but visual obscurations, especially on changing position, do occur and are often associated with lightheadedness and fainting spells. These episodes are probably due to ICP waves. Table 18–2 shows the various processes that have been associated with pseudotumor cerebri.

Table 18–2. PATHOLOGY ASSOCIATED WITH PSEUDOTUMOR CEREBRI

Vascular
  Major venous sinus obstruction
  Increased venous sinus pressure (e.g., secondary to AVM)
Hormonal
  Pregnancy, menarche, oral contraceptives
  Obesity
  Hypercortisolism
  Hypoparathyroidism
Toxic
  Hypo and hypervitaminosis A
  Drugs vs. steroids
    Tetracycline
    Nitrofurantoin
Anemia
Idiopathic Causes

When the patient is first seen with headache and papilledema, there is no way to make the diagnosis, since it is essentially one of exclusion. A CT scan, with and without contrast enhancement, is required to rule out hydrocephalus or a mass lesion. Evidence of sagittal or lateral sinus occlusion may be seen on the scan. Nuclear magnetic resonance imaging (NMRI) is especially useful in identifying sinus thrombosis. The ventricles may be normal in size, slightly enlarged, or slightly on the small side. Often, there are moderate amounts of CSF over the surface of the brain, but sometimes, this too is diminished. Occasionally, angiography may be required if the absolute status of the venous outflow needs to be evaluated.

Pathophysiology

There appear to be at least two of the intracranial compartments that are abnormal in this syndrome. CBF is normal, or slightly reduced, but CBV is elevated.[30, 35] This elevation in blood volume is greater than would be expected just from the elevated ICP but does not appear to be adequate to account for the entire rise in ICP. Studies of CSF dynamics have demonstrated an increase in outflow resistance of CSF, resulting from either an increase in venous sinus pressure or an increase in resistance to flow through the arachnoid villi.[20, 39] Why this situation of increased resistance appears to produce hydrocephalus in some patients and pseudotumor cerebri in others is unclear. Recent experimental work suggests that for hydrocephalus to occur, there must be a pressure gradient across the cerebral mantle.[12] Thus, when the absorption block is at the level of the villi, since there is no transmantle gradient, hydrocephalus does not develop. CSF absorption rates are abnormal in patients with pseudotumor cerebri, again confirming the potential pathologic role of increased outflow resistance in this syndrome.[11, 29] It is interesting that in experimental hypovitaminosis A,[16] fibrosis of the arachnoid villi has been found, and that in experimental hypoadrenalism, an increased resistance to CSF was noted.[22] These experimental findings further suggest that CSF reabsorption is a significant part of the pathophysiology of pseudotumor cerebri.

Recently, Hammer and colleagues[18] found elevated levels of vasopressin in the CSF in patients with pseudotumor cerebri, when compared with normal controls. They also found that in the pseudotumor cerebri patients, the CSF levels of vasopressin were higher than the blood levels. The reverse of this was true in the control population. They suggested that the increased vasopressin levels may alter capillary permeability and result in increased water content in the brain. Doczi and associates[15] have documented increased brain water content with the intraventricular administration of vasopressin in rats. However, since it is known that intracranial hypertension produces increases in vasopressin levels, it seems more probable that the elevated vasopressin levels are the result rather than the cause of the syndrome. However, this is an interesting hypothesis that will doubtless receive further study in the future.

Treatment

Since the reason for treatment is either relief of headache or protection of vision, many patients do not require any therapy. Once the papilledema is found, a CT scan is done. If this is normal, a spinal tap is performed to (1) measure the ICP and (2) examine the CSF, protein levels, and cells to rule out a chronic inflammatory process. The CSF should be clear and colorless, and the protein level should be normal or low. If visual acuity is normal and the blind spot only minimally enlarged, then weekly follow-up of visual fields to ensure that there is no visual deterioration may be all that is required. Frequently, the spinal tap produces resolution of the headache, as a result of lowering of the ICP. If headache continues despite stable vision, then acetazolamide (Diamox) may help by increasing CSF production rates. This syndrome is usually self-limiting, and thus, it is difficult to judge the results of therapy. If headaches persist, the papilledema increases, or both, or if there is evidence of further enlargement of the blind spot or decreasing visual acuity, then further therapy is necessary. The most effective agents are furosemide (Lasix) and corticosteroids. If either of these medications is used, because of the side effects of chronic usage, a firm plan of therapy should be outlined. The early drug dosage should be sufficient to produce resolution of the symptoms and signs, and once the papilledema has begun to resolve, the drug dosage is tapered off. During the tapering phase, continued examination of the visual fields and of visual acuity is necessary, since the swelling may recur as the dosage of medication is decreased.

In a small number of patients, the side effects of prolonged use of steroids make it impossible to continue their use (usually obesity and acne); the syndrome constantly recurs when medication is stopped; or severe visual loss or multiple obscurations of vision occur with change of position. In these patients, a lumboperitoneal shunt is indicated and is the best method to obtain resolution of the syndrome and recovery of vision.

SUMMARY

Intracranial hypertension is not a disease but a reflection of some imbalance between volume and pressure in the cranium. The clinical signs and symptoms of intracranial hypertension may be difficult to recognize in children. This is absolutely true in the unconscious child, and before instituting treatment of intracranial hypertension, it is necessary to establish what is producing the imbalance in the cranium and that the ICP is indeed elevated. This requires special neuroradiologic studies and measurement of the ICP. The various compartments of the intracranial space may contribute in different degrees to the cause of the raised ICP, and the selection of therapy has to be based on an understanding of the role of each compartment. The deleterious effects of ICP appear to be due to cerebral distortion and focal or global ischemia. While the normal brain can resist significantly elevated ICP, the damaged brain may not, and therapy is directed toward maintaining a normal ICP below 20 torr, if possible. Except in rare circumstances, it is possible with modern techniques to control the ICP in children. The benefit to the patient in terms of improved recovery, howver, depends upon the underlying pathologic processes. When there is a reversible underlying disease, the control of ICP can lead to dramatic recovery (e.g., head injury), whereas when the underlying disease leads to irreversible loss of neurons (e.g., anoxia, ischemia), control of ICP and preservation of life at a vegetative level may be a disservice to the patient and family.

There is no single therapy for increased ICP, and to select the most appropriate therapy, it is important to review constantly the various pathophysiologic mechanisms that may be active within the cranium. This therapy may be quite different from day to day in any one patient, depending upon the cause and the course of the disease process. In the unconscious patient, the use of ICP monitoring is an invaluable aid—and, the author feels, a necessity if therapy is to be given in a safe and controlled fashion.

References

1. Aarabi B, Long DM: Dynamics of cerebral edema. The role of an intact vascular bed in the production and propagation of vasogenic edema. J Neurosurg 51:779, 1979.
2. Bakay L: Radio-isotope studies in brain edema. In: Klatzo I, Seitelberger F (eds): Brain Edema. New York, Springer-Verlag, 1967, pp 517–529.
3. Bourke RS: Evidence for mediated transport of chloride in cat cerebral cortex in vitro. Exp Brain Res 8:219, 1969.
4. Bourke RS, Kimelberg HK, Daze MA, et al: Studies on the formation of astroglian swelling and its inhibition by clinically useful agents. In: Popp AJ, Bourke RS, Nelson LR, et al (eds): Neural Trauma. New York, Raven Press, 1979, pp 95–113.
5. Brock M, Zillig C, Weigand H, et al: The effects of dexamethasone in ICP in cases of posterior fossa tumors. In: Beks JWF, Bosch DA, Brock M (eds): Intracranial Pressure III. Berlin/Heidelberg/New York, Springer-Verlag, 1976, pp 236–246.
6. Bruce DA: CSF pressure dynamics and brain metabolism. In: Wood JH (ed): Neurobiology of Cerebrospinal Fluid. New York, Plenum Press, 1980.
7. Bruce DA, Bilaniuk LT, Dolinskas C, et al: Diffuse cerebral swelling following head injuries in children: The syndrome of "malignant brain edema." J Neurosurg 54:170, 1981.

8. Bruce DA, Langfitt TW, Miller JD, et al: Regional cerebral blood flow, intracranial pressure and brain metabolism in comatose patients. J Neurosurg 38:131, 1973.
9. Bruce DA, Raphaely RC, Goldberg AI, et al: The pathophysiology, treatment and outcome following severe head injury in children. Child's Brain 5:174, 1979.
10. Bruce DA, ter Weeme C, Kaiser G, et al: Mechanisms and time course for clearance of vasogenic cerebral edema. In: Popp AJ, Bourke RS, Nelson LR, et al (eds): Neural Trauma. New York, Raven Press, 1979, pp 155–171.
11. Calabrese VP, Selhorst JB, Harbeson JW: Cerebrospinal fluid infusion test in pseudo tumor cerebri. (Abstract.) Ann Neurol 4:173, 1978.
12. Conner ES, Foley L, Black PM: Experimental normal-pressure hydrocephalus is accompanied by increased transmantle pressure. J Neurosurg 61:322, 1984.
13. Cottrell JE, Robustelli A, Post K, et al: Furosemide- and mannitol-induced changes in intracranial pressure and serum osmolality and electrolytes. Anesthesiology 47:28, 1977.
14. Crocker EF, Zimmerman RA, Phelps ME, et al: The effects of steroids on the extravascular distribution of radiographic contrast material and technetium pertechnetate in brain tumors as determined by computer tomography. Radiology 199:471, 1976.
15. Doczi T, Szerdahelyl P, Gulya K, et al: Brain water accumulation after the central administration of vasopressin. Neurosurgery 11:402, 1982.
16. Eaton NP: Chronic bovine hypo and hypervitaminosis A and cerebrospinal fluid pressure. Am J Clin Nutr 22:1070, 1969.
17. Grubb RL, Jr., Raichle ME, Phelps ME, et al: Effects of increased intracranial pressure on cerebral blood volume, blood flow and oxygen utilization in monkeys. J Neurosurg 43:385, 1975.
18. Hammer M, Sorensen PS, Gjerris F, et al: Vasopressin in the cerebrospinal fluid of patients with normal pressure hydrocephalus and benign intracranial hypertension. Acta Endocrinol (Copenh) 100:211, 1982.
19. James HE, Bruce DA, Welsh F: Cytotoxic edema produced by 6-aminonicotinamide and its response to therapy. Neurosurgery 3:196, 1978.
20. Janny P, Chazal J, Colnet G, et al: Benign intracranial hypertension and disorders of CSF circulation. Surg Neurol 15:168, 1981.
21. Jefferson A, Clark J: Treatment of benign intracranial hypertension by dehydrating agents with particular reference to the measurements of the blind spot area as a means of recording improvement. J Neurol Neurosurg Psychiatry 39:627, 1976.
22. Johnston I: Reduced CSF absorption syndrome. Lancet 2:418, 1973.
23. Kuhl DE, Alavi A, Hoffman EJ, et al: Local cerebral blood volume in head-injured patients. Determination by emission computed tomography of [99]mTc-labeled red cells. J Neurosurg 52:309, 1980.
24. Kuhl DE, Reivich M, Alavi A, et al: Local cerebral blood volume determined by three-dimensional reconstruction of radionuclide scan data. Circ Res 36:610, 1978.
25. Laurent JP, Molinari GF, Oakley JC: Experimental model of cerebral hematoma. J Neuropathol Exp Neurol 35:560, 1976.
26. Lofgren J: Effects of variations in arterial pressure and arterial CO_2 tension on the cerebrospinal fluid pressure-volume relationships. Acta Neurol Scand 49:586, 1973.
27. Lorber J: Isosorbide in medical treatment of infantile hydrocephalus. J Neurosurg 49:702, 1973.
28. MacMillan V, Seisjö BK: The influence of hypocapnia upon intracellular pH and upon some carbohydrate substrates, amino acids and organic phosphates in the brain. J Neurochem 21:1283, 1973.
29. Martins AN: Resistance to drainage of cerebrospinal fluid: Clinical measurements and significance. J Neurol Neurosurg Psychiatry 36:313, 1973.
30. Mathew NT, Meyer JS, Ott ED: Increased cerebral blood volume in benign intracranial hypertension. Neurology 25:646, 1975.
31. Miller JD, Sakalas R, Ward JD, et al: Methyl prednisolone treatment in patients with brain tumors. Neurosurgery 1:114, 1977.
32. Millson C, James HE, Shapiro HM, et al: Intracranial hypertension and brain edema in albino rabbits. Part II. Effects of acute therapy with diuretics. Acta Neurochir 56:167, 1981.
33. Pappius HM, McCann WP: Effects of steroids on cerebral edema in cats. Arch Neurol 10:207, 1969.
34. Pollay M: Formation of CSF: Relation of studies of isolated choroid plexus to the standing gradient hypothesis. J Neurosurg 42:666, 1975.
35. Raichle ME, Grubb RL, Jr., Phelps ME, et al: Cerebral hemodynamics and metabolism in pseudotumor cerebri. Ann Neurol 4:104, 1978.
36. Reivich M: Arterial PCO_2 and cerebral hemodynamics. Am J Physiol 206:25, 1964.
37. Reulen HJ, Tsuyumie H, Tach A, et al: Clearance of edema fluid into cerebrospinal fluid. J Neurosurg 48:754, 1978.
38. Saunders ML, Miller JD, Stablain D, et al: The effects of graded experimental trauma on cerebral blood flow and responsiveness to CO_2. J Neurosurg 52:18, 1979.
39. Sklar FH, Beyer CN, Ramanathau M, et al: Cerebrospinal fluid dynamics in patients with pseudo tumor cerebri. Neurosurgery 5:208, 1979.
40. Swedlow D, Lewis L: Measurement of cerebral blood flow in children. Anesthesiology 53, 1980.
41. Teasdale G, Galbraith S, Jennett B: Operate or observe? ICP and the management of the "silent" traumatic intracranial hematoma. In: Shulman K, Marmarou A, Miller JD, et al (eds): Intracranial Pressure IV. New York, Springer-Verlag, 1980, pp 36–38.
42. Wei EP, Dietrich D, Povlishock JT, et al: Functional, morphological, and metabolic abnormalities of the cerebral microcirculation after concussive brain injury in cats. Cir Res 46:37, 1980.
43. Weis MH, Nulsen FE: The effect of glucocorticoids on CSF flow in dogs. J Neurosurg 32:452, 1970.
44. Zimmerman RA, Bilaniuk LT, Bruce DA, et al: Computed tomography of pediatric head trauma: Acute general cerebral swelling. J Radiol 126:403, 1978.

III Trauma

19
MANAGEMENT OF SCALP INJURIES

Louis C. Argenta, M.D.
Martin H. Adson, M.D.

The head is the most frequently injured area of the human body, and scalp lacerations are the most common type of head injury requiring operative care. In past centuries, loss of the scalp often led to life-threatening or fatal complications because of infection.[9] With refinement of appropriate treatment of these injuries, highly satisfactory results may now be obtained. The basic principles advocated by Cushing in 1918—thorough early cleansing, conservative débridement, primary closure, and use of scalp flaps—remain a cornerstone in the treatment of scalp injuries today.[8] Since no tissue in the human body mimics scalp in consistency or hair-bearing quality, injuries to this area still present a considerable technical and cosmetic challenge for reconstructive surgeons.

ANATOMY OF THE SCALP

The scalp is composed of five distinct layers, which can be remembered by using the mnemonic SCALP:

1. *S*kin is the most superficial layer of the scalp. It is densely hair-bearing, except in the forehead area. The scalp skin is the thickest skin on the human body (3 to 8 mm) and is an ideal source for skin grafts. It is thicker in the occiput and thins toward the anterior and temporal aspects of the skull.

2. The *c*onnective tissue subcutaneum is a thick cushioning layer of fat and connective tissue that attaches the skin to the underlying galea. It contains the adnexal tissues, lymphatics, nerves, and principal arteries and veins of the scalp. Within this layer, the major vessels extensively interconnect, a factor that often allows survival of comminuted narrowly based flaps that would otherwise be lost.

3. The *a*poneurotic layer, or epicranium, is a condensation of the fascia of the frontal and occipital muscles. It is the strongest layer of the scalp and is adherent to the skin by multiple fibrous septa. Considerable tension exists in this layer, so that when it is lacerated, gaping wounds result.

4. A *l*oose connective tissue layer lies between the epicranium and the pericranium. It is largely avascular, except for occasional emissary veins. Most of the mobility of the scalp is due to this loose layer.

5. The *p*ericranium, or periosteum of the skull, is the deepest layer of scalp. This layer is densely adherent to the skull and contains a rich vascular supply from the skull that will support skin grafts applied to it.

The blood supply of the scalp is relatively constant and is derived from five major paired blood vessels. All are end branches of the carotid system. They enter the scalp radially (Fig. 19–1) and then anastomose extensively in the subcutaneous tissue across the midline. Because of this wide-ranging intercommunication, extensive flaps covering large areas of the head can be developed on a single large axial vessel.[20] There are no significant perforating vessels of the scalp, except for occasional emissary

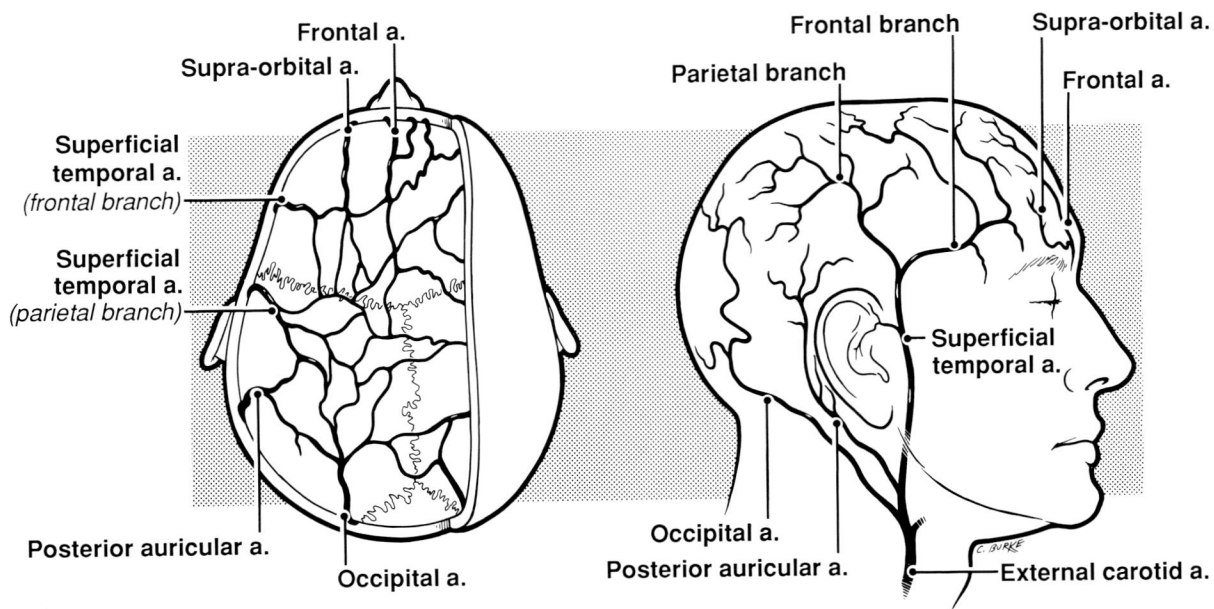

Figure 19–1. The blood supply to the scalp. Five major paired vessels perfuse the scalp. They interconnect extensively within the subcutaneous tissue. Consideration of these vessels is critical to planning successful flaps. (With permission of Clin Plast Surg 9:133, 1982.)

veins. Therefore, it is useless to delay skin flaps in the scalp. Collateral circulation of the scalp is so great that there is little impetus to develop new vessels through previous scars. Scalp flaps traversing previous scars are best avoided.

INITIAL TREATMENT OF SCALP INJURIES

Injuries to the scalp are frequently encountered in association with other major injuries. A complete and systematic evaluation of the patient with a scalp injury should be the same as for any victim of major trauma. Any injury that is grave enough to cause significant trauma to the scalp can also cause brain and spinal cord injuries, skull fracture, or major intra-abdominal and intrathoracic injury. Although trauma of the scalp and face may appear to be dramatic, the treatment of life-threatening injuries should always take precedence. Treatment of most scalp wounds can be safely deferred for up to 24 hours by wrapping the scalp with sterile dressings and applying pressure to achieve hemostasis. Clamping and ligation of partially severed major vessels must be accomplished in the emergency room, but such injuries are rare occurrences.

The basic principles of wound care apply to all wounds of the scalp:[11]

1. Gentle cleansing and removal of foreign material.
2. Hemostasis to avoid hematoma.
3. Conservative débridement of devitalized tissue.
4. Gentle manipulation of remnants, and suture closure without tension.

Tetanus prophylaxis should follow the guidelines of the American College of Surgeons.[7] Children up to age ten are usually covered by their initial diphtheria–pertussis–tetanus (DPT) immunizations. Systemic antibiotics should be administered judiciously in human bites,[12, 13] fetal scalp lacerations,[23] farm injuries, and wounds that are extensively contaminated or for which treatment has been delayed.

While many minor injuries of the scalp in children can be treated in the emergency room, significant wounds are preferably treated in the operating room, with the patient under general anesthesia. General anesthesia allows for careful exploration of the wound, hemostasis, and removal of foreign material. Devitalized portions of the temporal muscle should be débrided (Fig. 19–1). Radical débridement of the scalp is rarely indicated because of the extremely rich blood supply of the scalp. Many areas of scalp that appear compromised will survive fully. Even if superficial loss is later encountered, closure with a skin graft can be achieved successfully as a secondary procedure. Drains should be placed when there is excessive capillary oozing.

Lacerations

Simple or complex lacerations are closed by alignment of wound edges. Unhurried realignment of complex stellate lacerations usually allows primary closure. Single-layer closure with 3-0 or 4-0 monofilament permanent sutures achieves closure of the wound and hemostasis without extensive use of electrocautery. Sutures are usually left in place for 10 to 14 days to minimize retraction of the scalp, which will result in areas of alopecia. Following primary closure, children may shower and bathe almost immediately.

Lacerations secondary to fetal monitors or intravenous sloughs usually heal by simple dressing changes, without direct closure.[5, 26] Careful observation is mandatory in these cases, as abscess formation, sepsis, and death have been reported from these seemingly innocuous wounds.[4, 28]

Lacerations with a high risk for contamination, such as human bites and farmyard injuries, are probably best treated with secondary closure. Local wound care with frequent dressing changes with irrigation in combination with systemic antibiotics constitutes treatment for the first 24 to 48 hours. Clean wounds can then be loosely approximated with monofilament suture. Patients whose conditions remain questionable after 48 hours should have quantitative bacteriologic studies performed until counts drop below 10^5 bacteria per gram of tissue.[14, 24]

Partial-Thickness Loss of the Scalp

Scalp avulsions are almost always partial thickness, leaving the pericranium intact. Every attempt should made to replant surgically major segments of scalp that have been avulsed. A single successful artery and vein microvascular anastomosis can sustain the entire scalp.[20] If facilities for microsurgery are not available, the patient should be transferred to an appropriate hospital, if his or her general condition allows.

While primary scalp flaps can be acutely rotated over exposed pericranium, the most acceptable treatment is the application of partial-thickness skin grafts to the pericranium. These grafts may be taken from the avulsed scalp if it has not been severely damaged, but the buttock is the most frequent donor site. Skin grafts of thicknesses of ten thousandths to twelve thousandths of an inch are taken from any familiar dermatome and meshed. Younger infants require thinner grafts, since the donor area is thinner.[25] Grafts are sutured to the intact scalp margin, and tie-over bolsters are used to secure the graft for seven to ten days. Over the next six to eight months, these grafts will significantly contract, leaving a hairless defect that is 20 to 40 percent smaller. Areas of alopecia can later be serially excised or removed with the rotation of appropriate hair-bearing flaps.

Full-Thickness Loss of the Scalp

Full-thickness defects of the scalp are more difficult to manage because they involve loss of all layers, including the periosteum. Such injuries are often accompanied by damage to the skull and the underlying brain. Necrosis and sequestration of the calvarium occur when these wounds are not covered with viable tissue. Split- or full-thickness grafts do not survive on the outer table of the skull and should not be attempted. Usually, the scalp that remains is adequate to allow rotation of flaps to cover exposed bone. Very large defects of full-thickness loss rarely require the transfer of distant pedicled flaps if insufficient scalp remains. The development of microsurgery and musculocutaneous flaps has rendered the multiple-stage transfer of tubed flaps obsolete. The latissimus dorsi, trapezius, and pectoralis musculocutaneous flaps can be mobilized on their vascular pedicles to reach the temporal and forehead areas as pedicled flaps.[19] Free muscle or omental flaps can be transferred with microvascular anastomoses and can be covered with split-thickness skin grafts.[6, 15] The smaller the child, the more difficult the microvascular anastomoses. However, such anastomoses may be necessary in select cases.

Removal of the outer table of the skull allows development of granulation tissue, which will accept a skin graft. The entire exposed outer table is removed with a craniotome or sharp osteotome and is covered with moist saline dressings, frequently changed over the next seven to ten days. When adequate granulation tissue has developed, a skin graft is applied (Fig. 19–2). This procedure should be reserved for the older child whose skull has formed into two distinct tables. Such grafts are unstable over time because they shear readily from the skull with minimal trauma.

Scalp Flaps

Most wounds of the scalp are best treated using rotation flaps of remaining hair-bearing scalp. Such flaps restore the physiologic and anesthetic integrity of the scalp. Local flaps containing skin, subcutaneous tissue, and galea are utilized in one layer, leaving the periosteum of the donor site to accept a split-thickness skin graft. These flaps should be carefully planned by an experienced surgeon so that they are based peripherally to include at least one of the previously described major radiating vessels.[16] Use of Doppler ultrasonography may aid in the precise location and patency of these vessels. Before these flaps are mobilized, the surgeon should give careful consideration as to what hair-bearing tissue will remain after rotation of the flap. Flaps should be planned so that at a second operation, the area that is grafted in transfer of the original flap can be excised and closed primarily. Acute wounds are most safely treated with rotation of a single large flap and skin grafting of the donor site.

A large variety of scalp flaps are possible,[10, 17] as long as several technical points are observed. The inclusion of one of the major scalp vessels within these flaps almost ensures success (Fig. 19–3). Flaps should be slightly larger than the recipient area. It is sometimes helpful to use surgical towels to make

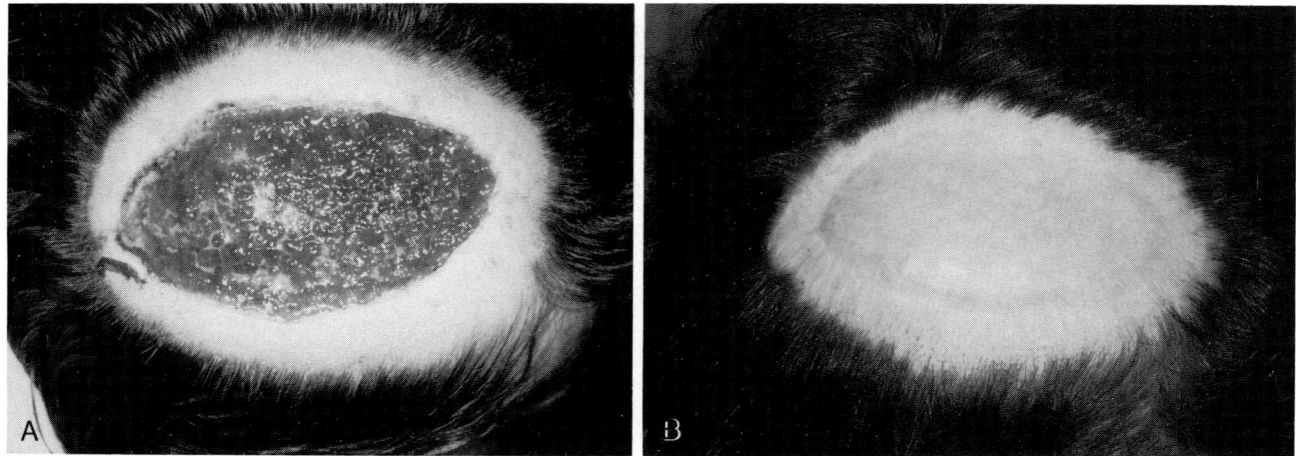

Figure 19–2. *A*, This 12-year-old boy suffered a 10 cm × 6 cm full-thickness avulsion of the scalp, including some of the outer table of the skull. The remaining outer table was treated with multiple burr holes. *B*, Within several weeks granulation tissue sufficient to support a graft was available, and a split-thickness graft was applied. (With permission from Clin Plast Surg 9:137, 1982.)

patterns. Towels are cut to the shape of each flap and are rotated into anticipated positions prior to making the actual cuts in the scalp.

Tourniquets and constricting bands are of minimal use. Incision lines are infiltrated with 0.5 percent lidocaine (Xylocaine) with epinephrine ten minutes before the incision is made. Electrocautery is used sparingly throughout the procedure, since damage to hair follicles may later result in areas of alopecia. Incisions are carried down to the pericranium, and the flap is peeled back from the skull at the avascular subgaleal plane.

The size of the flap can be increased by making multiple parallel incisions into the galea once the flap is elevated. Application of traction with a double hook on either side of the flap aids in determining the proper depth to which this incision should be made. The scalp can be felt to "give" when the proper depth of the galea is cut. Incisions can be made 3 to 5 mm apart. Care must be taken to avoid injury to major vessels of the flap when performing these incisions. The flaps are then transposed, and temporary fixation is achieved by the placement of staples. Once appropriate coverage of the defect has been accomplished, the wound should be closed with permanent monofilament sutures. A loose circumferential dressing is then placed, after the scalp has been copiously irrigated. This dressing should then be placed around the chin, to avoid removal of a turban type dressing by the child. Sutures are left in place for 10 to 14 days.

Types of Scalp Flaps

Rotation flaps containing an axial vessel may be used for coverage of most scalp defects. When small flaps are used, the adjacent scalp can be widely undermined and mobilized so that the donor defect

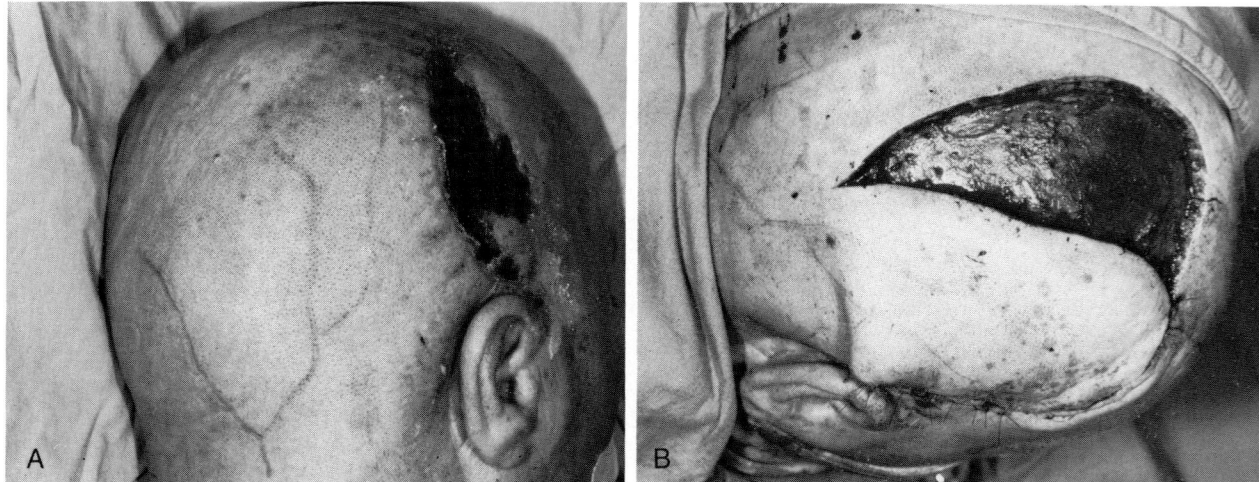

Figure 19–3. *A*, This 18-year-old male suffered full-thickness scalp loss three weeks after craniotomy for tumor. He had undergone extensive radiation preoperatively. The occipital vessels were marked out with Doppler ultrasonography and were incorporated into a large, posteriorly based flap. *B*, The flap was rotated without difficulty. The dog-ear resolved in six months and did not require further revision.

can sometimes be closed primarily. Defects of the vertex of the scalp can be closed with rotation flaps or pinwheel type patterns.[27]

Restoration of the anterior hairline is usually accomplished with a transposition flap brought anteriorly. Such flaps are most useful in correcting small or moderately sized defects. Bipedicle flaps are well suited for coverage of the forehead, temporal areas, or nape of the neck. Careful planning and the use of patterns should avoid errors in the use of these flaps. In the event of a mishap in planning, the bipedicle flap can be transected and used as two single pedicle flaps. "Dog-ears" that result after movement of a flap should be left intact. The surgeon should not attempt to exercise them and thus risk compromising the flap. These excesses in tissue usually smooth over with time, making secondary surgery unnecessary.

The technique of employing multiple large flaps to cover large areas of the scalp has been refined by Orticochea.[21, 22] By mobilizing all of the remaining scalp, forehead, and nape of the neck on three or four vascular pedicles, geometrically transposed flaps can achieve closure of very large defects (Fig. 19–4). Theoretically, it is possible to develop eight separate flaps, each based on an individual artery. However, in practice, the development of a smaller number of flaps is preferable.

The most versatile scalp flaps are those based on superficial temporal vessels and those based on the occipital vessels. Both of these vessels are of adequate size to support large areas of scalp beyond the midline. Flaps based on the temporal arteries offer an especially wide arc of rotation. It is important to realize that the width of the skull over the vertex is considerably greater than the width anteriorly or posteriorly. In the rotation of laterally based flaps to cover defects of the vertex, flaps must be designed so that their length on both sides extends beyond the midline. The flaps can be mobilized and brought to the vertex, where they will be sutured to one another in what will become the

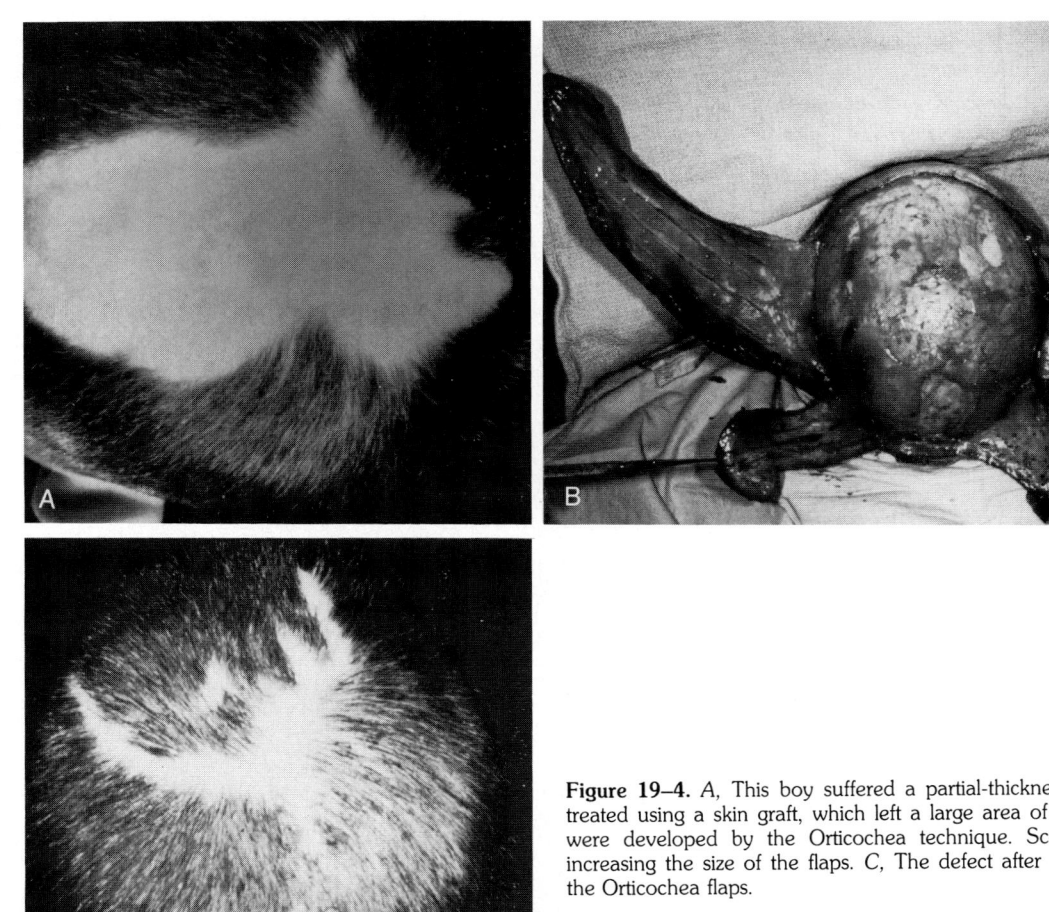

Figure 19–4. A, This boy suffered a partial-thickness avulsion and had been treated using a skin graft, which left a large area of alopecia. B, Multiple flaps were developed by the Orticochea technique. Scoring of the galea allows increasing the size of the flaps. C, The defect after geometric re-positioning of the Orticochea flaps.

midline. Conversely, flaps taken from the vertex and transferred anteriorly or posteriorly may be divided directly in the midline and then sutured side-to-side after transposition.

Controlled Tissue Expansion

Tissue expansion has proved a remarkable advancement in reconstruction of scalp defects.[1, 2, 18] For the first time, a method of creating new local tissue for reconstruction has become available. This is particularly valuable in scalp reconstruction, since the color, texture, and hair-bearing qualities of the scalp are unique in the body.

Tissue expansion is accomplished by the gradual enlargement of a silicone prothesis placed beneath the galea. This results in increased local tissue by the recruitment of adjacent scalp, the thinning of scalp, and the development of new skin by increasing the mitotic rate of the overlying tissue.[3] A wide variety of sizes and shapes of implants are available, and custom-made protheses can be manufactured.

No new hair follicles are created during the process of scalp expansion. Individual follicles are distracted from one another so that the existing hair follicles become more evenly distributed. Doubling of the distance between follicles is usually not perceptible. As much of the hair-bearing scalp as possible should be expanded to distribute evenly the follicles.

Protheses are placed through incisions that will be the edge of an advancing flap. This is usually at the edge of a defect. A surgical plane is developed beneath the galea that is large enough to allow the expansion prosthesis to rest several centimeters from the incision. The inflation reservoir is placed in an area where the child will not apply pressure to it while lying down. Multiple expanders around the scalp defect are a most effective way of generating adequate tissue for reconstruction.

After two weeks, the expander is filled with saline by percutaneous injection until tension of the overlying tissue is observed. Weekly or biweekly percutaneous instillation of saline is then carried out. Transient mild discomfort frequently accompanies initial inflation of the scalp, particularly in the forehead and temporal regions. However, after several inflations, there appears to be some loss of tone in the galea, and expansion proceeds more rapidly and is less painful. Children usually tolerate this procedure without difficulty (Fig. 19–5).

Filling of the prostheses usually takes six to eight weeks. Overexpansion of the remaining scalp is the rule, since too much tissue is rarely present in any reconstructive procedure (Fig. 19–6).

In a second procedure, the patient is returned to the operating room, where the prothesis is removed and the reconstruction completed. With the extra hair-bearing tissue created by controlled tissue expansion, it is usually possible to design relatively simple advancement or rotation flaps. The scalp flaps should be approximated with subcutaneous absorbable sutures and permanent monofilament sutures. The monofilament sutures are left in place at least two to three weeks.

Complications of tissue expansion include infection, deflation, extrusion of the prosthesis, and scarring. These complications are usually minor and are handled relatively easily. If deflation occurs, the

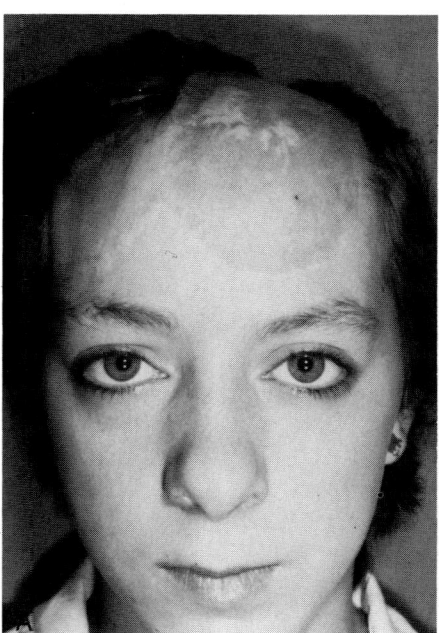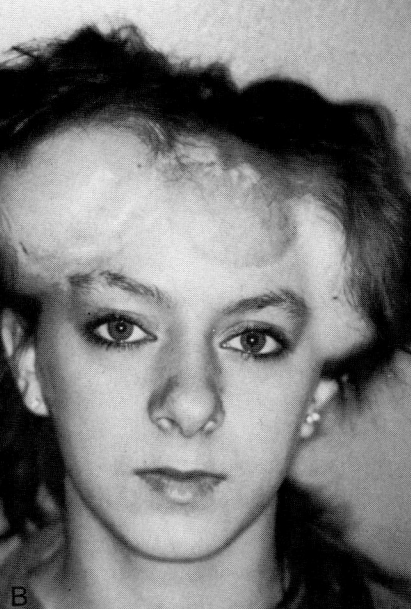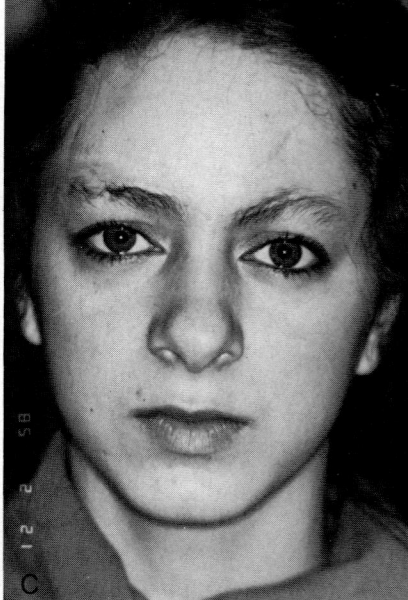

Figure 19–5. *A,* This 15-year-old girl suffered an avulsion injury of the forehead and scalp at the age of three. An unstable skin graft covered the scalp and forehead. *B,* Tissue expanders were placed on each side of the defect, and the normal scalp and forehead expanded to 450 cc over two months. *C,* The expanded tissue allowed complete removal of the graft and closure of the defect with anatomically correct tissue.

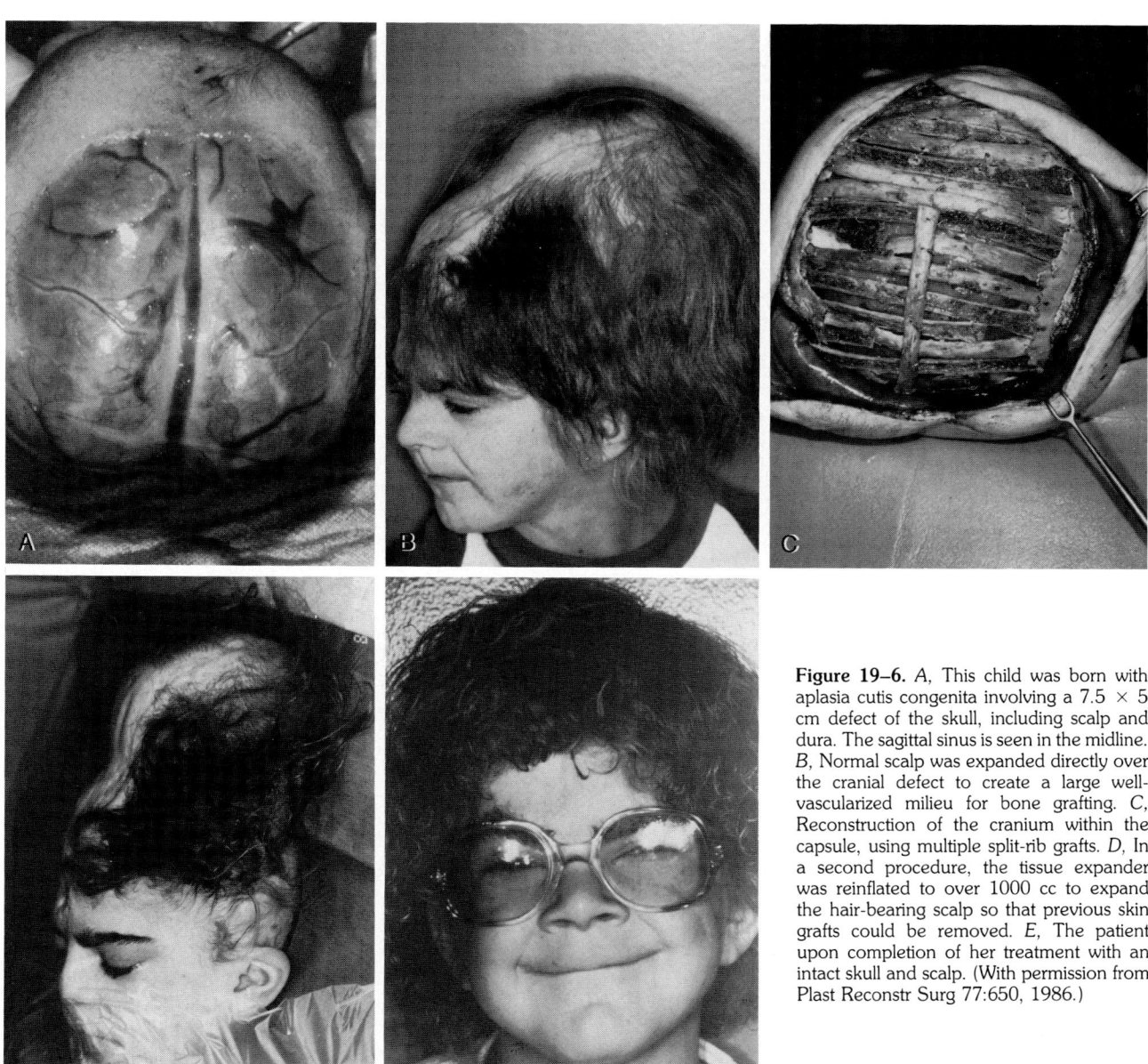

Figure 19–6. A, This child was born with aplasia cutis congenita involving a 7.5 × 5 cm defect of the skull, including scalp and dura. The sagittal sinus is seen in the midline. B, Normal scalp was expanded directly over the cranial defect to create a large well-vascularized milieu for bone grafting. C, Reconstruction of the cranium within the capsule, using multiple split-rib grafts. D, In a second procedure, the tissue expander was reinflated to over 1000 cc to expand the hair-bearing scalp so that previous skin grafts could be removed. E, The patient upon completion of her treatment with an intact skull and scalp. (With permission from Plast Reconstr Surg 77:650, 1986.)

prosthesis is simply replaced. Extrusion is usually the result of over zealous inflation or insufficient pocket size. If partial exposure of the prosthesis or minor infection occurs late in the course of expansion, the prosthesis may be removed, the wounds irrigated, and the flaps advanced. If infection occurs early after placement of the prosthesis, it is removed, and the second procedure is planned for two to three months later.

SUMMARY

In this century, the development of multiple techniques has allowed satisfactory reconstruction of even the most extensive scalp defects. Skin grafts, local rotation flaps, pedicled or free musculocutaneous flaps, and tissue expansion all have their appropriate places in reconstruction of scalp wounds. The correct use of each of these procedures depends on the extent of the injury and the experience of the surgeon. With proper planning and execution, reconstruction can be achieved with a high degree of success in children of any age.

References

1. Argenta LC, Dingman RO: Complete repair of aplasia cutis congenita involving scalp, skull and dura. Plast Reconstr Surg 77:650, 1986.
2. Argenta LC, Marks MW, Pasyk KA: Tissue expansion: New horizons in plastic surgery. Clin Plast Surg 12:159, 1985.

3. Austad ED, Thomas S, Pasyk KA: Tissue expansion: Dividend or loss. Plast Reconstr Surg 78:63, 1986.
4. Balfour HH, Block SH, Bowe ET, et al: Complications of fetal blood sampling. Am J Obstet Gynecol 107:288, 1970.
5. Brown AS, Huelzer DJ, Pierce SD: Skin necrosis from extravasation of IV fluids in children. Plast Reconstr Surg 64:145, 1979.
6. Chater NL, Buncke HJ, Alpert BS: Reconstruction of extensive tissue defects of the scalp by microsurgical composite tissue transplantation. Surg Neurol 7:343, 1977.
7. Committee on Trauma of the American College of Surgeons: Report Bull Am Coll Surg 64:20, 1979.
8. Cushing HC: A study of a series of wounds involving the brain and its enveloping structures. Br J Surg 5:558, 1918.
9. Davis JS: Scalping accidents. Bull Johns Hopkins Hosp 26:259, 1911.
10. Dingman RO: Surgical treatment of defects of the scalp. J Int Coll Surg 30:148, 1958.
11. Dingman RO, and Argenta LC: The surgical repair of traumatic defects of the scalp. Plast Reconstr Surg 9:131, 1982.
12. Goldstein E, Miller T, Citron D, et al: Infection following clenched-fist injury. A new perspective. J Hand Surg 3:455, 1978.
13. Guba A, Mulliken J, Hoopes J: Selection of antibiotics for human bites of the hand. Plast Reconstr Surg 56:538, 1975.
14. Heggers JP, Robson MC, Ristroph JD: A method of performing quantitative wound cultures. Milit Med 134:666, 1969.
15. Ikuta Y: Autotransplant of omentum to cover large denudation of the scalp. Plast Reconstr Surg 55:490, 1975.
16. Juri C, Juri J, Colnago A: Monopedicled transposition flaps for treatment of traumatic scalp alopecias. Ann Plast Surg 4:349, 1980.
17. Longacre JJ, Converse JM: Deformities of the forehead, scalp, and calvarium. *In:* Converse JM (ed): *Reconstructive Plastic Surgery*. Philadelphia, W.B. Saunders Co., 1977.
18. Manders EK, Graham WP, Schenden MJ, et al: Skin expansion to eliminate large scalp defects. Ann Plast Surg 2:305, 1984.
19. Maxwell GP, Leonard LG, Mason PD, et al: Craniofacial coverage using the latissimus dorsi musculocutaneous island flap. Ann Plast Surg 4:410, 1980.
20. Nahai F, Hurteau J, Vasconez L: Replantation of an entire scalp and ear by microvascular anastomosis of only one artery and one vein. Br J Plast Surg 31:339, 1978.
21. Orticochea M: Four-flap scalp reconstruction technique. Br J Plast Surg 20:159, 1967.
22. Orticochea, M.: New three-flap scalp reconstruction technique. Br J Plast Surg 24:184, 1971.
23. Plavidal F, Werch A: Fetal scalp abscess secondary to intrauterine monitoring. Am J Obstet Gynecol 125:65, 1976.
24. Robson MC, Heggeis JP: Delayed wound closure based on bacterial counts. J Surg Oncol 2:379, 1970.
25. Southwood WF: The thickness of skin. Plast Reconstr Surg 15:423, 1955.
26. Tuberville DF, Heath R, Bowen F, et al: Fetal complications of fetal scalp electrodes: A case report. Am J Obstet Gynecol 122:530, 1975.
27. Vecchione TR, Griffith L: Closure of scalp defects by using multiple flaps in a pinwheel design. Plast Reconstr Surg 62:74, 1978.
28. Winkel C, Synder D, Schlaerth J: Scalp abscess: A complication of the spiral fetal electrode. Am J Obstet Gynecol 126:720, 1976.

20
SKULL FRACTURES

John Mealey, Jr., M.D.

Skull fractures are found in over one quarter of all children who present at hospitals with head injuries[27] and in more than half of fatal cases of head trauma in childhood.[19] The nature and the physical forces of injury and the skull contour, thickness, and buttressing determine the type of fracture encountered. Compared with the adult skull, greater elastic deformation is probably necessary to produce tensile failure and skull fractures in young children, although experimental data are lacking in this age group.[22] Radiologic examinations are essential for the clinical diagnosis of skull fractures. Skull roentgenography and computed tomography (CT) tend to be complementary, and both may be advisable in selected cases.

LINEAR FRACTURES

Most of the skull fractures in children are linear and involve the cranial vault. Fracture lines may be single or complex, extend from suture to suture or buttress, or follow no predictable pattern. In infants and young children, fractures tend to be more separated or to be manifested in combination with suture diastasis. Falls and motor vehicle accidents account for most of these injuries. Skull fractures are also found in 30 to 70 percent of abused children with cranial trauma.[11, 56]

Roentgenographic diagnosis is difficult at times because of the variable developmental sutural patterns and synchondroses that may be found.[4] CT would be advisable in the obvious, more severe head injuries and whenever there is a clinical question of associated intracranial pathologic conditions. Although magnetic resonance imaging (MRI) does not ordinarily delineate skull fractures, it can provide an elegant elaboration of intracranial trauma.

Generally, children with head injuries of sufficient magnitude to cause a linear fracture of the calvarium are symptomatic and should be admitted to a hospital for observation. Skull roentgenograms are advisable at some time during such hospitalizations for dignosis and evaluation of skull fractures, but usually not as emergency procedures. Children with uncomplicated linear skull fractures generally resume normal activities within a few days. Most fractures heal by bony union and will no longer be evident roentgenographically after six months. An epicranial cerebrospinal fluid collection may sometimes develop acutely when the dura is lacerated at a linear fracture site. These lesions usually are transient and resolve spontaneously.[17] Early operative intervention is occasionally indicated when the scalp swelling is persistent or progressive (Fig. 20–1).

DEPRESSED SKULL FRACTURES

Depressed skull fractures in newborns are quite rare and have been associated with difficult births and forceps deliveries. An intrauterine etiology has also been documented with or without prior trauma to the maternal pelvis, notably from pressure on the fetal skull by the sacral promontory.[2, 21] Neonatal depressed skull fractures are ordinarily closed greenstick types of fractures in a parietal or frontal location. Most often, the infant appears well otherwise. Conventional treatment of these fractures in newborns has been surgical elevation when the depression is more than a 3 to 5 mm. Sponta-

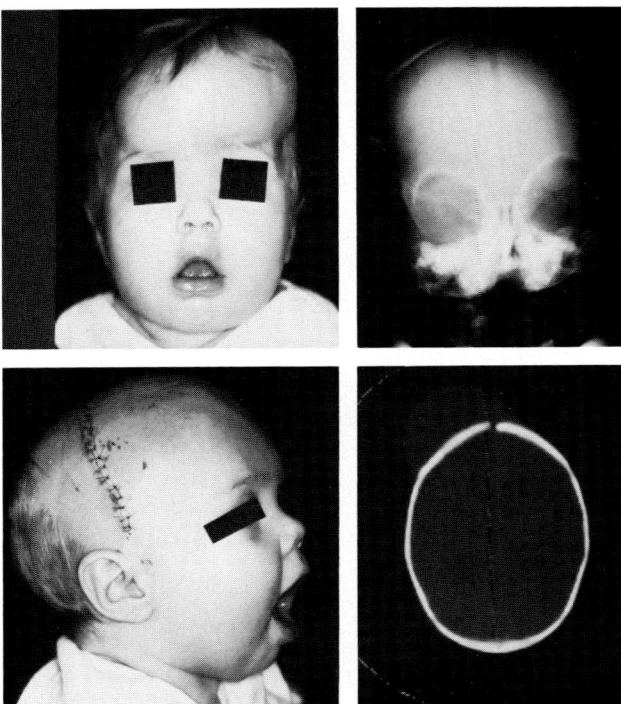

Figure 20–1. A seven-month-old infant with a progressive acute epicranial cerebrospinal fluid collection after closed head injury, linear and diastatic frontal fractures, and dural laceration. The infant was treated with craniotomy and duraplasty.

neous elevations have been reported within 24 hours and after several months without any intervention.[47] Skull indentations in the neonate have also been elevated by nonsurgical mechanical means.[73]

Depressed skull fractures account for 7 percent of the skull fractures found in children.[27] Around half of all depressed skull fractures seen in the population at large are found in infants and children.[34, 39] Fractures are considered to be depressed when the inner table is displaced by more than the thickness of the skull. These injuries are more apt to be found in the parietal and frontal bones than in temporal or occipital locations. Roughly a third of the depressed skull fractures in the pediatric age group are simple or closed. The most severe compound craniocerebral nonmissile wounds are found in victims of motor vehicle accidents. Focal neurologic deficits are usually secondary to localized brain contusion and hematoma and are noted in less than half of patients. Prolonged unconsciousness is exceptional. Roentgenographic diagnosis of depressed skull fractures may be improved by tangential views and the use of an image intensifier (Fig. 20–2). Cranial CT is generally advisable. This study provides an additional dimension of the degree of the cranial depression, an indication of the extent of any underlying fluid collection or hemorrhage, regional edema, or both and is a valuable adjunct for surgical treatment and follow-up. However, CT may not reliably delineate dural and dural sinus tears, small hematomas, or brain lacerations subjacent to the fracture. Nonetheless, this procedure may be diagnostic when skull roentgenograms appear normal (Fig. 20–3).

Compound depressed skull fractures should be débrided and elevated as soon as feasible. Débridement and elevation of the occasional one overlying the longitudinal or other major dural sinus in a neurologically normal patient would be exceptional, as surgery may precipitate severe hemorrhage. The principal goal of surgical treatment is prevention of infection, which makes operation within the first 24 hours after injury advisable. Restoration of the cranial contour follows as a secondary aim. Surgery may not be indicated for some closed fractures with only slight skull indentations that are not disfiguring or that are cosmetically concealed within the hairline. Surgical elevation might be considered in the majority of closed injuries where the fragments are depressed by more than 0.5 to 1.0 cm. However, since conventional x-ray films tend to underestimate the degree of depression and comminution, dural lacerations occur in at least a third of closed depressed skull fractures in young people, and brain lacerations in nearly a quarter.[34] The prognosis if left untreated is not well known.

For repair of compound wounds, the scalp laceration may be extended or incorporated in a scalp flap to gain adequate exposure. A conventional

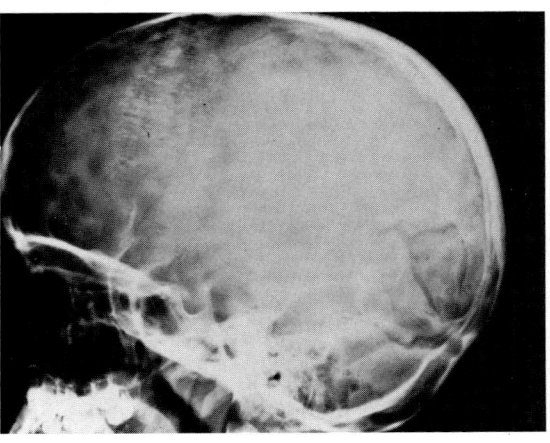
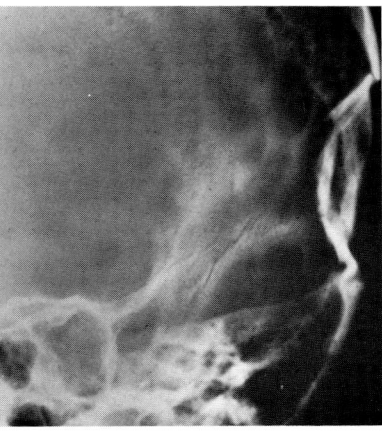

Figure 20–2. Depressed left parieto-occipital fracture, with the oblique roentgenogram demonstrating the extent of depression and comminution near the transverse dural sinus.

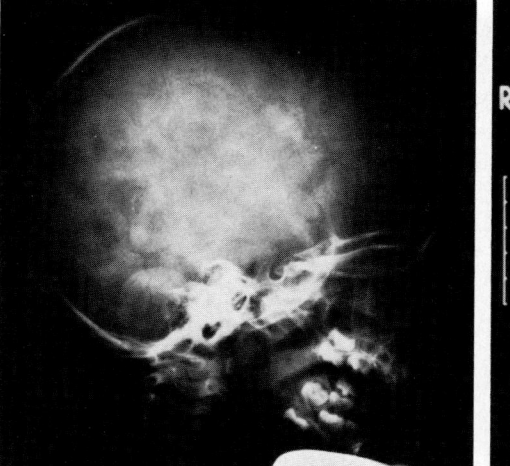 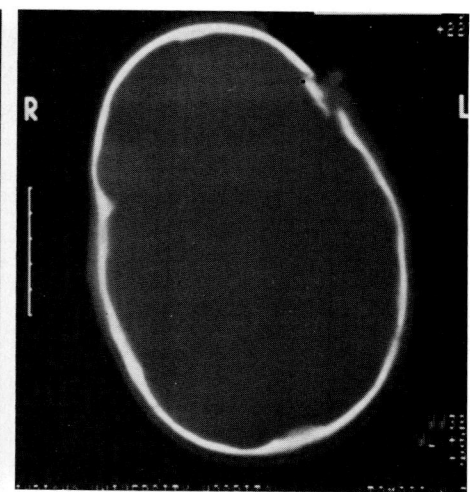

Figure 20-3. Compound depressed skull fracture evident on computed tomographic image of a two-year-old child with a laceration in the left temple and normal-appearing skull roentgenograms.

scalp flap preferably behind the hairline is appropriate for closed injuries. In young children with simple indentations, a burr hole or craniectomy at the margin of the depression may be used to lever the fragments into satisfactory position. However, in most cases, a craniectomy is advisable, encircling the periphery of the fracture, extracting the more central fragments, and elevating the margins of the defect. Elective subdural exploration is not indicated when CT is otherwise nonrevealing. When there is concomitant cerebral laceration, the dural defect should be extended for adequate hemostasis and débridement. Dural closure is desirable, using free pericranial or freeze-dried human cadaver dural grafts, where necessary. If the frontal sinus is exposed, the mucous membrane should be stripped away, the bone should be curetted, and the cavity should be packed with muscle or fat. The skull fragments are replaced as a primary mosaic cranioplasty, to reconstitute the desired contour prior to scalp closure. Skull roentgenography or CT should be repeated to confirm the completeness of the débridement and elevation.

Replacement of the bone fragments after a definitive surgical repair has become accepted practice.[43] Replacement of bone has been advocated even when it is not possible to close the dura.[38] Established infection in the wound would appear the only absolute contraindication. In most cases, there is a solid bone union that obviates the need for cranioplasty. The incidence of serious postoperative wound infection following definitive treatment of compound depressed skull fractures where the bone fragments have been replaced is less than 5 percent.

The value of prophylactic antibiotics in the perioperative management of compound depressed skull fracture has become more questionable, and the trend is away from their routine use.[12, 65] Antibiotic coverage would be considered when there is gross contamination or infection, when there is extension into the paranasal sinuses, and when methyl methacrylate has been inserted. Most children with blunt injuries resulting in depressed skull fractures recover without disabling neurologic and mental deficits, and the mortality rate observed is generally less than 10 percent.

PENETRATING CRANIOCEREBRAL TRAUMA

Gunshot wounds of the head are infrequently encountered in children. Early definitive surgery is advisable for optimal wound healing and prevention of infection.[24, 55] Cranial CT can define the extent of indriven bone and metal and complicating hematomas to facilitate surgical treatment. Devitalized tissue, clots, bone clusters, and accessible metal fragments should be removed. Primary dural and scalp closures are ordinarily indicated. Antibiotics, though no substitute for adequate wound débridement, are customarily administered. Retained bone and missile fragments are regularly found on follow-up CT in patients surviving gunshot wounds to the brain.[61] Despite concern about remote infection or abscess associated with intracerebral foreign bodies, these fragments are best left undisturbed in otherwise asymptomatic patients.[9, 64]

Penetrating craniocerebral wounds seem more prevalent in children and range from the inconspicuous or obscure to gross impalement of the head.[54, 68] In transorbital penetrations, the globe may be spared, with vision preserved. Skull x-ray films may not reveal the puncture. The compound craniocerebral nature of head wounds of this type and their potential for early or late infections and vascular complications should be recognized.[7, 14] With an obvious impalement, preparations for craniotomy should be completed or the débridement should be in progress prior to extraction of the foreign body. Orbital and other intracranial penetrations may be demonstrated by CT and direct early surgical treatment.[49]

BASAL SKULL FRACTURES

Fractures of the base of the skull have been diagnosed in 6 to 14 percent of head injuries in children.[15, 28, 54] Conventional skull roentgenograms were diagnostic in fewer than 10 percent of children with convincing clinical signs.[28] Multidirectional tomography with hypocycloidal blurring has greatly improved the detection of basal skull fractures. Cranial CT provides a further dimension for radiologic delineation of these fractures.[10]

Cerebrospinal Fluid Rhinorrhea

Anterior skull fractures that tear the meninges and extend into the paranasal sinus cavities or cribriform plate are the usual cause of traumatic cranionasal fistulas. Cerebrospinal fluid rhinorrhea has been diagnosed in 1 to 3 percent of civilian head injuries[23, 46, 66] and has been documented in less than 1 percent of head injuries reported in children.[15, 16, 28, 54] Traumatic cerebrospinal fluid rhinorrhea has been described in children as young as two years[8] but is seldom encountered in the first decade of life.[35, 36]

Cerebrospinal fluid rhinorrhea develops within 48 hours or by the end of the first week in 60 to 70 percent of patients.[46, 69] The onset may be more delayed in the remainder. However, within one month after injury, more than 90 percent of such cases will have occurred, and the condition is seldom first encountered beyond three months. Diagnostic determinations from glucose oxidase test tapes must be interpreted with caution, since false-positive results in nasal secretions and tears may occur in the majority of normal children.[32]

Since rhinorrhea ceases spontaneously in 80 percent or more of patients within a week or so after injury,[58, 66] initial management has been expectant. In still other patients, the leak resolves after several days of closed continuous lumbar cerebrospinal fluid drainage. Bacterial meningitis has been observed in 3 to 25 percent of patients with frontobasal skull fractures with cerebrospinal fluid rhinorrhea, generally early, and under conditions in which some form of antimicrobial therapy had been administered.[45, 46, 48] The natural risk of meningitis in unselected patients with post-traumatic rhinorrhea may be less than 10 percent.[42] The risk of remote meningitis is reportedly low in some series[6] and higher in others.[44] The mortality rate with this form of bacterial meningitis is comparatively low—6 percent in one study in adults.[25]

In both retrospective[50] and prospective[42] studies of acute traumatic cerebrospinal fluid fistulas, significant effectiveness of prophylactic antibiotics in preventing meningitis could not be demonstrated. Prophylactic antibiotic therapy does not prevent meningitis resulting from organisms supposedly sensitive to the antimicrobial drugs being administered.[58] The avoidance of antibiotic prophylaxis would also eliminate inherent drug complications and reduce the opportunity for more virulent supervening infections with resistant organisms. Accordingly, prophylactic antimicrobial therapy is no longer routinely advised in acute traumatic cerebrospinal fluid fistulas.[12, 48]

Surgical repair of traumatic cranionasal fistulas remains controversial in terms of selection of appropriate patients, localization of a causal dural defect, and timing of the operation. Surgical repair has been advocated in virtually every case in which traumatic cerebrospinal fluid rhinorrhea has ever been documented,[46] and this same policy of routine anterior fossa exploration has been advised in children.[8] The contrary and probably more widely followed practice has been to reserve surgical treatment for children with persistent or recurrent leaks beyond the acute phase of injury or for children in whom meningitis has supervened early or late. Rhinorrhea, pneumocephalus, or both associated with middle face fractures are ordinarily transient and resolve after facial fixation is done, without neurosurgical intervention.[36, 45]

Special diagnostic procedures have been used to confirm and localize cerebrospinal fluid leaks before surgical repair is undertaken. Colorimetric dye and fluorescein studies have generally been unsuccessful or frankly contraindicated because of neurotoxicity.[18, 51] Iophendylate (Pantopaque) has been helpful in some cases in the past.[3] Radionuclide infusion cisternography combined with nasal pledgets and radioactive counting may be of diagnostic value when the leaks are small, intermittent, or questionable.[13, 63] However, at present, the best means of diagnosis and localization of the anatomic site of an active cerebrospinal fluid fistula is by computed tomographic cisternography (Fig. 20–4). Thin axial and coronal scans are obtained before and after lumbar spinal infusion of the water-soluble contrast medium, to show the nature and extent of the pathologic processes.[1, 60, 62]

Surgery is usually done electively when traumatic brain swelling has largely subsided. An intradural approach is generally advisable initially through a unilateral or bifrontal bone flap, if necessary, according to the laterality of the rhinorrhea, the radiology, and the operative findings.[36, 46, 67] Magnification is helpful. Muscle, fat, flaps of dura and falx cerebelli, pericranium, temporalis fascia, fascia lata, and freeze-dried dura[70] all have been used in the repair of dural defects and are superior to grafts of synthetic materials. The graft is laid on intradurally with a generous overlap and is secured by several anchoring sutures. Tissue adhesives seem potentially useful, and isobutyl 2-cyanoacrylate is reportedly safe for this purpose.[52, 77] However, to date, none of the cyanoacrylate adhesives have been released for routine clinical use. Surgical repair by conventional craniotomy techniques obliterates

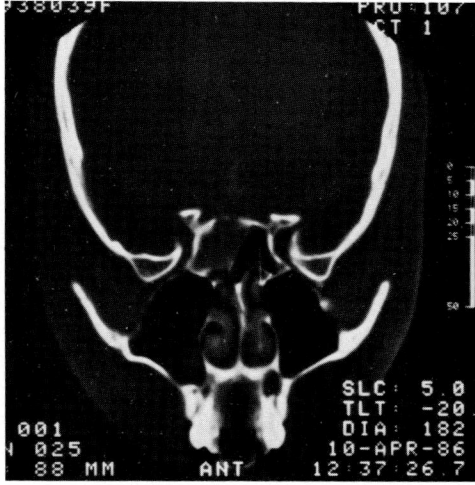 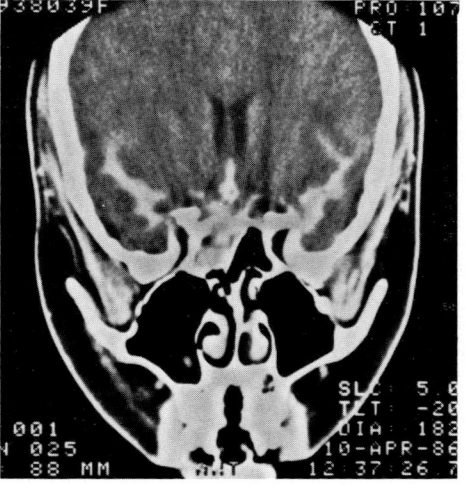

Figure 20–4. Cerebrospinal fluid rhinorrhea developed six months after this 16-year-old girl sustained multiple skull fractures in an automobile accident. There is an obvious defect in the planum and opacification of the left sphenoid sinus. Computed tomographic cisternography with water-soluble contrast medium demonstrates the fistula from the basal cisterns through this defect into the left sphenoid sinus. The leak was resolved after a sphenoidotomy was done to pack the sinus with subcutaneous fat, and a ventriculoperitoneal shunt was performed.

most of the anterior cerebrospinal fluid leaks. However, obliteration of the leak does not invariably prevent recurrent bouts of bacterial meningitis in children as well as in the adult population. Ventriculoperitoneal or lumboperitoneal shunts and sphenoidal packing have also been done to resolve recalcitrant cerebrospinal fluid rhinorrhea in patients with fistulas originating in the middle and posterior cranial fossas and after craniotomies had failed.[75]

Cerebrospinal Fluid Otorrhea

In cerebrospinal fluid otorrhea, the dural fistula is usually located in the middle cranial fossa through the thin tegmen tympani of the petrous bone, from longitudinal extensions of fractures of the temporal squama or parietal bone. A posterior fossa origin of cranioaural fistulas may be suspected in exceptional cases. Cerebrospinal fluid otorrhea has been diagnosed in 0.5 to 6 percent of pediatric head injuries.[15, 28, 54] Bleeding in the middle ear from a lacerated drum and hemotympanum without ensuing cerebrospinal fluid otorrhea are observed much more often.[16] Cranioaural fistulas are unusual in patients younger than five years of age because of underdevelopment of the mastoid air cells. Cerebrospinal fluid otorrhea is initially bloody and may be delayed in onset for several days by a blood clot. When the eardrum is not ruptured, the cerebrospinal fluid may be channeled into the nasopharynx via the eustachian tube and may be difficult to recognize. In most cases, cerebrospinal fluid otorrhea ceases spontaneously within a week,[45] and meningitis occurring early or late is uncommon.[6]

Prophylactic antibiotics are not routinely advisable for patients with basal skull fractures and blood in the middle ear or obvious cerebrospinal fluid otorrhea.[12, 16] The reported incidence of meningitis complicating acute traumatic cerebrospinal fluid otorrhea is less than 5 or 10 percent.[44, 50] *Streptococcus pneumoniae*, *Staphylococcus aureus*, and *Haemophilus influenzae*, which are frequently present in the nasopharynx and among the usual causes of post-traumatic bacterial meningitis, are not ordinarily found in the normal bacterial flora of the external auditory canal. In a prospective study of basal skull fractures in 50 patients, mostly with blood in the middle ear or cerebrospinal fluid otorrhea, antibiotics were not administered, and meningitis was not observed over a 3- to 24-month follow-up.[33]

Surgical repairs have been reported in 1 to 5 percent of patients when the otorrhea has been persistent, chronic, and intermittent or associated with meningeal infection[31, 46] and have been advocated for such sporadic cases in childhood.[8] Surgery has been performed in 9 of 24 children in whom the otorrhea seemed persistent.[26] Radiography is especially important when surgical exploration is considered, and hypocycloidal tomography is usually diagnostic. Computed tomography of the temporal bone can provide further complementary diagnostic information.[10, 79] Although endaural surgery and mastoidectomy have been employed to obliterate cranioaural fistulas, a transcranial intradural operation seems more appropriate for localization and grafting of the defect, particularly when there is useful hearing. A subtemporal approach, generally done first, can be extended to inspect the posterior aspect of the petrous bone by division of the tentorium.

Cranial Nerve Injuries

Olfactory Nerve. Partial, unilateral, or complete loss of the sense of smell has been described in 3 to 10 percent of patients with head injuries.[23, 31] This deficit would be difficult to ascertain in young children even if such examination was regularly attempted. There is no specific treatment.

Optic and Extraocular Nerves. Blunt head trauma may cause instantaneous blindness of one eye resulting from contusion or ischemia of the optic nerve in its intracranial and intracanalicular course.[78] Some spontaneous recovery of vision may be expected in up to 50 percent of patients, usually within days or weeks, but rarely is it complete.[29, 76] This condition has been reported in up to 5 percent of head injuries but is rare in children.[30, 74] Surgical treatment is ordinarily considered only in the isolated case, in which it can be ascertained that some vision is preserved initially, that further loss has since developed, usually over several days, and that light perception at least is retained. Under these circumstances, the orbit and the optic canal can be explored transcranially or transethmoidally to decompress the optic nerve. Good visual recovery following surgical treatment is generally unusual.[41] The extensive Japanese experience is exceptional; however, less than 15 percent of these patients were operated on during the first week after head injury.[20]

Fractures of the base of the skull, the orbit, or both may cause immediate primary palsies of the extraocular nerves. Blowout fractures of the orbits involving the floor or medial aspect may mimic a third nerve palsy.[78] Injury to the extraocular nerves has been reported in 1 to 9 percent of head injuries among the general population[31, 76] and, in decreasing order of frequency, to the sixth, third, and fourth cranial nerves.[72] Multiple partial injuries are observed more frequently than complete ophthalmoplegia. The sixth nerve is most apt to be involved bilaterally. Over 75 percent of patients with third and sixth nerve palsies recover spontaneously. The prognosis is poorer for isolated trochlear nerve contusional injuries resulting from blows to the vertex of the head.[78]

Facial Nerve. Facial paralysis, the commonest cranial nerve injury occurring at birth, tends to resolve promptly. Extracranial anastomosis of the facial nerve at the stylomastoid foramen to the phrenic or other cranial nerves may fail to restore facial function in young children with persistent paralysis. This observation probably reflects an intracanalicular causal etiology rather than the more conventional view of an extracranial origin of the nerve damage.[53]

Peripheral facial nerve palsies in general occur in about 1 percent of head injuries studied in children.[28, 54] The onset of the paralysis may be delayed in about 12 percent of the cases for several days and then gradually becomes more complete over two or three more days.[31, 40] Hypocycloidal tomography delineated a fracture in 75 percent of children with peripheral facial palsies associated with acute head injury.[26]

Satisfactory natural recovery may be expected in up to 90 percent of patients with facial palsies resulting from basal skull fractures.[57] Baseline and follow-up electrodiagnostic studies are of prognostic value. The outlook is especially favorable with expectant treatment when facial paralysis is incomplete or delayed in onset. Signs of spontaneous recovery are usually detected clinically and from electric testing within one to three months after injury. Beyond this time, exploration of the nerve should be considered if the paralysis remains complete. The timing and the role of various surgical procedures for facial nerve injuries remain controversial.[71]

Acoustic Nerve. Dizziness, hearing loss, and tinnitus have been noted in a third or more of patients after head injury.[5, 23] These symptoms are recognized in older children but may easily be overlooked in the very young. Conductive hearing deficits usually associated with longitudinal fractures of the petrous bone and ossicular chain disruption generally tend to improve. Significant partial or complete sensorineural deafness has been described in 1.5 percent of patients with head injuries occurring after either longitudinal or transverse fractures of the petrous bone in most instances, but also where there are no signs of fracture.[31] The actual incidence of this problem in children is unknown but is probably very low.[28]

Trigeminal and Lower Cranial Nerves. Intracranial damage to the trigeminal complex after head trauma in children is very rare, is associated with extensive basal skull fractures and penetrating injuries, and may be partial or complete.[37] Injuries to the ninth through the twelfth cranial nerves are not ordinarily observed in patients who survive after trauma to the head. Unilateral paralysis of these four nerves resulting from penetrating wounds around the jugular foramen is well documented.[59]

References

1. Admadi J, Weiss MH, Segall HD, et al: Evaluation of cerebrospinal fluid rhinorrhea by metrizamide computed tomographic cisternography. Neurosurgery 16:54, 1985.
2. Alexander E, Davis CH, Jr.: Intra-uterine fracture of the infant's skull. J Neurosurg 30:446, 1969.
3. Allen MB, Gammal TE, Ihnen M, et al: Fistula detection in cerebrospinal fluid leakage. J Neurol Neurosurg Psychiatr 35:664, 1972.
4. Allen WE, II, Kier EL, Rothman SL: Pitfalls in the evaluation of skull trauma. A review. Radiol Clin North Am 11:479, 1973.
5. Barber HO: The diagnosis and treatment of auditory and vestibular disorders after head injury. Clin Neurosurg 19:355, 1972.
6. Brawley BW, Kelly WA: Treatment of basal skull fractures with and without cerebrospinal fluid fistulae. J Neurosurg 26:57, 1967.
7. Bulluck MH, Baker, GS, Henderson JW: Injuries of the brain caused by penetration of the orbit. Minn Med 42:1408, 1959.
8. Caldicott WJH, North JB, Simpson DA: Traumatic cerebrospinal fluid fistulas in children. J Neurosurg 38:1, 1973.
9. Carey ME, Young HF, Rish BL, et al: Followup study of 103 American soldiers who sustained a brain wound in Vietnam. J Neurosurg 41:542, 1974.
10. Claussen CD, Lohkamp FW, Krastel A: Computed tomography of trauma involving brain and facial skull (craniofacial injuries). J Comput Assist Tomogr 1:472, 1977.
11. Cohen RA, Kaufman RA, Myers PA, et al: Cranial computed tomography in the abused child with head injury. Am J Roentgenol 146:97, 1986.

12. Cooper PR: Skull fracture and traumatic cerebrospinal fluid fistulas. *In:* Cooper PR (ed): Head Injury. Baltimore, Williams & Wilkins, 1982, pp 65–82.
13. Curnes JT, Vincent LM, Kowalsky RJ, et al: CSF rhinorrhea: Detection and localization using overpressure cisternography with Tc-99M-DTPA. Radiology 154:795, 1985.
14. Duffy GP, Bhandari YS: Intracranial complications following transorbital penetrating injuries. Br J Surg 56:685, 1969.
15. Dugger GS: Head injury. *In:* Farmer TW (ed): Pediatric Neurology. New York, Harper & Row, 1964, pp 392–442.
16. Einhorn A, Mizrahi EM: Basilar skull fractures in children. The incidence of CNS infection and the use of antibiotics. Am J Dis Child 132:1121, 1978.
17. Epstein JA, Epstein BA, Small M: Subepicranial hydroma. A complication of head injuries in infants and children. J Pediatr 59:562, 1961.
18. Evans JP, Keegan HR: Danger in the use of intrathecal methylene blue. JAMA 174:856, 1960.
19. Freytag E: Autopsy findings in head injuries from blunt forces. Statistical evaluation of 1,367 cases. Arch Pathol 75:402, 1963.
20. Fukado Y: Results in 400 cases of surgical decompression of the optic nerve. Mod Probl Ophthalmol 14:474, 1975.
21. Garza-Mercado R: Intrauterine depressed skull fractures of the newborn. Neurosurgery 10:694, 1982.
22. Gurdjian ES: Recent advances in the study of the mechanisms of impact injury of the head—a summary. Clin Neurosurg 19:355, 1972.
23. Gurdjian ES, Webster JE: Head Injuries. Mechanisms, Diagnosis and Management. Boston, Little, Brown & Co., 1958.
24. Hammon WH: Analysis of 2187 consecutive penetrating wounds of the brain from Vietnam. J Neurosurg 34:127, 1971.
25. Hand WL, Sanford JP: Posttraumatic bacterial meningitis. Ann Intern Med 72:869, 1970.
26. Harwood-Nash DC: Fractures of the petrous and tympanic parts of the temporal bone in children: A tomographic study of 35 cases. Am J Roentgenol Radium Ther Nucl Med 110:598, 1970.
27. Harwood-Nash DC, Hendrick EB, Hudson AR: The significance of skull fractures in children. A study of 1,187 patients. Radiology 101:151, 1971.
28. Hendrick EB, Harwood-Nash DCF, Hudson AR: Head injuries in children: A survey of 4465 consecutive cases at the Hospital for Sick Children, Toronto, Canada. Clin Neurosurg 11:46, 1964.
29. Hooper RS: Orbital complications of head injuries. Br J Surg 39:126, 1951.
30. Hooper R: Head injuries in childhood. Aust NZ J Surg 32:11, 1962.
31. Hughes BJ: The results of injury to special parts of the brain and skull. *In:* Rowbotham GF (ed): Acute Injuries of the Head. Their Diagnosis, Treatment, Complications and Sequels, 4th ed. Baltimore, Williams & Wilkins, 1964, pp 408–433.
32. Hull HF, Morrow G, III: Glucorrhea revisited. Prolonged promulgation of another plastic pearl. JAMA 234:1052, 1975.
33. Ignelzi RJ, VanderArk GD: Analysis of the treatment of basilar skull fractures with and without antibiotics. J Neurosurg 43:721, 1975.
34. Jamieson KG, Yelland JDN: Depressed skull fractures in Australia. J Neurosurg 37:150, 1972.
35. Jamieson KG, Yelland JDN: Surgical repair of the anterior fossa because of rhinorrhea, aerocele, or meningitis. J Neurosurg 39:328, 1973.
36. Jefferson A, Reilly G: Fractures of the floor of the anterior cranial fossa. The selection of patients for dural repair. Br J Surg 59:585, 1972.
37. Jefferson G, Schorstein J: Injuries of the trigeminal nerve, its ganglion and its divisions. Br J Surg 42:561, 1955.
38. Jennett B, Miller JD: Infection after depressed fracture of skull. Implications for management of nonmissile injuries. J Neurosurg 36:333, 1972.
39. Jennett B, Miller JD, Braakman R: Epilepsy after nonmissile depressed skull fracture. J Neurosurg 41:208, 1974.
40. Jongkees LBW: Facial paralysis complicating skull trauma. Arch Otolaryngol 81:518, 1965.
41. Kennerdell JS, Amsbaugh GA, Myers EN: Transantral-ethmoidal decompression of optic canal fracture. Arch Ophthalmol 94:1040, 1976.
42. Klastersky J, Sadeghi M, Brihaye J: Antimicrobial prophylaxis in patients with rhinorrhea or otorrhea: A double-blind study. Surg Neurol 6:111, 1976.
43. Kriss FC, Taren JA, Kahn EA: Primary repair of compound skull fractures by replacement of bone fragments. J Neurosurg 30:698, 1969.
44. Laun A: Traumatic cerebrospinal fluid fistulas in the anterior and middle cranial fossae. Acta Neurochir 60:215, 1982.
45. Leech PJ, Paterson A: Conservative and operative management for cerebrospinal-fluid leakage after closed head injury. Lancet 1:1013, 1973.
46. Lewin W: Cerebrospinal fluid rhinorrhea in non-missile head injuries. Clin Neurosurg 12:237, 1966.
47. Loeser JD, Kilburn HL, Jolley T: Management of depressed skull fracture in the newborn. J Neurosurg 44:62, 1976.
48. Loew F, Pertuiset B, Chaumier EE, et al: Traumatic, spontaneous and postoperative CSF rhinorrhea. Adv Tech Stand Neurosurg 11:169, 1984.
49. Lunsford LD, Woodford J, Drayer BP: Cranial computed tomographic demonstration of intracranial penetration by an orbital foreign body. Neurosurgery 1:57, 1977.
50. MacGee EE, Cauthen JC, Brackett CE: Meningitis following acute traumatic cerebrospinal fluid fistula. J Neurosurg 33:312, 1970.
51. Mahaley MS, Odom GL: Complication following intrathecal injection of fluorescein. J Neurosurg 25:298, 1966.
52. Maxwell JA, Goldware SI: Use of tissue adhesive in the surgical treatment of cerebrospinal fluid leaks. Experience with isobutyl 2-cyanoacrylate in 12 cases. J Neurosurg 39:332, 1973.
53. McHugh HE: Facial paralysis in birth injury and skull fractures. Arch Otolaryngol 78:443, 1963.
54. Mealey J, Jr.: Pediatric Head Injuries. Springfield, IL, Charles C Thomas, 1968.
55. Meirowsky Am: Penetrating craniocerebral trauma. Clin Neurosurg 12:253, 1966.
56. Merten DF, Osborne DRS, Radkowski MA, et al: Craniocerebral trauma in the child abuse syndrome: Radiological observations. Pediatr Radiol 14:272, 1984.
57. Miehlke A: Surgery of the Facial Nerve. Philadelphia, W.B. Saunders Co., 1973, pp 74–80.
58. Mincy JE: Posttraumatic cerebrospinal fluid fistula of the frontal fossa. J Trauma 6:618, 1966.
59. Mohanty SK. Barrios M, Fishbone H, et al: Irreversible injury of cranial nerves 9 through 12 (Collet-Sicard syndrome). Case report. J Neurosurg 38:86, 1973.
60. Nabawi P, MaFee M, Phillips J, et al: The success rate of metrizamide CT cisternography in the evaluation of cerebrospinal fluid (CSF) rhinorrhea. Comput Radiol 6:343, 1982.
61. Nagib MG, Rockswold GL, Sherman RS, et al: Civilian gunshot wounds to the brain: Prognosis and management. Neurosurgery 18:533, 1986.
62. Naidich TP, Moran CJ: Precise anatomic localization of atraumatic sphenoethmoidal cerebrospinal fluid rhinorrhea by metrizamide cisternography. J Neurosurg 53:222, 1980.
63. Park J, Strelzow VV, Friedman WH: Current management of cerebrospinal fluid rhinorrhea. Laryngoscope 93:1294, 1983.
64. Pitlyk PJ, Tolchin S, Stewart W: The experimental significance of retained intracranial bone fragments. J Neurosurg 33:19, 1970.
65. Plese JP, Humphreys RP: The use of prophylactic systemic antibiotics in compound depressed skull fractures in infancy and childhood. Arqu Neuropsiquiatr 39:286, 1981.
66. Raaf J: Posttraumatic cerebrospinal fluid leaks. Arch Surg 95:648, 1967.
67. Ray BS, Bergland RM: Cerebrospinal fluid fistula: Clinical

aspects, techniques of localization, and methods of closure. J Neurosurg 30:399, 1969.
68. Reeves DL: Penetrating craniocerebral injuries. Report of two unusual cases. J Neurosurg 23:204, 1965
69. Robinson RG: Cerebrospinal fluid rhinorrhea, meningitis and pneumocephalus due to non-missile injuries. Aust NZ J Surg 39:328, 1970.
70. Rosomoff HL: Ethylene oxide sterilized, freeze-dried dura mater for the repair of pachymeningeal defects. J Neurosurg 16:197, 1959.
71. Rovit RL, Murali R: Injuries of the cranial nerves. *In*: Cooper PR (ed): Head Injury. Baltimore, Williams & Wilkins, 1982, pp 99–114.
72. Rucker CW: The causes of paralysis of the third, fourth and sixth nerves. Am J Ophthalmol 61:1293, 1966.
73. Saunders BS, Lasoritz S, McArtor RD, et al: Depressed skull fracture in the neonate. J Neurosurg 50:512, 1979.
74. Schneider P: Perte de vision par traumatisme crânien fermé. Ophthalmologica 156:377, 1968.
75. Spetzler RF, Wilson CB: Management of recurrent CSF rhinorrhea of the middle and posterior fossa. J Neurosurg 48:393, 1978.
76. Turner JWA: Indirect injuries of the optic nerve. Brain 66:140, 1943.
77. VanderArk GD, Pitkethly DT, Ducker TB, et al: Repair of cerebrospinal fluid fistulas using a tissue adhesive. J Neurosurg 33:151, 1970.
78. Walsh FB, Hoyt WF: Craniocerebral trauma, hypoxia and injuries by other physical agents. *In*: Clinical Neuro-ophthalmology, Vol. 3. Baltimore, Williams & Wilkins, 1960, pp 2331–2537.
79. Wiet RJ, Valvassori GE, Kotsanis CA, et al: Temporal bone fractures. State of the art review. Am J Otolaryngol 6:207, 1985.

21
CONCUSSION AND CONTUSION FOLLOWING PEDIATRIC HEAD TRAUMA

Derek A. Bruce, M.D.
Luis Schut, M.D.

Concussion has been defined in its simplest, most restrictive sense as either "a temporary state of unconsciousness produced by trauma to the head"[18] or "the loss of consciousness and associated traumatic amnesia which occurs as the consequence of head trauma in the absence of physical damage to the brain."[19] These definitions imply (1) that concussion is transient, yet no time period is defined; and (2) that structural damage does not occur. In animal experiments, neuronal cell change in the brainstem reticular formation has been described following traumatic unconsciousness with recovery,[20, 21] suggesting that structural damage may indeed be part of the concussive process. A broader, less restrictive definition is that concussion is a clinical syndrome characterized by immediate and transient impairment of neuronal function, such as alterations of consciousness or disturbance of vision, resulting from mechanical forces (Committee to Study Head Injury Nomenclature, 1966). Again, the time period of the disturbance is not defined, and it is known that post-traumatic disturbances, such as deficits in short-term memory, may last for weeks following even minor trauma.[9] Symonds[17] proposed that concussion could not be restricted to transient states of unconsciousness, since the etiology was diffuse neuronal and axonal injury, and that a spread of injury must occur from mild and completely reversible to severe and irreversible. This hypothesis was expanded by Hooper[8] and, most recently, by Ommaya and Gennarelli,[12] who proposed the following hypothesis for concussion.

> Concussion represents a graded set of clinical syndromes following head injury wherein increasing severity of disturbance in level and content of consciousness is caused by mechanically-induced strains affecting the brain in a centripetal sequence of disruptive effect on function and structure. The effects of this sequence always begin at the surface of the brain in the mild cases and extend inwards to affect the diencephalic, mesencephalic core at the more severe levels of trauma.*

This concept of radial injury helps explain many of the clinical disturbances that are not associated with traumatic unconsciousness (e.g., amnesia). Further, it suggests that there may be a continuum of degree of injury that goes from mild amnesia to continued deep coma. The mechanism of concussion is believed to be shearing stresses set up within the brain substance.[7, 13] Linear acceleration alone

---

*Reprinted with permission from Ommaya AK, Gennarelli TA: Cerebral concussion and traumatic unconsciousness: Correlation of experimental and clinical observations on blunt head injuries. Brain 97:633–654, 1974.

does not appear to produce concussion, whereas rotational acceleration does.[13]

When consciousness is lost, the disruptive force has been sufficient to affect not only cortex and subcortical white matter function but also the brainstem reticular formation and the deep midthalamic nuclei. The loss of function may be due to physiologic blockade at the neuronal body, synapse, dendrite, axons, or some combination of these, that is associated with as yet unidentifiable pathologic damage or may be due to disruption of myelin sheaths and axons, with concomitant, irreversible structural damage. When the patient is seen, it may be impossible to decide how much underlying irreversible injury has occurred. This is particularly true if the patient is seen immediately following head injury. In human adult head injury autopsy material, major contusions or lacerations are present in 75 percent of patients,[5] and there is almost always evidence of structural damage to the brain. When primary brainstem hemorrhages are seen, there are usually accompanying changes in the supratentorial portion of the brain,[4] thus supporting the radial concept of injury. However, in children, no microscopic lesion may be found at autopsy, only severe, diffuse swelling of the brain.[111] This suggests that in this age group, concussion itself may cause death (e.g., by prolonged apnea) or may precipitate changes that cause death without producing identifiable structural change in the brain (e.g., acute swelling and vasodilatation). The clinical aspects of concussion in children will be discussed on the basis of the hypothesis of Ommaya and Gennarelli, as the authors feel that this is the best functional definition of concussion.

CLINICAL ASPECTS OF CONCUSSION

Any injury to the head that is associated with transient amnesia fulfills the criteria of concussion. In younger children, a history of amnesia may be very difficult to obtain, and in those younger than two years of age, concussion may be impossible to diagnose unless a period of traumatic unconsciousness has occurred. In older children and adults, there is good evidence[15] that the length of post-traumatic amnesia is a good measure of the severity of the concussive injury. The clinical syndrome of concussion is different at different ages in infancy and childhood, and the syndromes will be separately considered.

Traumatic unconsciousness is uncommon in children younger than one year of age. Many injuries to the head in this age group are the result of short falls (e.g., from the bed or changing table). Skull fractures are very frequently seen, but loss of consciousness is rarely reported. Occasionally, a history is obtained of a period of limpness with the eyes rolled up, but this is infrequent. The usual history is that of a child who is crying immediately after the fall and seems to be awake and alert without any identifiable traumatic unconsciousness. Minutes to hours after the injury, the child becomes irritable, pale, and often cold and clammy and begins to vomit. The vomiting may be quite intractable for a period of hours. The child's level of consciousness may also change, with increasing somnolence and general listlessness. This history in an adult would most probably be associated with an expanding mass lesion. This is rarely the case in infancy.

The physical examination shows a pale, somnolent child with rather floppy extremities. The fontanelle is generally soft, and the fundi clear. Plantar responses are generally extensive, which is normal to the end of the first year of life, and abdominal reflexes are usually absent. A localized subgaleal hematoma may be felt, and the remainder of the general physical examination is usually normal. The authors feel that skull x-ray films should be obtained in this group of children, since the frequency of linear skull fractures is high. A computerized axial tomography (CAT) scan has generally been normal, with the occasional appearance of subarachnoid hemorrhage. If the child can be roused by painful stimuli, and the fontanelle is soft, the authors do not routinely perform a CAT scan. If a full fontanelle is found or the sutures are split, suggesting elevated intracranial pressure (ICP), a CAT scan is necessary, since the rare epidural hematoma will be found. Occasionally, the deterioration in consciousness can be pinned down to a clear history of a seizure, but this is infrequent.

The majority of children require no special therapy. The vomiting in the milder cases may have stopped by the time the children present to the emergency room. Those with a fracture or continued vomiting are admitted, at least for overnight, and occasionally intravenous therapy is necessary to prevent dehydration. Prolonged somnolence or vomiting, the onset of seizures, the development of a full fontanelle, or bradycardia suggest the need for a CAT scan. The authors have not found that an electroencephalogram (EEG) or radionuclide scanning is helpful in this group of children. Seizures occurring at the time of injury, which do not recur, do not require therapy. Seizures that occur later (i.e., more than one hour after trauma) do, and the authors use phenobarbital. Phenobarbital is usually continued for a period of two years before it is stopped. There are no proven long-term effects on the brain of this type of trauma.

This pattern of delayed vomiting and somnolence is referred to as "the pediatric concussion syndrome,"[14, 16] but it does not fit in with the authors' theory of concussion as a sudden neurophysiologic malfunctioning. The injury that is usually sustained is low velocity and would not be expected to set up great shearing stresses within the brain. Experimentally Foltz and colleagues[6] showed that the reticular formation activity, which is absent following a concussive blow, could return and then disappear secondarily without any new trauma being delivered. It is possible that this delayed dysfunction in the reticular formation occurs in childhood and infancy and is responsible for the previously described clinical pattern. Frequently, however, there is no initial loss of consciousness, suggesting that this explanation is less than adequate. It is possible that subclinical seizures are occurring and producing the deteriorating pattern, but in this group of children, the EEG is usually normal. As is discussed later, sudden increases in intracranial blood volume might produce an increase in ICP with a similar symptomatology. That the ICP is high seems quite unlikely, since in general, the fontanelle is not full. This is a completely reversible process with no obvious pathology following a traumatic insult and, therefore, fulfills the criteria for concussion. The symptoms are similar to vagal stimulation and could be precipitated by chemical stimultion of the floor of the fourth ventricle as a result of neuroactive chemicals (e.g., histamine), which have been demonstrated in cerebrospinal fluid following trauma. The delay between injury and the onset of symptoms may be due to the diffusion time necessary for the chemicals to exit from the lateral and third ventricles and reach the floor of the fourth ventricle. The excellent recovery suggests that little or no pathologic damage is done to the brain, and it is clear that, as yet, there is no explanation for the delayed onset of symptoms.

Traumatic unconsciousness in the patient younger than one year of age is most commonly seen in the shaken child, in whom diffuse white matter injury; acute subarachnoid hemorrhage, subdural bleeding, or both; and acute brain swelling occur. The rarity of post-traumatic unconsciousness in the infant may be related to the immaturity of the brain, the poor myelination, or, more probably, the fact that the mechanisms of injury and the input forces are quite different in this age group. Whether or not the "pediatric concussion syndrome" is an aspect of concussion remains questionable.

In children older than one year, the various degrees of concussion to the brain can be more easily identified. The pattern of a minor injury without loss of consciousness that is followed by pallor, nausea, vomiting, and lethargy (pediatric concussion syndrome) is less common as age increases. The authors' experience is that this syndrome occurs most commonly with polar injuries after minor falls (e.g., from a swing or roller-skates) and most frequently follows blows to the occiput. With such injuries, transient cortical blindness may occur, and this is especially difficult to diagnose in the prespeech child. This blindness may be a cause of great anxiety, fear, and agitation, but no clear explanation for it can be found. Fortunately, traumatic blindness almost always resolves and is believed to represent some local concussive phenomenon. The CAT scan in these children is normal.

Minor episodes of concussion and brief periods of traumatic unconsciousness come to the attention of the physician less as the ages of patients increase, and in the teenager, many episodes of concussion occur on the sports field that pass unnoticed or are considered too minor to warrant medical attention. In children older than seven years of age, the most common pattern of behavior associated with concussion that requires hospitalization is one of marked fluctuation in the level of consciousness. Typically, this state is produced by a significant injury of the acceleration or deceleration type, usually in a pedestrian struck by an automobile. Consciousness usually is lost for less than an hour, and often the loss is only transient. There then follows a period of some recovery of consciousness, which is followed by marked waxing and waning of consciousness. The level of consciousness varies from talking and answering questions, or at least obeying commands, to deep stupor without any withdrawal to pain. Skull fracture may or may not be present, and the CAT scan is frequently normal, with the most common pathologic lesion being subarachnoid hemorrhage in approximately 20 percent of patients. The authors believe that it is valuable to obtain a CAT scan in these patients, especially if there is evidence of local trauma and skull fracture, as epidural hematomas may present in a similar fashion. The EEG is usually diffusely abnormal but without evidence of seizure discharges. Recovery occurs, and it is rare that any treatment other than intravenous fluids and supportive therapy is required. Because of the benign course of this syndrome, there is little information on the state of the ICP or other physiologic parameters. The authors have occasionally monitored the ICP in these children and have generally found it to be normal.

Recovery proceeds more slowly than would be expected from the admission state of the children, and seven to ten days is the average hospital stay. The period of post-traumatic amnesia, which is a measure of the severity of the concussion, usually lasts for much of the hospital stay and is frequently longer than a week. These children commonly exhibit minor personality changes, irritability, increased aggressiveness, and generally less controlled behavior for a period of weeks to months following injury. Further, they frequently experience minor difficulties in school and complain of difficulties with concentration and learning new information. Studies on short-term memory in children who have sustained head injuries have clearly demonstrated that these complaints have identifiable neuropsychologic correlates.[9] Therefore, it is important that all children sustaining this severity of concussion be followed for at least one year and that parents and teachers be properly alerted to the possible difficulties they may encounter. Follow-up CAT scans in this group of patients are usually entirely normal and show no evidence of focal or diffuse atrophy.

Another commonly seen clinical pattern of concussion follows more severe head injury in children. The children became unconscious immediately but fairly rapidly show signs of an improving neurologic state. While talking is rare, purposeful movements, occasional obeying of commands, and spontaneous eye opening may occur. This is followed within minutes to hours by the sudden deterioration of consciousness, with pallor, bradycardia, loss of purposeful pain responses, and spontaneous eye opening. In about 25 percent of these children, unilateral decerebrate posturing, alternating pupillary dilatation, and episodes of apnea occur. While this history and course are consistent with an expanding mass lesion, especially an epidural hematoma, and this must always be ruled out, the authors have found that such a lesion is rare. These children rarely have skull fractures, and the CAT scan usually shows evidence of diffuse swelling of the brain, with loss of cerebrospinal fluid spaces and no other specific focal lesion. The mechanism of this swelling appears to be mainly an increase in blood volume and not true cerebral edema.[10, 22] These children frequently require endotracheal intubation and mechanical hyperventilation to prevent the continued deterioration. With intensive supportive care, recovery occurs rapidly within two to three days, with little or no focal neurologic deficit. The period of post-traumatic amnesia tends to be shorter and the delayed memory defects less in this group of children than in those who present with a waxing and waning level of consciousness.

How does this pattern fit our hypothesis for concussion? The lack of a structural lesion on the CAT scan and the rapid, usually complete, recovery fulfill the criteria for concussive injury. It would appear that the acute brain swelling that occurs in this group either causes the secondary deterioration by causing increased ICP or is an accompaniment of a similar fourth ventricular stimulation, as was hypothesized to occur in the younger infants. In favor of the first hypothesis are the autopsy findings, in children, of severely swollen brains with minimal microscopic evidence of tissue injury and increased venous volume.[2, 11] If inadequately treated, this clinical pattern thus can result in death. Neither seizures nor shock appear to be responsible for the acute brain swelling.[1] Concentration and short-term memory appear to be less impaired in this group than in the previous group. This characteristic requires more intensive study but might be explained by a mechanism of injury that produces less shearing within the white matter but precipitates acute brain swelling.

The final pattern seen in children without identifiable mass lesions following trauma is that of the immediate onset of deep coma with alteration of pupillary responses and decorticate or decerebrate posturing or flaccidity. These children do not have a lucid period, and the injury represents a severe degree of shearing injury. The CAT scan most often shows diffuse swelling, but occasionally, deep white matter, corpus callosum, or brainstem hemorrhages are also seen, thus confirming the shearing injury.[23] With intensive care and rehabilitation, the majority of these patients recover, although 50 percent are left with neurologic or intellectual deficits. Although the severity of the injury implies that it is clearly associated with some irreversible structural lesions, the authors believe that this represents the most severe form, and transient amnesia the least severe form, of cerebral concussion.

It appears that the most useful clinical approach to the problem of concussion is to consider it as a spectrum of functional and pathologic changes in the brain produced by shear stress. The most minor result may be brief amnesia, and the most severe may be prolonged coma. In children, it appears that there are some delayed effects of the concussion that produce secondary nausea and vomiting, pallor, and, occasionally, deterioration in the level of consciousness some time following injury. At present, the mechanism of these changes is unclear, and an epidural mass lesion must always be considered. Further, with more severe degrees of concussion, a pattern of acute swelling of the brain can occur that appears to be due to acute suffusion of the brain with blood. Whether the increase in blood volume is responsible for an increase in ICP that produces secondary deterioration, or whether it is an accompaniment of some chemical or neuronally mediated brainstem or pontine irritation that produces deterioration and cerebral hyperemia at one time, is not yet clear. What is clear is that children may die from head injury as a result of acute brain swelling with little or no evidence of pathologic changes within the brain, and that therapy to support ventilation, decreased cerebral blood flow (CBF), and decreased cerebral blood volume (CBV) can prevent this. Therefore, in children, death may result from concussion, if the preceding hypothesis is correct. However, the authors have shown that even when diffuse shearing injury of the white matter has occurred, recovery may take place. Thus, death from concussion should always be preventable, unless the severe swelling is produced by prolonged apnea and anoxia such that there has been too much secondary injury to the brain for a recovery to occur.

It is clear that concussion of the brain no longer can be equated with a lack of pathologic damage but must be considered as a spectrum of injury. The postconcussive syndrome, while uncommon in children in its full-blown fashion, is seen associated with difficulties in short-term memory, learning, and behavior. As a result, concussion in its various degrees up to and including traumatic unconsciousness should not be taken lightly in the infant or the child, and parents should be made cognizant of the potential for future problems.

CONTUSION

Contusion implies bruising or microscopic hemorrhage within the cerebral substance, and it occurs as a result of two separate mechanisms. Local trauma to the static head may produce inbending and local depressed skull fracture, the impact being transferred to the underlying brain and thus resulting in bruising and contusion. In adults, contrecoup contusions in the area contralateral to the impact are quite common. In children, the authors have found such contusions to be rare. The second mechanism is associated with acceleration or deceleration injuries to the freely movable head. The inferior surfaces of the frontal lobes and the anterior surfaces of the temporal lobes are contused and sometimes lacerated by back-and-forth motion over the bony prominences of the orbital roof and the sphenoid wing, respectively. This latter mechanism is uncommon in children (10 percent of a series of 76 severe head injuries),[2] and the majority of contusions that the authors encounter are associated with local trauma to the scalp, bone, and underlying brain.

The CAT scan can readily identify hemorrhagic contusion and separate this from true intracerebral hemorrhage. The course of these lesions is one of progressive local cerebral edema and, frequently, progressive displacement of intracranial structures over several days (Fig. 21–1). There then follows slow resolution, usually with good recovery of function. Often, local areas of encephalomalacia are seen on follow-up CAT scan (Fig. 21–1C). The authors have seen in a number of patients, especially shaken babies, areas of focally decreased density on the CAT scan early after injury. Over time, these lesions behave like contusions, with an increase in local swelling and spreading edema, and are followed by resolution and residual encephalomalacia. While some of these local decreased density areas probably represent infarction, some appear to represent contusions but with minimal hemorrhage.

Contusions may be present clinically and may produce no symptoms at all. More frequently, there is gradual deterioration of local neurologic function over several days, with deterioration of level of consciousness. This is related to swelling and spreading edema from the focus (Fig. 21–1B). There is then a period of slow resolution with improving level of consciousness, and then later improvement in local neurologic dysfunction. The authors do not feel that these lesions, even when polar, should be surgically treated, as much of the involved brain may recover. If the swelling is severe, then ICP monitoring with control of the ICP to less than 20 mm Hg may be required to prevent herniation and to promote recovery. Occasionally, when a large hematoma accompanies the contusion, surgical evacuation may be required. Surgical intervention may be required more frequently when the lesions are in the temporal tip, but the authors believe that surgery should be postponed and medical therapy used whenever possible, since this regimen avoids the removal of any potentially viable brain. The authors treat the patients with steroids—dexamethasone, 1.5 mg/kg, or prednisolone, 5–10 mg/kg per 24 hours—immediately after the CAT scan diagnosis is made. However, there is no evidence that steroids have a significant effect on the outcome or time course of these lesions.

Pathologically, 75 percent of adults dying of head injury have evidence of contusion at autopsy. In children younger than four years of age, this percentage is very low, with an increase to almost the adult level by the age of five. In the authors' experience, the incidence of contusions in those children who die primary deaths following head injury has been only about 40 percent.

The responses of the child's brain to trauma are clearly different from those of the adult. The infant rarely is rendered unconscious unless severely shaken, and contusion is rarely present. The older child is easily rendered unconscious, with usually rapid recovery. In both these age groups, a delayed onset of lethargy, nausea, and vomiting frequently occurs. In the milder cases, this seems to be unassociated with elevated ICP, and the CAT scan is usually normal or shows mild swelling. The process is generally self-limiting, and therapy is supportive. In more severe cases, an increased CBV with diffuse brain swelling is often seen, and in these children the deterioration may be to deep coma. Recovery almost always occurs, but an increased level of intensive care support, including hyperventilation,

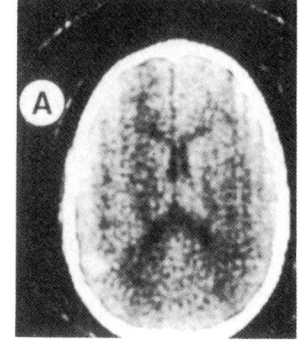
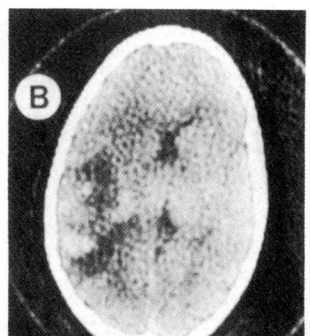
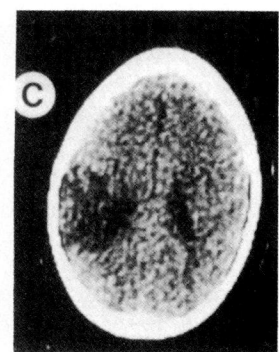

Figure 21–1. Serial CT scans following left parietal contusion. A, Immediate postinjury CT scan showing left parietal hemispheric contusion. B, Repeat CT scan seven days after trauma, showing spreading edema and midline displacement. C, Follow-up CT scan one month later, showing residual encephalomalacia.

may be necessary. However, this postconcussive brain swelling can be fatal and must always be taken seriously. Finally, even when evidence of early physical disruption of the white matter (shearing injury) is present, good functional recovery can be seen if early intensive care and late physiotherapy and rehabilitation are maximized.

Cerebral contusion in children is most frequently associated with direct trauma to the head and usually occurs under the site of a traumatic fracture. Contrecoup injuries are uncommon. Similarly, multiple contusions as a result of movement of the frontal and temporal lobes over the bony prominences of the orbital roof and temporal fossa are infrequent in children. The authors do not recommend surgical evacuation or removal of potentially viable brain unless other nonsurgical therapies have failed to control ICP. When a deteriorating level of consciousness or a significant midline shift is present, ICP monitoring is recommended as the only way of judging the need for decompressive medical therapy.

References

1. Bruce DA, Alavi A, Bilaniuk LT, et al: Diffuse cerebral swelling following head injuries in children. The syndrome of malignant brain edema. J Neurosurg 54:170, 1981.
2. Bruce DA, Raphaely RD, Goldberg AI, et al: The pathophysiology, treatment and outcome following severe head injury in children. Child's Brain 5:174, 1979.
3. Bruce DA, Schut L, Bruno L, et al: Outcome following severe head injuries in children. J Neurosurg 48:679, 1978.
4. Budzilovich GN: On pathogenesis of primary lesions in blunt head trauma with special reference to the brain stem injuries. In: McLaurin RL (ed): Head Injuries. New York, Grune & Stratton, 1976, pp 39–43.
5. Courville CB: Contrecoup injuries of the brain in infancy. Arch Surg 90:157, 1965.
6. Foltz EL, Jenkner FL, Ward AA: Experimental cerebral concussion. J Neurosurg 10:342, 1953.
7. Holbourn AHS: Mechanics of head injury. Lancet 2:438, 1943.
8. Hooper R: Patterns of Acute Head Injury. London, Edward Arnold, 1969.
9. Levin HS, Eisenberg HM: Neuropsychological outcome of closed head injury in children and adolescents. Child's Brain 5:281, 1979.
10. Lewis AJ: Mechanisms of Neurological Disease. Boston, Little, Brown & Co., 1976.
11. Lindenberg R, Fisher RS, Durlacher S, et al: The pathology of the brain in blunt head injuries of infants and children. In: Proceedings of the Second International Congress of Neuropathology, Vol. 1. Amsterdam, Excerpta Medica, 1955, pp 477–479.
12. Ommaya AK, Gennarelli TA: Cerebral concussion and traumatic unconsciousness: Correlation of experimental and clinical observations on blunt head injuries. Brain 97:633, 1974.
13. Ommaya AK, Gennarelli TA: Experimental head injury. In: Vinken PJ, Bruyn GW (eds): Handbook of Clinical Neurology, Vol. 23. New York, American Elsevier, 1975, pp 67–87.
14. Pickles W: Acute general edema of the brain in children with head injuries. N Engl J Med 242:607, 1950.
15. Russell WR, Smith A: Post-traumatic amnesia in closed head injury. Arch Neurol 5:4, 1961.
16. Schnitker MT: A syndrome of cerebral concussion in children. J Pediatr 35:557, 1949.
17. Symonds CP: Concussion and its sequelae. Lancet 1:5, 1962.
18. Tomlison BE: Pathology. In: Rowbotham GF (ed): Acute Injuries of the Head. Baltimore, Williams & Wilkins, 1964, p 99.
19. Ward AA, Jr.: The physiology of concussion. Clin Neurosurg 12:95, 1966.
20. Windle WF, Groat RA: Disappearance of nerve cells after concussion. Anat Rec 93:201, 1945.
21. Windle WF, Groat RA, Fox CA: Experimental structural alterations in brain during and after concussion. Surg Gynecol Obstet 79:561,. 1944.
22. Zimmerman RA, Bilaniuk LT, Bruce DA, et al: Computed tomography of pediatric head trauma: Acute general cerebral swelling. Radiology 126:403, 1978.
23. Zimmerman RA, Bilaniuk LT, Gennarelli T: Computed tomography of shearing injuries of the cerebral white matter. Radiology 127:393, 1978.

22
POST-TRAUMATIC HEMATOMAS

Robert L. McLaurin, M.D.
Richard Towbin, M.D.

Post-traumatic intracranial hemorrhage is usually a surgically correctable lesion that must be recognized early and treated with dispatch. Although the incidence of post-traumatic intracranial hematoma in children varies considerably in the different reported series, a minority of children with head injuries are candidates for surgical treatment. For example, in the largest series of consecutive cases of head injury, Hendrick and colleagues[17] noted an incidence of extra-axial hematomas of 6 percent. Despite this low incidence, failure to recognize the presence of a hematoma may transform an otherwise mild injury into a fatal or permanently disabling entity. Fortunately, the advent of computerized tomography (CT) has markedly simplified the process of recognition of a hematoma and also of monitoring postoperative intracranial changes. In the rare instance in which nonsurgical treatment is chosen, the CT scan is invaluable in following the progress of the intracranial hemorrhagic accumulation.

More recently, nuclear magnetic resonance imaging (NMRI) has added another dimension in the evaluation of intracranial hematomas, especially in the subacute and chronic stages. Gomori and associates[14] have defined the changes that occur in the images of intracranial hematomas during their evolution, resulting principally from progressive changes in hemoglobin. They described characteristics of acute (less than one week), subacute (one week to one month), and chronic (more than one month) hematomas. Snow and coworkers[29] found NMRI superior to CT in the diagnosis of small extra-axial collections and in distinguishing subdural hematomas from hydromas. However, they concluded that CT remains the procedure of choice in the evaluation of head injury during the first 72 hours.

It has been customary to subdivide post-traumatic intracranial hematomas into those that are extra-axial and those that involve the parenchyma of the neural tissue. The former are subdivided into extradural and subdural categories.

EXTRADURAL HEMORRHAGE

Extradural hemorrhage constitutes one of the most emergent sequelae of head trauma but at the same time is probably the most favorable type of traumatic intracranial bleeding that occurs in childhood, provided it is recognized and treated expeditiously. As a result of its moderately predictable clinical presentation and its characteristic appearance on CT scan, it is usually rather easily detected in the child under careful medical observation.

The incidence of extradural hemorrhage in pediatric patients is varied among reports by different authors. It appears to be less common in children than in adults and even more rare in infants. The cause of the lower incidence is unclear, since head injuries are actually more common in children than in adults. A reason that has been advanced for the lower incidence, particularly in infants, is that adherence between the dura and the cranial suture provides some fixation of dura to the calvarium and diminishes the likelihood of separation of the dura from the inner skull surface if bleeding occurs in the potential extradural space. Natelson and Sayers[24] reported no incidence of extradural hematoma in a series of 42 infants with severe head trauma at birth. The occurrence of extradural hematoma is less than 1 percent in the series of 4465 patients reported by Hendrick and colleagues.[17] In an extensive review of the literature as well as his own series of patients, Choux[9] found the incidence to be between 1.5 and 3.5 percent. However, it is noteworthy that this incidence is heavily weighted toward older children, so it must be concluded that extradural hematomas are rarely seen in newborns and that their incidence during infancy is very low.

The reason for the presumed low incidence of extradural hemorrhage in infancy (i.e., adherence of the dura to the overlying skull at the suture lines) has been challenged by Choux and associates.[10] They demonstrated the richness of the diploic and dural vascularization during infancy. In addition, these researchers found no indication, by injection of the extradural space, of attachment of the dura to suture lines, with the exception of the coronal suture.

Pathophysiology

The mechanism of the development of extradural hematomas has been the subject of much speculation and some investigation. Of historical interest, it was demonstrated by Bell in 1816 that a hammer blow delivered to a cadaver skull was capable of separating the dura from the skull without fracturing the skull.[4] He concluded that without such mechanical separation, the force of bleeding from the middle meningeal artery was incapable of causing hematoma accumulation. Subsequent experiments on dogs confirmed that some separation is, indeed, essential to the initiation of extradural bleeding.[12] The validity of Bell's observations regarding the lack of need for fracture has been substantiated by many subsequent observers. For example, Galbraith,[13] in reporting a series of 46 patients with extradural hemorrhage without skull fracture, found that 91 percent were younger than 31 years of age, and 28 percent were younger than 10 years of age. In the series of Hendrick and coworkers,[17] only 40 percent of the children with extradural hematomas had skull fracture, and half of these had depressed fractures.

The source of extradural hemorrhage may be arterial or venous, and it is believed that the incidence of venous bleeding in pediatric patients is higher than in adults. The classic epidural hematoma, occurring in the temporal fossa, results from a tear of the middle meningeal artery or one of its major branches (Fig. 22–1). The hematoma develops with separation of the dura from the inner skull table and a laceration of the arterial channel. The potential space created by inbending of the skull at the time of impact allows accumulation of the arterial hemorrhage, and this then results in further stripping of dura from the inner table. This process

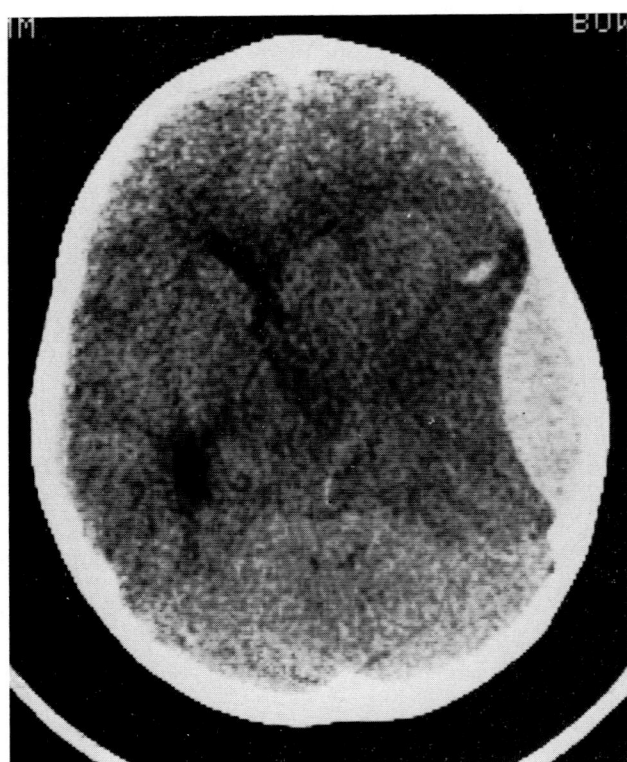

Figure 22–1. An eight-year-old with decreasing level of consciousness. A typical epidural hematoma appearing as a hyperdense, lentiform left temporoparietal collection exerting mass effect on adjacent brain. Focal hemorrhage coexists.

usually requires several hours and is accompanied by progressive displacement and molding of the underlying dura and brain. Conversely, there is no doubt that extradural bleeding may also result from direct injury to the major dural sinuses (e.g., a depressed fracture over the sagittal sinus) (Fig. 22–2). Therefore, it must be concluded that extradural hematoma may be arterial or venous in origin, but the unsettled issue is whether hematomas that are atypical in location, especially over the upper convexity of the cerebral hemisphere, are the result of venous or arterial bleeding. It is noteworthy that these hematomas in an atypical location generally run a more protracted clinical course, and it is principally for this reason that the assumption of a venous origin has been made. However, it seems equally logical to conclude that the atypical location is associated with bleeding from an arterial channel smaller than those in the temporal fossa, and also that the consequent brain molding from pressure in that location will result in transtentorial uncal herniation much more slowly than a similar expanding lesion in the temporal fossa.

Clinical Presentation

The classic clinical presentation of the child with extradural hematoma includes an initial injury of rather minor significance, but it should not be

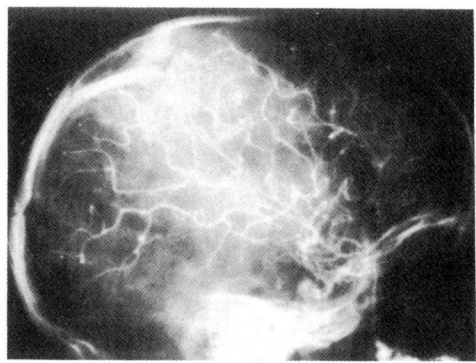
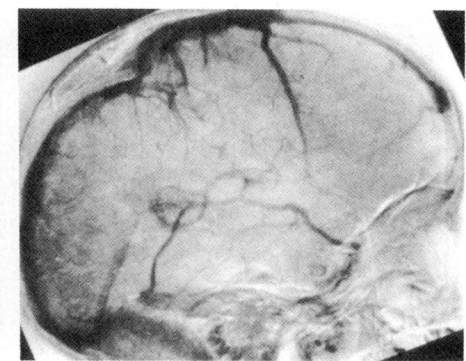

Figure 22–2. A depressed fracture over the sagittal sinus. Venogram shows depression of the sinus that was due to extradural hematoma beneath the fracture.

inferred that extradural hemorrhage may not follow more severe trauma. Choux,[9] in his series of 172 extradural hematomas in children, noted that only half of them had any initial disturbance of consciousness, whereas the remaining children had no history of any disturbed consciousness. The "lucid interval" described in traditional literature is the interval between recovery from the initial impact and later deterioration of consciousness. Although the lucid interval is usually a few hours long, in Choux's series, 60 percent of patients had lucid intervals lasting longer than 24 hours.

As indicated previously, the characteristically rapid course of deterioration is due not only to the arterial force of the bleeding point but also to the location in relation to the brainstem. A hematoma developing in the low temporal fossa causes herniation of the medial temporal lobe with displacement and compromise of the brainstem fairly rapidly. A similar hematoma occurring over the upper convexity of the cerebral hemisphere causes brainstem signs only later, since a greater degree of brain molding is necessary before the brainstem is affected.

If the child is seen shortly after the injury, some external evidence of trauma in the frontotemporal region is usually noted. This may include swelling and ecchymosis, although absence of bruising and swelling does not exclude an underlying extradural hematoma. If the child is lucid, there is usually the symptom of increasingly severe headache. This continues until the patient becomes more lethargic and confused. The stage of lethargy may be preceded by a period of hyperirritability. Vomiting is also a frequent occurrence in extradural hematomas and is said to be more common than with subdural hematomas or brain damage. Convulsions, usually focal in nature, may also be seen during this stage of cortical irritation. Nuchal stiffness may occur during the stage of early transtentorial herniation, and weakness of the opposite extremities that progresses to decerebrate extension and is accompanied by Babinski's response may also be noted. As uncal herniation progresses, there occurs rapid deterioration of consciousness, and the child's condition suddenly becomes critical. One of the earliest signs is anisocoria resulting from loss of the pupilloconstrictor innervation of the oculomotor nerve. Simultaneously, there usually occurs the classic Cushing triad of bradycardia, slowed and irregular respiration, and a widened pulse pressure. In infants and toddlers, the loss of blood volume to the extradural space may modify the cardiovascular signs.

Although seizures are an infrequent sign of extradural hemorrhage, their frequency has varied between 0 percent[21] and 10 percent.[8] In the largest series thus far reported, 172 patients, Choux[9] noted an incidence of 8.7 percent.[11]

The CT scan is, at present, the definitive diagnostic radiologic examination to verify the presence and location of an extradural hematoma. The absence of skull fracture by no means excludes the diagnosis. The CT image is quite easily interpreted in most instances, and characteristically the hematoma is seen in the frontotemporal region and assumes a lenticular configuration (Figs. 22–1 and 22–3). There may be some limitation of the hematoma by fixation of the dura at the coronal and lambdoid sutures. The underlying brain is depressed, and the midline structures are displaced to the contralateral side. During the early stages after injury, fresh blood in the extradural space may have undergone some degree of clotting and retraction, resulting in a nonhomogeneous appearance on the CT scan. Zimmerman and Bilaniuk[33] have described this as the "lucent swirl," and these authors have also provided detailed descriptions of the various stages through which an extradural hematoma passes in its radiologic progression (Fig. 22–4).

Treatment and Results

Treatment should actually begin at the first suspicion of a possible extradural hematoma and prior to obtaining the critical definitive CT scan. Initial management includes measures designed to reduce intracranial pressure. Patients should be immediately intubated if they are in obtunded or comatose states. Hyperventilation should be started to reduce arterial carbon dioxide partial pressure (pCO_2) to the range of 20 to 25 torr. In addition, hyperosmolar

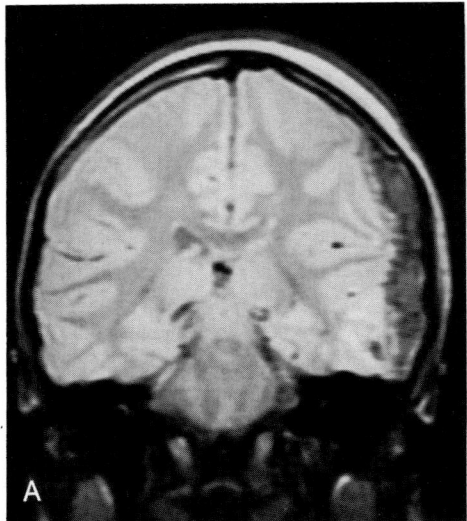
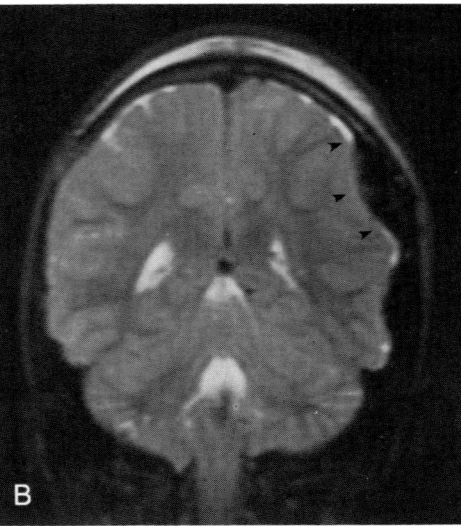

Figure 22-3. A 12-year-old who sustained left-sided head trauma 48 hours prior to admission and who reported progressive headache. A, Coronal T1-weighted (TR—800 msec, TE—20 msec) sequence demonstrates a slightly hypotensive, bilobulated epidural collection. B, On T2-weighted sequence (TR—2500 msec, TE—100 msec), the epidural collection becomes more hypotensive, indicating fresh blood. Extradural collection causes mass effect with minimal shift, white matter buckling, and effacement of subarachnoid space (arrowheads).

agents should be given immediately to effect some dehydration of the neural tissue.

Definitive treatment of the extradural hematoma should always be surgical removal, and delay of such treatment is unacceptable when the diagnosis has been established. Surgical treatment has, as its ultimate objectives, removal of the hematoma and control of the arterial bleeding points. Although a recent publication has reported successful management of extradural hematomas in children without surgery, this method of management is fraught with risks and should not be advocated in the presence of an acute extradural hemorrhage.[25]

When the hematoma occurs in the usual frontoparietal location, it is not necessary to perform an extensive bone flap. A subtemporal craniectomy can be done and enlarged to sufficient size to allow evacuation of the entire extradural hematoma. If

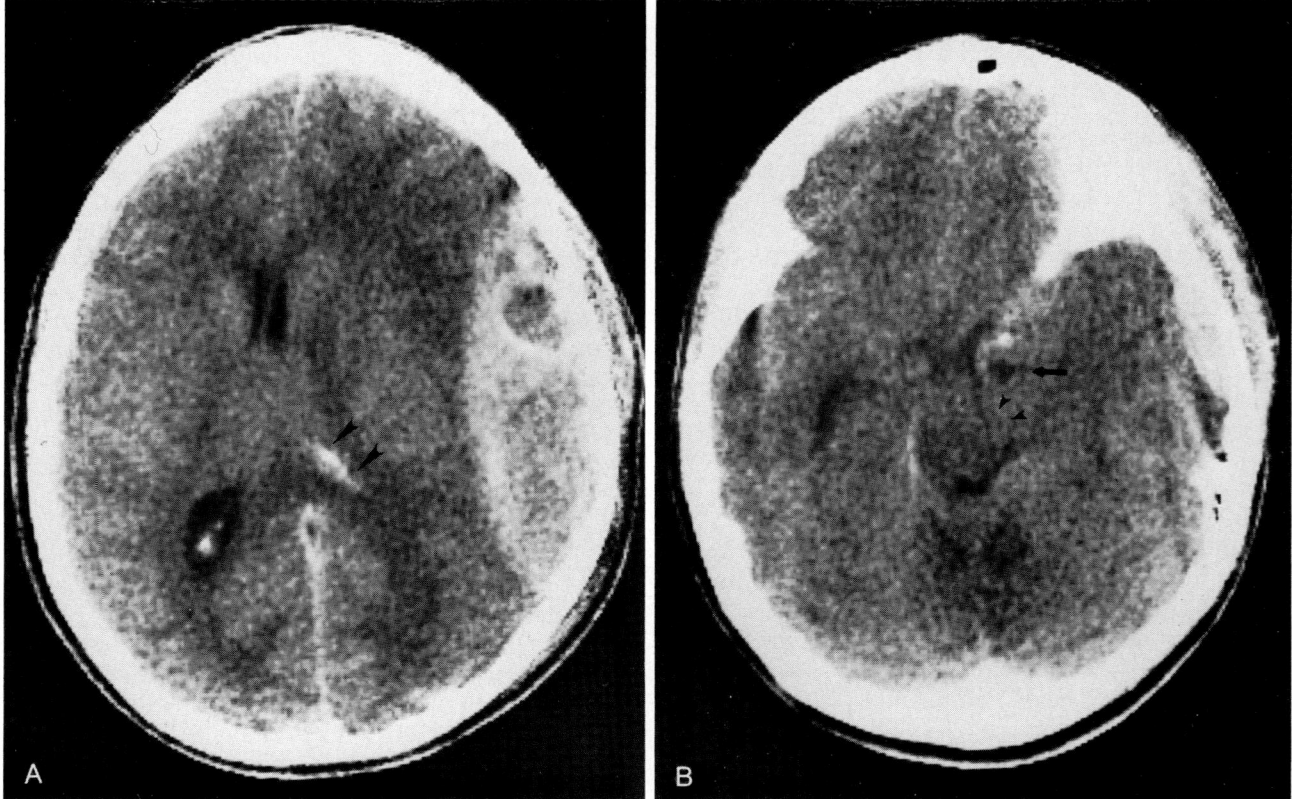

Figure 22-4. A head injury incurred from a fall off a bicycle. A, Large inhomogeneous temporoparietal epidural hematoma. Perilesional edema and deep hemorrhage (arrowheads), with ventricular compression and midline shift also present. B, Extradural hemorrhage causes effacement of suprasellar cistern, compression and medial displacement of the left temporal horn (arrow), and effacement of the left half of the ambient cistern (arrowheads), signs of downward herniation.

the hematoma is in some aberrant location, it may be necessary to perform a craniotomy over the central part of the hematoma in order to accomplish its evacuation. After removal of the surface hematoma, bleeding points can usually be easily identified and controlled by coagulation. Finally, the displaced dura should be sutured to adjacent extracranial tissues in order to obliterate the extradural space and prevent re-accumulation.

The results of treatment of arterial extradural hematomas in infancy and childhood are difficult to evaluate statistically because in many instances, the reported series have included patients with associated intradural hematomas or injury. For example, the series reported by Choux[9] in 1986 notes a 6 percent incidence of associated subdural hematoma, a 10 percent incidence of associated subdural hematoma and contusion, and a 9 percent incidence of associated contusion alone. However, in general, it is appropriate to conclude that the results of treatment of extradural hemorrhage are better than those relating to intradural hemorrhage, and the results depend largely on the speed of recognition and evacuation of the clot. Choux[9] reports a mortality rate of 14 percent.[11] As noted by previous researchers, the morbidity rate is significantly lower in children than in adults and particularly in patients younger than ten years of age. Factors that contribute to a poor prognosis include the absence of a lucid interval or a very brief lucid interval; the presence of an associated intracranial injury; and a delay in surgical evacuation.

Extradural hematomas of the posterior fossa are exceptionally rare. Takagi and associates[31] have reported the occurrence of extradural hemorrhage in the posterior fossa as a consequence of birth trauma. Arkins and coworkers[2] have reported three cases of acute posterior fossa epidural hematomas in children ranging from 16 months of age to four years. These researchers emphasize that the posterior fossa location is unique to children and that the mechanism is direct occipital trauma. Skull fracture is not necessary, as with supratentorial hematomas. The clinical picture may include a lucid period followed by decreasing consiousness and manifestations of brainstem impairment. The lateralized motor signs and anisocoria are missing. In emergency situations, the researchers suggested a ventricular tap, since part of the problem is an acute obstructive hydrocephalus. The definitive diagnosis again is made by the CT scan, and treatment by emergency craniotomy and clot removal is essential for survival (Fig. 22–5).

SUBDURAL HEMORRHAGE

Subdural hematomas have traditionally been classified as acute, subacute, or chronic. This classification may have merit in relation to pathophysiology but is somewhat artificial in that it delineates

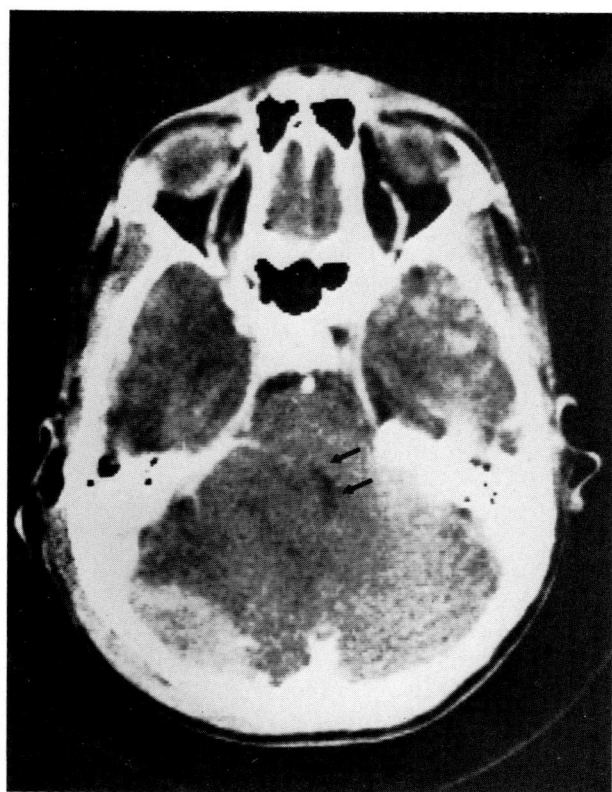

Figure 22–5. A teenage boy who fell out of a moving automobile and immediately lost consciousness. Right-sided posterior fossa epidural hematoma causing contralateral displacement and compression of fourth ventricle (arrows) and pons.

only the length of time the hematoma has been present before it becomes clinically manifest. For practical considerations, it is advisable to distinguish between acute and chronic hematomas because their clinical presentations are quite different. As noted in relation to extradural hemorrhage, bleeding into the subdural space may also be either arterial or venous in origin. If it originates from arterial sources, usually cortical arteries, the clinical presentation is rapid and occurs usually within the first 12 hours. If bleeding occurs from the venous structures, usually the bridging veins from cortex to dural sinuses, the clinical presentation probably is dependent on the severity of associated brain injury rather than on the bleeding itself. If there is significant neural damage, the clinical deterioration is rapid (acute), whereas if there is little or no brain damage initially, the presentation is protracted and delayed (chronic).

Acute Subdural Hemorrhage

According to the aforementioned pathophysiologic considerations, acute subdural hematomas may be of either arterial or venous origin. They are seen occasionally as a result of birth damage or later as a consequence of external impact, usually from vehicular accidents or falls.

The clinical picture of the newborn infant with acute supratentorial subdural bleeding has been described by Abroms and colleagues.[1] The newborn infant becomes acutely distressed within several hours after delivery, and this is usually accompanied by respiratory difficulty and occasionally by ipsilateral pupillary dilatation. It seems probable that the bleeding under these circumstances is due to arterial rather than venous cortical hemorrhage. The acute intracranial hypertension is manifested by increased tension of the fontanelle and also frequently by the presence of retinal hemorrhage. The diagnosis can be verified most easily by ultrasonography or CT. Tapping of the subdural space through the fontanelle or coronal suture may be misleading, since the hematoma is usually coagulated and solid. Emergency craniotomy is essential for the diagnosis to be established. Fortunately, perinatal acute subdural hematoma is becoming increasingly rare, and in the series reported by Gutierrez and Raimondi[16] 5 of 27 acute post-traumatic subdural hematomas were in newborns.

Acute subdural hemorrhage in older infants and children is relatively infrequent and, according to Zimmerman and Bilaniuk,[33] is four times more common in adults. Bruce and associates[6] reported acute subdural bleeding in only 8 percent of 85 children with severe head injury. Gutierrez and Raimondi[16] found that acute hematomas were six times as frequent in infants as in toddlers and that the most common age at which they occurred was between one and three months. Falls were the most frequent mechanism of injury, while abuse was the next most common cause in infancy.[16]

The source of bleeding in acute subdural hematomas has been a matter of some interest. Jellinger[18] has stated that the most common source is stretching and tearing of the bridging veins between the cortex and venous sinuses, and that these may occur without evidence of any direct damage to the brain. Tearing of major dural sinuses and torn vessels on the surface of the brain are less frequent causes. However, some observers have found it difficult to reconcile the occurrence of acute severe brain compression with purely venous bleeding, since the mere existence of a chronic subdural hematoma as a clinical entity attests to the likelihood that venous bleeding alone does not necessarily lead to acute symptoms.

Regardless of the mechanism of bleeding, the clinical setting in infants and children is one of a severe head injury. The presence of cerebral contusion, which usually accompanies an acute subdural hemorrhage, enhances the neurologic deterioration by providing an additional factor leading to cerebral edema, increased intracranial pressure, and shift of midline structures. The same galaxy of signs (e.g., motor and pupillary signs and consciousness) as were described with extradural hemorrhage may be seen. Although the occurrence of a lucid interval is rare in the presence of acute subdural bleeding, it may be seen in some instances. Indeed, in a review of 66 patients who experienced a lucid period and then died after head injury (not limited to children), Reilly and colleagues[27] found 41 intradural hematomas.

As in the newborn period, needle tapping of the subdural space is fraught with the possibility of error. The CT scan is the procedure of choice, although the surface lesion in infants younger than one year of age may be demonstrated by ultrasonography. The acute subdural hematoma is usually unilateral. The CT appearance has been described by Zimmerman and Bilaniuk.[33] Subdural blood presents as a hyperdense crescentic lesion overlying one or both hemispheres (Fig. 22–6). The hematoma may extend into the interhemispheric fissure, and evidence of an underlying cerebral contusion and hemorrhage may be associated with the surface lesion. Occasionally, the hematoma is not present on the original scan but occurs over a period of several days (Fig. 22–7).

Treatment of the acute subdural hematoma is a

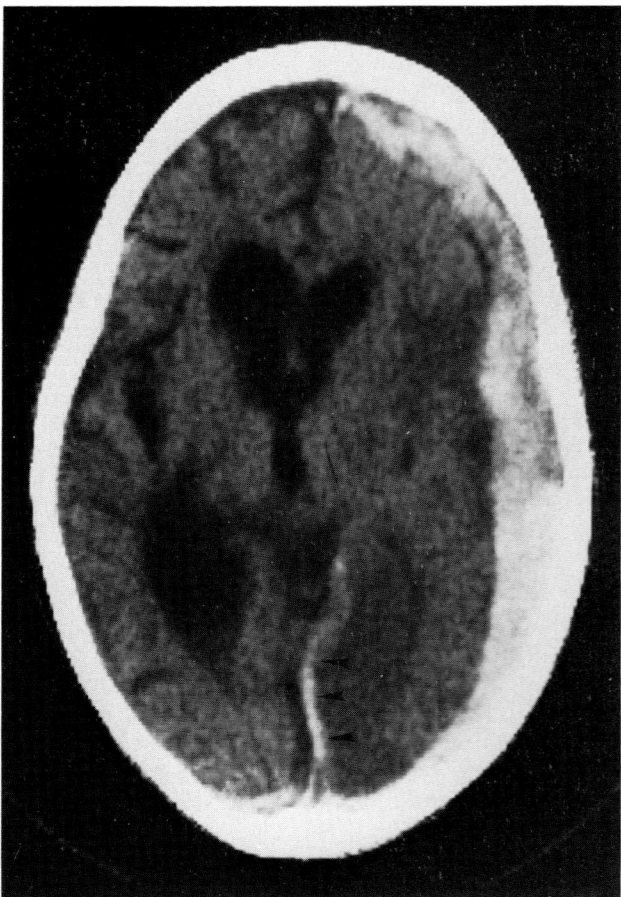

Figure 22–6. A 15-year-old with past anoxic insult resulting in brain atrophy was found unresponsive, with facial bruises and retinal hemorrhages. Axial CT scan demonstrates a large, hyperdense crescentric collection exerting mass effect on adjacent brain. The underlying atrophic changes are easily identified within the right cerebral hemisphere. Note the intrahemispheric subdural hematoma left of the falx cerebri (arrowheads).

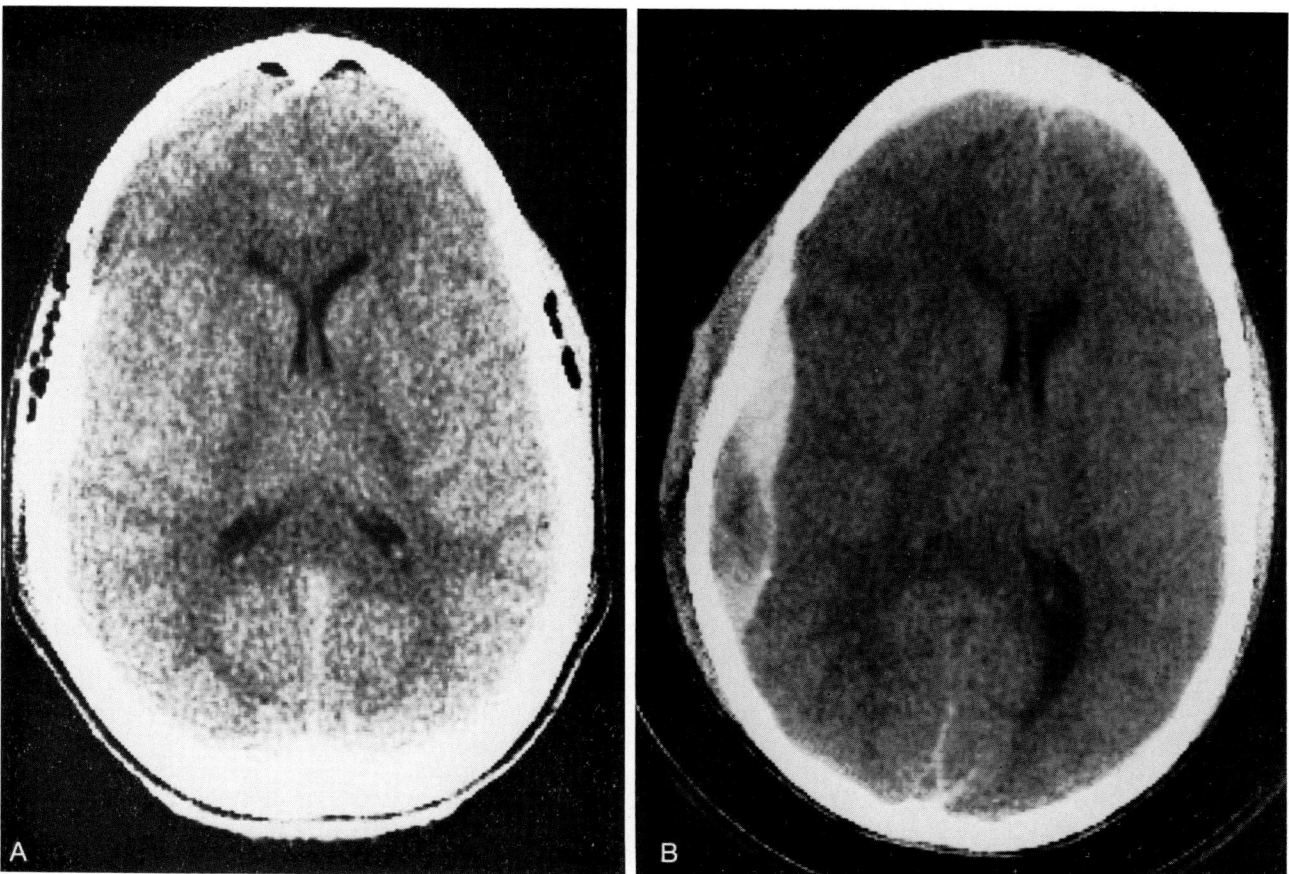

Figure 22–7. A teenage boy struck by a falling tree presented with focal neurologic signs and altered mental status. A, Several hours after injury, CT scan reveals minimal scalp swelling and no intracranial injury. B, Five days later, an acute subdural hematoma is identified.

true emergency, similar to extradural hemorrhage, if the hematoma is significantly contributing to the neurologic state. In this institution, the general policy has been to evacuate subdural hematomas that exceed 5 mm in thickness. The youngster should be treated with hyperventilation and hyperosmolar agents to decrease cerebral swelling. The craniotomy opening should be at least 3 inches in diameter. This permits removal of the solid surface hematoma and visualization of the cortex in order to allow control of bleeding points. The dura must be closed and the bone flap replaced after removal of the subdural clot. Following removal of the acute subdural hemorrhage, most children are candidates for intracranial pressure monitoring.

The results of treatment of children with acute subdural hematomas generally are less favorable than those with extradural bleeding. The residual deficit is probably more dependent on the severity of the brain contusion than on the compressive effect of the surface lesion.

Takagi and associates[30] have recently reviewed the problem of posterior fossa subdural hemorrhage in the newborn as a result of birth trauma. On the basis of a review of 25 patients, the researchers noted that the initial symptoms were respiratory abnormalities in 100 percent and cyanosis in one third of the patients. The average time of onset of symptoms was eight and a half hours after birth. The hematoma was most frequently located under the base of the brain and surrounding the brainstem but, in some instances, was present between the tentorium and the cerebellum. Posterior fossa subdural hematomas were more common in primipara deliveries. The origin of the bleeding in posterior fossa subdural hematomas is usually from tearing of the tentorium, with opening of the straight and lateral sinuses or tearing of the great vein of Galen. Less commonly, rupture of the bridging veins between the cerebellum and the major venous sinuses appeared to be the cause of bleeding. The authors concluded that the CT scan is the best diagnostic tool but that ultrasonography would probably be similarly effective in demonstrating the posterior fossa accumulation of blood. As with acute supratentorial hemorrhage, immediate surgery is indicated. It has also been noted that ventricular shunting may be necessary, even though the hematoma is evacuated.

Chronic Subdural Hemorrhage

Chronic subdural hematoma occurs rarely in pediatric patients older than two years of age, except as a complication of ventricular shunting. However, during infancy, it is seen frequently and is presumably the result of trauma. The incidence of chronic subdural hematoma is difficult to determine, since most authors have distinguished between acute and chronic subdural accumulations. As stated previously, the clinical distinction is based principally on the source of bleeding and the presence or absence of underlying brain damage. If subdural bleeding is of arterial origin, the presence of the hematoma is manifested earlier and will not then proceed to the chronic state. Likewise, if there is no associated brain damage, the accumulation of venous origin may occur slowly and may go undetected for a period of weeks or months. Nevertheless, in nearly all instances, the original basis of the hematomas is probably trauma. They may result from falls, such as those from a changing table or from the arms of parents. It was previously considered that the injury was frequently unobserved, since there was no definite history of a traumatic incident. This concept has lately been questioned because of the increasing awareness of the incidence of abused infants. Guthkelch[15] has pointed out that sudden acceleration and deceleration of the head without direct impact can cause tearing of the bridging veins in the adult. This mechanism occurs in the shaken infant. He reported 23 cases of proven or strongly suspected infant abuse, with subdural bleeding in 13 patients (57 percent). Many of the infants had no external evidence of trauma, and he therefore suggested that the presence of a chronic subdural hematoma, without a definite history of trauma, must be considered to have possibly resulted from a shaking movement.

The term "hematoma" is used somewhat loosely in describing this disease entity, since the content of the subdural accumulation may be thin and thus resemble hydroma fluid rather than the breakdown of a blood clot. It is reasonable to believe that the shaken baby may be equally susceptible to tears of the arachnoid and to avulsion of the bridging veins and that therefore the subdural accumulation may be a combination of cerebrospinal fluid and blood. It should be mentioned that birth injury is a very rare cause for chronic subdural hematoma. For reasons that are not totally clear, most reported series of infantile chronic subdural hematomas show a preponderance of male infants.

The original concept, accepted for many years, that a subdural hematoma gradually increases in size as a result of the breakdown of the hemoglobin and osmotic attraction of water across the membrane has very little support at present. The accumulation of blood in the potential subdural space may undergo either spontaneous resolution and reabsorption or organization with the formation of neomembranes lining and encapsulating the subdural accumulation. The neomembrane is derived from the inner layer of the dura. The outer membrane, which is in contact with the dura, is richly vascularized, whereas the inner membrane is poorly vascularized. The hematoma may become loculated and also may show evidence of stratification, suggesting repeated episodes of bleeding.

Clinical Presentation

The principal features of the clinical presentation are due to intracranial hypertension and to cortical irritation. The former results in enlargement of the cranial vault, abnormal width and tension of the fontanelle, irritability, and vomiting. A "sunset" appearance of the eyes is seen rarely, and papilledema has never been present, in the authors' experience. In approximately 60 percent of the cases, the presenting features include the signs of intracranial hypertension, while in the remaining 40 percent, seizures may be the original manifestation. The seizures may be generalized or localized, and any infant with onset of seizures after three months of age, in the absence of fever or apparent metabolic disturbances, must be considered as possibly harboring a subdural hematoma.

The macrocrania resulting from a chronic subdural hematoma is rarely greater than 2 cm above the ninetieth percentile, in contrast with more severe enlargement as a consequence of hydrocephalus. Matson[21] has stated that biparietal enlargement characterizes subdural accumulations, whereas hydrocephalus is more likely to cause fronto-occipital expansion. Low-grade intracranial hypertension may be detected by the presence of fullness of the fontanelles, palpable separation of the cranial sutures, and a "cracked-pot" percussion note to the skull. Transillumination of the infant's head may provide supportive information in the diagnosis of subdural hematoma, although the occurrence of excessive light transmission is not definitive diagnostically.

Retinal or subhyaloid hemorrhages may be seen, and if they are found in an infant with macrocrania, the diagnosis of subdural hematoma is very probable. However, it seems probable that the subhyaloid hemorrhages are not the consequence of the hematoma but perhaps reflect the type of trauma (e.g., shaken baby injury) that was responsible for the hematoma. The relationship of intraocular hemorrhage to the whiplash–shaken infant syndrome has been described by Caffey.[7]

Anemia may also be found in infants with subdural hematoma. In Matson's series,[21] it was noted in about one third of the patients, whereas Till[32] found a 40 percent incidence of hemoglobin of less than 10 gm. The cause of anemia is related partially to the nutritional deficit that may result from poor feeding and partially to the significant blood volume within the subdural space.

Although x-ray examination of the skull is not a definitive diagnostic tool for subdural hemorrhage, it should be done as part of the investigation if a subdural hematoma of unexplained etiology is sus-

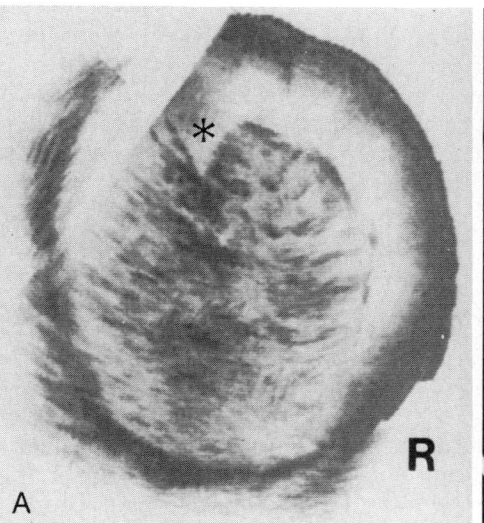
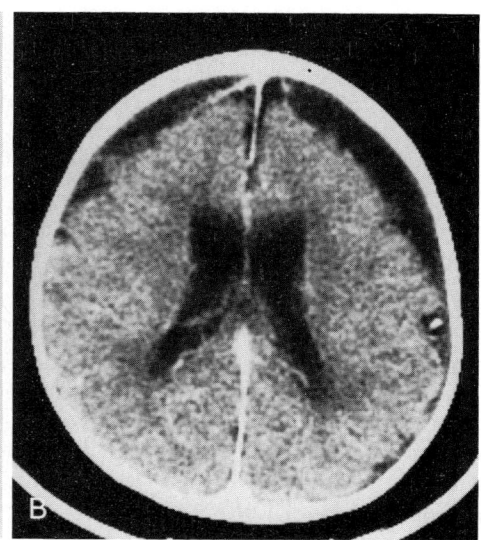

Figure 22–8. Coronal sonography on a three-week-old after a traumatic delivery. A, A hypoechoic chronic subdural hematoma widens the interhemispheric fissure(*) and flattens the brain surface. B, Axial computed tomography on a six-month-old abused infant reveals bilateral chronic subdural hematomas.

pected. The x-ray film may show suture separation and macrocrania and, only rarely, the presence of a skull fracture. However, it is more important that x-ray films of the long bones and thoracic cage be made, for evidence of more widespread injury.

The definitive diagnosis can be made by CT and usually by B-mode ultrasonography (Fig. 22–8). The characteristic CT appearance includes symmetric hypodense surface accumulations over the frontal lobes and extending variable distances backward. The subdural accumulation is slightly more dense than normal cerebrospinal fluid because of its blood and elevated protein content. There is usually effacement of the adjacent subarachnoid spaces. Generally, there is no shift or enlargement of the ventricular system. An enhancing membrane may be seen in very chronic hematomas (Fig. 22–9). The accumulations are crescentic, in contrast with the lenticular configuration of chronic subdural hematomas in adults. The subdural accumulation may appear as a layering of variable densities if there has been intermittent bleeding into the hematoma cavity. In contrast also with adult subdural hematomas, the cerebral sulci may be widened, suggesting atrophy, and there may be large sylvian cisterns and a wide interhemispheric fissure. The depth of the effusion is variable and may be a few millimeters or as much as 3 to 4 cm. In the latter circumstance, there is a strong likelihood of craniocerebral disproportion. With contrast enhancement, there may be increased density of the membranes separating the surface lesions from the underlying brain. Calcification may also occur in the membrane.

Ultrasonography, using the gray-scale B-mode technique, has become the other noninvasive method of imaging and definitive diagnosis.[22] Sonography generally has resolution adequate to determine the presence and the size of surface accumulations and, moreover, offers a relatively easy, harmless, and economical way to follow the size of chronic subdural hematomas during treatment. However, it should be noted that a small surface collection, particularly over the upper convexity of the brain, may escape ultrasonographic detection, but such lesions probably have no clinical significance.

Prior to the advent of CT and ultrasonography, the definitive method of diagnosis was by subdural tap, and this may still have some application at present. At this time, the principal reasons for

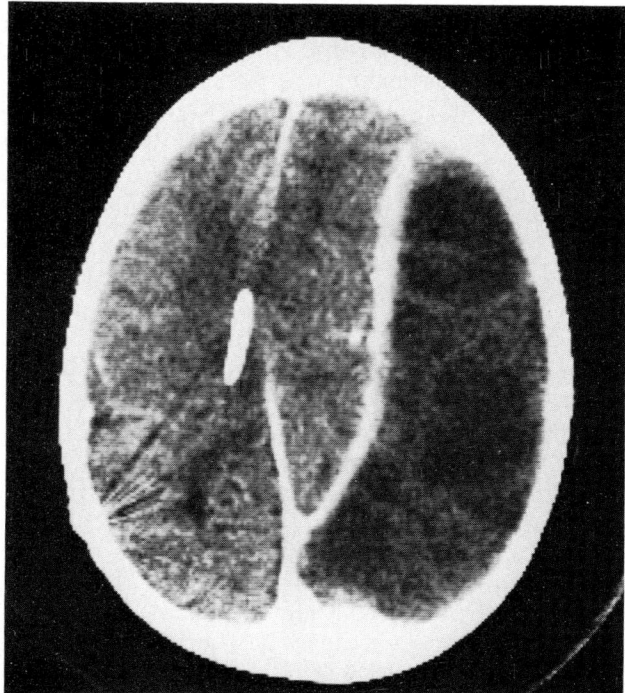

Figure 22–9. A five-year-old with intraventricular hemorrhage at birth, necessitating a ventriculoperitoneal shunt for hydrocephalus. There is a large left-sided chronic subdural hematoma with a thick, enhancing membrane.

tapping are to establish the character of the subdural fluid and to initiate treatment by partial removal of the subdural accumulation. The tapping procedure is done through the lateral border of the anterior fontanelle or the coronal suture and should be carried out only with meticulous attention to scalp preparation and sterile technique.

Treatment and Results

Treatment of the infantile subdural hematoma continues to be a controversial matter. There is not complete agreement regarding the proper management of either the liquid contents of the accumulation or the membranes that envelop those contents. It is generally accepted that the membranes begin to develop within one week of the subdural bleeding and increase in thickness over a period of several weeks. The membranes are known to contain delicate blood vessels, and these may contribute to the subdural accumulation. Although the practice of extensive craniotomy for removal of the membranes in order to prevent constriction of cerebral growth has not been completely abandoned, it would appear that there is very little evidence to support that method of surgical treatment. Thus, the methods of treatment that continue to be used include subdural tapping and shunting of the subdural effusion. A few neurosurgeons still prefer the use of cranial burr holes in order to evacuate the hematoma fluid and irrigate the subdural space.[9]

The experience in the Childrens Hospital Medical Center has generally favored treatment by tapping only, and it is believed that this is effective in the majority of infants.[23] Tapping of the subdural space is performed only in response to the presence of intracranial hypertension, manifested either by clinical features (e.g., irritability, vomiting) or by increased tension of the fontanelle. Seizures are not considered an indication of intracranial hypertension. Tapping is done by the method previously described. Fluid is allowed to drain from the subdural space as long as it flows spontaneously; it should never be aspirated. However, the cessation of flow of subdural fluid does not indicate that the subdural space has been emptied; it means only that the intracranial and ambient pressures have equilibrated. Characteristically, the interval between taps progressively increases as the fluid becomes less bloody. The total number of taps necessary may vary from one to ten, but if that number is exceeded, shunting probably should be considered.

An alternative method of treatment, as advocated by many experienced neurosurgeons, is early shunting after the diagnosis has been established. Shunting has been done into the pleural space[26] but more often into the peritoneal space.[11] While early shunting has the advantage of avoiding repeated taps and may in fact shorten hospitalization, it also has the disadvantage of subjecting the infant to a major surgical procedure and either permanent retention of the foreign body or a second procedure for its removal.

Craniocerebral disproportion is a common problem in the management of chronic subdural hematomas in infants. The disproportion results from the macrocrania that occurs slowly, particularly in early infancy, as a result of the subdural effusion. The underlying brain has not been constricted or compressed during this process and, therefore, has retained a relatively normal configuration and volume. The result, then, is a condition in which the brain no longer fills the intracranial space. It is the authors' opinion that unless this disproportion is quite severe, it does not constitute any significant hazard and is not harmful to brain development or growth. Various methods of dealing with the problem have been proposed, with the objective being to remodel the cranium and the dura to fit the brain. These methods of treatment are infrequently used and in the authors' judgment are not advisable.

While craniotomy for membrane removal is not generally performed at present, it still has occasional advocates. It was based on the belief that the membranes may contribute to persistence of subdural effusion and also may cause some constriction of the growing brain. Opponents of membrane removal note that the subdural membranes can hardly restrict brain growth, which nomally overcomes the restraints imposed by the dura, skull, and scalp. It has also been demonstrated that membranes spontaneously disappear after subdural effusion has been effectively evaluated by shunting.[28]

The results of treatment of chronic subdural hematomas in infants have demonstrated remarkable consistency, regardless of the method used. Most series have shown that approximately 75 percent of infants have normal development, whereas 5 percent have shown greater or lesser psychomotor retardation. What cannot be determined is whether the developmental delay is due to the presence of subdural effusion causing cerebral compression or to an associated parenchymal damage from the initial injury. The latter possibility seems more probable.

Subdural Hygroma

As indicated previously, there is no rigid distinction between subdural hygromas and subdural hematomas in infancy, since the extra-axial fluid accumulation is frequently a mixture of blood and cerebrospinal fluid. Although it is rather artificial, therefore, to discuss hygromas as a separate entity, the literature has traditionally divided these two pathologic sequelae to head injury. The commonly accepted explanation for the occurrence of a subdural hygroma is that a tear in the arachnoid results in an escape of cerebrospinal fluid into the subdural space, and, by a valvelike action, the arachnoid tear does not allow free communication between the subdural and subarachnoid compartments. This results in a loculated accumulation of fluid that may contain small amounts of blood. However, the subdural fluid accumulation acts as any other expanding lesion, with compression and displacement of the underlying brain tissue. It is noteworthy that subdural hygromas frequently are delayed in appearance and may not be seen by CT scan for days or weeks following a known injury.

Manifestation of subdural hygroma is similar to that of subdural hematoma. As noted previously, distinction between these lesions may be possible by NMRI scan.[29] Treatment is also similar in that tapping of the hygroma in the infant or burr hole drainage in the older child is indicated only in response to evidence of intracranial hypertension or progressive neurologic abnormality. The fluid contained within a subdural hygroma resorbs over a period of time and is not itself a source of neurologic deficit.

Intracerebral Hemorrhage

Intracerebral hemorrhage is an infrequent complication of trauma in infancy and childhood. In the series reported by Zimmerman and Bilaniuk,[34] 3 percent of pediatric head injury patients developed intracerebral hematomas, as compared with 10 percent in adults. It has been recognized for many years that intraparenchymal hematomas do occur in the tissue adjacent to the third ventricle as a consequence of bleeding from the germinal matrix in some newborn premature infants. These are not properly termed traumatic, in the sense of being due to mechanical forces.

True traumatic intracerebral hematomas, nevertheless, do rarely occur from the birth process.[24] These are located in the subcortical area and lead to significant damage to the developing brain. Such hematomas are distinctly less common than surface hemorrhages but may be demonstrated by ultrasonography or CT (Fig. 22–10). In addition, Martin and colleagues[20] have reported massive intracerebellar hemorrhage in low birth weight infants. Although the authors could not prove that it was traumatic in origin in all cases, they felt that the evidence indicated that molding and trauma to the suboccipital area and tentorium were the probable causes.

In older children, intracerebral hemorrhage is clearly seen as a consequence of trauma that may be mild or very severe. In the case of mild trauma, it is likely that it would not have been recognized prior to the CT era. The child may show progressive symptoms over a period of several days probably resulting from the actual delay in hematoma formation or the occurrence of perihematoma edema. The existence of delayed traumatic intracerebral hematoma has been documented by several researchers.[5] Atluru and associates[3] have recently described delayed intracerebral hemorrhage in five pediatric patients. The pathogenesis appears to remain undetermined, although the original theory was that hemorrhage resulted from direct damage to an arterial vessel, with later necrosis leading to rupture. It has also been proposed that local changes in blood flow or vessel wall integrity may cause a gradual diapedesis and oozing, with accu-

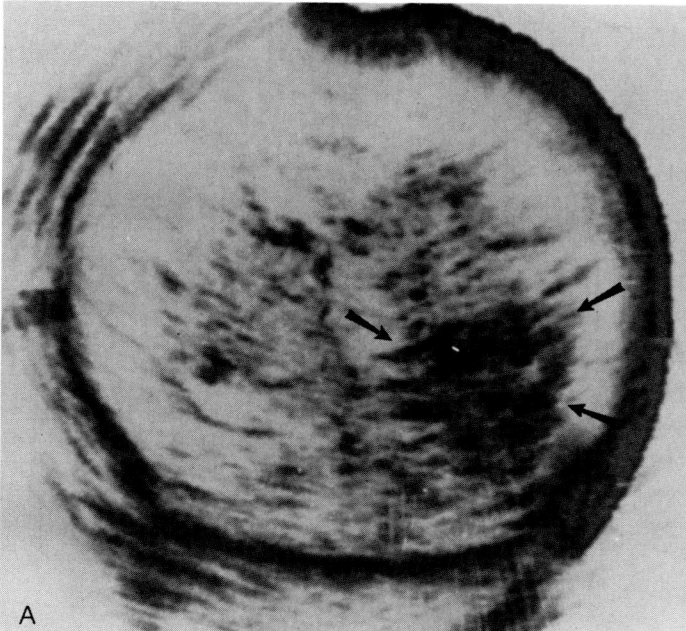
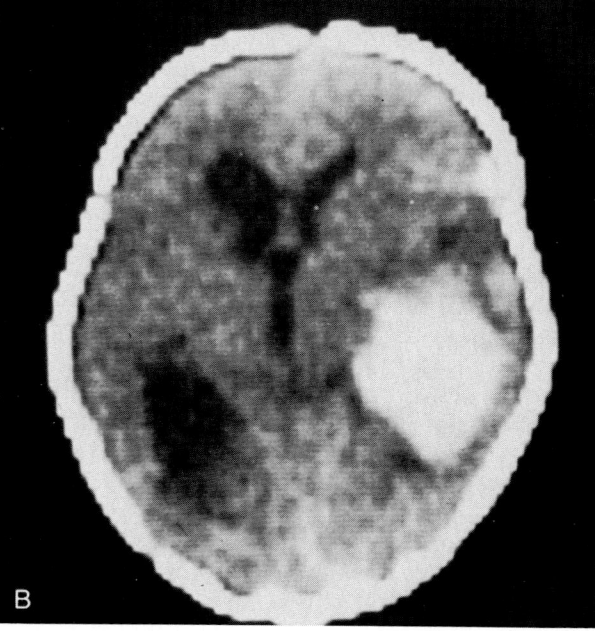

Figure 22–10. A 24-hour-old full-term infant after a traumatic delivery and experiencing seizures. A, Coronal sonography reveals focal hyperechoic lesion (arrows) in the left posterior parietal lobe. B, Non–contrast-enhanced CT scan confirms the parietal hemorrhage.

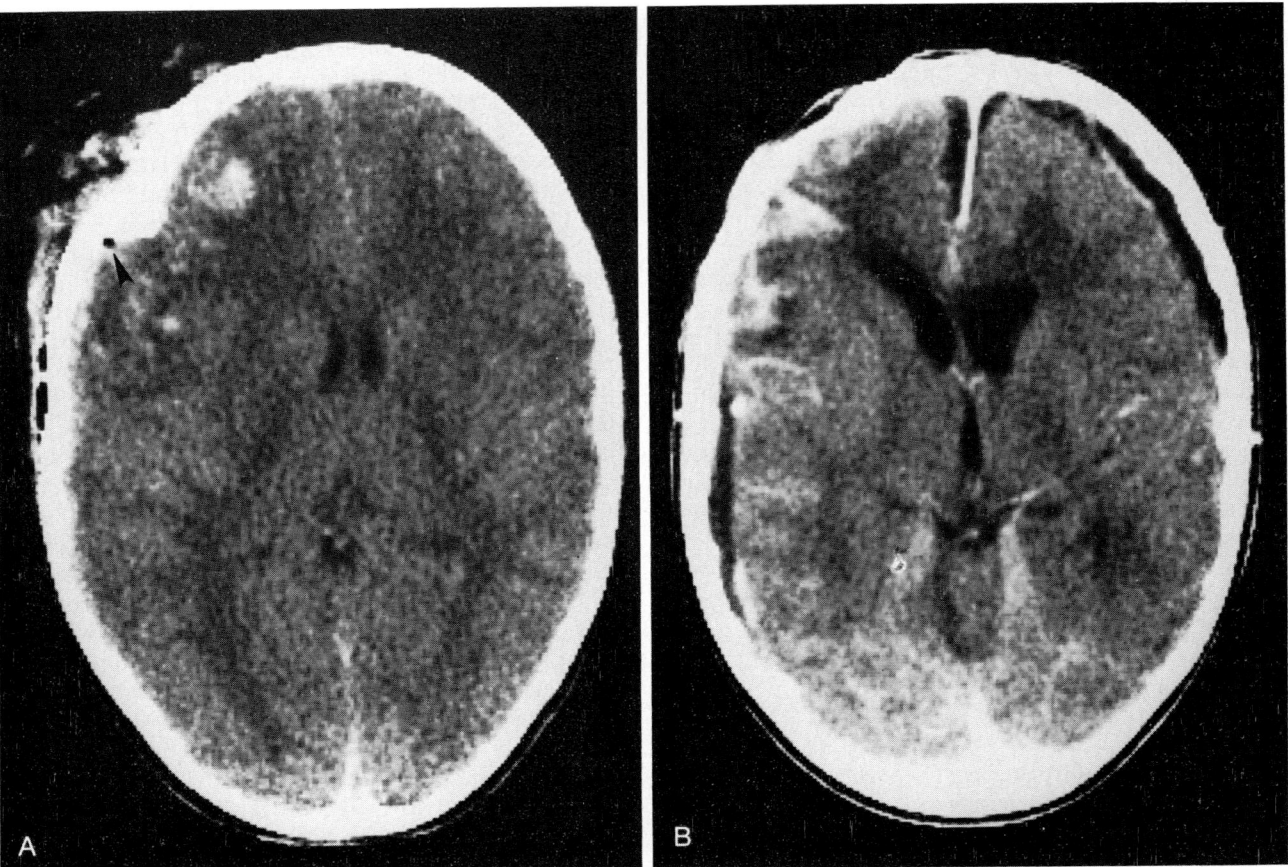

Figure 22–11. A ten-year-old struck by a truck, resulting in severe facial fractures, a depressed skull fracture, and hemorrhagic contusion. A, Hours after injury: a depressed frontal fracture with associated pneumocephalus (arrowhead) and hemorrhagic right frontal contusion. Perilesional edema and mild mass effect are present. B, Three weeks after injury: contrast-enhanced CT scan reveals aging infarct with gyral enhancement, ventricular enlargement and deformity, and widening of the extra-axial spaces.

mulation and coalescence to form a larger hemorrhage. This theory appears to be consistent with some experimental evidence showing hyperemia as the initial response to cerebral trauma. The loss of local autoregulation may allow an increase in blood pressure in the smaller vessels. Systemic hypertension, a frequent clinical correlate of brain injury, may also contribute to the occurrence of delayed hemorrhage.

Intracerebral hemorrhage may occur alone or in association with cerebral contusion or concomitant surface hemorrhage. The definitive diagnostic method in older children is the CT scan. The appearance of intracerebral hemorrhage depends to some extent on the mechanism of development of the circumscribed border and is frequently ovoid, with the axis oriented toward the brain surface. This is suggestive of a hematoma occurring in a shear cleft within the brain substance. The hematoma resulting from coalescence of hemorrhage at the site of contusion is more likely to be irregular and less distinct in its marginal definition (Fig. 22–11). In either event, the hematoma may be surrounded by an area of hypodensity that represents edema. Zimmerman and Bilaniuk[33] have stated that neovascularity was first apparent at the margins of the hematoma one to two weeks after injury. The loss of blood-brain barrier integrity permits a ring enhancement at the margin of the hematoma. Subsequently, the ring enhancement subsides, and the hematoma becomes isodense.

In contrast to the principle that extra-axial hematomas should always be removed when present, it is not always necessary or advisable to perform surgical evacuation of an intracerebral hematoma. Removal is indicated only if there is progressive clinical deterioration. If such deterioration does not occur, it is usually advisable to attempt management of the child in a manner similar to that of cerebral contusion without the presence of a hematoma. The relative rarity of an indication for surgery is illustrated by the absence of any surgically removed hematomas in the series of 85 severely injured childen analyzed by Bruce and associates.[6] Although four intracerebral hematomas were recognized, none were considered operable.

The late results of intracerebral hematomas are variable and are dependent on the size and the location of the hematoma and the presence of associated brain damage. An area of encephalomalacia or porencephalic cavitation may be present by CT scan. It is noteworthy that the incidence of post-traumatic seizures is quite high following intraparenchymal hematomas, but this is probably not diminished by early hematoma evacuation.[19]

References

1. Abroms IF, McLennan JE, Mandell F: Acute neonatal subdural hematoma following breech delivery. Am J Dis Child 131:192, 1977.
2. Arkins TJ, McLennan JE, Winston KR, et al: Acute posterior fossa epidural hematomas in children. Am J Dis Child 131:690, 1977.
3. Atluru V, Epstein LG, Zilka A: Delayed traumatic intracerebral hemorrhage in children. Pediatr Neurol 2:297, 1986.
4. Bell C, cited by Jacobson WHA: On middle meningeal hemorrhage. Guy's Hosp Rep 43:147, 1986.
5. Brown FD, Mullan S, Duda EE: Delayed traumatic intracerebral hematomas. J Neurosurg 48:1019, 1978.
6. Bruce DA, Raphaely RC, Goldberg AI, et al: Pathophysiology, treatment and outcome following severe head injury in children. Child's Brain 5:174–191, 1979.
7. Caffey J: The whiplash–shaken infant syndrome: Manual shaking by the extremities with whiplash-induced intracranial and intraocular bleedings, linked with residual permanent brain damage and mental retardation. Pediatrics 54:396, 1974.
8. Campbell JB, Cohen J: Epidural hemorrhage and the skull of children. Surg Gynecol Obstet 92:257, 1951.
9. Choux M: Extracerebral hematomas in children. In: McLaurin RL (ed): Advances in Neurotraumatology. Wien/New York, Springer-Verlag, 1986, pp 173–208.
10. Choux M, Grisoli F, Peragut J: Extradural hematomas in children. 104 cases. Child's Brain 1:337, 1975.
11. Collins WF, Pucci GL: Peritoneal drainage of subdural hematomas in infants. J Pediatr 58:482, 1961.
12. Ford LE, McLaurin RL: Mechanisms of extradural hematomas. J Neurosurg 20:76, 1963.
13. Galbraith S: Age distribution of extradural hemorrhage without skull fracture. Lancet 1:1217, 1973.
14. Gomori JM, Grossman RI, Goldberg HI, et al: Intracranial hematomas: Imaging by high-field MRI. Radiology 157:87, 1985.
15. Gutkelch AN: Infantile subdural hematoma and its relationship to whiplash injuries. Br Med J 2:430, 1971.
16. Gutierrez FA, Raimondi AJ: Acute subdural hematoma in infancy and childhood. Child's Brain 1:269, 1975.
17. Hendrick EB, Harwood-Nash MB, Hudson AR: Head injuries in children: A survey of 4465 consecutive cases at the Hospital for Sick Children, Toronto, Canada. Clin Neurosurg 11:46, 1964.
18. Jellinger K: The neuropathology of pediatric head injuries. In: Shapiro K (ed): Pediatric Head Trauma. Mt. Kisco, NY: Futura Publishing Company, Inc., 1983.
19. Jennett WB, Teasdale EG: Early assessment of the head injured patient. In: Jennett B, Teasdale G (eds): Management of Head Injuries. Philadelphia, F. A. Davis Co., 1981, pp 95–110.
20. Martin R, Roessmann U, Fanaroff A: Massive intracerebellar hemorrhage in low-birth-weight infants. J Pediatr 89:290, 1976.
21. Matson DD: Neurosurgery of Infancy and Childhood, 2nd ed. Springfield, IL, Charles C Thomas, 1969, p 934.
22. McLaurin RL, Babcock DS: Sonography of traumatic cranial hemorrhage. In: Vigouroux RP (ed): Advances in Neurotraumatology, Vol. 2. Wien, Springer-Verlag, 1987, pp 181–197.
23. McLaurin RL, Isaacs E, Lewis HP: Results of nonoperative treatment in 15 cases of infantile subdural hematoma. J Neurosurg 34:753, 1971.
24. Natelson SE, Sayers MP: The fate of children sustaining severe head trauma during birth. Pediatrics 51:169, 1973.
25. Pang D, Horton JA, Herron JM, et al: Nonsurgical management of extradural hematomas in children. J Neurosurg 59:958, 1983.
26. Ransohoff J: Chronic subdural hematoma treated by subdural-pleural shunt. Pediatrics 20:561, 1957.
27. Reilly PL, Adama JH, Graham DI, et al: Patients with head injury who talk and die. Lancet 2:375, 1975.
28. Shulman K, Ransohoff J: Subdural hematoma in children: The fate of children with retained membranes. J Neurosurg 18:175, 1961.
29. Snow RB, Zimmerman RD, Gandy SE, et al: Comparison of magnetic resonance imaging and computed tomography in the evaluation of head injury. Neurosurgery 18:45, 1986.
30. Takagi T, Fukuoka H, Wakabayashi S, et al: Posterior fossa subdural hemorrhage in the newborn as a result of birth trauma. Child's Brain 9:102, 1982.
31. Takagi T, Nagai R, Wakabayashi S, et al: Extradural hemorrhage in the newborn as a result of birth trauma. Child's Brain 4:306, 1978.
32. Till K: Subdural hematoma and effusion in infancy. Br Med J 3:400, 1968.
33. Zimmerman RA, Bilaniuk LT: Computed tomography in pediatric head trauma. J Neuroradiol 8:257, 1981.
34. Zimmerman RA, Bilaniuk LT: Radiology of pediatric craniocerebral trauma. In: Shapiro K (ed): Pediatric Head Trauma. Mt. Kisco, NY, Futura Publishing Co., Inc., 1983.

23
LATE COMPLICATIONS OF HEAD INJURY

Howard M. Eisenberg, M.D.
Rudy P. Briner, M.D.

In many cases, the ability of a child to reach full potential after head injury depends on the management of late or chronic sequelae and complications. The sequelae and complications discussed in this chapter include cranial defects, growing skull fracture, carotid-cavernous sinus fistula, seizure disorder, and persistent neuropsychologic dysfunction. Other important late complications such as hydrocephalus and cerebrospinal fluid rhinorrhea and otorrhea are reviewed in other chapters.

CRANIAL DEFECTS

Cranial defects are most often caused by operative removal of bone fragments after compound depressed fractures. Less commonly, they occur when a bone flap cannot be replaced because of severe brain swelling. The latter is less frequent now than in the past because of the more effective use of controlled respiration, osmotic diuretics, and other drugs to control brain swelling. Similarly, there now seems to be little enthusiasm for treating severe brain swelling by removing large portions of the skull.

The most common reasons to treat these defects are protection of the brain and improvement of the appearance of the patient. Other indications for surgery are the occasional presence of annoying symptoms attributed to these defects, including headache, throbbing sensations, and feelings of dizziness. Distortion of the brain by migration of the ventricles toward the bony defect has been observed in association with these skull defects;[36, 37] however, these changes are more probably the result of direct injury to the underlying brain and disruption of the dura than of the skull defect itself. Defects below the temporal or occipital muscles or small defects less than 2 to 3 cm in diameter often can be left untreated. The important considerations in the management of skull defects relate to the age of the patient, the time between the injury and reconstruction, and the choice of materials used to reconstruct the defect.

Cranioplasty can frequently be delayed in children younger than three years of age. Even large defects, particularly in children younger than two years, often close spontaneously. The newly formed bone generally conforms to the shape of the skull, providing a satisfactory cosmetic result. Another reason for delay of repair in young children is that the use of synthetic materials for reconstruction is unsatisfactory because of the rapid head growth that occurs during this period. This necessitates the use of autogenous bone, making the operation somewhat more difficult. Compound injuries should be considered contaminated, and when a synthetic graft is planned, a period of six to 12 months is recommended before repair of the defect. In these cases, an x-ray film of the skull should be made before reconstruction to rule out the presence of osteomyelitis.

The preference for different materials used for reconstruction varies among neurosurgeons. When reconstruction is done in children younger than three years of age, autogenous bone is the best material. Rib, the most commonly used graft, is split so that bony plates with one cortical surface can be placed edge to edge to cover the defect (Fig. 23–1).[33] Other sources of bone such as iliac crest or outer table from normal skull can also be used. The autogenous bone graft, once in place, becomes infiltrated with osteoblasts and acts as a scaffold for new bone formation. The graft can then compensate for growth of the skull. The disadvantages of autogenous grafts are the possibility of resorption before bone growth has closed the defect and the added difficulty of acquiring bone for grafting. In children older than three years, synthetic materials are generally satisfactory. All plastic grafts can be fashioned at the time of operation, when the skull defect is exposed, ensuring a good fit. Common complications of synthetic grafts are dislodgement and those complications associated with insertion of any foreign body, infection and breakdown of the overlying skin.

Repair of defects of the low forehead, particularly those that require reconstruction of an orbital rim or nasion, represent more difficult problems. Silastic prostheses are suitable for repair of these types of deficits. Silastic can be premolded over mesh into the complex curves that are required for a good cosmetic result. Although these grafts are not as rigid as other synthetic grafts, the protection provided is adequate. Other materials used to repair low forehead deficits with good cosmetic results are autogenous bone[34] and a combination of a polyurethane mesh and autogenous bone.[35]

GROWING SKULL FRACTURE

An infrequent complication of head injury is the formation of a skull defect at the site of a fracture (Fig. 23–2). The defect most often detected by visible or palpable swelling of the overlying scalp may also be associated with signs of brain injury such as hemiparesis and seizures. Although the condition was reported in the early 1800's,[27] the anatomy of the lesion, its pathogenesis, and even its natural history are still debated. The condition has been considered under several rubrics; traumatic leptomeningeal cyst or growing fracture are the most common.

Dyke[8] first used the term leptomeningeal cyst, and although this term has been perpetuated, it may be a misnomer, adding to the confusion about the anatomy of the lesion and its pathogenesis. It is agreed that the basic substrate for development of the condition is a skull fracture and an underlying dural tear. This has been repeatedly shown clinically and in animal experiments.[10, 26, 38] A popular concept of the pathogenesis was first stated by Taveras and Ransohoff.[42] They hypothesized that the condition developed initially as an outpouching of arachnoid through the lacerated dura. This arachnoid protrusion may increase in size because fluid that enters it is partially prevented from leaving by surrounding adhesions acting as one-way valves. The enlarging arachnoid cyst, aided by normal pulsations of the brain, gradually erodes the edges of the fracture and causes progressive enlargement of the skull defect. This popular concept, although appealing, has been questioned. Although there is clinical and anatomic evidence that a severe brain injury has taken place in many of these cases, the

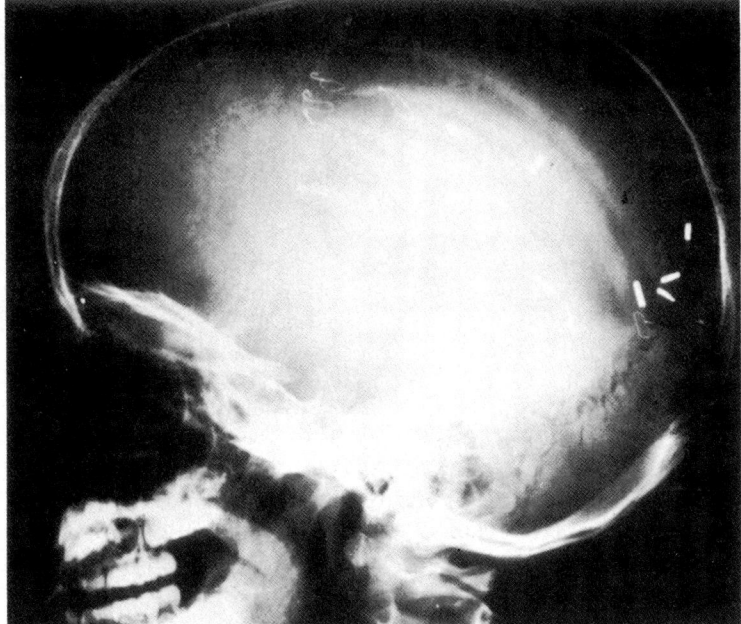

Figure 23–1. Cranioplasty using a rib graft in a three-year-old boy.

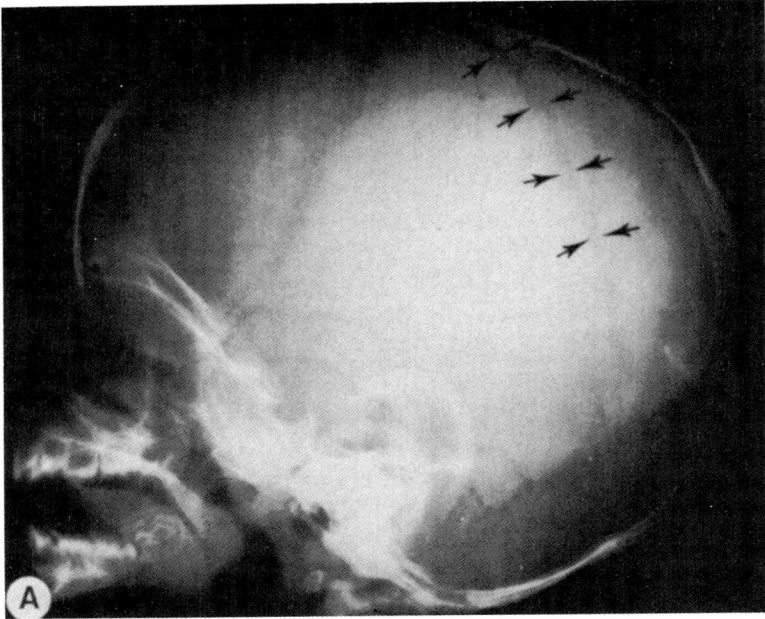
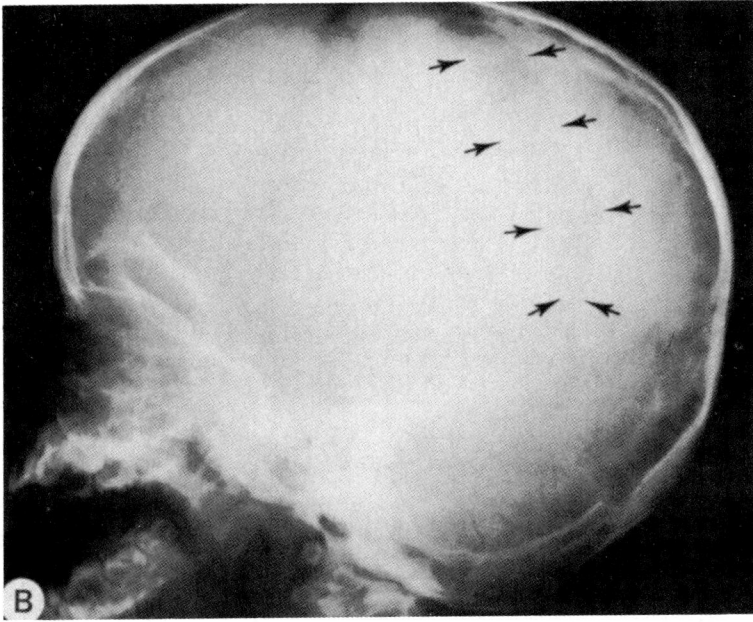

Figure 23-2. Evolution of a growing skull fracture. A, Diastatic parietal skull fracture in an eight-month-old girl. B, Widening of the fracture demonstrated five months later.

relationship between the cerebral injury and the skull defect is not clear. It is not known whether the cerebral injuries progress as a result of the defect or whether injury to the underlying brain aggravates the bony changes. Experiments in young dogs and cats have shown that discontinuity of the bone and dura was required to cause progressive skull defect, but adding an injury to the underlying brain did not appear to increase their incidence or size.[10, 26, 38] Winston and coworkers[47] reviewed four cases of enlarging dural defect that complicated operations for synostosis. In each case, there was an iatrogenic dural defect that was initially small, frequently unrecognized, and almost certainly without injury to the underlying brain. These researchers reasoned that there were only "two requirements for the entire syndrome of expanding dural defect, regardless of the mechanism of injury: 1) the dura must be disrupted; and 2) there must be an outward driving force, such as normally growing brain, hydrocephalus, cerebral edema, or neoplasm." Central in this scheme is the dura and its relationship to the growing brain. The laceration of the dura leads to an imbalance in the tensile forces of the dura surrounding growing brain (Fig. 23-3), and the result is a progressively enlarging dural defect. The sequelae of the enlarging dural defect can be brain herniation with resorption of bone, parenchymal injury, and arachnoid adhesion (Fig. 23-4). Pertinent in this regard is that Lende and

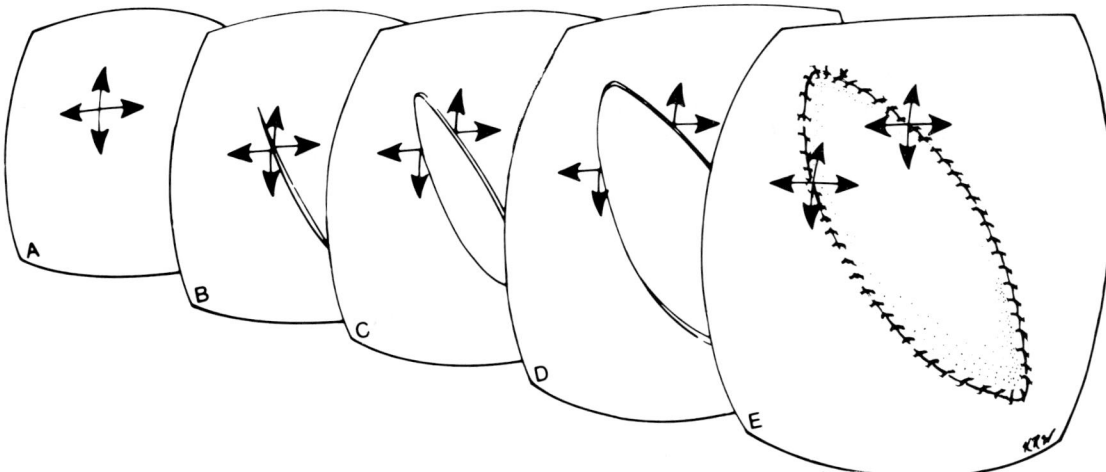

Figure 23–3. Diagram of tensile forces acting on the dura in an expanding defect. A, Intact dura, with forces in all tangential directions. B, Lacerated dura, with loss of centripetal tangential forces, thereby leaving the centrifugal forces unopposed. C and D, Progressive enlargement of the dural defect. E, Dural defect repaired and the normal state re-established (tensile forces again acting in all directions). (With permission from Winston K, et al.: J Neurosurg 59:847–853, 1983.)

Erickson[27] did not see an arachnoid or leptomeningeal cyst in any of their five reported cases. During surgery, they found fibrotic scar and gliotic brain between the edges of the bone. In one patient, a cyst was seen within this scar tissue, which they considered a porencephalic cyst. Similar operative findings have been described by Stein and Tenner.[41] They assumed that the leptomeningeal cysts seen in other reported cases were actually superficial porencephalic cysts covered by gliotic brain. Of ten patients treated at the Hospital for Sick Children in London,[22] seven were found to have cysts during surgery. Six of these cysts were clearly porencephalic; four communicated with the ipsilateral lateral ventricle. A leptomeningeal cyst was not seen in any of these patients. A true leptomeningeal cyst occurring in a patient who has suffered trauma must then be considered a rare finding. The pathologic finding most frequently seen during surgery is a fibrotic and gliotic scar insinuated between the edges of the bony defect.

Growing skull fractures occur virtually only in

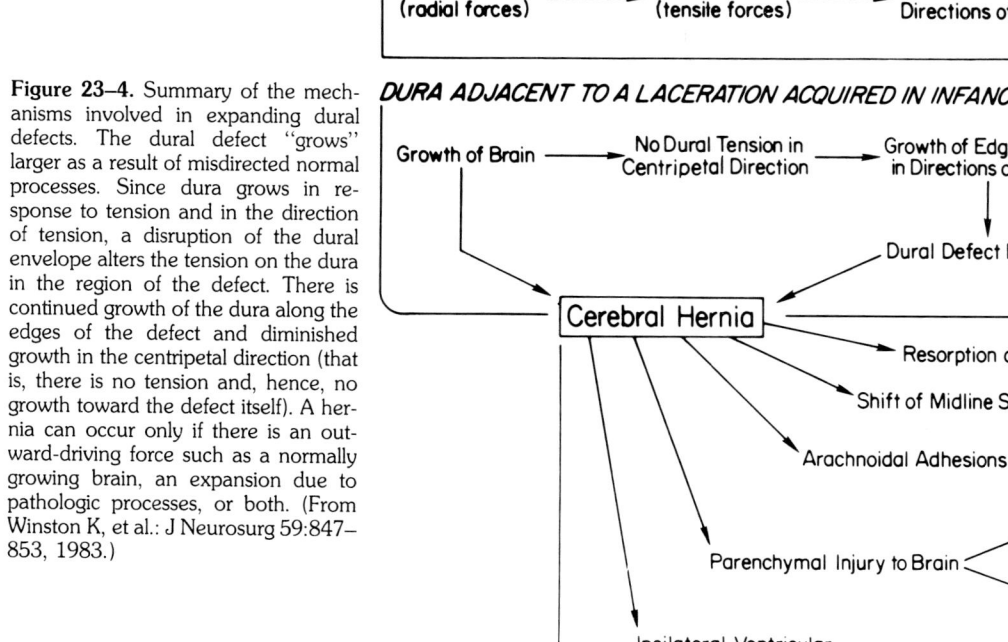

Figure 23–4. Summary of the mechanisms involved in expanding dural defects. The dural defect "grows" larger as a result of misdirected normal processes. Since dura grows in response to tension and in the direction of tension, a disruption of the dural envelope alters the tension on the dura in the region of the defect. There is continued growth of the dura along the edges of the defect and diminished growth in the centripetal direction (that is, there is no tension and, hence, no growth toward the defect itself). A hernia can occur only if there is an outward-driving force such as a normally growing brain, an expansion due to pathologic processes, or both. (From Winston K, et al.: J Neurosurg 59:847–853, 1983.)

infants and children. In a review of the world literature up to 1960,[27] the initial injury in half of the patients occurred before 12 months of age, and in 90 percent of cases before three years of age. Matson's oldest patient was 12 years of age at the time of injury, but the next oldest in his series was less than four years of age.[36] Excluding the oldest patient, the mean age of the remaining 16 patients in his series was ten and a half months. All other reports also emphasize the early age at the time of the initial injury. In another series,[15] the oldest child was two years of age at the time of injury. The remaining eight were injured at one year of age or younger. Similarly, of ten other patients, seven were injured when they were younger than one year of age.[22]

The most common presenting symptom is a scalp mass. Other symptoms are those that can be attributed to an associated brain injury, the most common being seizures and focal weakness. The condition is almost always first noticed by finding scalp swelling or a palpable skull defect after a head injury. X-ray films show a characteristic bony defect lying in the course of a skull fracture (Fig. 23–2). Frequently, the pre-existing fracture is diastatic. The bony defect is irregular, with saucerized margins. Sometimes, the edges are everted, and the inner table frequently appears eroded. However, erosion of the outer table has also been described. In many cases, the bony defect has been noted to cross the suture lines.[22] An almost universal finding is dilatation of the ipsilateral lateral ventricle. This has been found in almost every instance in which the lateral ventricles were studied.[15, 22, 36] The cause of the ventricular dilatation is not certain. It has been hypothesized that it may be related to pressure in the ventricle unopposed by the resistance of a normally intact dura.[39] A more probable explanation is that it is caused by atrophy. The frequent finding that the midline is shifted toward the side of the dilated lateral ventricle supports this idea. In many cases, there is an obvious porencephalic cyst, which not infrequently communicates with the lateral ventricle.[22, 36]

The natural history of the condition has not been clearly defined. There is probably a period of early rapid progression. Some defects reach a very large size in relatively short periods of time, one or two months. This rapid progression is probably followed by a period of slower change or even stability. However, it is unlikely that the condition ever spontaneously improves with resolution of the swelling and new bone formation. Occasionally, a skull defect in a fracture line is found in an adult with a history of head injury in childhood.[43] Several untreated patients have been described. In most of these,[1, 38, 43] the defect once found did not appear to progress. No new neurologic findings occurred, and change in the skull defect was not apparent in serial x-ray films. However, in one reported untreated patient,[38] the skull defect increased in size over a year, and a neurologic deficit progressed from a monoparesis to a hemiparesis. In view of this potential for change after detection, these defects should be repaired when they are discovered in early childhood. When they are found in adults or adolescents as an incidental finding, and when small, the necessity for surgery may be questioned.

The surgical repair of these lesions can be more difficult than imagined by those who are inexperienced. The dural defect may be considerably larger than the bony defect. This feature should be kept in mind when planning a scalp flap. When the bony defect is exposed, a fibrotic and gliotic scar is frequently seen between the bone edges. Occasionally, there are visible or palpable cysts in the scar or below the scar. The scar is dissected from the bone edges, and bone is removed until the dura is visible circumferentially. Occasionally 3 to 4 cm of bone on each side must be removed to allow visualization of the dural edges. Usually, it is not necessary to remove the scar, but occasionally, a superficial cyst may be encountered and should be removed or fenestrated. The most important part of the repair is closure of the dura; a tight dural closure with autograft is preferable. Although a cranioplasty is generally done at the time of dural repair, it may be postponed without jeopardizing the repair.[36]

CAROTID–CAVERNOUS SINUS FISTULA

This is a rare complication of head injury in adults, and there is little doubt that it is even less common in children. Even in large series, the number of patients younger than 20 years of age are few. The details of three cases occurring in childhood have been reported. The youngest patient was two and a half years old,[6] and the other two were seven years of age.[2, 4] Considering these cases, it is likely that the lesion and its effects and treatment are similar in adults and children. The treatment of choice is transarterial placement of a detachable balloon under radiographic guidance; the carotid artery remains patent.[5, 9, 44]

POST-TRAUMATIC SEIZURES

A distinction must be made between early post-traumatic seizures and post-traumatic epilepsy. The goal is to identify those children in whom long-term antiepileptic medication is needed. There is some disagreement on the nomenclature. Early post-traumatic seizures have been defined as seizures occurring within 24 hours of injury to within two weeks of injury. On the other hand, late post-traumatic epilepsy has been defined as occurring as early as eight days after injury. However, since the proportion of seizures initially appearing between the end of one week and four weeks after trauma is very small, studies with differing definitions of early seizures and post-traumatic epilepsy can be compared.

The incidence of early post-traumatic seizures ranges from 2 to 5 percent.[11, 13, 19] The effect of age on incidence is uncertain. Jennett[16, 19, 20] found that with severe injury, adults and children have an equal frequency of post-traumatic seizures, but there was an excess of early seizures in children with only minor head injuries. However, Annegers and colleagues[3] and Kollevold[24] predict a higher incidence of early post-traumatic seizures among children at all levels of injury, from mild to severe. Annegers and coworkers,[3] Jennett,[17] and Kollevold[24] agree that serious injuries, especially those involving hematomas and depressed skull fracture, are much more likely to be accompanied by early post-traumatic seizures. Post-traumatic seizures also seem to be more common when there is a history of birth injury.[13, 40] In Kollevold's series,[25] patients with a family history of epilepsy had an increased frequency of early post-traumatic seizures. However, Jennett failed to find an increased frequency of early seizures in patients with a family history of epilepsy. That early post-traumatic seizures are a significant problem associated with head injury in children is not in dispute; however, the prediction and management of post-traumatic epilepsy is not nearly so clear.

While the incidence reported for post-traumatic epilepsy in children is about the same as the incidence of early post-traumatic seizures,[12, 17] the relationship of early post-traumatic seizures to post-traumatic epilepsy is not clear. In Jennett's series,[17, 19] children with early post-traumatic seizures were at increased risk for post-traumatic epilepsy when compared with children without early post-traumatic seizures. However, Annegers and associates[3] and Hendrick and Harris[12] found no association between children with early post-traumatic seizures and those who develop post-traumatic epilepsy. The frequency of post-traumatic epilepsy has generally been reported to be higher in adults than in children.[11] Children with depressed fractures and hematomas, prolonged loss of consciousness, or both have an increased incidence of post-traumatic epilepsy.[3, 20, 21]

In the only study of a head injury cohort compared with the general population, Annegers and coworkers[3] found that within one year after head injury, children with head injuries had a risk of epilepsy five times that of the general population. During the five years following head trauma, the risk of epilepsy was three times that of the general population. However, after five years, no clear increase in risk could be demonstrated.[3] In a review of prophylactic anticonvulsant treatment of head trauma patients, Hauser[11] found no good evidence that prophylactic anticonvulsants decrease the frequency of post-traumatic epilepsy (when patients of all ages were considered). However, the efficacy of prophylactic anticonvulsants in patients with head injuries (the risk-benefit ratio) is currently being studied in two NIH-supported randomized clinical trials.

Determining who is at increased risk and, therefore, should be treated with anticonvulsants is obviously, at least for the present, imprecise. Only approximately 50 percent of children who develop post-traumatic epilepsy do so in the first year after injury.[3, 11, 21, 46] A child who has one late post-traumatic seizure has about a 45 percent chance of having a second, and in these patients, anticonvulsant therapy should be strongly considered.[11] In addition, patients with severe injuries are at increased risk for post-traumatic epilepsy, and anticonvulsant treatment should also be discussed as an option. At present, there is less clear evidence to recommend anticonvulsant treatment in children with only early post-traumatic seizures. Patients who receive anticonvulsant therapy should probably be treated for one to two years. There is a significant rate of remission in post-traumatic epilepsy; 20 to 50 percent of patients with post-traumatic epilepsy may eventually become seizure-free without medicine.[11] On the other hand, patients who take medicine for two to three years probably have about a 25 percent chance of relapse when medication is stopped. Changes found by electroencephalography have only limited predictive value for the occurrence of seizures. When children with epilepsy resulting from all causes were studied after their medication was discontinued, those with severe electroencephalogram (EEG) abnormalities relapsed at a higher rate than those who had no or only mild abnormalities. However, patients with severe EEG abnormalities made up a small fraction of the total group at risk.[14] No similar study has been made of children with head injuries who never had a seizure or who only had a seizure in the first week after injury but were given prophylactic anticonvulsants. The attendant risks of anticonvulsant therapy and the relatively imprecise risks of post-traumatic epilepsy should be balanced by physician, patient, and family in coming to a decision on starting and stopping therapy. Many patients and their families may accept the risk of seizures when presented with the choices.

NEUROPSYCHOLOGIC DEFICITS

A serious and pervasive sequela of head injury is neuropsychologic deficit. Although not only a late complication, these deficits may persist and present problems in long-term management. The concept that neural plasticity generally confers a special advantage to young children in recovery from head injury is not supported by data.[9, 30–32] While there are many examples of recovery after focal injury in young children beyond what could be expected for adults, particularly regarding language deficits, the evidence does not support greater recovery in children after diffuse injury including severe head trauma. Levin and colleagues,[31] comparing groups of adolescents and children matched in severity and type of injury, found that the children were not less but maybe even more vulnerable to the deleterious effects of diffuse injury on memory and cognition. In addition, residual psychologic impairment has been found in children with even brief periods of coma, sometimes after only momentary loss of consciousness.[23] Further, some functions seem more at risk than do others. When a group that included both children and adolescents was assessed after head injury by testing multiple indices,[29] impairment of memory was the most commonly found abnormality, exceeding linguistic deficits or visual-spatial impairment. When these memory deficits were more closely analyzed, retrieval of information was found to be more severely affected than storage. The occurrence of retrieval deficits has been emphasized in the memory disorders associated with Korsakoff's syndrome.[45] In view of the importance of temporal lobe structures for memory and their vulnerability in head injury,[18] it may be inferred that involvement of these regions is partially responsible for impaired retrieval in patients with head injuries. When the memory deficits were related to specific areas of injuries, it was found that patients with left temporal lobe lesions had impairment of verbal memory that was not found in patients with right temporal lobe lesions, whereas those patients with a right temporal lobe lesion had impairment of visual memory.[28]

The degree of neuropsychologic impairment generally correlated well with the duration of coma and the severity of acute neurologic impairment.[29] General intelligence assessed by measuring intelligence quotient (IQ) showed that global intelligence was generally in the normal range in all but the most severely injured patients.[29] However, when postinjury measurements were compared with premorbid ability, it was found that only partial intellectual recovery was generally achieved.[23] Although global IQ measurements may return to the normal range, other performance scores are frequently abnormal.[9, 30, 32] Further, while patients often can compensate for learning impairment secondary to decreased intellectual functions, the impairment in learning and socialization caused by behavioral disturbances are often the most troublesome sequelae of head injury in children. The identification of specific neuropsychologic deficits is important in fostering the maximum rehabilitation. Therefore, neuropsychologic evaluations are needed in planning the resumption of schooling and determining the need for special education and rehabilitative services, and should be part of the follow-up of any child who has sustained a head injury, particularly one associated with loss of consciousness.

References

1. Addy DP: Expanding skull fracture of childhood. Br Med J 4:338, 1973.
2. Agnetti V, Pav A, Pinna L, et al: Cerebral pseudo-angiomatous pattern in a case of carotid-cavernous fistula. J Neurosurg Sci 18:75, 1974.
3. Annegers JF, Grabon JD, Groover RV, et al: Seizures after head trauma: A population study. Neurology 30:683, 1980.
4. Arseni C, Horvath L, Caurea V, et al: Carotid-cavernous fistula in the child. Rev Roum Med Neurol Psychiatr 16:29, 1978.
5. Barrow DL, Fleischer AS, Hoffman JC: Complications of detachable balloon catheter technique in the treatment of traumatic intracranial arteriovenous fistulas. J Neurosurg 56:396, 1982.
6. Broughton WL, Gee W, Doppman J, et al: Nonpulsatile exophthalmos in carotid–cavernous sinus fistula. J Pediatr Ophthalmol 14:221, 1977.
7. Debrun G, Lacour P, Caron JP, et al: Detachable balloon and calibrated-leak balloon techniques in the treatment of cerebral vascular lesions. J Neurosurg 49:635, 1978.
8. Dyke CG: The roentgen-ray diagnosis of the skull and intracranial contents. In Golden R (ed): Diagnostic Roentgenology. New York, T Nelson and Sons, 1938, p 7.
9. Goldstein FC, Levin HS: Intellectual and academic outcome following CHI in children and adolescents: Research strategies and empirical findings. Developmental Neuropsychol 1:195, 1985.
10. Goldstein F, Sakoda T, Kepes JJ, et al: Enlarging skull fractures: an experimental study. J Neurosurg 27:541, 1967.
11. Hauser WA: Posttraumatic epilepsy in children. In: Shapiro K (ed): Pediatric Head Trauma. New York, Futura Publishing Co., Inc., 1983, pp 271–287.
12. Hendrick EB, Harris L: Post-traumatic epilepsy in children. J Trauma 8:547, 1968.
13. Hendrick EB, Harwood-Nash DC, Hudson, AR: Head injuries in children: A survey of 4465 consecutive cases at the Hospital for Sick Children, Toronto, Canada. Clin Neurosurg 11:46, 1964.
14. Holowach J, Thurston DL, O'Leary J: Prognosis in childhood epilepsy follow-up study of 148 cases in which therapy had been suspended after prolonged anticonvulsant control. N Engl J Med 286:169, 1972.
15. Ito H, Miwa T, Onodra Y: Growing skull fracture of childhood with reference to the importance of brain injury and its pathogenetic consideration. Child's Brain 3:116, 1977.
16. Jennett WB: Early traumatic epilepsy. Lancet 1:1023, 1969.
17. Jennett WB: Epilepsy After Nonmissile Head Injuries. Chicago, Wm. Heinemann, 1975.
18. Jennett WB: Head injuries and the temporal lobe. In: Herrington RN (ed): Current Problems in Neuropsychiatry. Br J Psychiatry (special publ), No. 4, Asford, Headley Bros Ltd., 1969.
19. Jennett WB: Trauma as a cause of epilepsy in childhood. Dev Med Child Neurol 15:56, 1973.
20. Jennett WB, Miller JD, Braakman R: Epilepsy after nonmissile depressed skull fracture. J Neurosurg 41:208, 1974.
21. Jennett WB, Teather D, Bennie S: Epilepsy after head injury. Residual risk after varying fit-free intervals since injury. Lancet 2:652, 1973.
22. Kingsley D, Till K, Hoare R: Growing fractures of the skull. J Neurol Neurosurg Psychiatry 41:312, 1978.
23. Klonoff H, Low MD, Clark C: Head injuries in children with a prospective five year follow-up. J Neurol Neurosurg Psychiatry 40:1211, 1977.
24. Kollevold T: Immediate and early cerebral seizures after head injuries. Part I. J Oslo City Hosp 26:99, 1976.
25. Kollevold T: Immediate and early cerebral seizures after head injuries. Part IV. J Oslo City Hosp 29:35, 1979.
26. Lende RA: Enlarging skull fractures of childhood. Neuroradiology 7:119, 1974.
27. Lende RA, Erickson RC: Growing skull fractures of childhood. J Neurosurg 18:479, 1961.

28. Levin HS, Eisenberg HM: Neuropsychological impairment after closed head injury in children and adolescents. J Pediatr Psychol 4:389, 1979.
29. Levin HS, Eisenberg HM: Neuropsychological outcome of closed head injury in children and adolescents. Child's Brain 5:281, 1979.
30. Levin HS, Eisenberg HM, Miner ME: Neuropsychologic findings in head injured children. In Shapiro K (ed): Pediatric Head Trauma. New York, Futura Publishing Co., Inc., 1983.
31. Levin HS, Eisenberg HM. Wigg NR, et al: Memory and intellectual ability after head injury in children and adolescents. Neurosurgery 11:668, 1982.
32. Levin HS, Ewing-Cobbs L, Benton AL: Age and recovery from brain damage. In: Scheff SW (ed): Aging and Recovery of Function in the Central Nervous System. New York, Plenum Press, 1984, pp 169–205.
33. Longacre JJ, DeStefano GA: Further observations of the behavior of autogenous split-rib grafts in reconstruction of extensive defects of the cranium and face. Plast Reconstr Surg 20:281, 1957.
34. Longacre JJ, Kahl JB, Wood RW: Reconstruction of extensive defects in and about the orbit. Am J Ophthalmol 61:763, 1966.
35. Maniscalco JE, Leake D, Habal MB: Cranioplasty. Use of a combination graft. J Fla Med Assoc 63:869, 1976.
36. Matson DD: Neurosurgery of Infancy and Childhood, 2nd ed. Springfield, IL, Charles C Thomas, 1969.
37. Milhorat TH: Pediatric Neurosurgery. Philadelphia, F. A. Davis, 1978.
38. Ramamurthi B, Kalyanaraman S: Rationale for surgery in growing fractures of the skull. J Neurosurg 32:427, 1970.
39. Sato O, Tsugane R, Kageyama N: Growing skull fractures of childhood. Possible mechanism of its focal ventricular dilatation. Child's Brain 1:148, 1975.
40. Snoek JW, Minderhoud JM, Wilmink JT: Delayed determination following mild head injury in children. Brain 107:15, 1984.
41. Stein BM, Tenner MS: Enlargement of skull fracture in childhood due to cerebral herniation. Arch Neurol 26:137, 1972.
42. Taveras JM, Ransohoff J: Leptomeningeal cysts of the brain following trauma with erosion of the skull. A study of seven cases treated by surgery. J Neurosurg 10:233, 1953.
43. Vas CJ, Winn JM: Growing skull fractures. Dev Med Child Neurol 8:735, 1966.
44. Vinuela F, Fox A: Interventional neuroradiology. In: Wilkins RH, Rengachary SS (eds): Neurosurgery. New York, McGraw-Hill, 1985.
45. Warrington EK, Weiskrantz L: Amnesic syndrome. Consolidation or retrieval? Nature (Lond) 228:628, 1970.
46. Weiss GH, Caverness WF: Prognostic factors in the persistence of posttraumatic epilepsy. J Neurosurg 37:164, 1972.
47. Winston K, Beatty RM, Fischer EG: Consequences of dural defects acquired in infancy. J Neurosurg 59:839, 1983.

24
SPINAL CORD INJURY

Arnold H. Menezes, M.D.
John C. Godersky, M.D.
Wendy R. K. Smoker, M.D.

Injury to the spinal column and the spinal cord is relatively infrequent in the pediatric population. The incidence of hospitalization for acute spinal cord injury in the United States (1970–1977), for individuals 19 years of age or younger, was 21.2 per million, whereas the highest incidence was in the 20 to 24 year age group, being 68.0 per million.[20, 23, 73] This does not take into account the large numbers of patients who die at the scene of the accident or prior to admission. Kewalramani and colleagues,[73] in a population survey in northern California, reported 58 children younger than 15 years of age who suffered a spinal cord injury during a one-year span. Twenty-eight of these died at the scene of the accident or prior to hospitalization. Autopsies revealed severe spinal cord injury in the majority and associated multisystem trauma. Most series reporting on pediatric spinal cord and spinal column injuries discuss only the incidence of hospitalization rather than the true incidence of injuries.

The anatomy and biomechanics of the spine change from birth through adolescence. This produces alterations in the bony and ligamentous relationships and leads to variations in the etiology and the pathophysiology of the injury with age.[6, 53, 57, 61, 69, 90, 101] When taken as a whole, motor vehicle accidents account for 45 percent of pediatric spinal injuries; diving injuries, 23 percent; falls, 12 percent; football and other sports, 5 percent; gymnastics, 7 percent; and miscellaneous, 8 percent.[66] Between 20 and 25 percent suffer from multisystem injuries.*

As with the adult population, a large proportion of spinal fractures result in no neurologic deficits. Of 74 cervical spine fractures encountered in children younger than 18 years of age, only 27 were accompanied by a neurologic deficit.[66] In an eight-year review, Zabramski and coworkers[119] encountered a total of 52 patients younger than 16 years of age with acute traumatic spinal cord or spinal column injuries. Of this group, 24 children were identified as neurologically intact.

Anderson and Schutt[5] reviewed the Mayo Clinic experience in all children, younger than 14 years of age when admitted, with spinal column and spinal cord injuries. There were 156 children treated between 1950 and 1978.[12] Forty-four of these had a neurologic deficit. The neurologic deficit was complete in 16, and 11 of these died. None of the patients with complete injuries showed any recovery. Of the 28 patients with incomplete spinal cord injuries, two died. Within this series, lesions above the fourth cervical level occurred in 39 of 156 (25 percent), and half of these had a neurologic deficit. Twenty-two children (14 percent) had a lesion between the fourth and seventh cervical segments, and seven had neurologic dysfunction. Cervical injuries accounted for 39 percent of patients in their series. In 15 children, the injury was between T1 and T5, and in 42 children, it was between T6 and T12. Twenty-seven children had localization of their injury between L1 and L4, and in nine it was below this level. McPhee[81] reported on 42 children younger than 15 years of age with fractures or dislocations of the spine admitted to the Royal Brisbane Hospital Complex. Males accounted for 63

---
*References 5, 6, 9, 20, 23, 25, 64, 66, 81, 86, 101, 119

percent of patients with these injuries. Half the injuries occurred in the cervical spine, while injuries at more than one level occurred in 35 percent of the patients. Spinal cord injuries occurred in 14 percent of these patients. Lesoin and coworkers[77] had a similar experience, with 50 percent of injuries being in the cervical spine.

Various authors have stressed the frequent occurrence of spinal cord injury without evidence of radiographic abnormality in the pediatric population.[10, 20, 64, 89, 114, 119] Burke reviewed 29 infants and children younger than 13 years of age admitted over an 18-year span with spinal cord injuries.[25] Five were due to birth injuries (four were breech delivery), and in 16 no fracture was visualized. Of 52 patients reported by Zabramski and coworkers,[119] nine had no evidence of fracture or subluxation. Melzak,[83] in reviewing The Stoke-Mandivelle hospital series of the National Spinal Injury Center in Buckinghamshire, found 29 patients who were admitted with spinal cord injuries, and only 16 had fractures. At the Hospital for Sick Children in Toronto, 95 children were admitted with spinal cord injuries over a 15-year period.[32] No x-ray evidence of injury was found in 34 patients; 8 of these 34 had traumatic infarction of the spinal cord.

It is evident that certain areas of the pediatric spine and spinal cord are more susceptible to injury, and this varies with age. Injuries to the upper cervical spine and the cervical-thoracic junction are common with birth trauma.* Subsequent to the neonatal period, 75 percent of injuries between infancy and eight years occur in the cervical spine, with a predilection for the upper cervical spine.† Between the ages of 8 and 14, 60 percent of injuries occur in the cervical spine; 20 percent, in the thoracic region; and the remainder, in the thoracolumbar junction and the lumbar spine.[5, 69, 81, 119] In adolescents aged 14 to 16 years, the pattern of injuries parallels that of the adult population.

PECULIAR FEATURES OF THE PEDIATRIC SPINE

The normal cervical spine in children differs considerably from that in adults. By the age of eight to ten years, most individuals have achieved an adult configuration. When injury occurs in childhood, fractures and dislocations of the upper cervical spine occur with relatively greater incidence than in other locations. The youngest patients with these lesions have been newborns, in whom autopsies have revealed atlanto-occipital and atlantoaxial dislocation, fracture of the odontoid, and transsection of the spinal cord.[1, 8, 107]

The newborn spine is elastic, and the supporting ligamentous structures allow longitudinal distraction up to 2 inches.[78] However, the spinal cord can stretch only a quarter of an inch. A longitudinal traction force caused by the difference between the inherent elasticity of the spinal column and the lesser elasticity of the dura and its contents may cause disruption over several cord segments. About 70 percent of spinal injuries at birth occur with breech deliveries, and 30 percent with cephalic presentations.[4, 18, 49, 70, 103, 107] In breech delivery, traction force is applied to the torso, while uterine contraction grips the aftercoming head. This is worsened in the extended position. The spinal cord is fixed by the lumbar and cervical roots, and the delicate thoracocervical junction or the upper cervical spinal cord bears the brunt of traction injuries. Multisegment stretching can cause injury to the ligaments, producing prevertebral soft-tissue injury and cord damage without fracture. This was seen in the 12 autopsies reported by Aufdermaur.[8]

The unique structural characteristics of the infantile vertebral column allow traction and elongation of the spinal column to occur.[56, 76, 78] In a study on occipitoatlantal mobility in 17 newborn cadavers, hyperextension in ten allowed the posterior atlantal arch to invaginate into the foramen magnum, causing dorsal cervicomedullary compression.[55] In 4 of these 17 infant cadavers, vertical translation of the odontoid occurred in hyperflexion with ventral compression on the lower medulla oblongata. Momentary distortion or compression of the spinal cord may occur with displacement of vertebrae or stretching of the spinal column by cervical hyperflexion. This can also lead to selective compromise of the segmental cord blood supply.[96, 108] Cadaveric studies have shown that forceful traction applied to the infant tends to produce injuries of the brainstem, with the medulla oblongata being drawn into the foramen magnum.[1, 107] The cerebellum and the medulla oblongata both are at risk to be impaled by bony structures, as previously described, as well as subject to pressure and laceration by the edge of the foramen magnum. The findings of Yates,[118] that distortional trauma to the cervical spine can occur at birth and can result in damage to the cervical portions of the vertebral arteries, was further investigated by Jones.[70] Of 320 necropsies preformed at Birmingham Children's Hospital during 1967, 78 were stillbirths and 114 neonatal deaths.[70] A random selection of 30 fetuses was made, and the spinal cord and vertebral arteries were carefully examined. In 19 patients, there was evidence of hemorrhage around one or both vertebral arteries or crescentic adventitial hematoma.[24] These stretch injuries affect the dura and the spinal cord as well as the vertebral arteries and may account for the perinatal mortality and morbidity rates reported.

There is a preponderance of atlas and axis injuries in infants and young children that is related to the developmental anatomy of the high cervical region.[11, 110, 111] A large infantile head on a small body results in high torques being applied to the neck

---

*References 1, 8, 26, 49, 70, 75, 78, 107
†References 5, 29, 39, 42, 51, 66, 79, 89, 90, 100, 115, 119

with acceleration and stress.[102] The cervical musculature only becomes supportive at puberty. The ligaments and joint capsules are lax in small children, allowing for mobility at the cost of stability.[27, 101, 111, 119] The facets in the upper three cervical vertebrae have a horizontal orientation to the articular surfaces, and this permits increased translation motion.[11, 31, 111] These facets never become as oblique as in the lower cervical spine. There is an incomplete development and flattening of the uncinate processes in children younger than ten years of age, making them ineffective in withstanding flexion-rotation forces.[20, 85, 116] Finally, the fulcrum of cervical movement may be located higher in young children than in adolescents and adults.[73] Because the immature spine is progressively ossifying, the injuries in patients younger than eight years of age tend to be avulsions, epiphyseal separations, or fractures of the growth plate rather than true fractures. This mechanism pertains to all spinal injuries in this age group but is most commonly seen in odontoid fractures. Here, the line of separation is through the basal synchrondrosis, which is below the level of the superior facets.[31, 60, 100, 115]

Minor trauma has precipitated instability in children who already have a structural defect in their bony elements (e.g., assimilation of the atlas, os odontoideum) or ligamentous complex (e.g., inflammatory states, Down's syndrome).[68, 84, 85, 116] Absence of the posterior elements of the upper cervical spine may lead to soft-tissue wedging into the upper cervical canal during neck extension. This may indent the unprotected spinal cord.[51, 85] Hangman's fractures may also occur with violent forces.[115]

Cattell and Filtzer[31] studied the normal cervical spine in 160 children between the ages of 1 and 16 years. Ten children were grouped at each year. Flexion-extension lateral cervical spine x-ray films were done in a standardized manner. Twenty percent of the children in all age groups had a predental space (space between the anterior arch of the atlas and the odontoid process) of 3 to 5 mm (Fig. 24–1). An overriding of the atlas anterior arch on the odontoid process occurred in 20 percent during extension. A pseudosubluxation between the second and third cervical vertebrae was visualized in 45 percent of normal children. There was an absence of uniform angulation between the adjacent vertebrae in 16 percent during neck flexion. The neurocentral synchrondrosis of the axis was present in 100 percent of individuals younger than three years of age, in 50 percent of those three to six years of age, and in extremely few older than eight years of age. The pseudosubluxations that occur in the cerical spine in the infant and young child are due to the anterior wedging of the vertebral bodies, poorly developed joints of Luschka, ligamentous laxity, and the relative horizontal plane of the articular processes.[11, 31, 68, 116]

PATHOLOGY AND PATHOPHYSIOLOGY OF SPINE AND SPINAL CORD INJURY

Spinal Column Trauma

The special anatomic features of the immature spine that predispose to certain types of injury have

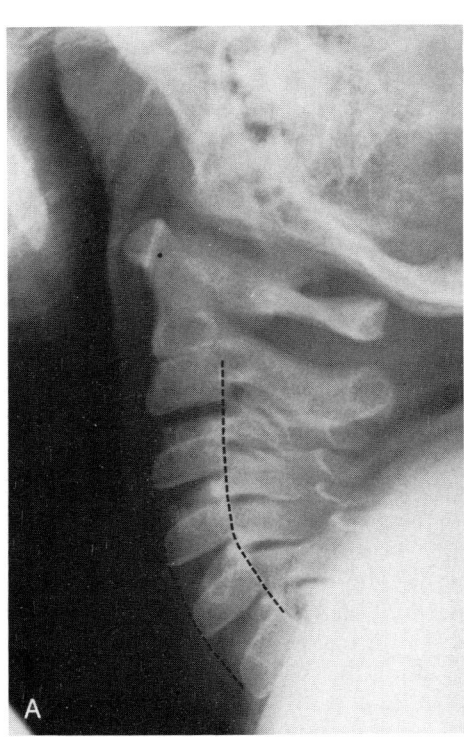
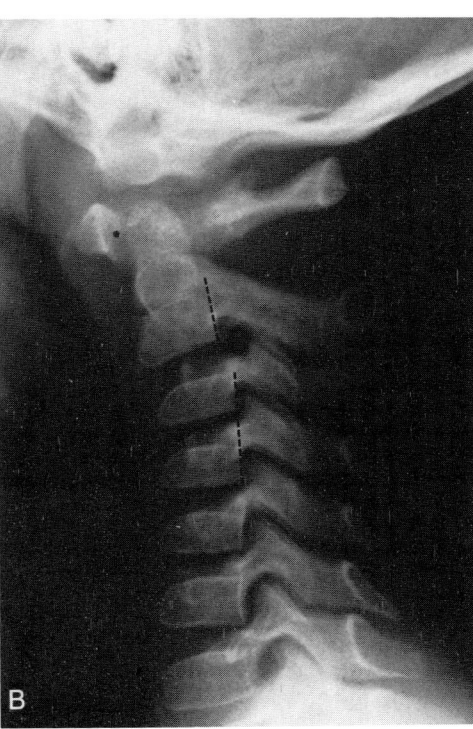

Figure 24–1. Normal laxity of the cervical spine in a four-year-old child. A, Extension position. Lines drawn tangent to the anterior and posterior margins of the vertebral bodies are smooth (broken lines). The predental space measures 2 mm (dot). B, Flexion position. There is anterior subluxation of C2 on C3, with interruption of the tangent lines (broken lines). The predental space has widened to 5 mm (dot).

already been mentioned. The pathologic findings share some characteristics with those in adults, but others are unique to the pediatric population. In a series of 100 spinal autopsies, there were 12 children, and cervical epidural hematoma was the most common finding along with ligamentous disruption in these.[8] The injuries consisted of severance of the cartilaginous end-plate, with fracture of the growth plate. Seven cord injuries were located in the cervical spine, four in the thoracic region, and one in the lumbar spine. Birth injuries accounted for two cord injuries, and motor vehicle accidents the remaining ten.

Ten percent of all neonatal deaths are attributed to a spinal cord injury.[4, 47, 70] The injuries occur with breech presentation, transverse lie, and internal podalic version. In the "star-gazing position" of breech presentation[1, 15, 103] or the "flying fetus" position[74] of transverse lie, the hyperextended neck is particularly prone to injury with vaginal delivery. No case of cesarean birth has had permanent spinal cord injury. The lower cervical and upper thoracic spine are particularly vulnerable to longitudinal stress leading to epidural hemorrhage, cord injury, and hematomyelia. LeBlanc and Nadell[76] operated on three children younger than three years of age, who had disruptions of the lower cervical and upper thoracic dural sacs with severe cord injury and disruption. Fractures were seen in this situation.

Trauma to the upper cervical spine has resulted in occipitoatlantal and atlantoaxial dislocations, rotatory luxations, and, in some instances, the delayed development of an os odontoideum (Fig. 24–2).[41, 46, 65, 72, 84, 85, 88, 94] A total of 15 to 70 percent of spinal cord injuries in the pediatric population have no demonstrable fracture or dislocation. Present investigations into the syndrome of spinal cord injury without radiographic abnormalities in children is being undertaken with nuclear magnetic resonance imaging (NMRI) and positron-emission tomography (PET).

The mechanics of spinal trauma can be classified into five categories:[10, 19, 38, 67, 98, 109] (1) flexion dislocation, (2) flexion compression, (3) compression burst, (4) extension, and (5) gunshot and penetrating injuries. In addition, a rare distraction injury may occur that is coupled with rotational phenomenon. Flexion dislocations are associated with maximal ligamentous damage with minimum bone pathology, unilateral or bilateral locked facets, and severe neurologic deficits. In flexion-compression injuries, the most anterior aspect of the vertebral body is reduced in height, with associated posterior ligmentous disruptions (Fig. 24–3). In compression burst fractures resulting from axial loading, the vertebral bodies may be shattered, but the ligaments are commonly preserved. In severe extension injuries, there may be fractures of the spinous processes, laminae, and the interarticular facets and avulsion fractures of the anterior portions of the vertebral bodies. In penetrating injuries, the damage to the nervous system constitutes the most serious problem, and the spinal column is usually stable. The penetrating object and the resultant shock wave combine to result in various degrees of neurologic deficit. Distraction injuries are especially prominent at the occipitoatlantal and atlantoaxial joints.

Holdsworth[67] classified fractures of the vertebral column into stable and unstable varieties. Fracture dislocations, accompanied by rupture of the ligamentous complex and facet interlock, are unstable. Rotational fracture dislocations are the most unstable of all vertebral fractures and are the result of rotational flexion force, disruption of the posterior ligament complex, and lateral displacement of the upper vertebral body on the lower. Burst fractures associated with fractures of the neural arch, referred

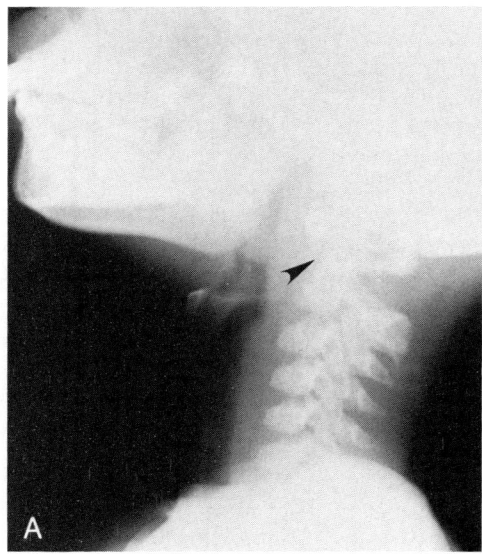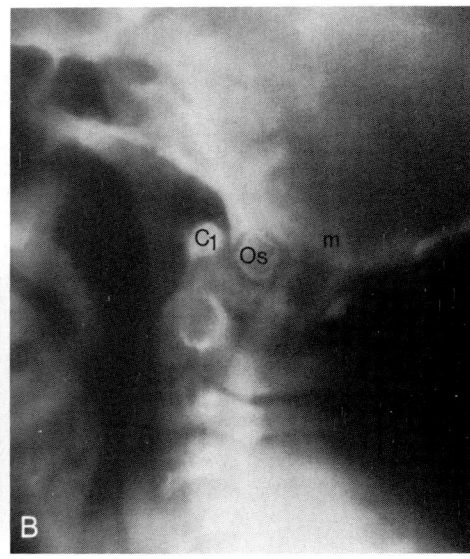

Figure 24–2. A, Traumatic atlantoaxial dislocation in the sagittal plane (arrowhead) with an associated rotary component. Note that the odontoid process is intact in this four-year-old girl. B, Metrizamide-enhanced myelotomogram of craniovertebral junction at age 14 years (same patient as in A). An os odontoideum has developed (Os), indenting the ventral medulla (M).

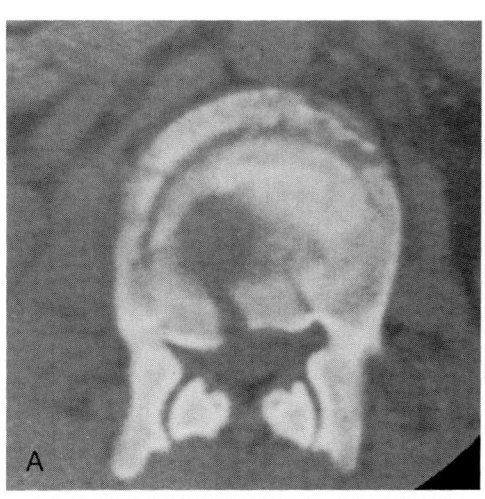
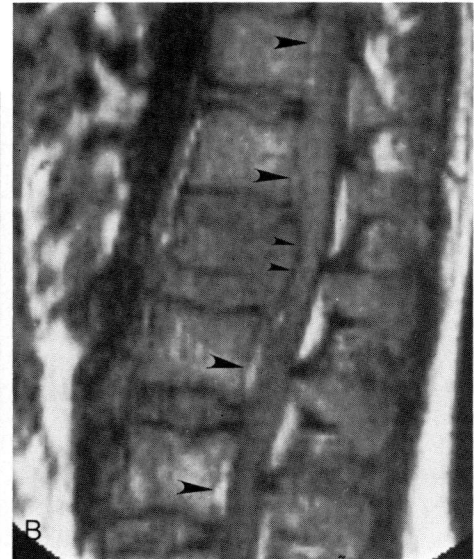
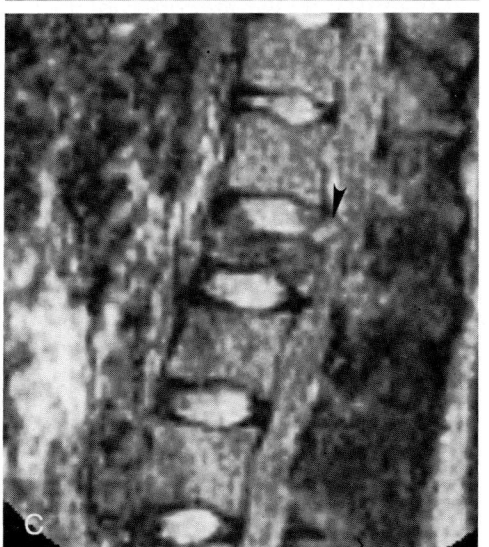

Figure 24–3. *A*, CT scan reveals a burst fracture of T12, with posterior displacement of the fracture fragments, compromising the AP diameter of the spinal canal. No anterior epidural fat is visualized. *B*, Midsagittal T1-weighted nuclear magnetic resonance (NMR) image reveals cord compression at T12 (small arrowheads). The bright signal intensity of normal epidural fat, well seen above and below (large arrowheads), is obliterated at T12. (TR/TE = 450/40). *C*, Midsagittal T2-weighted NMR image better demonstrates the T12 collapse. A small fragment of bone is displaced posteriorly into the spinal canal (arrowhead). (TR/TE = 1700/80).

to as "shear" fractures, are limited to the lower thoracic and the lumbar regions and frequently occur as a result of seatbelt injuries. Such fractures are unstable. The stable fractures are simple wedge fractures of flexion, with impaction of fractures fragments, and extension fractures localized to the cervical spine. Here, the posterior ligaments are intact, maintaining stability in neutral and flexed positions. Burst fractures have to be considered unstable unless there is impaction of the fracture fragments, as in the lumbar spine.[7] However, in the cervical spine, they may be frequently associated with severe neurologic deficit and instability.

In the upper thoracic spine (second to the tenth thoracic vertebrae), considerable violence is necessary to produce a fracture or dislocation. The narrow spinal canal makes it almost inevitable that these children will sustain neurologic injury. These fractures are stable as a result of the support of the rib cage, but the major consideration is the degree of spinal cord compromise. The axial loading or wedge compression fractures, as well as anterior subluxations, are stable.[19, 38] Because there is very little rotatory motion of the upper part of the thoracic spine, most of the injuries occur in flexion, with axial loading. The "sagittal slice fracture" occurs when the vertebra above slices in the sagittal plane through the vertebra below, displacing half of the lower vertebra to a lateral position. Spinal dislocation here results from total disruption of the posterior and anterior ligaments as well as the disk. The resultant instability may be further compounded by an inappropriate laminectomy removing the posterior supporting elements, when an anterior compression fracture is present. In this situation, surgical intervention with decompression and internal fixation and arthrodesis is essential for neurologic recovery and prevention of kyphosis.[19, 81, 98]

Most fractures of the thoracic and lumbar spine occur at the fulcrum of motion where the thoracic and lumbar portions of the spine meet. Neurologic injury here may affect the conus medullaris or the cauda equina (Fig. 24–4). The five types of fractures previously described can occur here. Acute fractures of the thoracolumbar spine should be considered initially unstable and should be immobilized. Vertebral compression fractures with reduction of more than 40 percent of the normal height require posterior stabilization.[19] The most unstable fracture in this region is the rotatory fracture-dislocation. Here, early reduction with internal fixation and arthrodesis is preferred.

Spinal Cord Injury

The majority of spinal cord injuries resulting in permanent loss of sensory and motor function do not involve initial physical transsection, but rather compression and contusion.[36] As a result, during the initial few hours after injury, impulse generation and conduction cease, blood flow to the injured segment decreases, and consequent ischemia or hypoxia triggers extensive tissue destruction.* Experimental studies have demonstrated the presence of central hemorrhages and edema in the spinal cord, during the first few hours after injury. It is felt that ischemia plays a significant role in the continuum of pathologic processes leading to spinal cord dysfunction. The greatest neurologic loss occurs at impact, and the deficit may improve with time. However, the pathologic picture is the reverse. Even in the face of improved neurologic function, the gross pathologic picture evolves over five to seven days, from a small central necrotic area to extensive central and peripheral necrosis, dependent on the severity of the trauma. Studies of early alterations in the traumatized spinal cord have included pial circulation, histopathology, electric conduction, biochemical changes, and circulatory changes within the intrinsic vasculature.*

Seconds following traumatic impact of the cord, small flame hemorrhages appear in the gray matter and beneath the pia-arachnoid membrane. Within ten minutes, the hemorrhage spreads to the white matter. As this develops, it affects the general cord

---

*References 30, 34, 36, 37, 44, 48, 54, 82, 99, 106, 112, 113

*References 18, 20, 34, 35, 37, 38, 43, 87, 92, 96, 99, 105, 108, 112, 113

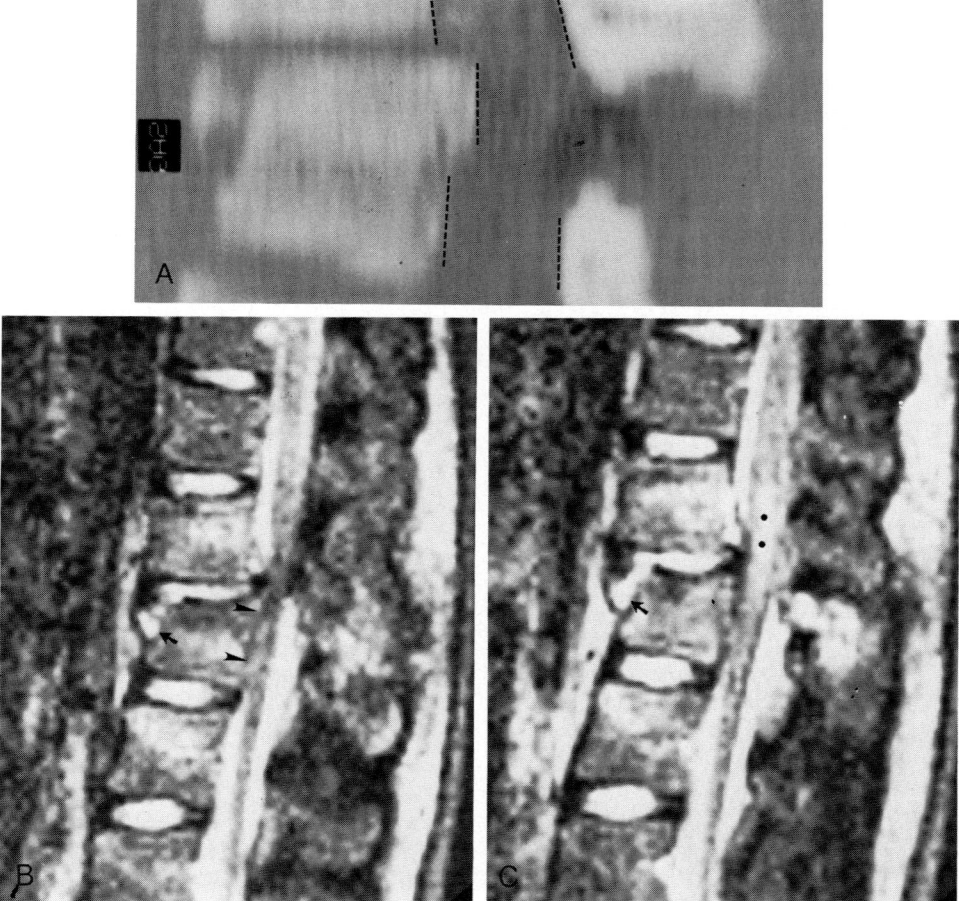

Figure 24–4. A, L1 fracture with cord compression. Midsagittal reformatted CT scan demonstrates a fracture of the L1 vertebral body, with posterior displacement into the spinal canal (the spinal canal is indicated by the broken lines). Midsagittal (B) and left parasagittal (C) T2-weighted NMR images reveal obliteration of the high signal intensity CSF at the L1 level anteriorly (arrowheads). There is hemorrhage under the anterior longitudinal ligament (arrows) and a suggestion of hemorrhage in the distal spinal cord (C, dots). (TR/TE = 1700/120.)

microcirculation, as evidenced by capillary wall thickening, extravasation of blood and fluid from the vessel lumen, and morphologic alterations of the myelin sheath and the periaxonal space. The predominant pattern is a central to peripheral spread of the pathologic condition. The central gray matter is involved before the peripheral gray matter, the more central white matter changes before the peripheral white matter. Significant formation of edema is noted by the end of the second day following a moderately severe concussion injury (Fig. 24–5). The appearance of edema is related to the time elapsed following trauma and the severity of the injury. In severe compression injuries, edema may be seen as early as four hours, followed by tissue necrosis. This is characterized by the shrinkage of neurons, cytolysis, and glial scar formation at the injury site. The initial hemorrhagic infarction is followed by removal of necrotic parenchyma and the development of adhesive arachnoiditis and intramedullary cavitation (Fig. 24–6).

Ultrastructural pathology following moderately acute impact lesions in monkeys correlates with the light microscopic changes. Within several hours, varying degrees of damage are seen, ending in shrunken axons and excessive tissue necrosis. Electron microscopic examinations have shown that microcysts develop from the myelin, forming sacs filled with fluid under tension and containing a swollen axon. These rupture into the extracellular space, creating larger cavities in the spinal tissue, presumably by release of lytic enzymes. There is platelet and red cell infiltration into the perivascular

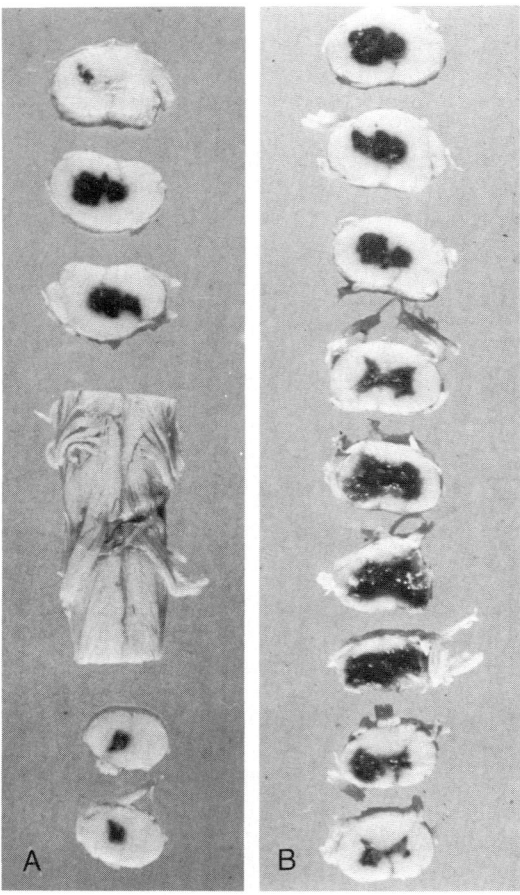

Figure 24–6. A, Autopsy specimen of cervical spinal cord from a 16-year-old male with C6–C7 fracture-dislocation occurring five weeks previously. The impact to the external surface is seen in the center of the unsectioned segment. Hematomyelia is seen in the central gray matter above and below the injury site. B, Sections through the injured spinal cord. Early cavitation and white matter disruption are seen in the center sections, which correspond to the impact site. Note the ascending and descending central cord hemorrhagic changes.

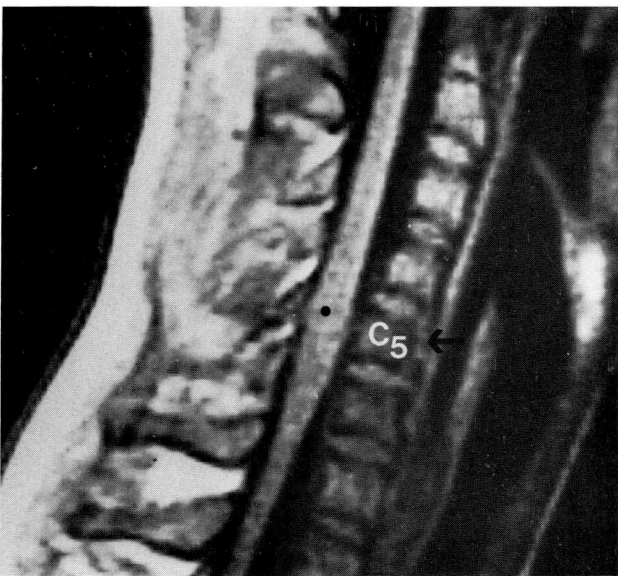

Figure 24–5. Midsagittal NMR image of the cervical canal made 28 hours after cervical spinal cord injury in a 13-year-old male. There is focal cord swelling (dot) at the C5–C6 level. The C6 vertebral body is compressed. There is hematoma beneath the anterior longitudinal ligament at the C5 level (arrow). No disk herniation or epidural clot is seen.

spaces, adding to the cellular necrosis. Damage to the vascular endothelium reduces the synthesis and release of prostacyclin and promotes additional platelet aggregation, resulting in decrease in blood flow to that region of the tissue. Changes in spinal cord blood flow (SCBF) begin shortly after impact. This decrease in SCBF is due to vasospasm, stasis, and thrombosis of vessels of the gray matter. There is a rapid decrease in the spinal cord oxygen partial pressure (pO_2) over the first 30 to 60 minutes following trauma, and a persistent state of hypoxia for several hours thereafter.

A significant and common finding in traumatized spinal cord tissue is accumulation of lactate at some distance distal and proximal to the area of the lesion. Lactic acidosis negatively affects the glucose and oxygen consumption in aerobic metabolism, as well as the ionic sodium–potassium adenosine triphosphate-dependent (ATP-dependent) cell pump. The decrease in cellular oxidative phosphorylation sets in motion chemical transformations, involving membrane phospholipids and production of circulating prostaglandins, along with stimulation of adenosine diphosphate (ADP). Prostaglandins of the F series (which have vasoconstrictive properties) are increased in the acutely contused spinal cord of the cat.[62] Of greater significance is the injury-induced release of prostaglandin precursor, arachidonic acid, which increases the formation of thromboxanes (TXA_2 and TXB_2). Thromboxane A_2 is an important vasoconstrictor and promoter of platelet aggregation. Under normal circumstances, its actions are counteracted by the production of prostacyclin in the vascular endothelium. However, in injured spinal cords, endothelial lipid peroxidation leads to a selective decrease in prostacyclin production, and the primary action of thromboxane A_2 goes unopposed.

Free radicals generated as a result of the injury-induced tissue hypoxia initiate peroxidative reactions within the lipid bilayer of cell and organelle membranes. These lipid peroxidation reactions are catalyzed by the extravasated blood or hemoglobin and the contents of disrupted organelles. The free radicals attack unsaturated lipids in the membranes, leading to inhibition of key neuronal enzymes and ultimately to the disruption of membrane function to the point that impulse generation cannot take place. Free radicals may arise in the injured spinal cord, secondary to synthesis of prostaglandins or thromboxanes. Interestingly, calcium ions accumulate rapidly in the injured spinal cord, favoring prostaglandin production. The lipid peroxides inhibit production of prostacyclin and indirectly enhance platelet and granulocyte adhesiveness and free radical production. The end result is a self-perpetuating process resulting in tissue death.

Spinal cord injuries are classified as[37, 105, 109]

1. Complete lesions with loss of motor, sensory, and autonomic function distal to the injury.
2. Posterior cord syndrome, in which only crude touch sensation is present.
3. Anterior cord syndrome, akin to the syndrome of the anterior spinal artery. Here touch and proprioception are preserved, although there is loss of all other cord functions. This is an indication for myelography to exclude the presence of disk or bony fragments compressing the spinal cord.
4. Central cord syndrome; children with this problem may go on to significant recovery.
5. Partial spinal cord syndrome of Brown-Séquard.
6. Root syndrome; pain in a radicular distribution may indicate reversible injury to the root at that level, even when associated with sensory, motor, or reflex loss. One cannot overemphasize the value of functional recovery of even a single nerve root at the level of the brachial plexus or thoracolumbar junction.

Current Applied Research in Spinal Cord Injury

There are six steps in the care of a child with spinal cord injury and neurologic deficit.[34, 37, 98] Each phase of treatment may influence the final neurologic outcome. The steps are (1) splinting and immobilization, (2) medical stabilization, (3) alignment of the spine, (4) diagnostic procedures, (5) decompression of compressed neural elements, and (6) stabilization of the spine. Once medical stabilization is accomplished, realignment of the spinal column is of paramount importance. The initial anatomic integrity of the spinal cord observed following some types of injury suggests that recovery could be facilitated if appropriate therapy were aimed at (1) preventing ischemia-related tissue degeneration, (2) supporting excitability of surviving spinal neurons, and (3) enhancing blood flow within the injured spinal segment. To this end, various surgical and pharmacologic therapies have been tried, with relatively poor success.

Laminectomy to "decompress the swollen spinal cord" has proved ineffectual and, at times, detrimental to the patient.[37, 66] Midline myelotomy to relieve the "tension and pressure" within the spinal cord and to prevent the progression of the ischemic hemorrhagic tissue destruction has not proved efficacious. Dorsal rhizotomy above the level of the injury and myelotomy as proposed by Osterholm[87] in the early 1970's have not changed the final outcome in these patients.

Corticosteroids. The use of corticosteroids in patients with spinal cord injury remains controversial.[21, 22, 45, 62, 82] The rationale for using steroids in traumatic myelopathy is that they are useful in preserving cellular and vascular membrane integrity and in preventing the disruption of intracellular lysosomes. High-dose glucocorticoid treatment has improved the blood flow to the injured spinal cord by interfering with the injury-induced activation of the prostaglandin system.[82] The National Acute Spinal Cord Injury Study, using high doses of methylprednisolone compared with the standard dose, showed no significant difference in observed neurologic recovery.[22]

Osmotic Diuretics. Aside from their potential hazards, there is no compelling clinical evidence that osmotic diuretics are effective in arresting sensorimotor paralysis or that they can affect the outcome of hemorrhage or ischemia in spinal cord tissue.[34, 37]

Antiadrenergic Compounds. Noradrenalin is released from spinal cord tissue following trauma and accumulates in toxic quantities.[87] This observation prompted the suggestion that inhibitors of the synthesis of noradrenalin might block or diminish the pathologic sequelae following spinal cord injury. These compounds were tested and shown to be ineffective.[34, 61, 109] In addition, the proposal that norepinephrine was responsible for the secondary pathologic changes in the injured spinal cord has not been borne out.

Naloxone. Naloxone, a narcotic antagonist, was used with success in animals subjected to spinal cord injury.[43] Motor function returned earlier in those treated with naloxone than in control subjects. Faden and colleagues[44] demonstrated that naloxone reversed the hypotension caused by transsection of the cervical spinal cord, implicating endorphins in the pathophysiology of spinal shock. It was felt that restoration of blood pressure augmented the spinal cord blood flow and reduced subsequent ischemia.[44, 45, 48, 63] The phase I trial of naloxone treatment in acute spinal cord injury in a clinical setting has shown that patients treated with naloxone showed a greater trend to recovery of evoked potentials over a period of six weeks to six months after injury.[48] The most promising agent to have emerged from recent experimental research has been naloxone.

Thyrotrophin-Releasing Hormone (TRH). Thyrotrophin-releasing hormone may act in vivo as a partial physiologic opiate antagonist. Faden and associates[45] reported on early pharmacologic treatment with TRH, providing significant improvement in neurologic recovery after experimental spinal injury. This is still under investigation.

Hyperbaric Oxygenation. It is believed that exposure of the subject to high atmospheric pressures in a closed chamber may reduce cellular hypoxia and vessel constriction. This treatment has not been widely adopted because of conflicting results, lack of availability, and the various claims that oxygenation at high pressures can induce pulmonary and CNS toxic manifestations.[37]

Hypothermia. This therapeutic approach consists of local spinal cord perfusion to reduce temperature for a period of three to four hours. The rationale was based on its ability to lower metabolic and oxygen requirements of damaged tissue, to reduce swelling, and to allow vasoconstriction of vessels at the site of injury.[34, 87] It was also suggested that local cooling of the spinal cord could block the metabolic acidosis resulting from trauma. Its effectiveness has not been borne out clinically.

Omental Transposition. An intriguing surgical approach to the problem of spinal cord ischemia following trauma involves partial detachment and transposition of the omentum so that it lies on the dura of the part of the cord with the lesion. Goldsmith[59] feels that the omentum is a source of potent angiogenesis factor, which is lipid in structure and voluminous in amount. Goldsmith has observed that vascularization of the omental–spinal cord interface occurs rapidly when the cord is injured. Absorption of fluid by the omentum is believed to be the reason for the preservation of somatosensory evoked potentials and motor function in spinal cord–injured animals, as long as the omentum is applied to the spinal cord within three hours of injury, a finding not observed in control animals. Further experience and experimentation are required.

Despite all these efforts, the mortality rate in spinal cord–injured patients ranges from 11 to 14 percent.[20, 37, 45, 48]

Clinical Diagnosis

The diagnosis of spinal cord injury in the general population is usually made on the basis of recognized trauma, followed by immediate rapid development of the classic clinical syndrome of paralysis and spinal cord shock. However, this is not the case in children. The peculiar features of the pediatric spine allow for longitudinal distraction and rotational forces to cause injuries in the spinal cord at various levels without fracture or dislocation. A significant number may have a delayed onset of neurologic deficits. The time interval between injury and the appearance of objective sensorimotor dysfunction, termed "latent," can range from a few minutes to three to four days.[89, 102]

The leading cause of neonatal spinal cord injury is delivery of the fetus with a hyperextended head from either a transverse lie or a breech presentation. On initial physical examination, the infant is often hypotonic, and there is difficulty in establishing respiration. The infants are noted to have abdominal breathing chronically and to move the arms and legs infrequently. In the immediate newborn period, a weak cry, poor feeding, and floppy lower extremities are clues to the presence of spinal cord injury. Repeated bouts of pneumonia, urinary tract infection, the development of spasticity in the lower extremities, and Horner's syndrome point to a cervicothoracic junction spinal cord lesion. Allen[4] found on re-examination of 31 infants initially diagnosed as having Werdnig-Hoffmann disease, that 19 were suffering from spinal cord injuries. Transverse myelitis and spinal cord tumors should be considered in children who had a normal neonatal period followed by paralysis. A diagnostic dilemma occurs in infants with bilateral brachial plexus palsy, who may also have motor or sensory loss or a Horner's syndrome and fit into the criteria for central cord injury. Spinal radiographs are usually normal in this group, although the chest radiograph is abnormal, with a bell-shaped chest appearance indicative of loss of the external muscles of respiration.[49] Visualization of the spinal cord with opacification of the cerebral spinal fluid, utilizing plain radiography, computed tomography (CT), or NMRI, is important because it usually demonstrates a block in the subarachnoid space.[18, 26, 49, 56, 103] Infrequently, localized spinal cord atrophy may be identified.

A high index of suspicion is required for the diagnosis of spinal injury in the acutely injured, unconscious child. Vertebral column or spinal cord injury should be suspected in the conscious individual with symptoms of neck or back pain or localized tenderness and in the child in whom an asymmetric response to stimulation is obtained. Frontal or occipital head trauma and limitation of neck movement should alert the clinician to possible hyperflexion or hyperextension injuries to the cervical spine. Bruising over the thoracic, cervical, or lumbar spine may indicate underlying bony trauma. Abdominal distention with hypotonia in the lower extremities is a clue to spinal cord injury in the young child. An underlying pre-existing pathologic condition, such as inflammatory disease of the upper respiratory system, may make the cervical spine prone to atlantoaxial instability with minor trauma.

An additional complication in the evaluation of the child with a spinal injury is that 15 to 70 percent of patients with major neurologic involvement have normal radiographs. Therefore, accurate diagnosis may depend upon serial observations and examinations. In the awake, cooperative child, sensory, motor, and reflex examination allows one to assess reliably the level of cord injury. In spinal shock, there is flaccid paralysis below the level of the lesion, and the deep tendon reflexes are lost. There is urinary retention and autonomic imbalance resulting in hypotension. If the injury is not too severe, voluntary control is re-established, and recovery begins within a few hours of injury. However, if the injury is severe, the spinal cord distal to the level of injury is isolated, and mass reflexes set in unaccompanied by any evidence of improvement in voluntary motor activity or sensory perception. Assessment of reflexes is helpful in determining the level of the lesion in infants and children with cervical spinal cord and cauda equina injuries. The reflex loss is generally appropriate to the degree of motor involvement. Thus, spinal cord injury may result in a complete loss of function, a partial loss of function with or without cauda equina sparing, or root dysfunction. Neurotrauma motor index scoring is useful in comparing patients and results from various treatment regimens.[37] The authors have found it extremely useful in the day-to-day treatment of a patient and helpful in assessing efficacy of treatment.

In regard to prognosis for children with traumatic quadriplegia, 85 percent of all patients who were initially "complete" will remain complete, and a small percentage regain some motor function in their legs.[37] The few patients who improve may do so because of aggressive therapy or because the initial examination reflected a shock or concussive effect. In severe partial lesions, 8 to 25 percent recover. In central cord lesions with relatively preserved function in the legs, recovery of lost motor power occurs between 75 and 80 percent of the time.

Paraplegia has been similarly analyzed. In thoracic lesions, the data is practically identical to that in cervical lesions. However, in the thoracolumbar junction area, it appears that as many as 30 percent of those with initially complete lesions will regain motor function.[37]

Radiographic Evaluation. The integrity of the posterior osseoligamentous complex of the spinal canal is essential for spinal column stability.[7, 10] Consequently, anterior vertebral injuries involving the vertebral bodies, ligaments, and disks are relatively more stable than those that involve the posterior and lateral complex. Conventional radiography encompasses spine films in the frontal, lateral, and oblique positions, especially in the cervical spine. An open-mouth odontoid view is difficult to obtain in a young child or infant. Pleuridirectional tomography and computerized axial tomography are important diagnostic tools to assess the degree of bony and soft-tissue disruption and the maintenance of midline and lateral column alignment. Suspicion of spinal cord injury, in the absence of fracture or dislocation on plain radiographs, requires the visualization of the spinal cord, using water-soluble contrast-enhanced myelography or, if possible, NMRI.[84, 85, 109] The peculiarities of the pediatric cervical spine and their radiographic interpretation have already been discussed. With cervical spine injuries, the absence of a neurologic deficit and the presence of a stable cervical spine necessitates dynamic views in flexion and extension to assess stability. At times, paraspinal muscle spasm is protective in nature, and studies need to be repeated once the spasm has been relieved. Immobilization may be required until the spasm resolves.

In a patient with an unstable fracture of the cervical spine, skeletal traction with increasing weight may be required to reduce the deformity. The effects of the traction are documented with appropriate radiographs. In 5 percent of individuals, a symptomatic disk herniation may be present, and this must be identified so that appropriate treatment measures may be followed.[12, 37]

Pleuridirectional tomography and CT have greatly enhanced our understanding of the bony pathology.[7, 19, 47, 84] Combined with visualization of the cerebrospinal fluid spaces and the spinal cord, this provides information regarding the size of the spinal cord, the amount of subarachnoid space, the presence of disk herniation or intraspinal hematoma, and the alignment of the spinal canal. NMRI in the T1- and T2-weighted phases provides a good understanding of the pathophysiology of spinal cord injuries (Fig. 24–7). Spinal cord transsection, hemorrhagic myelomalacia, ligamentous and bony disruptions as well as subperiosteal injuries are well visualized. The authors recommend immediate identification of bony pathology with plain radiographs and CT, to be followed by NMRI as soon as possible in all cases of spinal cord and spine injuries (Fig. 24–7).

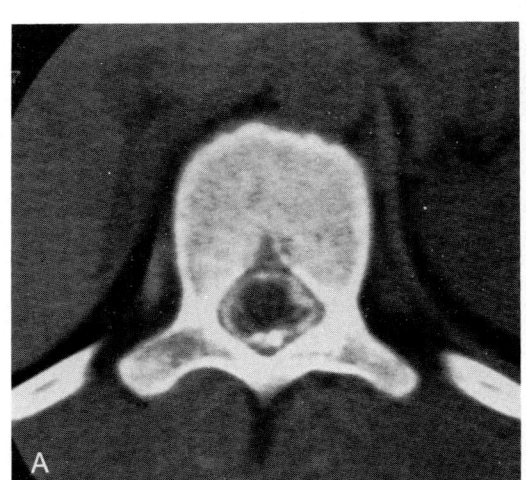
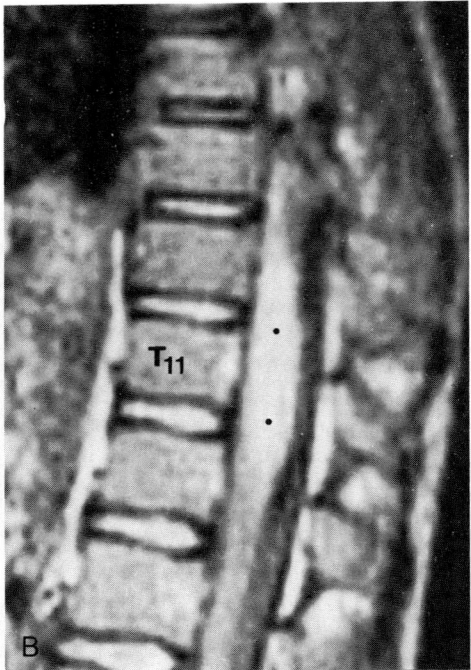
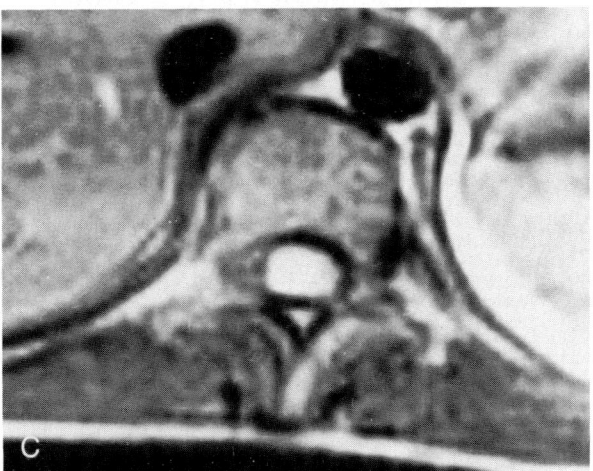

Figure 24–7. A, Spinal cord hematoma; 1 cc of Pantopaque was introduced via lumbar puncture. There was a complete block to the cranial flow of contrast material at the T11–T12 level. CT metrizamide-enhanced myelogram reveals enlargement of the spinal cord at the T11 level and a diminutive subarachnoid space. Two droplets of Pantopaque are trapped within the posterior subarachnoid space. Midsagittal (B) and transverse (C) T1-weighted NMR images demonstrate high signal intensity within the spinal cord, consistent with hemorrhage (dots). (TR/TE = 1000/40).

Age-Related Problems

Spinal Cord Injuries During Birth. Intrapartum injuries to the fetal spinal cord have been described. Certain factors stand out as being important. These are longitudinal stretching of the vertebral column in breech presentation, tortional forces applied in rotating the head in cephalic deliveries, shoulder distortion with traction on the cord, and hyperextension of the head in breech delivery.

A state of shock and difficulty in initiating respiration are common with these lesions. The motor manifestations vary with the site of the injury. Those above the C3–4, level are promptly fatal, unless the infant is given constant respiratory support. Damage to the lower cervical and upper thoracic cord, often associated with brachial plexus injury, produces flaccidity of the arms and hands, respiratory embarrassment with paradoxical respiration, and occasionally Horner's syndrome (Fig. 24–8). Varying degrees of flaccidity of the legs follow injuries to the lubosacral segments. Bladder paralysis is common, but a newborn's problems can usually be managed without catheterization. Radiographs of the spine are usually normal. However, they are useful in excluding congenital anomalies, especially spina bifida, and they may occasionally demonstrate vertebral dislocations. In these instances, myelography or NMRI demonstrates soft-tissue disruption of the neural tissue at the site of injury and hematoma in the extradural space.

"Spinal shock" subsides within a few weeks, and it then becomes possible to establish a reasonably accurate and durable assessment of the infant's neurologic status. The infant is alert, with very few, if any, cranial nerve abnormalities, unless the brainstem was injured with traction. Reflex movements develop in response to noxious stimuli over a wide receptive area in the arms and the legs. Spasticity leading to contractures is unusual and is seen only

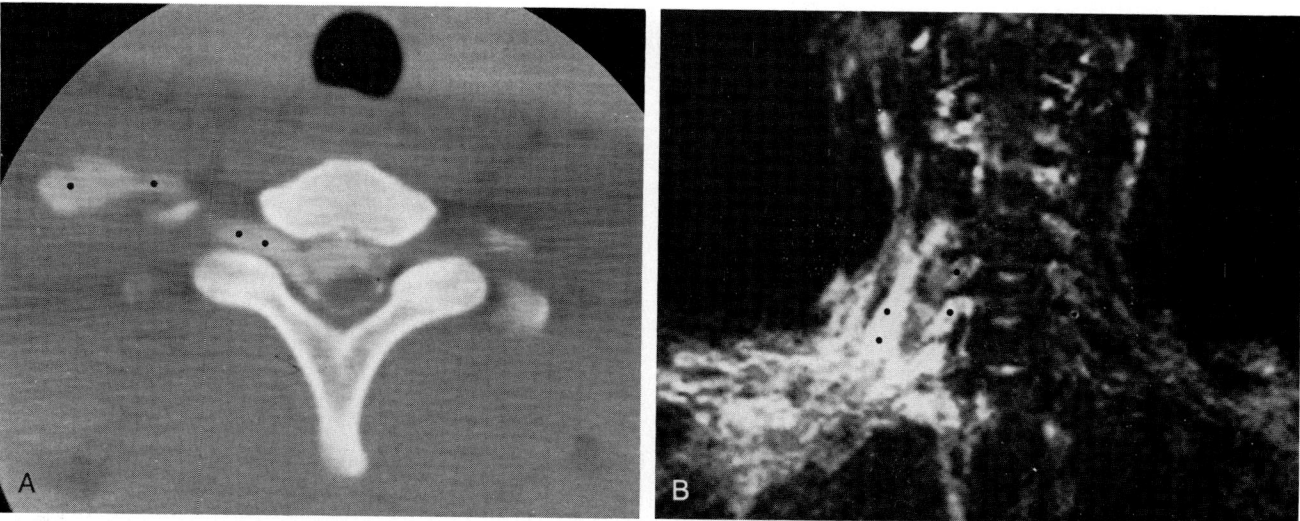

Figure 24–8. A, Brachial plexus root avulsion. CT metrizamide-enhanced myelogram at C7 reveals extravasation of contrast material outside of the spinal canal, along the tract of the avulsed C8 nerve root (dots). (An identical pattern of extravasation was also present one level higher, involving the C7 nerve root.) B, T2-weighted coronal NMR image demonstrates CSF extravasation at the C7 and C8 levels into the soft tissues of the neck (dots). (TR/TE = 1700/120).

in the hips and the femoral muscles. Koch and Eng[75] reviewed the long-term prognosis of 14 infants with neonatal spinal cord injuries. Eight of the 14 patients died: four patients at less than three months of age, three patients between three months and one year of age, and one patient at three and a half years. Six children survived for more than two years for a follow-up examination. The quality of survival for those with functional levels of C8–T1 and below depends on the presence and severity of medical complications. Supportive measures for such patients include bracing of the thoracolumbar spine as the infant grows.

Trauma Occurring to Patients Younger than Eight Years of Age. This is limited to the cervical spine. In patients younger than six years of age, most injuries occur above the C3 level.* A significant proportion are referable to the odontoid process, where separation occurs at the neurocentral synchondrosis. The superior segment angulates and is displaced forward with the atlas (Fig. 24–9). In the youngest infant in the authors' series in whom this occurred, the injury was the result of birth trauma, and this infant had an associated epidural intracranial hematoma. Radiographs may also reveal fractures of the pedicles, with anterior subluxation of the atlas and the body of C2 on C3, typical of hangman's fracture. These are unstable. Reduction is best achieved with the head and neck placed in a hyperextended position over the edge of a mattress. Should positioning not succeed in reduction, braided wire is placed between two burr holes on each side of the skull to maintain traction in the infant whose skull does not tolerate the insertion of tongs. The weight should not exceed 2 pounds in children younger than two years of age. In the slightly older child, once adequate reduction of spinal deformity has been achieved, rigid external fixation can be obtained by the use of the halo vest. This offers the advantage of prolonged immobilization and early active rehabilitation. Careful attention is paid to the cleanliness of the pins and the tong sites. Symptoms of local pain and headache may indicate penetration of the skull, leading to osteomyelitis or even cerebritis.

In the older child, cervical spine fractures are managed by reduction and immobilization. The presence of disk herniation, bone fragments, or hematoma impinging on the spinal cord requires decompression and, in this instance, fusion. Fusion can be accomplished from either the anterior approach or the posterior route. This is followed by external immobilization and early rehabilitation. The authors have performed an anterior cervical diskectomy at the C3–4 level in four patients aged six and eight years, with good results. Thus, surgery is indicated only for stabilization of an unstable fracture, reduction of locked facets that are irreducible, débridement of a compound wound, and removal of bone fragments and disk material from the spinal canal.[33, 95, 109, 117] When posterior fusion is necessary in the cervical spine, wire fixation alone does not serve the purpose. This is because bone stability is not achieved as in adults. The wire may cut through the thin unossified spinous process or lamina, and as the child grows, a position of hyperextension may occur or subsequent disruption of the wire with impingement on the spinal cord. Hence, bony fusion is recommended.[64, 84, 85]

The treatment of choice is wiring of bone to each individual lamina or facet so that once incorporation of bone has taken place, the bone will grow with

---

*References 6, 13, 17, 25, 42, 60, 71, 76, 100, 115

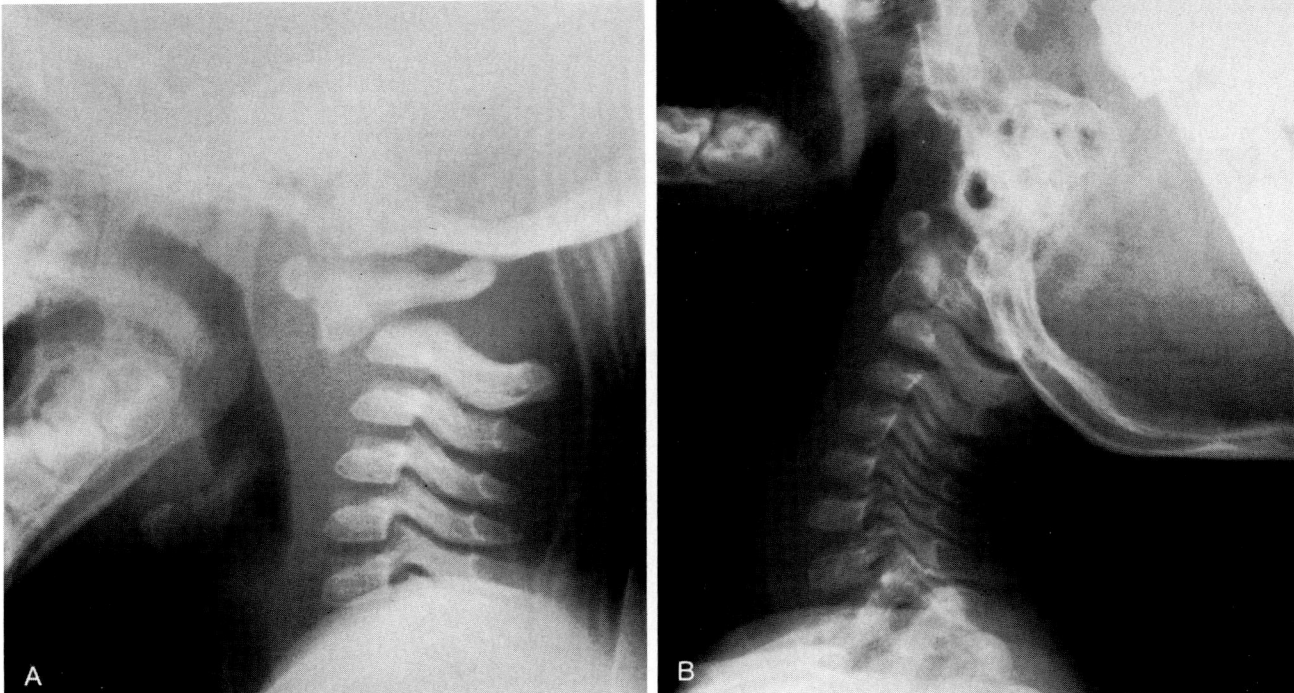

Figure 24–9. *A,* Lateral cervical spine radiograph in a 14-month-old male with odontoid fracture-dislocation. There is avulsion at the neurocentral synchondrosis. *B,* Radiograph of the subject in A, done ten weeks after halo traction and immobilization. There is healing at the axis-odontoid fracture site, with good alignment.

the child. The authors' experience with 96 such cervical fusions over the past ten years has shown no decrease in the growth potential or exaggerated cervical lordosis. Bone is harvested from rib, posterior iliac crest, or the tibia. The authors prefer using rib for posterior cervical fusions.

Spinal Cord Trauma in Patients Aged Eight to Sixteen Years of Age. Cervical injuries predominate in this age group and account for about 60 to 70 percent of injuries. Thoracic and thoracolumbar junction injuries are related to severe violent forces, as with crush injuries, sports injuries, falls from heights, and automobile accidents.* The principles of management of unstable cervical spine injuries are the same as previously described. Unstable thoracic or thoracolumbar spine fractures, whether complete or incomplete, require stabilization. This should be accomplished via the anterior route, after appropriate diagnostic procedures have delineated the soft tissue and bony pathology.[19, 91, 98] The transthoracic anterior approach to resect the involved vertebral body and disk allows visualization of the ventral dural sac and confirmation of decompression. A rib graft with attached vascular pedicle is then rotated into position and wedged between the vertebra above and the vertebra below the level of injury. This allows for the removal of the compressed, disrupted bony segment involved. This allows for the removal of the compressed, disrupted bony segment involved (Fig. 24–10). The removal of the segment prevents kyphosis, and the vascularized rib graft shows incorporation into the recipient site within six to eight weeks. It is the author's view that thoracolumbar junction fractures are best approached via a posterolateral decompressive route, which allows visualization of the dura mater and the spinal cord, via a hemilaminectomy. A concomitant transpedicular approach to the ventral spinal canal permits the anterior bony decompression to be performed. Stabilization, using either Luque or Harrington rods and bone fusion, is then done. Surgical intervention in this fashion has allowed immediate stabilization and rehabilitative measures to be instituted.

In summary, the care of the child and the young adult with spinal injury and neurologic deficit is divided into six phases. These are comprised of immobilization, medical stabilization, restitution of alignment of the spine, diagnostic procedures, surgical decompression if there is compression of the neural elements, and stabilization of the spine. Rehabilitation must be instituted from the time of admission following the acute spinal insult.

SPECIAL CONSIDERATIONS

Lesions of the Craniovertebral Junction

The cervical spine is the most mobile portion of the spine. The relative motion of the occipito-at-

---

*References 8, 23, 25, 29, 40, 50, 53, 66

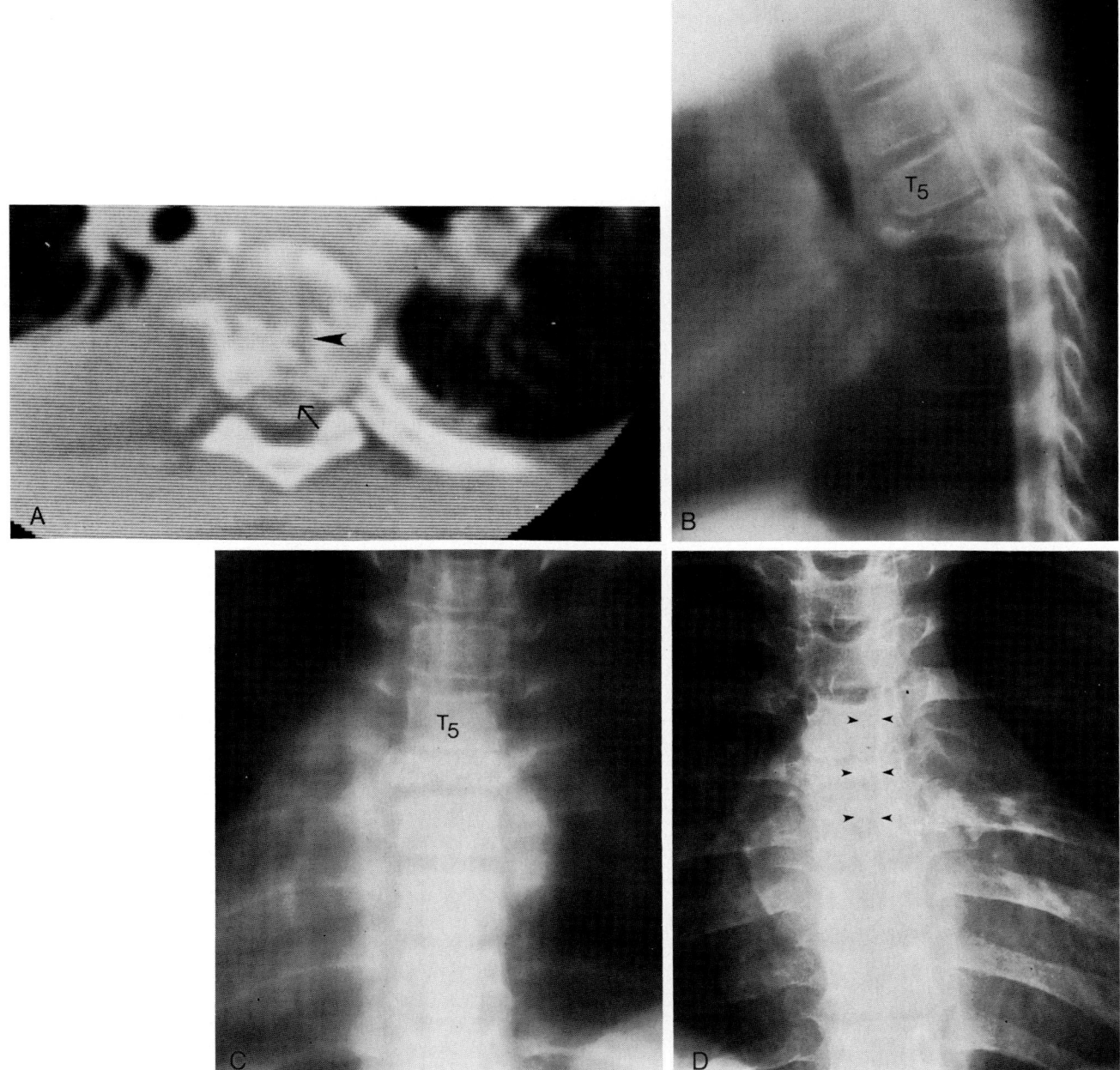

Figure 24-10. *A*, Axial CT scan of T6 vertebra in a 12-year-old male with incomplete spinal cord injury. The spinal cord (arrow), outlined with metrizamide in the CSF, is ventrally located against the comminuted vertebral body (arrowhead). *B*, Metrizamide-enhanced myelotomogram of thoracic spine in lateral projection. There is compression of the T6 vertebral body. The posterior fragment is retropulsed into the spinal canal, impinging onto the spinal cord. *C*, Metrizamide-enhanced thoracic myelotomogram reveals the burst compression fracture at T6. *D*, Thoracic spine, anteroposterior view, done three months after transthoracic anterior vertebral decompression of spinal cord at T6. A vascularized T6 rib graft bridged T5-T7 for fusion (small arrowheads).

lanto-axial region is controlled by the geometry of the articular surfaces and ligaments and their elastic properties. This complex serves as a transition zone between the standard vertebral joint structures and the completely different skull. It functions as a single unit, with the atlas serving as a washer or bearing between the occipital condyles and the axis vertebrae.

Atlanto-Occipital Dislocation

The true incidence of atlanto-occipital dislocation is obscured by the devastating nature of the injury itself. In a review of 112 victims of trauma who died at the scene of the injury, Bucholz and Burkhead[24] discovered that 26 had a cervical spine injury. Of these 26 patients, nine had a traumatic atlanto-occipital dislocation, and five had an odontoid fracture. Alker and coworkers,[3] in a similar experience, found that 19 percent had altanto-occipital dislocation. The most frequent mechanism of injury appears to be hyperflexion and distraction force applied to the skull.[41, 84, 88, 93] The authors' neurosurgical experience encompasses six patients, three of whom were children. The injury resulted in disruption of the atlanto-occipital ligament, tectorial membrane, and alar ligaments of the occipitoatlantal joints, allowing forward dislocation of the cranium on the spine (Fig. 24–11). Traumatic dislocations of the occipitoatlantal articulation may place the cranium forward in relation to the atlas. Avulsion of the cranial nerves as well as transsection of the medulla oblongata and upper cervical cord have been reported in postmortem studies. Infants and young children who survive are usually comatose with a hemiparesis, quadriparesis, or diaphragmatic breathing. A retropharyngeal hematoma is the first clue. Displacement of the atlas from the occipital condyles and separation may also be seen. Significant anterior and posterior displacement of the odontoid from beneath the basion is highly suggestive of occipitoatlantal dislocation.[93] Frontal and lateral CT reconstructions as well as pleuridirectional tomography reveal the separation of the occipital condyles from the lateral masses of the atlas.[84] Arteriography may reveal stenosis or occlusion of the vertebral arteries. The therapeutic objective is skeletal fixation rather than axial skeletal traction. Most patients who survive have undergone an occipitoatlantal fixation with wire and autogenous bone graft, supplemented with methyl methacrylate.

Atlantoaxial Luxation

Luxation refers to a complete and lasting disruption of the articular facets of the synovial joint. Examples of this are interlocking of articular facets or the marked diastasis that occurs with hyperflexion fracture luxation. The C1–2 luxations can be divided into anterior, posterior, and rotational types. Fielding and Hawkins,[46] in a biomechanical study of the strength of the atlantoaxial ligament complex, showed that the force required to fracture the odontoid process was much less than the force required to cause failure of all the ligaments in the same specimen. In the clinical setting, the frequency of fracture of the odontoid process in children is much greater than atlantoaxial luxation secondary to trauma.

The rotatory atlantoaxial luxation is not an uncommon finding in patients with infections of the upper respiratory system or other inflammatory conditions.[46, 52, 104] In normal patients, rotation of the atlas and the axis is within the range of 35 degrees.[97] This may also occur in a traumatic situation, but if the rotation exceeds 40 degrees, facet interlock occurs (Fig. 24–12).[46, 97] In the authors' series of 16 adolescent patients with rotatory luxation beyond 40 degrees, trauma was the causative factor in each and every one. Football spearing injury occurred in 8 of 16 children, motor vehicle accidents in four, and wrestling injury in three others. One ten-year-old girl sustained her injury with a fall on the ice. In three patients, an associated occipitoatlantal rotatory luxation was also present, leading to a characteristic "cock robin" appearance of the head.[111] This abnormality had been reported following surgical repair of cleft lip and cleft palate and removal of orthodontic devices and a body cast. It may go unrecognized if the symptoms are minor or may be diagnosed when associated with brainstem dysfunction or cervical myelopathy. Children with this lesion have been erroneously diagnosed as having a brainstem vascular insult, cerebellar tumor, Chiari malformation, cervical migraine, syringomyelia, and ocular palsies. All patients present with a torticollis and diminished range of motion of the neck. Facial flattening is prominent, and symptoms of neural compression occur when the atlas is separated from the odontoid process by

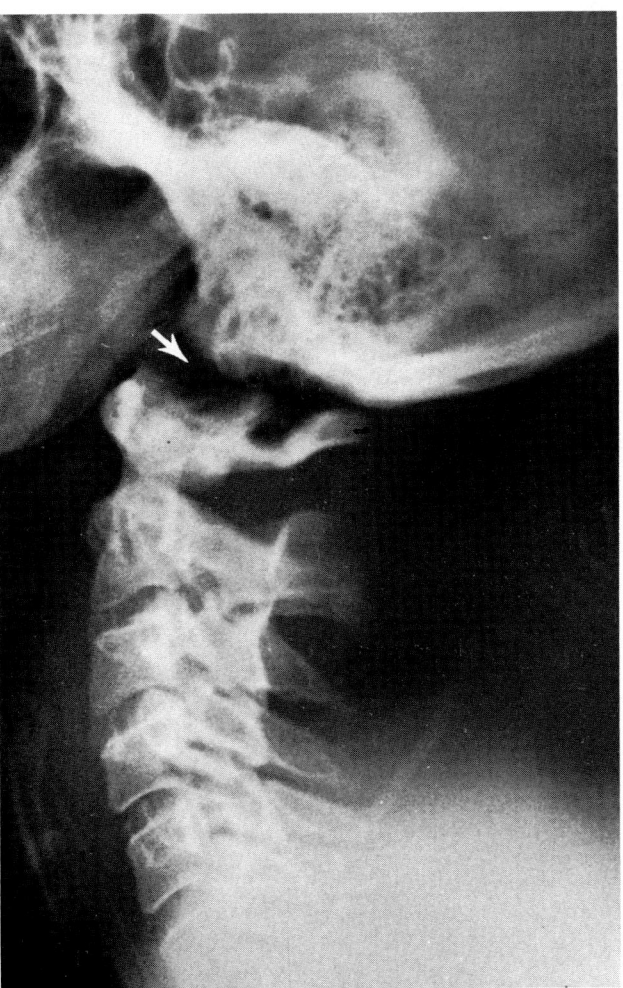

Figure 24–11. Lateral cervical radiograph reveals disruption of atlas from its occipital articulation (arrow).

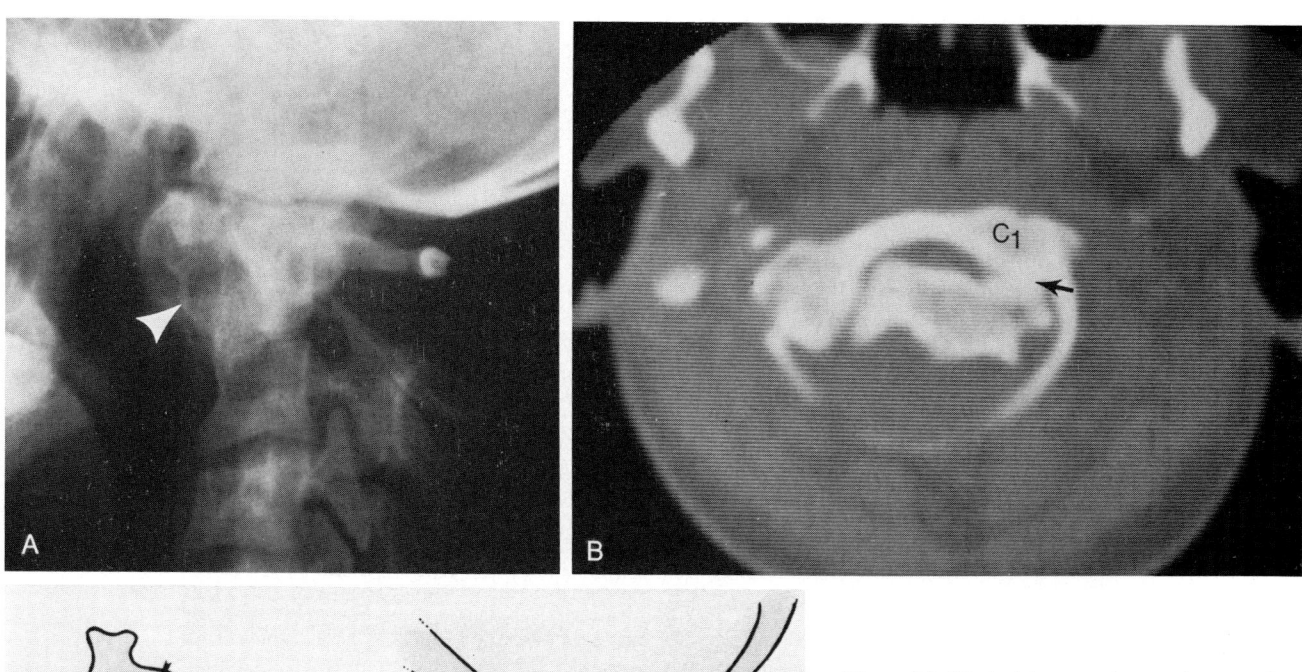

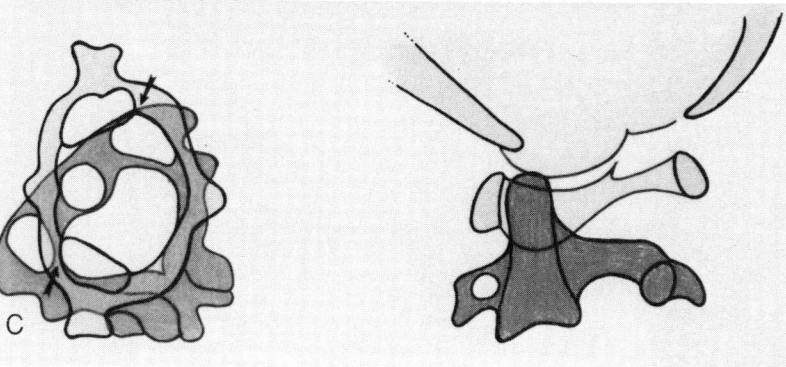

Figure 24–12. A, Atlantoaxial rotary luxation. Lateral radiograph of skull and upper cervical spine. There is rotation of the atlas in relation to the axis, with forward projection of lateral atlantal mass (arrowhead). B, Axial CT scan through atlas (C1) reveals the facet interlock (arrow) with the axis superior facet (C2). Note the compromised canal. C, Line drawings to illustrate the pathology.

more than 5 mm, allowing a rotation of the atlas on the axis and, thus, canal compromise. Diagnostic procedures utilized are lateral cervical radiographs, cine roentgenographs, tomograms, CT scans, and, recently, NMR images (Fig. 24–13).

Fielding and Hawkins[46] attempted to classify atlantoaxial rotatory fixation into four types. This is dependent upon the integrity of the transverse ligament and the secondary support ligament complex. If the transverse ligament is intact, and the dens acts as a pivot, the rotation is within 35 to 40 degrees and is correctable with traction and realignment. It is seen in minor trauma and infections and is associated with inflammatory conditions at the craniovertebral region. It is the most common of pediatric rotatory atlantoaxial displacements. When the transverse ligament ruptures, the atlas arch is displaced forward, causing compromise of the canal diameter. In this circumstance, rotation may exceed 40 degrees, with atlas displacement forward more than 5 mm, indicating rupture of both the transverse ligament complex and the alar and accessory check ligaments. This requires reduction and surgical immobilization.

Spinal Cord Injury Without Radiographic Abnormalities in Children

This lesion has been compared with the acute central cord syndrome in adults.[2, 25, 32, 66, 89, 114] In this syndrome of spinal cord injury, the mechanisms of neural damage include flexion, hyperextension, longitudinal distraction, and ischemia. Children younger than eight years of age suffer a greater degree of neurologic dysfunction than those who are older. In 52 percent of the children with this form of injury, the onset of paralysis is delayed up to four days after injury, and most of these children recall transient paresthesias, numbness, and subjective motor loss. The neurologic examination at the time of initial evaluation reveals four individual syndromes: complete physiologic transsection, central cord syndrome, Brown-Séquard syndrome, and a partial dysfunction of the cord. The long-term prognosis is unfavorable.

The anatomic features peculiar to children permit transient subluxation without bony injury. An acute reversible disk prolapse might be the cause of the pathology. The other factors taken into considera-

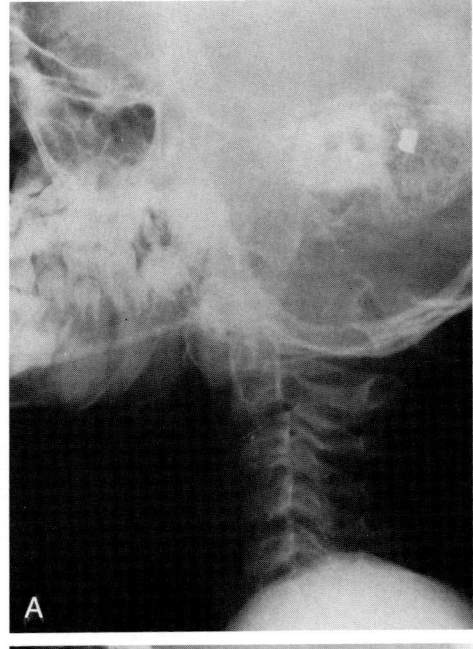
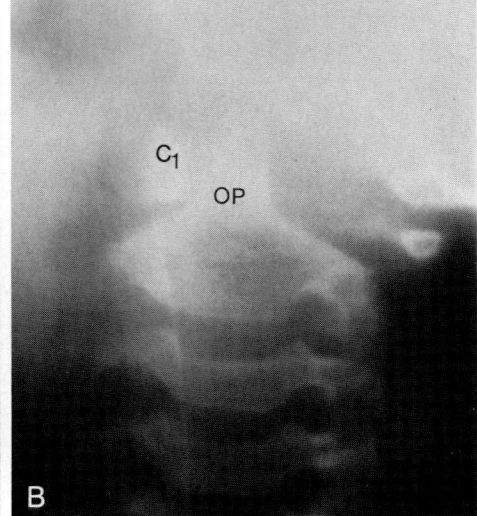
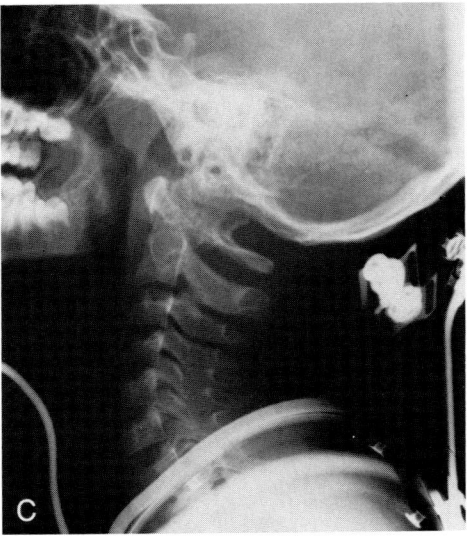

Figure 24–13. A, Lateral head and neck radiograph in an eight-year-old male wrestler reveals rotational luxation of atlas on axis. B, Frontal polytomogram of the upper cervical spine in the same patient as in A. The anterior atlantal arch has moved to a lateral position (C1) in relation to the odontoid process (OP). C, Lateral radiograph of the cervical spine in a brace, following reduction of atlantoaxial rotary luxation.

tion are the longitudinal distraction of the cord, which may occur without fracture, and also interference with the microvasculature of the spinal cord. In this context, compression or spasm of the anterior spinal artery system has been a consideration. Choi and associates[32] reported on eight such patients and postulated a vascular occlusion of the radicular vessels by trauma, or aortic-mediastinal insult. An occlusion of the anterior spinal artery was demonstrated in their series. In a significant number of football[80] and gymnastic injuries, a burning sensation was described by affected patients.

SUMMARY

The pediatric spine and its supporting structures are in a process of progressive development and ossification.[16, 102] Specific pathologic states occur at different ages, and it is essential that one be familiar with this when treating a young individual with spine or spinal cord injury. The long-term management of paraplegic and quadriplegic children shares many of the problems seen in adults so affected. Careful assessment of urinary function, control of urinary infection, and intermittent catheterization has proved a valuable means of achieving social continence.[14] Pharmacologic agents and various surgical procedures have wide application.[28, 37, 58] It is important to pay close attention to nutrition, protein, and electrolyte balance from the acute phase into the chronic rehabilitation of such children. Decubitus ulcers are rarely a significant problem in the bedridden child, whose small size makes frequent turning easier than in the adult. However, the ambulatory child in braces is at risk for the development of decubitus ulcers over the bony prominences, and regular inspection is mandatory. Scoliosis is more common in a growing paraplegic child than in the adult with paraplegia. Attention to posture, bracing, and strengthening of weakened muscles decreases the asymmetric pull on the spinal column and can prevent or retard the development of scoliosis. Early recognition and treatment is the best method of avoiding functional deformity.

References

1. Abroms IF, Bresnan MJ, Zukerman JE, et al: Cervical cord injuries secondary to hyperextension of the head in breech presentation. Obstet Gynecol 41:369, 1973.
2. Ahmann PA, Smith SA, Schwartz JF, et al: Spinal cord infarction due to minor trauma in children. Neurology 25:301, 1975.
3. Alker GJ, Oh YS, Leslie EV: High cervical spine and craniocervical junction injuries in fatal traffic accidents. A radiological study. Ortho Clin North Am 9:1005, 1978.
4. Allen JP: Birth injury to spinal cord. Northwest Med 69:323, 1970.
5. Anderson JM, Schutt AH: Spinal injury in children. A review of 156 cases seen from 1950 through 1980. Mayo Clinic Proc 55:499, 1980.
6. Andrews LA, Jung SK: Spinal injury in children in British Columbia. Paraplegia 17:442, 1979.
7. Atlas SW, Regenbogen V, Rogers LF, et al: The radiographic characterization of burst fractures of the spine. AJR 7:675, 1986.
8. Aufdermaur M: Spinal injuries in juveniles. J Bone Joint Surg [Br] 3:513, 1974.
9. Babcock JL: Spinal injuries in children. Pediatr Clin North Am 22:487, 1975.
10. Babcock JL: Cervical spine injuries. Diagnosis and classification. Arch Surg 111:646, 1976.
11. Bailey DK: The normal cervical spine in infants and chidren. Radiology 59:712, 1952.
12. Bailey RW, Badgeby CE: Stabilization of the cervical spine by anterior fusion. J Bone Joint Surg 42:565, 1960.
13. Baker DH, Berdon WE: Special trauma problems in children. Radiol Clin North Am 4:289, 1966.
14. Barkin M, Dolfin D, Herschorn S, et al: The urologic care of the spinal cord injury patient. J Urol 129:335, 1983.
15. Barnett E, Nairn A: A study of fetal attitude. Br J Radiol 38:338, 1965.
16. Barson AJ: The vertebral level of termination of the spinal cord during normal and abnormal development. J Anat 106:489, 1970.
17. Battacharyya SK: Fracture and displacement of the odontoid process in a child. A case report. J Bone Joint Surg [Am] 56:1071, 1974.
18. Bell HJ, Dykstra DO: Somatosensory evoked potentials as an adjunct to diagnosis of neonatal spinal cord injury. J Pediatr 106:298, 1985.
19. Bohlman H: Treatment of fractures and dislocations of the thoracic and lumbar spine. J Bone Joint Surg 57 [Am] 1:165, 1985.
20. Bracken MB, Freeman DH, Jr, Hellendrand KA: Incidence of acute traumatic hospitalized spinal cord injury in the United States, 1970–1977. Am J Epidemiol 113:615, 1981.
21. Bracken MB, Collins WF, Freeman DF, et al: Efficacy of methylprednisolone in acute spinal cord injury. JAMA 251:45, 1984.
22. Bracken MB, Shepard MJ, Hellendrand KA, et al: Methylprednisolone and neurological function 1 year after spinal cord injury. Results of the National Acute Spinal Cord Injury Study. J Neurosurg 63:704, 1985.
23. Bruce DA, Schut L, Sutton L: Brain and cervical spine injuries occurring during organized sports activities in children and adolescents. Primary Care 11:175, 1984.
24. Bucholz RW, Burkhead WF: The pathological anatomy of fatal atlanto-occipital dislocations. J Bone Joint Surg [Am] 61:248, 1979.
25. Burke DC: Traumatic spinal paralysis in children. Paraplegia 11:268, 1974.
26. Byers RK: Spinal cord injuries during birth. Dev Med Child Neurol 17:103, 1975.
27. Caffey J: The whiplash–shaken infant syndrome. Manual shaking by the extremities with whiplash-induced intracranial and intraocular bleedings, linked with residual permanent brain damage and mental retardation. Pediatrics 54:396, 1974.
28. Cahill JL, Okamoto GA, Higgins T, et al: Experiences with phrenic nerve pacing in children. J Pediatr Surg 18:851, 1983.
29. Campbell J, Bonnett C: Spinal cord injury in children. Clin Orthop 112:114, 1975.
30. Campbell JB, DeCrescito V, Tomasula JJ, et al: Effects of antifibrinolytic and steroid therapy on the contused spinal cord of cats. J Neurosurg 40:726, 1974.
31. Cattell HS, Filtzer DL: Pseudosubluxation and other normal variations in the cervical spine in children. J Bone Joint Surg 47:1295, 1965.
32. Choi JU, Hoffman HJ, Hendrick EB, et al: Traumatic infarction of the spinal cord in children. J Neurosurg 65:608, 1986.
33. Cloward RB: Treatment of acute fractures and fracture-dislocations of the cervical spine by vertebral bony fusion. J Neurosurg 18:201, 1961.
34. de La Torre JC: Spinal cord injury: Review of basic and applied research. Spine 6:315, 1981.
35. Dohrmann GJ, Wick KM, Bucy PC: Spinal cord blood flow patterns in experimental traumatic paraplegia. J Neurosurg 38:52, 1973.
36. Ducker TB, Kindt GW, Kempe LG: Pathological findings in acute experimental spinal cord trauma. J Neurosurg 35:700, 1971.
37. Ducker TB, Lucas J, Wallace CA: Recovery from spinal cord injury. Clin Neurosurg 30:495, 1983.
38. Ducker TB, Perot PL, Jr.: Spinal cord oxygen and blood flow in trauma. Surg Forum 22:413, 1971.
39. Dunlap JP, Morris M, Thompson RG: Cervical spine injuries in children. J Bone Joint Surg [Am] 40:681, 1958.
40. Dzilba RB, Gervin AI: Irreversible spinal deformity in Olympic gymnasts. Annual meeting, American Orthopaedic Society for Sports Medicine, Anaheim, California, March, 1983.
41. Evarts CM: Traumatic occipito-atlantal dislocation. Report of a case with survival. J Bone Joint Surg [Am] 52:1653, 1970.
42. Ewald FC: Fracture of the odontoid process in a seventeen month infant treated with a Halo. J Bone Joint Surg [Am] 53:1636, 1971.
43. Faden AI, Jacobs TP, Mougey E, et al: Endorphins in experimental spinal injury: Therapeutic effect of naloxone. Ann Neurol 10:326, 1981.
44. Faden AI, Jacobs TP, Mougey E, et al: Opiate antagonist improves neurological recovery after spinal injury. Science 211:493, 1981.
45. Faden AI, Jacobs TP, Smith MT, et al: Comparison of thyrotropin-releasing hormone (TRH), naloxone and dexamethasone treatments in experimental spinal injury. Neurology 33:673, 1983.
46. Fielding JW, Hawkins RJ: Atlanto-axial rotatory fixation. J Bone Joint Surg [Am] 59:37, 1977.
47. Fielding JW, Stillwell WT, Chynn KY, et al: Use of computed tomography for the diagnosis of atlanto-axial rotatory fixation. A case report. J Bone Joint Surg [Am] 60:1102, 1978.
48. Flamm ES, Young W, Collins WF, et al: A phase I trial of

naloxone treatment in acute spinal cord injury. J Neurosurg 63:390, 1985.
49. Franken EA: Spinal cord injury in the newborn infant. Pediatr Radiol 3:101, 1975.
50. Garrick JA, Requa RK: Injuries in high school sports. Pediatrics 61:465, 1978.
51. Gaufin LM, Goodman SJ: Cervical spine injuries in infants. Problems in management. J Neurosurg 42:179, 1975.
52. Gehweiler JA, Osborne RL, Becker RF: Atlantoaxial rotatory fixation. In Gehweiler JA, et al: The Radiology of Vertebral Trauma. Philadelphia, W. B. Saunders Co., 1980, pp 145–147.
53. Gelehrter G: Fracture of the vertebrae in children and adolescents. Arch Orthop Unfallchir 49:253, 1957.
54. Gerber AM, Olson WL, Harris JH: Effect of phenytoin on functional recovery after experimental spinal cord injury in dogs. Neurosurgery 7:472, 1980.
55. Gilles FH, Bina M, Sotrel A: Infantile atlantooccipital instability. Am J Dis Child 133:30, 1979.
56. Glasauer FE, Cares HL: Traumatic paraplegia in infancy. JAMA 219:38, 1972.
57. Glasauer FE, Cares HL: Biomechanical features of traumatic paraplegia in infancy. J Trauma 13:166, 1973.
58. Glenn WWL, Hogan J, Phelps ML: Ventilatory support of the quadriplegic patient with respiratory paralysis of diaphragm pacing. Surg Clin North Am 60:1055, 1980.
59. Goldsmith HS: Omental transposition to the brain and spinal cord. Surg Rounds June, 1986, pp 22–33.
60. Griffiths SC: Fracture of the odontoid process in children. J Pediatr Surg 7:680, 1972.
61. Hachen HJ: Spinal cord injury in children and adolescents. Diagnostic pitfalls in therapeutic considerations in the acute state. Paraplegia 15:55, 1977–1978.
62. Hall ED, Braughler JM: Glucocorticoid mechanism in acute spinal cord injury. A review and therapeutic rationale. Surg Neurol 18:320, 1982.
63. Hamilton AJ, McBlack P, Carr DB: Contrasting actions of naloxone in experimental spinal cord trauma and cerebral ischemia: A review. Neurosurgery 17:845, 1985.
64. Hause M, Hoshino R, Omata S, et al: Cervical spine injuries in children. Fukushima J Med Sci 20:114, 1974.
65. Hawkins RJ, Fielding JW, Thompson WJ: Os odontoideum: Congenital or acquired. J Bone Joint Surg [Am] 58:413, 1976.
66. Hill SA, Miller CA, Kosnik EJ, et al: Pediatric neck injuries: A clinical study. J Neurosurg 60:700, 1984.
67. Holdsworth F: Fractures, dislocations and fracture-dislocations of the spine. J Bone Joint Surg [Am] 52:1534, 1971.
68. Holmes JC, Hall JE: Fusion for instability and potential instability of the cervical spine in children and adolescents. Orthop Clin North Am 9:923, 1978.
69. Hubbard DD: Injuries of the spine in children and adolescents. Clin Orthop 100:56, 1974.
70. Jones EL: Birth trauma and the cervical spine. Arch Dis Child 45:147, 1970.
71. Jones ET, Hensinger RN: C2-C3 dislocation in a child. J Pediatr Orthop 1:419, 1981.
72. Kalsbeck WD, McLaurin RL, Harris BS, III, et al: The national spinal cord injury survey: Major findings. J Neurosurg 53:19, 1980.
73. Kewalramani LS, Kraus JF, Sterling HIN: Acute spinal cord lesions in a pediatric population: Epidemiological and clinical features. Paraplegia 18:206, 1980.
74. Knowlton RW: A flying faetus. J Obstet Gynaecol Br Emp 45:834, 1938.
75. Koch BM, Eng GM: Neonatal spinal cord injury. Arch Phys Med Rehabil 60:378, 1979.
76. LeBlanc JH, Nadell J: Spinal cord injuries in children. Surg Neurol 2:411, 1974.
77. Lesoin F, Kabbaj K, Dhellemmes P, et al: Fractures du rachis chez l'enfant. Problèmes diagnostiques et thérapeutiques. A propos de 67 observations. Neurochirurgie 30:289, 1984.
78. Leventhal HR: Birth injuries of the spinal cord. J Pediatr 56:447, 1960.
79. Marlin AE, Williams GR, Lee JF: Jefferson fractures in children. Case report. J Neurosurg 58:277, 1983.
80. Maroon JC: "Burning hands" in football spinal cord injuries. JAMA 238:2049, 1977.
81. McPhee IB: Spinal fractures and dislocations in children and adolescents. Spine 6:533, 1981.
82. Means ED, Anderson DK, Waters TR, et al: Effect of methylprednisolone in compression trauma to the feline spinal cord. J Neurosurg 55:200, 1981.
83. Melzak J: Paraplegia among children. Lancet 2:45, 1969.
84. Menezes AH: Traumatic lesions of the craniovertebral junction. In: VanGilder JC, Menezes AH, Dolan K (eds): Textbook of Craniovertebral Junction Abnormalities. Mt. Kisco, NY, Futura Publishing Co., Inc., 1987.
85. Menezes AH, VanGilder JC: Craniovertebral abnormalities. In: Youman J (ed): Neurological Surgery, 3rd ed. Philadelphia, W. B. Saunders Co., 1987.
86. Micheli LJ: Back injuries in gymnastics. Clin Sports Med 4:85, 1985.
87. Osterholm JL: The pathophysiological response to spinal cord injury. J Neurosurg 40:5, 1974.
88. Pang D, Wilberger JE: Traumatic atlanto-occipital dislocation with survival: Case report and review. Neurosurgery 7:503, 1980.
89. Pang D, Wilberger JE, Jr.: Spinal cord injury without radiographic abnormalities in children. J Neurosurg 57:114, 1982.
90. Papavasiliou V: Traumatic subluxation of the cervical spine during childhood. Orthop Clin North Am 9:945, 1978.
91. Paul RL, Michael RH, Dunn JE, et al: Anterior transthoracic surgical decompression of acute spinal cord injuries. J Neurosurg 43: 299, 1975.
92. Pincus JH, Lee S: Diphenylhydantoin and calcium: Relation to norepinephrine release from brain slices. Arch Neurol 29:239, 1973.
93. Powers B, Miller MD, Kramer RS, et al: Traumatic anterior atlanto-occipital dislocation. Neurosurgery 4:12, 1979.
94. Riccardi JE, Kaufer H, Louis DS: Acquired os odontoideum following acute ligament injury. J Bone Joint Surg (A) 58:410, 1976.
95. Roy L, Gibson A: Cervical spine fusions in children. Clin Orthop 73:146, 1970.
96. Schneider RC, Crosby EC: Vascular insufficiency of brain stem and spinal cord in spinal trauma. Neurology (Minneap) 9:643, 1959.
97. Selecki BR: The effects of rotation of the atlas on the axis. Experimental work. Med J Aust 1:1012, 1969.
98. Seljeskog EL: Thoracolumbar injuries. Clin Neurosurg 30:626, 1983.
99. Senter JH, Venes JL: Loss of autoregulation and post-traumatic ischemia following experimental spinal cord trauma. J Neurosurg 50:198, 1979.
100. Sherk HH: Fractures of the odontoid process in young children. J Bone Joint Surg [Am] 60:921, 1978.
101. Sherk HH, Schut L, Lane JM: Fractures and dislocations of the cervical spine in children. Orthop Clin North Am 7:593, 1976.
102. Silverman FN, Kaltan KR: "Trauma" and "no-trauma" of the cervical spine in pediatric patients. In: Kattan KR (ed): Trauma and No Trauma of the Cervical Spine. Springfield, IL, Charles C Thomas, 1975, pp 206–241.
103. Stern WE, Rand RW: Birth injuries to the spinal cord. A report of 2 cases and review of the literature. Am J Obstet Gynecol 78:498, 1959.
104. Sullivan CR, Bruwer AJ, Harris LE: Hypermobility of the cervical spine in children. A pitfall in the diagnosis of cervical dislocation. Am J Surg 95:636, 1958.
105. Tator CH: Spine–spinal cord relationships in spinal cord trauma. Clin Neurosurg 30:479, 1983.
106. Taylor S, Ashby P, Verrier M: Neurophysiological changes following traumatic spinal lesions in man. J Neurol Neurosurg Psychiatry 47:1102, 1984.

107. Towbin A: Latent spinal cord and brain stem injury in newborn infants. Dev Med Child Neurol 11:54, 1969.
108. Turnbull LM: Microvasculature of the human spinal cord. J Neurosurg 35:141, 1971.
109. Venes JL: Spinal cord injury. *In*: McLaurin RL (ed): Pediatric Neurosurgery. New York, Grune & Stratton, 1982, pp 333–343.
110. Vigouroux RP, Baurand C, Choux M, et al: Les traumatismes du rachis cervical chez l'enfant. Neurochirurgie 14:689, 1968.
111. Von Torklus D, Gehle W: The upper cervical spine. Regional anatomy, pathology and traumatology. *In*: Verlag GT (ed): A Systemic Radiological Atlas and Textbook. New York, Grune & Stratton, 1972, pp 2–91.
112. Wagner FC, VanGilder JC, Dohrmann GJ: Pathological changes from acute to chronic in experimental spinal cord trauma. J Neurosurg 48:92, 1978.
113. Wallace MC, Tator CH, Frazee P: Relationship between posttraumatic ischemia and hemorrhage in the injured rat spinal cord as shown by colloidal carbon angiography. Neurosurgery 18:43, 1986.
114. Walsh JW, Stevens DB, Young BA: Traumatic paraplegia in children without contiguous spinal fracture or dislocation. Neurosurgery 12:439, 1983.
115. Weiss MH, Kaufman B: Hangman's fracture in an infant. Am J Dis Child 126:268, 1973.
116. White AA, III, Panjabi MM: The clinical biomechanics of the occipito-atlantoaxial complex. Orthop Clin North Am 9:867, 1978.
117. Wickboldt J, Sorensen N: Anterior cervical fusion after traumatic dislocation of the cervical spine in childhood and adolescence. Child's Brain 4:120, 1978.
118. Yates DO: Birth trauma to the vertebral arteries. Arch Dis Child 311:436, 1959.
119. Zabramski JM, Hadley MN, Browner CM, et al: Pediatric spinal cord and vertebral column injuries. BNI Q 2:11, 1986.

ized. # 25

PERIPHERAL NERVE INJURIES IN CHILDREN

Alan R. Hudson, M.B.
David D. Kline, M.D.
Joseph Piatt, Jr., M.D.
Susan E. Mackinnon, M.D.
Harold J. Hoffman, M.D.

The management of children suffering from peripheral nerve injuries has been modified by recent advances in neurobiology and neurotechnology. Nerve grafting was introduced to the clinical arena approximately one hundred years ago, and a series of major wars has allowed surgeons the opportunity of gaining considerable clinical experience in the field of peripheral nerve surgery. In the last decade, understanding of the basic neurobiology of the peripheral nerve has evolved to the level that this scientific information is more directly influencing the art of clinical practice. Thus, it is essential that the peripheral nerve surgeon have a firm grasp of cellular and subcellular morphology and physiology of the neuron, Schwann's cells, muscle, and supporting tissues. The operating microscope, microinstrumentation, and intraoperative electrophysiologic techniques are a few examples of the manner in which neurotechnology has influenced the field of peripheral nerve surgery, and the master neurosurgeon must understand both the principles and the practical application of these techniques.

THE NORMAL NERVE

Gross Anatomy

Mastery of gross anatomy is absolutely required prior to the management of any child suffering from a peripheral nerve injury. In recent years, medical school curricula have reduced the intensity of courses on gross anatomy. During residency training, most young surgeons are attracted to the intricacies of brain and spinal cord anatomy, and they are exposed to little formal training in the anatomy of the peripheral and autonomic nervous systems. The fascination of the normal and variable anatomy of the brachial and lumbar sacral plexuses, the anatomic relationships of the nerves to surrounding tendons and vessels, and the detailed innervation patterns of all peripheral nerves are facts that are not easily retained by neurosurgeons caring for only the occasional patient with peripheral nerve injury.[15, 44] Brushing up on regional anatomy, never mastered by the surgeon as either an undergraduate or a postgraduate student, the night before surgery is inadequate preparation in both the practical and the medical legal senses. Neurosurgeons are ideally suited to care for peripheral nerve problems, by virtue of their experience in assessing motor and sensory abnormalities, experience with microtechniques, and basic understanding of neurophysiology. Surgeons who intend to care for children with nerve injuries must take the additional step of becoming master anatomists. Those who enjoy reading classic anatomic texts, take delight in paging through beautifully illustrated atlases, and marvel at the anatomic portrayal of classical sculpture are likely to enjoy caring for patients with nerve injuries. Those for whom such pursuits have little fascination should concentrate on other areas of neurosurgery.

Microscopic Anatomy

Peripheral nerve neurosurgeons cannot make management decisions (e.g., whether or not to resect a lesion incontinuity) unless they understand the detailed anatomy of the nerve fiber and its supporting structures (Fig. 25–1). Concepts of morphology are best mastered by studying electron microscopic sections.[17] This should be the starting point. Once such information has been acquired, it is far easier for the observer to interpret tissues prepared with light microscopy preparation techniques.[18] The electron microscopic level comes close to marrying structure and function, and the electron microscope did much to dispel the confusion of nomenclature that arose following the introduction of various light microscopy staining techniques.[19] The reaction of peripheral nerve to injury is fairly typical, regardless of the nature of the injuring agent.[2] These sequential changes are also most easily understood if the surgeon uses the electron microscopy evidence as a starting point. Subsequently, the neurosurgeon will be able to interpret standard quick sections and paraffin-mounted sections more easily, even though the infinite detail of electron microscopy is not revealed by the sections prepared in a routine laboratory.

Physiology

Most neurosurgeons have had an elementary grounding in concepts of nerve impulse generation and transmission. An appreciation of cellular pathology then sets the stage for easy understanding of alterations of normal physiology. For example, the absence of nerve conduction following significant segmental demyelination and the fairly rapid resumption of function following segmental remyelination are easily appreciated once it is understood that the axon remains intact to the periphery throughout that particular pathologic sequence.

A modern electrophysiologic clinical laboratory is an arena of sophistication and expertise. Normal and altered physiology are frequently assessed by various stimulation and recording techniques. These basic principles are employed during nerve operations both on experimental animals and on humans.[30, 33] The peripheral nerve surgeon need not acquire absolute mastery of these techniques to the degree that is required in the area of gross anatomy and operative technique, but the clinician must understand the principles involved and be able to interpret the results of the studies. Thus, any surgeon caring for children with nerve injuries must visit the electromyography (EMG) laboratory from time to time, to determine the accuracy of electrode placement in frightened children, the certainty or lack of certainty of oscilloscope wave form production, and, thus, the validity of the interpretation of the overall results.

PERIPHERAL NERVE PATHOLOGY

During surgery, the surgeon will be confronted with normal- and abnormal-appearing peripheral nerves. The surgeon should have a mental picture of the internal structure of the nerve.[32] On this rest the fundamental concepts of technical decision making. A useful and practical way of gaining this facility is to use single nerve fiber pathology as a base and to build from that starting point the probable fascicular and gross peripheral nerve pathology. Therefore, surgeons should be familiar with the concepts of interruptions of axonal flow, alterations in blood-nerve barrier function, paranodal and segmental demyelination, and wallerian degeneration.[37] The fundamental mechanisms of peripheral nerve sprouting and regeneration were elegantly described by Ramon y Cajal, and details of these concepts have subsequently been added as

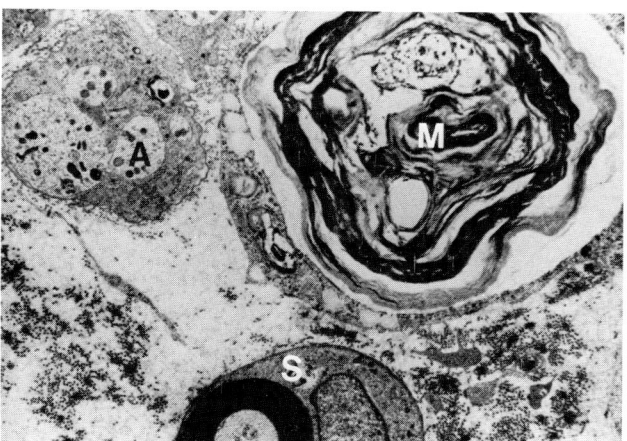

Figure 25–1. This electron micrograph shows a normal myelinated fiber (S) adjacent to a fiber undergoing wallerian degeneration (M). The tips of regenerating axon sprouts (A) are seen, with their attendant Schwann cells.

a result of electron microscopic study. The surgeon should think of the pathology of the lesion confronting him or her in terms of degeneration and regeneration, as these concepts form the detailed basis of the standard grading schemes recorded in classic texts.[9, 42, 44] Kline[25] has emphasized that the common pathology that will confront the peripheral nerve surgeon is lesion incontinuity and not the severed nerve. The concept of the varying structure of lesion incontinuity was beautifully illustrated in Tinel's classic text.[49] Kline[30] has emphasized intraoperative electrophysiologic techniques, and Millesi[36] the microsurgical techniques that can be used to allow the surgeon to assess the mixed pathology of peripheral nerve lesion incontinuities. Understanding the pathology of a severed peripheral nerve is, of course, important but fairly easy. Understanding the pathology of lesion incontinuity entails a knowledge of all grades of nerve fiber pathology and, thus, represents a far greater challenge to the surgeon.

The sequential degenerative and regenerative changes of sensory and motor end organs have been relatively less stressed than the changes occurring in the nerve fiber. Nevertheless, irreparable damage to denervated target organs may well be the most significant limiting variable in the final clinical outcome following nerve repair. It seems well established that sprouting of regenerative axons can be induced by sectioning back on an injured peripheral nerve many years following the original injury. What is equally apparent is the fact that prolonged delay between the injury and repair vitiates the end result. It is probable that one of the major factors underlying this anomaly is that end organs, deprived of neurotrophic influences over a prolonged period of time, are unable subsequently to react to the reappearance of new axonal sprouts.

TIMING OF INTERVENTION

The practical rules guiding the timing of intervention in the management of the child with a peripheral nerve injury have evolved from a variety of sources. These sources include small animal and large animal experimentation as well as vast clinical experience. In part, they are based on science. In part, they stem from pragmatic considerations. These rules form the touchstone around which the clinician fashions the management of an individual case. Thus, it is unlikely that any particular case will be treated exactly according to the proposed schedule. In some instances, the prognosis for a good or a poor result rests much more heavily on some other variable (e.g., the exact element of the brachial plexus injured or the age of the patient). Nevertheless, the authors believe that end results are frequently vitiated by a lack of understanding of the critical importance of timing in decision making in peripheral nerve surgery.

Day One. The peripheral nerve should be repaired on the day of injury, provided the following criteria are observed: (1) the nerve is sharply transected (e.g., by glass or knife); (2) there is no or minimal bruising, crushing, or traction as a component of the injury; (3) an expert microsurgeon and a fully equipped operating room are available; and (4) there are no contraindications because of the general condition of the patient. If these circumstances exist, all current evidence suggests that the best results will follow immediate nerve repair.[29]

Two Weeks. If any of the criteria outlined in the preceding section do not pertain, the wounds should be closed and surgery postponed until the time of wound healing. It is reasonable to atraumatically tack the ends of damaged nerves to adjacent tissues to prevent retraction.

At the time of surgical exploration, the longitudinal and transverse extents of the nerve pathology will be much more easily appreciated. Sewing damaged nerve to damaged nerve guarantees a poor result. This is much less likely to be the case if surgery is delayed as suggested.

Three Months. As a general rule, intervention should be delayed for three months in cases in which the exact nature of the nerve pathology is uncertain. The purpose of waiting is to allow the true pathology to manifest itself. Lesser forms of nerve injury advertise their presence by partial motor or sensory recovery during this period. This timing rule applies to the commonly encountered situation of stretch injuries, nerve injuries complicating bone fracture, nerve injuries complicating other operations in which the nerve is thought not to have been severed, and compression injuries by cast or tourniquet.

This simple plan of timing of intervention is a guide, and exceptions will be made to the rule. For example, in major crushing and tissue-losing injuries to a limb, once bony and vascular stability have been achieved, it might be appropriate to graft an avulsed peripheral nerve, provided the limit of normal, undamaged nerve is clearly defined. This type of maneuver should be carried out only by an experienced peripheral nerve surgeon and may be advantageous in that it does not require subsequent nerve surgery in the presence of recently placed venous grafts and internal bone fixation. Such a maneuver commits the surgeon to prolonged observation of the patient, awaiting nerve recovery. In the absence of appropriate recovery following the appropriate time interval, the surgeon then faces the very difficult decision of making a diagnosis of inadequate nerve repair, which would then require reoperation, resection of the previous suture lines, and subsequent nerve repair after a costly delay of many months.

The "three-month" rule is primarily applied to postadolescent patients. One of the commonest factors vitiating useful recovery is delay in referral. Patients harboring irreparable nerve injuries are watched for extended periods of time in the hope that there will be some form of miraculous recovery. This is particularly apparent in medical legal cases, in which situation the surgeon then faces the double charge of initial mismanagement of the patient and subsequent further mismanagement of the patient by failure to refer the individual to an appropriate specialist (Fig. 25–2).[20, 27, 28]

The younger the patient, the longer the three-month interval may be extended in nerve lesions of unknown pathology. In neonatal nerve stretch injuries, for example, the period of conservative treatment may be extended as long as eight months. In an adult, a nerve injury that results in absolutely no motor or sensory recovery within three months is very unlikely to ultimately display spontaneous recovery to the extent of allowing useful limb function. In a young child, this is not the case, so greater leeway is allowed. However, the managing surgeon must be acutely aware of the fact that he or she may be allowing valuable months to tick by while observing a nerve injury that may be totally incapable of spontaneous recovery.

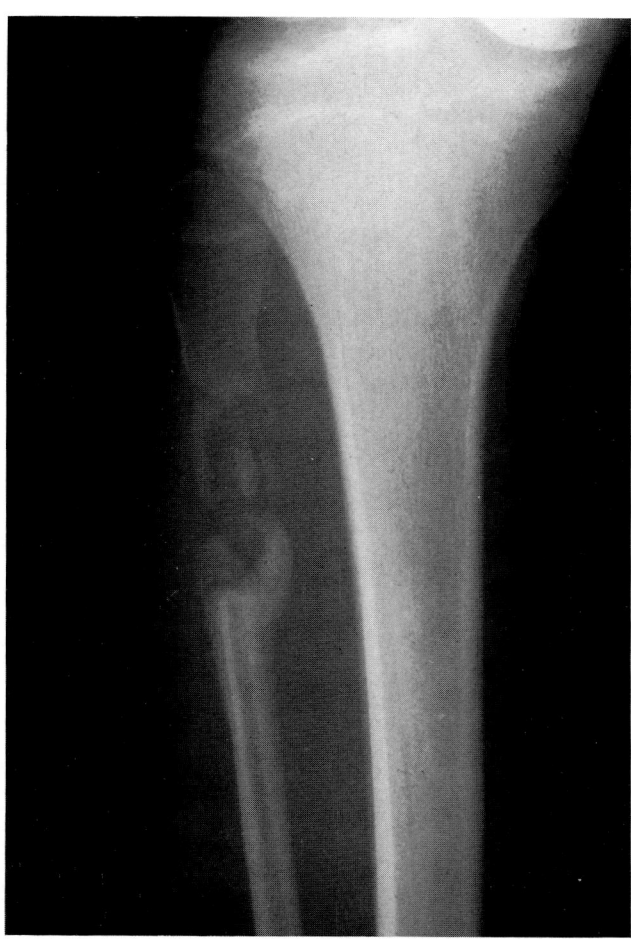

Figure 25–2. This adolescent patient awoke with a footdrop following surgery for this fibular lesion. Failure of subsequent motor sensory recovery led to exploration, which revealed that the peroneal nerve had been completely transected.

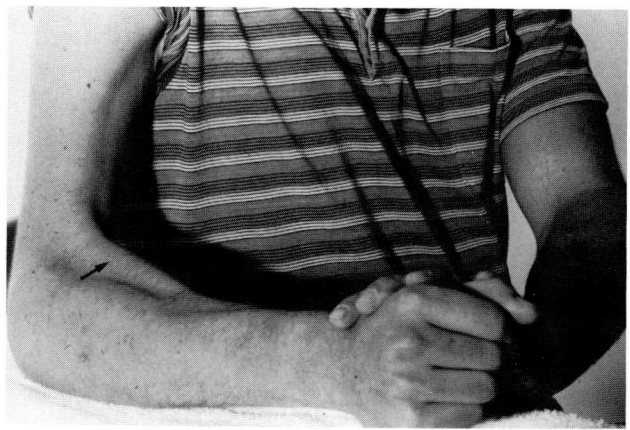

Figure 25–3. Return of radial nerve function allows the patient to flex the elbow via the brachioradialis (arrow). There is no return of musculocutaneous function and, hence, no power in the biceps or the brachialis.

The clinician must be on guard particularly for the clinical situation in which there is recovery of some elements of injured nerves and not of others. Usually, the early recovery of one element is greeted with the confident hope that this implies that all injured elements will recover. This may not be the case. Thus, each injured element must be observed independently, and independent decision-making rules applied. For example, the return of function of a brachioradialis muscle in a patient with a radial nerve palsy within the three-month period would argue for continued conservative management of that nerve injury. Failure of concomitant recovery of musculocutaneous function and, hence, failure of resumption of elbow flexion by the biceps argue for exploration of the musculocutaneous nerve (Fig. 25–3).

The central theme that applies during the three-month period of waiting is that of repeated clinical examination. The observer is seeking evidence of early motor or sensory recovery in the first appropriate target organs.

CLINICAL EXAMINATION

In older children, the clinical examination is along conventional lines, and few difficulties should be experienced.[21] The majority of the crucial management steps are based on standard clinical maneuvers.[29] The sophistication of detailed sensory testing, with relative weight being given to small increments of stimulus, is of great importance in understanding the sensory nervous system but of little importance in practical day-to-day decision making. This is indeed fortunate, because, obviously, such cooperation is denied in younger children and in infants. The clinician should be confident that, with care, the crucial management decisions can be made in the office without sophisticated technology. It is essential that young children be examined in a warm and pleasant environment. The parent should gently and slowly undress the child while the history is being taken. While the parent is giving a history of what movements the child could or could not perform in the past and what movements are now possible, the observer records spontaneous movements made by the child in the security of the parent's lap. The parent should then gently restrain the unaffected limb while appropriate cookies, toys, and other objects are dangled in front of the child so that the patient is forced to reach for the object with the affected limb. In the majority of cases, the diagnosis can be made by combining the information being given by the parent to the clinician with observations made of the patient from a distance of three to four feet. Finally, the finer points of examination are completed by a hands-on examination of the child.

Tinel's sign is of extremely limited value in the management of the child with peripheral nerve injury. The desired end point is sensorimotor recovery, not an advancing Tinel's sign. Fifty percent of World War II nerve injury patients who had advancing Tinel's sign ultimately required peripheral nerve surgery. The clinician is aided primarily by the absence of the sign. Lack of an advancing Tinel's sign in an anticipated time frame suggests that not even a few fine axons have traversed the lesion, a fact that is usually quite obvious by the paralysis and anesthesia subtended by that injured nerve.

INVESTIGATIONS

Electrophysiologic Studies

The appropriate use of electrophysiologic studies is one of the least understood features of the management of children with nerve injuries. The judicious and appropriate electrophysiologic study by experts results in data that is extremely helpful in the overall management of the child.[26] This being the case, why is it that there is so much confusion regarding this particular test?

Electrophysiologic studies are supplemental to repeated clinical examination. In the vast majority of cases, the electrophysiologic data merely confirm what has already been demonstrated by clinical examination. It is most unusual for the course of clinical management to be altered by new information supplied by the electromyographer. The end result of the management program is measured by the return of function of the affected limb in the injured child. The end point is not an alteration of wave forms on an oscilloscope. One of the commonest errors is to maintain conservative treatment because there is a suggestion of electrophysiologic improvement, even though there is clearly no clinical advance. By the time the clinician appreciates the fact that the few axons that were the basis of the electrophysiologic improvement are not of sufficient number to allow return of movement or sensation, the crucial postinjury time period has extended, to the detriment of the patient. For the electrical data to be of any benefit, anatomic accuracy of electrode placement is essential. The decision as to which sites to sample requires an intelligent appraisal of the clinical problem. Thus, the actual performance of the studies has to be done by an expert and not by a poorly prepared technical assistant.

In certain situations, the electrophysiologic data can be very helpful. For example, the function of the rhomboid muscle might be of considerable significance to the anatomic placement of the lesion.[21] In some children, this muscle may be difficult to evaluate and an electrophysiologic report stating that the muscle is definitely or definitely not innervated may be most useful. Similarly, careful testing of the brachioradialis muscle in cases of radial nerve palsy may reveal excellent evidence of significant re-innervation prior to clinical contraction of the muscle. In such a situation, it is appropriate to wait a few more weeks, anticipating evidence of clinical recovery.

An appropriate electrical study at one month and at three months following injury may provide valuable data. However, this is usually not the case, as the data merely confirm what is perfectly obvious on clinical examination. The tests may be either uncomfortable or, occasionally, painful, and both the number and the extent of tests should be determined by an expert accustomed to performing these tests in children. Such an expert is totally familiar with the variety of percutaneous and transcutaneous techniques, and the electromyographer uses evoked sensory potential studies in an appropriate fashion. Repeated clinical evaluations by an expert should be combined with occasional electrophysiologic studies conducted by an expert. This results in optimal care for the child. Repeated electrophysiologic studies conducted by those less than truly expert, combined with superficial and infrequent clinical examinations, usually result in inappropriate management decisions.

Radiology

All experienced neurosurgeons have seen patients with obvious pseudomeningoceles displayed by myelography who have reasonably good function subtended by that spinal nerve. Conversely, nerve roots may be avulsed without the production of pseudomeningoceles. For a myelogram to be of any use in the assessment of a brachial plexus stretch injury in the child, it is preferable to use water-soluble contrast material. Using this technique, it is possible to evaluate the presence or absence of individual rootlets (Fig. 25–4). Subse-

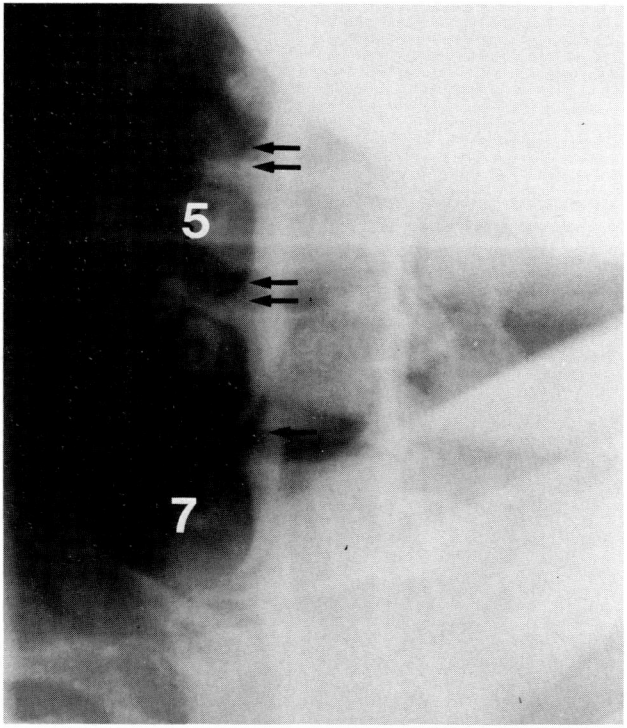

Figure 25–4. Root avulsion. The single arrow points to intact nerve rootlets. Note the absence of nerve roots at more proximal levels and associated pseudomeningoceles (double arrows).

quent computed tomography (CT) may provide good pictures of pseudomeningoceles but does little to add to the overall evaluation of the patient (Fig. 25–5). Rarely, arachnoid cysts may coincide with pseudomeningocele formation and cause spinal cord compression (Fig. 25–6). The authors have considered abandoning myelography as part of the routine work-up in patients with complex brachial plexus stretch injuries because of the false-negative and false-positive information obtained. However, on balance, it is felt that the information gained is still worth obtaining, so the authors still routinely perform myelography at three months, when a final decision is being made for or against operative intervention. Routine CT scanning may be very helpful in defining tumor boundaries (Figs. 25–7 and 25–8), and occasionally, routine x-ray films may help settle the diagnosis (Fig. 25–9). The authors have insufficient experience with the use of nuclear magnetic resonance imaging (NMRI) to comment on its usefulness in imaging either meningoceles or the plexus elements.

OPERATIVE TECHNIQUE

The anesthetist should be warned that stimulation and recording techniques will be utilized dur-

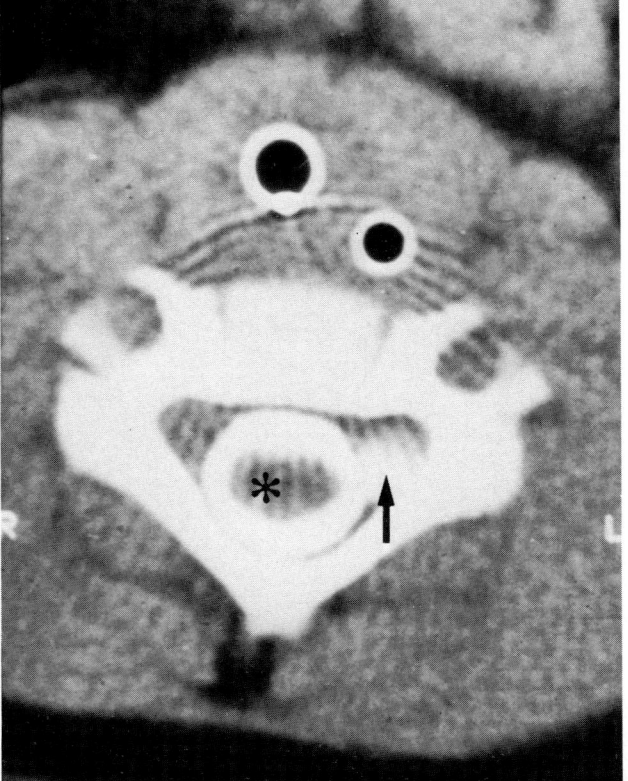

Figure 25–5. Root avulsion. The arrow points to contrast material in the pseudomeningocele. The asterisk indicates the spinal cord.

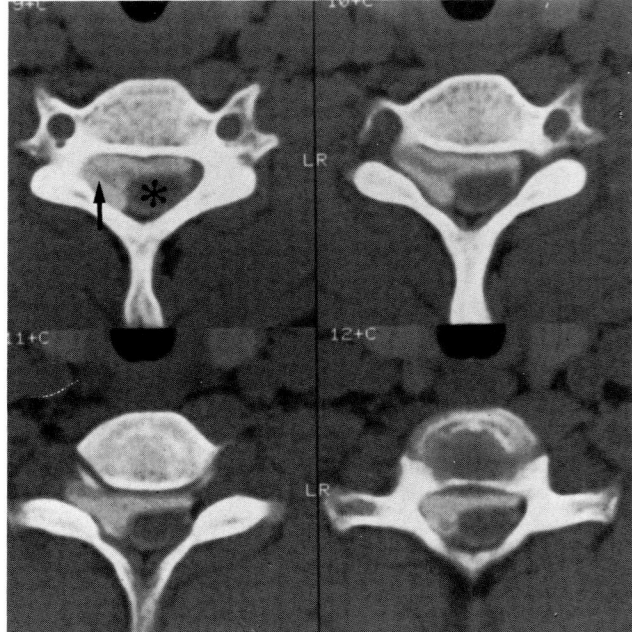

Figure 25–6. Traumatic arachnoid cyst (asterisk) associated with the pseudomeningocele (arrow) formation. This patient required laminectomy for spinal cord decompression, prior to brachial plexus surgery.

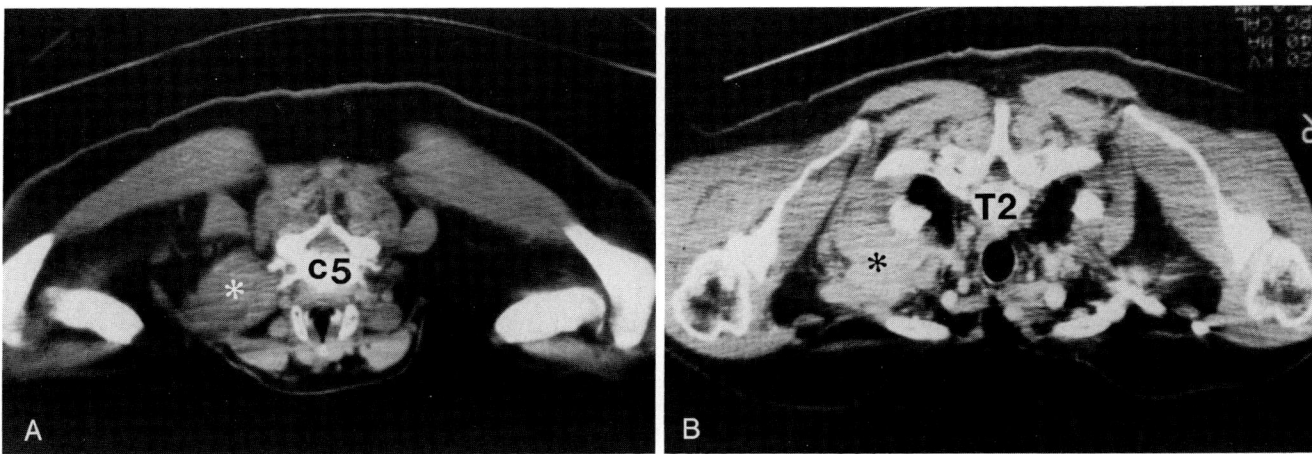

Figure 25–7. *A* and *B,* CT scan following contrast enhancement of the cerebral spinal fluid allowed delineation of the medial extent of this neurofibroma in the upper cuts and definition of the lower pole of the tumor (shown here) (asterisk). Most lower brachial plexus tumors that impinge on the pleural cavity can be resected by operations from above, without resorting to thoracotomy.

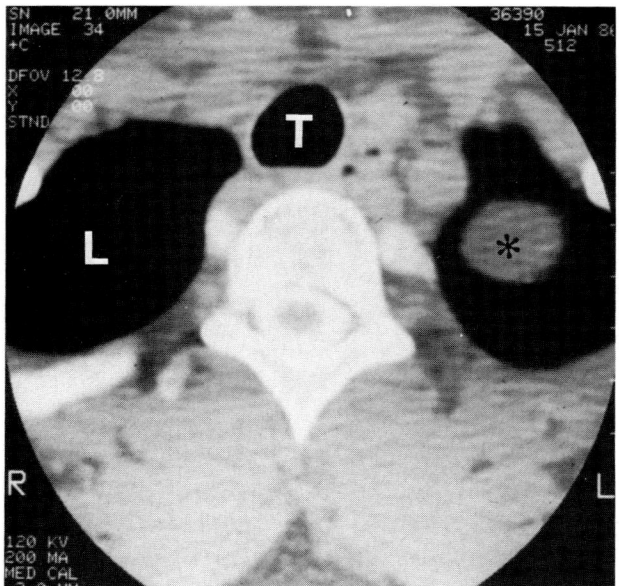

Figure 25–8. CT scanning may be helpful in determining the extent of tumors. In this case of fibromatosis, the mass extends from the transverse process at C5 to the midaxilla. T, trachea; L, lung.

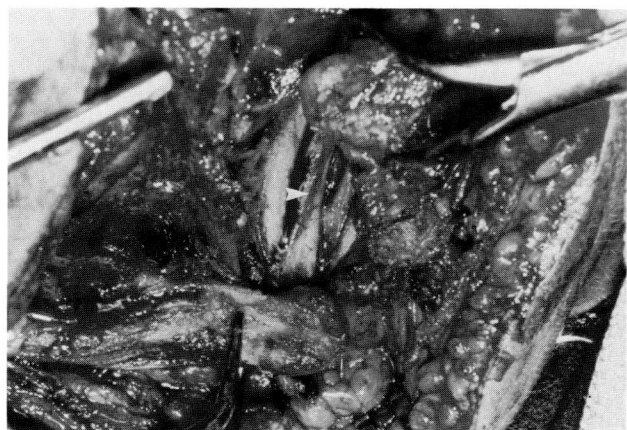

Figure 25–9. This congenital pseudoarthrosis of the clavicle eventually led to brachial plexus compression. The proximal and distal fragments of the clavicle have been pulled apart and are held by towel clips. Arrowhead points to the underlying brachial plexus.

ing the operation, so prolonged neuromuscular blockade is inappropriate. Access for intravenous lines may be limited if one arm is the site of the operation, and both legs are the sites of potential nerve graft harvesting. The majority of patients with peripheral nerve injuries do not require blood transfusion. The child should be positioned and draped so that the affected limbs can be freely moved. For example, in posterior triangle dissection, the arm is pulled firmly down to the patient's side, whereas in an axillary dissection, the arm is brought out at a right angle to the body. This allows a significant sweep of the clavicle, and hence, it is very unlikely that clavicular division will be required in operations on children. The affected limb should be totally exposed so that the results of direct nerve stimulation during the operation can be recorded.

Control of blood loss should be meticulous in all patients, particularly in infants. Virtually all bleeding can be controlled with bipolar cautery.

In complex injuries, the duration of surgery requires that careful attention be given to maintenance of body temperature in young children.

Such fundamental techniques as external neurolysis, internal neurolysis, nerve suture, and grouped fascicular and fascicular grafting are identical to those used in operations on adults.[11, 16, 24] These techniques have been well described (Fig. 25–10).[48] It is emphasized that these microtechniques offer an opportunity for significant damage to peripheral nerve when performed by less-than-expert surgeons. The issue is not so much that of exceptional difficulty as the need for specific training in the handling of tissues of the peripheral nerves. Practice on rodent sciatic nerve gives a lifelike model and should routinely be the experience of the surgeon training in peripheral nerve techniques. Similarly, the laboratory is an excellent place to practice the various stimulation and recording techniques so that the various practical problems that arise during the course of an operation will have been previously experienced in the animal dissection room.

PHYSIOTHERAPY

The purpose of physiotherapy should be fully appreciated by the physiotherapist, the parents, and the patient, if he or she is old enough. The purpose of physiotherapy is not to aid nerve regeneration. Unfortunately, at present there is no technique that the surgeon, physiotherapist, or patient can use to improve nerve regeneration. Once the surgery is completed and the period of postoperative immobilization is past, the die is cast and regeneration either will or will not occur. Physiotherapy is not performed by the physiotherapist but by the patient, aided by the parents, in the case of very young children. What is, in fact, the role of the physiotherapist? The physiotherapist prescribes a progressive program to ensure the maintenance of a full range of passive movement of all affected

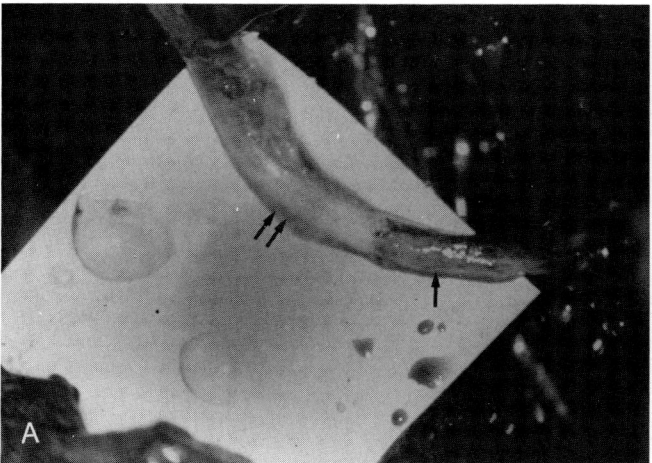 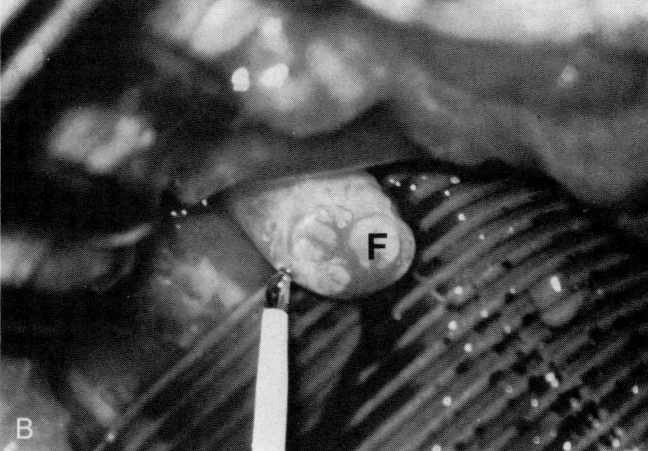

Figure 25–10. *A*, Microsurgical technique allows accurate apposition to be achieved between an intercostal nerve (double arrows) and a sural nerve graft (arrow). *B*, The stump of the musculocutaneous nerve (F) is carefully prepared so that a normal fascicular pattern is seen and no epineurial tissue caps the stump.

joints. Subsequently, specific exercises are taught to maximize the strength of re-innervated muscles. A second critical function is that of supportive psychologist. Many months may intervene between nerve injury or nerve surgery and ultimate recovery. It is essential that the patient and the parents understand the overall time course of the program. Following a major nerve injury, this time course is usually two years, and quite frequently, very little by way of encouraging return occurs in the first six months. The physiotherapist checks to see that the exercise program is being followed at home and refers the patient back to the supervising surgeon should problems arise. In many instances, it is apparent that a significant neurologic deficit will occur, regardless of the degree of recovery. Both psychologic and physical adaptation are required, and the physiotherapist has a major role to play in this regard.

The authors are unaware of any evidence proving that electrostimulation therapy alters the outcome following nerve injury. If such therapy is employed, care must be taken not to burn the areas where electrodes are placed on anesthetized skin.

A common problem is that patients or parents think that the exercise program is the responsibility of the physiotherapist and is conducted in a departmental setting. Nothing could be further from the truth. The exercise program is conducted at home and is the responsibility of the patient or the parents. Modern materials are available for the construction of static or dynamic splints. These devices are reasonably inexpensive and could be made according to a design sufficiently rugged to withstand the wear and tear imposed by a child.

Sensory re-education is of unproven value and is currently under critical study.[5] This technique may prove to be useful, and again, the emphasis should be on exercises performed at home by the patient.

In many ways, the place of physiotherapy is analogous to the place of electromyography in the overall management plan. Collaboration with experts can be of great benefit to the patient and the managing surgeon. Misdirected and inexpert work leads to confusion and poor patient management.

RECONSTRUCTIVE SURGERY

Pediatric surgeons who had to deal with the aftereffects of polio developed a wide range of soft-tissue and bony operations designed to overcome the disadvantage of paralyzed muscle groups. As a general rule, it is appropriate to allow 18 months to two years for full recovery from nerve injury or nerve surgery before assessing the patient for further appropriate reconstructive surgery.[41] On occasion, the initial exploration reveals a hopeless and inoperable situation, in which case, it is clearly appropriate to move to reconstructive procedures in a shorter time frame.

As a general statement, most peripheral nerve surgeons prefer to operate on children rather than adults. The magnitude of the operation is diminished by virtue of the smaller subject. Small blood vessels contract well, and tissues heal nicely. Although absolute proof is lacking, it is the general consensus among experienced peripheral nerve surgeons that the prognosis for an identical injury is far better in children than in adults.

SPECIFIC NERVE INJURIES

As a general statement, specific nerve injuries in children require management strategies similar to those well described for adults with similar injuries.[29] However, three specific nerve injuries require specific comment.

Neonatal Brachial Plexus Injuries

Neonatal brachial plexus injuries are similar to stretch injuries occurring in adults.[40] Therefore, the pathology may be at a root, spinal nerve, trunk, or cord level. As in adults, the pathologic condition may characteristically involve more than one of these anatomic subdivisions. Thus, the topic encompasses far more than the classic root avulsion syndromes, long described (Fig. 25–11). As in adults, the management of pediatric patients with multiple root avulsions is an extremely challenging endeavor (Figs. 25–12 and 25–13). The reparative techniques employed are similar to those recommended for adults. However, the authors are impressed by how much can be accomplished by operations on extraforaminal plexus elements in young children suffering from neonatal stretch injuries.[40]

Interest in the direct repair of birth injuries to the brachial plexus is not new. In 1903, Kennedy[22] reported exploration of the brachial plexus in three patients with conditions similar to Erb's birth palsy. In each case, he found lesions involving the C5 and C6 nerve roots and the upper trunk. He resected neuromata proximally and distally until normal fascicular patterns appeared, and he re-established continuity by direct suture. A subsequent report, in which he mentioned two new cases, described encouraging examples of functional improvement. Kennedy recommended operation at age two months if muscle responsiveness to faradic stimulation had not begun to return by then.

Kennedy's papers[22, 23] stimulated several contemporary surgeons to attempt to reproduce his findings and results. Not all were successful. In 1913, Fairbank[8] reported five patients treated by exploration of the plexus. In only one of them did he find lesions of C5, C6, and the upper trunk amenable to resection of neuromata and direct nerve suture. In two patients, after resection of neuromata, the re-

Figure 25–11. Bilateral Erb's palsy in an eleven-month-old child. The patient is unable to abduct the shoulder, flex the elbow, or extend the wrist on either side.

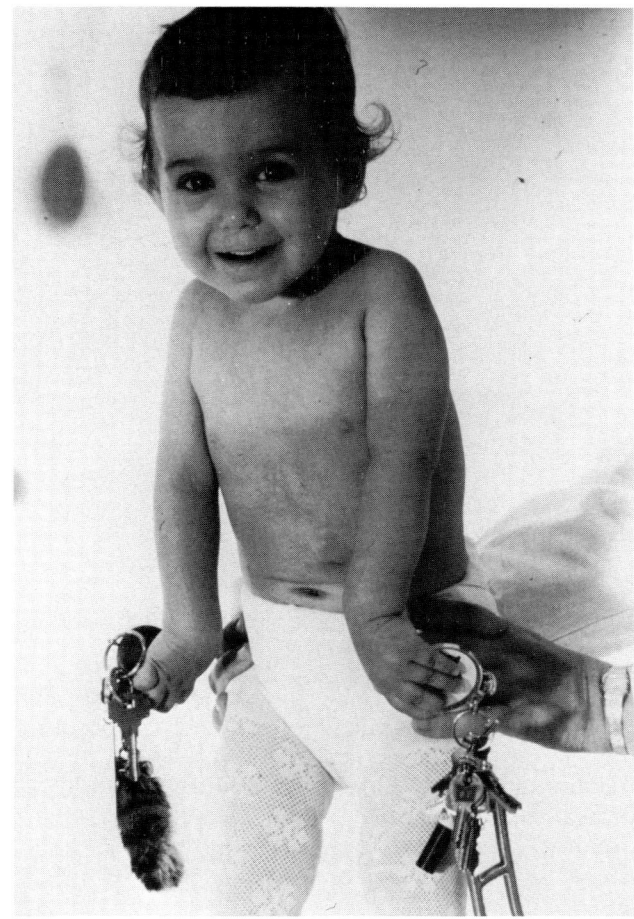

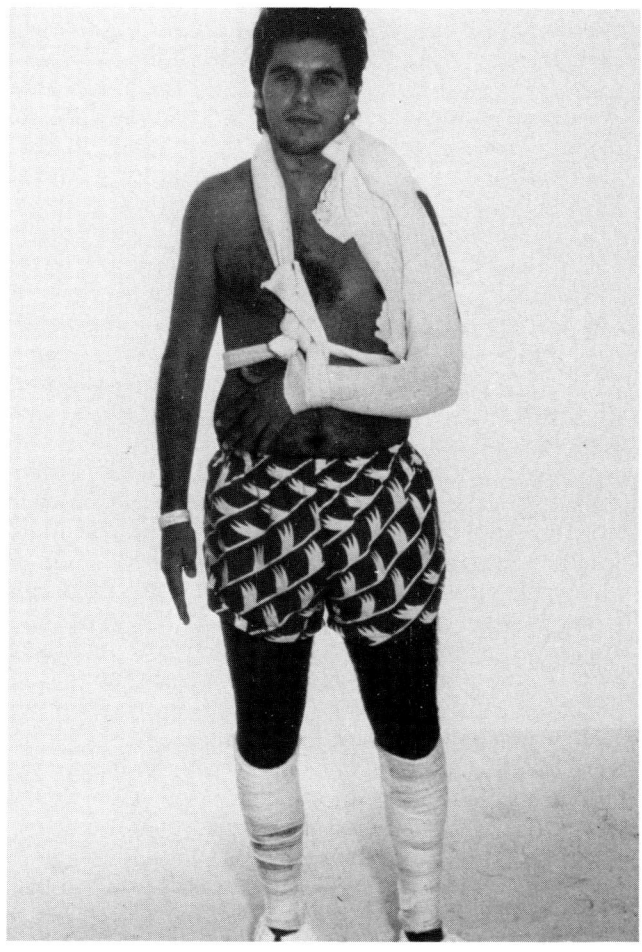

Figure 25–12. Two days after intercostal transfer for multiple root avulsion. Both sural nerves have been harvested. These grafts are in apposition with intercostal nerves and with the musculocutaneous nerve on the left side.

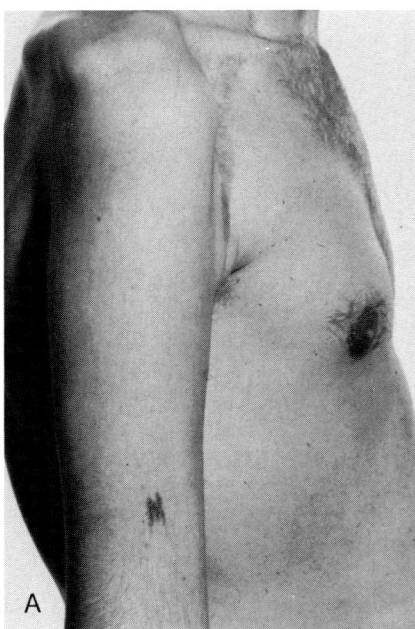
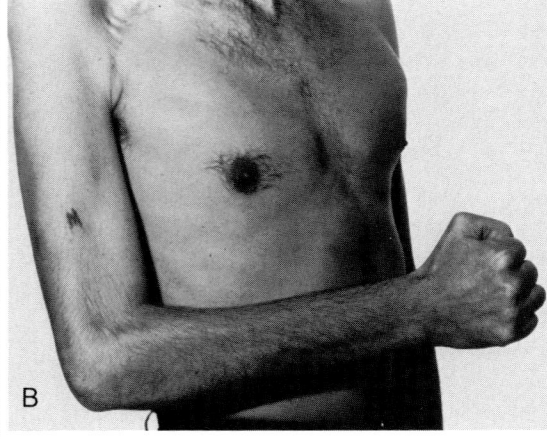

Figure 25–13. Eighteen months following intercostal transfer. A, At rest. B, The patient takes a deep breath and flexes his elbow by contracting his biceps via the intercostal grafts. Note that this patient has a normally enervated forearm and hand and is thus an excellent subject for this type of operation.

maining proximal stumps were inadequate for suture, and he was forced to graft the distal portions of C5 and C6 into slits in the C7 root. In the remaining two patients, only neurolysis could be performed. Discouraged, Fairbank wrote, "Undoubtedly the best thing . . . is to excise and suture the ends together. Unfortunately, to find such a condition, on exposure of the plexus, suitable for such treatment is the exception rather than the rule." His dissatisfaction with the intractability of the lesions uncovered at operation carried over to the long-term results of treatment, which he felt to be so poor as not to justify surgery.

Preparatory to undertaking the surgical management of patients with brachial plexus birth injury, Clark, Taylor, and Prout,[4] in 1905, published a cadaver study of the mechanisms of injury. They demonstrated that the critical event was distraction of the head and neck away from the shoulder, refuting an alternative hypothesis popular at the time that compression of the plexus by the clavicle played an important role. In their specimens, there was sequential fraying and rupture of the roots from C5 down to T1; as in clinical experience, the mildest injuries affected C5 alone or C5 and C6 together. In this same report, they describe their first clinical efforts: They explored seven patients, six of whom exhibited the same pathology as Kennedy's patients, rupture of C5, C6, or the upper trunk amenable to resection of neuromata and direct suture. Two of their seven patients died in the immediate postoperative period, but despite what should have been a staggering operative mortality rate for such a benign condition, Taylor persevered.[45, 46] In addition to rupture of the upper elements of the plexus, which had been the exclusive focus of operative management, he recognized the occurrence of intraforaminal injuries and avulsions from the cord, and he proposed grafting of the distal portion of the avulsed root into a slit in an adjacent healthy nerve. By 1920, he had accumulated a series of 70 cases,[47] and his operative mortality rate had dropped to 4.3 percent. He believed that recovery, when it did occur, was usually complete by three months, and if recovery was incomplete at that point in time, he advocated exploration. While conceding that there were no perfect arms among his patients, he asserted that his results were better than what could be hoped for otherwise.

In their 1917 review of the discipline, Wyeth and Sharpe[51] set the surgical management of plexus birth injury squarely within the borders of the nascent field of neurosurgery. They reported 81 explorations of the plexus, and like their contemporaries, they found a preponderance of ruptures of the C5 and C6 roots. Surgical technique and results were not discussed.

Other authors of that era who described experiences with the direct repair of brachial plexus birth injuries were rather less enthusiastic, and the attention of physicians caring for such children turned elsewhere. Because the doctrine of the favorable prognosis of brachial plexus birth injury was accepted widely, early referral for surgical treatment was believed unnecessary. Furthermore, as the occurrence of intraforaminal root ruptures and nerve root avulsions came to be recognized, surgeons, who at this time did not have the technical means to deal with such lesions, abandoned nerve repair and concerned themselves with release of contractures and muscle transfers.

The modern resurgence of interest in the neurosurgical management of brachial plexus birth injury has depended on two relatively recent developments: (1) an understanding of the natural history of this lesion founded on prospective, population-based studies and (2) a variety of technologic advances affecting the safety and precision of peripheral nerve surgery.

In addition to several modern, well-described series of patients with brachial plexus birth injury, there have been a number of recent reports examining the epidemiology and natural history of this condition founded on vigorous ascertainment of cases for a given population base and on long-term follow-up of affected patients. The stated incidence of brachial plexus birth injury in these reports varies between 0.38 and 2 per 1000 live births, and some authors believe that improved obstetric techniques are causing this figure to fall. Maternal diabetes, high birth weight for other reasons, breech presentation, and shoulder dystocia all are risk factors for plexus injury. Some authors have noted a preponderance of right-sided injuries, attributable to the common left occiput anterior presentation, which places the right shoulder at risk for impaction against the pubic bone. Plexus injury is bilateral in 8.3 to 23 percent of patients. Bilateral lesions are highly associated with breech presentation, in which excessive traction on both shoulders may be utilized to deliver the aftercoming head. Injuries to the upper portion of the plexus are more common than complete injuries, and isolated birth injuries to the lower plexus of the Klumpke type are decidedly uncommon.

The wide variance in estimations of the prognosis of brachial plexus birth injury seems to be a function of varying causative mechanisms: Reports based on referral practices or on surveys of referral hospitals are more pessimistic than are prospective reports from obstetric units. On the basis of patients seen in orthopedic or rehabilitative referral practices, Adler and Patterson,[1] Wickstrom,[50] and Eng and colleagues[6,7] cite gloomy full recovery rates ranging from 6 to 13.4 percent. Gjorup's patient population[13] was a mix, derived both from the obstetric department of a general hospital and from an orthopedic hospital; he found that one third of his patients ultimately obtained a usable arm. In contrast, surveys of cases culled from obstetric units report full recovery rates ranging from 75 to 95 percent, and in the only prospective examination of this issue that has come to the authors' attention, Gordon and coworkers[14] reported complete recovery in 53 of 56 children (95 percent) identified through the Collaborative Perinatal Study.

In patients destined to make a satisfactory recovery, return of strength begins early. Bennet and Harrold[3] found that all their patients who achieved complete recoveries had begun to show improvement by two weeks of age. In the report of their prospective study, Gordon and coworkers[14] indicated that 93 percent of patients destined to attain complete recovery had done so by four months. Metaizeau and colleagues[35] have found that patients who exhibit no sign of recovery by three months ultimately have unsatisfactory functional outcomes; with regard to individual muscle groups, they assert that if there is no progress toward recovery between three and six months, then the ultimate likelihood of spontaneous improvement is essentially nil. Similarly, Gilbert and Tassin[12] have found that all patients with satisfactory recoveries have detectable deltoid and biceps contractions by three months. Spontaneous recoveries are complete by 12 to 18 months.

The modern, published experience with the microsurgical treatment of brachial plexus birth injury has been largely European, and the leader has been Gilbert in Paris. In their 1980 report, Gilbert and colleagues describe in some detail the operative management and final results of 21 apparently consecutive cases. It is of interest that in none of their patients could all the elements of the brachial plexus be stimulated successfully; in every patient, they found avulsions, frank ruptures, or ruptures in pseudocontinuity. In a more recent paper,[12] the researchers discuss the management of the first 100 of the 152 cases that they had explored by that time. Ruptures were the predominant lesion in the upper plexus. Gaps of greater than 3 cm were managed with grafts. Resection of neuroma was dictated by failure of stimulation across the lesion or by failure of conduction of evoked potentials. Avulsions were managed by neurotization from proximal stumps of adjacent ruptured roots or from intercostal nerves. Among 38 children with sufficient follow-up for evaluation, the biceps was normal or almost normal by 24 months in 85 percent. The deltoid recovered in 82 percent, but the external rotators of the shoulder exhibited good or fair results in only 72 percent of patients. The researchers mention that in cases of C7, C8, and T1 root avulsion, they neurotized the ulnar nerve in preference to the posterior cord, claiming that in children as distinguished from adults there is potential for functional recovery of the hand.

Several other authors have reported similar but more limited experiences. In a general review of brachial plexus surgery, Narakas[38,39] mentioned exploration of seven children with birth injury to the plexus. He advocated exploration in the event that no improvement had occurred by the third month of life. He indicated that the pattern of plexus injury found in children is identical to that found in adults. Solonen and coworkers[43] described reconstruction of the plexus in three patients with birth injury. In their first patient, they found ruptures of C5, C6, and C7; in the remaining two patients, there was rupture of C5 and avulsion of C6. Treatment was by nerve grafting of the ruptured roots, and in each patient, there was some degree of functional recovery referable to the roots that had been repaired. Metaizeau and colleagues[35] have reviewed their experimental and clinical work with obstetric paralysis. The researchers cite their own previous studies of shoulder dystocia in cadavers, demonstrating the propensity of the C5 and C6 roots for rupture and that of the C7, C8, and T1 roots for avulsion from the spinal cord. They discuss 14 apparently consecutive cases of plexus exploration. Nerve roots that they found to be in continuity they did not disturb, whether the root could be stimulated or not. Roots found to be ruptured were repaired with saphenous nerve grafts after resection of neuroma. Avulsed roots were neurotized from deep branches of C4 or from intercostal nerves. As in their experimental studies, during surgery they found a preponderance of ruptures affecting the upper roots and of avulsions affecting the lower roots, and it seems that in every case, microsurgical reconstruction using nerve grafts was required. They reported good to fair results in 8 of their 14 cases. In the only North American contribution, Terzis[48] has reported 11 plexus explorations. Operative details were provided for only two patients, for whom sural nerve interposition grafts were necessary.

In summary, there is consensus in the surgical literature concerning two broad issues critical to the microsurgical management of brachial plexus birth injuries. First, if there is no sign of recovery by the end of three months after birth, the ultimate functional outcome is unsatisfactory. Second, among patients explored at this age, the lesions exposed during surgery are predominantly stretch injuries of elements of the upper plexus and are thus eminently suitable for neurolysis or short nerve grafts. Avulsions, though somewhat less common, can now be repaired by neurotization from any of several healthy, expendable nerves in the region. The surgical pessimism that prevailed through the middle decades of this century, entrenched in uncertainty about the natural history of plexus injury and skeptical of the amenability of plexus lesions to treatment, no longer seems justified.

Controversy still exists as to the timing of intervention.[31] In adult stretch injury cases, the authors believe that the final decision-making process should start three months after the injury and that patients should ideally come to surgery within four months of the original injury. Some neurosurgeons recommend that children suffering from congenital injuries not come to surgery before 11 months because of the high rate of spontaneous recovery of infants suffering from birth injuries. It is felt that the superior regenerative ability of young children would still allow for a successful outcome following nerve grafting at this late stage. Other experts favor a more aggressive attitude following a timetable more akin to that employed in adult patients. The authors are emphatically against very early surgery in these children, as they then have no way of deciding whether or not to resect a lesion incontinuity at that stage. Resection of a plexus element that would ultimately spontaneously recover does the patient a great disservice; on the other hand, leaving an irreparably damaged element is scarcely in the patient's best interest. As the vast majority of brachial plexus stretch injuries leave the nerve elements intact and one is, therefore, dealing with a lesion incontinuity, sufficient time must elapse to allow for the spontaneous regeneration of axons through the lesion, a feature which can be recorded by stimulation and recording techniques on the table, before exploration is undertaken. Therefore, as a general statement, the authors would be against exploration at less than three months of age, and they tend to adopt a more conservative time frame in the management of these injuries.

Compartment Syndrome

The occurrence of nerve damage coupled with nerve and general tissue ischemia is well described in various closed compartment syndromes. Such syndromes, coupled with possible direct injury to the median nerve, may be seen in children suffering from supracondylar fractures. Management de-

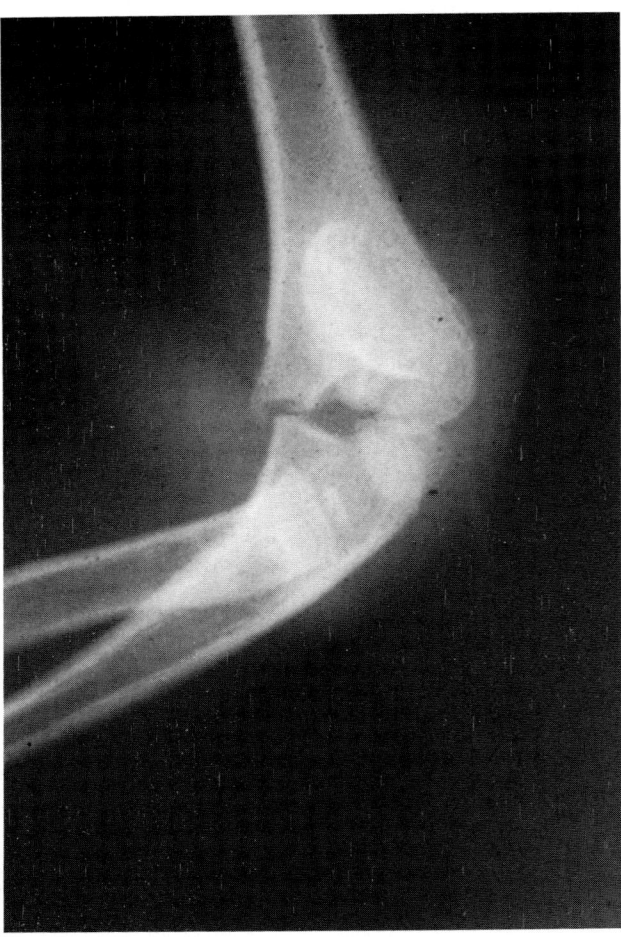

Figure 25–14. Children suffering from fractures in the area around the elbow joint should immediately have their radial pulse and median nerve function assessed. Absence of either requires extremely prompt attention by a specialist orthopaedic surgeon, if the dreaded long-term complication of Volkmann's ischemic contracture is to be avoided.

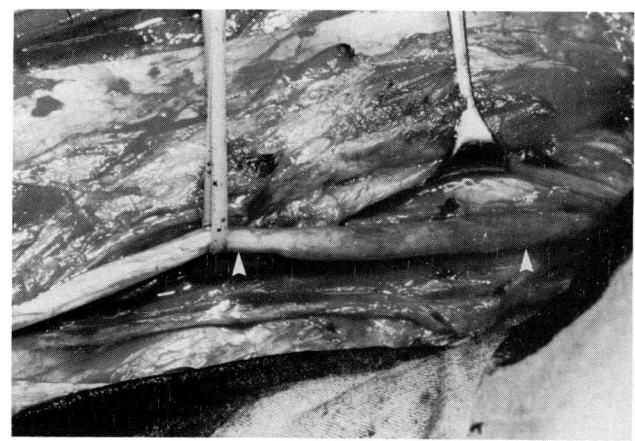

Figure 25–15. A nerve-injection injury has resulted in this typical elongated lesion incontinuity (arrowheads). This type of injury requires extensive resection and subsequent grafting.

pends primarily on early diagnosis and appropriate orthopedic management of the injured limb (Fig. 25–14). The peripheral nerve surgeon subsequently exploring what is thought to be a median nerve entrapment will be dismayed to find woody, discolored, fibrotic tissues and will appreciate that external neurolysis of the median nerve alone, itself the previous object of pressure and ischemia, is likely to be of small benefit to the patient.

Parents should encourage young children to reach for objects with the affected limb, while gently restraining the normal arm. Children should be encouraged to grasp objects with the affected hand even if they subsequently transfer them to the normal hand for further manipulation.

Nerve Injection Injuries

Children are susceptible to nerve injection injuries. The sciatic nerve may have a relatively thin covering of gluteal musculature in younger children. Children may move just as an intramuscular injection is about to be made. The key to this situation is clearly prevention, and injection into the lateral aspect of the thigh is probably the safest

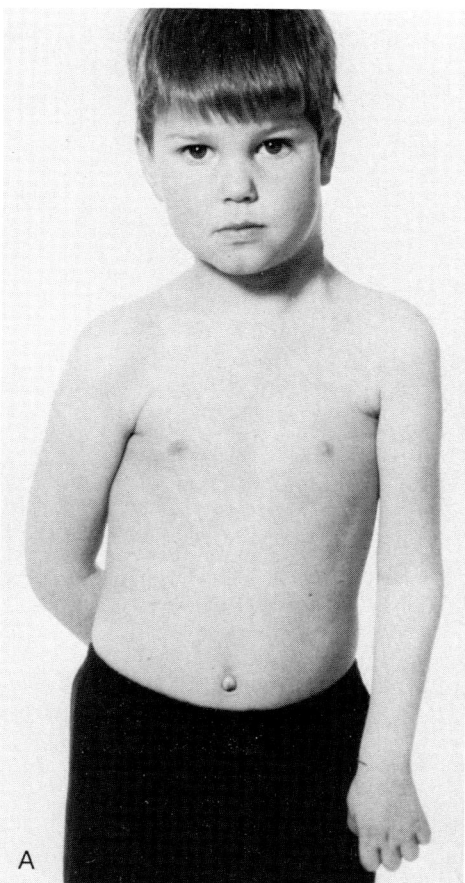
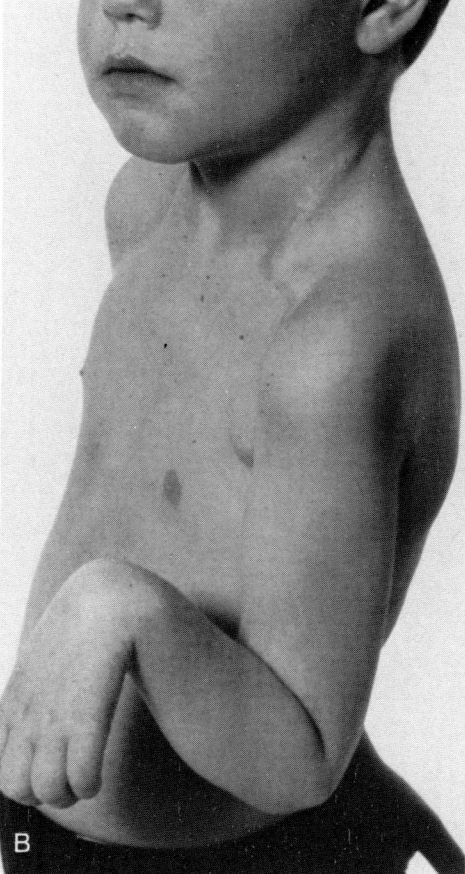

Figure 25–16. A, This patient suffered a devastating and extensive plexus injury. A decision was made to attempt to regain proximal control, and B demonstrates the return of elbow flexion, which is accomplished by an ulnar nerve graft placed between his accessory nerve and the musculocutaneous nerve.

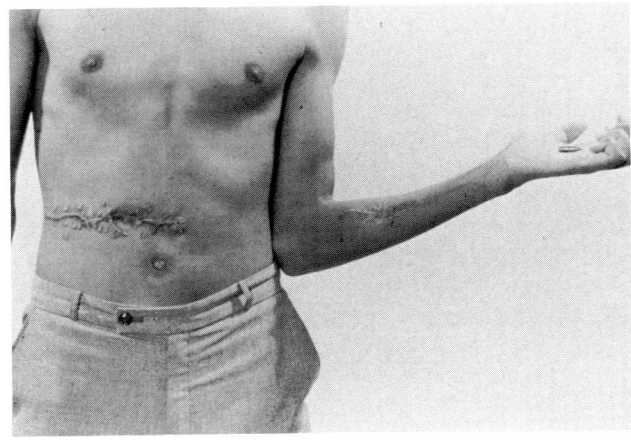

Figure 25–17. The rifle bullet (held in the patient's hand) traversed a friend, killing him, and then traversed the anterior abdominal wall of this patient, subsequently dividing the median and ulnar nerve.

site. The pathology of these lesions has been carefully investigated, and they represent the classic lesion incontinuity. However, a peculiar feature is that the injury is to the nerve fibers, and the fascicular structure may be intact. Thus, it is essential that these lesions be very carefully evaluated with electrophysiologic recordings during surgery and not solely by microsurgical techniques (Fig. 25–15).[10, 34]

SUMMARY

Peripheral nerve injury in children may result in extremely severe motor and sensory disability, and in young children, may affect growth potential of the limb. Restoration of such function following peripheral nerve surgery is an extremely rewarding experience. To accomplish such a pleasing result, the supervising surgeon must have a thorough knowledge of anatomy at both gross and microscopic levels as well as of appropriate physiology and pathology of peripheral nerve (Figs. 25–16 and 25–17). Rules regarding the timing of surgical intervention in adults are modified to a greater degree, the younger the patient. Intraoperative microsurgical and electrodiagnostic techniques are similar to those employed in adult surgery, and the surgeon operates with a greater hope of a successful outcome (Fig. 25–18).

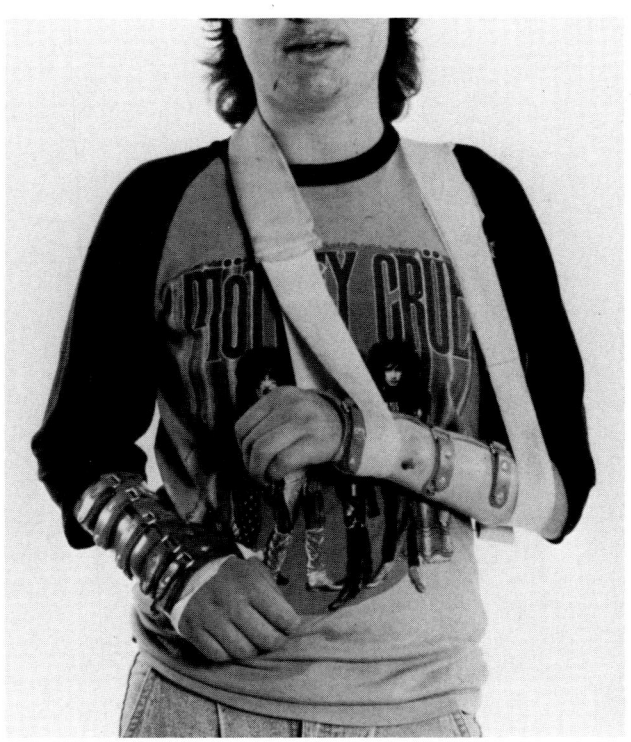

Figure 25–18. This adolescent fractured his right humerus and sustained a radial nerve palsy. On the left, he has a severe plexus injury and probably a radial nerve palsy complicating a fractured midshaft humerus on the left side. This patient is embarking on a two-year program of, initially, nerve surgery and, subsequently, reconstructive operations.

References

1. Adler B, Patterson RL, Jr.: Erb's palsy: Long-term results of treatment in eighty-eight cases. J Bone Joint Surg [Am] 49A:1052, 1967.
2. Asbury A, Johnson P: Pathology of Peripheral Nerve, Vol. 9. Philadelphia, W. B. Saunders Co., 1978.
3. Bennet GC, Harrold AJ: Prognosis and early management of birth injuries to the brachial plexus. Br Med J 1:1520, 1976.
4. Clark LP, Taylor AS, Prout TP: A study on brachial birth palsy. Am J Med Sci 130:670, 1905.
5. Dellon AL: Evaluation of Sensibility and Re-education of Sensation in the Hand. Baltimore, Williams & Wilkins, 1981.
6. Eng GD: Brachial plexus palsy in newborn infants. Pediatrics 48:18, 1971.
7. Eng GD, Kock B, Smokvina MD: Brachial plexus palsy in neonates and children. Arch Phys Med Rehabil 59:458, 1978.
8. Fairbank HAT: Birth palsy: Subluxation of the shoulder joint in infants and young children. Lancet 1:1217, 1913.
9. Gentili F, Hudson AR: Peripheral nerve injuries: Types, causes, grading. In: Wilkins RH, Rengachary SS (eds): Neurosurgery. New York, McGraw-Hill Book Co., 1985, pp 1802–1812.
10. Gentili F, Hudson AR, Hunter DA, et al: Nerve injection injury with local anaesthetic agents: A light and electron microscopic, fluorescent microscopic and horseradish peroxidase study. Neurosurgery 6:263, 1980.
11. Gentili F, Hudson AR, Kline DG, et al: Morphological and physiological alterations following internal neurolysis of normal rat sciatic nerve. In: Gorio A, Millesi H, Mingrino S (eds): Posttraumatic Peripheral Nerve Regeneration: Experimental Basis and Clinical Implications. New York, Raven Press, 1981, pp 183–196.
12. Gilbert A, Tassin J-L: Obstetrical palsy: A clinical, pathologic, and surgical review. In: Terzis JK (ed): Microreconstruction of Nerve Injuries. Philadelphia, W.B. Saunders, 1987, pp 529–553.
12a. Gilbert A, Khouri N, Carliozz H: Birth palsy of the brachial plexus: Surgical exploration and attempted repair in 21 cases. Rev Chir Orthop 66:33, 1980.
13. Gjorup L: Obstetrical lesion of the brachial plexus. Acta Neurol Scand 42:9, 1965.
14. Gordon M, Rich H, Deutschberger J, et al: The immediate and long-term outcome of obstetric birth trauma: I. Brachial plexus paralysis. Am J Obstet Gynecol 117:51, 1973.
15. Henry AK: Extensile Exposure. Edinburgh, E. & S. Livingstone Ltd., 1962.
16. Hudson AR: Peripheral nerve surgery. In: Bunge R, Dyck PJ, Lambert EH, Thomas PK (eds): Peripheral Neuropathy, Vol. 2. Philadelphia, W. B. Saunders Co., 1984, pp 420–438.
17. Hudson AR, Berry H, Mayfield F: Chronic injuries of peripheral nerves by entrapment. In: Youmans YR (ed): Neurological Surgery, 2nd ed. Philadelphia, W. B. Saunders Co., 1982, pp 2430–2474.
18. Hudson AR, Hunter DA, Kline D, et al: Histological studies of experimental interfascicular nerve graft repairs. Neurosurg 51:333, 1979.
19. Hudson AR, Kline D, Bratton B, et al: Electron microscopy. Axonal transmission. In: Jewett DL, McCarroll HR, Jr. (eds): Nerve Repair and Regeneration: Its Clinical and Experimental Basis. St. Louis, C. B. Mosby, 1979, pp 220–227.
20. Hudson AR, Kline DG, Mackinnon SE: Entrapment neuropathies. In: Horwitz NH, Rizzoli, HV (eds): Postoperative Complications of Extracranial Neurological Surgery. Baltimore, Williams & Wilkins, 1987, pp 260–282.
21. Hudson AR, Tranmer B: Brachial plexus injuries. In: Wilkins RH, Rengachary SS (eds): Neurosurgery. New York, McGraw-Hill Book Co., 1985, pp 1817–1832.
22. Kennedy R: Suture of the brachial plexus in birth paralysis of the upper extremity. Br Med J 1:298, 1903.
23. Kennedy R: Further notes on the treatment of birth paralysis of the upper extremity by suture of the fifth and sixth cervical nerves. Br Med J 2:1065, 1904.
24. Kline DG: "Operative experience with major lower extremity lower lesions, including the lumbosacral plexus and the sciatic nerve. In: Omer GE, Spinner M (eds): Management of Peripheral Nerve Problems. Philadelphia, W. B. Saunders Co., 1980.
25. Kline DG: Evaluation of neuroma in continuity. In: Omer G, Spinner M (eds): Management of Peripheral Nerve Problems. Philadelphia, W. B. Saunders Co., 1980, pp 450–462.
26. Kline DG: Diagnostic approach to individual nerve injuries. In: Wilkins RH, Rengachary SS (eds): Neurosurgery, Vol. 2. New York, McGraw-Hill Book Co., 1984, pp 1833–1845.
27. Kline DG, Hudson AR: Complications of nerve injury and nerve repair. In: Lazar S, Greenfield J (eds): Complications in Surgery and Trauma. Philadelphia, J. B. Lippincott, 1983, pp 695–708.
28. Kline DG, Hudson AR: Nerve injuries. In: Horwitz NH, Rizzoli HV (eds): Postoperative Complications of Extracranial Neurological Surgery. Baltimore, Wilkins & Williams, 1987, pp 245–259.
29. Kline DG, Hudson AR: Peripheral nerve injuries. In: Youmans JR (ed): Neurological Surgery, 2nd ed. Philadelphia, W. B. Saunders Co., 1987 (in press).
30. Kline DG, Hudson AR, Bratton BR: Experimental study of fascicular nerve repair with and without epineurial closure. J Neurosurg 54:513, 1980.
31. Leffert RD: Brachial Plexus Injuries. New York, Churchill Livingstone, 1985.
32. Mackinnon SE, Dellon AL, Hudson AR, et al: Alteration of neuroma formation by manipulation of its microenvironment. Plast Reconstr Surg 76:345, 1985.
33. Mackinnon SE, Hudson AR, Falk RE, et al: Peripheral nerve allografts: An assessment of regeneration across pretreated nerve allografts. Neurosurgery 15:690, 1984.
34. Mackinnon SE, Hudson AR, Gentili F, et al: Peripheral nerve injection injury with steroid agents. Plast Reconstr Surg 69:482, 1982.
35. Metaizeau JP, Prevot J, Lascombes P: Les paralysies obstétricales: Evolution spontanée et résultats du traitement précoce par microchirurgie. Ann Pediatr (Paris) 31:93, 1984.
36. Millesi H: Brachial plexus injuries: Management and results. In: Terzis JK (ed): Microreconstruction of Nerve Injuries. Philadelphia, W.B. Saunders, 1987, pp 347–360.
37. Morris J, Hudson AR, Weddell G: A study of degeneration and regeneration in the divided rat—sciatic nerve based on electron microscopy. Z Zellforsch Mikrosk Anat 124:165, 1972.
38. Narakas A: Brachial plexus surgery. Orthop Clin North Am 12:303, 1981.
39. Narakas AO: The surgical treatment of traumatic brachial plexus lesions. Int Surg 65:521, 1980.
40. Piatt JH, Hudson AR, Hoffman HJ: Preliminary experiences with brachial plexus exploration in children: Birth injury and vehicular trauma. Neurosurgery 22:715, 1988.
41. Richards RR, Waddell JP, Hudson AR: Shoulder arthrodesis for the treatment of brachial plexus palsy. Clin Orthop 188:250, 1985.
42. Seddon H: Surgical Disorders of the Peripheral Nerves. New York, Churchill Livingstone, 1972.
43. Solonen KA, Telaranta T, Ryoppy S: Early reconstruction of birth injuries of the brachial plexus. J Pediatr Orthop 1:367, 1981.
44. Sunderland S: Nerves and Nerve Injuries, 2nd ed. New York, Churchill Livingstone, 1979.
45. Taylor AS: Results from the surgical treatment of brachial birth palsy. JAMA 48:96, 1907.
46. Taylor AS: Conclusions derived from further experience in the surgical treatment of brachial birth palsy. Am J Med Sci 146:836, 1913.
47. Taylor AS: Brachial birth palsy and injuries of similar type in adults. Surg Gynecol Obstet 30:494, 1920.
48. Terzis JK: Microreconstruction of Nerve Injuries. Philadelphia, W. B. Saunders Co., 1987.
49. Tinel J: Nerve Wounds. London, Ballière, Tindall and Cox, 1918.
50. Wickstrom J: Birth injuries of the brachial plexus: Treatment of defects in the shoulder. Clin Orthop 23:187, 1962.
51. Wyeth JA, Sharpe W: The field of neurological surgery in a general hospital. Surg Gynecol Obstet 24:29, 1917.

IV Neoplasms

26
INTRODUCTORY SURVEY OF PEDIATRIC BRAIN TUMORS

Lucy Balian Rorke, M.D.
Luis Schut, M.D.

Neoplasms of the central nervous system (CNS) account for a major proportion of all solid tumors in children younger than 15 years of age[2, 6] and, in fact, constitute the second most common cancer in childhood.[8] The incidence figures from population studies in the United States[26] and other countries[5, 9, 11, 12] are remarkably consistent from one population group to another, averaging two to five cases per 100,000 per year.

Tumor incidence is slightly higher for males than females (1.2:1), but this sexual predominance merely reflects the normal population sex ratio at any point in time.[7, 9, 22] On the other hand, there are variations between the sexes for specific tumor types. Although the incidence in males is slightly higher than in females in almost all varieties, there are two exceptions to this. Ependymomas and optic nerve gliomas are more common in females; in fact, there are almost three times as many optic nerve gliomas in girls as in boys (Table 26–1).

The incidence among the major racial groups is remarkably similar,* although histologic subtypes differ widely from one group to another.[5, 19, 25] For example, cerebellar astrocytomas and primitive neuroectodermal tumors (medulloblastomas) are more common in North America and Europe, whereas craniopharyngiomas and tumors of the pineal region occur more frequently in Africa and Japan. Ependymomas are most common in India.[5]

If all primary CNS tumors in children are tabulated by location, over 90 percent are located within the brain or surrounding structures (i.e., meninges, pineal gland, optic nerves, and parasellar region). The majority of statistical studies analyzing distribution of tumors within the brain emphasize their more frequent location in the posterior fossa, in comparison with the supratentorial compartment.† A total of 54 to 70 percent of pediatric brain tumors are said to be located in the posterior fossa, with an average of 60 percent. However, analysis of 382 consecutive CNS tumors and hamartomas diagnosed, treated, or both at The Children's Hospital of Philadelphia (CHOP) over a seven-year period (July 1, 1979, to June 30, 1986) disclosed that only 40.8 percent were in the posterior fossa, whereas 53.7 percent were supratentorial. A total of 5.5 percent were located in the spinal cord and filum terminale (Table 26–2).

These figures may reflect a change in clinical practice rather than a shift in growth of CNS tumors in children in one region versus another, a change consequent to remarkable advances in surgical technique, anesthesia, and postoperative intensive care of pediatric neurosurgical patients over the past 20 years. For example, prior to the use of the dissecting microscope, many surgeons were reluctant to operate on neoplasms in the pineal region. Thus, statistics derived from an old surgical series would

---

*References 5, 9, 11, 12, 14, 17, 22, 23, 26

†References 1, 4, 6, 10, 13, 16, 21, 24

Table 26–1. RATIO OF MAJOR CHILDHOOD BRAIN TUMORS AMONG BOYS AND GIRLS*

Tumor	Ratio
Astrocytoma	
Cerebellar	1.45:1 (M:F)
Cerebral	1.16:1 (M:F)
Brainstem	1:1 (M:F)
Optic system	2.67:1 (F:M)
Primitive neuroectodermal tumor	1.34:1 (M:F)
Ependymoma	1.25:1 (F:M)
Craniopharyngioma	1.2:1 (M:F)
Germ cell tumor	1.57:1 (M:F)

*Based upon analysis of 382 CNS tumors diagnosed, treated, or both at The Children's Hospital of Philadelphia.

have provided a spuriously low incidence for this group of tumors. In addition, widespread use of computed tomography (CT) and, more recently, nuclear magnetic resonance imaging (NMRI) have allowed earlier clinical diagnosis of and surgery on a larger number of so-called "low-grade" cerebral tumors, such as ganglioglioma and gliomatosis cerebri.

It has long been known that although all histologic varieties of CNS tumors may be found at any age, certain types are more common among infants and children than among older individuals. These include primitive neuroectodermal tumors (e.g., medulloblastoma, pineoblastoma); astrocytomas of the cerebellum, brainstem, and optic nerve; ganglioglioma; craniopharyngioma; ependymoma; germ cell tumors; mixed glioma; oligodendroglioma; choroid plexus tumors; and pineocytoma (Table 26–3).

Whereas almost 50 percent of brain tumors in adults are astrocytomas, only about one third of brain tumors in children fall into this category. Moreover, the majority of astrocytic tumors in adults are histologically malignant (38.2 percent),[20] in contrast with only 6.1 percent in children.

Two tumor types not reported in the adult series[20] include ganglioglioma and mixed glioma. Ganglioglioma is as common in children as craniopharyngioma and, in fact, is more common than ependymoma. The majority are located within the cerebrum (21 of 26, or 81 percent), and all except one in the authors' series were histologically benign at the time of diagnosis.

Table 26–2. DISTRIBUTION OF 382 PRIMARY CNS TUMORS AND HAMARTOMAS IN CHILDREN DIAGNOSED AT CHOP DURING A SEVEN-YEAR PERIOD, JULY 1, 1979, TO JUNE 30, 1986

Location	Number	Percentage
Supratentorial	205	53.7
Cerebral, optic nerve, intraventricular, and meningeal	140	
Supra-parasellar	31	
Pineal or ectopic	34	
Infratentorial	156	40.8
Spinal Cord	21	5.5

In contrast, the mixed gliomas are more frequently located in the cerebellum (12 of 18, or 67 percent), and in the authors' series, all were histologically benign. The most common combination of glial cells forming these tumors consisted of a mixture of astrocytes and oligodendroglia; 12 of the 18 tumors (67 percent) fell into this category.

An inescapable problem in diagnosis of CNS tumors in individuals of all ages has been histologic variation within certain broad diagnostic categories, most notoriously gliomas and primitive neuroepithelial tumors.

The most familiar classification of glial tumors is that introduced by Bailey and Cushing in 1926.[3] Since that time, the classification has been subjected to a number of modifications and has been expanded to include nonglial tumors as well. The most recent modification is that proposed by a select group of internationally renowned neuropathologists convened by the World Health Organization (WHO).[27] With the exception of a classification proposed by the Japanese Society of Neuropathologists in 1983, none of the systems of nomenclature in use throughout the world have specifically focused on the problem of classifying CNS tumors in children. A small group of pediatric neuropathologists recently addressed this problem and proposed a modification of the WHO classification for diagnosis of childhood CNS tumors.[18]

It is important to note that no classification system currently in use is ideal, and in fact, all are subject to change. This is a consequence partly of fundamental differences among pathologists, the biology of the neoplasms, and continuing expansion of our knowledge of the composition of these tumors. Pathologists who are called upon to diagnose relatively large numbers of childhood CNS neoplasms and who use a variety of routine and sophisticated techniques are sometimes confronted with histo-

Table 26–3. COMPARATIVE FREQUENCY OF SPECIFIC TUMOR TYPES IN BRAINS OF CHILDREN AND ADULTS IN SURGICAL SERIES

Diagnosis	Children (%)* (N = 361)	Adults (%)† (N = 358)
Astrocytoma (all types)	32.1	46.9
Primitive neuroectodermal tumor (medulloblastoma)	19.4	3.3
Ganglioglioma	6.7	—
Craniopharyngioma	6.7	1.1
Ependymoma	5.5	2.5
Germ cell tumors	5.3	1.4
Mixed glioma	4.7	—
Oligodendroglioma	2.8	1.9
Meningioma	2.8	13.4
Choroid plexus tumors	2.2	1.4
Pineocytoma	1.4	0.8
Pituitary adenoma	0.5	8.7
Metastatic disease	0.5	10.6

*Data from CHOP series
†Data from Salcman M: The morbidity and mortality of brain tumors. Neurol Clin 3:229, 1985.

logic patterns and cellular variations hitherto unrecognized. This does not necessarily mean that the biologic nature of the tumors is changing, although that remains a possibility. Rather, it may reflect a change in the practice of neurosurgeons.

In past years, there was a tendency to submit a tiny specimen for pathologic examination and to suction away the major part of the tumor. Thus, the pathologist was forced to make a diagnosis on a minute scrap of tissue. This diagnosis was used as a guide for both prognosis and selection of a treatment regimen for a tumor that may have occupied a volume 10 to 30 times the size of the biopsy. Therefore, it is not surprising that the view of the histologic features of some tumors has been incomplete, the prognoses sometimes incorrect, and the treatment inappropriate.

In the ideal situation, the surgeon removes as much tumor as is safely possible, and none is discarded. If tissue is not to be used for research purposes (e.g., tissue culture studies, development of genetic probes, production of monoclonal antibodies), it should be sent in its entirety to the pathologist. Only through intensive study of the histology and the biology of these neoplasms that threaten the lives of children can we hope to treat and ultimately cure them.

References

1. Allen JC: Chemotherapy for primary brain tumors. Pediatr Ann 7:81, 1978.
2. Annual Report, Tumor Registry, The Children's Hospital of Philadelphia, 1982.
3. Bailey P, Cushing H: A Classification of Tumors of the Glioma Group on a Histologic Basis with a Correlated Study of Prognosis. Philadelphia, J. B. Lippincott, 1926.
4. Cushing H: The intracranial tumors of preadolescence. Am J Dis Child 33:551, 1927.
5. Dohnmann GJ, Farwell JR: Intracranial neoplasms in children: A comparison of North America, Europe, Africa and Asia. Dis Nerv Syst 37:696, 1976.
6. Duffner PK, Cohen ME, Freeman AI: Pediatric brain tumors: An overview. CA 35:287, 1985.
7. Farwell JR, Dohnmann GJ, Flannery JT: Central nervous system tumors in children. Cancer 40:3123, 1977.
8. Freeman AI: Introduction. Cancer 56:1743, 1985.
9. Gjerris F, Harmsen A, Klinken L, et al: Incidence and long-term survival of children with intracranial tumors treated in Denmark, 1935–1959. Br J Cancer 38:442, 1978.
10. Gold JA, Smith KR: Childhood brain tumors: A 15-year survey of treatment in a university pediatric hospital. South Med J 68:1337, 1975.
11. Heiskanen O: Intracranial tumors of children. Child's Brain 3:69, 1977.
12. Hooper R: Intracranial tumors in childhood. Child's Brain 1:136, 1975.
13. Keith HM, Craig WM, Kernohan JW: Brain tumors in children. Pediatrics 3:839, 1949.
14. Levy LF, Auchterlouie MB: Primary cerebral neoplasia in Rhodesia. Int Surg 60:286, 1975.
15. Matson DD: Surgery of posterior fossa tumors in childhood. Clin Neurosurg 15:247, 1968.
16. Matson DD: Neurosurgery in Infancy and Childhood. Springfield, IL, Charles C Thomas, 1969.
17. Pasteur DK, Lalitha VS: Pathological analysis of intracranial space–occupying lesions in 100 cases including children. Part 2. Incidence, types and unusual cases of glioma. J Neurol Sci 8:143, 1968.
18. Rorke LB, Gilles FH, Davis RL, et al: Revision of the World Health Organization classification of brain tumors for childhood brain tumors. Cancer 56:1869, 1985.
19. Rubinstein LJ: Tumors of the central nervous system, fasc. 6. In: Atlas of Tumor Pathology. Washington, DC, Armed Forces Institute of Pathology, 1972.
20. Salcman M: The morbidity and mortality of brain tumors. Neurol Clin 3:229, 1985.
21. Schiffer D: Morbid anatomy of the tumors of the posterior fossa in childhood. Mod Probl Pediatr 18:3, 1977.
22. Schoenberg BS, Schoenberg DG, Christine BW, et al: The epidemiology of primary intracranial neoplasms of childhood. Mayo Clin Proc 51:51, 1976.
23. Templeton AC, Tumours of the brain. Recent Prog Cancer Res 41:200, 1973.
24. Walker MD: Diagnosis and treatment of brain tumors. Pediatr Clin North Am 23:131, 1976.
25. Walker AE, Hopple TL: Brain tumors in children. J Pediatr 35:671, 1949.
26. Young JL, Miller RW: Incidence of malignant tumors in U.S. children. J Pediatr 86:254, 1975.
27. Zülch KG: Histological Typing of Tumors of the Central Nervous System. Geneva, World Health Organization, 1979.

27
CEREBELLAR ASTROCYTOMAS

Leslie N. Sutton, M.D.
Luis Schut, M.D.

> When to take great risks; when to withdraw in the face of unexpected difficulties; whether to face an attempted enucleation of a pathologically favourable tumor to its completion with the prospect of an operative fatality or to abandon the procedure short of completeness with the certainty that after months or years even greater risks may have to be faced at a subsequent session—all this takes surgical judgement which is a matter of long experience and which can scarcely be transmitted by the written word.
>
> HARVEY CUSHING

The cerebellar astrocytoma is at once one of the most common neoplasms of childhood and one of the most rewarding for the neurosurgeon to treat. Recent series place the incidence of this tumor between 12 and 28 percent of all pediatric brain tumors.[15, 16] If only those neoplasms arising within the posterior fossa are included, the cerebellar astrocytoma accounts for about a third and is approximately equal in incidence to medulloblastoma. It is a disease almost exclusively of children and young adults, but cases have been reported in adults of 60 years or more of age.[16, 28] In Cushing's landmark series[9] published in 1931, the mean age at presentation was 13 years, but most of his patients had been symptomatic for two years or more and presented with blindness secondary to chronic papilledema. Cushing himself suggested that improved diagnostic techniques would probably allow diagnosis at a younger age, and this prediction has been fulfilled. By 1971, the average age upon initial admission to the hospital was 8.9 years.[13] The authors' own series of 59 patients at the Children's Hospital of Philadelphia, collected since the advent of computed tomography (CT) scanning, shows a mean age of 8.9 ± 4.2 at presentation (Fig. 27–1). The etiology of these tumors remains obscure. The predominance of the lesion during childhood prompted Cushing to suggest a congenital origin, and in fact, infants under one year of age have been reported with cerebellar astrocytomas.[16] Although many patients give a history of some antecedent trauma, this is hardly surprising in a population composed of children. It is likely that the injury merely calls attention to a pre-existing deficit; no link between trauma or any other external etiologic factor and cerebellar astrocytoma has ever been established. The sex incidence in most series is approximately equal, providing no additional clues.

CLINICAL PRESENTATION

With this disease, the typical history is characteristic and indistinguishable from that of other extrinsic posterior fossa masses. For the most part, the symptoms are those of increased intracranial pressure arising from obstructive hydrocephalus or from the mass itself. They are frequently insidious and, retrospectively, may have been present, on and off, for years. The slow growth of these tumors allows for gradual displacement of the adjacent cerebellum and brainstem, and alarming symptoms usually await the development of massive tumors and hydrocephalus. In small children, the cranium can expand, accommodating the increased intracranial volume with little increase in pressure. The early symptoms that do occur are often nonspecific and are often attributed to viral illness, migraine, gastrointestinal upset, or psychiatric disease.

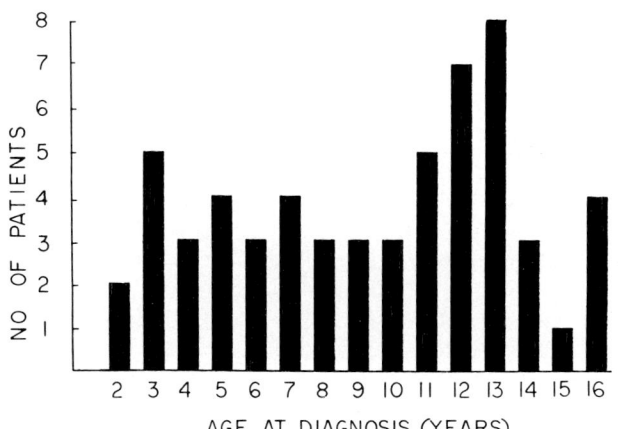

Figure 27-1. Age distribution of 59 patients with cerebellar astrocytomas seen at Children's Hospital of Philadelphia between 1975 and 1986. The mean age at presentation was 8.9 years.

The most frequent signs and symptoms are shown in Figure 27-2. The average duration of symptoms before diagnosis was seven months, varying from one day to three years. Symptoms are frequently recurrent rather than progressive, and there may be weeks or even months of remission. A long history of headaches or vomiting in the context of a posterior fossa mass suggests the diagnosis of astrocytoma, whereas a history of only a few days or weeks makes a more rapid growing tumor, such as a medulloblastoma, more probable.

Headache is perhaps the most common symptom in children with posterior fossa tumors and occurs in virtually 100 percent of patients in some series.[13] Nonspecific headache occurs with surprising frequency in children, but the headache of a posterior fossa tumor is characteristic. It is more often frontal than suboccipital, at first.[9] When headache becomes localized to the suboccipital region, it is frequently described along with neck pain or stiffness, suggesting tonsillar herniation. Headaches occurring only in the morning and subsiding with activity are particularly ominous. The combination of hypoventilation associated with sleep and the increased intracranial pressure associated with recumbency conspire to provoke the headache upon awakening, and pain may awaken the child from sleep. Coughing, sneezing, or straining at stool may result in headache, and some children develop constipation in order to avoid discomfort. Long-standing or recurring headaches of this type in a child demand a CT scan, with contrast enhancement, or a nuclear magnetic resonance imaging (NMRI) scan.

Vomiting is a common symptom and is frequently limited to the morning. The persistence of vomiting throughout the day suggests direct involvement of the lower brainstem with the tumor. The vomiting is described as projectile and is often unassociated with antecedent nausea. If it is accompanied by headache, the associated vomiting-induced hyperventilation may relieve the latter. Persistent vomiting without other signs or symptoms is often investigated by extensive gastrointestinal (GI) evaluations or is ascribed merely to psychogenic factors, with the tumor being discovered months or years later. The work-up of persistent vomiting in a child should include an evaluation for a posterior fossa tumor.

The third characteristic symptom is ataxia or other gait disturbance, and older children with cerebellar astrocytomas are often described as having "always been a clumsy child." Examination may reveal nystagmus, dysmetria, or simply a broad-based gait. A child with presumed "viral cerebellitis" or "acute cerebellar ataxia of childhood" should have a CT or an NMRI scan prior to diagnostic lumbar puncture, to avoid a catastrophe from misdiagnosis.

Other symptoms and signs occur less frequently, and later in the evolution of the symptom complex.

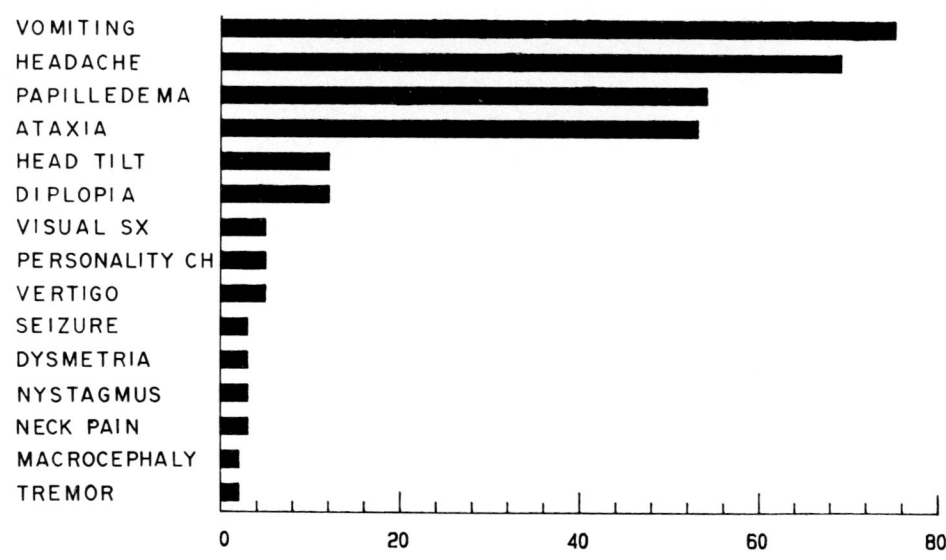

Figure 27-2. Signs and symptoms at presentation seen in children with cerebellar astrocytomas.

Diplopia secondary to sixth nerve palsies may arise from hydrocephalus. Visual obscurations or frank blindness from chronic papilledema still occur, but with less frequency than in Cushing's day. Neck pain and torticollis may be confused with spinal conditions and arise from tonsillar impaction. Dizziness is nonspecific but is frequently mentioned by patients. Small children and infants may present only with macrocephaly.

Tumors in the midline (vermis) tend to present at a younger age, and patients complain predominantly of headache and vomiting. Laterally placed tumors (cerebellar hemisphere) are more likely to occur in older patients and are more likely to be associated with appendicular cerebellar signs.[16]

DIAGNOSTIC EVALUATION

The initial evaluation of the child suspected of harboring a posterior fossa tumor should include a CT scan with and without the injection of intravenous contrast material. Young children require sedation with chloral hydrate or intramuscular pentobarbital to avoid motion artifact. This study is highly accurate, with a diagnostic accuracy in the range of 96 to 98 percent.[27, 40] Difficulties are occasionally experienced in the region of the inferior vermis, where bone artifacts from the foramen magnum and petrous bones can obscure the lesion.

Cerebellar astrocytomas have a characteristic appearance on CT, but it is not entirely specific. Most solid cerebellar astrocytomas appear as low-density, midline masses within the vermis that enhance uniformly (Fig. 27–3).[8] Medulloblastomas also enhance uniformly but are usually of increased density on the precontrast study,[41] and ependymomas tend to enhance irregularly and often contain calcifications. Cystic astrocytomas are more often eccentrically placed within the cerebellar hemisphere and are frequently quite large, measuring 4 to 5 cm across (Fig. 27–4). They are hypodense on the precontrast scan but have a density about twice that of cerebrospinal fluid,[40] the result of increased protein content. This helps distinguish these lesions from other cystic lesions, such as arachnoid cysts or Dandy-Walker cysts. If there is a mural nodule, it may or may not enhance. The cyst wall enhances when it is composed of active tumor, but not when it is formed of reactive non-neoplastic glial tissue. This is of concern to the surgeon, as the cyst wall must be excised when it is neoplastic. However, it is necessary to remove only the mural nodule when the cyst wall is composed of nonenhancing gliosis. Hydrocephalus is present in almost all cases, whether the tumor is located within the vermis or the cerebellar hemisphere.

CT scanning is particularly valuable in the postoperative follow-up period. Since the tumors are usually quite large, the postoperative tumor bed is also quite large, and recurrent tumors have a large space to fill before becoming symptomatic. Small recurrences can be detected by CT long before they become symptomatic; thus, a program of systematic monitoring of patients after surgery is essential. Any residual contrast enhancement seen in a scan done more than a few weeks postoperatively suggests recurrent or residual tumor, as does persistent distortion and asymmetry of the fourth ventricle. The postoperative defect should have the density of cerebrospinal fluid, and density higher than this

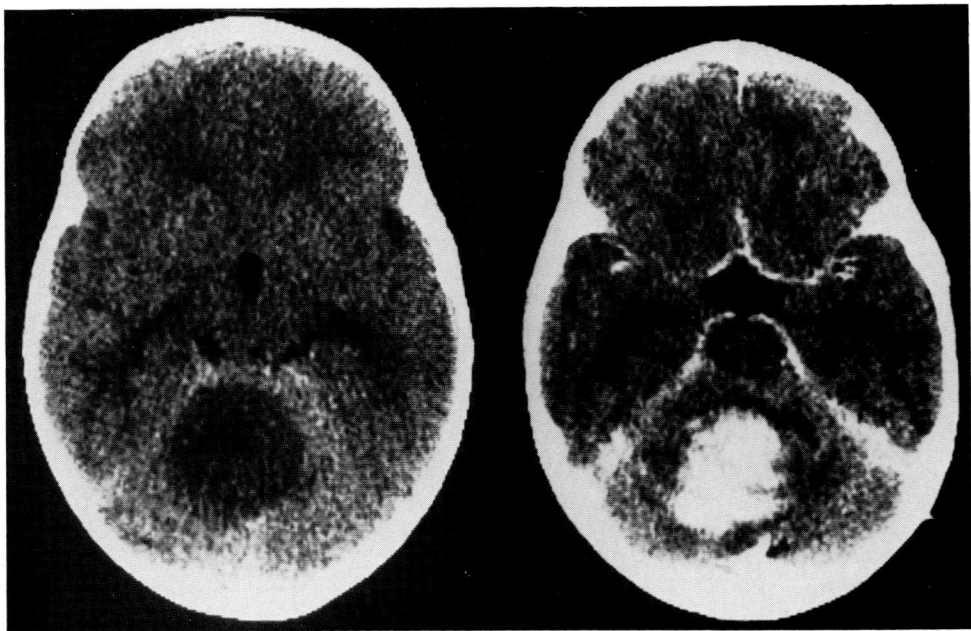

Figure 27–3. Unenhanced (left) and contrast-enhanced (right) CT scans of a typical child with a solid vermian astrocytoma. These tumors are usually of decreased density and enhance homogenously.

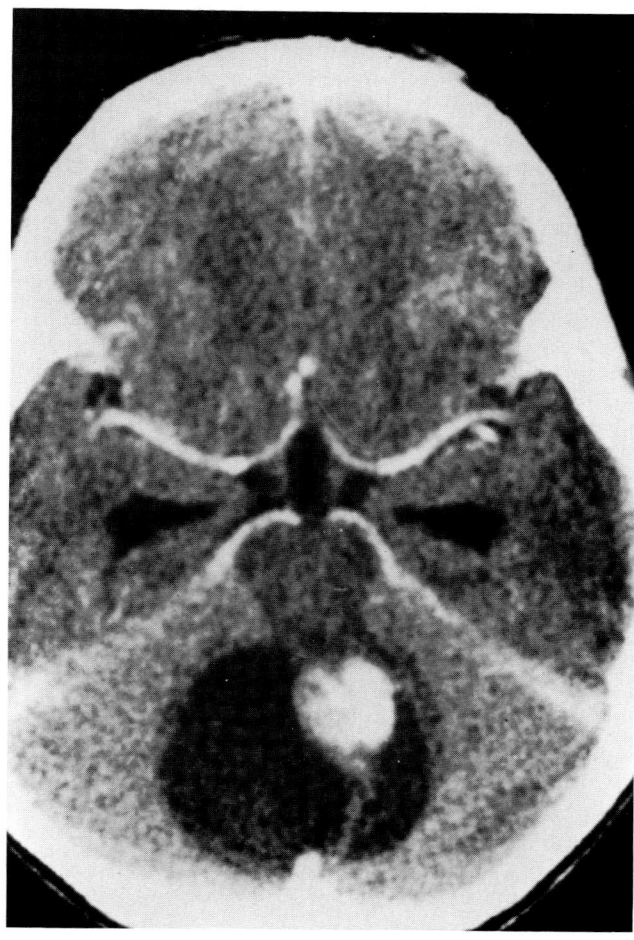

Figure 27–4. Contrast-enhanced CT scan of a cystic cerebellar astrocytoma. At surgery, the lesion was comprised of a fluid-filled cyst and a solid mural nodule.

within the cavity suggests recurrence of a tumor cyst.

NMRI is gaining in popularity as a screening test because it avoids having to irradiate the patient. Cerebellar astrocytomas are well seen on this study (Fig. 27–5) but, in general, are not distinguishable from other types of posterior fossa tumors. Midsagittal cuts may aid in establishing preoperatively whether or not there is attachment to the brainstem. It is unclear what place NMRI will have in the follow-up management of these patients. Our limited experience suggests that NMRI is extremely sensitive to any abnormality, including postoperative scarring and edema, but it is not particularly specific for tumor recurrence. Perhaps this will change when paramagnetic contrast agents are approved for use in children.

MANAGEMENT

Frequently, children with posterior fossa tumors are extremely ill at presentation, are vomiting, and are complaining of severe headache. These symptoms are usually the result of obstructive hydrocephalus rather than the mass itself, and considerable debate has centered on the mangement of this hydrocephalus: Options include preoperative steroids followed by tumor removal;[24, 38] external ventricular drainage;[21] and placement of a CSF shunt before tumor removal.[1, 2, 11, 18, 19, 31, 34] Advocates of preoperative shunting point out advantages: (1) time is afforded to prepare the patient and the family, perform diagnostic tests, and schedule major surgery electively, and (2) a safer surgical pro-

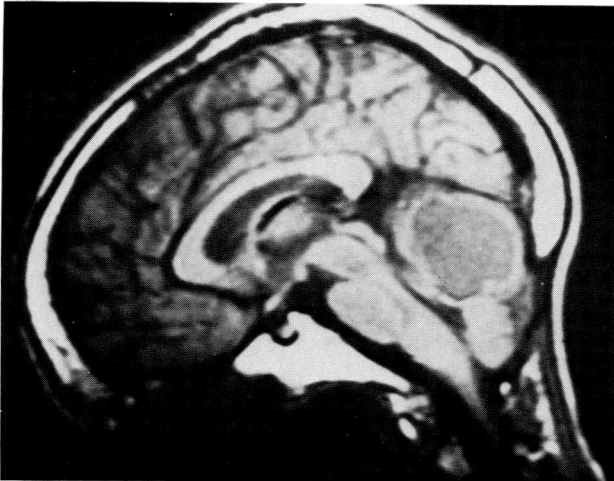

Figure 27–5. T1-weighted NMR image of a cystic vermian astrocytoma taken in the midsagittal plane. The lesion is seen to be entirely confined to the cerebellum and is separate from the fourth ventricle and brainstem.

cedure is potentially allowed in the posterior fossa after the intracranial pressure is decreased. In one series, the operative mortality rate was decreased with preoperative shunting.[2] Other authors point out potential disadvantages: (1) only about 20 to 30 percent of patients with cerebellar astrocytomas ultimately require shunts postoperatively[16, 29, 34] (30 percent in the authors' series), and preoperative shunts condemn the entire group to the possibility of shunt-related complications; (2) a preoperative shunt delays definitive treatment; (3) shunts serve as a potential route for dissemination should the tumor prove to be malignant;[2, 21] and (4) upward transtentorial herniation has been reported after acute decompression of the supratentorial compartment when the posterior fossa mass is left behind.[26]

McLaurin[26] has suggested that these risks and benefits probably balance each other in the end and that either approach is acceptable. It is the policy of the authors to begin dexamethasone, 1 mg/kg/day upon admission, avoid preoperative shunting, and perform surgery on the next elective operating room day. If the child deteriorates suddenly, the tumor is removed on an emergency basis.

Proper anesthetic management is crucial to the safe conduct of posterior fossa surgery. Patients with posterior fossa tumors should be assumed to have a "full stomach and tight head,"[36] meaning that precautions should be taken to fit the conditions of a full stomach and reduced intracranial compliance. The patient is *lightly* premedicated or is not premedicated at all, and narcotics are avoided. Atropine is given to dry up oral secretions. Induction of anesthesia is accomplished once a secure intravenous line is inserted. The patient is pre-oxygenated using a bag and mask, then pancuronium is given, followed by thiopental. As the patient loses consciousness, cricoid pressure is given to occlude the esophagus and prevent regurgitation, and hyperventilation is instituted. When paralysis ensues, the endotracheal tube is inserted, and the stomach is emptied via a nasogastric tube. Monitoring consists of electrocardiography, end-tidal carbon dioxide analysis, and analysis of other exhaled gases, using mass spectrometry, arterial blood pressure by cuff and arterial line, stethoscope, and frequent blood gas analysis. Maintenance anesthesia employs the technique of nitrous-narcotic-relaxant-barbiturate.

For surgery on posterior fossa tumors, the prone position is recommended (Fig. 27–6). The risks of air emboli attendant with the sitting position are largely eliminated, and the surgeon's arms become less fatigued. Children two years of age or older are flexed and held in three-point pin fixation, and infants are supported in flexion by a padded cerebellar head rest. If the operating surgeon places himself at the side of the patient's neck facing the head, a surprising good visualization of the high vermian region and the tentorial notch is achieved.

In all patients, surgery is begun by placing an

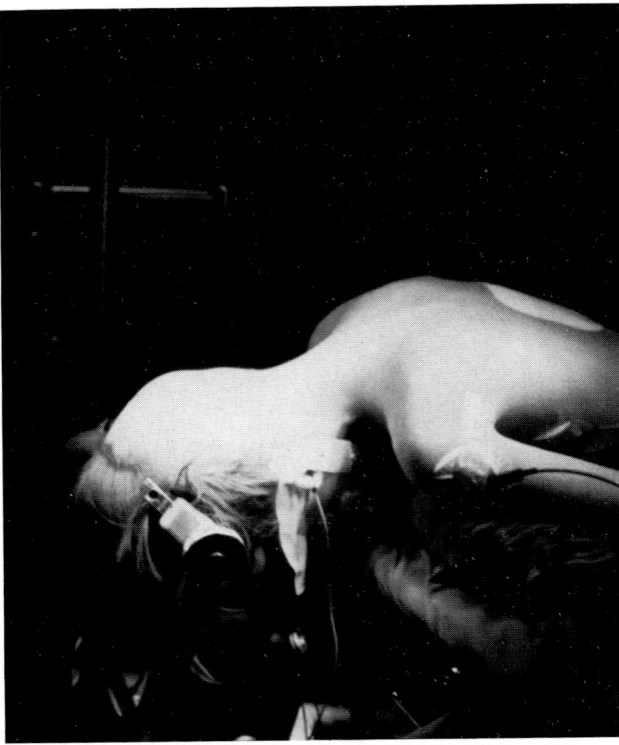

Figure 27–6. Position favored for posterior fossa surgery at Children's Hospital of Philadelphia. The head is flexed and supported by a three-point pin headholder. The prone position diminishes the risk of air embolus.

occipital burr hole to provide access to the ventricle and by cannulating the ventricle with a Silastic ventriculostomy catheter, in patients with hydrocephalus. This is tunneled subcutaneously and is left in place during the immediate postoperative period. A midline incision is made from the inion to the midportion of the neck, and the craniectomy extends from the transverse sinuses to the foramen magnum. Free craniotomy flaps for posterior fossa procedures have been described[37] but have not gained wide acceptance. The arch of C1 is usually removed. The dura is opened with a Y-shaped incision, extending below the tonsils, and cerebrospinal fluid is vented through the ventriculostomy to reduce the tension in the posterior fossa. If the CT scan reveals a lesion in the midline, the vermis is gently opened in the midline, using bipolar cautery and gentle suction. Self-retaining retractors are inserted, and the tumor is identified as a generally firm, avascular mass surrounded by a soft layer of gliotic brain. The dissection is carried out in this plane, circumferentially around the tumor, using bipolar cautery, suction, and cottonoid sponges, and the retractor depth is gradually deepened. This should be done gently and under direct vision—shoving cotton sponges blindly into the depths of the dissection may injure the brainstem below, resulting in prolonged coma or respiratory disturbances. It is not necessary to remove large solid tumors as a single specimen. It is often safer to gut the tumor and to remove superficial portions piecemeal, once the margin is dissected, to permit better visualization of the important deep attachments. If the tumor is attached to the cerebellar peduncles or brainstem, this portion is left for the end of the procedure, when the operating microscope and carbon dioxide laser may be of value. Special attention must be paid to bridging veins draining the superior vermis to the sagittal sinus when operating on tumors in the superior vermis. They may be inadvertently torn and should be coagulated and sharply divided, when possible. The goal of surgery is total removal of the tumor. Large fragments left behind may swell or hemorrhage, and rarely is a planned staged resection of value.[25]

Laterally placed tumors are approached through the cerebellar hemisphere. Often, there is a cystic component, and yellowish-brown fluid can be aspirated through a cannula to provide relaxation prior to identifying the tumor itself. If the CT scan shows an enhancing cyst wall, this is presumed to be part of the tumor and must be removed.[24, 40]

Wound closure is difficult, at best. The posterior fossa dura shrinks during the procedure, and a watertight closure is often impossible without a graft. It is the policy at the Children's Hospital of Philadelphia to close the dura as well as possible to prevent a cerebellar hernia, and to lay a gelatin sponge over any defects.

Postoperative Management and Complications

Patients are usually maintained on high doses of corticosteroids for a week, and then the doses are slowly tapered, over an additional week. The children are observed in the intensive care unit for at least 24 hours. The ventriculostomy is either clamped or left open at a height of 100 mm CSF for the first 24 hours and, then, is gradually raised. If the patient tolerates this without developing signs of increased intracranial pressure or a large subcutaneous cerebrospinal fluid collection under the craniectomy incision, the ventriculostomy is removed at the bedside, preferably within 48 hours, to decrease the likelihood of infection. If the patient's level of consciousness deteriorates in the early postoperative period, the ventriculostomy is immediately opened. If this does not result in prompt improvement, a repeat CT scan is obtained, with the objective of identifying a hematoma in the operative site, a subdural hematoma in the supratentorial compartment from rapid decompression of the ventricular system, or an epidural hematoma from one of the head-rest pins perforating the skull.

Children who have undergone removal of huge solid vermian lesions often exhibit severe truncal ataxia, extreme irritability, high-pitched nasal speech, and abnormalities of ocular motility immediately postoperatively. These problems usually resolve over several days. A picture of aseptic meningitis often develops in patients about a week after surgery, characterized by fever, headache, nuchal rigidity, increased irritability, and cerebrospinal fluid pleocytosis.[9] This is presumably due to a chemical irritation from spilled cyst fluid or blood in the cerebrospinal fluid and is treated by serial lumbar punctures to remove fluid and by increasing the steroid dosage. However, a cerebrospinal fluid sample should always be sent for culture and Gram stain, since bacterial meningitis also may occur in the postoperative period.

Perforation of a gastric or duodenal ulcer[9] is a rare but serious complication that, in the authors' experience, has occurred in the young child harboring a tumor with brainstem involvement. Massive hemorrhage is usual, and early abdominal surgery is usually required.

Subcutaneous collections of cerebrospinal fluid under the incision (pseudomeningoceles) are not uncommon.[34] These may be treated initially with intermittent lumbar puncture and removal of 20 cc of cerebrospinal fluid daily and wrapping the head with an elastic bandage. If a follow-up CT scan shows persistent hydrocephalus and if the wound is threatened, or the child develops persistent headache or worsening gait difficulty, a shunting procedure is required. In the authors' series, 30 percent of children with cerebellar astrocytomas eventually required shunts.

Postoperative CT scans without and with contrast enhancement are obtained prior to discharge of the patient from the hospital, at six months, and at yearly intervals thereafter, for at least five years. Recurrent or substantial residual tumor is an indication for reoperation, since most partially resected lesions progress.[17] Small residual tumors may be followed with serial scans. The value of surveillance testing in cerebellar astrocytomas is difficult to prove, but it seems logical that small recurrences would be easier to reoperate on than large, symptomatic ones.[22, 23]

Considerable controversy remains regarding the indications for radiation therapy for juvenile cerebellar astrocytomas. It is generally agreed that totally resected lesions should not be irradiated,[24, 25] and numerous reports have described late malignant transformations of recurrent astrocytomas that had been irradiated 10 to 48 years previously.[3, 5, 7, 25, 30, 33, 35] Recurrences generally arise from partially resected lesions,[17] and in many cases the recurrent tumor can be totally resected at reoperation.[24] Radiation therapy does appear to improve outcome with partially resected lesions, boosting relapse-free survival rates from 36 percent for patients not irradiated to 83 percent for patients who were, in one series.[17] Radiation therapy seems reasonable when tumors have recurred despite an apparent total excision, when there is brainstem involvement precluding total excision at reoperation, or in frankly malignant lesions that have not been previously irradiated.

PATHOLOGY

Astrocytomas in the cerebellum arise either laterally in the hemispheres or medially in the vermis. Tumors arising from the cerebellar peduncles or from the floor of the brainstem with large exophytic portions extending into the cerebellum or fourth ventricle are considered primary brainstem tumors rather than true cerebellar astrocytomas, and carry a less favorable prognosis. Cerebellar astrocytomas may be entirely solid, with a fleshy, gray cut surface and readily defined margins or may contain numerous small cysts. The classic tumor (uncommon in the authors' experience) consists of a large, laterally located cyst containing yellow fluid, with a well-defined mural nodule. In the authors' series, approximately half the tumors had a cyst visible on CT scan or at surgery, and the majority arose from the vermis rather than the hemisphere. Other reported series note vermis involvement in 40 to 100 percent of tumors.[10, 16, 29] Hemorrhagic tumors have been reported.[39]

HISTOLOGY

Until recently, the most common histologic subtype of cerebellar glioma was called a "juvenile" astrocytoma, but for reasons that are unclear, the modifying adjective was changed to "pilocytic."[42] This term was originally introduced to describe elongated, bipolar astrocytes that literally look hairlike, consequent to their growth within fiber tracts such as the corpus callosum.[32] However, the majority of astrocytes that make up cerebellar tumors in children simply do not display such morphologic features.

The neoplastic cells most often look like astrocytes of the fibrillary variety; they have round to oval nuclei and a variably sized perikaryon, from which processes extend. These are sometimes coarse and unipolar or bipolar, or they may be delicate and multipolar, producing a stellate pattern. Rosenthal's fibers are often abundant in regions of dense growth.

The characteristic histologic pattern of the pilocytic astrocytoma consists of a biphasic growth in which islands of densely packed astrocytes with the coarse processes alternate with fields in which a honeycombed pattern is formed by the delicate, anastomosing branches of the stellate forms (Fig. 27-7).

In a group of 361 brain tumors diagnosed, treated, or both at the Children's Hospital of Philadelphia from mid-1979 to mid-1986, a total of 43 "pure" cerebellar astrocytomas were diagnosed. Sixty-one percent of these were of the pilocytic variety (Table 27-1). Those tumors manifesting a monophasic population of astrocytes with the coarser processes and, usually, an abundance of Rosenthal's fibers were called fibrillary astrocytomas and make up almost 30 percent of the group. Anaplastic astrocytomas are the least common but, nonetheless, account for slightly more than 10 percent of the tumors.

Mixed glial tumors, which were more common in the cerebellum than in the cerebrum in children

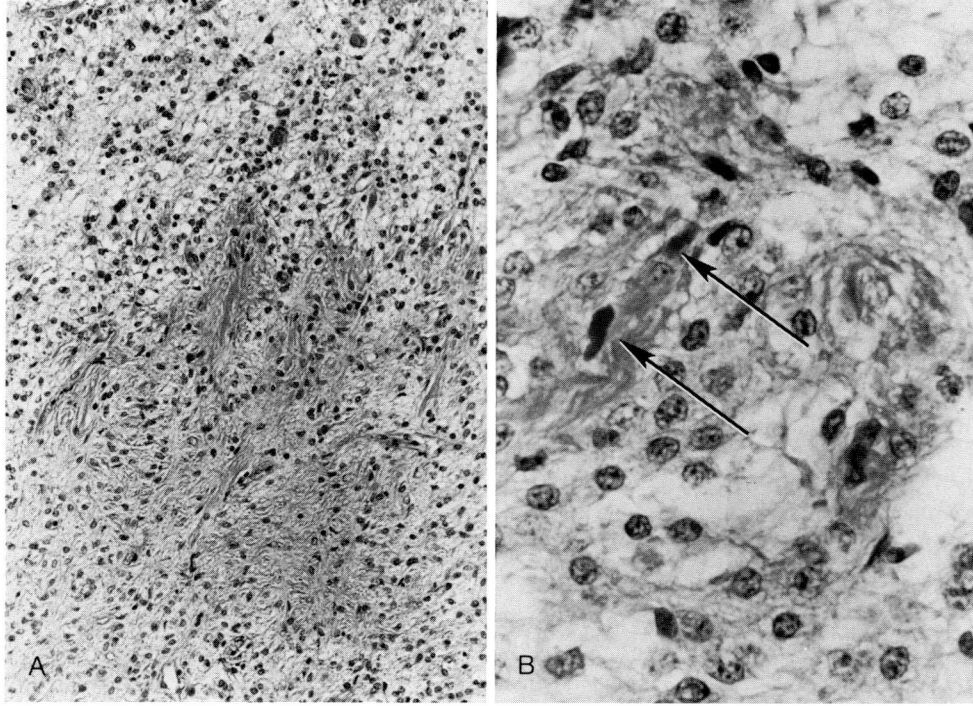

Figure 27–7. *A*, Typical biphasic pattern of cerebellar astrocytoma of the pilocytic type from a four-year-old child. Note the island of dense fibrillar growth surrounded by a looser, microcystic arrangement (H & E × 250). *B*, Higher magnification of the same tumor, showing astrocytes with wavy processes and two Rosenthal fibers (arrows). Note mature character of the astrocytic nuclei (H & E × 400).

Table 27-1. ASTROCYTIC TUMORS IN CEREBELLUM OF 361 CHILDREN WITH BRAIN TUMORS DIAGNOSED AT THE CHILDREN'S HOSPITAL OF PHILADELPHIA JULY 1, 1979, TO JUNE 30, 1986

Histologic Type	Number	Percentage
"Pure" astrocytomas	43/361	11.9
Pilocytic	26/43	61.0
Fibrillary	12/43	28.0
Anaplastic	5/43	11.0
Mixed glioma	11/361	3.0
Astrocytoma-oligodendroglioma	9/11	82.0
Astrocytoma-ependymoma	1/11	9.0
Astrocytoma-ependymoma-oligodendroglioma-ganglioglioma	1/11	9.0

(12 cerebellar, 5 cerebral), are most frequently composed of a mixture of neoplastic astrocytes and oligodendroglia, ependymal cells, or both as well as sometimes even ganglion cells (Table 27-1). None, in the authors' series, manifested anaplastic features.

The wall of those cerebellar astrocytomas that have a cystic component is generally richly vascularized and bears a resemblance to granulation tissue. The vessels often have the structure of capillaries (i.e., they consist of a single layer of endothelial cells). These delicate vessels are apparently vulnerable to injury, as it is not rare to find free hemosiderin or hemosiderin-laden macrophages, occasionally in large numbers, within these tumors (Fig. 27-8).

Although nuclei in the neoplastic astrocytes are sometimes pleomorphic and hyperchromatic and may even form small morulalike clusters, the bulk of these tumors do not seem to undergo the same type of biologic evolution or dedifferentiation characteristic of cerebellar astrocytomas. Moreover, they typically extend into contiguous subarachnoid space but rarely disseminate more widely throughout cerebrospinal fluid pathways.

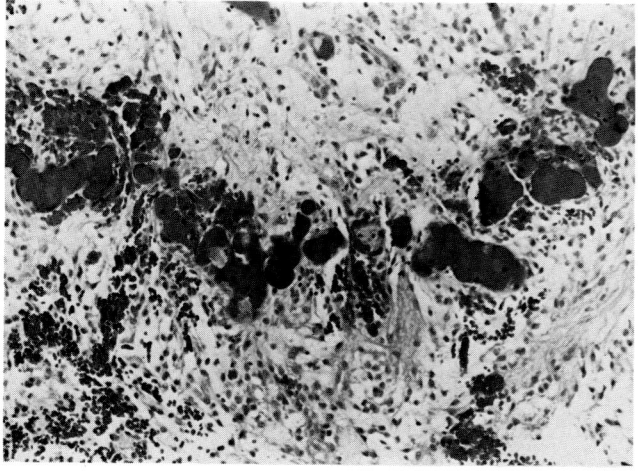

Figure 27-8. Numerous dilated capillarylike blood vessels with acute adjacent hemorrhage in a portion of cyst wall of a cerebellar astrocytoma from a four-year-old child (H & E × 250).

OUTCOME

Cerebellar astrocytoma is the pediatric brain neoplasm with the most favorable prognosis. The operative mortality rate should be less than 4 percent in patients undergoing initial surgery,[10, 13] although a higher operative mortality rate is expected with reoperation.[10, 24] Operative deaths have been due to acute hydrocephalus, respiratory compromise resulting from brainstem manipulation,[13] and sudden cardiac arrest.[29]

Several authors have reported lengthy follow-up of patients with benign cerebellar astrocytomas.[6, 9, 13, 15, 17] A 20-year survival rate of 80 percent may be expected for the group as a whole,[15] and 12 patients from Bailey's original series have been followed for 28 to 50 years without showing recurrence.[6]

Several attempts have been made to correlate histologic pattern with outcome, beginning with Cushing, who found that the distinction between protoplasmic and fibrillary astrocytomas was not useful in predicting outcome.[9] Gjerris and Klinken[15] divided childhood cerebellar astrocytomas into juvenile and diffuse types and reported a 94 percent 25-year cumulative survival rate for the former compared with 38 percent for the latter. Davis and Joglekar[10] found that the diffuse group was more likely to show recurrence early (within four years) but that later recurrence was unrelated to histologic group.[10] Gilles and coworkers[14] found that in cases in which microcysts, leptomeningeal deposits, Rosenthal's fibers, and foci of oligodendroglia clustered together (glioma A) there was an extremely favorable prognosis, and in cases with pseudorosettes, high cell density, mitoses, and calcification (glioma B) there was only a 29 percent ten-year survival rate. Malignant astrocytic tumors of the cerebellum have been reported and are usually fatal.[12, 29, 35] Rarely, histologically benign tumors may behave in a malignant fashion.[4, 20]

Partial resection is associated with recurrence, despite reports of prolonged symptom-free survival in a few patients whose tumors were only subtotally removed or biopsied.[6] Griffin and colleagues[17] reported a 100 percent survival rate in patients whose tumors were totally resected, compared with only a 36 percent recurrence-free survival rate in the partially resected group. In the authors' series of 59 patients, where CT scanning was available to assess completeness of resection, 16 tumors were subtotally resected, and of these, ten recurred at a mean interval of 3.2 years. Eight of these tumors were subsequently totally resected at the time of recurrence. Only one patient with an apparent total resection had a recurrence. If extent of resection is removed as a variable, there appears to be no difference in prognosis for solid versus cystic tumors or for vermian lesions as opposed to those in the hemispheres.[6, 29]

As the outlook for pediatric brain tumors has improved, more attention has been paid to functional outcome, in addition to simply survival rates. Anecdotally, children treated for cerebellar astrocytomas may expect full and productive lives.[6] Formal neuropsychologic testing has been performed on 18 of the authors' patients, and the average full-scale IQ was found to be 98.2. Verbal IQ (101.2) was slightly higher, on average, than performance IQ (95.0), and achievements in specific educational areas, social maturity, and memory were average for the group. Poor neuropsychologic outcome was apparent in two patients and was clearly related to a difficult postoperative course.

References

1. Abraham J, Chandy J: Ventriculo-atrial shunt in the management of posterior fossa tumors. Preliminary report. J Neurosurg 20:252, 1963.
2. Albright L, Reigel DH: Management of hydrocephalus secondary to posterior fossa tumors. J Neurosurg 46:52, 1977.
3. Alpers CE, Davis RL, Wilson CB: Persistence and late malignant transformation of childhood cerebellar astrocytoma. J Neurosurg 57:548, 1982.
4. Auer RN, Rice GPA, Hinton GG, et al: Cerebellar astrocytoma with benign histologic and malignant clinical course. J Neurosurg 54:128, 1981.
5. Berwell WR, Kepes JJ, Seitz EP: Late malignant recurrence of childhood cerebellar astrocytoma. J Neurosurg 37:470, 1972.
6. Bucy PC, Thieman PW: Astrocytomas of the cerebellum. Arch Neurol 18:14, 1968.
7. Budka H: Partially resected and irradiated cerebellar astrocytoma of childhood: Malignant evolution after 28 years. Acta Neurochir 32:139, 1975.
8. Butler AR, Horji SC, Kricheff II, et al: Computed tomography in astrocytomas. Neuroradiology 129:433, 1978.
9. Cushing H: Experiences with the cerebellar astrocytomas. A critical review of seventy-six cases. Surg Gynecol Obstet 52:129, 1931.
10. Davis CH, Joglekar VM: Cerebellar astrocytomas in children and young adults. J Neurol Neurosurg Psychiatry 44:820, 1981.
11. Elkins CW, Fonseca JE: Ventriculovenous anastomosis in obstructive and acquired communicating hydrocephalus. J Neurosurg 18:134, 1961.
12. Fresh CB, Takei Y, O'Brien MS: Cerebellar glioblastoma in childhood. J Neurosurg 45:705, 1976.
13. Geissinger JD, Bucy PC: Astrocytomas of the cerebellum in children. Arch Neurol 24:125, 1971.
14. Gilles FH, Winston K, Fulchiero A, et al: Histologic features and observational variation in cerebellar gliomas in children. J Natl Cancer Inst 58:175, 1977.
15. Gjerris F, Klinken L: Long-term prognosis in children with benign cerebellar astrocytoma. J Neurosurg 49:179, 1978.
16. Gol A, McKissock W: The cerebellar astrocytomas. A report on 98 verified cases. J Neurosurg 16:287, 1959.
17. Griffin TW, Beaufait D, Blasko JC: Cystic cerebellar astrocytomas in childhood. Cancer 44:276, 1979.
18. Hekmatpanah J, Mullan S: Ventriculo-caval shunt in the management of posterior fossa tumors. J Neurosurg 26:609, 1967.
19. Jane JA, Kaufman B, Nulsen F, et al: The role of angiography and ventriculovenous shunting in the treatment of posterior fossa tumors. Acta Neurochir 28:13, 1973.
20. Kepes JJ, Lewis RC, Vergara GG: Cerebellar astrocytoma invading the musculature and soft tissues of the neck. J Neurosurg 52:414, 1980.
21. Kessler LA, Dugan P, Concannon JP: Systemic metastases of medulloblastoma promoted by shunting. Surg Neurol 3:147, 1975.
22. Klein DM, McCullough DC: Surgical staging of cerebellar astrocytomas in childhood. Cancer 56:1810, 1985.
23. Kun LE, D'Souza B, Tefft M: The value of surveillance testing in childhood brain tumors. Cancer 56:1818, 1985.
24. Lapras C, Palet JD, Lapras Ch. J, et al: Cerebellar astrocytomas in childhood. Child's Nerv Syst 2:55, 1986.
25. Matson DD: Surgery of posterior fossa tumors in childhood. Clin Neurosurg 15:247, 1968.
26. McLaurin RL: On the use of precraniotomy shunting in the management of posterior fossa tumors in children. A cooperative study. In: Chapman P (ed): Concepts in Pediatric Neurosurgery, Vol. 6. Basel, S Karger, 1985, pp 1–5.
27. Naidich TP, Lin JP, Leeds NE, et al: Primary tumors and other masses of the cerebellum and fourth ventricle: Differential diagnosis by computed tomography. Neuroradiology 14:153, 1977.
28. Obrador S, Blazquez MG: Benign cystic tumors of the cerebellum. Acta Neurochir (Wien) 32:55, 1975.
29. Page LK: Astrocytomas involving the cerebellar midline. In: Marlin A (ed): Concepts in Pediatric Neurosurgery, Vol. 7. Basel, S Karger, in press.
30. Raffel C, Edwards MSB, Davis RL, et al: Post-irradiation cerebellar glioma. J Neurosurg 62:300, 1985.
31. Raimondi AJ, Yashon D, Matsumoto S, et al: Increased intracranial pressure without lateralizing signs: The midline syndrome. Neurochirurgia 10:197, 1967.
32. Russell DS, Rubinstein LJ: Pathway of tumors of the nervous system. London, Arnold, 1977, pp 156–157.
33. Scott RM, Ballantine HT: Cerebellar astrocytoma: Malignant recurrence after prolonged postoperative survival. J Neurosurg 39:777, 1973.
34. Stein BM, Tenner MS, Fraser RA: Hydrocephalus following removal of cerebellar astrocytomas in children. J Neurosurg 36:763, 1972.
35. Steinberg GK, Shuer LM, Conley FK, et al: Evolution and outcome in malignant astroglial neoplasms of the cerebellum. J Neurosurg 62:9, 1985.
36. Swedlow DB: Anesthesia for neurosurgical procedures. In: Gregory G (ed): Pediatric Anesthesia. New York, Churchill Livingstone, 1983, pp 679–705.
37. Tomita T, Raimondi AJ: Fourth ventricle tumors. In: Pediatric Neurosurgery of the Developing Nervous System. New York, Grune & Stratton, 1982, pp 383–393.
38. Wilson CB: Diagnosis and surgical treatment of childhood brain tumors. Cancer 35:950, 1975.
39. Young RE: Cerebellar astrocytoma presenting as a cerebellar hemorrhage in a child. Neurology 30:1020, 1980.
40. Zimmerman RA, Bilaniuk LT, Bruno L, et al: Computed tomography of cerebellar astrocytoma. Am J Roentgenol 130:929, 1978.
41. Zimmerman RA, Bilaniuk LT, Pahlajani H: Spectrum of medulloblastomas as demonstrated by computed tomography. Radiology 126:137, 1977.
42. Zulch KJ: Histological Typing of Tumors of the Central Nervous System. Geneva, World Health Organization, 1979, p 44.

28
MEDULLOBLASTOMAS AND PRIMITIVE NEUROECTODERMAL TUMORS OF THE POSTERIOR FOSSA

Michael S. B. Edwards, M.D.
Roger J. Hudgins, M.D.

In 1925, Bailey and Cushing described 34 patients, most of them children, with a tumor they designated medulloblastoma to distinguish it pathologically from other tumors of the posterior fossa.[2] Five years later, Cushing published his experience with the surgical treatment of this tumor: Three years after surgery, only one of 61 patients was alive.[16] In 1953, the value of radiation therapy for medulloblastoma was emphasized by Patterson and Farr,[54] who reported a three-year survival rate of 53 percent in children treated with surgery and craniospinal irradiation. With the recent improvements in diagnostic capabilities, surgical techniques and technology, and adjuvant therapies, five-year survival rates of 60 percent or more can be expected in hospitals specializing in the care of children with central nervous system (CNS) cancer.

EPIDEMIOLOGY

Medulloblastoma is one of the most commonly occurring tumors of the posterior fossa and accounts for 4 to 10 percent of all primary brain tumors[61] and 15 to 20 percent of tumors in children.[53, 61] It occurs most frequently in children. The incidence curve reaches a plateau between ages three to eight years, with a peak at age eight,[14] but the tumor has been found in patients of all ages, from newborns to adults in the seventh decade.[61] There is a 2:1 predominance in males.[14, 60, 61] Familial occurrence is rare; only seven confirmed and six probable instances have been reported.[14] The authors treated two siblings who harbored medulloblastoma.

PATHOLOGY AND ETIOLOGY

The name medulloblastoma is derived from "pluripotential medulloblast," which Bailey and Cushing proposed as the cell of origin. However, this primitive cell has never been identified, and most neuroembryologists believe that it does not exist. Medulloblastoma most often occurs in the midline and arises in the inferior medullary velum of the cerebellum. The tumor grows to occupy the fourth ventricle and tends to infiltrate surrounding areas. In their review of 135 cases, Park and associates[53] found that the tumor infiltrated the vermis alone in

We thank Cindy Huff for typing the manuscript in draft and Neil Buckley for editing it.

30 percent of cases, and the brainstem in 32 percent; extended into the cerebellar hemisphere in 31 percent; and was limited to one cerebellar hemisphere in 7 percent.[53] Grossly, the tumors are soft and friable and may have central areas of necrosis. Focal hemorrhage occurs in 15 percent of these tumors.[39] Calcification is uncommon.

Medulloblastoma commonly spreads along cerebrospinal fluid (CSF) pathways, and metastatic lesions have been identified in over half the cases seen at autopsy.[60] Myelographic evidence of spinal metastases with no clinical evidence of cord involvement is found at the time of first surgery in 11 to 43 percent of patients.[20, 21] Spinal metastases are most commonly found in children younger than five years of age. Extraneural metastases occur much less frequently. Kessler and coworkers[36] reviewed the literature up to 1975 and identified 53 cases of extraneural metastases, many of which appeared to be related to preoperative shunting. Remote metastases most frequently involve the bone marrow and cervical lymph nodes.

Histologically, medulloblastoma is a highly cellular tumor composed of round to oval cells with hyperchromatic nuclei and scant cytoplasm (Fig. 28–1). A large number of mitotic figures are usually present. Homer-Wright rosettes, which suggest neuronal differentiation, are found in less than one third of cases, but the "pseudorosettes" described by Bailey and Cushing are characteristic of and diagnostic for medulloblastoma.[60] "Pseudorosettes" are composed of carrot-shaped cells surrounding an eosinophilic center. A desmoplastic variant that has been identified usually occurs in the cerebellar hemispheres of young adults.[35, 60] It is characteristically well-demarcated from the surrounding cerebellum, is firm, almost woody on cut surface, and has a propensity to involve the meninges.[8]

In 1934, Stevenson and Echlin[65] proposed that medulloblastoma arises from remnants of the fetal external granular layer, which is present in the infant cerebellum and then moves through the molecular layer to form the internal granular layer. This theory can be reconciled with the proposal of Raaf and Kernohan[57] that medulloblastoma arises from cell nests in the inferior medullary velum; there is evidence that the external granular cells originate in the neuroepithelial roof of the fourth ventricle and migrate laterally to form the external granular layer.

Recently, Rorke[59] proposed that medulloblastomas be included in the group of tumors designated primitive neuroectodermal tumors (PNET) by Hart and Earle.[31] This reclassification is based on the tenet that medulloblastoma is not unique to the cerebellum but is similar histologically to other CNS tumors that arise from neoplastic transformation of primitive neuroepithelial cells. In Rorke's model, origination from the external granular cell implies that differentiation would occur along neuronal lines only, which does not explain the frequent tendency of medulloblastoma to differentiate along spongioblastic and glial lines. However, Rorke proposes that all PNETs, including medulloblastoma, arise from the pool of undifferentiated cells found in the subependymal region of the fetus. This model implies that tumors may differentiate along multiple cell lines and thus provides an embryologic justification for grouping together the primary intracranial, small, round cell tumors such as medulloblastoma, pineoblastoma, and ependymoblastomas.

CLINICAL FEATURES

Because medulloblastomas grow rapidly, the duration of symptoms before presentation is usually short, averaging two months in the series of Choux and Lena.[13] The first signs and symptoms are usually related to hydrocephalus caused by the tumor obstructing the CSF pathways. In their review of 676 children with medulloblastoma, Choux and Lena found headache, vomiting, and papilledema in 80 percent of patients. Infants with open sutures usually have no signs of increased intracranial pres-

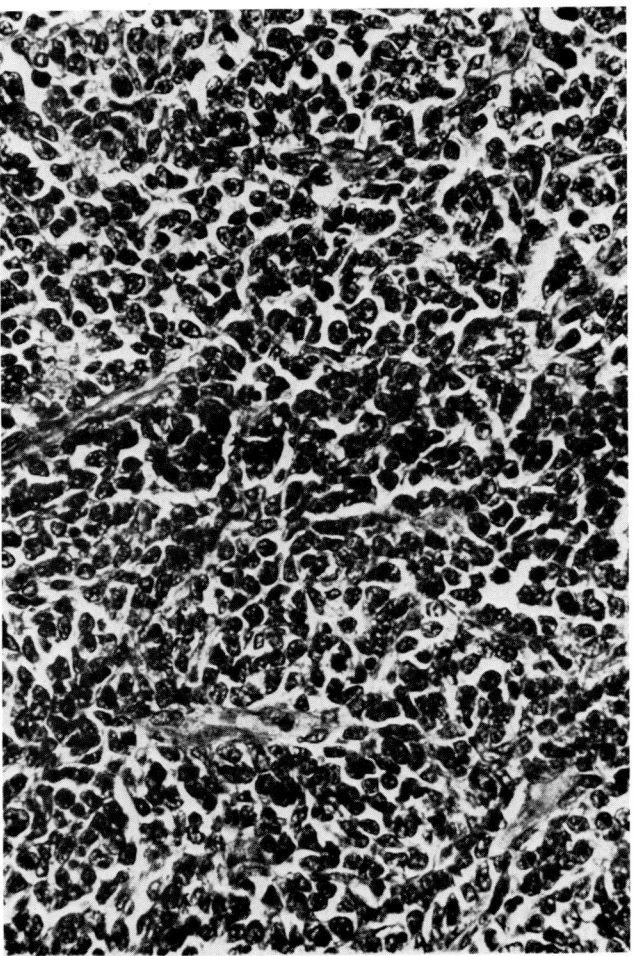

Figure 28–1. Typical medulloblastoma pathology showing highly cellular tumor with small, round uniform cells and numerous vascular channels (× 160).

sure but may present with accelerated head growth and irritability. Transient intracranial pressure waves may be associated with episodes of stiffening and extension of the neck and extremities, apnea, and bradycardia secondary to cerebellar tonsillar herniation.[48]

Ataxia is the symptom that most frequently leads to a diagnostic radiographic study. Truncal ataxia, which is the result of the midline position of the tumor, is commonly found, and coordination in the extremities is usually relatively spared. Except for an abducens palsy secondary to increased intracranial pressure, cranial nerve deficits are uncommon. Long tract findings may be present if there is pressure on the brainstem caused by the tumor, hydrocephalus, or chronic tonsillar herniation. Impaction of the cerebellar tonsils may also cause neck pain, a head tilt, or both. Although the duration of symptoms is usually shorter for medulloblastoma, there are no reliable findings in the history or neurologic examination that can be used to differentiate between medulloblastoma and other tumors that arise in the posterior fossa.

RADIOLOGY

During the last ten years, computed tomography (CT) has supplanted ventriculography and angiography as the radiologic procedure of choice for the diagnosis and postoperative follow-up of medulloblastoma. CT findings that characterize medulloblastoma are a midline mass lesion, the density of which is slightly increased compared with that of normal brain and that enhances homogeneously after administration of contrast material (Fig. 28–2).[42, 50, 74] Atypical features such as the presence of a cystic or necrotic component, calcification, hemorrhage, lack of contrast enhancement, and eccentric position may occur in up to 47 percent of patients.[72, 73] The tumor frequently fills the fourth ventricle, extending inferiorly to the obex or cisterna magna and superiorly to the aqueduct of Sylvius. It may grow through the foramen of Luschka and invade the cerebellopontine angle. Hydrocephalus that is usually present is caused by the tumor filling and obstructing the fourth ventricle or the aqueduct.

Since it became available, nuclear magnetic resonance imaging (NMRI) has replaced CT as the primary modality for imaging medulloblastoma.[7, 37] NMRI provides high-resolution images of the tumor and associated abnormalities such as hydrocephalus in sagittal, coronal, and axial planes without the use of intravenous contrast material or ionizing radiation (Fig. 28–3). Medulloblastoma characteristically has T1-weighted images with low signal intensities but has high signal intensities on T2-weighted images.

Because NMRI does not produce images of bone, the problem of partial volume averaging that occurs

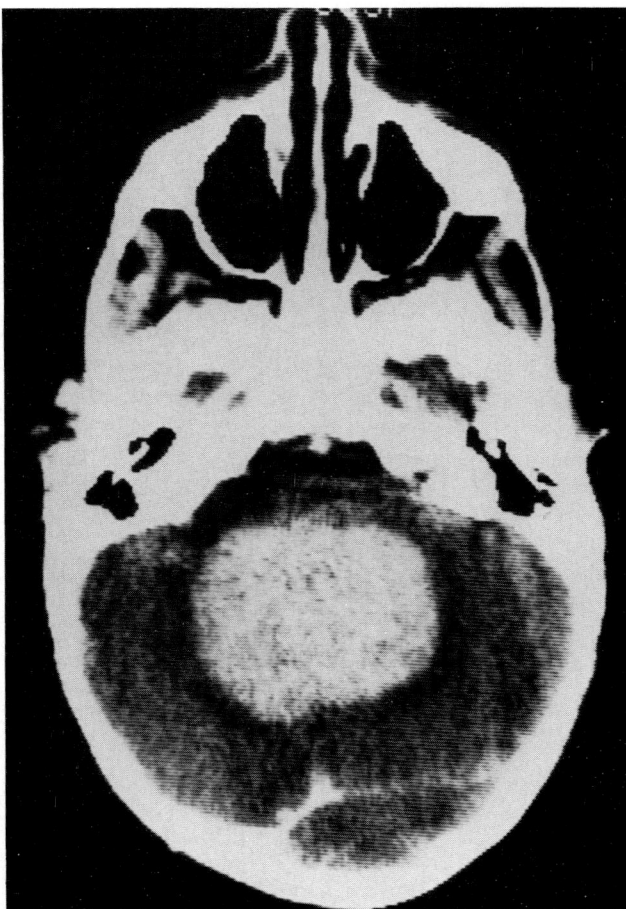

Figure 28–2. Axial, contrast-enhanced CT scan shows a large contrast-enhancing medulloblastoma in the midline that fills the fourth ventricle.

with CT and limits studies of the posterior fossa is avoided. However, NMRI is limited because calcium within a tumor cannot be identified and because it is difficult to differentiate between tumor and edema on the basis of relaxation times. Calcification and edema can be seen readily on CT scans, and it may be necessary to obtain both studies. The use of surface coils should improve the resolution of NMRI, and it may eventually supersede myelography for postoperative staging. However, it is unfortunate that there is no radiologic modality that can, with certainty, distinguish medulloblastoma from other posterior fossa tumors.

SURGERY

A complete history must be taken, and thorough physical and neurologic examinations must be performed. Although a child is usually stable enough to allow a complete assessment to be made, in some patients rapid progression of tumor or a significant rate of neurologic deterioration may dictate emergency intervention. Deterioration is usually caused by the associated hydrocephalus. After hydrocephalus is confirmed by radiologic studies, it can be

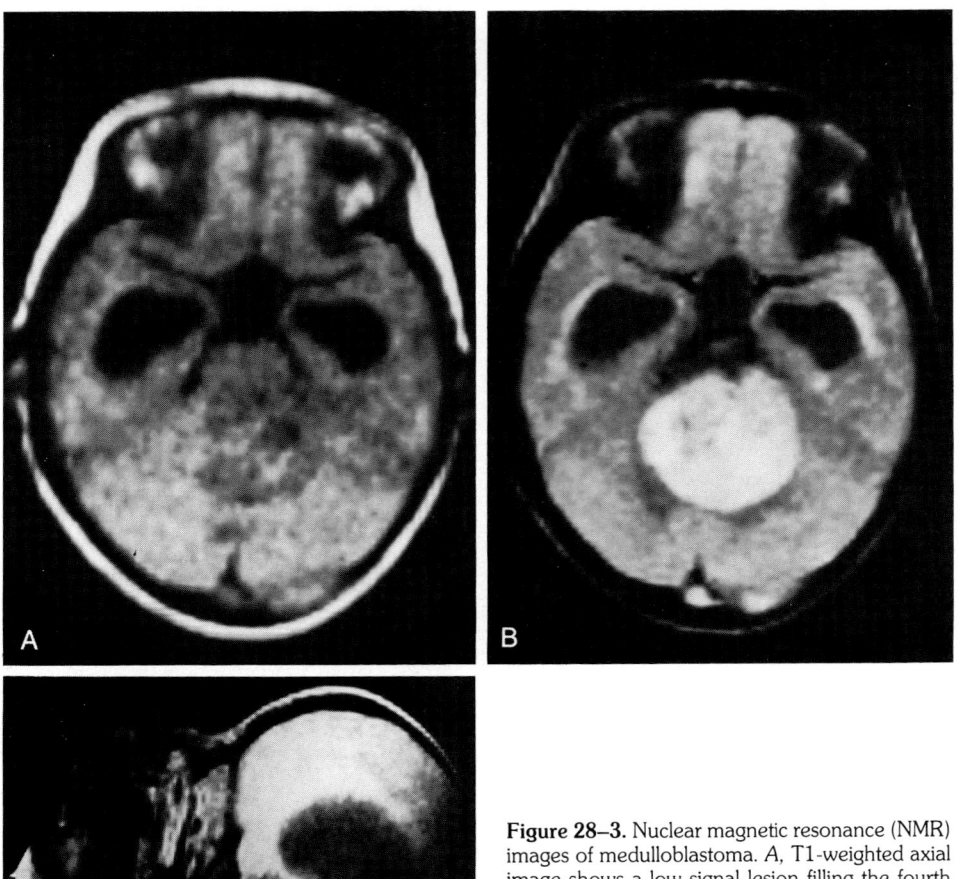

Figure 28–3. Nuclear magnetic resonance (NMR) images of medulloblastoma. *A*, T1-weighted axial image shows a low signal lesion filling the fourth ventricle. Temporal horns are dilated from obstructive hydrocephalus. *B*, A T2-weighted axial image; increasing the weight makes the lesion more visible. *C*, Sagittal NMR image shows a medulloblastoma that fills the fourth ventricle and bows the brainstem forward and the cerebellum posteriorly. The lesion extends from the tentorium, superiorly, to the midmedulla, inferiorly.

reversed or stabilized by external ventricular drainage, treatment with corticosteroids, or both. In the presence of a posterior fossa mass, upward herniation[32] and intratumoral hemorrhage[69, 70] may occur upon draining the ventricles. This risk can be lessened by continuously monitoring intracranial pressure and draining only that volume of CSF necessary to maintain intracranial pressure within normal ranges. Other measures that might be employed include intubation and hyperventilation, administration of steroids, and intravenous infusion of mannitol. It is fortunate that emergency measures are usually not necessary, and there is usually time for a complete work-up before surgery.

The authors prefer to operate with the patient in the prone position because it reduces the risk of air embolus, frontal pneumocephalus, and hypotension associated with the sitting position.[34] If hydrocephalus is present, an occipital burr hole is placed, and a catheter is passed into the ventricle. The authors avoid the risk of upward herniation by delaying drainage of CSF until they are ready to open the dura over the posterior fossa.

A vertical, midline incision beginning just above the inion and extending into the upper cervical region is made. Blood loss may be minimized by using the Shaw hemostatic scalpel. A generous craniectomy is performed to ensure exposure and to minimize the need to retract the cerebellum. Most medulloblastomas extend caudally to the obex and even beyond, and it is necessary to remove the posterior arch of C1 to maximize exposure. It should be remembered that the C1 ring is cartilaginous in infants and young children, and care should be taken not to cut through it with the scalpel.

If the dura is tight even with hyperventilation (pCO_2 = 25 mm Hg), intracranial pressure is lowered by draining CSF via the ventricular catheter. The authors prefer to control intracranial pressure by CSF drainage only, and not by administration of mannitol; in combination, the two approaches may cause an increased incidence of postoperative pneumocephalus and subdural hematoma. Mannitol is used only if there is no hydrocephalus.

Because of the large, midline occipital sinus in children, the dura is opened with a Y-shaped incision, trapping the sinus between hemoclips at the junction of the upper limbs of the Y.[34] The lower limb is then opened in a paramedian fashion to avoid opening the sinus further.

The cisterna magna is opened, and a cotton patty is placed to prevent blood, tumor, or both from collecting in the cistern. The operating microscope is brought into the field. Frequently, the tumor is visible at the vallecula, protruding into the cisterna magna. Tomita and McClone[66] have shown that CSF or arachnoid from the cisterna magna almost invariably has evidence of seeding of medulloblastoma cells. The significance of this finding is unknown, but it is not a contraindication for radical resection of tumor.

The floor of the fourth ventricle is identified and a cotton patty is placed between the tumor and the brainstem. The vermis is then split, and tumor debulking is begun. Frequently, the tumor is friable, and a constant oozing of blood occurs until the majority of tumor has been removed. It is usually easy to control bleeding with bipolar coagulation and by applying gentle pressure with cotton balls soaked in warm saline. By using the Cavitron Ultrasonic Aspirator (CUSA), the CO_2 laser, or both, tumor can be removed rapidly without moving or causing traction on adjacent vital neural structures.

As internal debulking of the tumor is continued, it becomes possible to dissect the edge of the tumor free from the floor of the fourth ventricle; this area and the cerebellar peduncles are occasionally invaded by tumor. The laser is useful for the excision of small fragments of tumor from these areas.[23] Total tumor resection should be accomplished whenever possible to reduce the tumor burden for subsequent therapy.

Meticulous hemostasis is achieved before closure. An absorbable hemostat (Surgicel or Avitene) may be used to line the tumor bed, but care should be taken that these substances are secure and will not float free and block CSF pathways. The bone edges and mastoid air cells are then rewaxed thoroughly to avoid postoperative CSF otorrhea. The dura is closed in a watertight fashion; if the dura is inadequate for a tight closure, pericranium, muscle fascia, or artificial substances can be used.

If careful technique is used and there is meticulous attention to detail, the operative mortality rate should approach zero,[33] and the morbidity rate should be 5 to 10 percent. Children commonly have increased ataxia, mild facial paresis, or oculomotor dysfunction in the immediate postoperative period, but these usually clear with time. Postoperative aphasia that lasts days to weeks is a rare finding that is the result in part of decompression of hydrocephalus.

Postoperatively, intracranial pressure is controlled by drainage of CSF through the external ventricular drain. Intracranial pressure is maintained at 15 mm Hg for the first 24 hours and, in an attempt to open CSF pathways, is allowed to rise to 20 mm Hg for the next 24 hours, after which the drain is shut off. If the child tolerates this well, the catheter is removed; if not, a ventriculoperitoneal shunt is inserted. With this protocol and with surgical unblocking of the aqueduct, the authors have found that 60 percent of children do not require placement of a ventriculoperitoneal shunt. Because of the high percentage of children who will not require shunting and because of the risk of shunt-related metastases,[32, 36] the authors prefer not to place a shunt preoperatively.

A slow steroid taper is begun four to seven days after surgery and is continued for two to six weeks. A small maintenance dose of steroids is continued during radiation therapy, to ameliorate the side effects of radiation. A slow steroid taper may reduce the incidence of aseptic meningitis associated with surgery in the posterior fossa, seen with more rapid tapers.[9]

POSTOPERATIVE STAGING AND FOLLOW-UP

CT scans with and without contrast enhancement are obtained within the first 72 hours after surgery to assess the extent of tumor resection. Areas of contrast enhancement seen within this period probably represent residual tumor, and a noncontrast CT scan is obtained to differentiate blood from enhancing tumor. A myelogram is obtained two weeks after surgery to assess possible spinal subarachnoid seeding (Fig. 28–4). Spinal disease is confirmed by myelography in 11 to 43 percent of cases.[19, 21]

Cytologic studies and levels of the polyamines putrescine and spermidine are determined in CSF collected at myelography two weeks after surgery; for the first full year after surgery, CSF is collected every two to three months for cytologic studies and determination of polyamine levels. Elevation of polyamine levels (especially putrescine) above the postoperative baseline is predictive of recurrence, occasionally before there is clinical or radiographic evidence.[45, 46] Myelography, which is repeated at intervals of four to six months during the first year, may be supplanted by spinal NMRI for the assess-

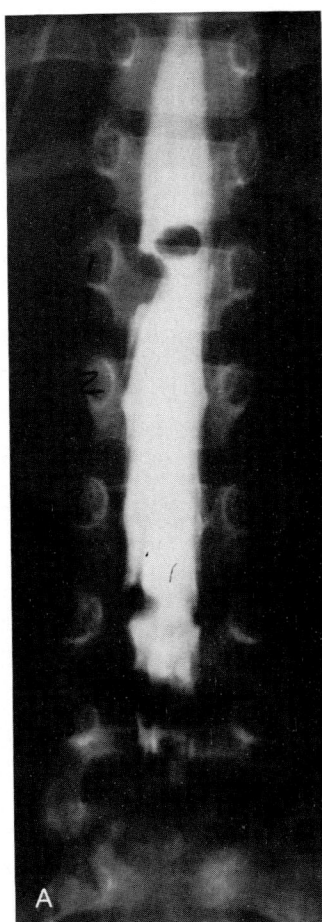
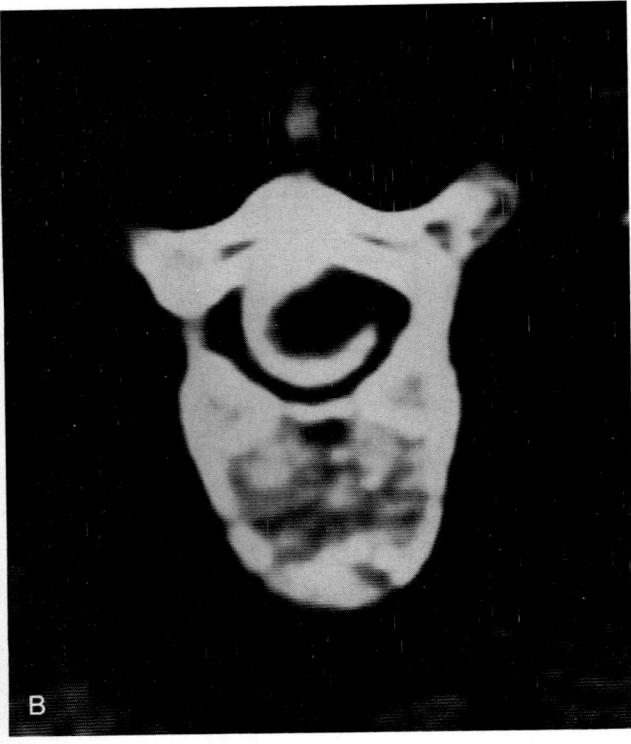

Figure 28–4. *A*, Postoperative staging myelogram shows multiple filling defects in the lumbar region that are consistent with disseminated medulloblastoma. *B*, Metrizamide-enhanced CT scan confirms the presence of medulloblastoma in the lumbar subarachnoid space.

ment of the presence or absence of spinal metastases. Studies are currently under way at the School of Medicine of the University of California, San Francisco, to determine the relative sensitivities of NMRI and myelography. CT or, if available, NMRI of the brain and posterior fossa is performed every two or three months for the first two years.

POSTOPERATIVE TREATMENT AND RESULTS

Although Cushing's early attempt to irradiate medulloblastoma postoperatively was ineffective, the efficacy of using larger fields and higher doses was firmly established by Cutler and colleagues,[17] Lampe and MacIntyre,[40] and Penfield and Feindel[55] in the 1930's and 1940's. In 1953, Patterson and Farr[54] reported that craniospinal irradiation improved survival rate.

In current practice, the whole brain is irradiated through lateral opposing ports to a dose of 3500 to 4500 rad, with a boost to the posterior fossa to deliver 5000 to 5500 rad to the tumor bed. The spinal cord is irradiated to 3000 to 4000 rad through a posterior port.[4, 5, 15, 29, 44, 49, 63] It is well-documented[4, 5, 15, 63] that irradiation of the posterior fossa to at least 5000 rad produces a much lower incidence of both posterior fossa recurrence and CNS and extra-CNS metastases.

Recurrent medulloblastoma is responsive to a wide variety of drugs, including nitrosoureas, procarbazine, vincristine, cyclophosphamide, aziridinylbenzoquinone, cisplatin, and dibromodulcitol.[43] Despite this known sensitivity to chemotherapeutic intervention, most studies have found either no difinite efficacy of adjuvant chemotherapy[62, 68] or a benefit only for poor-risk patients.[27] Two large, randomized studies have evaluated the efficacy of adjuvant chemotherapy in the treatment of medulloblastoma.[27] In the study conducted by the International Society of Pediatric Oncology (SIOP), surgery and irradiation alone were compared with surgery, irradiation, and adjuvant chemotherapy with vincristine-CCNU (lomustine). Vincristine was given weekly during irradiation, and both drugs were continued over a one-year maintenance period. Adjuvant chemotherapy showed no clear benefit compared with surgery and irradiation alone in the 287 patients entered into the study. Children who have undergone subtotal resection, those under two years of age, and those with brainstem involvement did appear to benefit, however. The Children's Cancer Study Group (CCSG) used a similar randomized protocol with the addition of prednisone in 198 children. The only benefit of chemotherapy found was for children with more advanced disease such as tumors that invade the brainstem or metastatic lesions from the primary tumor.

The use of modern techniques including microneurosurgical tumor resection, megavoltage radiation therapy, and possibly chemotherapy has significantly increased the survival rate in children with medulloblastoma. In the 1930's, the five-year survival rate was essentially zero; many centers now report five-year survival rates of 60 percent or greater in good-risk patients.[12, 49, 53]

PROGNOSIS

Several factors that affect the incidence of recurrence and the survival rate of children with medulloblastoma are discussed in the following.

Age. The survival rate for children younger than three years of age is very low. Chin and Marvyama[11] found a survival rate of 17 percent in children three years of age or younger, compared with a survival rate of 63 percent for children aged three to six years. This dismal outcome in infants appears to be related to dissemination of disease by the time of presentation and to the lower tolerance of the infant brain to the effects of radiation;[1, 12] therefore, radiation doses are compromised.

Sex. There are many reports that females have better survival rates than do males.[6, 30, 51, 58] Others have reported that there is no difference in survival rate according to sex,[5, 47] while still others have reported longer survivals in males.[13] Females appear to have little, if any, survival advantage.

Tumor Location and Extent. At presentation, myelography has demonstrated spinal subarachnoid seeding of medulloblastoma in 11 to 30 percent of patients.[19, 21] It is readily apparent that dissemination of disease either within the CNS or systemically is a poor prognostic factor, which was confirmed by the findings of both the SIOP and CCSG trials. For this reason, postoperative staging of myelography is essential to planning of subsequent therapy and to determining the prognosis.

Tumor Histology. Although it has been stated that the lateralized desmoplastic variant of medulloblastoma has a better prognosis,[10, 35] Hoffman and coworkers[33] and Choux and Lena[13] have reported that patients with this variant have poorer survival rates than that found for patients with midline lesions. Results reported recently by the Childhood Brain Tumor Consortium for a series of 512 patients with medulloblastoma show that survival of the 87 patients with the desmoplastic variant was not significantly different from survival for the other patients with midline tumors. Information that is currently available suggests that patients who harbor the laterally placed desmoplastic variant lesion have poorer survivals.[28]

Based on Rorke's PNET classification, Packer and associates[52] divided medulloblastomas into two groups, those that show differentiation along glial, neuronal, or ependymal cell lines (PNET-D) and those that are undifferentiated (PNET-U). They found four-year survival rates of 72 percent for patients with PNET-U and 32 percent for patients with PNET-D ($p = 0.004$). They felt that undifferentiated tumors did better either because they are more sensitive to radiation or because differentiated tumors, which may have a longer period of growth, are more likely to disseminate.

Extent of Surgical Resection. Radical or aggressive subtotal resection is preferable to partial resection or biopsy. Hoffman and colleagues[33] reported five-year survival rates of 59 percent for radical excision, 49 percent for subtotal excision, and 30 percent for partial excision or biopsy. Raimondi and Tomita[58] reported five-year survival rates of 42 percent for patients with total resection versus 30 percent for patients with partial resection or biopsy. The SIOP and the CCSG studies found no difference in survival rate between patients with total and patients with subtotal (80 percent) removal of tumor mass.[12]

Based on this information, we can define two prognostic groups of children with medulloblastoma. The high-risk group is defined by the presence of any one of the following criteria: (1) age less than two years, (2) less than 75 percent tumor resected, (3) leptomeningeal spread, (4) metastatic disease, and (5) tumor cells in the CSF more than two weeks after surgery. The low-risk group is defined by (1) age greater than two years, (2) more than 75 percent of tumor resected, (3) no evidence of tumor spread from the primary site. Based on these criteria, appropriate treatment and surveillance for recurrence can be determined. Children in the high-risk group are treated with chemotherapy before and after craniospinal irradiation; children in the low-risk group are not treated with chemotherapy, and the dose of radiation to the whole brain and spinal cord is decreased to 2400 rad in an attempt to decrease the effects of late sequelae.

TREATMENT SEQUELAE

Although radiation therapy and chemotherapy are obviously critical to the treatment of medulloblastoma, these modalities may adversely affect the developing brains of children. There is growing interest in the sequelae of lowered intelligence, endocrine dysfunction, and poor social behavior in patients treated with these modalities.[3, 18, 22, 64] Duffner and coworkers[22] evaluated the effects of radiation therapy on the intelligence of ten children with posterior fossa tumors, six of whom had medulloblastoma. Each patient had a deterioration of at least 25 points in a full-scale intelligence quotient test. All children had evidence of dementia, learning disabilities, or intellectual retardation. Radiation can also cause endocrine dysfunction, especially decreased growth hormone production,[12, 14] and spinal irradiation may cause myelotoxicity and reduced axial growth.[56, 67]

Because of the high-risk of whole brain and spinal irradiation and because most recurrences of medulloblastoma occur in the posterior fossa,[63] the authors have reduced the radiation dose to the whole brain and spinal cord to 2500 rad but continue to boost the dose to the posterior fossa to 5500 rad in patients who have no evidence of CNS metastatic disease. Since 1979, 37 patients have been irradiated on this protocol, which includes combination therapy with procarbazine, 100 mg/m²/day for two weeks before irradiation, and hydroxyurea administered three times a week during irradiation (Brain Tumor Research Center Protocol 7922). There were 13 recurrences during this period, with only one recurrence in the spinal cord. Tomita and McClone[67] have reported control of medulloblastoma, using a similar low-dose neuroaxis irradiation protocol.[67] The authors feel that decreasing the dose of radiation to the whole brain and spinal cord in low-risk patients has little or no effect on the failure rate but may lessen the severity of radiation sequelae.

MANAGEMENT OF RECURRENCE

Latchaw and associates[41] have reviewed the period of risk for recurrence of medulloblastoma and have concluded that Collin's law of congenital tumors is applicable to medulloblastoma. This law, originally proposed for Wilms's tumor, states that patients may be considered cured if they survive for a period of time exceeding the sum of their age at diagnosis plus nine months (gestational age). They found that less than 2 percent of patients with medulloblastomas violate Collin's law. Kun and coworkers[38] found that 70 percent of recurrences occur within two years of initial therapy. Unfortunately, late recurrences, some of which appear more than ten years after initial treatment, are well-documented.

If tumor recurs in the posterior fossa of a child who is doing well and who has no evidence of metastatic disease, reoperation may be considered. Resection of bulky recurrent tumor reduces the tumor burden for subsequent radiation therapy and chemotherapy.

Both single-agent and combination chemotherapy have been used extensively to treat recurrent medulloblastoma.[27] Unfortunately, responses to many of these regimens have been transient, but Levin and colleagues[44] recently reported long-term survival in patients treated sequentially with various combinations of either or both systemic and intraventricular chemotherapeutic agents. When these agents failed or when myelosuppression became so severe that chemotherapy was not possible, the patients were reirradiated.[44] This treatment led to a median survival after recurrence of two years, and 25 percent quartile survivals of 2.9 years. (Chemotherapy of recurrent medulloblastoma is discussed in the works by Edwards and coworkers,[24-26] and Friedman and Schold.[27])

Reirradiation and chemotherapy are considered for patients who have undergone resection of bulky recurrent tumors in the posterior fossa or for patients with metastatic disease outside the posterior fossa. The authors recently reported results of a phase I/II study of reirradiation for recurrent malignant brain tumors in children.[71] Included in the study group were 16 children with recurrent medulloblastoma, all of whom had previously received what is currently believed to be the maximum safe dose of radiation. All received a focal tumor boost of 3000 rad, and 15 of 16 underwent reirradiation of the spine. Misonidazole was given as a radiosensitizing agent but produced no apparent benefit. Median survival after treatment was 20 months, with a median time to progression of 11 months. Twenty-one percent of the 29 patients in the study group developed radiation toxicity; this toxicity proved fatal in two children. The results are comparable with those reported for children receiving salvage chemotherapy for recurrent brain tumors.

Despite the primitive, aggressive nature of medulloblastoma, it is now a "curable" tumor in a significant number of affected children. The use of modern techniques, including NMRI, microneurosurgical radical tumor excision, megavoltage radiation therapy, and appropriate chemotherapy, has significantly improved survival. Improvements in survival have been gained at the expense of disorders of endocrine function and intellectual and psychosocial development in some children. The treatment of recurrent disease remains palliative in almost all children. Present studies have been designed to improve survival and to decrease the late effects of therapy.

References

1. Allen JC, Epstein F: Medulloblastoma and other primary malignant neuroectodermal tumors of the CNS. J Neurosurg 57:446, 1982.
2. Bailey P, Cushing H: Medulloblastoma cerebelli, a common type of mid-cerebellar glioma of childhood. Arch Neurol 14:192, 1925.
3. Bamford FN, Jones PM, Pearson D, et al: Residual disabilities in children treated for intracranial space-occupying lesions. Cancer 37:1149, 1976.
4. Bellani FF, Gasparini M, Lombardi F, et al: Medulloblastoma: Results of a sequential combined treatment. Cancer 54:1956, 1984.
5. Berry MP, Jenkin DT, Keen CW, et al: Radiation treatment for medulloblastoma. J Neurosurg 55:43, 1981.

6. Bloom HIG, Wallace Enic, Henk JM: The treatment and prognosis of medulloblastoma in children: A study of 82 verified cases. Am J Roentgenol 105:43, 1969.
7. Brant-Zawadzki M, Badarni JP, Mills CM, et al: Primary intracranial tumor imaging: A comparison of magnetic resonance and CT. Radiology 150:435, 1984.
8. Burger PC, Vogel FS: Surgical pathology of the nervous system and its coverings. New York, John Wiley and Sons, 1976, pp 292–299.
9. Carmel PW, Fraser AR, Stein BM: Aseptic meningitis following posterior fossa surgery in children. J Neurosurg 41:44, 1974.
10. Chatty EM, Earle KM: Medulloblastoma: A report of 201 cases with emphasis on the relationship of histologic variants to survival. Cancer 28:977, 1971.
11. Chin HW, Marvyama Y: Early response—long-term results in the radiotherapy of childhood medulloblastoma. J Neurol Oncol 1:53, 1983.
12. Chin HW, Marvyama Y, Young AB: Medulloblastoma: Recent advances and directions in diagnosis and management, Part II. Curr Probl Cancer 8:1, 1984.
13. Choux M, Lena G: Medulloblastoma. Neurochirurgie 28:13, 1982.
14. Choux M, Lena MD, Hassoun JH: Prognosis and long-term follow-up in patients with medulloblastoma. Clin Neurosurg 13:246, 1983.
15. Cuberlin RL, Luk KH, Wara WM, et al: Medulloblastoma: Treatment results and effects in normal tissue. Cancer 43:1014, 1979.
16. Cushing H: Experience with cerebellar medulloblastoma: Critical review. Acta Pathol Microbiol Immunol Scand 7:1, 1930.
17. Cutler E, Sosman M, Vaughn W: The place of radiation in the treatment of medulloblastoma: Report of 20 cases. Am J Roentgenol 35:429, 1936.
18. Danoff BF, Cowchock FS, Marquette C, et al: Assessment of the long-term effects of primary radiation therapy for brain tumors in children. Cancer 49:1580, 1982.
19. Deutsch M: The impact of myelography on the treatment results for medulloblastoma. Int J Rad Oncol 10:999, 1984.
20. Deutsch M, Reigel DH: The value of myelography in the management of childhood medulloblastoma. Cancer 45:2194, 1980.
21. Dorwart RH, Wara WM, Norman D, et al: Complete myelographic evaluation of spinal metastases from medulloblastoma. Radiology 139:403, 1981.
22. Duffner PK, Cohen ME, Thomas P: Late effects of treatment on the intelligence of children with posterior fossa tumors. Cancer 51:233, 1983.
23. Edwards MSB, Boggan JE, Fuller T: The laser in neurological surgery. J Neurosurg 59:555, 1983.
24. Edwards MS, Levin VA, Seager ML, et al: Intrathecal chemotherapy for leptomeningeal dissemination of medulloblastoma. Child's Brain 8:444, 1981.
25. Edwards MS, Levin VA, Wilson CB: Brain tumor chemotherapy: An evaluation of agents in current use for Phase II and III trials. Cancer Treat Rep 64:1179, 1980.
26. Edwards MSB, Levin VA, Wilson CB: Chemotherapy of recurrent posterior fossa tumors. Clin Neurosurg 30:209, 1983.
27. Friedman HS, Schold SC: Rational approaches to the chemotherapy of medulloblastoma. Neurol Clin 3:843, 1985.
28. Gillis F: Personal communication, 1986.
29. Halpern EL, Burger PC: Conventional external beam radiotherapy for central nervous system malignancies. Neurol Clin 3:867, 1985.
30. Harisiadis L, Chang CH: Medulloblastoma in children: A correlation between staging and results of treatment. Int J Radiat Oncol Biol Phys 2:833, 1977.
31. Hart MN, Earle KM: Primitive neuroectodermal tumors of the brain in children. Cancer 32:890, 1973.
32. Hoffman HJ, Hendrick EB, Humphreys RP: Metastasis via ventriculoperitoneal shunt in patients with medulloblastoma. J Neurosurg 32:83, 1970.
33. Hoffman HJ, Hendricks EB, Humphreys RP: Management of medulloblastoma in childhood. Clin Neurosurg 30:226, 1982.
34. Hudgins RJ, Edwards MSB: Infratentorial brain tumors. Rev Neurosurg (in press).
35. Hughes PG: Cerebellar medulloblastoma in adults. J Neurosurg 60:994, 1984.
36. Kessler CA, Dugan P, Concannon JP: Systemic metastases of medulloblastoma promoted by shunting. Surg Neurol 3:147, 1975.
37. Kulkarni MV, Kirchner SG, Price RR, et al: Magnetic resonance imaging in pediatrics. Pediatr Clin North Am 32:1509, 1985.
38. Kun LE, D'Souza B, Tefft M: The value of surveillance testing in childhood brain tumors. Cancer 56:1818, 1985.
39. Lament JP, Bruce DA, Schut L: Hemorrhagic brain tumors in pediatric patients. Child's Brain 8:263, 1981.
40. Lampe I, MacIntyre RS: Medulloblastoma of cerebellum. Arch Neurol 62:322, 1949.
41. Latchaw JP, Hahn J, Moylan DJ, et al: Medulloblastoma: Period of risk reviewed. Cancer 55:186, 1985.
42. Lee Y-Y, Glass JP, Eys J, et al: Medulloblastoma in infants and children: Computed tomographic follow-up after treatment. Radiology 154:677, 1985.
43. Levin VA: Chemotherapy of primary brain tumors. Neurol Clin 3:855, 1985.
44. Levin VA, Vestnys PS, Edwards MS, et al: Improvement in survival produced by sequential therapies in the treatment of recurrent medulloblastoma. Cancer 51:1364, 1983.
45. Marton LJ, Edwards MS, Levin VA: Predictive value of cerebrospinal fluid polyamines in medulloblastoma. Cancer Res 39:993, 1979.
46. Marton LJ, Edwards MS, Levin VA, et al: CSF polyamines: A new and important means of monitoring patients with medulloblastoma. Cancer 47:757, 1981.
47. Mealey J, Hall PV: Medulloblastoma in children: Survival and treatment. J Neurosurg 46:56, 1977.
48. Milhorat TH: Pediatric Neurosurgery. Philadelphia, F.A. Davis, 1979, pp 216–223.
49. Norris DG, Bruce C, Byrd RL, et al: Improved relapse-free survival in medulloblastoma utilizing modern techniques. Neurosurgery 9:661, 1981.
50. North C, Segall HD, Stanley P, et al: Early CT detection of intracranial seeding from medulloblastoma. AJNR 6:11, 1985.
51. Nuchel B, Anderson AP: Medulloblastoma: Treatment and results. Acta Radiol Ther Phys Biol 17:305, 1978.
52. Packer RJ, Sutton LN, Rorke LB, et al: Prognostic importance of cellular differentiation in medulloblastoma of childhood. J Neurosurg 61:296, 1984.
53. Park TS, Hoffman HJ, Hendricks EB, et al: Medulloblastoma: Clinical presentation and management. J Neurosurg 58:543, 1983.
54. Patterson E, Farr RF: Cerebellar medulloblastoma treated by irradiation of the whole CNS. Acta Radiol 39:323, 1953.
55. Penfield W, Feindel J: Medulloblastoma of cerebellum with survival for seventeen years. Arch Neurol 57:481, 1947.
56. Probert JC, Parker BR, Kaplan HS: Growth retardation in children after megavoltage irradiation of the spine. Cancer 32:634, 1973.
57. Raaf J, Kernohan JW: Relation of abnormal collections of cells in posterior medullary velum of cerebellum to origin of medulloblastoma. Arch Neurol 52:163, 1944.
58. Raimondi AJ, Tomita T: Medulloblastoma in childhood: Comparative results of partial and total resection. Child's Brain 5:310, 1979.
59. Rorke LB: The cerebellar medulloblastoma and its relationship to primitive neuroectodermal tumors. J Neuropathol Exp Neurol 42:1, 1983.
60. Rubenstein LJ: Tumors of the Central Nervous System, fasc. 6. In: Atlas of Tumor Pathology. Washington, DC, Armed Forces Institute of Pathology, 1972, pp 130–153.
61. Schut L, Bruce DA, Sutton LN: Medulloblastoma. In: Wilkins RH, Rengachary SS (eds): Neurosurgery. New York, McGraw-Hill, 1985, pp 758–762.

62. Seiler RW, Bernasconi S, Berchtold W, et al: Swiss pediatric oncology group: Adjuvant chemotherapy with procarbazine, vincristine and prednisone for medulloblastoma: A preliminary report. Helv Paediatr Acta 36:249, 1981.
63. Silverman CL, Simpson JR: Cerebellar medulloblastoma: The importance of posterior fossa dose to survival and patterns of failure. Int J Radiat Oncol Biol Phys 8:1869, 1982.
64. Spunberg JJ, Chang CH, Goldman M, et al: Quality of long-term survival following radiation for intracranial tumors in children under the age of two. Int J Radiat Oncol Biol Phys 7:727, 1981.
65. Stevenson L, Echlin F: Nature and origin of some tumors of the cerebellum-medulloblastoma. Arch Neurol 31:93, 1934.
66. Tomita T, McClone DG: Spontaneous seeding of medulloblastoma: Results of cerebrospinal fluid cytology and arachnoid biopsy from the cisterna magna. Neurosurgery 12:265, 1983.
67. Tomita T, McClone DG: Medulloblastoma in childhood: Results of radical resection and low-dose neuroaxis radiation therapy. J Neurosurg 64:238, 1986.
68. Van Eys J, Chen T, Moure T, et al: Adjuvant treatment for medulloblastoma and ependymoma using IV vincristine, intrathecal methotrexate and intrathecal hydrocortisone: A Southwest Oncology Group study. Cancer Treat Rep 65:681, 1981.
69. Vaquero J, Cabezudo JM, DeSola RG: Intratumoral hemorrhage in posterior fossa tumors after ventricular drainage. J Neurosurg 54:406, 1981.
70. Waga S, Shimizo T, Shimosaka S, et al: Intratumoral hemorrhage after a ventriculo-peritoneal shunting procedure. Neurosurgery 9:249, 1981.
71. Wara WM, Wallner KE, Levin VA, et al: Retreatment of pediatric brain tumors with radiation and misonidazole: Results of CCSG/RTOG phase I/II study. Cancer 58:1636, 1986.
72. Weinstein ZR, Downey EF: Spontaneous hemorrhage in medulloblastoma. AJNR 4:986, 1983.
73. Zee C-S, Segall HD, Miller C, et al: Less common CT features of medulloblastoma. Radiology 144:97, 1982.
74. Zimmerman RA, Bilawick CT, Pahlajani H: Spectrum of medulloblastoma demonstrated by computed tomography. Radiology 126:137, 1978.

29
BRAINSTEM TUMORS IN CHILDHOOD: SURGICAL INDICATIONS

Fred J. Epstein, M.D.
Jeffrey H. Wisoff, M.D.

Intrinsic brainstem tumors have traditionally been treated with radiation therapy and adjunctive chemotherapy, with relatively little success. Although the neurologic course transiently improves after therapy, it invariably progresses after a relatively short remission, and children rarely survive more than one or two years after the primary diagnosis.[2] Prior to the availability of computerized tomography (CT), the neuroradiologic diagnosis was made by pneumoencephalography, which characteristically disclosed a widened brainstem. There was no early technology that permitted visualization of the neural tissues, and for this reason, there was a tendency to "lump" all brainstem tumors together.

With the availability of more sophisticated neurodiagnostic modalities, such as CT and nuclear magnetic resonance imaging (NMRI), it has become obvious that brainstem tumors are relatively heterogeneous and may be classified according to location within the brainstem and gross anatomic appearance, and probable pathologic diagnosis. It is also becoming evident that the decision of whether or not to recommend surgery may be based on the integration of the neurodiagnostic evaluation with the clinical course and neurologic examination.[3-5]

Over the past five years (1981 to 1986), the senior author has operated on 79 brainstem tumors, and all of the material presented in this chapter was derived from this surgical experience (Table 29–1). Included in this material is a simple system for classification of brainstem tumors and surgical recommendations concerning which of these neoplasms should or should not be operated on.

NEURODIAGNOSTIC CATEGORIES

Anatomic Classifications

Brainstem tumors may be classified into five general categories: (1) diffuse, (2) focal, (3) cystic, (4) exophytic, and (5) cervicomedullary.

Diffuse Tumors (24 Patients)

The diffuse brainstem tumor is the most common, having the appearance, on CT scan, of a hypodense area throughout much of the pons (Fig. 29–1), and often extending rostrally into the midbrain. There is usually little or no enhancement, and the NMRI scan characteristically discloses that the neoplasm is more extensive than the CT scan suggests, involving medulla, pons, midbrain, and even thalamus.

Table 29–1. TUMOR CLASSIFICATION AND MICROSCOPIC PATHOLOGY

Type	Number	Pathology	Result
Diffuse	24	Grade IV Astrocytomas	Dead, 6 to 12 months postoperatively, from tumor progression
Cystic	6	Grade I–II Astrocytomas	Alive and clinically stable or improved 9 to 60 months postoperatively
Cervicomedullary	20	14 Grade I–II Astrocytomas 3 Gangliogliomas 3 Grade IV Astrocytomas	Twelve or 14 "benign" tumors alive and clinically stable. Three malignant tumors, dead 8 to 14 months postoperatively
Dorsally exophytic	6	Grade I–II Astrocytomas	Alive and improved 12–60 months postoperatively
Anterolaterally and posterolaterally exophytic	18	1 Ganglioglioma 2 Grade I–II Astrocytomas	Three "benign" tumors alive and stable 12 to 60 months postoperatively
		15 Grade III–IV Astrocytomas	Fifteen grade III–IV tumors, dead 6 to 24 months postoperatively
Focal	5	3 Grade I–II Astrocytomas 2 Grade IV Astrocytomas	Three "benign tumors," improved or stable Two malignant tumors, dead from tumor progression 6–12 months postoperatively

Focal Tumors (5 Patients)

Focal brainstem tumors are defined by an area of contrast enhancement on the CT scan (Fig. 29–2) and the absence of associated hypodensity. In addition, the NMRI scan discloses a focal lesion less than 2.5 cm in diameter without significant associated edema. It is important to emphasize that in many cases the NMRI will disclose that a tumor that appeared to be focal on the CT scan is much more extensive and, in fact, is diffuse. In other words, a true focal tumor does not appear significantly larger on the NMRI scan than the CT scan.

Cystic Astrocytomas (6 Patients)

The appearance of cystic astrocytoma of the brainstem is very similar to cystic astrocytoma of the cerebellum. The CT scan discloses a mural nodule (Fig. 29–3) that enhances with contrast material and is often associated with a large cyst that may excavate much of the brainstem. These tumors are commonly in the cerebral peduncle or pons, and both the CT and the NMRI scans provide satisfactory imaging.

Exophytic Tumors

Dorsally Exophytic Tumors (6 Patients). Dorsally exophytic neoplasms grow from the subependymal surface of the brainstem posteriorly into the fourth ventricle (Fig. 29–4A). From a neuroradiologic perspective, the CT scan discloses a neoplasm that may appear similar or identical to a medulloblastoma. However, the NMRI scan often discloses that the neoplasm is in fact an exophytic brainstem tumor.

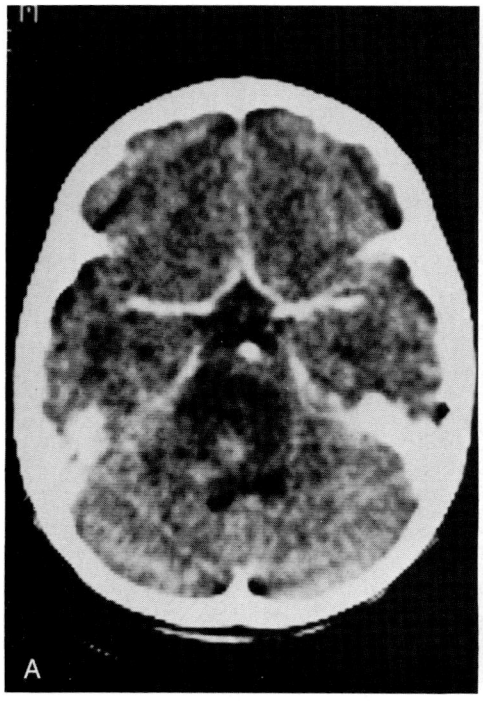
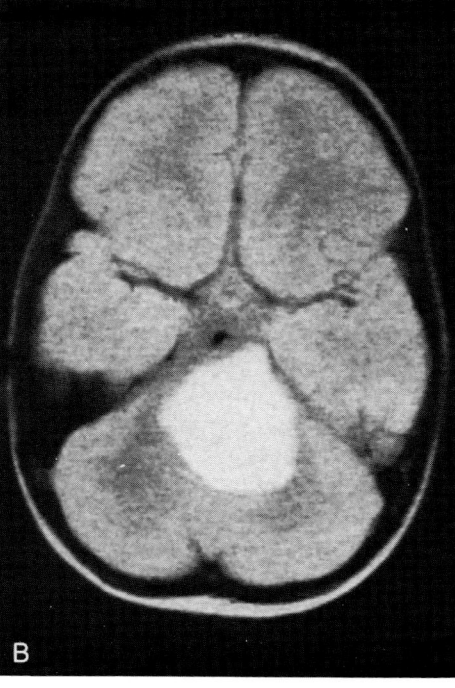

Figure 29–1. Diffuse brainstem tumor. A, Contrast-enhanced CT scan shows enlarged, hypodense pons, with posterior displacement of fourth ventricle. B, T2-weighted nuclear magnetic resonance (NMR) image demonstrates the total extent of tumor, not apparent on CT.

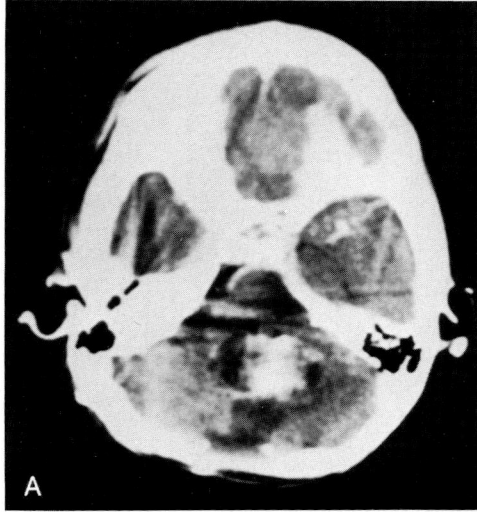
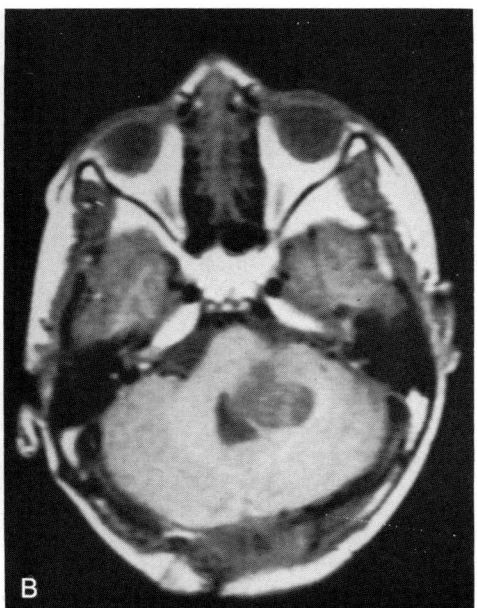

Figure 29–2. Focal brainstem tumor. A, Contrast-enhanced CT scan shows focal enhancing lesion in dorsolateral pons. B, NMR image reveals low-signal focal lesion congruent with the lesion shown on CT scan in A.

Posterolaterally and Anterolaterally Exophytic Tumors (18 Patients). Posterolaterally exophytic tumors grow through the brachium pontis into the cerebellum (Fig. 29–4B). The CT scan commonly discloses that the bulk of the tumor is within the hemisphere, and the relationship to the brainstem may be overlooked. This is because these tumors are often in the region of the pontomedullary junction and bone artifacts may obscure the image. The NMRI scan usually defines the relationship of the tumor to the brainstem and, in these cases, is a valuable surgical adjunct. In occasional cases, the relationship of an anterolaterally exophytic tumor to the brainstem is not obvious, and a preoperative diagnosis of acoustic neuroma or meningioma may be considered.

Cervicomedullary Tumors (20 Patients)

Tumors of the cervicomedullary junction extend rostrally into the medulla and caudally into the cervical spinal cord (Fig. 29–5). Although the rostral caudal length of the tumor may vary, these neoplasms rarely extend above the pontomedullary junction. The CT scan is not reliable in delineating these neoplasms, as bone artifacts in the region of the foramen magnum distort the image. While a spinal CT scan with subarachnoid metrizamide is

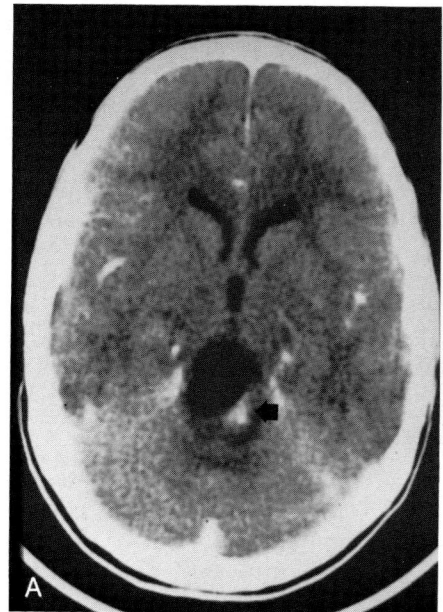
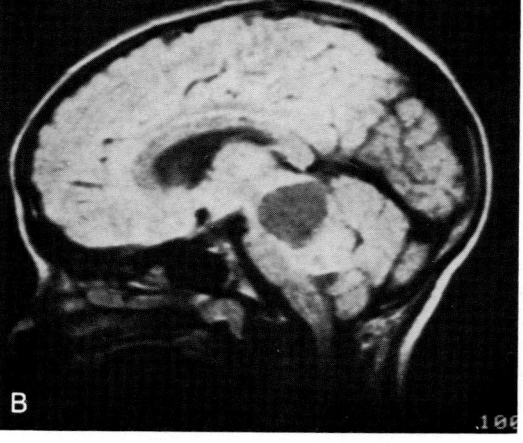

Figure 29–3. Cystic brainstem tumor. A, Contrast-enhanced CT scan: Note enhancing tumor nodule (arrow). B, T1-weighted NMR image of midsagittal plane demonstrates a cyst.

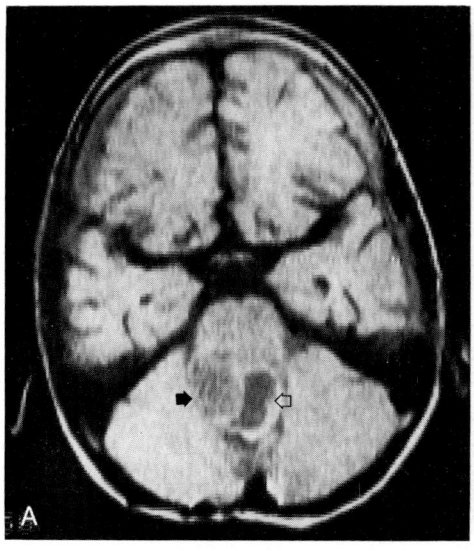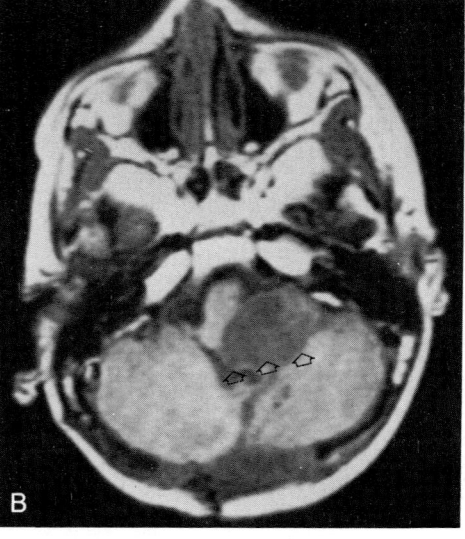

Figure 29-4. Exophytic brainstem tumor. A, T1-weighted NMR image of dorsally exophytic tumor (black arrow) with cyst (open arrow). B, T1-weighted NMR image of exophytic tumor (arrows) in the cerebellopontine angle.

an excellent adjunct for imaging of these neoplasms, the NMRI obviates the need for all these studies because the sagittal image clearly demonstrates the rostral-caudal extent of the neoplasm.

Clinical Manifestations

The clinical manifestations of brainstem neoplasms may be correlated with the anatomic classification, as noted on the neurodiagnostic studies.

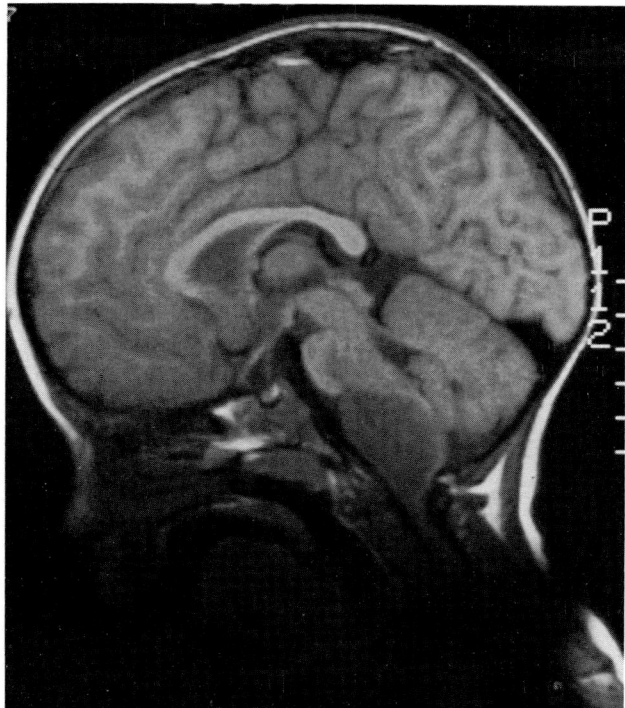

Figure 29-5. Cervicomedullary tumor. NMR image demonstrating expanded medulla. Note normal pons.

Diffuse Tumors

The diffuse tumor is the most common brainstem tumor and the one that is the historical stereotype for brainstem neoplasm. The clinical evolution of the diffuse tumor is relatively rapid: Oculomotor imbalance and diplopia, with or without obvious facial weakness, is a common primary complaint. Neurologic examination often discloses bilateral cranial nerve dysfunction in the presence of ataxia and spasticity in the lower extremities.

Focal Tumors

The focal tumor may present in a way identical to the diffuse neoplasm, or in some cases, the course is more insidious, with the neurologic examination suggesting that the tumor is restricted to a relatively small region of the brainstem. In the authors' experience, a tumor that appears focal on the CT scan but is associated with typical bilateral signs and symptoms is re-classified as diffuse, following the NMRI scan, which discloses that the neoplasm is much more extensive than the CT scan suggested. Focal tumors have an atypical history, as neurologic symptoms are commonly present for months or, rarely, years prior to definitive diagnosis. In addition, the neurologic examination commonly discloses that signs and symptoms are referable to a single focus in the brainstem (i.e., unilateral cranial nerve dysfunction and contralateral hemiparesis).

Cystic Astrocytoma

Cystic astrocytomas are rare neoplasms. In most circumstances, the mural nodule is relatively small, and the cystic component of the tumor is responsible for the symptoms. The clinical course is variable, and occasionally, months or even a year or two may pass between the first symptoms and the definitive diagnosis. In the authors' experience, hemiparesis, with or without oculomotor dysfunction, was the earliest symptom.

Exophytic Tumors

Dorsally Exophytic Tumors. These neoplasms extend posteriorly into the fourth ventricle and obstruct cerebrospinal fluid pathways. For this reason, the clinical manifestations are secondary to hydrocephalus, and these children often have long histories of headaches. Ataxia and nystagmus are commonly noted on neurologic examination or generally appear sometime after the first manifestations of headache. In some cases, these neoplasms may be clinically differentiated from medulloblastoma by the long antecedent history and the chronicity of the symptoms at the time of definitive diagnosis.

Anterolaterally and Posterolaterally Exophytic Tumors. These tumors often become manifest as a result of compression and infiltration of the brachium pontis, and intention tremors associated with focal brainstem dysfunction are common. As the tumor grows and extends posteriorly into the cerebellum, the fourth ventricle and aqueduct are displaced, and hydrocephalus commonly evolves sometime during the clinical course.

The magnitude of brainstem dysfunction is quite variable and is related to whether or not the "bulk" of the neoplasm is extending into the cerebellum or into the brainstem.

Cervicomedullary Tumors

Lower cranial nerve dysfunction associated with quadriparesis or hemiparesis is the primary symptom. Occasionally, intractable neck pain and torticollis are the only complaints. Symptoms are commonly present for many months or even years prior to definitive diagnosis.

SURGERY

Options

In considering the surgical option, the first and most obvious issue is whether or not surgery should be carried out at all. Retrospective analysis has made it clear that surgery is only potentially beneficial for low-grade gliomas, and therefore, it is essential to utilize clinical and neurodiagnostic studies to identify these patients.

The most common brainstem tumor is the diffuse type, and these neoplasms are invariably malignant astrocytomas. It has become obvious that the characteristic hypodensity that is noted on the CT scan is not edema, but infiltrating malignant tumor. Although these patients were not injured by the surgery, none was better as a result of it, and all died as a result of tumor progression within six to nine months.

It must be emphasized that there is no indication or justification for carrying out a biopsy, as the diagnosis is obvious, and therapeutic options are extremely limited (see discussion).

General Principles

Surgery is only potentially beneficial for patients with focal, cystic, exophytic, and cervicomedullary tumors of the brainstem. Prior to discussing these groups individually, it is important to recognize some general principles of brainstem tumor surgery. Perhaps the first and most important is that the surgeon must recognize that it is impossible to excise completely a glioma and potentially catastrophic to attempt it.

The goal of surgery is to reduce the "tumor burden," and the amount of neoplastic tissue that is actually removed may be variable. It has been the authors' experience that 50 to 80 percent of the volume of the brainstem mass was removed. There were a few cases in which the intraoperative assessment suggested gross total excision, but the postoperative neurodiagnostic evaluation invariably disclosed that, in reality, there was at least some residual tumor. This is clearly, at least in part, the reason that patients with malignant neoplasms did not benefit from surgery. Obviously, radical though subtotal excision of a slowly growing tumor offers the possibility of long-term clinical remission, while the same operation for a malignant tumor does not favorably affect the dismal prognosis.

The second important principle is that there is never a cleavage plane between a glioma and the surrounding brainstem. For this reason, the surgeon must not attempt to define a tumor-brain interface, as this invariably damages functioning neural tissue. Rather, these neoplasms must be debulked "bit by bit," from inside out, until the surgeon believes that the periphery of the tumor is near or visible. At times normal white matter may be appreciated, but it is rarely possible to remove the entire mass and visualize normal white matter circumferentially around the entire tumor cavity. Tumors may be removed with relative safety only if all instruments are within the mass. This is because low-grade gliomas displace functioning neural elements but do not infiltrate to the same degree as malignant astrocytomas.

Evoked Potential Monitoring

Monitoring brainstem evoked potentials is a valuable surgical adjunct, because the electrical activity becomes relatively disordered as the interface between tumor and normal neural tissue is approached. It is essential to use a monitoring system that updates information every few seconds. It is of very little practical use to be informed that something in the dissection disrupted the potentials sometime in the previous 30 to 120 seconds, as by then it is too late for corrective measures (i.e., temporarily halting the tumor excision).

Focal Tumors

A focal tumor located beneath the ependymal surface of the fourth ventricle (Fig. 29–6) may be partially or totally excised at surgery. However, it is important to emphasize that the surgical indication for operating on such a tumor is based on not only the appearance of the CT scan but also the NMRI scan and the clinical presentation. A child who has a focal tumor but whose clinical examination discloses typical signs and symptoms of a diffuse brainstem tumor undoubtedly harbors an infiltrating, malignant tumor, and the enhancing focal component is only the "tip of the iceberg." In these circumstances, the NMRI scan invariably discloses a diffuse, infiltrating neoplasm that is not obvious on the CT scan. For this reason, if surgery is to be considered for any focal tumor of the brainstem, it is essential that the NMRI scan be obtained to be certain that this is indeed a focal and not a diffuse neoplasm.

In the authors' experience, a low-grade focal astrocytoma causes very focal neurologic dysfunction, and the authors re-emphasize that the surgeon be cognizant that it is the combination of the neurodiagnostic studies and the clinical manifestations that will suggest consideration of a surgical option.

The focal tumor beneath the floor of the fourth ventricle is approached through a posterior fossa craniectomy, with a small incision in the caudal 1 cm of the cerebellar vermis. The tonsils and vermis are retracted laterally, which offers a generous exposure of the floor of the fourth ventricle. Inspection of the ependymal surface of the fourth ventricle makes the location of the tumor obvious, as the median raphe is invariably displaced to the contralateral side and the ependymal surface is very often disrupted over that part of the neoplasm closest to the surface. The laser is the ideal instrument to make an incision into the tumor through the floor of the fourth ventricle. Following this, laser dissection, ultrasonic dissection, or both may be employed to carry out a radical tumor excision. It must be re-emphasized that it is not generally possible to identify normal white matter circumferentially around a brainstem tumor, and the surgeon must have some concept as to where the tumor abuts or infiltrates normal brainstem structures. Intraoperative brainstem potentials become disordered as the periphery of the tumor is excised, and when this occurs, the procedure must be interrupted or terminated.

Focal tumors beneath the floor of the fourth ventricle are relatively simple to expose, whereas the same neoplasm occurring in the region of the basis pontis is not easily visualized during surgery. This is because the focal tumor does not grow exophytically into the cerebellopontine angle, and in the absence of a massively expanded pons, there is very little room for surgical manipulation between the fifth and the seventh cranial nerves as they exit from the brainstem. For this reason, while it is possible to obtain a tissue biopsy, it is generally not feasible to carry out a radical tumor excision. Therefore, only under rare circumstances should tumors be approached when they are confined to the basis pontis.

Cystic Astrocytomas

Cystic astrocytomas may occur in either the pons or the midbrain. In the former location, the mass bulges posteriorly into the ventricle, and surgical

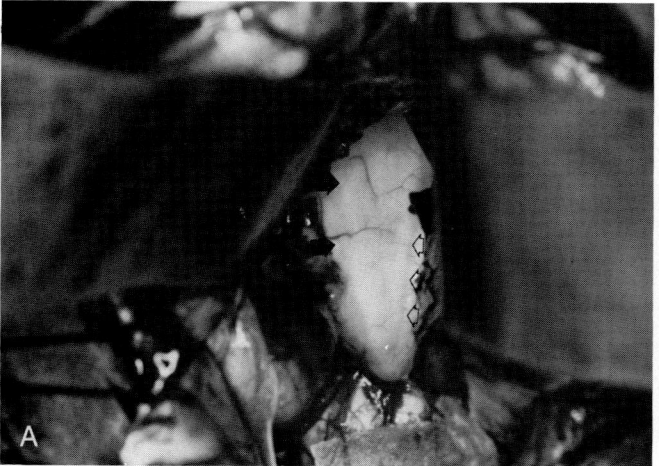 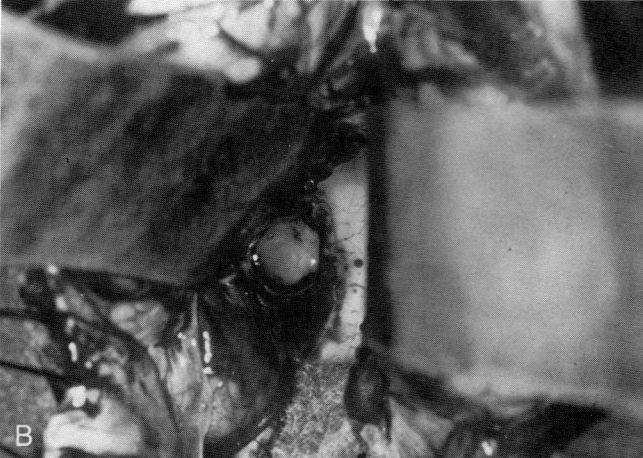

Figure 29–6. Operative approach—focal tumor. A, Exposure of floor of fourth ventricle median raphe (open arrows), displaced to right. Tumor (black arrows) causes floor to bulge. B, Tumor removed. Glial walls present.

exposure is through the inferior vermis. The laser may be utilized to incise the overlying ependyma and enter the cyst. The mural nodule may be at least partially excised through the large cyst cavity. Because the exposure is invariably relatively limited, the laser is the ideal instrument for excising as much of the solid nodular component of the neoplasm as possible. Black "laser char" invariably obscures the interface between the tumor and the brainstem, and it is necessary to interrupt the dissection at regular intervals to remove the blackened tissue.

In cases in which the solid component of the neoplasm is in the peduncle, surgical exposure is via a temporal craniotomy and subtemporal exposure of the incisural notch. Following removal of the arachnoid, the bulging peduncle is immediately obvious. It is necessary to incise the tentorium to expose fully the cerebral peduncle in the anteroposterior dimension. An incision is made over the point at which the neoplasm is closest to the surface of the peduncle. Once tumor tissue is recognized, the incision must be extended over the full length of the tumor. It is important to recognize that the dissection must be carried out within the bulk of the tumor, and there is never an attempt to define the interface between the tumor and the brainstem prior to debulking the neoplasm. The bulk of the mass is removed with laser or ultrasonic dissecting systems, and as in the pons, it is generally not possible to define normal white matter circumferentially around the tumor. The surgical goal is to obtain a radical, though subtotal excision, and where white matter may be observed in a few areas in the periphery of the neoplasm, there must be no great effort to obtain a gross total excision. It has been the authors' experience that between 50 and 95 percent of the solid component of the neoplasm may be removed; it is essential that the entire cyst be evacuated. There are cases in which the cyst is multiloculated, and although the surgical impression may suggest that they have been adequately drained, compartments of the cyst may remain. It is for this reason that ultrasonography is an invaluable surgical adjunct, and it may be utilized to monitor the extent of tumor removal and cyst drainage. In some cases, ultrasonography may disclose that a portion of the cyst remains, in which case, it may be appropriate to make an additional surgical effort to drain it.

Cervicomedullary Tumors

Tumors of the cervicomedullary junction extend rostrally into the medulla and caudally into the spinal cord (Fig. 29–7). They are exposed through a small, suboccipital craniectomy and upper cervical laminectomy. Operations are carried out with the patient in the prone position, which facilitates utilization of intraoperative ultrasonography. The latter is most helpful in identifying the rostral and caudal poles of the neoplasm prior to opening the dura. The cerebellar tonsils are gently separated, exposing the rostral area of the neoplasm. In some circumstances, the medullary component of the tumor is a cyst, whereas in others it is a solid tumor. In any event, the myelotomy is started in the middle of the tumor rather than over the rostral or caudal poles, where there is a greater hazard of injuring normal spinal cord or brainstem tissue. Following exposure of the tumor, the laser and Cavitron ultrasonic aspirator are utilized to debulk the neoplasm. In most circumstances, it is possible to obtain a gross total excision of the cervical component of the tumor and a radical subtotal removal of the medullary component. Once again, a more conservative approach in the brainstem is necessary, as there is a greater hazard of injuring the surrounding gray matter in this area as opposed to the lesser hazard of injuring white matter, which largely surrounds the spinal component of the tumor. In cases in which there are rostral, caudal, or intratumor cysts, ultrasonography, once again, con-

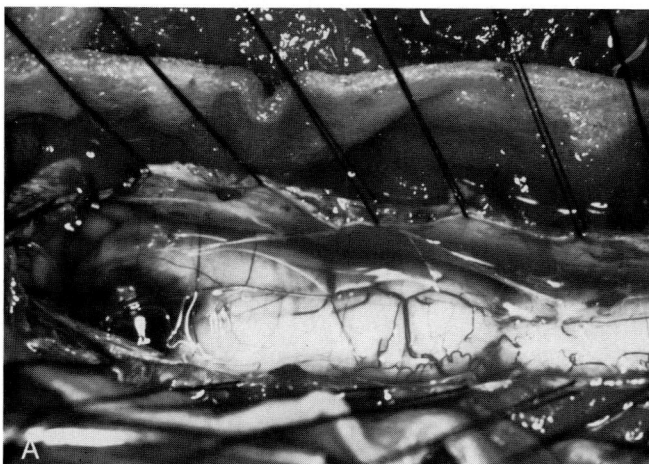
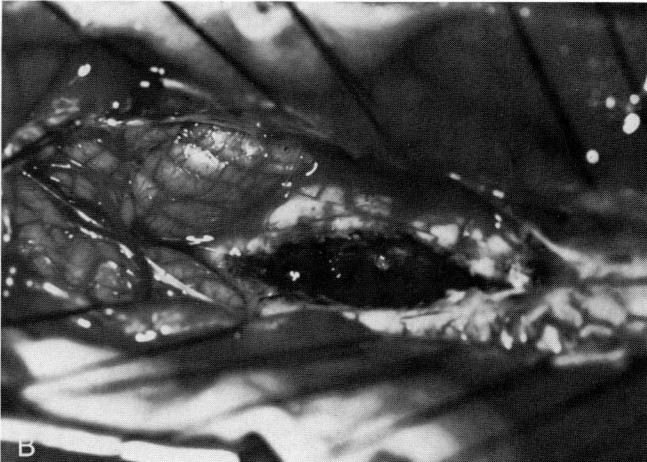

Figure 29–7. Operative approach—cervicomedullary tumor. A, Swollen medulla and cervical spinal cord. B, Tumor removed.

tributes to monitoring the dissection and identifying residual cysts that may have been overlooked as the surgery proceeded. It is important to drain all the cyst cavities, as in some circumstances, these contribute to the evolving symptoms.

Exophytic Tumors

Dorsal Exophytic Tumors

Tumors in this location are approached as midline cerebellar neoplasms. In fact, there are many circumstances in which either medulloblastoma or vermis astrocytoma is the preoperative diagnosis. The relationship of the tumor to the brainstem may be recognized only as the tumor is removed, when it becomes obvious that the tumor is growing from the brainstem along the floor of the fourth ventricle. Invariably a thin "shelf of tumor" is left in situ. It is important to emphasize that there must be no effort to excise totally the part of the neoplasm that is coming from the floor of the fourth ventricle, since the normal brainstem structures are just anterior to it. Therefore, any effort to excavate the dorsal surface of the brainstem results in significant damage to the vital brainstem tissues. This is in contradistinction to other brainstem tumors in which the neoplasm has displaced brainstem structures around it, and for this reason, the dissection may be continued as long as it is carried out within the centrum of the neoplasm.

Posterolaterally Exophytic Tumors

Posterolaterally exophytic tumors are exposed through a cortical incision lateral to the vermis. In most cases, the tumor is encountered between 2 and 3 cm beneath the surface of the cerebellum. The hemispheric component of the neoplasm may be removed as any cerebellar tumor. In most circumstances, the origin of the tumor is recognized prior to surgery, though there are cases in which the anatomy is obvious only in the operating room. In any event, it is safe to remove all of the hemispheric component of the tumor and to pursue it into, and even through, the brachium pontis. There is little danger to functioning neural tissue as long as the deeper component of the neoplasm is removed from inside out, and it is safe to identify the glia-tumor interface within the brachium pontis. These neoplasms do not generally extend anteriorly into the substance of the brainstem, and for this reason, the surgeon must have a clear concept of where the dissection must be terminated.

Anterolaterally Exophytic Tumors

These tumors are exposed through retromastoid craniectomy. In most cases, the exophytic component of the neoplasm separates the fifth and the seventh cranial nerves, which facilitates removal of the tumor between them. Only the exophytic component of the neoplasm must be removed, as pursuing it into the brainstem almost invariably damages or destroys the fifth and the seventh cranial nerves, which results in serious cosmetic and functional disability.

DISCUSSION

Perhaps the most important contribution to the management of brainstem neoplasms is the recognition that they are not a single entity but, in fact, consist of different tumors that may be classified according to location and probable pathology. While diffuse neoplasms are the most common, accounting for 70 percent of brainstem tumors, the other categories are not rare, and surgical options may be considered for all of them.[5]

It has been the authors' experience that surgery is only potentially beneficial for benign astrocytomas or gangliogliomas of the brainstem. No patient with a malignant tumor has derived significant benefit, and in the authors' experience, all have died within 12 months of surgery. Therefore, if the surgical option is to be seriously considered, it is essential that there be some relatively reliable preoperative assessment of tumor pathology. The relationship of pathology to the clinical course and neurodiagnostic demonstration of the location and extent of the tumor is important in making this determination.

All diffuse brainstem tumors are malignant. The characteristic hypodensity that is noted on the CT scan is not edema but infiltrating neoplasm. There is no justification for attempting surgical excision or biopsy, as the pathology and prognosis are obvious, and the only proven therapeutic option is radiation therapy.

Focal tumors may be low-grade astrocytomas. However, in the presence of a clinical course that is typical of a diffuse brainstem astrocytoma, one may assume that the apparent focal component is the "tip of the iceberg" and that, in reality, the patient harbors a diffusely infiltrating malignant tumor. Therefore, the only focal tumor that may be considered a surgical candidate must have both a CT scan and an NMRI scan appearance that suggests a "benign" neoplasm and must be associated with an atypical clinical presentation manifested by a paucity of signs and symptoms arising from a relatively distinct region of the brainstem. The same neoplasm that is associated with bilateral cranial nerve dysfunction and long tract signs must be regarded as malignant, with no surgical option.

Cervicomedullary neoplasms are commonly low-grade astrocytomas or gangliogliomas and are often favorably affected by radical surgical excision. It is possible that a few of these neoplasms may be cervical spinal cord tumors that have grown rostrally into the medulla, as the microscopic pathology is often similar to typical low-grade astrocytomas that occur in the spinal cord. In other words, whereas the great majority of spinal cord astrocytomas of childhood are benign, the converse seems to be the situation with neoplasms of the pons or midbrain, where the overwhelming number of tumors are diffuse and malignant. Tumors of the cervicomedullary junction may represent a "melting pot" in terms of pathology, and primary surgical extirpation may be most appropriate for tumors in this location.

The dorsally exophytic brainstem tumor is also a surgical lesion amenable to radical excision. It is of importance to recognize that these tumors are commonly low-grade astrocytomas and that long-term survival may be expected with or without radiation therapy.

Some researchers have suggested that it is important to perform routine biopsies of brainstem tumors to make an accurate pathologic diagnosis prior to recommending a course of treatment.[1,6] The authors take strong exception to this because there is no consistent useful information to be obtained from biopsy, and the fact that a procedure may be carried out with little morbidity and mortality does not justify inflicting it on an already ill child. It must be recognized that the microscopic pathology of a brainstem tumor is not homogeneous. Glioblastomas commonly have a large component that, if examined alone, would be diagnosed as grade II astrocytoma. The only time that a brainstem biopsy is meaningful is when it discloses a highly malignant tumor, in which case, the biology of the neoplasm will be related to its most malignant component and the dismal prognosis will be obvious. However, in cases in which biopsy discloses a low-grade tumor, there is no way of assessing whether or not this reflects the microscopic pathology of the centrum of the neoplasm, and it is not logical to recommend a treatment course based on that examination. In fact, in the authors' experience with radical excision of brainstem tumors, surgery performed on two patients yielded a relatively large specimen that revealed a grade II astrocytoma, whereas the autopsy specimen (12 days and 36 days postoperatively) disclosed a glioblastoma with wide neuraxis dissemination.

It is intriguing that a few patients with apparent brainstem neoplasms continue to survive many years after diagnosis. It seems probable that in some of these cases, the diagnosis was made prior to the availability of CT, and some of these good results were in children who had an incorrect diagnosis. The authors' own experience supports this hypothesis inasmuch as we have encountered two pontine hematomas secondary to occult angiomas, and one arachnoid cyst of the clivus, all of which were misinterpreted as intrinsic brainstem neoplasms. This emphasizes the necessity of expert review of technically satisfactory neurodiagnostic studies, as the correct diagnosis was obvious retrospectively, and with proper neuroradiologic attention, misinterpretation would not have occurred.

SUMMARY

Brainstem tumors are a heterogeneous group of neoplasms that may be classified according to clinical and neurodiagnostic criteria. The authors have described simple anatomic categories that include diffuse, focal, exophytic, cystic, and cervicomedullary tumors. While there is no surgical option for the most common diffuse brainstem neoplasms, the others may be operated on if the clinical and radiographic assessment suggests the possibility of a benign neoplasm. Although surgery has been well-tolerated and often beneficial, it would be premature to comment as to the duration of remission or the possibility of permanent cure.

References

1. Albright AL, Price RA, Guthkelch AN: Brain stem gliomas of children. A clinicopathologic study. Cancer 52:2313, 1983.
2. Allen JC: Brain stem glioma. Neurol Neurosurg 4:2, 1983.
3. Berger MS, Edwards MSB, LaMasters D, et al: Pediatric brain stem tumors: Radiographic, pathological and clinical correlations. Neurosurgery 12:298, 1983.
4. Entzian W: Removal of intraponto-mesencephalic spongioblastoma. Neurosurg Rev 6:67, 1983.
5. Epstein F, McCleary EL: Intrinsic brain-stem tumors of childhood: Surgical indications. J Neurosurg 64:11, 1986.
6. Reigel DH, Scarff TB, Woodford JE: Biopsy of pediatric brain stem tumors. Child's Brain 5:329, 1979.

30
TUMORS OF THE FOURTH VENTRICLE: EPENDYMOMAS, CHOROID PLEXUS PAPILLOMAS, AND DERMOID CYSTS

E. Bruce Hendrick, M.D.
Corey Raffel, M.D., Ph.D.

Tumors occurring in the fourth ventricle in children may arise from the contents of the ventricle (choroid plexus), from the lining of the fourth ventricle (ependymoma), or from cells not normally found in the ventricle (dermoid tumors). Ependymomas are tumors arising from the ependymal cells lining the ventricles. Choroid plexus papillomas arise from the choroid plexus. Other tumors that do not arise in the fourth ventricle but may project into it, such as medulloblastoma and astrocytoma, are not discussed in this review.

ANATOMY OF THE FOURTH VENTRICLE

The fourth ventricle lies entirely within the posterior fossa. Its floor is formed by the tegmentum of the upper half of the medulla and the tegmentum of the pons. Its roof is formed by the superior and inferior medullary velum (tela choroidea of the fourth ventricle). The cerebellar peduncles form the lateral margin. The cerebral aqueduct (of Sylvius) enters the rostral termination of the fourth ventricle, and the foramen of Magendie opens into the vallecula inferiorly. Each lateral recess opens into a medullocerebellar cistern via a foramen of Luschka. The striae medullares divide the floor into a superior and an inferior half. Lying on either side of the midline in the superior half are the facial colliculi, overlying the abducens nuclei and facial nerves. Lateral to the colliculi are the vestibular areas. Inferior are the medial hypoglossal trigones and the lateral vagal trigones. It should be quite apparent that these important structures in the floor of the ventricle limit tumor resection in this direction.

EPENDYMOMAS

Ependymomas are tumors derived from, and having the features of, differentiated ependymal cells. About one half of these tumors present before the age of 18 years.[10] In children, the fourth ventricle is the most common location, accounting for about 60 percent of the intracranial tumors in most series.[7, 10, 20, 25, 38] The posterior fossa tumors tend to occur in young children, while lateral ventricle tumors predominate in older children and adolescents.[29] Ependymomas tend to occur in young patients, with 50 percent presenting before the age of three years.[7, 10, 20, 25, 38] At the Hospital for Sick Children (HSC), 67 patients with ependymomas have been treated between 1950 and 1983. The age at presentation ranged from seven weeks through 16 years, with a mean of 3.76 years. The tumors are rarely congenital.[1] Ependymomas have no sex predilection. Of the 67 HSC patients, 38 were boys and 29 were girls (1.3:1).

The most common presenting symptoms are related to hydrocephalus, caused by obstruction of the fourth ventricle. Nausea and vomiting were present in 41 patients (61 percent), and headaches in 35 patients (52 percent). Signs of a posterior fossa mass were also common. The presenting symptoms in the HSC series are in Table 30–1.

The clinical signs present at initial evaluation in the series of HSC patients are shown in Table 30–2. Again, the most common findings are related to raised intracranial pressure (ICP) (papilledema, in 58 percent of patients) and the posterior fossa (ataxia, in 45 percent).

As with any tumor in the very young, a high index of suspicion must be maintained, as some of the presenting symptoms and signs are quite nonspecific (i.e., developmental delay, irritability, and weight loss).

Many schemes have been proposed for the histologic classification of ependymomas.[17, 18, 33] At the Hospital for Sick Children, the tumors are divided into ependymomas and malignant ependymomas or ependymoblastomas. Ependymomas are characterized by three features.[1] The uniform cells are arranged around vascular structures and extend in cell process to the wall of the vessel, forming perivascular pseudorosettes. The cells may form true ependymal rosettes, in which a group of cells is arranged around a lumen, reminiscent of the central canal of the spinal cord. Lastly, the cells contain blepharoplasts, which are the basal bodies of cilia. These small intracellular structures are best demonstrated with special silver stains. Even under high power, they are hard to identify, but their presence confirms the ependymal nature of the tumor.[34] Rarely, elements of subependymoma are admixed with ependymomas of the fourth ventricle in children.[1] Subependymomas without admixed ependymoma have not been reported in children.

Ependymoblastomas may contain any of the structures just mentioned, but in addition, they have nuclear hyperchromatism, cytoplasmic and nuclear pleomorphism, more disorganized cytoarchitecture, mitosis, necrosis, or other features of anaplasia. The authors do not restrict the term ependymoblastoma to a rare tumor, as suggested by Rubinstein.[25]

The relationship of histopathology to outcome is not clear. In some series, the median survival is unaltered by this factor,[2, 13] but in most other series, patients with ependymoma do better than those with ependymoblastoma.[18, 32, 35] In the HSC series, patients with ependymoma, of which there were 51, had a five-year survival rate of 20 percent, whereas the 16 patients with ependymoblastoma had a mean five-year survival rate of 6 percent.

The radiographic modality of choice in the evaluation of a patient suspected of harboring a posterior fossa mass is computed tomography (CT).[44] Ependymomas may be high in density, isodense with brain, or of mixed density on precontrast CT scan. They usually show some enhancement after intravenous infusion of contrast material. Calcification is common, occurring in about 50 percent of the tumors (Figs. 30–1 and 30–2). The hallmark of ependymomas is extension through the vallecula and below the foramen magnum (Fig. 30–3). Sagittal or coronal images are helpful in demonstrating this extension. Hydrocephalus, with the obstruction at the level of the fourth ventricle, is also commonly seen.

Table 30–1. SYMPTOMS OF INTRACRANIAL EPENDYMOMA IN 67 PATIENTS AT THE HOSPITAL FOR SICK CHILDREN

Symptom	No. of Patients	Percentage
Nausea and vomiting	41	61
Headache	35	52
Ataxia	22	33
Visual symptoms	13	19
Decreased appetite/weight loss	9	13
Dizziness	7	10
Head tilt	5	8
Irritability	5	8
Lethargy	4	6
Neck pain	3	5
Fever	3	5
Difficulty in swallowing	1	2
Voice change	1	2
Back pain	1	2
Hemiparesis	1	2
Developmental delay	1	2
Seizures	1	2

Table 30–2. SIGNS OF INTRACRANIAL EPENDYMOMA IN 67 PATIENTS AT THE HOSPITAL FOR SICK CHILDREN

Signs	No. of Patients	Percentage
Papilledema	39	58
Ataxia	30	45
Nystagmus	24	36
Gaze palsy	18	27
Lower cranial nerve palsy	7	11
Weakness	5	8
Irritability	5	8
Macrocephaly	4	6
Meningismus	3	5
Opisthotonos	2	3
Lethargy	2	3
Dehydration	2	3
Comatose	2	3
Respiratory changes	2	3
Emaciation	1	2
Loss of head control	1	2
Scoliosis	1	2

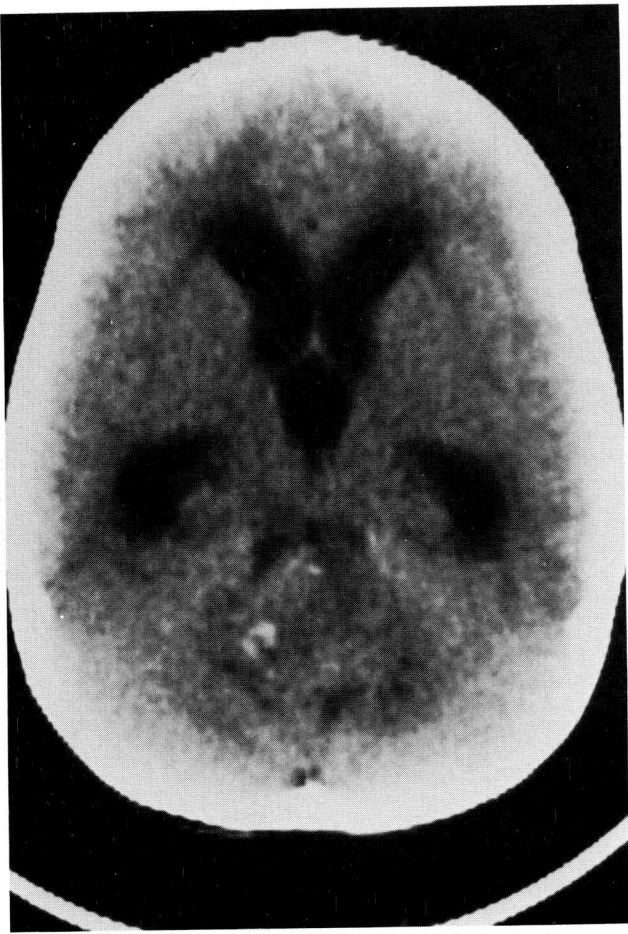

Figure 30–1. Unenhanced CT scan shows ependymoma with scattered areas of calcification.

Nuclear magnetic resonance imaging (NMRI) may supplement CT under the circumstances just described. The anatomic detail obtained is spectacular, and the beam-hardening artifacts common in the posterior fossa with CT scanning are not present.

The authors would stress, however, that no imaging finding is pathognomonic of ependymomas; histologic diagnosis cannot be made on the basis of the images obtained.

The authors do not feel that angiography is necessary in the preoperative evaluation of a patient with a posterior fossa mass, unless hemangioblastoma is a possibility.

The differential diagnosis of a mass in the fourth ventricle in children includes tumors arising in the fourth ventricle (ependymomas, meningiomas, choroid plexus papillomas) and tumors that arise near the ventricle and are exophytic into it (medulloblastomas, astrocytomas, brainstem gliomas).

Surgical therapy has three goals: (1) establishing the diagnosis, (2) re-establishing normal cerebrospinal fluid (CSF) flow, and (3) total removal of the tumor. The authors believe that preoperative shunting is not necessary in these patients, as adequate room in the posterior fossa can be obtained by a combination of preoperative steroids, hyperventilation, and osmotic diuresis. If these measures prove inadequate, an occipital burr hole is placed and a catheter passed into the lateral ventricle. The catheter is removed at the end of the operation. By avoiding placement of a shunt, the authors do not have to be concerned about upward herniation (occurring in 5 percent of patients) or intratumoral hemorrhage.[2]

The operative approach starts with the patient prone and the neck flexed. A midline incision is made, extending from just above the inion to the spinous process of C6. After reflection of muscle off the occiput and C1 and C2, a suboccipital craniectomy is performed. The craniectomy extends to the transverse sinus superiorly and widely laterally, and includes the foramen magnum inferiorly. The arch of C1 is removed, and additional cervical laminectomies are performed as indicated by tumor extension. The dura is opened with Y-shaped incision. The tumor can usually be identified in the vallecula. The foramen of Magendie is identified. The tumor is removed with the Cavitron ultrasonic aspirator (CUSA) or other technique, as indicated. The vermis is split early in the procedure to give wide access to the tumor in the fourth ventricle.

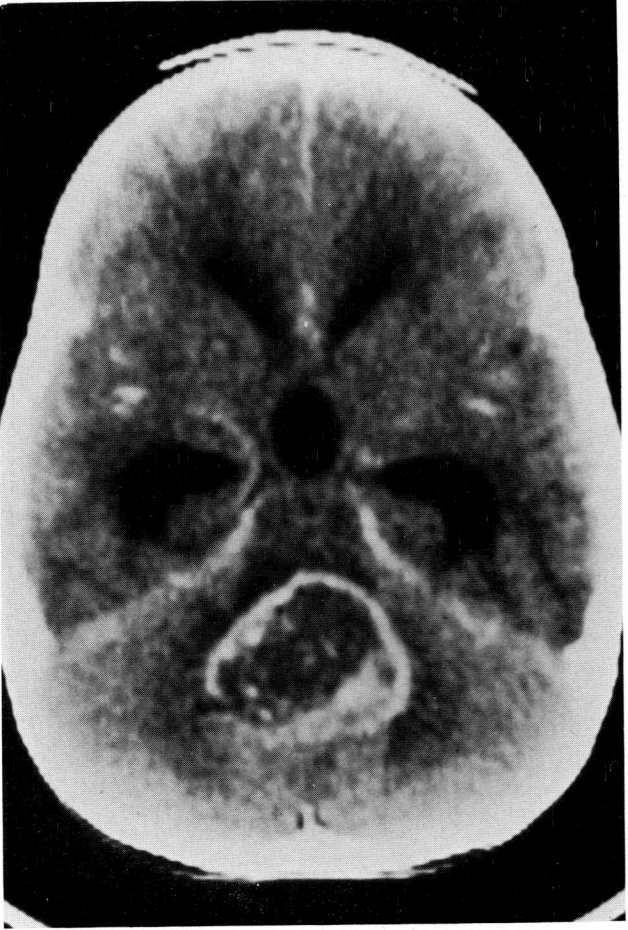

Figure 30–2. Enhanced CT scan of same patient as in Figure 30–1.

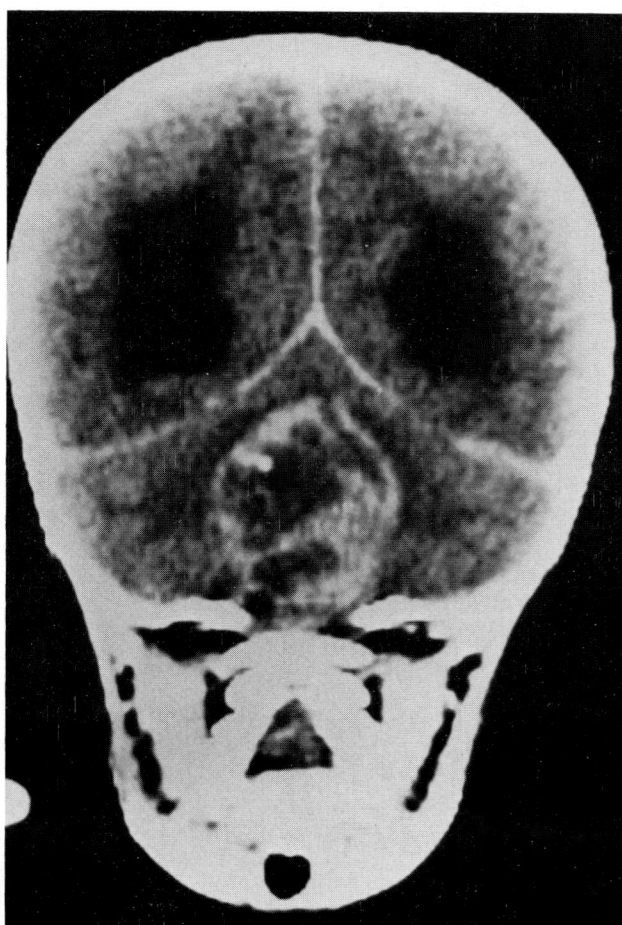

Figure 30–3. Coronal image showing extension of ependymoma through the vallecula and through the foramen magnum.

Usually, the tumor is easily removed, as it is not adherent to the walls of the ventricle except at the site of origin. Care is taken to remove all tumor in the lateral recesses of the ventricle and to follow an extension out the foramina of Luschka, if present. The tumor occasionally molds itself into available spaces, without being adherent to them, a condition termed "plastic ependymoma."[8] The major difficulty seems to occur near the end of the operation, when the tumor's site of origin can be identified. This is most frequently the floor of the fourth ventricle, and a small amount of tumor extending into the floor must be left behind. Additionally, extension up the aqueduct of Sylvius is sometimes difficult to resect but, usually, can be removed. Overall, attempts at removal should be nearly complete. At the Hospital for Sick Children, 46 of 66 operations accomplished removal of all tumor, except that presenting in the floor of the ventricle. Closure is performed in layers; a water-tight dural closure is obtained. Cadaver, freeze-dried dura is used if a graft is necessary to achieve an adequate dural closure.

Postoperative therapy should include radiation to the posterior fossa, as such therapy has been demonstrated to improve the survival rate.[3, 10, 38, 40] The use of additional whole brain and spinal irradiation is controversial. The rationale for craniospinal irradiation relates to the occurrence of CSF metastases. These have been shown to occur more frequently with poorly differentiated lesions and with fourth ventricle versus lateral ventricle lesions.[19, 30] However, the rate of metastasis varies, from 0 to 68 percent in different series, and the factors influencing metastasis are not entirely clear. The authors reserve craniospinal irradiation for those patients over two years of age with positive postoperative myelography or with malignant tumors. It has been suggested that craniospinal irradiation may not prevent CSF spread of tumor,[29] but others disagree.[30]

At the Hospital for Sick Children, of 62 patients operated upon, there was one intraoperative death and six deaths in the first postoperative month. There were no five-year survivors among 15 patients who underwent biopsy or subtotal resection. The five-year survival was 11 of 38 patients with nearly total or total resection. Postoperative radiation therapy was given routinely. Chemotherapy was usually reserved for recurrences. Currently, no chemotherapeutic regimen has been clearly demonstrated to be of benefit in the treatment of ependymomas, although anecdotal reports on the efficacy of bischloroethylnitrosourea (BCNU) have appeared.[22, 23, 43]

In the literature, the five-year survival rate for ependymomas in children ranged from 16 to 58 percent. Multiple studies have demonstrated a worse prognosis with tumors of the fourth ventricle versus supratentorial tumors.[10, 29, 30] The prognosis may also be worse in children younger than two years of age.[30] While some studies suggest that the histopathology is unrelated to survival, other studies have suggested worse prognoses for those patients with ependymoblastoma.[2, 10, 13, 32, 35]

CHOROID PLEXUS PAPILLOMAS

Tumors of the choroid plexus are relatively uncommon, accounting for 0.4 to 0.6 percent of all intracranial tumors in large series.[9, 37] The tumors are more common in children than adults. They account for about 3 percent of intracranial tumors in the pediatric age group.[26, 27] In children, 40 percent occur in patients younger than one year of age, and 86 percent of the tumors appear in children five years of age and younger.[15] Thus, the incidence of choroid plexus papillomas is higher in children.

In children, 60 to 70 percent of the tumors occur in the lateral ventricles, and about 20 to 30 percent occur in the fourth ventricle.[27, 31] The remaining tumors occur in the third ventricle and cerebellopontine angle. Interestingly, in adults, the fourth ventricle is the most common site. The tumors are as common in boys as in girls.[26, 31]

Clinically, the vast majority (70 percent) present with signs and symptoms of hydrocephalus, with enlargement of the head or irritability, headache, nausea and vomiting, and papilledema.[26, 27] Overproduction of CSF by the tumors has been well documented and can be as much as four times the normal rate.[11, 12, 27] In some cases, this overproduction probably contributes to the hydrocephalus. Tumors of the fourth ventricle are frequently accompanied by localizing signs.[16]

Plain skull x-ray films show evidence of increased ICP (split sutures, sellar changes) and, occasionally, tumor calcification. CT scanning is currently the radiologic examination of choice.[15] Usually, a lobulated mass of varying density in the fourth ventricle is seen. Occasionally, the tumor extends through the vallecula into the cisterna magna. The mass usually enhances brightly with intravenous contrast material. The authors do not routinely use preoperative angiography, but characteristic findings on angiography include symmetric hydrocephalus, a mass filling the fourth ventricle that has a granular vascular stain, and hypertrophy and tortuosity of either or both the medullary and vermian branches of the posterior inferior cerebellar artery.[14]

The CSF is abnormal in 60 percent of cases; the most common abnormalities are increased protein levels, xanthochromia, or both.[16, 26]

Grossly, the choroid plexus papilloma is a reddish tumor with an irregular surface. Under the microscope, it is seen to be composed of cuboidal cells arranged in fronds, resembling in every way normal choroid plexus.[28] No choroid plexus carcinoma (malignant papilloma) has been reported as arising in the fourth ventricle of a child.

The initial steps in the surgical approach are the same as those described for ependymoma, although the craniectomy need not be carried up to the transverse sinus. After opening the dura, the initial step is dissecting the tumor from the nodulus and uvula of the vermis. After lateral retraction of the tonsils, the tumor's blood supply can be isolated, coagulated, and divided. The opening into the fourth ventricle is enlarged by splitting the inferior vermis. The tumor, which does not invade brain tissue, is then carefully dissected free of the walls of the fourth ventricle. Before removing the tumor, one must be especially careful that all vessels have been coagulated and cut; midline feeding vessels from the precentral system must not be overlooked. Total tumor removal is the goal.

Because of their benign, noninvasive nature, patient survival after excision of these tumors is excellent. The operative mortality rate should be low, and long-term survival should approach 100 percent. The survival is influenced by the presence of subarachnoid seeding. Such tumor spread has been documented with benign histologic appearance. Radiation therapy has been given in cases of CSF spread; its efficacy has not been demonstrated.[16, 28]

DERMOID CYSTS

Dermoid cysts are rare lesions in the fourth ventricle. Although they can occur anywhere in the skull, they are most common in the posterior fossa, near or at the midline. Many of the tumors are associated with a complete or incomplete dermal sinus.[24] The fourth ventricle may not have an associated sinus; in the posterior fossa, the tumors may be extradural, in the vermis, or in the fourth ventricle.

These tumors arise from incomplete separation of the epithelial ectoderm from the neuroectoderm in the region of the anterior neuropore at about the fourth week of development. As would be expected, the cyst wall is composed of epidermis and dermis, including hair follicles, sweat glands, sebaceous glands, or all three. The tumors enlarge slowly and become filled with desquamated epithelium, sweat, and sebaceous materials.[21] Rarely, the lesions rupture and give rise to an aseptic meningitis. More frequently, repeated bouts of septic meningitis lead to the discovery of an occipital dimple with a sinus tract. Usually, the infecting organism is *Staphylococcus epidermidis*. The patient

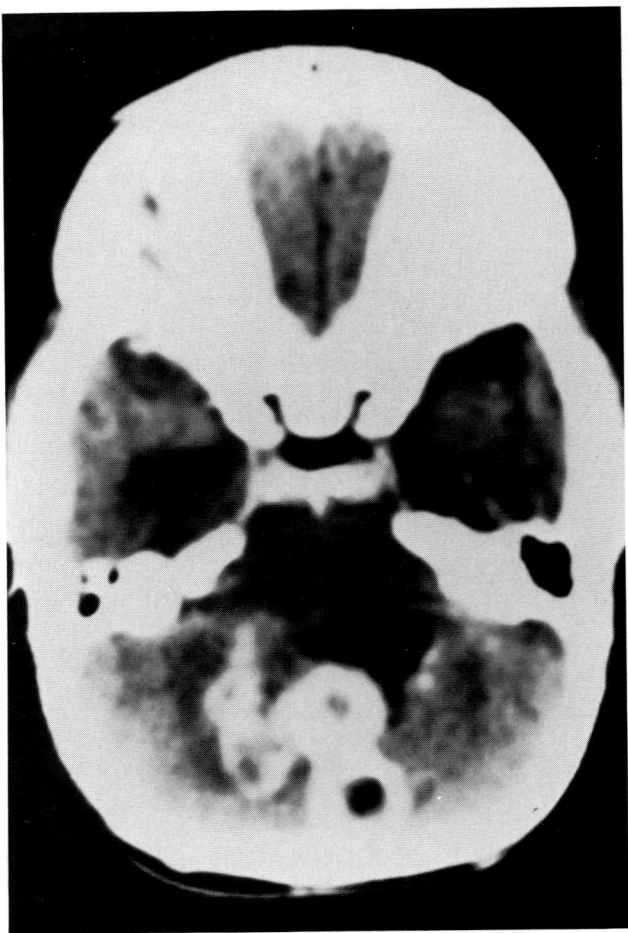

Figure 30–4. Dermoid cyst in the posterior fossa.

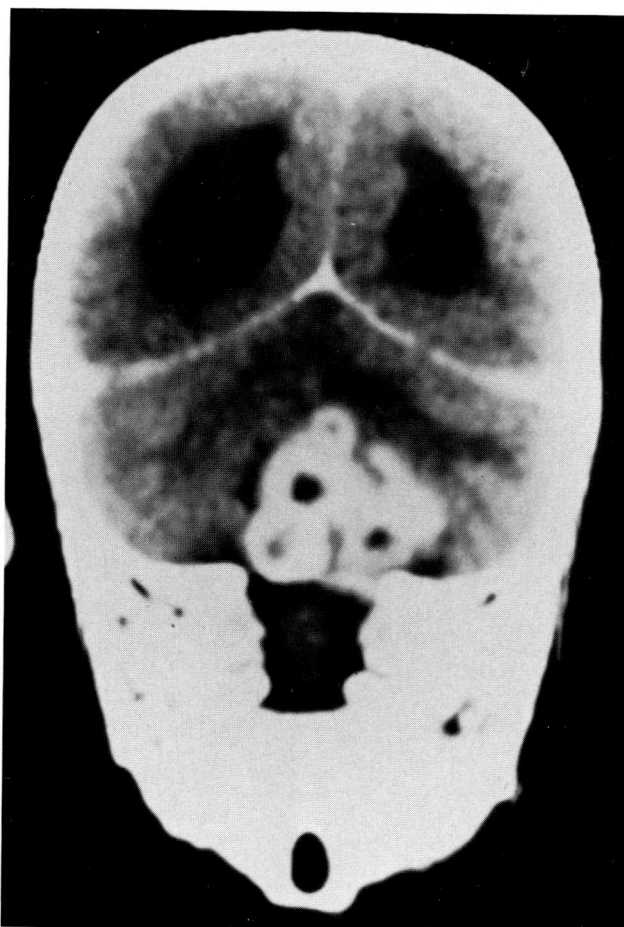

Figure 30–5. Coronal image of a dermoid cyst in the posterior fossa.

may also present only with a sinus tract, with purulent drainage from the sinus tract in the absence of meningitis, or with hydrocephalus, which may be obstructive, secondary to the mass in the fourth ventricle, or communicating, secondary to arachnoiditis caused by repetitive bouts of septic or aseptic meningitis. The sinus tract may be difficult to see, and one may have to comb hair up or shave the occiput when a sinus is suspected.

Radiographically, plain skull films may reveal an occipital bony defect with densely sclerotic margins.[6] If no sinus is present, the plain films are normal. CT scanning is the examination of choice. Dermoid tumors are low-density lesions. The capsule may enhance after intravenous contrast injection (Figs. 30–4 and 30–5). The contents of the cyst have a CT density between CSF and fat. NMR scanning may supplant CT scanning as the study of choice in the future.

These are benign tumors, and operative approaches should achieve total excision. This includes total resection of any sinus tract. The tumors usually separate easily from the substance of the brain, but scarring after repeated surgery may give rise to dense adhesions. Nevertheless, careful microscopic dissection should allow total removal. In light of the additional difficulty caused by adhesions, operative intervention should take place at the time of sinus discovery. One should plan on a major posterior fossa exploration when operating upon a child with a sinus tract. If the cutaneous tract is excised without following it to its termination, the result is frequently a continuous draining, nonhealing wound.

References

1. Abbott M, Namiki H: Congenital ependymoma. Case report. J Neurosurg 28:162, 1968.
2. Barone BM, Elbidge AR: Ependymomas. A clinical survey. J Neurosurg 33:428, 1970.
3. Bloom HJG: Intracranial tumors: Response and resistance to therapeutic endeavors, 1970–1980. Int J Radiat Oncol Biol Phys 8:1083, 1982.
4. Bloom HJG: Recent concepts in the conservative treatment of intracranial tumors in children. Acta Neurochir 50:103, 1979.
5. Chin HW, Manyama Y, Markesbery W: Intracranial ependymoma. Results of radiotherapy at the University of Kentucky. Cancer 49:2276, 1982.
6. Corkill G, McCullough GAJ, Tonge RE: Cranial dermal sinus: Value of plain skull x-ray examination and early diagnosis. Med J Aust 1:885, 1974.
7. Coulon RA, Till K: Intracranial ependymomas in children. Child's Brain 3:154, 1977.
8. Courville CB, Broussalian SL: Plastic ependymoma of the lateral recesses. Report of eight verified cases. J Neurosurg 18:792, 1961.
9. Cushing H: Intracranial Tumors: Notes upon a Series of Two Thousand Verified Cases with Surgical-mortality Figures Pertaining Thereto. Springfield, IL, Charles C Thomas, 1932.
10. Dohrman GJ, Farwell JR, Flannery JT: Ependymomas and ependymoblastomas in children. J Neurosurg 45:273, 1976.
11. Eisenberg HM, McComb JG, Lorenzo AV: Cerebrospinal fluid overproduction and hydrocephalus associated with choroid plexus papilloma. J Neurosurg 40:381, 1974.
12. Fairburn B: Choroid plexus papilloma and its relation to hydrocephalus. J Neurosurg 17:166, 1960.
13. Fokes EC, Jr., Earle KM: Ependymomas: Clinical and pathological aspects. J Neurosurg 30:585, 1969.
14. Hammon WK, Kempe LG, Hayes GJ: Angiographic appearance of a papilloma of the choroid plexus of the lateral ventricle. J Neurosurg 20:711, 1963.
15. Harwood-Nash DC, Fitz CR: Neuroradiology in Infants and Children, Vol. 2. St. Louis, MO, C.V. Mosby Co., 1976, pp 750–754.
16. Hawkins JC: Treatment of choroid plexus papillomas in children: A brief analysis of twenty years' experience. Neurosurgery 6:380, 1980.
17. Kernohan JW, Fletcher-Kernohan EM: Ependymomas. A study of 109 cases. Res Publ Assoc Res Nerv Ment Dis 16:182, 1937.
18. Kernohan JW, Sayre GP: Tumors of the central nervous system, fasc 35. In: Atlas of Tumor Pathology, Sect. X, facs. 35. Washington, DC, Armed Forces Institute of Pathology, 1952, p 129.
19. Kim YH, Fayos JV: Intracranial ependymoma. Radiology 124:805, 1977.
20. Koss WT, Miller MH: Intracranial Tumors of Infants and Children. Stuttgart, George Thieme, 1971.
21. Lekias J, Stokes B: Dermoid lesions of the central nervous system in children. Aust NZ J Surg 39:335, 1970.
22. Levin VA: Chemotherapy of recurrent brain tumors. In: Prestayko AW, Crooke ST (eds): Nitrosoureas: Current Status and New Developments. New York, Academic Press, 1981, pp 159–167.

23. Levin VA, Edwards MSB, Gutin PH, et al: Phase II evaluation of dibromodulcitol in the treatment of recurrent medulloblastoma, ependymoma and malignant astrocytoma. J Neurosurg 61:1065, 1984.
24. Logue V, Till K: Posterior fossa dermoid cysts with special reference to intracranial infection. J Neurol Neurosurg Psychiatry 15:1, 1952.
25. Matson DD: Neurosurgery of Infancy and Childhood. Springfield, IL, Charles C Thomas, 1969.
26. Matson DD, Crofton FDL: Papilloma of the choroid plexus in childhood. J Neurosurg 17:1002, 1960.
27. Milhorat TH, Hammock MK, Davis DA, et al: Choroid plexus papilloma. I. Proof of cerebrospinal fluid overproduction. Child's Brain 2:273, 1976.
28. Nasser SI, Mount LA: Papillomas of the choroid plexus. J Neurosurg 29:73, 1968.
29. Oi S, Raimondi AJ: Ependymoma in children. In: Pediatric Neurosurgery. Surgery of the Developing Nervous System. New York, Grune & Stratton, 1982, pp 419–428.
30. Pierre-Khan A, Hirsch JF, Roux FX, et al: Intracranial ependymomas in childhood. Survival and functional results of 47 cases. Child's Brain 10:145, 1983.
31. Raimondi AJ, Gutierrez FA: Diagnosis and surgical treatment of choroid plexus papilloma. Child's Brain 1:81, 1975.
32. Renaudin JW, DiTullio MV, Brown WJ: Seeding of intracranial ependymomas in children. Child's Brain 5:408, 1979.
33. Ringertz N, Reymond A: Ependymomas and choroid plexus papillomas. J Neuropathol Exp Neurol 8:355, 1949.
34. Rubinstein LJ: Tumors of the central nervous system. In: Atlas of Tumor Pathology, Series II, fasc. 6. Washington, DC, Armed Forces Institute of Pathology, 1972, pp 104–126
35. Rubinstein LJ: The definition of ependymoblastoma. Arch Pathol 90:35, 1970.
36. Rubinstein LJ: Tumors of the central nervous system. In: Atlas of Tumor Pathology, Series II, fasc. 6. Washington, DC, Armed Forces Institute of Pathology, 1972, pp 257–262.
37. Russell DS, Rubinstein LJ: Pathology of tumors of the nervous system. London, Edward Arnold, 1959, pp 139–142.
38. Salazar OM, Castro-Vita H, Van Houtie P, et al: Improved survival in cases of ependymoma after radiation therapy. J Neurosurg 59:652, 1983.
39. Scheithauer BW: Symptomatic subependymoma. Report of 21 cases with review of the literature. J Neurosurg 49:689, 1978.
40. Sheline GE: Radiation therapy of tumors of the central nervous system in childhood. Cancer 35:957, 1975.
41. Tomita T, Raimondi AJ: Fourth ventricular tumors. In: Pediatric Neurosurgery. Surgery of the Developing Nervous System. New York, Grune & Stratton, 1982.
42. Velasco-Siles JM, Raimondi AJ: Choroid plexus papilloma. In: Pediatric Neurosurgery. Surgery of the Developing Nervous System. New York, Grune & Stratton, 1982, pp 451–460.
43. Wilson CB, Gutin P, Boldrey EB: Single-agent chemotherapy of brain tumors. A five-year review. Arch Neurol 33:739, 1976.
44. Zee CS, Segall HD, Ahmadi J, et al: Computed tomography of posterior fossa ependymomas in childhood. Surg Neurol 20:221, 1983.

31
TUMORS OF THE CEREBRAL HEMISPHERES IN CHILDREN

Marion L. Walker, M.D.
Arno Fried, M.D.
Jogi Pattisapu, M.D.

It has long been recognized that tumors of the central nervous system (CNS) constitute a significant portion of all tumors seen in childhood. Brain tumors are second only to leukemia as the most common malignancy in children, and they are the most frequently occurring solid tumors seen in this age group. Several aspects of the management of pediatric brain tumors are distinctly different from those of tumors in the adult population. The mode of presentation, diagnostic evaluation, surgical treatment, and perioperative management may be vastly different in pediatric patients compared with adult patients. This chapter focuses on childhood tumors that occur in the cerebral hemispheres. Other intracranial supratentorial tumors, and tumors in the posterior fossa, are addressed in other chapters of this textbook.

Although childhood supratentorial tumors occur more frequently than previously recognized, they are often overshadowed by the attention given to those occurring in the posterior fossa. Matsori[23] estimated a 30 percent incidence of supratentorial tumors in children, but more recent reports indicate a higher percentage of supratentorial tumors than posterior fossa tumors in children younger than two years of age (55 percent versus 45 percent).[2, 14, 15, 16, 29, 37] This younger age group also has an increased incidence of tumors of the cerebral hemispheres. After the age of eight years, there is again a slight majority of supratentorial neoplasms.[14, 18]

Undoubtedly, referral patterns affect the distribution of tumors, along with the overall incidence of cerebral hemisphere tumors seen at any given center. A pediatric neurosurgical service with a higher proportion of younger children may accordingly report higher incidences of supratentorial and hemispheric tumors than has been previously appreciated.[37]

Tumors involving the cerebral hemispheres represent approximately 35 percent of the total supratentorial tumors seen in childhood.[14, 15] Although supratentorial tumors may be more common in the first two years of life, the incidence of cerebral hemisphere neoplasms is not different from that seen in children of all ages.[16, 27] Interestingly, several authors report a 2:1 ratio of boys to girls in their series of children with cerebral hemisphere tumors.[14, 15, 18, 23] In Hoffman's series,[15] 10 percent of the lesions were located in the occipital lobe, and the remainder were distributed almost equally among the frontal, parietal, and temporal lobes.

Childhood tumors may also be categorized by the age of presentation. Congenital neoplasms (discovered before two months of age) are often teratomas, astrocytomas, or tumors of neuroectodermal origin.[1, 16, 35] In the infant group (two months to two

CLINICAL PRESENTATION

Seizures

Epilepsy is seen in approximately 40 percent of children with cerebral hemisphere tumors,[15, 16] which is consistent with the experience of the authors. A variety of seizure patterns may result from hemispheric tumors, including grand mal, petit mal, focal, psychomotor, sensory epilepsy, or any combination of the preceding.

In recent years, unsuspected CNS tumors have been identified in epileptic children with suspected metabolic abnormalities or static structural lesions (arachnoid cysts) (Fig. 31–1). Using newer diagnostic modalities such as nuclear magnetic resonance imaging (NMRI), tumors of the cerebral hemispheres may be diagnosed earlier in their clinical course. Since epilepsy is often present for many years before a hemispheric tumor is discovered, it seems appropriate to evaluate all children with seizures, using NMRI, except those with the most

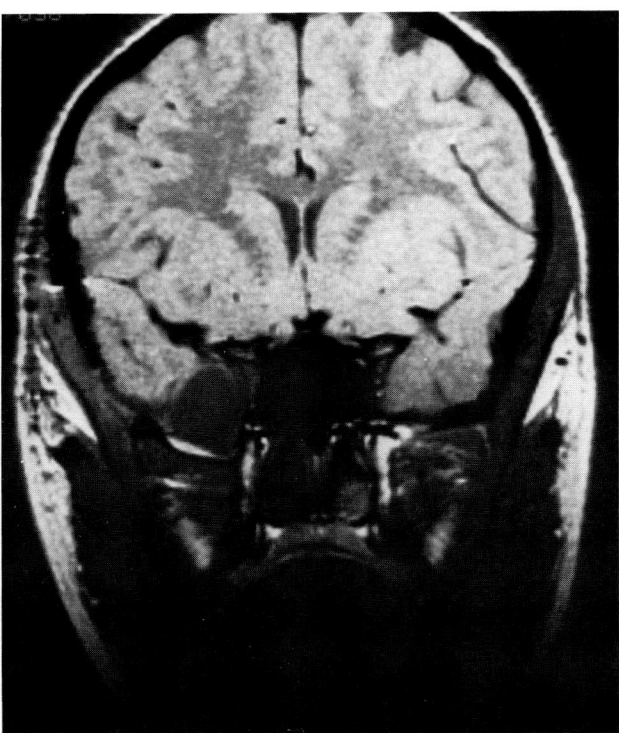

Figure 31–1. A coronal NMR showing a right temporal lobe lesion. This patient had been followed for seven years because of seizures and was thought to have an arachnoid cyst. This study suggests a small rim of brain tissue surrounding the area of low signal. At surgery, this was found to be a solid low-grade astrocytoma. No cystic component was encountered.

years), astrocytomas, ependymomas, and neuroectodermal tumors are frequently encountered. In children older than two years of age, astrocytomas and ependymomas are the most commonly seen intrahemispheric neoplasms.[1]

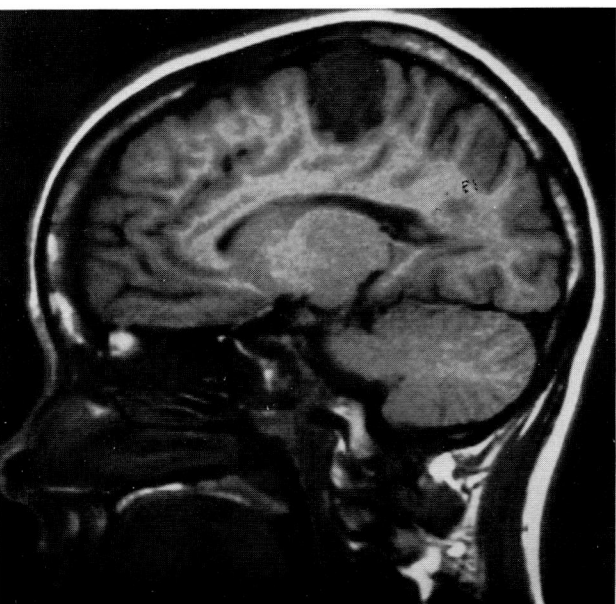

Figure 31–2. This 12-year-old female had been followed for right-sided focal seizures. Her CT scans were interpreted as normal. This NMR image easily identifies a lesion in the left motor cortex. This lesion proved to be a low-grade astrocytoma.

obvious and straightforward seizure types (e.g., febrile convulsions). NMRI often identifies cerebral lesions better and earlier than conventional computed tomography (CT),[40] and earlier diagnosis lessens the interval between the onset of seizures and surgical intervention. Many children with epilepsy have been followed through much of their childhood before a hemispheric lesion became apparent on diagnostic imaging studies (Fig. 31–2).

Increased Intracranial Pressure

Macrocrania is frequently seen in infants presenting with increased intracranial pressure from hemispheric tumors. A 60 to 80 percent incidence of macrocrania is reported in several series of infants with congenital CNS neoplasms.[1, 16, 29, 35] In younger children with an expansile skull, the rapidly growing neoplasm sometimes occupies an entire hemisphere and results in skull asymmetry. In addition to the direct mass effect, hemispheric tumors may also obstruct cerebrospinal fluid (CSF) pathways, resulting in hydrocephalus and increased intracranial pressure. Hydrocephalus is seen in 82 percent of children younger than one year of age with hemispheric tumors, although macrocrania sometimes occurs in the absence of hydrocephalus.[27]

Other signs of increased intracranial pressure include papilledema, sixth cranial nerve palsy, and a bulging fontanelle in infants. However, the infant fontanelle may be surprisingly soft, even in the presence of a large hemispheric lesion, and is often an unreliable indicator of increased intracranial pressure. The expansibility of the infant skull results in macrocrania and reduces the intracranial pressure. Papilledema is reported in 40 to 60 percent of older children, and sixth nerve palsy is seen in approximately 20 percent of children with hemispheric tumors.[15,16]

At least half the children with cerebral tumors complain of headache at presentation.[15,24] The headaches may be severe and are usually the result of increased intracranial pressure or of direct pressure on pain-sensitive structures. While older children often complain of headache, the discomfort may be identified as irritability, head holding, or head banging in younger children.[16] Headaches from increased intracranial pressure are frequently more severe in the morning and usually improve when the patient is active. Vomiting often accompanies the headache, especially when the patient awakens.[1,24]

Occasionally, patients with chronically increased intracranial pressure may present with visual loss or intermittent visual obscurations. Children who are too young to complain have visual inattention, are unable to grasp toys, and frequently collide with walls or furniture. It is especially important to document visual loss in children, since profound visual loss from increased intracranial pressure is rarely recovered (Fig. 31–3). Therefore, children who present with loss of vision require urgent neurosurgical intervention.

Focal Deficits

Tumors of the cerebral hemispheres may cause variable focal neurologic deficits, depending on their location. They may include monoparesis or hemiparesis, sensory loss, personality change, or worsening school performance. Most children with hemispheric tumors have impairment of the motor cortex or the internal capsule.[15] Superficially located tumors may cause deficits involving only the face, arm, or leg, and deep tumors often involve the internal capsule and result in contralateral hemiparesis. Lesions of the parietal lobe tend to present with focal deficits earlier in their clinical course than tumors located distant to the motor cortex.

Phakomatoses

Children with tumors of the hemispheres may also have one of the phakomatoses.[2,22] Tuberous sclerosis is often noted in patients with subependymal giant cell astrocytomas.[17,22] An increased operative complication rate has been reported in these children, resulting mainly from tumors involving the cardiac conduction pathways or an intracardiac rhabdomyosarcoma.[1,2,22] Von Recklinghausen's disease (neurofibromatosis) may be present in children with low-grade astrocytomas of the hemispheres as well as in children who present

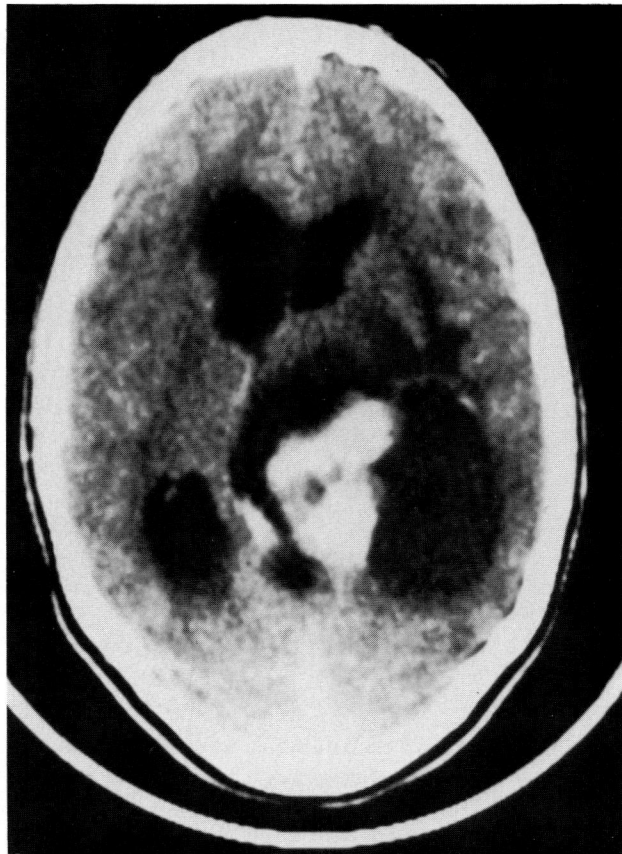

Figure 31–3. This eight-year-old girl presented with a long-standing history of symptoms compatible with increased intracranial pressure. She had papilledema on examination and was found to be completely blind.

with large hamartomas of the hemispheres.[2,22,30] In children with neurofibromatosis, hamartomas involving the visual pathway are demonstrated more clearly with NMRI than with CT (Fig. 31–4).

Hemorrhage

Spontaneous intracranial hematomas in children are infrequent, and tumors should be suspected when a child presents in this manner.[16,39] Wakai and colleagues[36] noted a 14 percent incidence of hemorrhage in congenital CNS tumors, most frequently occurring in astrocytomas and ependymomas.[36] Although the tumor is suspected on radiologic evaluation, it may not be recognized until surgery or postoperative studies.

DIAGNOSTIC STUDIES

Over the past decade, rapid improvement in neuroimaging techniques has resulted in a greatly increased ability to diagnose intracranial abnormalities. With the advent of CT and NMRI, studies that were once common and indispensable (such as

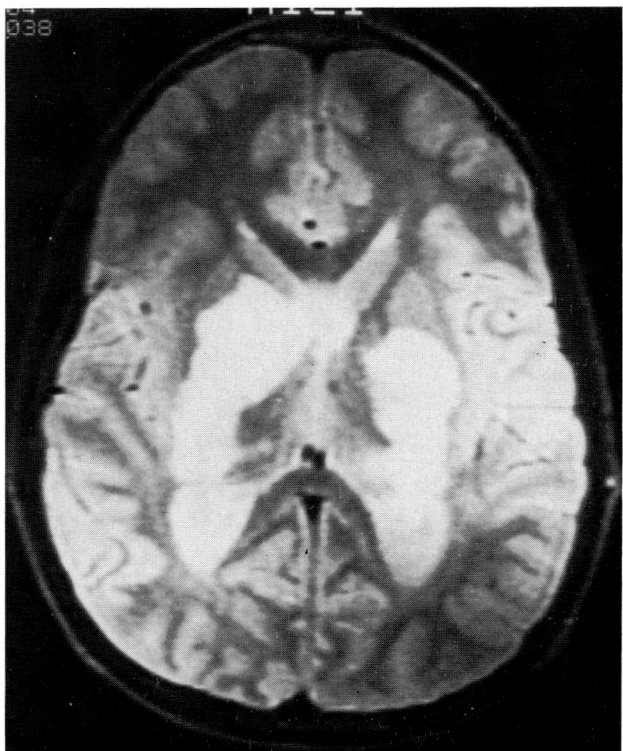

Figure 31–4. This NMR image shows increased signal along the optic radiations in a patient with neurofibromatosis. These lesions, on stereotaxic biopsy, proved to be hamartomas.

pneumoencephalography, ventriculography, and radioisotope scanning) are now of historical interest only.

Plain Skull Radiography

Much valuable information may be obtained from routine skull radiographs when evaluating a child for an intracranial neoplasm. Focal skull deformities, calcification, erosion of the dorsum sella, and splitting of the cranial sutures may be identified, and this sometimes aids in the differential diagnosis of hemisphere lesions. It is reported that approximately 80 percent of tumors in infants are associated with abnormal findings on plain skull x-ray films (Fig. 31–5).[16]

Computerized Tomography

Computerized tomography (CT) has revolutionized the diagnosis of intracranial neoplasms, and today it is the method of choice for evaluating the child with a suspected brain tumor. The newer generation of scanners provide excellent detail of tumor location, vasculature, and surrounding edema. Hemorrhage, calcification, and tumor necrosis are easily identified on CT scans, often providing valuable information regarding the histology of the lesion. For example, following contrast enhancement, the mural nodule of a cystic astrocytoma characteristically enhances density without enhancement of the cyst wall, which often suggests the diagnosis. Solid astrocytomas, oligodendrogliomas, ependymomas, and teratomas are often patchy in appearance, with irregular contrast enhancement. Today, the CT scan is essential during the initial evaluation of patients presenting with signs and symptoms of CNS pathology.

Cerebral Angiography

The recent emergence of high-quality CT and NMRI has made cerebral angiography unnecessary in many patients. However, angiography frequently offers valuable information in children suspected of harboring cerebral hemisphere tumors. Although the importance of this diagnostic modality has faded dramatically over the past ten years, it is essential when an aneurysm or an arteriovenous malformation is included in the differential diagnosis. The angiogram often defines increased vascularity (vascular blush) in hemangioblastomas, teratomas, and certain gliomas. Today, angiography is reserved for atypical cases or lesions with large blood vessels adjacent to or within the tumor mass.

Nuclear Magnetic Resonance Imaging

Similar to the case with CT a decade ago, nuclear magnetic resonance imaging (NMRI) has in recent years revolutionized the diagnostic approach to intracranial tumors.[40] Today, the high-quality images from state-of-the-art NMRI units provide a wealth of diagnostic information. NMRI is more sensitive to most, if not all, neoplastic tissue and is especially valuable in the evaluation of cerebral hemispheric lesions. The ability to differentiate between CSF and fluid within a tumor cyst is of special importance when evaluating hemisphere lesions. Frequently, patients are diagnosed with CNS lesions that were not recognized on previous CT scans.

Since NMRI is a much more valuable diagnostic tool, all patients with persistent seizures should be evaluated using this modality, even if the CT scan is normal. The authors have treated several epileptic patients in whom NMRI identified hemispheric tumors as the cause of the seizures. Multiple prior diagnostic evaluations (including two or more CT scans) had failed to identify the small lesions, which were often located in the temporal or parietal regions.

Electroencephalography

Electroencephalography (EEG) is not a diagnostic test routinely used in most cases of CNS neoplasms.

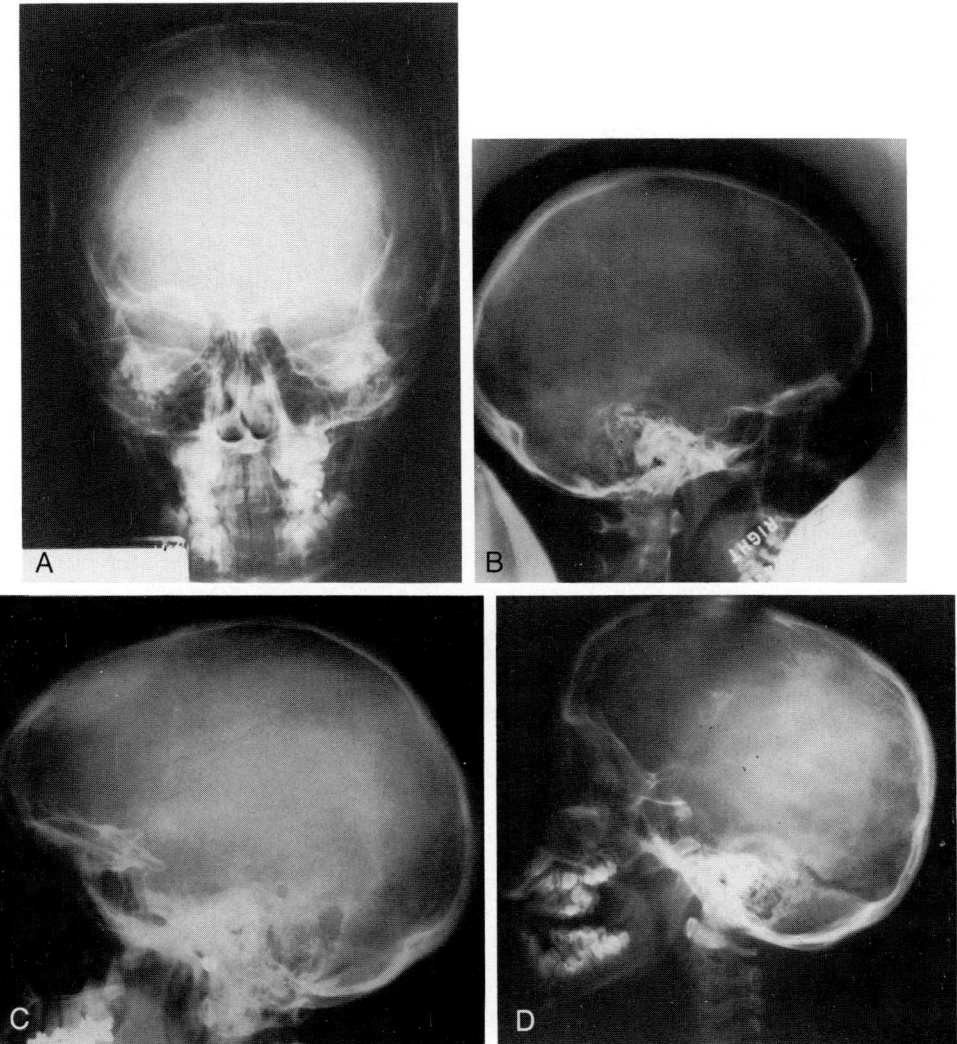

Figure 31–5. Common findings on plain skull radiographs in patients with intracranial tumors. *A*, Focal skull erosion. *B*, Calcification. *C*, Erosion of the dorsum sella. *D*, Splitting of the cranial sutures.

However, it is sometimes helpful in evaluating children with hemispheric lesions by identifying a focal abnormality and indicating the need for further studies. An epileptic patient with a focally abnormal electroencephalogram should be evaluated with NMRI, even if the CT scan is negative.

TREATMENT

Just as in the area of diagnostic evaluation, the surgical management of childhood tumors is rapidly evolving. Over two decades ago, Matson[23] recognized the grim prognosis of children with CNS neoplasms. However, technologic advancement in operative and perioperative management in recent years has resulted in lower mortality and morbidity rates, thus significantly improving the prognosis in these children.[10, 19, 38]

Surgery

Timely surgical intervention is the mainstay of improved prognosis in children with hemispheric tumors. With the currently available surgical methods and with the postsurgical mortality rate approaching zero, most patients with hemispheric lesions can be operated upon successfully. Because many of these tumors are malignant, and since the side effects of radiation therapy are harmful to the developing brain, an attempt at safe and gross total surgical excision is mandatory. This takes on even more importance in the very young, since the patient often is treated with surgery, with efforts made to maintain or control tumor recurrence with chemotherapy. Radiation therapy is usually administered to children older than four years of age or to those who have limited options for treatment.

Today, near-total resections of hemispheric lesions are possible with the surgical microscope, laser, Cavitron ultrasonic aspirator, and other new components of the surgical armamentarium. The microscope offers the magnification and illumination necessary to discern tumor tissue from the surrounding normal brain. Although lasers have been important in posterior fossa surgery, the authors have not found it to be especially useful in tumors involving the cerebral hemispheres.[38] In the authors' experience, the Cavitron ultrasonic aspirator is more useful than the laser in resecting hemispheric tumors, except when the lesions are adjacent to vital brain structures, where the laser is more precise for removing the last small portions. However, tumors in children are frequently soft, and standard surgical suction often is all that is needed for complete tumor removal.

Radiation Therapy

Although radiation therapy plays an important role in controlling tumor growth and preventing recurrence, there is no question that it is harmful to the developing brain.[19, 27, 33] Although there is no definite age at which time the brain is no longer vulnerable to radiation therapy, it is generally believed that the infant is especially vulnerable. Children younger than four years of age who receive whole-brain irradiation suffer some lowering of intelligence and have a high risk of learning disabilities. Beyond four years of age, the child is much less likely to suffer deleterious effects from whole-brain irradiation. If only local radiation therapy is required, the risk to the developing brain is significantly reduced. In some cases, the child may be followed closely using serial CT or NMRI studies, and tumor recurrence is documented prior to radiation therapy.

Not all tumors of the cerebral hemispheres need immediate postoperative radiation therapy.[31] Malignant astrocytomas, oligoastrocytomas, ependymomas, metastases, and primitive neuroectodermal tumors are some of the common hemispheric tumors that require radiation therapy. The authors' approach includes repeat craniotomy for debulking or total resection of recurrent tumors prior to radiation therapy.

Chemotherapy

Very little is known regarding chemotherapy of intracranial neoplasms in children, and most of the experience concerning its efficacy is derived primarily from treatment of other childhood cancers. Chemotherapy appears to benefit patients with malignant neoplasms, but which drug combinations are most effective is as yet undetermined. Available evidence suggests that the developing brain is less affected by chemotherapeutic agents than by radiation therapy, and for this reason, malignant tumors of infancy may be initially treated with chemotherapy until the patient is three or four years of age, when radiation therapy is better tolerated.

At present, two chemotherapy regimens are often used: (1) lomustine (CCNU), vincristine, and prednisone, and (2) the 8 in 1 drug regimen. Both protocols require meticulous attention to bone marrow suppression and to renal damage and, therefore, are administered by an experienced pediatric oncologist.

Repeat Craniotomy

In recent years, reoperation for benign and malignant recurrent brain tumors has proved to be a viable treatment alternative in properly selected patients. Barrer and associates[3] reported a 4 percent mortality rate and a 9 percent morbidity rate in children undergoing repeat craniotomies for a variety of CNS neoplasms. This is in line with the risks of the initial craniotomy, and the results from this small group of patients seem promising. The child with a good functional status and a surgically accessible lesion would benefit from a second surgical procedure prior to chemotherapy.

SPECIFIC TUMOR TYPES

Astrocytomas of the Cerebral Hemisphere

The most common tumors of the cerebral hemisphere are astrocytomas, and 50 percent of the supratentorial astrocytomas occur in the cerebral hemisphere.[15] Most other series report a 14 to 64 percent incidence of hemispheric astrocytomas in children younger than 16 years of age.[4, 14, 20, 21, 23, 25, 37] There is no sex predilection, and they occur in all age groups, with a peak incidence between 8 and 12 years.[9, 24, 25] Approximately half the cases are benign (grade I or II), and half are malignant (grade III or IV).[4, 16, 20, 21, 23]

The majority (50 to 70 percent) of supratentorial gliomas are associated with a tumor cyst, and unlike the cerebellar cystic astrocytomas, the cyst wall is lined by neoplastic tissue in 70 percent of cases.[15, 23-26] The tumor is contiguous with the ventricle in most cases, with the mural nodule located at the medial aspect of the lesion.[25] This factor must be remembered during surgical intervention, since the cyst wall should be resected in an attempt to prevent recurrence.[15] In addition, when the lesion involves the frontal, temporal, or occipital lobes, an en bloc resection via a lobectomy should be considered. Hoffman[15] noted a slight improvement in survival rate in the frontal pole gliomas, possibly due to the lobectomy, although this was not confirmed by others.[20, 21]

Histologically, the pilocytic type is seen in the majority of hemispheric supratentorial astrocytomas in childhood.[24] Of these lesions, the cystic type predominates (65 percent) and is associated with the most favorable prognosis (mean survival of 16 years in 15 patients).[24] This tumor resembles the cerebellar spongioblastoma and has an extremely benign clinical course.[24, 25]

It is well known that the prognosis with hemispheric low-grade gliomas is better in children than in adults. In a recent report by Laws and coworkers,[20, 21] the five-year survival rate in patients with supratentorial low-grade gliomas was 83 percent for those less than 20 years of age, 35 percent for those aged 20 to 49, and 12 percent for those older than 50 years of age.[20, 21] Dohrmann and colleagues[9] reported the probability of survival with cerebral hemisphere astrocytomas at one, two, five, and ten years as 0.779, 0.748, 0.678, and 0.628, respectively. Several features that predispose to a favorable outcome have been identified, including age, total resection, postoperative neurologic deficit, altered consciousness, personality changes, and the presence of a tumor cyst.[20, 21]

Malignant transformation may occur in low-grade astrocytomas, and they may present as malignant gliomas or glioblastoma multiforme. Glioblastomas account for about 7 percent of all intracranial neoplasms in childhood, and their behavior in children is similar to that in adults. The male to female ratio is 3:2, with a peak incidence at 12.7 years.[9] Approximately half the lesions occur in the cerebral hemispheres, mostly involving the frontal lobe.

Oligodendrogliomas

Approximately 1 to 3 percent of all primary intrahemispheric neoplasms in children are oligodendroglial in origin, if mixed gliomas are excluded.[8] However, the incidence is much higher (9 to 30 percent), if tumors with an astrocytic component are included (e.g., oligoastrocytomas).[12] These slowly growing lesions occur most often in the cerebral cortex, with the mean age between 10 and 13 years and a male predominance (2:1).[8] Although seizures are the presenting complaint in most children (75 to 100 percent), headaches, behavioral changes, nausea, and vomiting are also frequently noted.

Calcification is often seen on plain skull x-ray films, and CT scans identify an irregularly defined lesion with patchy contrast enhancement. Angiography shows an avascular mass but, sometimes, reveals abnormal tumor vessels and a vascular "blush."

Pathologically, most oligodendrogliomas contain a mixture of astrocytes and oligodendroglia. In some cases, the astrocytic component of the tumor predominates, and the tumor is referred to as an oligoastrocytoma. It is not known if these tumors are more likely to undergo malignant degeneration than the oligodendroglioma.

Surgical resection offers the best prognosis in these children, with a five-year survival rate of 75 to 85 percent in one series.[8] Radiation therapy is of questionable benefit in "pure" oligodendrogliomas but may improve outcome in patients with a mixed glial tumor (oligoastrocytoma). Children with oligodendrogliomas must be followed closely for late recurrence or malignant degeneration and should be considered for multiple operations, as necessary. Dohrmann and associates[8] noted a slightly increased survival rate with repeat craniotomies for recurrent oligodendroglioma.

Ependymomas

Ependymomas constitute approximately 9 percent of all intracranial tumors in childhood. They usually occur in children younger than six years of age, with the mean age between two and three years.[5, 7] Again, there is a male predominance, and the lesion is located in the supratentorial compartment in 30 to 50 percent of cases. The children present with headache, vomiting, and increased head circumference, and seizures occur in approximately 30 to 40 percent of the hemispheric lesions. Coulon and Till[5] noted that macrocysts occur in one half of the supratentorial lesions, but they are usually not associated with a benign histology (Fig. 31–

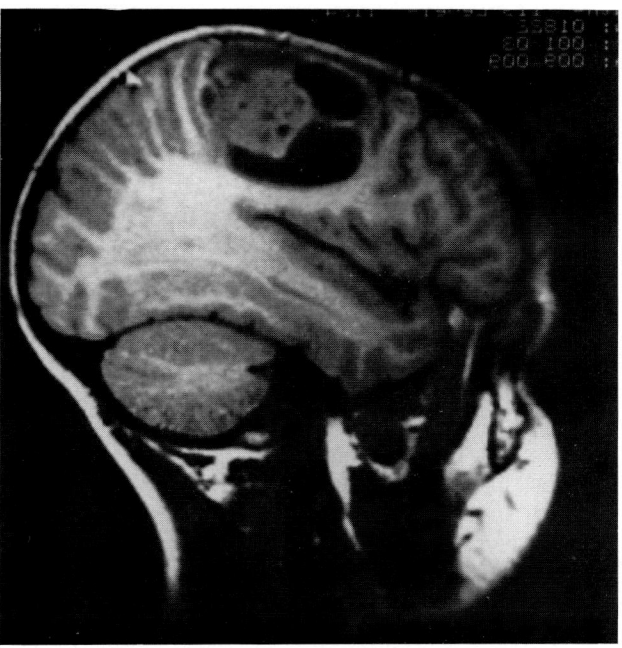

Figure 31–6. This NMR image shows the large macrocysts that often occur in ependymomas. These lesions can occupy much of one cerebral hemisphere. This lesion proved to be a malignant ependymoma.

6). Histologically, the hemispheric ependymomas are similar to the posterior fossa lesions, and they occasionally undergo malignant degeneration into ependymoblastomas.

Surgical excision, with postoperative radiation therapy, offers the best prognosis in the child with an ependymoma. It is well recognized that the supratentorial ependymoma has a much better prognosis than the posterior fossa lesion.[5, 7, 16] The five-year survival rate for hemispheric ependymomas is approximately 60 percent with gross total removal and radiation therapy, compared with a 10 percent survival rate for the infratentorial tumor.[7] Distal metastases and spinal seeding occur in 25 percent of patients and require meticulous searching and treatment.[28]

Gangliogliomas

Gangliogliomas comprise 0 to 7.6 percent of all childhood brain neoplasms.[13, 32] Since the extensive review by Courville[6] in 1930, much has been learned about these interesting tumors. They most often occur in patients younger than 30 years of age and show a slight male predominance. Gangliogliomas are usually diagnosed in children with poorly controlled seizures, progressive headaches, or behavioral changes.[13, 32] Although they may occur at any location, they are frequently located in the temporal lobe or the floor of the third ventricle.

Radiographically, plain skull x-ray films identify calcification in approximately 10 percent of cases, possibly with areas of skull thinning or erosion when the tumor is superficially located. The CT scan frequently demonstrates a well-demarcated, low-density area that often enhances with contrast administration (Fig. 31–7). On angiography, they appear as avascular masses, with vessel displacement and mass effect.

Pathologically, the tumor contains a mixture of ganglion cells (neurons) and a glial stroma (astrocytes). However, the diagnosis may be difficult in locations where ganglion cells occur normally.

The slowly growing and nonaggressive nature of gangliogliomas makes surgical resection the treatment of choice in children with accessible lesions. They are relatively radioresistant, and radiation therapy after surgical removal has not been proved to be of added benefit. In one study, the survival rate for patients with gangliogliomas has been estimated at 75 percent at seven years, and most authors note a benign course in children with surgically treated lesions.[6, 13, 32] Rarely, the astrocytic component of the tumor may undergo malignant degeneration and present as an anaplastic ganglioglioma.[13] Recurrent tumors should be re-explored if they are surgically accessible and should be considered for postoperative radiation therapy.

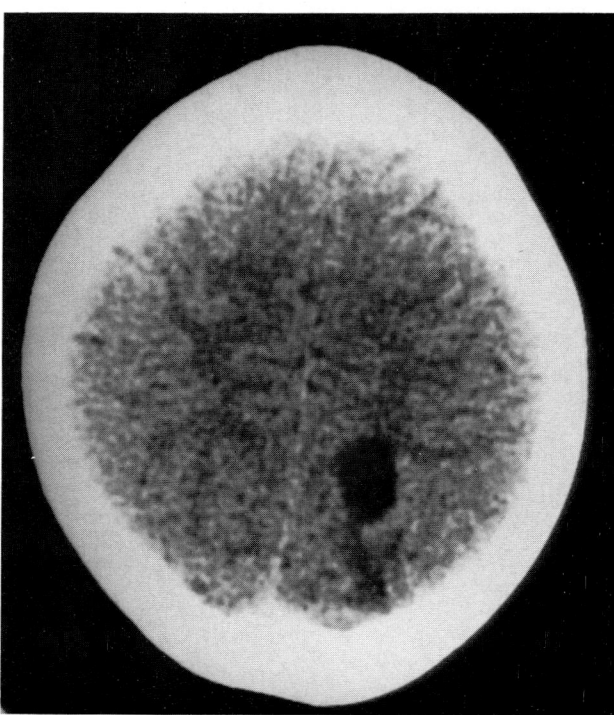

Figure 31–7. The CT scan demonstrates a low dense lesion that is often seen in gangliogliomas. Local skull erosion is quite common.

Teratomas

Teratomas are the most commonly diagnosed intrahemispheric tumor in neonates and infants younger than two years of age. They constitute approximately 40 percent of congenital tumors, and the majority occur in the pineal region.[11, 35] Most infants present with macrocrania and signs of increased intracranial pressure. Interestingly, the teratoma is the most common CNS neoplasm in stillborn babies, and many neonates with a teratoma are stillborn. The tumors often attain huge sizes and occupy most of the supratentorial space in the newborn patients (Fig. 31–8).

Surgical intervention in patients in this age group carries a significant risk to the neonate. Operative mortality rates of 20 to 40 percent have been reported in neonates with congenital brain tumors.[1, 35] Therefore, initial management of hydrocephalus with a delayed craniotomy should be considered in most instances.

Pathologically, teratomas contain elements derived from all three germ cell layers. Occasionally, the larger tumors may show evidence of malignant degeneration and necrosis. The prognosis in children with benign teratomas is very favorable after complete surgical excision.[15] However, a 7 percent one-year survival rate was noted by Wakai and associates[35] in infants with malignant teratomas.

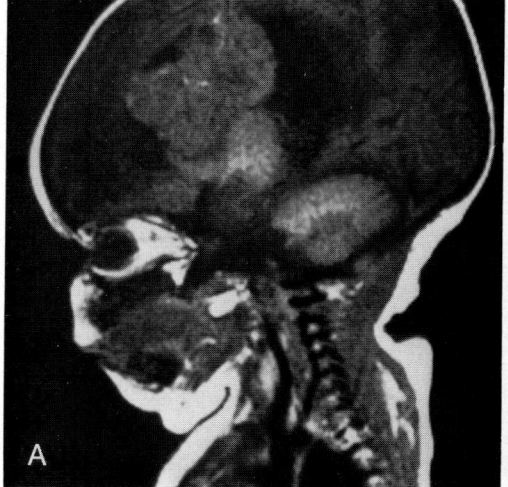 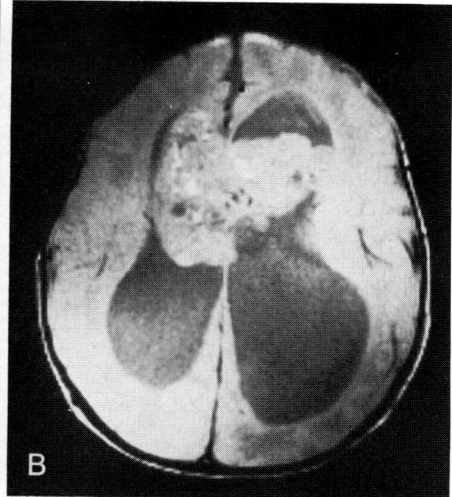

Figure 31–8. Sagittal (A) and axial (B) NMR images demonstrate a large tumor in the neonate, surgically proven to be a teratoma.

Cerebral Metastases

Cerebral metastasis is a well-known complication of malignant disease, yet there are inadequate data concerning the problem in childhood. It is estimated that approximately 2 to 8 percent of intracranial neoplasms in children are metastases.[16, 34] Neuroblastoma, embryonal rhabdomyosarcoma, and nephroblastoma (Wilms's tumor) are the most common primary sources of metastases to the CNS.[16, 18, 34] Vannucci and Baten[34] reported on 14 cases in a series of 231 autopsies performed on pediatric patients with solid malignant tumors. Excluding leukemias, lymphomas, primary CNS neoplasms, and invasion of the brain from contiguous structures, they found a 6 percent incidence of hemispheric metastasis. All the patients had pulmonary metastatic disease at the time of diagnosis of cerebral involvement. The prognosis for children with CNS lesions was poor, with survival between 2.5 and 20 months, depending on the primary malignancy and the location of the metastasis. Multiple lesions were noted in half the patients in their series.

SUMMARY

Tumors of the cerebral hemispheres constitute approximately 35 percent of the total supratentorial neoplasms seen in childhood. Boys are affected more commonly than girls, and the lesions are distributed evenly throughout the cerebral hemispheres. They present with seizures, headache, and other symptoms of increased intracranial pressure. The most common tumors of the cerebral hemispheres are astrocytomas, except in the newborn, in whom teratomas are most frequently seen.

Over the past three decades, significantly improved operative and anesthetic management has afforded a positive outlook for the pediatric patient, resulting in decreased overall mortality rates and a better quality of life. However, there are many unanswered questions regarding pediatric brain tumors. Further improvement in the outcome of these patients will someday accompany our advances in understanding the biology of these tumors.

References

1. Albright AL: Brain tumors in neonates, infants, and toddlers. Contemp Neurosurg 7:1, 1985.
2. Allen JC: Tumors of the central nervous system in infants. In: Hoffman HJ, Epstein FJ (eds): Disorders of the Developing Nervous System. Boston, Blackwell Scientific Publications, 1986, pp 751–766.
3. Barrer SJ, Schut L, Sutton LN, et al: Re-operation for recurrent brain tumors in children. Child's Brain 11:375, 1984.
4. Bruno L, Schut L: Survey of pediatric brain tumors. In: Pediatric Neurosurgery. Surgery of the Developing Nervous System. New York, Grune & Stratton, 1982, pp 361–365.
5. Coulon RA, Till K: Intracranial ependymomas in children. A review of 43 cases. Child's Brain 3:154, 1977.
6. Courville CB: Ganglioglioma: Tumor of the central nervous system: Review of the literature and report of two cases. Arch Neurol Psychiatry 24:434, 1930.
7. Dohrmann GJ, Farwell JR, Flannery JT: Ependymomas and ependymoblastomas in children. J Neurosurg 45:273, 1976.
8. Dohrmann GJ, Farwell JR, Flannery JT: Oligodendrogliomas in children. Surg Neurol 10:21, 1978.
9. Dohrmann GJ, Farwell JR, Flannery JT: Astrocytomas in childhood: A population-based study. Surg Neurol 23:64, 1985.
10. Duffner PK, Cohen ME, Myers MH, et al: Survival of children with brain tumors: SEER Program, 1973–1980. Neurology 36:597, 1986.
11. Ellams ID, Neuhauser G, Agnoli AL: Congenital intracranial neoplasms. Child's Nerv Syst 2:165, 1986.
12. Favier J, Pizzolato GP, Berney J: Oligodendroglial tumors in childhood. Child's Nerv Syst 1:33, 1985.
13. Hall WA, Yunis EJ, Albright AL: Anaplastic ganglioglioma in an infant: Case report and review of the literature. Neurosurgery 19:1016, 1986.
14. Harwood-Nash D, Fitz C: Brain neoplasms. In: Harwood-Nash D, Fitz C (eds): Neuroradiology in Infants and Children. St. Louis, C.V. Mosby, 1976, pp 668–788.

15. Hoffman HJ: Supratentorial brain tumors in children. *In*: Youmans JR (ed): Neurological Surgery, 2nd ed. Philadelphia, W.B. Saunders Co., 1982, pp 2702–2732.
16. Jooma R, Hayward RD, Grant DN: Intracranial neoplasms during the first year of life: Analysis of one hundred consecutive cases. Neurosurgery 14:31, 1984.
17. Kapp JP, Paulson GW, Odom GL: Brain tumors with tuberous sclerosis. J Neurosurg 26:191, 1967.
18. Koos WT, Miller MH: Intracranial Tumors of Infants and Children. St. Louis, C.V. Mosby, 1971, pp 89–146.
19. Kun LE, Mulhern RK, Crisco JJ: Quality of life in children treated for brain tumors. J Neurosurg 58:1, 1983.
20. Laws ER, Taylor WF, Clifton MB, et al: Neurosurgical management of low-grade astrocytoma of the cerebral hemispheres. J Neurosurg 61:665, 1984.
21. Laws ER, Taylor WF, Bergstralh EJ, et al: The neurosurgical management of low-grade astrocytoma. *In*: Little JR (ed): Clinical Neurosurgery. Baltimore, Williams & Wilkins, 1986, pp 575–588.
22. Martuza RL: Neurofibromatosis and other phakomatoses. *In*: Wilkins RH, Rengachary SS (eds): Neurosurgery. New York, McGraw-Hill, 1985, pp 511–521.
23. Matson DD: Gliomas of the cerebral hemispheres. *In*: Matson DD, Ingraham FD (eds): Neurosurgery of Infancy and Childhood, 2nd ed. Springfield, IL, Charles C Thomas Publishers, 1969, pp 480–522.
24. Mercuri S, Russo A, Palma L: Hemispheric supratentorial astrocytomas in children. J Neurosurg 55:170, 1981.
25. Palma L, Guidetti B: Cystic pilocytic astrocytomas of the cerebral hemispheres. J Neurosurg 62:811, 1985.
26. Palma L, Russo A, Mercuri S: Cystic cerebral astrocytomas in infancy and childhood: Long-term results. Child's Brain 10:79, 1983.
27. Raimondi AJ, Tomita T: Brain tumors during the first year of life. Child's Brain 10:193, 1983.
28. Renaudin JW, DiTullio MV, Brown WJ: Seeding of intracranial ependymomas in children. Child's Brain 5:408, 1979.
29. Sato O, Tamura A, Sano K: Brain tumors in early infants. Child's Brain 1:121, 1975.
30. Schut L, Duhaime AC, Rorke L, et al: Von Recklinghausen's disease. *In*: Hoffman HJ, Epstein FJ (eds): Disorders of the Developing Nervous System. Boston, Blackwell, 1986, pp 591–607.
31. Sheline GE: The role of radiation therapy in the treatment of low-grade gliomas. *In*: Little JR (ed): Clinical Neurosurgery. Baltimore, Williams & Wilkins, 1986.
32. Sutton LN, Packer RJ, Rorke LB, et al: Cerebral gangliogliomas during childhood. Neurosurgery 13:124, 1983.
33. Tiberin P, Moar E, Zaizov R, et al: Brain sarcoma of meningeal origin after cranial irradiation in childhood acute lymphocytic leukemia. J Neurosurg 61:772, 1984.
34. Vannucci RC, Baten M: Cerebral metastatic disease in childhood. Neurology 24:981, 1974.
35. Wakai S, Arai T, Nagai M: Congenital brain tumors. Surg Neurol 21:597, 1984.
36. Wakai S, Yamakawa K, Manaka S, et al: Spontaneous intracranial hemorrhage caused by brain tumor: Its incidence and clinical significance. Neurosurgery 10:437, 1982.
37. Walker ML, Storrs BB: Use of the CO_2 lasers for surgical excision of primary brain tumors in children. Concepts Pediatr Neurosurg 3:207, 1983.
38. Walker ML, Storrs BB: Lasers in pediatric neurosurgery. Pediatr Neurosci 12:23, 1985.
39. Wyler AR, Hered J, Smith JR, et al: Subarachnoid hemorrhage in infancy due to brain tumor. Arch Neurol 29:447, 1973.
40. Zimmerman RA, Bilaniuk LT: Magnetic resonance imaging of pediatric brain tumors. Neurosurgery 1:1, 1986.

32
INTRAVENTRICULAR TUMORS

Anthony J. Raimondi, M.D.

One may consider intraventricular tumors to be ependymal, glial, or mesenchymal in origin, with the ependymal tumors arising from the ependymal lining and the glial tumors arising from the subependymal tissue. The mesenchymal tumors originate from either the vascular component or the tela choroidea of the choroid plexus. The incidence of ependymal tumors is greatest in the fourth ventricle. The lateral ventricles are the commonest site of glial tumors and the choroid plexus papilloma. The incidence ratio of lateral ventricle choroid plexus papillomas to third ventricle papillomas is approximately 7 to 1, whereas fourth ventricle papillomas, practically speaking, do not occur in childhood. One may say much the same for intraventricular meningiomas, strange though it may seem, even considering the high incidence of meningioma in children with von Recklinghausen's disease.

Gliomas, teratomas, and papillomas tend to expand circumferentially within the ventricular system, displacing neural structures and obstructing cerebrospinal fluid flow (CSF). Similarly, ependymomas have a tendency to expand within the ventricular system until they fill it completely, dilating it uniformly, thereby justifying the name often given to these tumors: plastic ependymomas. Whether dilated irregularly or uniformly, whether filling completely or partially the ventricular system, intraventricular tumors almost invariably produce hydrocephalus. Therefore, one of the first tasks that a clinician must undertake when treating a child with an intraventricular tumor is the determination of the presence and the type of hydrocephalus. Specifically, does the child have monoventricular, biventricular, or triventricular hydrocephalus? The extent and the type of vascularization of the pedicle of the tumor is also important, as is the determination of whether one of the ventricular horns has become entrapped. Lastly, it is important to evaluate the presence and the extent of parenchymal invasion—generally, basal ganglia—by intraventricular tumors. The ependymoma, the glioma, and the mesenchymal tumor all have a tendency to invade, to damage, or to destroy the parenchymal tissue by compression.

EPENDYMOMAS

The texture of lateral ventricle ependymomas is generally gelatinous, with varying degrees of softness and liquefaction compartmentalized throughout the mass. The transitional areas to parenchymal tissue are denser, and extension of the tumor into the parenchyma itself may be identified as an increase in density similar to what one observes in a glioma. Ependymomas generally have a sessile base, only seldom are pedunculated, and very often extend from one lateral ventricle into the third ventricle and then across into the contralateral ventricle. It is important for surgeons to remember this pathoanatomic characteristic of the ependymoma, so that they may exercise great caution in pursuing the extent of the tumor from the lateral ventricle into the third ventricle. It is not advisable to attempt to pursue these tumors directly, or through the septum pellucidum, with the intent to resect them totally: Their natural history is not affected favorably by radical resection. The worst prognosis among ependymomas is for those bordering the CSF pathways.

It is preferable to resect an ependymoma with either the laser or the Cavitron ultrasonic aspirator, though aspiration is quite effective when the tumor is gelatinous. However, the use of aspiration to resect the intraparenchymal extension of an ependymoma is discouraged, especially if the extension is into the basal ganglia. When the laser is used, fluffy cotton pads should be rolled from one edge of the neoplasm to the other and they should be wet continuously to avoid applying undue pressure to the parenchymal surfaces and then should be suctioned dry with aspiration so as to draw the pedicle of the tumor into the fluffy cotton. One should not attempt to identify individual bleeding vessels or try to coagulate them, since this results only in extending the area of dissection into the brain substance. These minuscule bleeding vessels should be stopped by applying fluffy cotton and suctioning the cotton dry. Using the laser to attempt to stop the bleeding is futile, since although the blood is coagulated by the carbon dioxide laser beam, the subjacent vessels continue to bleed. The ependymoma should be vaporized initially at approximately 5 to 6 watts in the pulse mode, and the wattage should be increased steadily as the continuous mode is used. Broad sweeps of vaporization over the surface of the tumor avoid the formation of gutters or craters.

As previously stated, no purpose is served by attempting to resect completely an intraventricular ependymoma, because of the biologically malignant nature of this tumor. It is adequate to resect what comes away easily.

GLIAL TUMORS

In discussing glial tumors, it is necessary first to call attention to the fact that parenchymal gliomas very often may bulge or fungate into a ventricular chamber, certainly inadequate anatomic evidence to justify classifying these as intraventricular tumors. On the other hand, the subependymal glioma is a tumor that expands almost exclusively within the ventricular system, irrespective of whether its growth is primarily from the subependymal glial tissue of the lateral ventricle wall or the septum pellucidum. Pathoanatomically and clinically, these tumors behave in a manner that is indistinguishable from ependymoma or choroid plexus papilloma. Of course, each of these three intraventricular tumors has its own characteristic biologic activity. Conversely, the clinical behavior of the subependymal glioma is indistinguishable from that of either the ependymal or mesenchymal tumors just described. Children present with a midline syndrome, and neuroradiologically one identifies symmetric or asymmetric biventricular hydrocephalus and an enhancing intraventricular mass. It is most unusual for a subependymal glioma of the lateral ventricle to extend from one lateral ventricle into the third ventricle or the opposite lateral ventricle, unless the mass grows from the septum pellucidum. These lobular, glistening, grayish yellow tumors do not obliterate the centrencephalic draining veins, permitting the surgeon to recognize the fact that the tumor is subependymal in origin and glial in nature.

Because of the fact that these tumors are very benign, seldom invade the basal ganglia or thalamus, never seed, are not radiosensitive, and tend to be well circumscribed, the surgeon is urged to attempt a complete resection. This resection should be directed only to the removal of the intraventricular portion of the tumor, to the extent of unblocking the obstructed CSF pathways. Again, the laser or the Cavitron ultrasonic aspirator is very much preferred to aspiration for removal of the neoplasm. The use of biopsy forceps to remove the tumor piecemeal is strongly discouraged. Laser or Cavitron resection may be performed either by destroying all of the tumor in situ, beginning at the dome of the lesion and then gradually "shaving" layers of tumor away from the central mass, or by "cutting" the tumor at its pedicle (Fig. 32–1). In either event, the surgeon should use either telfa strips or fluffy cotton to protect the ventricular wall, and then long fluffy cotton should be placed around the pedicle of the tumor. Subsequent to this, the laser or Cavitron ultrasonic aspirator may be used to cut the globular mass or tumor from its pedicle at a level close to and parallel with the ventricular surface. This procedure permits en bloc removal of the globular mass.

In light of the fact that *gliomas of the septum pellucidum* generally occlude both foramina of Monro and often extend asymmetrically into the lateral ventricles, it is best to approach these tumors through a convexity cerebrotomy or through the corpus callosum. The cerebrotomy permits excellent exposure of one lateral ventricle and allows the surgeon the option of opening the septum pelluci-

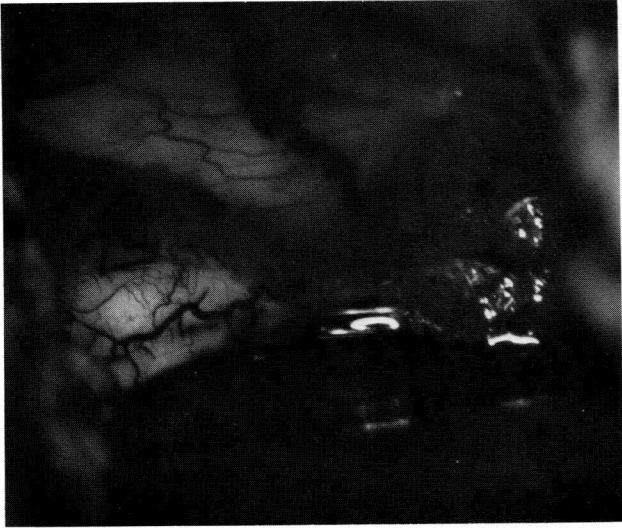

Figure 32–1. Intraventricular tumor. The choroid plexus papilloma is at the right of the figure, and the moderately neoplastic choroid plexus extends from it to the left. There is discoloration of the ependymal surface.

dum for entrance into the other lateral ventricle, or of teasing the body of the fornix from the surface of the thalamus for access to the third ventricle. The approach through the corpus callosum is more versatile in that it permits direct access to both lateral ventricles and the third ventricle but has the disadvantage of increased risk of memory impairment because of potential damage to the entirety of the corpus callosum and the fornices.

Consequently, if an approach through the corpus callosum is used, the surgeon should incise this commissure minimally, making the incision just long enough to permit exposure of the tumor anteriorly. This incision may be made in the portion of the corpus callosum that is most flattened, since it is immediately overlying the tumor mass. After the corpus callosum is incised, CSF flows into the field, permitting the surgeon to retract the ventricles and identify the terminal veins at their point of entry into the internal cerebral veins. Immediately after this is done, the surgeon must precisely identify the fornix. Do not incise more than one third the length of the corpus callosum!

As for all other lesions described in this chapter, the laser or the Cavitron ultrasonic aspirator is strongly recommended for tumor removal. Since the use of aspiration is unavoidably accompanied by traction of the tumor mass in one direction or another, it exposes the child to undue risks of damage to the fornices. Consequently, suction is to be avoided. All of the intraventricular extension of this type of tumor should be resected, though the surgeon need not pursue each last millimeter of tumor because of the extremely benign nature of this neoplasm. It is sufficient to remove the intraventricular excrescences of tumor and to unblock the CSF pathways.

CHOROID PLEXUS PAPILLOMA

Before considering resection of a choroid plexus papilloma of the lateral ventricle, one is advised to look for secondary surgical lesions, complications of expansion of this highly vascular tumor at the trigone, since they both complicate the clinical condition of the child and render the surgical procedure more involved. Secondary, asymmetric hydrocephalus is the most common, and most deceptive, of such complications. The pathogenesis of this asymmetric hydrocephalus is a combination of (1) an expansile and pulsatile mass located within one lateral ventricle; (2) obstruction of the foramen of Monro by extension of neoplastic tissue along the choroid plexus, from the glomus into the third ventricle; and (3) the extraordinarily high protein level of the CSF. Obstruction of the foramen of Monro needs no specific comment; however, the elevated CSF protein level and the pulsatile tumor provoke an inflammatory process, sterile to be sure, within the arachnoid membranes of the basal cisterns and the cerebral convexity. The mechanisms by which an intraventricular pulsatile mass produces ventricular dilation are eloquently described in the work by Di Rocco.[1]

Another major complication, with very specific surgical implications, is the expansion of the papilloma within the body and trigone of the lateral ventricle, thereby causing obstruction of the temporal horn and subsequent cystic transformation of this chamber. The ependymal lining of the trigone may permanently be converted into a fibrocollagenous material, adhering to the surface of the tumor and taking on the appearance of a capsule. This results in the formation of a cystic cavity over the body of the trigone mass. At times, secondary to occlusion of the occipital horn and continued secretion of CSF (with very high protein levels) into this trapped occipital horn, cystic transformation of this chamber may result. Therefore, the surgeon may be confronted with the clinical picture of a neoplastic lesion at the trigone (Fig. 32–2) and one to three cystic lesions within the same hemisphere (temporal, occipital, supraneoplastic).

Management of the choroid plexus papilloma at the trigone that is complicated by secondary cysts is best effected by direct surgical attack through a temporal parietal flap, one that is large enough to permit access to the greater wing of the sphenoid anteroinferiorly and the area of the transverse sinus at the sigmoid sinus posterolaterally. Once the bone flap has been reflected, it is best not to open the dura until after the cyst or cysts have been drained.

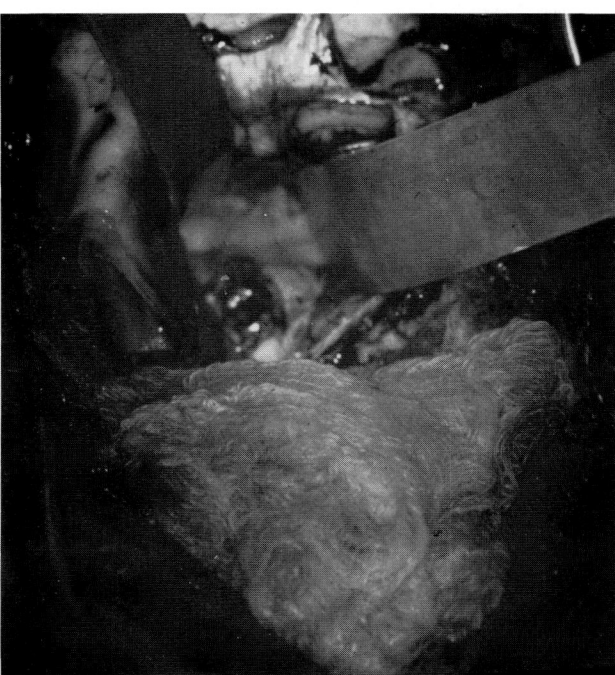

Figure 32–2. A tumor within the third ventricle has been approached by the parasagittal transcorpus callosal route. Cotton has been placed beneath the tumor to elevate it into the operative field. Notice the yellowish discoloration of the roof of the third ventricle.

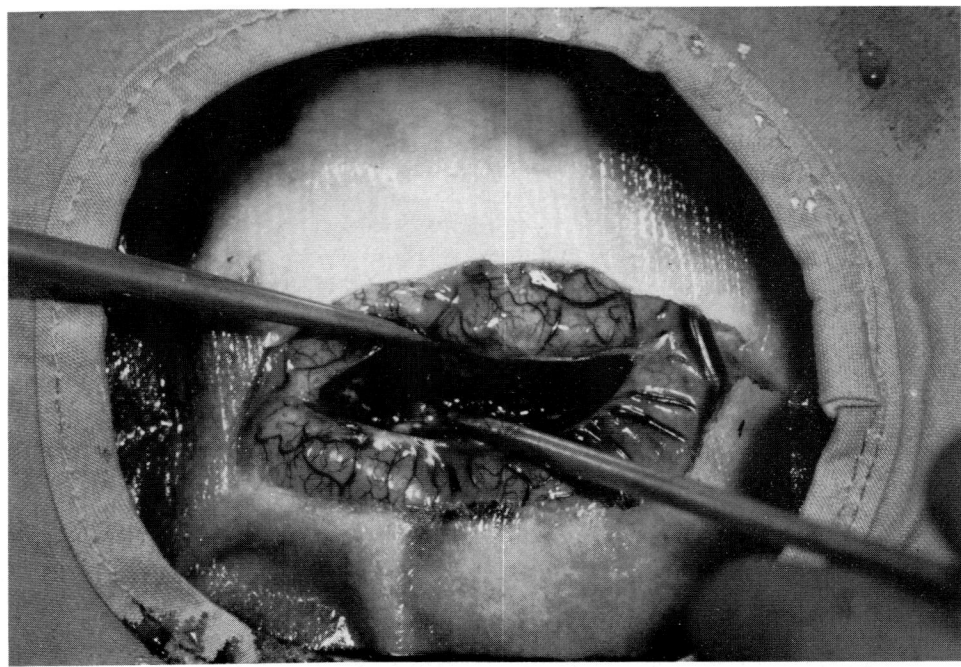

Figure 32–3. Linear cerebrotomy. This illustrates the technique for performing a sulcal linear cerebrotomy. The arachnoid was cut with microscissors after it had been coagulated with bipolar forceps. Laser was not used because it makes a wider area of destruction than do scissors and bipolar forceps. After the cortical surface was coagulated, the sulcus was opened with no. 15 blade for incision. Then the dissection through the cortex and white matter was performed with coagulation and microsuction.

Stab incisions of the dura permit insertion of a ventricular cannula into the cystic chamber so that the densely xanthochromic fluid may be drained, resulting in cystic collapse and remarkably diminished intracranial pressure. The dura is opened afterwards.

Irrespective of drainage of the cystic fluid, once the dura is opened, the surgeon notes flattening of the gyri. A linear cerebrotomy, 3 to 4 cm, within a sulcus located behind the angular gyrus provides generous access to the trigone (Fig. 32–3). It is best to perform the cerebrotomy in the most flattened, most pathologic portion of the cortex overlying the tumor, so that one is not obliged to resect a cone of cerebral tissue. A long, linear incision provides more than adequate exposure of the ventricular system immediately overlying the trigone tumor mass, especially when secondary cystic formation has resulted. The cerebral mantle is already maximally compressed from the underlying tumor and cyst. Therefore, the surgeon should take great care in ascertaining that this parenchyma is protected with both fluffy cotton and telfa strips prior to inserting self-retaining retractors to hold the parenchyma away from the tumor mass, adjacent to the dura. All the while, the cerebral convexity should be maintained in the most anatomic state possible (Fig. 32–4). Bipolar coagulation and then sectioning of the arachnoid with microscissors, followed by bipolar coagulation of the cerebral mantle, ensure complete hemostasis of this highly vascular area at the time of cortical incision.

Either laser cerebrotomy or the use of two spatulae to separate the white matter along the paths of the cortical spinal tracts permits surgical access to the ventricle and cystic areas. Prior to performing the cerebrotomy, bipolar coagulation and sectioning of the arachnoid with microscissors, followed by bipolar coagulation of the microvasculature at the base of the sulcus, ensure complete hemostasis and clean access to the underlying white matter. It is stressed that laser cerebrotomy not only is not more efficient but also, in fact, is less precise; it opens a wider cut than divarication and is fundamentally

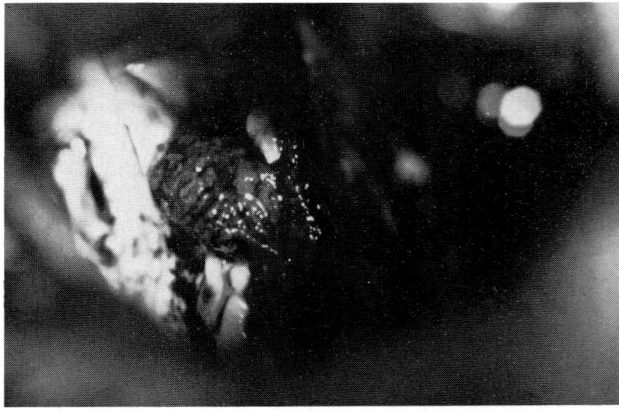

Figure 32–4. This papillary tumor of the anterior portion of the third ventricle, with a digital extension through the foramen of Monro, is visualized bulging into the right lateral ventricle. After performance of a right frontal craniotomy and transfrontal lobe approach to the dilated right lateral ventricle, this tumor was visualized. Removal was performed by coagulating, and shrinking the tumor with bipolar forceps.

destructive. After the dissection through the centrum semiovale has been completed and the ependyma identified, this latter cell layer is coagulated with bipolar cautery. It is then sectioned with microscissors, unsheathing the tumor proper and exposing the fibrocollagenous tissue stratified between xanthochromic ependyma and the surface of the choroid plexus papilloma.

The surface of the tumor is separated from the surrounding ependyma and parenchyma by cotton fluffies, which are pulled into the desired size and form and then are freshly soaked in normal saline that has been kept at body temperature. These fluffies are used to separate the tumor from surrounding tissue, to which it may have become adherent by the formation of fibrocollagenous and proteinaceous bridges. A layer of cotton or telfa strips is then placed between the tumor and the ependyma of the ventricular wall, as cotton fluffies are snuggled around the tumor and then are gently placed along the pedicle of the tumor, at the point of adherence of choroid plexus to the ventricular surface at both the trigone and the choroidal fissure. In this manner, the tumor is completely separated from the wall of the ventricle, and one is able to define the pedicle so as to identify the line of entry of choroidal arteries and the exit of draining veins.

Ideally, the technique of tumor removal consists of vaporizing it in situ with a laser or gradually shrinking it with bipolar forceps. Carbon dioxide laser vaporization works very well if the tumor is not highly vascularized but is both laborious and dangerous if vascularization is extensive. In the event that the tumor consists of a multitude of microcystic chambers containing CSF, carbon dioxide vaporization may take an extraordinarily long period of time. Consequently, shrinking the tumor with bipolar forceps is the single most desirable and reliable technique for removal of choroid plexus papilloma.

The correct use of bipolar forceps for such coagulation consists of placing the forceps blades along the surface of the tumor and closing them until they are approximately 6 to 7 mm apart, trapping between them a small segment of the papilloma. The bipolar forceps are then activated, causing shrinkage of the tumor. This technique is repeated rapidly and continuously along the entire surface of the tumor, first working in isolated areas and then extending the surface of coagulation over larger surface areas, thereby both shrinking the tumor and diminishing the circulation of blood within it. One occasionally hears pops resulting from explosion of microcysts of CSF. Progressive use of coagulation to shrink the tumor increases steadily one's vision of the surrounding tissue as the tumor becomes smaller, until the pedicle is identified. It is best to resist the temptation to coagulate the pedicle as soon as it is identified, since more effective and safer coagulation may be obtained when the tumor bulk has been very much diminished. As a consequence of the introduction of the laser and the increased efficiency of electrocautery, it is no longer acceptable to use "blind" application of hemostatic clips to the pedicle. Extension of the tumor mass along the floor of the ventricle, over the choroidal fissure, represents insertion of the vascular pedicle, which may reach anteroinferiorly from the trigone, toward the hippocampus, and then superomedially toward the terminal sulcus and the foramen of Monro. The entire extension of tumor along this tract is along the normal anatomic line of the choroid plexus of the lateral ventricle. The subependymal system represents entry of the draining veins, which penetrate the choroidal fissure to enter the quadrigeminal and galenic systems. Another drainage pathway is into the supraculminate system. These draining veins, and the small, at times almost microscopic, feeding arteries should be coagulated and transected, using the operating microscope, proceeding a millimeter at a time. Coagulation and transection of larger feeding arteries is dangerous, so small hemoclips should be applied to them after they have been coagulated and before they are suctioned. In this manner, the surgeon may proceed to separate the entirety of the tumor mass from its adherence to the junction of the cerebral hemisphere with the thalami along the choroidal fissure.

Once the tumor has been completely removed, the ventricular chamber should be filled with physiologic solution to permit inspection for microscopic bleeders. It is best to wait a period of ten minutes before proceeding to closure. As a postscript to this section, it is emphasized that total removal of the lateral ventricle choroid plexus papilloma, in one piece, without shrinking it, was acceptable in the era before bipolar coagulation and the laser but is very much discouraged at this time. In fact, one is hard pressed to justify such undertakings, since there is always adequate time to refer the child to a major center for tumor removal with appropriate instruments.

Both papillary tumors originating within the third ventricle and those extending into the third ventricle through the foramen of Monro are operated on with the same techniques. A choroid plexus papilloma of the lateral ventricle may extend along the choroid plexus into the terminal sulcus, and anteriorly as far as the foramen of Monro, entering the third ventricle. When this occurs and the foramen of Monro is occluded, one may encounter encysted occipital and frontal horns as the mass occludes the trigone and enters the third ventricle. When the tumor is limited to the third ventricle, biventricular hydrocephalus resulting from occlusion of both foramina of Monro develops.

A temporofrontoparietal flap is necessary for such a procedure to be effective. Before opening the dura, any encysted ventricular chambers are punctured, allowing the egress of fluid. A cerebrotomy of 3 to 4 cm in length is made behind the angular gyrus, and the tumor is isolated prior to sectioning of its vascular pedicle. Vaporization or bipolar coagulation of the tumor facilitates its isolation and the identification of the pedicle. The pedicle should be coagulated or clipped prior to sectioning. Then, advancing toward the foramen of Monro and coagulating minute perforating feeders along the bed, one may either vaporize the tumor or lift it from its bed within the terminal sulcus. This anteromedial dissection is not carried beyond the point at which the body of the fornix continues into the crus fornices. The foramen of Monro is identified, and obliteration of the perforating feeders to the tumor is carried out by proceeding posteriorly from the foramen of Monro to approximately the point at which the body of the fornix ends. This frees the tumor from its attachment to the floor of the trigone and the body of the lateral ventricle. Extension of tumor from the lateral into the third ventricle, through the foramen of Monro, is variable in amount, vascularity, and adhesion (to the foramen of Monro, the roof of the third ventricle, the anterior surface of the third ventricle). However, there is always a constricted area at the foramen. If the surgeon chooses the transforaminal entry into the third ventricle, this must be enlarged, after coagulation and clipping of the neoplastic extension through the foramen.

An alternative technique for entering the third ventricle, one that is equally complete in exposing the third ventricle and that has the advantage of avoiding completely dissection along the columns of the fornix, entails stripping of the tela choroidea of the roof of the third ventricle from its insertion onto the superior surface of the thalamus at the terminal sulcus. At this point, the tela choroidea of the roof of the third ventricle is continuous with the choroid plexus of the lateral ventricle. The dissection is carried out with fluffy cotton, rolling it backward over the surface of the thalamus, from lateral to medial. This strips choroid plexus of the roof of the third ventricle from the thalamus, laying open the entirety of the third ventricle, establishing a continuity between it and the lateral ventricle. In essence, the compartmentalization of the lateral and the third ventricles is taken down; the fornix is rolled back over the superior aspect of the thalamus where the horizontal surface of the thalamus (floor of the body of the lateral ventricle) turns inferiorly to become the vertical surface of the thalamus (lateral wall of the third ventricle). When this is done, any lesion within the third ventricle is visualized immediately.

If the surgeon chooses to use the septothalamic approach, he or she must first ascertain that the tumor is not growing through this potential space directly into the third ventricle. If it is not, the tela choroidea of the roof of the third ventricle is stripped from its attachment to the superior surface of the thalamus medial to the terminal sulcus, along the floor of the lateral ventricle, with great care being taken not to damage the body of the fornix! A wide and free communication between the lateral and the third ventricles is thus established, permitting separation of the main tumor mass from its extension into the third ventricle, and subsequent removal of the tumor in two (lateral and third ventricular) portions, rather than one. It is not wise to attempt to lift the tumor from the lateral and the third ventricles as one piece: The lateral ventricular mass "blinds" the surgeon to the vascular supply of the third ventricle mass.

After the tumor has been removed from the lateral ventricle, the surgeon may inspect the tumor within the third ventricle, taking care to ascertain that the anterior septal, terminal, and internal cerebral veins are freed from the tumor and adhesions to it.

Appropriately fashioned telfa strips are then inserted along the superior surface of the tumor, separating it from the roof of the third ventricle and the internal cerebral vein within this latter structure. Similarly, telfa strips are placed along the lateral surfaces of the tumor and then along its anterior surface as far inferiorly as the floor of the third ventricle. When this is done, gently, and with telfas that are soaking wet, one avoids damaging the vascular or nuclear structures bordering on the third ventricle and ensures freeing of the intraventricular mass.

At this time, a large fluffy piece of cotton is placed in the lateral ventricle, at the foramen of Monro, and the line of dissection is moved from transventricular to parasagittal by retracting the frontal lobe laterally. This gives access first to the genu and rostrum of the corpus callosum and then to the lamina terminalis (anterior border of the third ventricle), as far inferiorly as the supraoptic recess. If the tumor has lobulated inferiorly and is adherent to the walls of the third ventricle, one may choose to enter this chamber through its anterior margin. This requires performing a cerebrotomy from the rostrum of the corpus callosum inferomedially along the fornix, and then through the lamina terminalis as far inferiorly as the supraoptic recess. Complete visualization of the anterior and superior portions of the third ventricle, of the anterior septal vein, and of the foramen of Monro is achieved! Since all vascular supply and drainage to the third ventricular portion of these tumors is along the tela choroidea, one need not be concerned that there may be vessels within the area of the floor of the third ventricle or the lamina terminalis.

Lateral ventricle papillomas may also extend through the choroidal fissure into the quadrigeminal cistern and, at times, even into the contralateral ventricle. Those papillomas extending directly medially through the choroid fissure, and into the quadrigeminal cistern, may either expand "dumbbell fashion" on either side of the choroid fissure or into a nodule within the quadrigeminal cistern. They may then penetrate the contralateral ventricle through its choroid fissure, thereby becoming indistinguishably intermingled with its columns. In either event, the tumor compresses the quadrigeminal plate, becomes adherent to the commissure of the fornix, and elevates the splenium of the corpus callosum. There is obstruction to the passage of CSF from the ambient cistern into the quadrigeminal cistern, forward displacement of the pineal gland and the suprapineal recess of the third ventricle, and, to some degree, extension of the tumor along the anterior surfaces of the culmen monticuli and the lobulus centralis of the cerebellar vermis.

Access to the angular gyri on both sides and to the region of the quadrigeminal cistern is achieved through a biparietal craniotomy and an S-shaped skin flap. After puncture of the temporal horn (bilaterally, when the tumor is expanding in both trigones), the dura is opened. The tumor is dissected from its ventricular adhesions down to its pedicle at the choroidal fissure, from the pes hippocampus anteriorly to the collateral eminence posteriorly, through a cerebrotomy posterior to the angular gyrus.

After the intraventricular (on both sides, when the tumor extends into the contralateral ventricle) portion or portions of the tumor have been removed, the line of dissection is changed from transventricular to parasagittal. Fluffy cotton should already have been positioned in the lateral ventricle, along the choroidal fissure. The dissection of the tumor within the quadrigeminal cistern is performed after the parasagittal approach, coming down bilaterally on either side of the falx cerebri. The anterior and posterior branches of the lateral posterior choroidal artery, going to the tumor with the quadrigeminal and inferior retrosplenial arteries, are identified as a group, occluded, and transected. It is necessary to identify the anterior choroidal arteries, by coming posterolaterally through and over the tela choroidea of the third ventricle. Venous drainage into the lesser and greater galenic systems, and their tributaries, diminishes considerably once these last feeding vessels are transected. Removal of the tumor without identifying, occluding, and transecting the bridging veins results in the opening of these major normal venous structures.

Consequently, the tumor may be removed in two or three pieces, depending upon whether it has extended in dumbbell fashion into the quadrigeminal cistern or has entered the contralateral ventricle.

Pineal region tumors may (1) expand superior to the roof of the third ventricle, in which case they are approached in the same way as tumors of the roof of the third ventricle (Fig. 32–5); (2) remain within the pineal and quadrigeminal cisterns, in which case they are approached in the same way as tumors of the posterior third ventricle; or (3) extend into the posterior fossa by growing primarily within the superior cerebellar cisterns and displacing the lobulus centralis of the vermis posteriorly,

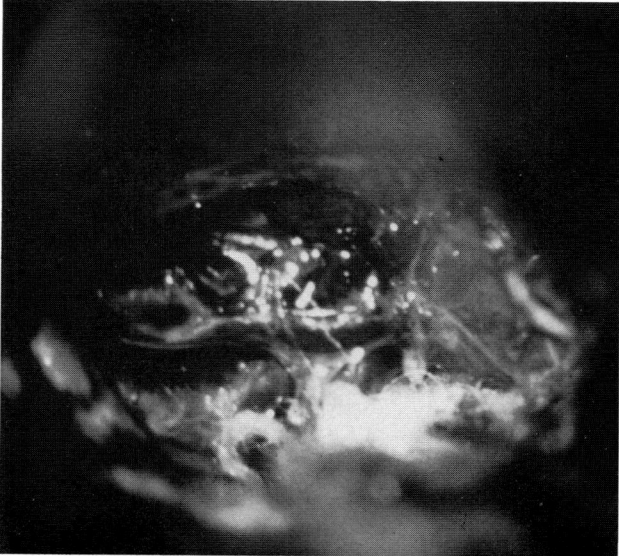

Figure 32–5. Intraventricular papillary tumor. This is a papilloma of the choroid plexus of the body of the lateral ventricle, which is visualized immediately upon opening the ependyma of the lateral ventricle. The surgical approach was through the right frontal lobe.

in which case they are approached through a suboccipital-supracerebellar craniotomy. The incidence of expansion of pineal tumors into the third ventricle, between the third ventricle and the body of the corpus callosum, or into the posterior fossa is equal. The criteria upon which one may base a decision concerning which of these approaches is best for pineal tumors have been published elsewhere.[2] For this chapter, suffice it to state that this decision is predicated entirely upon the direction of tumor displacement of the deep venous structures (i.e., the lesser and greater galenic systems). Downward displacement of the lesser galenic system indicates a parasagittal-transcallosal approach. Upward displacement of the lesser galenic system indicates an occipital craniotomy and a parasagittal-supracerebellar approach to the pineal region. Elevation of the greater galenic vein indicates a suboccipital craniotomy and a supracerebellar-infratentorial approach to the tumor. The specifics of the pineal region tumor, whether entirely extraventricular or with intraventricular extension, are presented elsewhere in this text.

When discussing tumors of the third ventricle, it is best to consider them from a surgical anatomic point of view as anterior, superior, or posterior third ventricular tumors, a consideration that assists the surgeon in determining which approach to the third ventricle is most opportune. For anterior third ventricle tumors, a transcerebral approach to one lateral ventricle and then entrance into the third ventricle through the foramen of Monro, or a subfrontal approach to the lamina terminalis and then midline entrance directly into the third ventricle are preferable. The transparenchymal–translateral ventricle approach to identify the body of the fornix and tease this structure from the thalamus is ideal for access to tumors of the superior third ventricle, whether pedunculated into the third ventricle from the roof of this chamber or lobulating superiorly and superolaterally above the roof. For masses extending into the region of the posterior third ventricle, the author prefers the occipital–parasagittal–transtentorial approach.

From an anatomic point of view, the third ventricle should be visualized as a very irregular structure in both its vertical and horizontal planes. Anteroinferiorly are the suprachiasmatic and infundibular recesses. Posteroinferiorly is the superior surface of the mesencephalon. Directly posteriorly one encounters the iter (aqueduct of Sylvius). Posterosuperiorly are the pineal and suprapineal recesses. Superiorly is the roof of the third ventricle with its choroid plexus. Anterosuperiorly are the two foramina of Monro and the point at which the terminal veins are tributary to the internal cerebral veins. Directly anteriorly is the lamina terminalis. Wedged between the thalami and hypothalami laterally, the mesencephalon and optic chiasm inferiorly, and the internal cerebral veins superomedially, the third venticle is accessible only directly anteriorly, directly posteriorly, or superolaterally.

The subfrontal approach, sectioning the lamina terminalis, is quite adequate if one wishes to perform only a third ventriculostomy. However, such an approach is strongly discouraged by the author for exposure and proper removal of a tumor, since it does not provide adequate exposure of the vascular structures in the roof of the third ventricle. This approach is quite satisfactory for removal of *colloid cysts* of the third ventricle, a not uncommon tumor in adults, but a very uncommon tumor in children. Once identified, the colloid cyst of the third ventricle should be separated from the surrounding walls of the third ventricle by a blunt-edged microdissector until it is seen to float freely within the third ventricle after this chamber is filled with irrigating solution. Then, its attachment to the paraphysis, if not already, inadvertently, sectioned, should be identified, coagulated, and transected with microscissors. The colloid cyst is then simply lifted from the field. The reader is urged, at this point, to be certain that the cyst is not attached to the anterior septal, the terminal, or the internal cerebral veins before lifting it form the third ventricle.

For tumors of the *roof of the third ventricle* (in light of the fact that these tumors are, with the rarest of exceptions, choroid plexus papillomas), the reader is referred to the section of this chapter concerning the choroid plexus papilloma of the third ventricle. Here, suffice it to say that this tumor is best removed through the septal-interthalamic route because of its enormous size and its attachment to the undersurface of the roof of the third ventricle. However, either the transcallosal or transforaminal route may be used.

The only tumor of the posterior third ventricle is the pineal region tumor (see Chapter 35). For a discussion of fourth ventricular tumors, see Chapter 30.

References

1. Di Rocco C: Communicating hydrocephalus induced by mechanically increased amplitude of the intraventricular cerebrospinal fluid pulse pressure: Experimental studies. Exp Neurol 59:40, 1978.
2. Raimondi AJ, Tomita T: Pineal tumors in childhood: Epidemiology, pathophysiology, and surgical approaches. Child's Brain 9:329, 1982.

33
OPTIC NERVE GLIOMAS AND OTHER TUMORS INVOLVING THE OPTIC NERVE AND CHIASM

David C. McCullough, M.D.
Dennis L. Johnson, M.D.

Optic nerve gliomas are not common. In Martin and Cushing's series[37] of 2000 brain tumors, only 1 percent were optic nerve gliomas. Since 75 percent of these tumors occur in the first decade of life, the series reported from major pediatric neurosurgical centers reflect a higher incidence. Optic gliomas make up 4 percent of the brain tumors seen at Children's Hospital National Medical Center, as compared with 3.6 percent reported by Matson,[39] 4 percent by Sayers,[48] and 6 percent by Hoffman.[26]

PATHOLOGY

Pathologically, the tumors may be solid, may be gelatinous, or may contain large cysts. Tumors may appear as fusiform enlargement of the optic nerve, with secondary involvement of the chiasm, or may envelop primarily the chiasm and spread secondarily to the optic nerves or into the hypothalamus. "Skip" lesions, or segmental nodules of glioma, may also be seen in the optic pathway.[11, 42, 50] The microscopic appearance (Fig. 33–1) is that of a low-grade astrocytoma with simple bipolar, pilocytic astrocytes and numerous Rosenthal's fibers.[2, 3, 8, 50, 56, 57] Although Hoyt and Baghadassarian[28] suggested that optic gliomas are non-neoplastic, tissue culture studies have confirmed the neoplastic character of these tumors.[38] Evidence of histologic malignancy is extremely unusual in children but has been described in adults.[6, 22, 29, 51] Malignant transformation of optic gliomas is uncommon.[6, 59] An association with neurofibromatosis is seen in 30 to 50 percent of patients with optic gliomas.[7, 26, 36, 43]

BIOLOGIC BEHAVIOR

Since it was first described in the early nineteenth century,[30, 34] the treatment of children with optic glioma has been controversial. The indolent biologic behavior of most optic gliomas, combined with the progressive visual loss, has intensified the controversy. Martin and Cushing[37] concluded that any treatment of optic gliomas was presumptuous. Fowler and Matson[19] reported that the biologic behavior of these tumors was difficult to predict. Some tumors progress inexorably despite aggressive treatment. However, many patients have survived over 20 years in spite of incomplete tumor removal and no radiation therapy.[15, 28, 39, 41, 44, 48, 54] Taveras and colleagues[53] reported cases of long-term survival with radiation therapy alone. Spontaneous tumor regression and visual improvement have also been cited.

In 1969, the dilemma of optic pathway gliomas was heightened with Hoyt and Baghadassarian's assertion[28] that the biologic behavior of these tumors

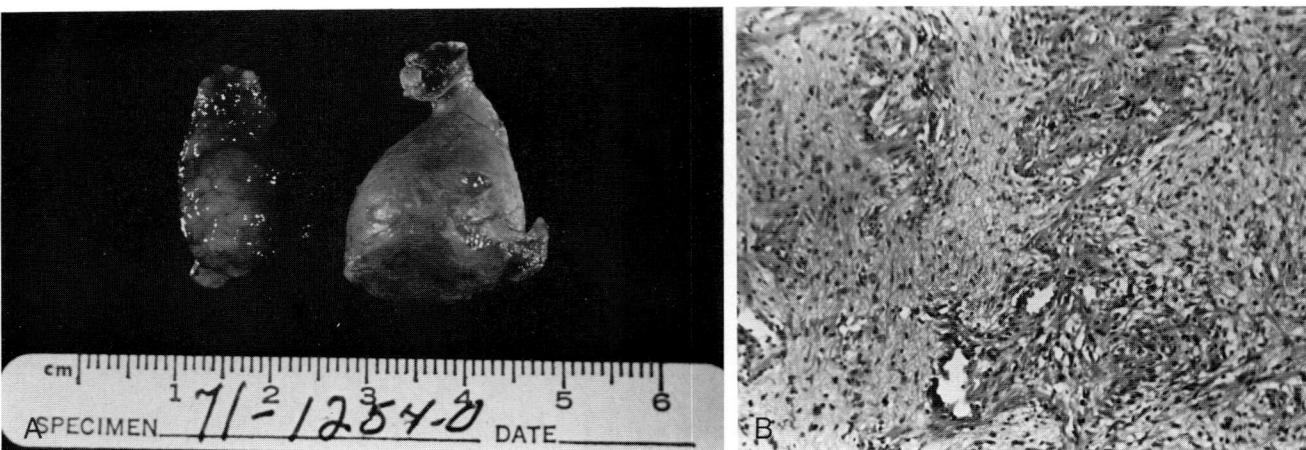

Figure 33–1. A, Optic glioma confined to optic nerve. B, Characteristic microscopic appearance, with bipolar, pilocytic astrocytes enmeshed in optic nerve.

was not frankly neoplastic but rather hamartomatous. In a long-term study of visual fields in nonirradiated and irradiated patients, Glaser and associates[20] found no beneficial effect from radiation. They also condemned surgical morbidity as unwarranted. In contrast, Hoffman[26] and others [5, 13, 16, 35, 44] have documented the relentlessly aggressive biologic behavior of some optic gliomas that is at least slowed by radiation therapy.

Although arguable, the biologic behavior of optic gliomas is usually indolent, and survival for longer than ten years can be expected. Slow but progressive visual loss is the rule, but the protracted morbidity and the quality of long-term survival has not been well-documented.

DIAGNOSTIC TESTS

Computed tomography (CT) and nuclear magnetic resonance imaging (NMRI) provide accurate localization and narrow the spectrum of possible diagnoses. Optic gliomas are usually isodense, and many are enhanced by intravenous contrast material, especially the more posterior lesions. Calcifications have been described in lesions that involve the optic tract.[18] With modern neuroimaging, there is seldom a need for plain skull x-ray films, which classically demonstrate a J-shaped sella; optic foraminal views showing an optic foramen > 7 mm or a difference of more than 2 mm between the right and the left foramina;[48] tomography; arteriography; or pneumoencephalography. Visual evoked responses may help document a change in an individual patient but have limited usefulness in screening or diagnosis.[10]

CLASSIFICATION, PRESENTATION, AND THERAPY

Optic pathway gliomas and other tumors from which they must be differentiated can be classified by anatomic location. The clinical presentation, differential diagnosis, treatment, and prognosis of tumors that are confined to (1) the optic nerve, (2) the optic nerve and chiasm, and (3) the chiasm and the hypothalamus are distinctly different.

Tumors of the Optic Nerve

Presentation and Diagnosis

Tumors of the optic nerve commonly present in childhood, with proptosis, visual loss, papilledema, or optic atrophy.[58] The proptotic eye is displaced downward and outward. In the very young, visual loss may be manifested by strabismus, nystagmus, or both. Papilledema is seen more often than optic atrophy and is probably due to perineurial venous obstruction. These tumors are commonly found when asymptomatic children with neurofibromatosis are screened with CT or NMRI scans (Fig. 33–2).

Differential Diagnosis. The differential diagnosis in children with neurofibromatosis who present with proptosis includes neurofibromas of the orbit and congenital defects of the sphenoid wing. In this group of patients, disfiguring proptosis is usually caused by a diffuse neurofibroma that is virtually impossible to remove. Pulsating exophthalmus is more characteristic of congenital defects in the sphenoid bone. In patients known to have neurofibromatosis, the diagnosis of optic glioma can usually be made on neuroradiologic grounds alone.

Other tumors that must be differentiated (Table 33–1) from optic nerve gliomas include hemangioma, lymphoma, rhabdomyosarcoma, and metastases from neuroblastoma, leukemia, or Ewing's sarcoma. Fibrous dysplasia, paranasal mucocele, and meningioma are rarely seen.

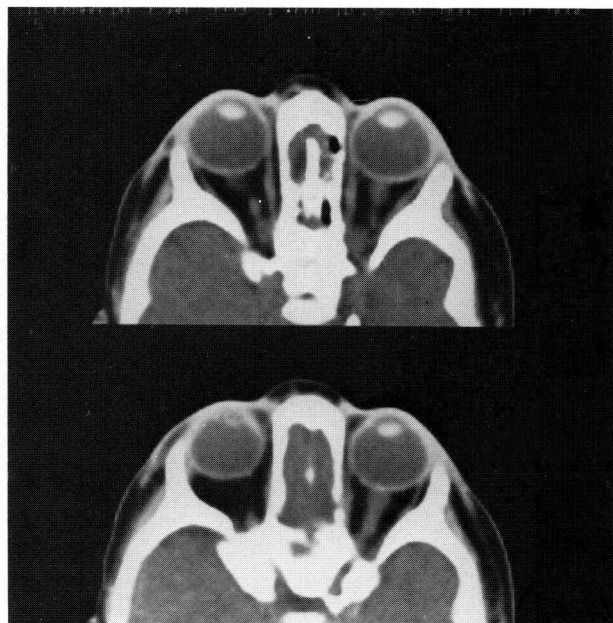

Figure 33–2. Optic nerve glioma with fusiform enlargement of both optic nerves in a four-month-old infant with nystagmus.

Treatment

Optic gliomas limited to the intraorbital or intracranial optic nerve that do not include the chiasm and that are associated with no vision are resected. These tumors do not recur, and normal vision is preserved in the contralateral eye. The approach to children with impaired visual acuity or a visual field defect is more problematic. The authors recommend surgical resection in children younger than five years of age in whom acuity is impaired but cannot be quantitated and in whom visual fields cannot be accurately traced. In the older child with normal visual acuity or in the child with neurofibromatosis, the surgeon and family may wish to follow the lesion carefully by clinical examination (visual acuity and fields) and by NMRI or CT at six-month intervals. Optic nerve gliomas may spread to the chiasm and even into the opposite nerve.[32, 46]

Tumors of the Optic Nerve and Chiasm

Presentation and Diagnosis

Tumors that involve the optic chiasm and the posterior optic nerve present more commonly with optic atrophy than with papilledema. Loss of visual acuity is not as profound as with the tumors that involve the nerve more anteriorly, but a visual field deficit can usually be identified in both eyes. CT demonstrates fusiform enlargement of one or both optic nerves and the optic chiasm (Fig. 33–3).

Differential Diagnosis. If a fusiform enlargement of the optic nerve and chiasm can be identified on CT, the differential diagnosis, especially in the patient with von Recklinghausen's disease, is very limited. In the patient without neurofibromatosis, germinoma and sarcoidosis should be considered.

Clinical Prognosis and Therapy

Although many authors do not differentiate this group of tumors from neoplasms of the chiasm extending into the hypothalamus, tumors localized to the nerve and chiasm do not cause pituitary dysfunction, hydrocephalus, or clinical evidence of hypothalamic dysfunction. Tym[55] reported four cases of optic glioma confined to the chiasm and optic nerve that were verified histologically. All patients were alive and well 9 to 18 years following diagnosis. Three of the four patients had neurofibromatosis, and none received radiation therapy. Heiskanen and coworkers[23] reported 14 patients, nine of whom were biopsied. Follow-up was 4 to 18 years, with a mean of ten years. Nine patients received radiation therapy. All but one was alive at follow-up, but two patients developed panhypopituitarism following radiation therapy. Three patients received no radiation therapy, and visual acuity was "stable" in all survivors. Thirty percent of these patients had neurofibromatosis. In Hoyt and Baghadassarian's series,[28] nine patients had tumors confined to the optic nerve and chiasm. Thirty percent of those patients had deterioration of vision, but there was no difference in the visual morbidity of patients who received radiation therapy and those who did not receive radiation ther-

Table 33–1. DIFFERENTIAL DIAGNOSIS OF OPTIC GLIOMAS

Optic Nerve Glioma
  Hemangioma
  Lymphoma
  Rhabdomyosarcoma
  Metastases
    Neuroblastoma
    Leukemia
    Ewing's sarcoma
  Fibrous dysplasia
  Paranasal mucocele
  Meningioma
  Neurofibromatosis
    Orbital neurofibroma
    Congenital defect in sphenoid bone
Optic Nerve and Chiasm Glioma
  Germinoma
  Sarcoidosis
Optic Chiasm Glioma Extending into the Hypothalamus
  Pituitary adenoma
  Craniopharyngioma
  Malignant astrocytoma
  Epidermoid and dermoid tumors
  Chordoma
  Colloid cyst
  Fibrous dyplasia
  Sarcoidosis
  Histiocytosis X
  Tuberculous granuloma
  Hemangioendothelioma

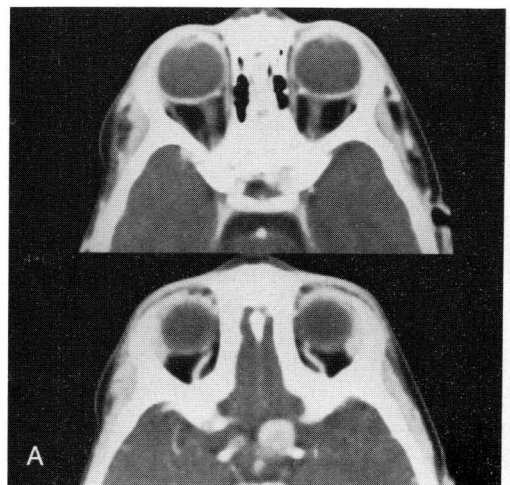 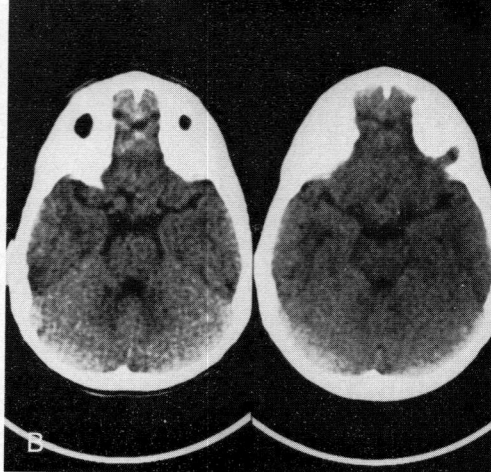 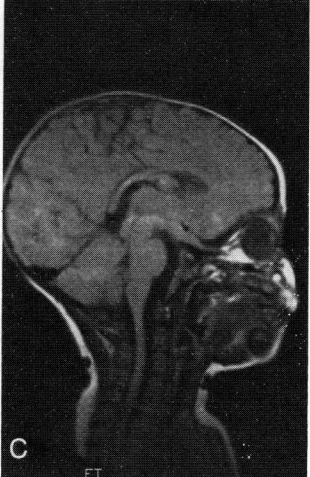

Figure 33–3. Optic nerve glioma extending into optic chiasm in a seven-month-old infant with spasmus nutans. A, With contrast enhancement. B, Without contrast enhancement. C, Sagittal nuclear magnetic resonance (NMR) image through optic nerve and chiasm tumor.

apy. All patients were alive at follow-up, but the length of follow-up was not well-documented.

Children with optic gliomas confined to the chiasm should be followed carefully every six months for clinical or radiographic evidence of progression. Radiation therapy is reserved for patients with documented progression.

Tumors of the Optic Chiasm Extending into the Hypothalamus

Presentation

Gliomas that originate primarily from the chiasm and extend posteriorly and superiorly into the hypothalamus are distinctive for symptoms and signs of increased intracranial pressure as well as hypothalamic dysfunction. Increased intracranial pressure is caused by hydrocephalus secondary to occlusion of the foramina of Monro. Headaches, vomiting, and obtundation are more commonly seen in this group. The tumor diffusely infiltrates the chiasm and the walls of the third ventricle as well as the hypothalamus, but it is not known to invade the dura. Signs of hypothalamic invasion include the diencephalic syndrome,[14] diabetes insipidus, anorexia, obesity, hypersomnia, and precocious puberty. Spasmus nutans (head bobbing, head tilt, and nystagmus) has been described in association with optic glioma,[1, 32] and in the authors' experience, most of these infants have chiasmatic tumors extending into the hypothalamus. Hemiplegia has also been reported.[26, 40]

Diagnosis

Radiographically, these tumors are often large, may be cystic, and are associated with ventriculomegaly (Figs. 33–4 and 33–5). In the patient with neurofibromatosis, the tumor is most probably an optic glioma. However, in the absence of neurofibromatosis, the differential diagnosis is diverse and includes pituitary adenoma, craniopharyngioma, germinoma (Fig. 33–6),[9] malignant astrocytoma (Fig. 33–7), metastatic medulloblastoma from the posterior fossa, epidermoid and dermoid tumors, chordoma, colloid cyst, fibrous dysplasia, sarcoi-

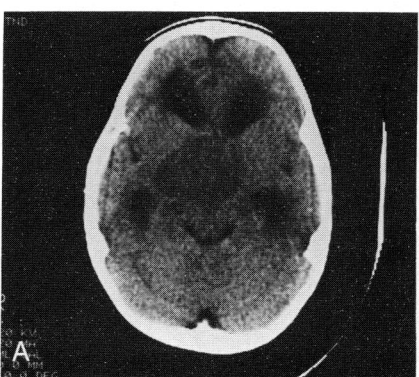 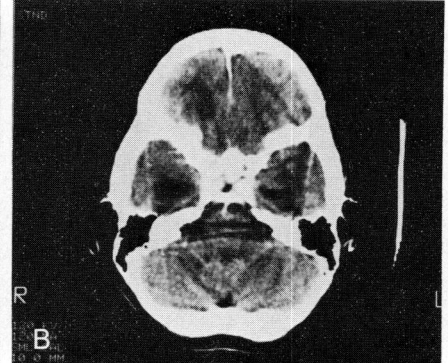 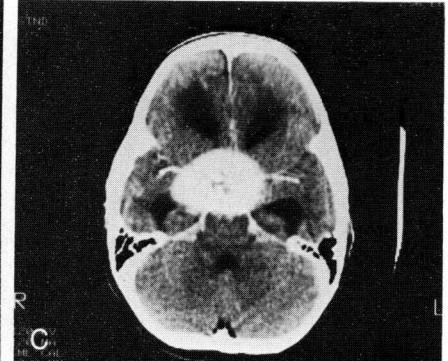

Figure 33–4. Optic glioma involving chiasm in a five-year-old with headaches, vomiting, and visual loss in the right eye. A, Without contrast enhancement. B, With contrast enhancement. C, With contrast enhancement demonstrating hydrocephalus.

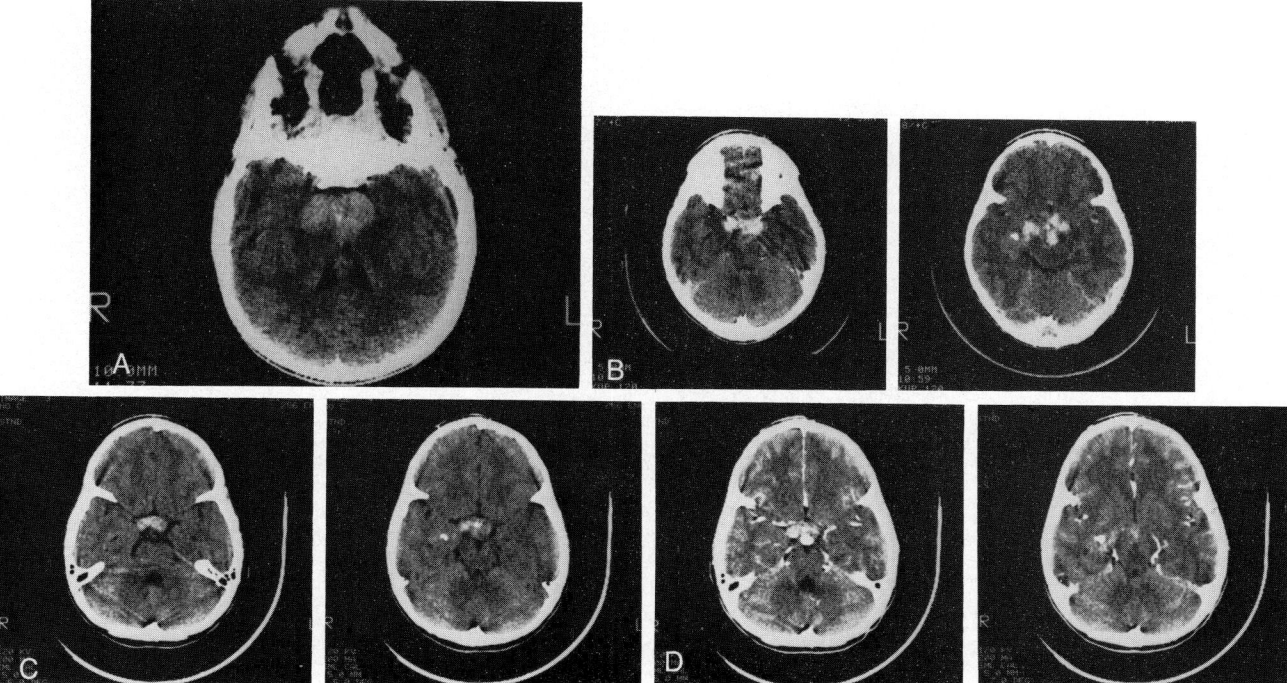

Figure 33–5. Optic chiasm–hypothalamus glioma in a six-year-old child with neurofibromatosis, right esotropia, and right hemianopsia. *A*, Coronal plane film before irradiation with contrast enhancement. *B*, Before irradiation with contrast enhancement. *C*, Without contrast enhancement, three and a half years after irradiation. *D*, With contrast enhancement, three and a half years after irradiation.

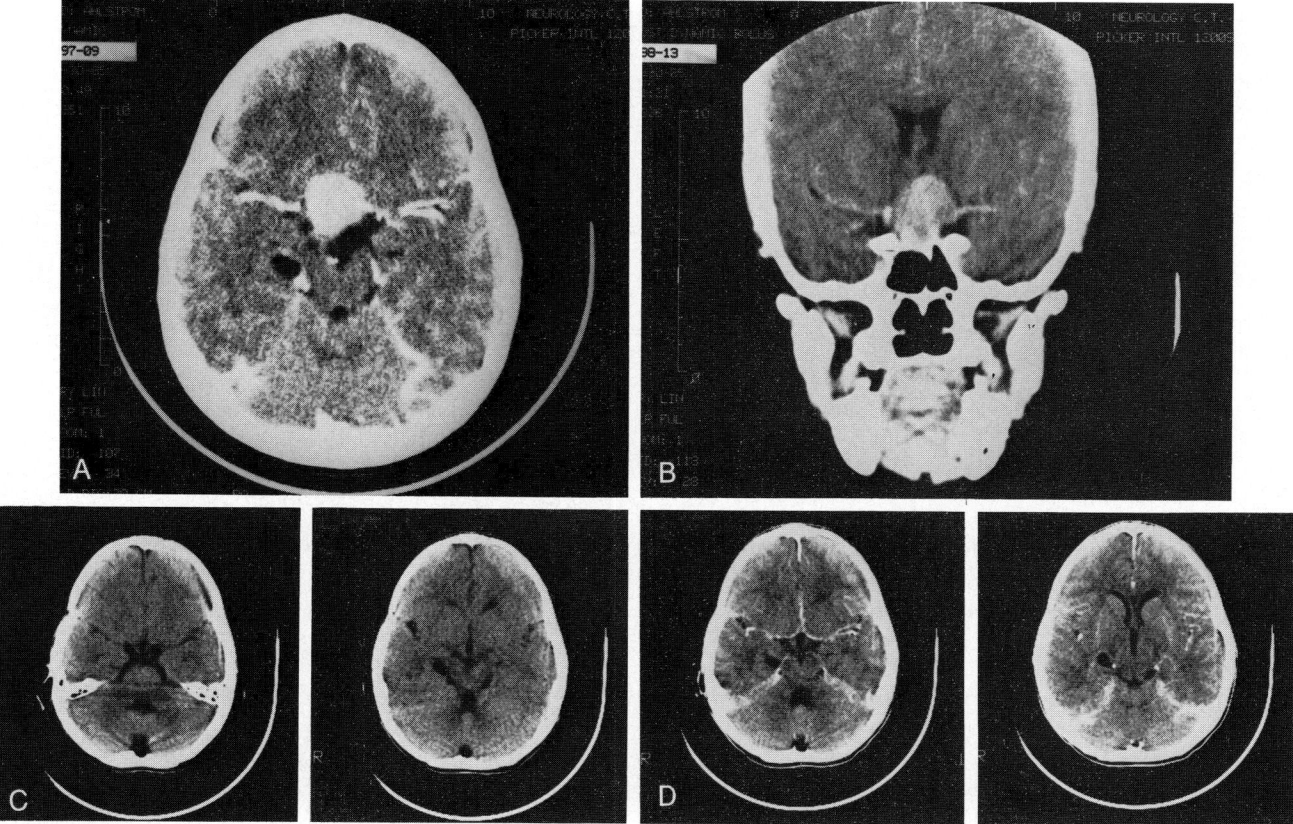

Figure 33–6. Germinoma in an eight-year-old boy with severe headaches, rapidly progressive visual loss, and long-standing emotional problems. *A*, Before irradiation. *B*, Before irradiation in coronal plane. *C*, Without contrast enhancement, 18 months after irradiation. *D*, With contrast enhancement, 18 months after irradiation.

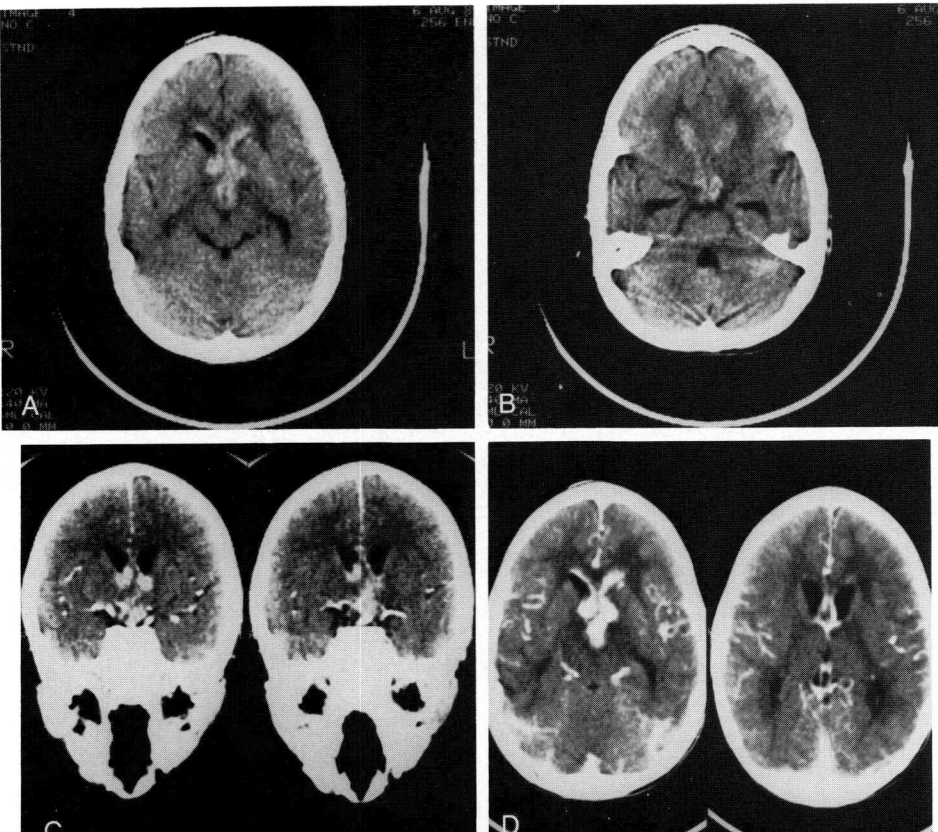

Figure 33–7. Malignant glioma in a six-year-old boy with diabetes insipidus. A and B, Without contrast enhancement. C, Coronal view, with contrast enhancement. D, With contrast enhancement.

dosis, histiocytosis X (Fig. 33–8), tuberculous granuloma, and hemangioendothelioma (Table 33–1).

Clinical Prognosis and Therapy

Most authors do not clearly distinguish optic chiasmatic–hypothalamic gliomas from other optic pathway gliomas. Heiskanen and colleagues[23] reported five patients who would qualify for this group. One patient died following ventriculography. Three patients died within three years of surgery, and one patient died 15 years after surgery and radiation therapy.

Lloyd[34] reported 20 patients with tumors at this site. Six patients died, and in the five that were autopsied, extension into the hypothalamus was confirmed. Visual acuity decreased in all but one patient. Fourteen patients in this group received radiation therapy. Three of the patients who died had radiation therapy. The follow-up period varied from 2 to 13 years.

Hoyt and Baghadassarian[28] reported a total of 19 patients with tumor extending into the hypothalamus. Twenty-five percent of those patients who were irradiated experienced deterioration of their visual acuity. Thirty-three percent of those who were not treated with radiation deteriorated. Four of their patients died, but the follow-up of the other patients in this categroy is not documented.

Although outcome statistics stress survival and disregard quality of life, the poor prognosis in this group has been confirmed by other authors.[5, 13, 44]

In light of the diverse differential diagnosis and the ominous natural history of optic chiasmatic–hypothalamic tumors, a surgical approach is indicated. Indeed, surgical removal is possible for pituitary adenomas, craniopharyngiomas, epidermoid and dermoid tumors, colloid cysts, granulomas, and hemangioendotheliomas. Histio-

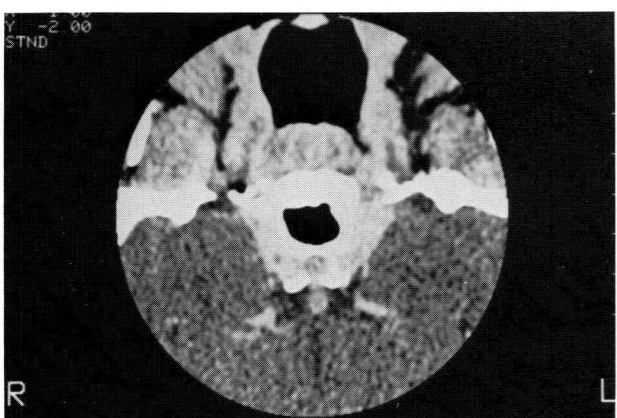

Figure 33–8. Seventeen-year-old girl with histiocytosis X, presenting with diabetes insipidus.

cytosis X is treated with low-dose radiation. In contrast, other suprasellar and sellar lesions are less amenable to treatment. Germinomas are responsive to radiation, although suprasellar germinomas carry a worse prognosis than those in the pineal region[27] and may recur outside the field of irradiation. A combination of surgical debulking and radiation therapy is the best treatment for progressive optic gliomas, malignant astrocytomas, and chordomas. Supervoltage radiation therapy with tumor doses of 5500 to 6000 rad in over 6 to 6.5 weeks is administered with rotational fields.[13]

Recent reports suggest that chemotherapy has at least a palliative effect on optic gliomas. Rosenstock and associates[47] reported 16 patients treated with vincristine and actinomycin D. The diagnosis was confirmed by biopsy in 14 of the patients. Four children with recurrent tumors who had previously been treated with radiation therapy had "stable" visual acuity 13 to 115 months following chemotherapy. Of the 12 newly diagnosed children, four progressed while under drug therapy but stabilized after radiation therapy. Three were still under treatment, and the remaining five children are stable 1 to 60 months following chemotherapy.

Intellectual retardation and delayed endocrinopathies associated with radiation therapy are correlated with the age of the child at treatment.* In children younger than five years of age, chemotherapy may delay tumor progression until an age when radiation would have less risk of disabling, long-term side effects. Moreover, Sayers[48] has suggested that tumor growth may slow after the first 15 years of life.

CONCLUSION

Considerable controversy has arisen over optic pathway gliomas, partly because the tumors are relatively rare, but largely because they have not been adequately classified and categorized. However, it is clear that the presentation, treatment, and prognosis are distinctly different for tumors that involve primarily the nerve, the nerve and optic chiasm, and the optic chiasm extending into the hypothalamus.

Tumors involving the nerve that present with visual loss should be resected. Children with neurofibromatosis who have no apparent visual loss may be followed. Great care must be exercised in following the very young patient with no demonstrable visual loss but with a tumor confined to the optic nerve.

Tumors of the optic nerve and chiasm are more likely to present with visual field loss in both eyes. When the CT scan demonstrates fusiform enlargement of one or both optic nerves, including the chiasm, an optic glioma is most probably present. Since no beneficial effect of radiation therapy has yet been demonstrated in this group, radiation therapy should be reserved for clinical and radiographic progression. Visual acuity often remains stable over long periods and may even improve spontaneously.

In contrast, tumors that involve primarily the chiasm, with extension into the hypothalamus, present with signs of increased intracranial pressure and hypothalamic dysfunction. Even though the prognosis in this group of children is poor, a surgical approach is warranted. Benign lesions that may masquerade as optic gliomas can be removed, whereas more malignant tumors such as germinoma are responsive to radiation therapy. Since children younger than five years of age are not good candidates for radiation therapy even if there is radiologic evidence of progression, chemotherapy may be a reasonable alternative.

Although the natural history of optic gliomas does not appear to be different in patients with neurofibromatosis, the differential diagnosis is more restricted. Furthermore, these patients tend to develop other tumors that may undergo sarcomatous degeneration and may result in their demise. Radiation therapy should be undertaken with considerable forethought.

The dilemma of optic glioma has been narrowed by CT and NMRI. In addition to precise morphologic localization and accurate diagnosis, modern radiographic imaging could allow documentation of the natural history of optic gliomas. If radiographic progression of the tumor can be clearly demonstrated, children with optic chiasm–hypothalamic tumors and gliomas confined to one or both optic nerves and the chiasm might be randomized, to study the effects of radiation therapy versus no radiation therapy. Then the controversy over the treatment of optic gliomas may be resolved.

References

1. Albright AL, Sclabassi RJ, Slamovits TL, et al: Spasmus nutans associated with optic gliomas in infants. J Pediatr 105:778, 1984.
2. Anderson DR, Spencer WH: Ultrastructural and histochemical observations of optic nerve gliomas. Arch Ophthalmol 83:324, 1970.
3. Arkhangelsky VN: Neoplasms of the optic nerve. Ophthalmologica 151:260, 1966.
4. Bamford FN, Jones PM, Pearson D, et al: Residual disabilities in children treated for intracranial space-occupying lesions. Cancer 37:1149, 1976.
5. Brand WN, Hoover SV: Optic gliomas in children: Review of 16 cases given megavoltage radiation therapy. Child's Brain 5:459, 1979.
6. Brooks WH, Parker JC, Jr., Young AB, et al: Malignant gliomas of the optic chiasm in adolescents. Clin Pediatr 15:557, 1976.
7. Christensen E, Andersen SR: Primary tumors of the optic nerve and chiasm. Acta Psychiatr Neurol Scand 27:5, 1952.
8. Chutorian AM, Schwartz JF, Evans RA, et al: Optic gliomas in children. Neurology (Minneap) 14:83, 1964.

---

*References 4, 12, 17, 21, 24, 25, 33, 42, 45, 49, 52

9. Cohen DH, Steinberg M, Buchwald R: Suprasellar germinomas: Diagnostic confusion with optic gliomas. Case report. J Neurosurg 41:490, 1974.
10. Cohen ME, Duffner PK: Visual evoked responses in children with optic gliomas with and without neurofibromatosis. Child's Brain 10:99, 1983.
11. Condon JR, Rose FC: Optic nerve glioma. Br J Ophthalmol 51:703, 1967.
12. Danoff BF, Cowchock FS, Marquette C, et al: Assessment of the long-term effects of primary radiation therapy for brain tumors in children. Cancer 49:1580, 1982.
13. Danoff BF, Kramer S, Thompson N: The radiotherapeutic management of optic nerve gliomas in children. Int J Radiat Oncol Biol Phys 6:45, 1980.
14. DeSousa AL, Kalsbeck JE, Mealey J, Jr., et al: Diencephalic syndrome and its relation to opticochiasmatic glioma: Review of twelve cases. Neurosurgery 4:207, 1979
15. Dodge HW, Love JG, Craig WM, et al: Gliomas of the optic nerves. Arch Neurol Psychiatry 79:607, 1958.
16. Eggers H, Jakobiec FA, Jones IS: Tumors of the optic nerve. Doc Ophthalmol 41:43, 1976.
17. Eiser C: Intellectual abilities among survivors of childhood leukemia as a function of CNS radiation. Arch Dis Child 53:391, 1978.
18. Fletcher WA, Imes RK, Hoyt WF: Chiasmal gliomas: Appearance and long-term changes demonstrated by computerized tomography. J Neurosurg 65:154, 1986.
19. Fowler FD, Matson DD: Gliomas of the optic pathways in childhood. J Neurosurg 14:515, 1957.
20. Glaser JS, Hoyt WF, Corbett J: Visual morbidity with chiasmal glioma. Arch Ophthalmol 85:3, 1971.
21. Goff JR, Anderson HR, Jr., Cooper PF: Distractibility and memory deficits in long-term survivors of acute lymphoblastic leukemia. J Dev Behav Pediatr 1:158, 1980.
22. Harper CG, Stewart-Wynne EG: Malignant optic gliomas in adults. Arch Neurol 35:731, 1978.
23. Heiskanen O, Raitta C, Torsti R: Management and prognosis of gliomas of the optic pathways in children. Mod Probl Paediatr 18:216, 1977.
24. Hirsch JF, Renier D, Czernichow P, et al: Medulloblastoma in childhood. Survival and functional results. Acta Neurol Chir 48:1, 1979.
25. Hochberg FH, Slotnick B: Neuropsychologic impairment in astrocytoma survivors. Neurology 30:172, 1980.
26. Hoffman HJ: Optic pathway gliomas. In: Amador L (ed): Brain Tumors in the Young. Springfield, IL, Charles C Thomas, 1983, pp 622–633.
27. Hoffman HJ: Suprasellar germinomas. In: McLaurin RL (ed): Pediatric Neurosurgery. Surgery of the Developing Nervous System. New York, Grune & Stratton, 1982, pp 487–491.
28. Hoyt WF, Baghadassarian SA: Optic glioma of childhood. Br J Ophthalmol 53:793, 1969.
29. Hoyt WF, Meshel LG, Lessel S, et al: Malignant optic glioma of adulthood. Brain 96:121, 1973.
30. Hudson AD: Primary tumors of the optic nerve. R Lond Ophthalmol Hosp Rep 18:317, 1912.
31. Jain NS: Optic gliomas. Br J Ophthalmol 45:54, 1961.
32. Kelly TW: Optic glioma presenting as spasmus nutans. Pediatrics 45:295, 1970.
33. Kun LE, Mulhern RK, Crisco JJ: Quality of life in children treated for brain tumors. Intellectual, emotional, and academic function. J Neurosurg 58:1, 1983.
34. Lloyd LA: Gliomas of the optic nerve and chiasm in childhood. Trans Am Ophthalmol Soc 71:488, 1973.
35. MacCarty CS, Boyd AS, Jr., Childs DS: Tumors of the optic nerve and optic chiasm. J Neurosurg 33:439, 1970.
36. Marshall D: Glioma of the optic nerve, as a manifestation of von Recklinghausen's disease. Am J Ophthalmol 37:15, 1954.
37. Martin P, Cushing H: Primary gliomas of the chiasm and optic nerves in their intracranial portion. Arch Ophthalmol 52:209, 1923.
38. Martuza RL, Kornblith PL, Liszczak TM: Characteristics of human optic gliomas in tissue culture. J Neurosurg 46:78, 1977.
39. Matson DD: Neurosurgery of Infancy and Childhood. Springfield, IL, Charles C Thomas, 1969, pp 436–448.
40. McCullough DC, Epstein F: Optic pathway tumors. A review with proposals for clinical staging. Cancer 56:1789, 1985.
41. Miller NR, Iliff WJ, Green WR: Evaluation and management of gliomas of the anterior visual pathways. Brain 97:743, 1974.
42. Myles ST, Murphy SB: Gliomas of the optic nerve and chiasm. Can J Ophthalmol 8:508, 1973.
43. Oxenhandler DC, Sayers MP: The dilemma of childhood optic gliomas. J Neurosurg 48:340, 1978.
44. Packer RJ, Savino PJ, Bilaniuk LT, et al: Chiasmatic gliomas of childhood. A reappraisal of natural history and effectiveness of cranial irradiation. Child's Brain 10:393, 1983.
45. Raimondi AJ, Tomita T: Advantages of "total" resection of medulloblastoma and disadvantages of full head postoperative radiation therapy. Child's Brain 5:550, 1979.
46. Rand CW, Irvine R, Reeves DL: Primary glioma of the optic nerve. Arch Ophthalmol 21:799, 1939.
47. Rosenstock JG, Packer RJ, Bilaniuk L, et al: Chiasmatic optic glioma treated with chemotherapy. J Neurosurg 63:862, 1985.
48. Sayers MP: Optic nerve gliomas. In: McLaurin RL (ed): Pediatric Neurosurgery. Surgery of the Developing Nervous System. New York, Grune & Stratton, 1982, pp 513–522.
49. Shalet SM, Beardwell CG, Aarons BM, et al: Growth impairment in children treated for brain tumours. Arch Dis Child 5:491, 1978.
50. Spender WH: Primary neoplasms of the optic nerve and its sheaths: Clinical features and current concepts of pathogenetic mechanisms. Trans Am Ophthalmol Soc 70:490, 1972.
51. Spoor TC, Kennerdell VS, Martinez AJ, et al: Malignant gliomas of the optic pathway. Am J Ophthalmol 89:284, 1980.
52. Spunberg JJ, Chang CH, Goldman M, et al: Quality of long-term survival following irradiation for intracranial tumors in children under the age of two. Int J Radiat Oncol Biol Phys 7:727, 1981.
53. Taveras JJ, Mount LA, Wood EH: The value of radiation therapy in the management of glioma of the optic nerves and chiasm. Radiation 66:518, 1956.
54. Tenny RT, Laws ER, Jr., Younge BR, et al: The neurosurgical management of optic glioma. Results in 104 patients. J Neurosurg 57:452, 1982.
55. Tym R: Piloid gliomas of the anterior optic pathways. Br J Surg 49:322, 1961.
56. Verhoeff FH: Primary intraneural tumors (gliomas) of the optic nerve, a histological study of eleven cases, including a case showing cystic involvement of the optic disc, with demonstration of the origin of cytoid bodies of the retina and cavernous atrophy of the optic nerve. Arch Ophthalmol 51:120, 1922.
57. Verhoeff FH: Tumors of the optic nerve. In: Penfield W (ed): Cytology and Cellular Pathology of the Nervous System, Vol. 3. New York, Paul B. Hoeber, 1932, pp 1029–1039.
58. Walsh FB: The ocular signs of tumors involving the anterior visual pathways. Am J Ophthalmol 42:347, 1956.
59. Wilson CB, Feinsod M, Hoyt WF, et al: Malignant evolution of childhood chiasmal pilocytic astrocytoma. Neurology (Minneap) 26:322, 1976.

34
CRANIOPHARYNGIOMAS

Harold J. Hoffman, M.D., B.Sc. (Med.)
Corey Raffel, M.D., Ph.D.

Craniopharyngiomas are the most common suprasellar tumor in children. In Matson's large series[25] of brain tumors, craniopharyngiomas constituted 9 percent. At the Hospital for Sick Children, these tumors account for 6 percent of brain tumors and 14 percent of supratentorial tumors.[15] The benign histologic features of the tumor are in discordance with their malignant clinical behavior. Because these extra-axial lesions insinuate themselves into adjacent neurologic structures, total removal is considered hazardous by some surgeons,[2, 22, 28] whereas others advocate total extirpation.[16, 26, 34] The role of radiation therapy in the treatment of craniopharyngiomas is also debated.[2] At the Hospital for Sick Children, the authors approach each patient with total excision as the goal and believe total removal can be achieved safely in the vast majority of children with craniopharyngiomas.

PATHOLOGY

Erdheim[12] was the first to propose the well-accepted hypothesis that craniopharyngiomas arise from embryonic squamous cell rests of an incompletely involuted hypophyseal-pharyngeal duct. These rests lie in the pituitary stalk, extending from the tuber cinereum to the pituitary gland. Therefore, the tumor is adherent to the tuber cinereum and can insinuate itself into the substance of the hypothalamus. Elsewhere, the tumor is covered by meninges and is easily separated from neural and vascular structures. Because of the infiltrative nature of the tumor in the tuber cinereum, concern has been expressed that surgical removal may leave nests of tumor cells behind in this region.[2] The nests of tumor seen in sections through the anterior hypothalamus are, in reality, fingers of tumor that have been sectioned transversely and thus appear to be isolated cell rests. As pointed out by Sweet,[34] an intense astrogliosis is induced by the tumor in the tuber cinereum. The layer of gliosis separates the tumor from the functional hypothalamic neurons and provides a plane of separation when the tumor capsule is pulled off the brain in this region.

Grossly, the tumors are largely or partially cystic. Because of their location, craniopharyngiomas compress the optic chiasm anteriorly, the diaphragma sellae inferiorly, and the third ventricle superiorly; they may fill the anterior third ventricle and cause hydrocephalus. If the diaphragma sella is deficient, the tumor can infiltrate pituitary gland and expand the sellae. The tumor may also extend posteriorly down the clivus, ventral to the pons. The solid portions of the tumor frequently contain either or both small granular and large craggy foci of calcifications. The cystic portion contains yellow-green fluid in which glittering cholesterol crystals are seen.

The cyst walls are composed of columnar or stratified squamous epithelium resting on a collagenous basement membrane that separates the tumor from the surrounding meninges. In the solid portion, the epithelial elements are separated by loosely arranged stellate cells, giving rise to the "adamantinomatous" pattern. Calcification of the keratin is common, and as the masses of keratin coalesce, large foci of calcification may occur.

CLINICAL FEATURES

One half to slightly more than one half of all craniopharyngiomas occur in patients younger than 18 years of age.[6,9] The tumors are rarely seen in patients younger than five years of age, although occurrences as early as the neonatal period have been reported.[3] In large series of craniopharyngiomas, a slight male predominance or an equal distribution between the sexes has been shown.

The time between onset of symptoms and diagnosis is typically short, a majority of patients being treated within one year of onset of symptoms.[16] At the Hospital for Sick Children, visual complaints were most common at presentation.[16,31] Of 72 patients with craniopharyngiomas, 45 had visual field defects, either bitemporal hemianopia or homonymous hemianopia; 24 had papilledema; and 24 had a significant decrease in visual acuity, frequently affecting one eye more than the other. Headache was a common symptom, usually related to obstructive hydrocephalus. See-saw nystagmus, in which one eye moves upward and rotates inward while the other eye moves downward and rotates outward, was seen in four patients. This type of nystagmus, which is diagnostic of lesions of the diencephalon, upper midbrain, parasellar region, or all three can be found in 5 to 10 percent of patients with craniopharyngiomas.[11]

Symptoms and signs of hypothalamic-pituitary dysfunction are present in over 50 percent of patients at presentation. The most common symptom is shortness of stature, present in 20 of the 72 patients seen at the Hospital for Sick Children. In some series, growth delay is the most common presenting sign in children, occurring in over 90 percent of patients.[8] Diabetes insipidus is a presenting endocrinologic syndrome in about 20 percent of patients. Obesity, hypothyroidism, and hypocortisolism are other endocrinologic syndromes found in children with craniopharyngiomas.

PREOPERATIVE EVALUATION

The preoperative evaluation of the patient with a suspected craniopharyngioma consists of three parts: (1) radiologic, (2) visual, and (3) endocrinologic.

Plain skull radiographs are abnormal in more than one half of children with craniopharyngioma. The most common finding is abnormal calcification in the suprasellar region. Enlargement of the sella may also be seen.

Computed tomography. (CT) scanning is currently the study of choice for evaluating patients suspected of harboring a craniopharyngioma. The CT scan is sensitive and has allowed for identification of small tumors in patients with no other symptoms besides headache. The typical craniopharyngioma has a low-density cyst surrounded by a partially calcified contrast-enhancing capsule. There may be an associated partially calcified, contrast-enhancing solid tumor. Occasionally, solid tumors without cyst formation are seen. The tumor is centered in the suprasellar cistern and may extend in any direction, although most commonly extension is anterior, superior, posterior, or all three. Fine coronal CT images enhanced with intravenous contrast material may show the relationship of the tumor to surrounding vascular structures in sufficient detail to make angiography unnecessary.

Angiography has proved useful in demonstrating the direction of growth of craniopharyngiomas (Fig. 34–1).

Magnetic resonance imaging (MRI) supplements CT scanning and angiography in assessing the patient with a craniopharyngioma and determining the relationship of the tumor to surrounding structures. The sagittal format of the MRI scan shows the direction of growth of the craniopharyngioma (Fig. 34–2).

Craniopharyngiomas can be divided into three groups. The small sellar tumors show no displacement of vessels and do not impinge on optic apparatus (Fig. 34–3). The prechiasmatic tumors are seen to extend anteriorly. They typically elevate the A1 segment of the anterior cerebral artery. They rarely displace the basilar artery. They impinge on optic nerves, and affected children frequently present with visual impairment (Fig. 34–4). The retrochiasmatic tumors extend posteriorly. They typically fill the third ventricle and encroach on the foramina of Monro, thus causing hydrocephalus.

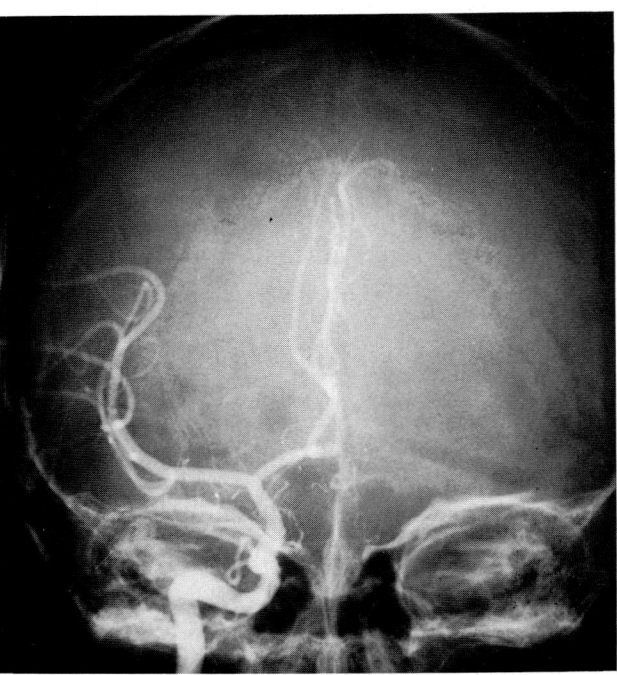

Figure 34–1. Anteroposterior carotid angiogram in a patient with prechiasmatic craniopharyngioma, showing elevation of A1 segment of anterior cerebral artery.

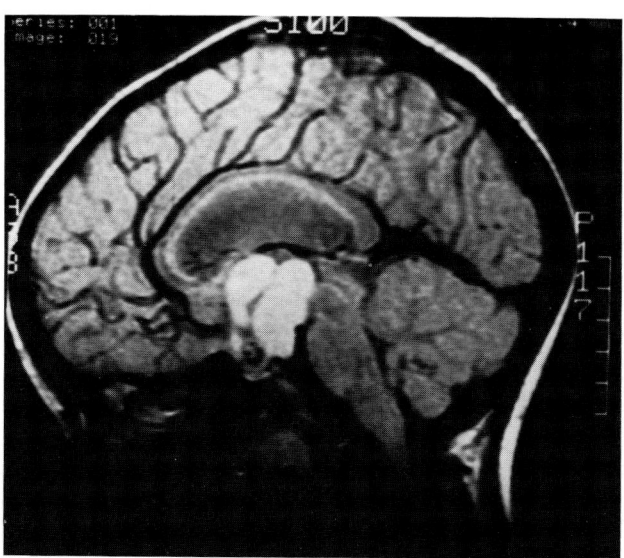

Figure 34–2. Nuclear magnetic resonance (NMR) image of a patient with retrochiasmatic craniopharyngioma, showing upward and posterior direction of tumor growth.

Such tumors do not impinge on the optic apparatus, but affected patients frequently have papilledema due to their hydrocephalus. Retrochiasmatic tumors do not impinge on the A1 segment of the anterior cerebral artery, but they do displace the basilar artery posteriorly, off the clivus (Fig. 34–5).

All patients with a craniopharyngioma should have a thorough visual examination preoperatively. Visual acuity and tangent screen visual field testing should be included in the preoperative visual assessment.

Patients with craniopharyngiomas can have distortion of the columns of the fornix and consequently may have a memory disorder. Furthermore, in removing a craniopharyngioma, one may disturb the fornices and create a memory disorder. Consequently, all patients with craniopharyngioma should have accurate, neuropsychologic testing prior to surgery.

Neuroendocrinologic testing performed preoperatively should include tests for diabetes insipidus, impairment of the pituitary-adrenal axis, and impairment of the pituitary-thyroid axis. Even patients with no symptoms referable to pituitary dysfunction should be tested, as careful evaluation reveals some endocrine deficiency in most patients.[35]

Serum cortisol levels should be measured in the morning and in the evening. Impairment of adrenocorticotrophic hormone may affect the absolute levels of serum cortisol but may also be reflected only in a loss of the normal diurnal variation in serum cortisol levels. Because many of these patients have no adrenal reserve preoperatively, they must be given exogenous steroid supplements (dexamethasone, 0.2 mg/kg to a maximum of 10 mg, as a loading dose, then 0.1 mg/kg q6h, to a maximum of 4 mg, maintenance) prior to any stressful procedure, such as angiography or surgery.

Thyroid function should be assessed with serum thyroxine (T_4) and triiodothyronine (T_3) or T_3 radioactive uptake levels. Patients with hypothyroidism should be given replacement therapy with L-thyroxine.

Assessment for diabetes insipidus includes questioning the patient about urinary frequency, new onset of nocturia, or new onset of enuresis. Serum electrolytes should be checked and, of course, corrected if abnormal. Water deprivation with serial serum and urine osmolarities is the most sensitive test for confirming the presence of diabetes insipidus.

Serum growth hormone levels, and luteinizing hormone (LH) and follicle-stimulating hormone (FSH) levels in pubertal and postpubertal patients, complete the endocrine work-up.

SURGICAL MANAGEMENT

Three types of surgical procedures have been recommended for the treatment of craniopharyngiomas: (1) cyst drainage and biopsy, (2) subtotal resection, and (3) total removal. The first two options are usually followed by radiation therapy.

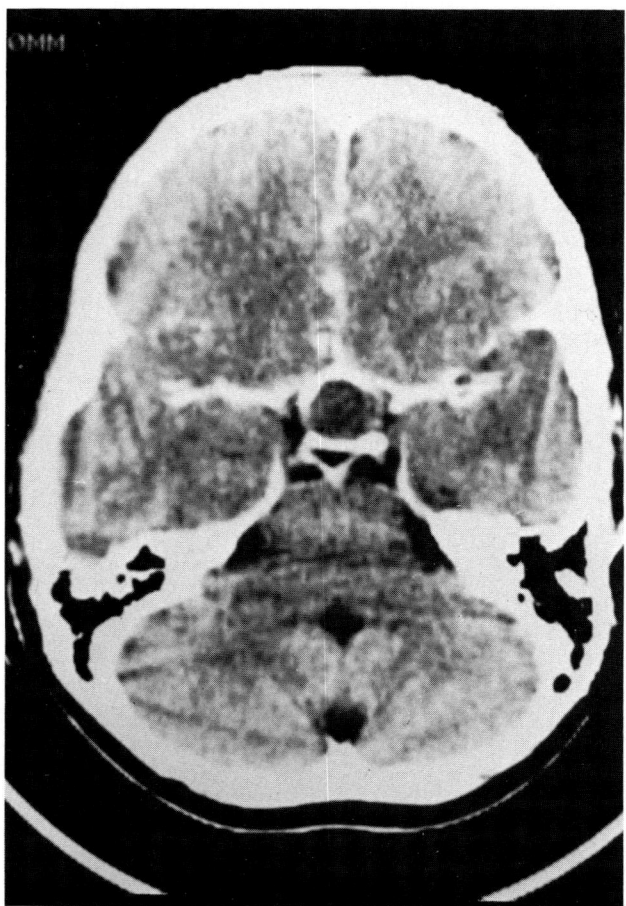

Figure 34–3. Axial CT scan of a patient with a sellar craniopharyngioma.

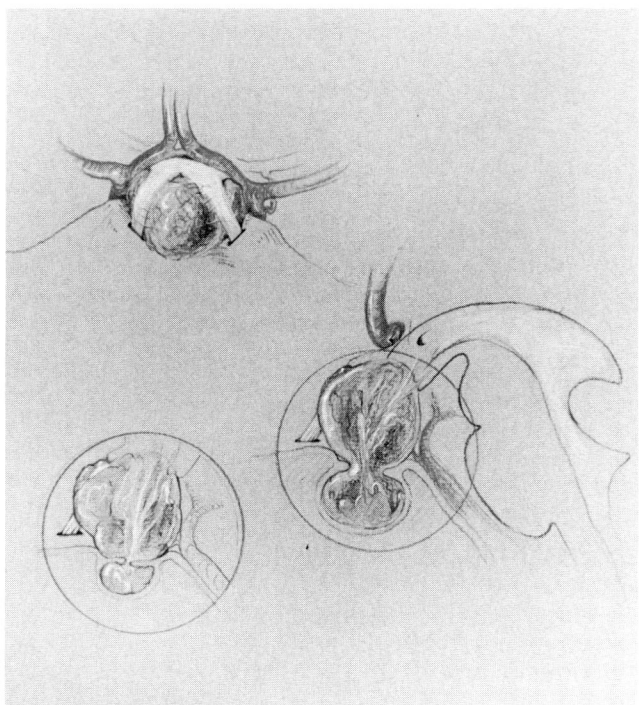

Figure 34–4. Diagrammatic depiction of prechiasmatic craniopharyngioma. (With permission from Hoffman HJ: Craniopharyngiomas. Can J Neurol Sci 12:348–352, 1985.)

Advocates of conservative surgical treatment of craniopharyngiomas have suggested many approaches, including open biopsy with or without placement of an indwelling intracystic catheter for later repeated percutaneous drainage; stereotactic biopsy and cyst damage;[4, 23, 24, 28] and subtotal resection via a variety of approaches.[6, 8, 9] The rationale for a conservative approach is the belief that total removal of a craniopharyngioma is impossible.[7, 23, 24] However, this supposition is clearly false. With the advent of steroid therapy, Matson began to attempt total removal of these tumors in 1950.[26] His long-term results indicate that 18 of 34 children (53 percent) were alive and tumor free; an additional four patients were alive and tumor free after one recurrence. Thus, without the aid of the operating

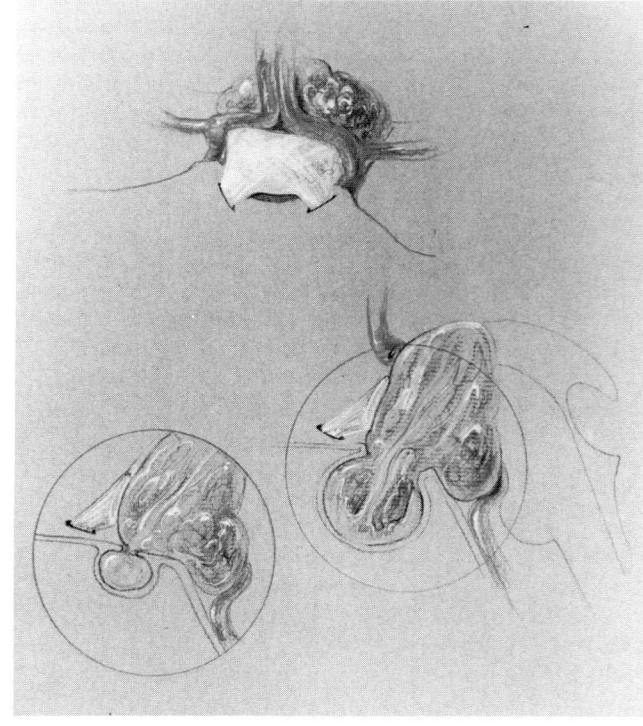

Figure 34–5. Diagrammatic depiction of retrochiasmatic craniopharyngioma. (With permission from Hoffman HJ: Craniopharyngiomas. Can J Neurol Sci 12:348–352, 1985.)

microscope, 63 percent of Matson's patients had an apparent surgical cure.[20]

One reason that some surgeons believe that conservative approaches to craniopharyngiomas are appropriate relates to the erroneous belief that tumor removal will lead to irreparable damage to the hypothalamus or to the optic apparatus.[7, 19, 29, 33] In his 1976 exposition, Sweet[34] showed that craniopharyngiomas are separated from functional brain by an intense astrogliosis that provides a margin of safety between the tumor and functioning neural tissue. The experience at the Hospital for Sick Children supports this view. During surgery, there appears to be a safe plane of cleavage between the tumor and surrounding neural structures; adherence of the solid portion of the tumor to neighboring blood vessels can be encountered that occasionally leads to a subtotal resection.

An attempt to show a worse neuropsychologic outcome in patients undergoing attempted total resection as compared with those undergoing biopsy, cyst aspiration, and radiation therapy has been reported.[13] However, only three of the 14 patients in whom a total resection was attempted had postoperative neuroradiologic studies documenting total removal. Eleven of the 14 received postoperative radiation therapy. The authors believe that this report emphasizes the hazards of attempted total excision of craniopharyngiomas without the use of the operating microscope and without careful determination of total resection postoperatively.

Major morbidity and mortality as a result of damage to the hypothalamus or optic apparatus has not been seen in the author's patients with totally removed tumors. In a recent review of totally removed craniopharyngiomas at the Hospital for Sick Children, it was found that in two thirds, vision was improved postoperatively.[16] Hypothalamic dysfunction occurred in most patients postoperatively. Diabetes insipidus was present in 23 of 24 patients. An eating disorder resulting in obesity was present in eight patients. Almost all patients with craniopharyngiomas have dysfunction of the hypothalamic-pituitary axis preoperatively, when tested carefully.[35] In the Hospital for Sick Children series, patients with totally removed tumors continued to have hypopituitarism and commonly required exogenous thyroid hormone (23 of 24), hydrocortisone (22 of 24), and human growth hormone (12 of 24). Normal growth may occur without exogenous growth hormone, even in the face of low serum growth hormone levels.[18] Sex hormone replacement may be necessary as the children reach puberty. These endocrine deficits, with the exception of diabetes insipidus, differ little from those seen in patients undergoing less radical procedures.[8, 16, 31] No patient had a significant decrease in intellectual performance, as determined by IQ testing. No operative mortality has occurred at the Hospital for Sick Children since the use of the operating microscope has become routine. Thus, the complications predicted with total removal by those who favor less radical procedures have failed to materialize.

There is some evidence in the literature that craniopharyngiomas are more aggressive in children than in adults. In Kahn's report[19] of a 45-year experience with craniopharyngiomas, an excellent result was achieved in 21 percent of children and 67 percent of adults. Both Kramer[22] and Hoff and Patterson[14] have concluded that craniopharyngiomas grow faster and are more likely to recur in children than in adults. The authors feel that the more aggressive nature of craniopharyngiomas in children argues for attempted total removal, as this offers the best chance for cure.

Many surgical approaches to craniopharyngiomas have been described, including subfrontal, transpterional, subtemporal, transcallosal, transsphenoidal, and transpalatal. However, in order to remove the tumor totally, the surgeon must have easy access to both optic nerves and both internal carotid arteries as well as the overlying lamina terminalis, to allow access to the third ventricle. For sellar and prechiasmatic tumors, these criteria are met by the subfrontal approach alone (Fig. 34–6A). For retrochiasmatic tumors, the pterional approach to allow access to the posterior portion of the tumor is combined with the subfrontal approach (Fig. 34–6B).

In cases in which the craniopharyngioma was large enough to produce obstruction of the third ventricle and hydrocephalus, the authors have found that insertion of a shunt as a preliminary step has improved the patient's functional status and tolerance to the surgical removal of the tumor.

Craniopharyngiomas require careful dissection from adjacent optic apparatus and internal carotid arteries as well as from the overlying hypothalamus. Therefore, they must be approached so that all these structures are in view and can be safely separated from tumor.

The sellar tumors and the prechiasmatic tumors can be very satisfactorily approached by a subfrontal route. The patients are put in a supine position, with the neck extended and the nose pointing directly upward in anatomic position. A right-sided approach is preferred, as the right hemisphere is typically nondominant.

The incision in the scalp is made behind the hairline, and the bone flap extends from the midline medially, down to the supraorbital margin inferiorly, out to the pterion laterally, and back to just in front of the coronal suture posteriorly. The dural opening is along the supraorbital ridge. Draining veins from the frontal pole to the sagittal sinus are coagulated and divided, and the olfactory nerve is coagulated and divided just behind the olfactory bulb to avoid avulsion of the bulb from the cribriform plate.

Using microsurgical techniques, the chiasmatic cistern is exposed and opened, and the frontal lobe

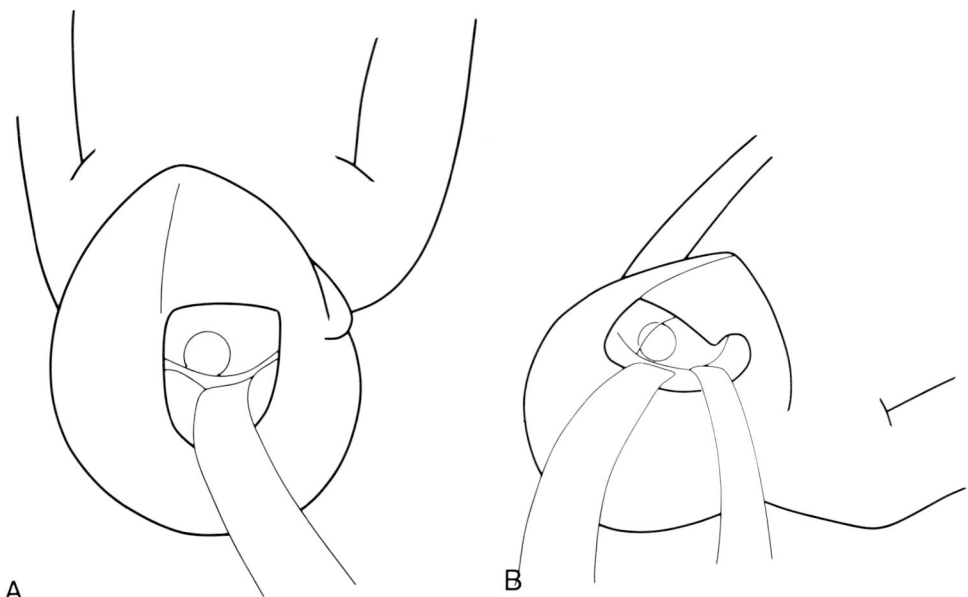

Figure 34–6. *A,* Subfrontal approach to sellar and prechiasmatic craniopharyngiomas. *B,* Subfrontal and transpterional approach to retrochiasmatic craniopharyngiomas.

is retracted off the chiasm and the optic nerves, allowing full visualization of optic nerves, chiasm, and internal carotid artery.

This brings the tumor into clear view. The capsule is pierced with a fine needle, and the tumor contents are aspirated to ensure that one is dealing with tumor rather than a vascular structure. The capsule of the tumor is then coagulated and incised. The fluid contents are aspirated, and the solid contents are removed with the ultrasonic aspirator. Once the tumor is decompressed, traction can be applied to the capsule and the filamentous adhesions between the tumor and adjacent structures are freed up. The glial reaction between tumor and tuber cinereum allows one to pull tumor capsule free of the hypothalamus. With an intact diaphragma sellae, the tumor can be easily separated from the pituitary fossa. The pituitary stalk, if visualized, should be preserved. If the diaphragma sellae is deficient, the craniopharyngioma will invade the pituitary gland, and traction of the tumor will free it up from this structure. With a deficient diaphragma sellae, the craniopharyngioma may be intimately adherent to the side wall of the sellae, and as one pulls the tumor free, one may get venous bleeding from the cavernous sinus. This can be controlled easily with gentle pressure. With the tumor removed, there is a clear view of both optic nerves, both internal carotid arteries, and the intact membrane of Liliequist posteriorly.

In the case of a retrochiasmatic tumor, the bone flap is extended to include the pterion and the anterior temporal squama. The dura is opened over the frontal pole, down through the sylvian region, and over the temporal pole. The frontal lobe is retracted upward, and the temporal lobe is retracted posteriorly, which brings the bifurcation of the internal carotid artery, and the optic nerve and chiasm, into view. The optic nerve and chiasm are separated from the internal carotid artery, which exposes the craniopharyngioma capsule. This is then coagulated and incised, and the craniopharyngioma contents are emptied by suction and the ultrasonic aspirator. With this done, the tumor typically collapses. The chiasm moves back away from tuberculum sellae, allowing the tumor to be extracted between the two optic nerves. If the tumor cannot be totally removed between the internal carotid artery and the optic nerve, one can, by elevating the frontal lobe, expose the lamina terminalis. By opening the lamina terminalis, one can enter the third ventricle, where the craniopharyngioma capsule can be seen invaginating the very thinned-out floor of the third ventricle. Thus, the tumor can be delivered through the lamina terminalis, between the two optic nerves, and between the internal carotid artery and the optic nerve. Again, with the tumor removed, one is exposed to a beautiful view of the suprasellar anatomy, including an intact membrane of Liliequist.

Postoperatively, the patient must be monitored closely. Surgical retraction of the frontal lobe may result in seizure activity, and prophylactic doses of phenytoin should accordingly be administered for a period of seven to ten days (5–7 mg/kg/24 hr). Preoperative doses of dexamethasone are continued for 48 to 72 hours postoperatively, at which point, maintenance doses of cortisone (25 mg/m^2) are substituted. Eventually, the cortisone should be reduced to the lowest effective level, with a warning to the patient that an increase in dosage may be necessary to avoid possible addisonian crises during periods of stress or infection.

If the sphenoid sinus has been entered during a surgical approach through the tuberculum sellae, then prophylactic antibiotics should be administered to prevent postoperative meningitis.

Total removal of a craniopharyngioma almost invariably leads to diabetes insipidus. This condition normally becomes manifest during the first 24 to 48 hours postoperatively. Treatment is now very simple and effective. Desmopressin (DDAVP) is administered by nasal instillation in doses of 5 to 20 mg (contained in 0.05 to 0.2 cc) every 12 to 24 hours. This material is extremely effective for postoperative as well as long-term management.

Thyroid studies should be repeated after surgery; if there is evidence of hypothyroidism, thyroid treatment should be instituted. Similarly, gonadotrophic hormones should be assessed in pubertal children, and appropriate replacement therapy should be begun if the hormone levels are found to be depressed.

Finally, clinical monitoring of the patient's growth, together with growth hormone studies, should begin six months postoperatively. If growth slows or halts entirely, and if growth hormone levels are significantly depressed, replacement therapy is begun. However, in some cases, normal growth continues despite the absence of growth hormones.[18] Therapeutic intervention in such cases is obviously unnecessary.

Despite an intraoperative appearance of total removal, craniopharyngiomas can recur. In the era before CT, the estimation of the extent of tumor removal depended on the surgeon's impression. In Matson's series,[20] the recurrence rate was 26.5 percent, and in Sweet's series[34] of 23 patients, the rate of recurrence was 8.7 percent. With the advent of CT scanning, the amount of tumor remaining postoperatively can be more accurately determined.[16] In the author's experience, total excision can be achieved in two thirds to three fourths of patients.[16, 17] When the postoperative CT scan showed no tumor, or remaining calcium with no enhancing tumor, no tumor recurrence was observed (Figs. 34–7 and 34–8).[16] However, if tumor must be left behind, then recurrent symptoms are inevitable.[16] In such situations, the authors would recommend postoperative radiation therapy.

In patients in whom the surgeon believes that total tumor removal has been achieved but in whom postoperative imaging shows residual tumor, reoperation is indicated. Without reoperation, recurrent symptoms are inevitable.[16]

RADIATION THERAPY

Radiation therapy has been demonstrated to have a destructive effect on craniopharyngiomas, even though the brain parenchyma would be expected to be harmed by doses high enough to affect the stratified squamous epithelium of the tumor. In the

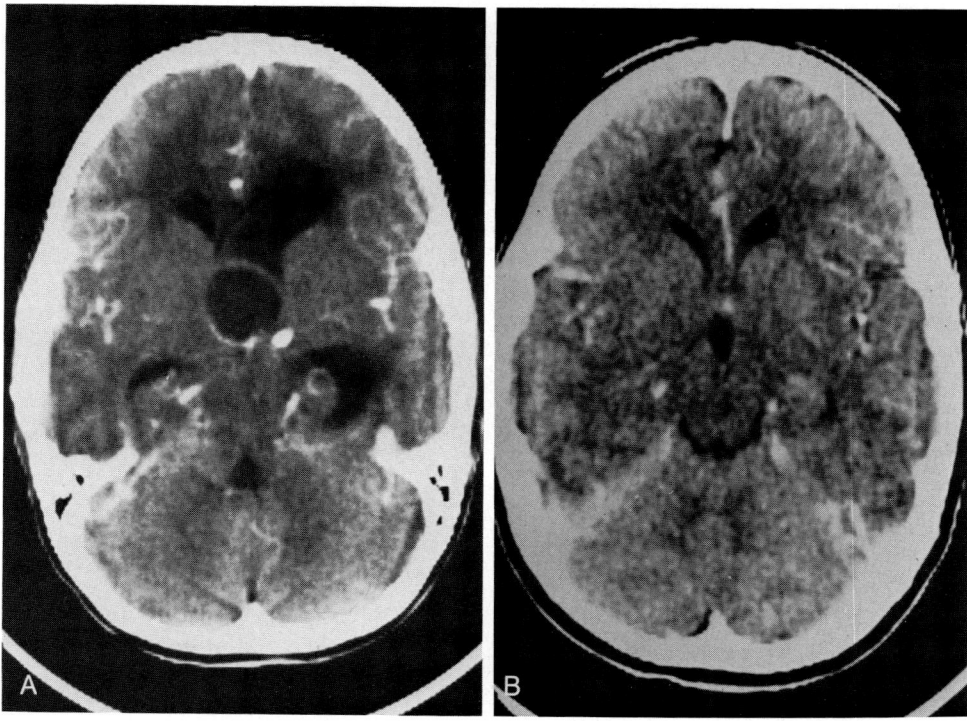

Figure 34–7. *A*, Axial CT scan of cystic retrochiasmatic craniopharyngioma that has produced hydrocephalus. *B*, Postoperative axial CT scan on the same patient as in *A*, showing total resection of the tumor and resolution of hydrocephalus.

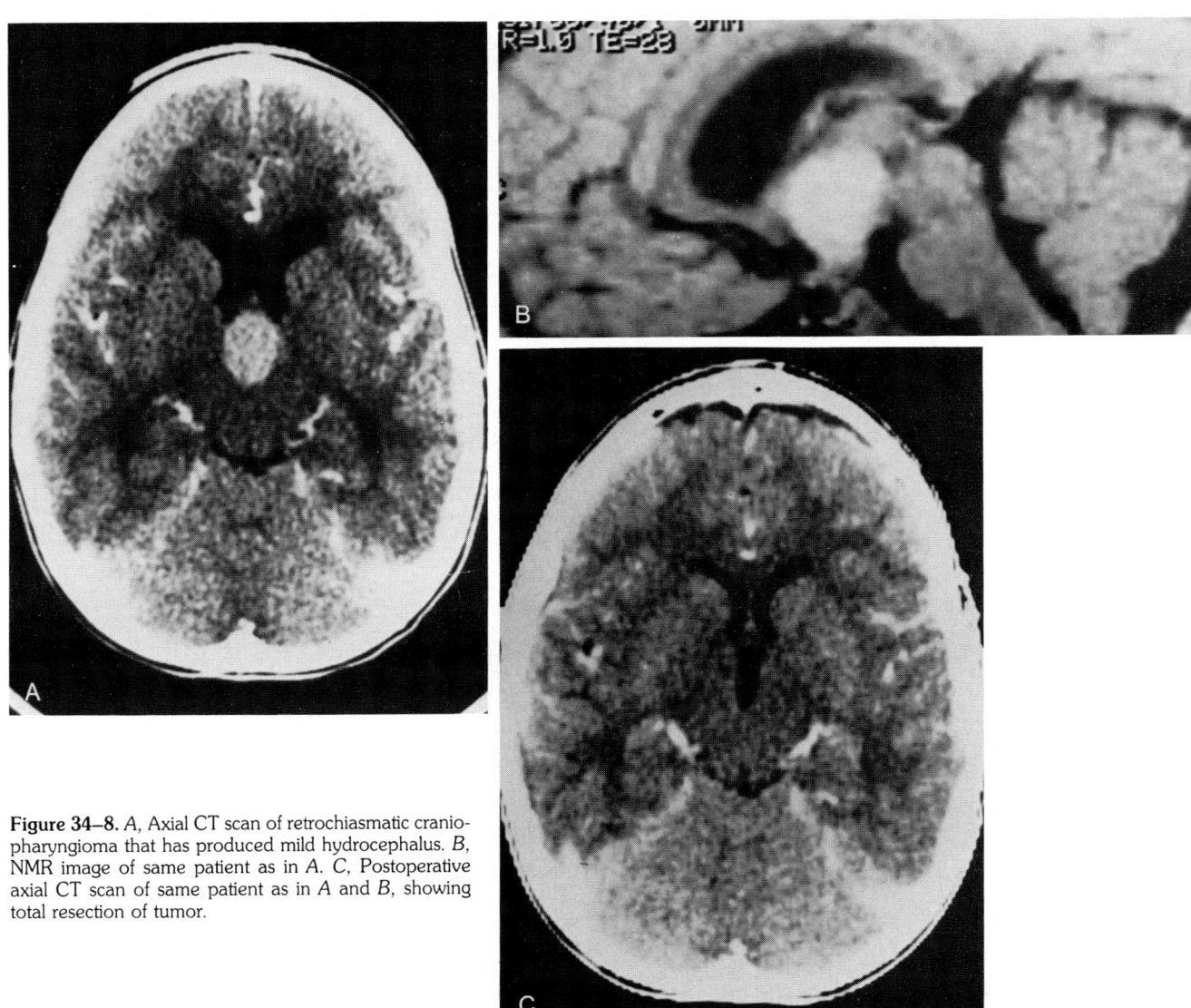

Figure 34–8. *A*, Axial CT scan of retrochiasmatic craniopharyngioma that has produced mild hydrocephalus. *B*, NMR image of same patient as in *A*. *C*, Postoperative axial CT scan of same patient as in *A* and *B*, showing total resection of tumor.

Cleveland Clinic series, 78 percent of patients treated with subtotal resection alone have died, compared with 18 percent of patients receiving postoperative radiation therapy. Similar improvements in reduction in recurrence has been achieved by the addition of radiation therapy to subtotal resection in other series.[27]

However, radiation therapy does have risks. Calcification of the basal ganglia is commonly seen in patients irradiated for parasellar lesions (Fig. 34–9). Furthermore, radiation therapy is not always effective, and craniopharyngiomas can continue their relentless growth despite radiation therapy (Fig. 34–10). Furthermore, in such cases, the radiation therapy creates an intense reaction that makes any further curative surgery an impossibility.

The major risks are radiation necrosis of the brain and optic nerves.[2, 10, 32] This delayed reaction of the brain to radiation may result from too large a total dose, too short an interval between fractions, or too few fractions. Current recommendations are 5000 to 6000 rad given with rotating ports, 6×6 cm maximum, and no more than 200 rad per day.[2] In addition to radiation necrosis, parasellar irradiation may give rise to meningeal sarcomas, meningiomas, and bilateral carotid occlusion.[1, 5, 21] In children, exposure of the brain to radiation may lead to a decline in intellect.

To avoid the complications of external beam radiation therapy, the intracystic injection of radio-

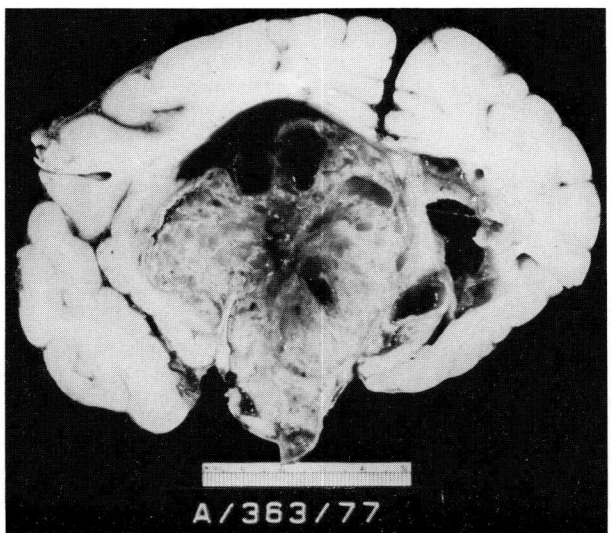

Figure 34–10. Post-mortem specimen showing large craniopharyngioma eight years after biopsy and radiotherapy.

active isotopes has been proposed.[5, 21] The radionuclide can be placed into the tumor cyst stereotactically or via an indwelling catheter connected to an Ommaya reservoir. These techniques have been shown to reduce the size of the cyst and to prevent further tumor growth. They are limited to use in tumors made up of one or two large cysts with a minor solid component.

SUMMARY

Craniopharyngiomas are benign tumors arising from squamous cell rests in the pituitary stalk. They give rise to symptoms by compressing nearby neural structures. The goal of surgical therapy is total excision; this goal can be reached in more than 70 percent of patients, with minimal morbidity. If total removal is ascertained by postoperative neuroimaging, the recurrence rate is less than 10 percent.

The authors feel that if after total excision there is obvious tumor left behind, reoperation is indicated to remove such residual tumor. If only a subtotal excision can be performed because of the nature of the tumor and its relationship to surrounding structures, postoperative radiation therapy should be carried out. Without such therapy, recurrence of symptoms will become evident within a matter of months.

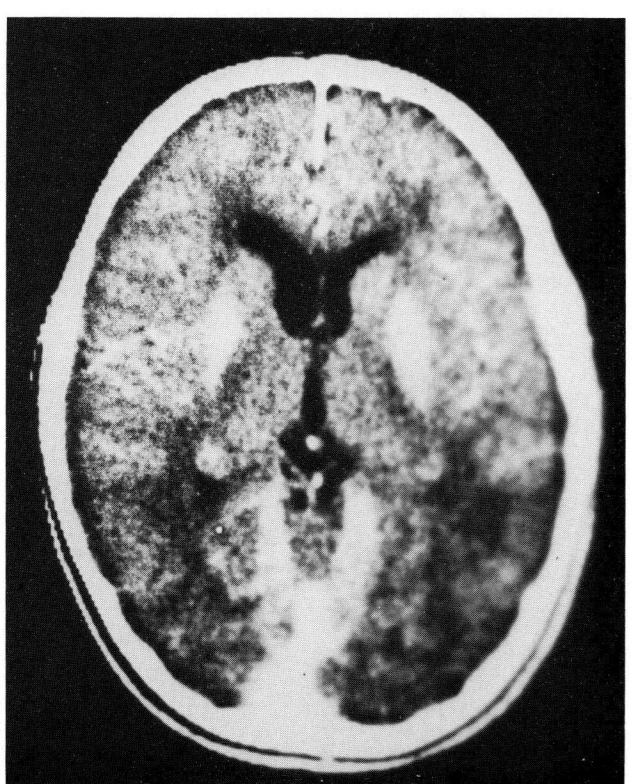

Figure 34–9. Calcification of basal ganglia in a patient irradiated for a craniopharyngioma.

References

1. Allen J: The effects of cancer therapy on the nervous system. J Pediatr 93:903, 1978.
2. Amacher AL: Craniopharyngioma: The controversy regarding radiotherapy. Child's Brain 6:57, 1980.
3. Azar-Kia B, Kreskman VR, Schecter MM: Neonatal craniopharyngioma: Case report. J Neurosurg 42:91, 1975.

4. Backlund E-O: Studies on craniopharyngiomas. I. Treatment, past and present. Acta Chir Scand 138:743, 1972.
5. Backlund E-O: Studies on craniopharyngiomas. III. Stereotaxic treatment with intracystic yttrium-90. Acta Chir Scand 139:237, 1973.
6. Bannr M, Hoare RD, Stanley P, et al: Craniopharyngiomas in children. J Pediatr 983:781, 1973.
7. Bartlett JR: Craniopharyngiomas. A summary of 85 cases. J Neurol Neurosurg Psychiatry 34:37, 1971.
8. Baskin DS, Wilson CB: Surgical management of craniopharyngiomas. A review of 74 cases. J Neurosurg 65:22, 1986.
9. Bloom HJ, Tumors of the central nervous system. In: Voute PA, et al (eds): Cancer in Children, 2nd ed. New York, Springer-Verlag, 1986, pp 197–222.
10. D'Lorenzo N, Nolletti A, Palma L: Late cerebral radionecrosis. Surg Neurol 10:281, 1978.
11. Drachman DA: See-saw nystagmus. J Neurol Neurosurg Psychiatry 29:356, 1966.
12. Erdheim J: Uber hypophysengangsyeschwulste und Hirncholesteatome. Sitzungsb Akad Wissensch 113:537, 1904.
13. Fischer EG, Welch K, Belli JA, et al: Treatment of craniopharyngiomas in children, 1972–1981. J Neurosurg 62:496, 1985.
14. Hoff JT, Patterson RH, Jr.: Craniopharyngiomas in children and adults. J Neurosurg 36:299, 1972.
15. Hoffman HJ: Supratentorial tumors in childhood. In: Youmans J (ed): Neurological Surgery, 2nd ed. Philadelphia, W.B. Saunders Co., 1982, pp 2702–2732.
16. Hoffman HJ, Chuang S, Ehrlich R, et al: The microsurgical removal of craniopharyngiomas in childhood. In: Chapman PH (ed): Concepts in Pediatric Neurosurgery, Vol. 6. New York, S Karger, 1985, pp 52–62.
17. Hoffman HJ, Hendrick EB, Humphreys RP, et al: Management of craniopharyngiomas in children. J Neurosurg 47:218, 1977.
18. Holmes LB, Frantz AG, Rabkin MT, et al: Normal growth with subnormal growth hormone levels. N Engl J Med 279:559, 1968.
19. Kahn EA, Gosch HH, Seeger JF, et al: Forty-five years experience with craniopharyngiomas. Surg Neurol 1:5, 1973.
20. Katz EL: The late results of radical excision of craniopharyngiomas. J Neurosurg 42:86, 1975.
21. Kobayashi T, Kageyama N, Ohara K: Internal irradiation for cystic craniopharyngioma. J Neurosurg 55:896, 1981.
22. Kramer S: Craniopharyngioma. The best treatment in conservative surgery and post-operative radiation therapy. In: Morley TP (ed): Current Controversies in Neurosurgery. Philadelphia, W.B. Saunders Co., 1976, pp 336–343.
23. Kramer S, McKissock W, Concannon JP: Craniopharyngiomas. Treatment by combined surgery and radiation therapy. J Neurosurg 18:217, 1961.
24. Leksell L, Backlund E-O, Johansson L: Treatment of craniopharyngiomas. Acta Chir Scand 133:345, 1967.
25. Matson DD: Neurosurgery of Infancy and Childhood, 2nd ed. Springfield, IL, Charles C Thomas, 1969, p 545.
26. Matson DD, Crigler JF: Management of craniopharyngioma in childhood. J Neurosurg 30:377, 1969.
27. McMurry FG, Hardy RW, Dohn DF, et al: Long-term results in the management of craniopharyngiomas. Neurosurgery 1:238, 1977.
28. Mori K, Handa H, Murata T, et al: Results of treatment for craniopharyngioma. Child's Brain 6:302, 1980.
29. Northfield DWL: Surgery of the Central Nervous System. Oxford, Blackwell, 1973, pp 314–327.
30. Patterson R, Danylevich A: Surgical removal of craniopharyngiomas by a transcallosal approach through the lamina terminalis and sphenoid sinus. Neurosurgery 7:111, 1980.
31. Richmond IL, Wara WM, Wilson CB: Role of radiation therapy in the management of craniopharyngiomas in children. Neurosurgery 6:513, 1980.
32. Ross HS, Rosenberg S, Friedman AH: Delayed radiation necrosis of the optic nerve. Am J Ophthalmol 76:683, 1973.
33. Rougerie J: What can be expected from the surgical treatment of craniopharyngiomas in children? Child's Brain 5:433, 1979.
34. Sweet WH: Radical surgical treatment of craniopharyngioma. Clin Neurosurg 23:52, 1976.
35. Thomsett MJ, Conte FA, Kaplan SL, et al: Endocrine and neurologic outcome in childhood craniopharyngioma: Review of effect of treatment in 42 patients. J Pediatr 97:728, 1980.
36. Waga S, Handa H: Radiation-induced meningioma: With review of literature. Surg Neurol 5:215, 1976.
37. Waltz TA, Browneil B: Sarcoma: A possible late result of effective radiation therapy for pituitary adenoma. Report of two cases. J Neurosurg 24:901, 1966.

35
PINEAL REGION TUMORS

Derek A. Bruce, M.B., Ch.B.
Luis Schut, M.D.
Leslie N. Sutton, M.D.

Pineal region tumors are reported to constitute 3 to 8 percent of children's brain tumors. Prior to improvements in neuroimaging techniques, for example, computed tomography (CT) and nuclear magnetic resonance imaging (NMRI), it is certain that a fair number of these tumors were overlooked. In a series of 300 consecutive brain tumors at Children's Hospital of Philadelphia (CHOP), 10 percent were pineal region tumors. Because of the high mortality rate associated with surgery in this area of the brain in the 1920's and 1930's[7, 12, 22] many tumors were not biopsied, and the standard treatment was cerebrospinal fluid (CSF) shunting and radiation therapy.[13] While the results of reported series using this approach have been quite encouraging,[1, 23] with a 60 to 70 percent five-year survival rate and a 50 to 60 percent ten-year survival rate, the older children did best and most of the children younger than six years of age either died or had tumor recurrence. If the survival rate of the younger children is to improve, with the best possible quality of life, it is clear that individual therapy depending on the tumor type is the only possible way of obtaining this result.

PINEAL GLAND

The pineal gland sits in the posterior superior portion of the third ventricle, deep to the pineal recess of the ventricle and superior to the habenular commissure. On silver stain, the pineocyte, a specialized neuron, is identified by its club-shaped cell process. Scattered astrocytes are present in the normal gland, which has a somewhat acinar appearance. Adrenergic nerve terminals have been identified, although their function is not clear. It has been hypothesized that they represent the pathways by which photic stimulation from the retina reaches the pineal gland and that their site of origin is the postganglionic sympathetic nerves from the superior cervical ganglion. In animals, there is an association between light and dark exposure and the amount of melanin secreted in the pineal cells.[15] There also is a suggested relationship between the amount of melatonin and sexual activity. High melatonin levels resulting from prolonged darkness may suppress sexual activity during hibernation. Thus, in mammals, the pineal gland appears to be a secretory organ. An active role for the pineal gland in humans has not yet been defined. Precocious puberty is occasionally reported in prepubertal males, but these children usually have germinomas. Since these tumors are known to seed down the third ventricle and to arise also in the pineal and suprasellar regions, it is not at all certain that the pineal tumor is the cause of the precocious puberty. The authors have seen only one patient present with precocious puberty in 30 pineal region tumors.

PATHOLOGY

The pineal region has the widest variety of tumors of any region of the brain because of the many types of tissues that are present within this single small area. The pineal gland is bounded by the tentorial margins and the vein of Galen posteriorly; the vermis of the cerebellum inferiorly; the pulvinars of the thalami laterally; the posterior midbrain and superior colliculi directly inferiorly; and the third ventricular ependyma anteriorly. Superior in position is the cavum velum interpositum, its vessels, and the corpus callosum. The vascular supply to the pineal gland is via the posterior medial choroidal arteries, and the venous drainage is, at least partially, into the great vein of Galen. Tumors may arise from any of the intrinsic pineal gland cells or surrounding tissues. In addition, because of its position in the midline, cell rests that give rise to epidermoid, dermoid, and germ cell tumors and teratomas have the potential for occurring in this area. Table 35–1 shows the possible lesions of the pineal region that are most commonly found. Tumors in this area are of multiple pathologies, ranging from benign surgically curable lesions through lesions that require only local radiation therapy to lesions that require craniospinal radiation therapy and chemotherapy. Because the region is intimately in contact with CSF spaces to the third ventricle, cavum velum interpositum, choroid fissure, and quadrigeminal plate cisterns, the potential for CSF seeding of tumors in this area is high. Some of the tumors that occur here seem to have a high propensity for early spread, whereas others do not. Besides the actual tumor pathology, the propensity for spread must be considered when therapy is undertaken. Because of the multiplicity of tumors and, as we shall see, the inability to define tumor pathology without biopsy, it is increasingly accepted that tumor tissue should be obtained prior to therapy.

PRESENTATION

Pineal region tumors can present at any age; the youngest child the authors have seen was five months old. Most series of pineal tumors include adults and children or are heavily weighted toward teenage males. It is probable that the accepted pathology of these tumors in children has been misstated because of the inclusion of the older patients. Because of the anatomy of this area of the brain, the most frequent presentation of a pineal region tumor is that of intracranial hypertension. Seventy percent of children present with signs and symptoms referable to CSF pathway obstruction. Increasing head circumference and bulging fontanelles in infants and headaches in older children are the usual presentation. The classic morning headache that is relieved by activity should not be dismissed as school phobia. Intracranial pressure (ICP) reaches its peak in the morning hours just prior to waking. This is a result of (1) the prone position, (2) rises in arterial carbon dioxide pressure (Pa_{CO_2}) during sleep, and (3) dreaming that occurs just prior to waking and is accompanied by increases in cerebral blood flow and cerebral blood volume. Thus, the ICP is at its peak at the time of waking. Other common symptoms and signs are disturbance of concentration, diplopia, and, occasionally, personality change or disturbance of sleeping patterns. In some children, frank disturbances in emotional content are seen. This may be the result either of elevated ICP or of invasion of the tumor into the fimbria and limbic circuits. Precocious puberty, while reported, is very rare and probably occurs in only 3 percent or less of pineal region tumors.

Clinical signs may be limited to those of intracranial hypertension, positive Macewen's sign, papilledema, or sixth nerve palsy. The most frequent localizing finding is the presence of Parinaud's syndrome, retraction nystagmus, difficulty with upward gaze, and disocciation of pupillary response to light and distance. Fourth nerve palsies have been seen in several children. Long-tract involvement, with hemiparesis or sensory disturbances, are usually due to brainstem lesions. Cerebellar symptoms of ataxia and nystagmus may be seen in large tumors that grow and compress the cerebellar vermis or may be the result of hydrocephalus. Occasionally, a visual field cut may be seen from direct invasion of the tumor into the lateral geniculate bodies.

Occasionally, as a result of diffuse early CSF seeding, a complex picture of multifocal transient neurologic symptoms, often associated with headaches of a migrainous pattern, is seen. This consists of seizures, transient hemiparesis, sensory changes, and visual field cuts and may initially be difficult to distinguish from complex migraine or from a seizure disorder. The finding of a frank pineal region mass is not always evident on the first CT scan, and several scans may be required before such a lesion is identified. Unless there is involvement of the pituitary stalk or the hypothalamus, as occasionally

Table 35–1. COMMON LESIONS OF THE PINEAL REGION

Neoplastic
  Germ cell tumors
  Ependymomas
  Primitive neuroectodermal tumor (PNET)
  Glioma
  Choroid plexus papilloma
  Lipoma
  Pineal cell tumor
  Epidermoid tumor
  Dermoid tumor
  Meningioma
  Ganglioneuroblastoma

Developmental
  Arachnoid cyst
  Cyst of cavum velum interpositum
  Pineal cyst

Vascular
  Arteriovenous malformation
  Arterial aneurysm
  Vein of Galen aneurysm

occurs with germinomas, hormonal disturbances are rare. The most frequent endocrine disturbance is a syndrome of inappropriate antidiuretic hormone release, which probably occurs as a result of hydrocephalus of the third ventricle. The clinical presentation has not been diagnostic of tumor type, although in the Children's Hospital of Philadelphia series,[18] tegmental dysfunction was more common in children with germ cell tumors, focal motor deficits were more frequent in children with glial tumors, and signs of intracranial hypertension alone occurred more often in patients with primary pineal parenchymal tumors.

SPECIAL STUDIES

Plain skull films may show split sutures, sellar erosion, or pineal calcification, their role in diagnosis is of decreasing importance. The CT scan is currently the most commonly used diagnostic test. Tumors are easily seen, and other non-neoplastic lesions in the area can be differentiated (Fig. 35–1).[25] The presence of CSF pathway seeding by tumor can be recognized by the absence of clear CSF spaces and by the diffuse enhancement of the subarachnoid space and tentorial edges. The extent of hydrocephalus is easily measured. However, the CT scan has not proved to be an adequate modality

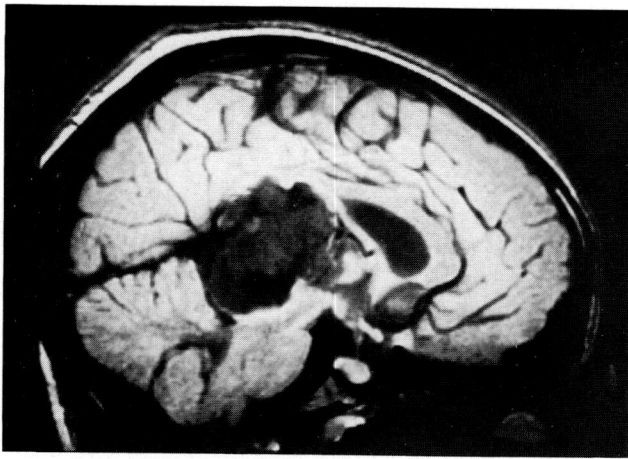

Figure 35–2. Nuclear magnetic resonance (NMR) image showing pineal tumor.

for pathologic diagnosis of tumor type.[24, 25] Certain criteria were more common, depending on the tumor type, but there was too much overlap for certainty of pathologic diagnosis.

Germ cell tumors are irregular, usually are of increased or mixed density on the uninjected scan, and tend to enhance in a heterogeneous fashion. The presence of calcification is variable. Primary parenchymal lesions are similar to the germinomas but more frequently enhance diffusely and homogeneously. Glial tumors are of variable contour and can be either isodense or hypodense on the uninjected scan. The enhancement pattern of the glial tumors is very variable. NMRI scan has proved very useful in defining the location of the vascular structures, especially the internal cerebral veins and the great vein of Galen. It gives an excellent three-dimensional image of the tumor (Fig. 35–2) and surrounding brain and has rendered angiography unnecessary in most cases. The location of the tumor, the brainstem, and the aqueduct are especially well seen in the sagittal images. NMRI has not yet been of any help in separating the various tumor pathologies, but it does differentiate well epidermoid tumors, teratomas, and vascular lesions from the other types of pathologic conditions. Angiography is now reserved for those patients in whom large venous dilatations appear to be present or in whom the lesion is clearly an arteriovenous malformation or an aneurysm.

CSF STUDIES

Germ cell tumors have been demonstrated to produce a variety of identifiable proteins: alpha-fetoprotein, and beta-human chorionic gonadotropin (HCG), which may be present in blood or in CSF. Since at least 70 percent of children with pineal region tumors present with symptoms of elevated ICP and hydrocephalus, it is rare that spinal tap is

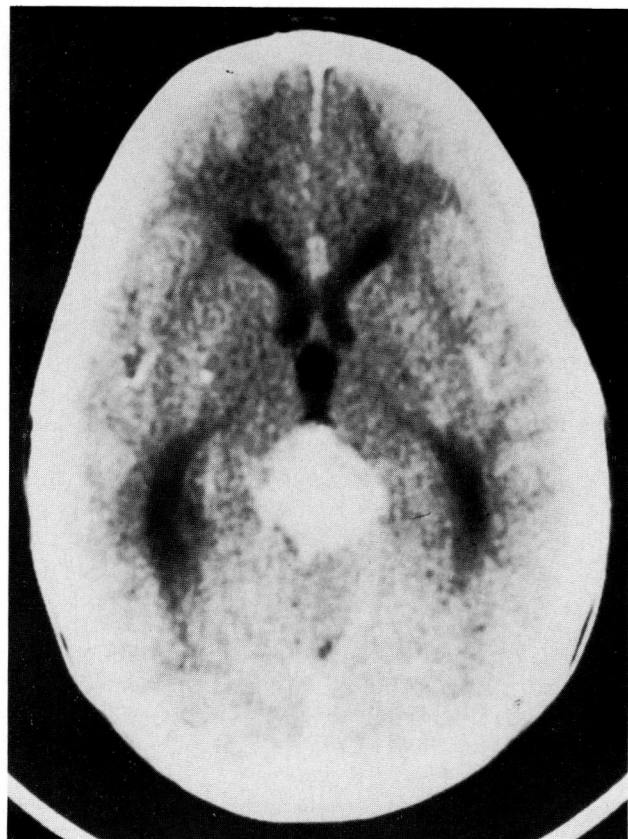

Figure 35–1. CT scan showing pineal region tumor.

an appropriate early study prior to tumor removal, thus, limiting the value of CSF studies. If a ventriculoperitoneal shunt is inserted prior to tumor removal, ventricular CSF can easily and safely be obtained. Unfortunately, it appears quite rare that the levels of alpha-fetoprotein or beta-HCG are elevated. Further, an elevated level of alpha-fetoprotein alone appears not to be diagnostic of tumor type,[8,10] although when CSF levels of both alpha-fetoprotein and beta-HCG are elevated, the diagnosis of a malignant germ cell tumor (e.g., embryonal carcinoma or choriocarcinoma) is nearly certain. Thus, for primary diagnosis, CSF markers are of little help. The role of these same markers as early indicators of clinical recurrence of tumor is being studied, and in two of five patients with recurrent embryonal cell carcinoma, elevated alpha-fetoprotein levels were found.[18] There is continued controversy about the specificity of alpha-fetoprotein and HCG. While it has generally been assumed that their presence indicates germ cell tumors, these compounds have been reported in primary pineal cell tumors and gliomas of the pineal region.[10]

It is apparent that biopsy of pineal region tumors is an important first step in diagnosis. It is imperative, if a rational treatment is to be selected, that the tumor type be identified. Table 35–2 shows the incidence of the different tumor types that have been identified in a series of 35 consecutive pineal tumors at Children's Hospital of Philadelphia (all biopsied). This is quite different from previously reported series. This experience is unique because of the much younger mean age of the patients (six years) than any previously reported series and because of the realization that in the literature, the recurrence rate in children of this age is approximately 100 percent. This is also the age group below which the maximum side effects from chemotherapy and radiation occur and, therefore, the age group for whom it is most important to pick the therapy that is most likely to cure the tumor and least likely to damage the child.

SURGERY

Stereotactic Biopsy

With the use of stereotactic frames that can be placed in the CT scanner, stereotactic biopsy is becoming increasingly popular. It has been demonstrated to be a safe technique for deep-seated tumors, including those in the brainstem. This technique is certainly applicable to pineal region tumors. One of the concerns about such closed biopsy in this area is the number of vascular structures that surround the pineal gland. However, with current two-dimensional arteriography and CT techniques, it is becoming possible to feed into the computer digitized information on the location of the main vascular structures and to pick a pathway for the biopsy needle that avoids the vessels. Biopsy technique has been used safely in patients with pineal tumors, with a positive biopsy rate of up to 80 percent.[6,14] Even if specimens can now be safely obtained, there is a second concern. Are the tissue samples obtained adequate for certain diagnosis of tumor type? The authors have seen mixed germ cell tumors in which one area appears to be germinoma, whereas other areas exhibit evidence of embryonal cell or yolk-sac tumor. Similarly, the importance of differentiation in the primitive neuroectodermal tumor (PNET; pineoblastoma) probably should play a role in therapeutic planning.[16] Thus, adequate amounts of tissue must be obtained for accurate diagnosis. Currently, the best approach in experienced hands is still open surgical biopsy and debulking.

Table 35–2. INCIDENCE OF PINEAL REGION TUMORS: CHOP (1975–1985)

Pineal germ cell tumors	
Germinoma	7 (20%)
Mixed germ cell tumor	5 (14%)
Teratoma	1 (3%)
Pineal Parenchymal	
Pineoblastoma (PNET)	6 (17%)
Pineocytoma	4 (11%)
Glial Tumors	9 (26%)
Others	3 (9%)
	35

Direct Surgical Approaches

A number of different approaches to the pineal region of the brain have been described.[4,5,19] The best approach is that with which the surgeon is most familiar and comfortable. If the surgeon has no experience in this area, it is advisable to refer these children to a center with the necessary experience.

The most popular current approach is that proposed by Stein,[19] the supracerebellar intratentorial technique. This is performed with the patient in the sitting position but can be performed with the patient in the prone position and achieves access to the pineal region over the vermis of the cerebellum. The problems with this approach in the small child are

1. The sitting position is often difficult to achieve in the child under one year of age.
2. There is a high risk of overdrainage of CSF and, if the ventricles are very large prior to surgery, collapse of the hemispheres and subdural bleeding.
3. It is difficult to maintain temperature control.
4. There is the definite risk of air embolism.

Because of these, the authors have favored a modification of the supratentorial interhemispheric approach preferred by Dandy.[7] The child is placed prone, either in the pin headrest or the cerebellar headrest, depending on age. The neck is in the neutral position. This position makes temperature control easy, avoids the risk of air embolism, and prevents the problem of overdrainage of CSF. This position has the additional benefit that as the operation progresses, less and less retraction is required because gravity tends to pull the occipital lobes laterally away from the tumor. It is occasionally necessary to take a bridging vein, and this produces no complications, provided it is done sufficiently far posteriorly. The craniotomy flap is located posterior to the rolandic vein and is centered around the lambda (Fig. 35–3). The posterior corpus callosum and the vein of Galen are readily identified. If the tumor is anteriorly located in the posterior third ventricle, a small portion of the corpus callosum, usually 2 to 3 cm, is opened. If the tumor is large and more posteriorly located, it is frequently not necessary to divide the corpus callosum. The internal cerebral vein on the side of the dural opening is easily defined, running in the cavum velum interpositum, and if, as occasionally happens, it is buried in tumor, this can readily be ascertained. Another advantage of this approach is that it permits the surgeon to evaluate the degree of involvement of the internal cerebral vein and the great vein of Galen at the beginning of the operation and, thus, to decide if total resection appears feasible.[4]

If the ventricles are enlarged, a ventricular catheter is inserted through the most lateral of the burr holes and is attached to a Rickham's reservoir. This is left in situ postoperatively and allows for acute decompression of the ventricular system in the immediate postoperative period but can also act as a site for intrathecal chemotherapy or for obtaining CSF for cytologic studies or CSF markers through the course of the disease. With intraoperative ventricular decompression, minimal retraction to approach the pineal area is usually required. In children who have been previously shunted or in whom the ventricles are not enlarged, brain retraction may be improved by the use of a lumbar CSF drain, hyperventilation, or osmotic dehydrating agents. The authors have used this operative approach in over 30 children with pineal region tumors. There have been no deaths and only one significant morbidity, in a child with a large multicystic astrocytoma.

Germinomas often appear to be well-circumscribed and have an apparent plane between tumor and brain, even as they penetrate the upper brainstem. Frequently, these tumors can be grossly resected, and the tumor bulk can always be diminished to only microscopic disease, thus decreasing the risk of CSF spread from residual tumor and effectively opening the CSF pathways by opening the suprapineal recess of the third ventricle. The plane of the tumor is easiest to identify by opening the pineal recess early in the course of surgery and entering the third ventricle. The tumor, covered by ependyma, is easily identified and can be followed posteriorly out of the third ventricle into the region of the superior collicular plate and the brainstem. These tumors are usually soft and suctionable, with vascularity close to the tumor capsule but with relatively little vascularity within the tumor itself. Bleeding is rarely a problem and is quite easy to control. The surgical carbon dioxide laser can be helpful in debulking these lesions.

The embryonal cell carcinoma, choriocarcinoma, and yolk-sac tumors are a difficult surgical problem. They are often quite large, usually firm and fibrous, and usually very vascular. They grow around the major veins and often have to be removed using several approaches between the internal cerebral veins lateral to them, and from posterior to the vein of Galen. The carbon dioxide laser is quite helpful in dealing with these tumors. Gross total resection is very difficult, except in the smaller ones. The major goals are (1) to obtain adequate pathologic tissue to be certain of diagnosis, and (2) if possible, to debulk the tumor to open the suprapineal recess, decompress the ventricle, and avoid the need for a shunt. Surgery on these lesions is often quite unsatisfactory, if only the amount of tumor resected is considered. The authors have seen choriocarcinoma that had the angiographic appearance of arteriovenous malformation (AVM).

Teratomas (Fig. 35–4), dermoid tumors, and epidermoid tumors all are potentially resectable, surgically curable tumors. Often, they are large. Thus, to achieve adequate exposure of the far inside of the tumor, it may be necessary to open the tentorium, divide or make a window through the falx, or open the dura on both sides of the midline to approach the tumor bilaterally. With the bone flap over the midline, this is quite simple to do. Trying to make a window in the falx often leads to troublesome bleeding and is an approach the authors rarely use. Opening the tentorium is easily accomplished from the interhemispheric approach, and usually, this is done about 1.5 to 2 cm from the midline insertion of the vein of Galen. The remain-

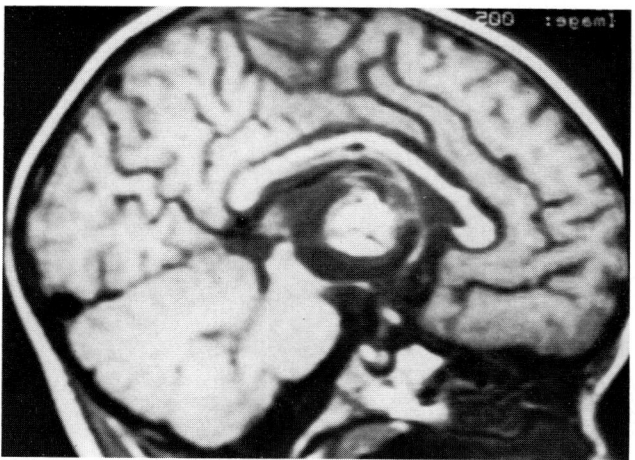

Figure 35–3. NMR image showing pineal teratoma.

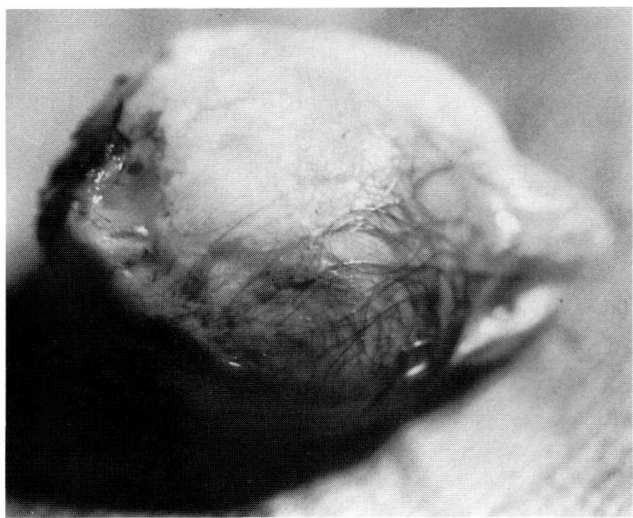

Figure 35–4. Specimen of pineal teratoma.

der of the surgical technique is the standard one of debulking the internal portion of the tumor and then delivering the capsule into the field and removing it.

Pineocytomas have a variable consistency: some appear quite scirrhous and tough, whereas others are fairly friable and soft. For the tougher tumors, the carbon dioxide laser is helpful in the debulking process. Rarely is there a true capsule, but an interface between brain and tumor is often quite clear, allowing gross total resection to be accomplished. An unusual type, the papillary pineocytoma,[21] has been seen in two children, both teenage boys, who presented with hydrocephalus one to two years prior to the finding of a pineal mass. These tumors clearly arose in the posterior midbrain, close to the aqueduct. Pineal cell rests have been identified in this region and may be the site of origin for these tumors. The pineal gland arises as an outpouching of the embryonic diencephalon. These tumors are usually soft and grossly resectable.

Pineoblastomas have the consistency of PNETs anywhere else in the nerous system. The major vascularity is at the surface at the tumor interface and, therefore, is easily controlled. The tumors are usually soft and easily aspirated. Once again, gross total removal can frequently be accomplished. It is advisable to try to diminish the tumor bulk to avoid the risk of CSF seeding.

Glial tumors in this area are usually grayish and semifirm and often do not suction easily. Again, the carbon dioxide laser has proved valuable for the glial tumors. They are rarely very vascular, and quite extensive resection can often be accomplished without worsening the patient's signs and symptoms.

Thus, the goals of surgery on all these lesions are
1. Obtaining adequate tissue for accurate diagnosis.

Table 35–3. OPERATIVE MORBIDITY WITH INTERHEMISPHERIC APPROACH

Number of patients undergoing surgery	30
Transient worsening of Parinaud's syndrome	4 (13%)
Transient hemianopsia	6 (20%)
Permanent visual field cut	2 (8%)
Prolonged coma, delayed development	1 (1%)

2. Diminishing tumor bulk to the smallest safely achievable size.
3. Opening up the posterior third ventricle and achieving resolution of hydrocephalus.
4. Totally removing the tumor, in benign lesions.

The operative morbidity is shown in Table 35–3. Table 35–4 demonstrates another advantage of the interhemispheric approach. Only 5 of 20 children operated on by this route required postoperative shunts. This then markedly diminishes the complications of shunt malfunction and decreases the risk of systemic spread of these tumors.

PATHOLOGY

The classification of the pathology of the pineal region tumors has been confusing. The accepted pathologic classification is shown in Table 35–2. The incidence of the various types of tumors in a consecutive series of children with pineal tumors seen at the Children's Hospital of Philadelphia since 1975 is shown in the same table. Primary pineal cell neoplasms are most frequently diagnosed, accounting for a third of all tumors. The second most common group of tumors are the germ cell tumors, but more than 70 percent of these have been embryonal cell tumors, and less than 30 percent, germinomas. The third largest group has been glial tumors. The age range of patients with these tumors was from 0.6 to 16 years, and the mean age was six years. There were slightly more males than females, this being most obvious in the patients with embryonal cell carcinomas, of whom six of seven were males. During the same time period of 1975, the authors saw 20 other pineal lesions, AVMs, aneurysms, or cysts. Two of the pineoblastomas were in children who had had retinoblastoma of the familial variety.

TREATMENT

Except for the totally resectable lesions (teratomas, dermoid tumors, and epidermoid tumors),

Table 35–4. CHILDREN WITH HYDROCEPHALUS AND PINEAL TUMORS TREATED BY POST-INTERHEMISPHERIC APPROACH

Postoperative shunt	5
No shunt	15
	20

some therapy other than surgery is required to prevent tumor recurrence. Radiation therapy is the major therapeutic modality. The standard local dose is 5000 to 5500 rad over six weeks. In children with germinomas, it may be possible to decrease the local radiation to 4000 to 4500 rad because of the radiosensitivity of the tumor. Gliomas require only local radiation therapy, without axis therapy. However, germinomas, embryonal cell tumors, and the primary pineal lesions all have been recorded to produce CSF spread. Indeed, two children, one with a pineocytoma and one with a pineoblastoma, had evidence of diffuse CSF spread at the time of diagnosis. Craniospinal radiation doses are usually 3500 to 4000 rad. Once again, it may be possible to decrease the dose of spinal axis radiation without running the increased risk of tumor recurrence. This is currently being investigated in children with PNETs. The rapid response of germinomas to radiation therapy has been noted, and this has been proposed as a diagnostic test for tumor pathology. If the tumor dramatically shrinks with 2000 rad of radiation, it can be assumed to be a germinoma, and surgical biopsy can be avoided. However, the authors feel that this is not a reliable way of making a pathologic diagnosis, since they have seen rapid shrinkage of germinomas that have had embryonal cell carcinoma within them and with PNETs. CSF shunting has been previously discussed, and in many children, this is not necessary after debulking. Many of the tumors found in this area of the brain are not primary neuroectodermal tumors, and the germ cell family of tumors can spread easily in the abdominal cavity or the blood stream. Thus, if a shunt can be avoided, the chances of such spread are minimized.

Radiation therapy, both local and spinal axis, is associated with good survival rates for patients with germinomas. Five-year survival rates range from 25 percent[3] to 70 to 79 percent,[1,20] and ten-year survival rates range from 12.5 to 64 percent. However, in most of these reports, not all the tumors were proven germinomas. The authors' own experience is that not one germinoma has recurred after axis irradiation, with a follow-up of eight years. The other tumors of the germ cell line, embryonal cell carcinoma and choriocarcinoma, have very high mortality and recurrence rates despite radiation therapy.[17] The mortality rate approaches 100 percent, over five years. Chemotherapy has been demonstrated to be effective in the treatment of embryonal cell carcinoma of the testes and ovaries.[11] The use of vincristine, actinomycin-D, and cyclophosphamide (Cytoxan) has been proved effective.[17] Cis-platinum (CPDC) has been proved to be an effective agent against embryonal cell carcinoma of testicular origin[9] but has not been shown to be effective against the intracranial tumor in the few reported cases. The combination of cis-platinum, vinblastine, and bleomycin has also been shown to be effective against noncerebral embryonal cell carcinoma and is being tested against intracranial lesions. Methotrexate prior to radiation therapy has been effective in decreasing tumor size in germinomas but has not yet been demonstrated to be effective in the other germ cell tumors. Also, since germinomas appear to be very radiosensitive and potentially curable tumors with irradiation, it is not clear that chemotherapy is necessary. Radiation therapy alone does appear to be adequate to cure potentially a high percentage of germinomas but is ineffective therapy alone against the more common embryonal cell carcinoma or choriocarcinoma. The latter tumors require a combination of radiation therapy and chemotherapy. The ideal chemotherapeutic regimen has not yet been established. When germ cell tumors have recurred, they have done so locally, followed ultimately by CSF dissemination. Fifty percent or more of pineocytomas recur despite radiation therapy, and these tumors are prone to seeding the CSF pathways either prior to diagnosis or at the time of recurrence. Thus, axis irradiation is necessary. Fifty percent of these tumors appear to recur despite axis irradiation, and at least in children, adjuvant chemotherapy may be required if the results are to be improved. No information is available as to what the best drug regimen might be. Currently, at the Children's Hospital of Philadelphia, the authors are using a combination of CPDC, vincristine, and lomustine (CCNU). PNET (pineoblastoma) is treated in the pineal region as it is in the posterior fossa.[16] This tumor also recurs, usually with diffuse CSF spread as well as locally. Fifty percent of these tumors are likely to recur over a three-year period. The majority of glial tumors that occur in the pineal region are low grade, and local radiation therapy is usually adequate to control growth for prolonged periods of time. Malignant gliomas, when found, are treated with a combination of radiation therapy and chemotherapy. The selection of chemotherapy varies from CPDC, vincristine, and CCNU to methotrexate, cyclophosphamide, carboplatinum to 8-in-1 therapy. There is good evidence that the addition of chemotherapy in malignant glial tumors of childhood significantly lengthens the time to relapse and improves possible cure rates.

CONCLUSION

In young children, the incidence of tumors in the pineal region is high, 9 to 10 percent of all brain tumors. Many different types of pathologic tumors occur in this area. In children younger than ten years of age, the incidence of the different types of tumors is different from what has been reported for adults. Germ cell tumors and primary pineal parenchymal tumors occur with equal incidence and are the most frequently seen tumors. Further, only 25 percent of the germ cell tumors appear to be germinomas. Thus, because of the hazards of unnecessary therapy to the young brain and the necessity of tailoring the chemotherapy and radiation therapy to the particular tumor type, it is appropriate that tumor tissue be obtained prior to therapy. Ideally, in experienced hands, this can be accomplished at the same time that tumor removal or debulking is performed. Surgery in this area should carry a mortality rate no greater than that with other tumor surgery in childhood, with which expected mortality rates are 1 to 2 percent.[2] Morbidity depends on the surgical approach selected. There are benefits and drawbacks to all the various approaches described. The authors prefer the interhemispheric approach with the patient prone, for the reasons described previously and because it avoids CSF shunting in many cases.

Surgical therapy is curative in only a small proportion, possibly 30 percent of cases. The other tumors require local or axis radiation therapy, and some also require chemotherapy. Chemotherapeutic regimens are not yet established and are still in trial stages.

While good long-term results are reported (70 percent, five-year survival rate; 64 percent, ten-year survival rate) with shunting and irradiation, the mean age of the patients in this series was 13.7 years. There were 21 boys and only 6 girls. Of the six children younger than six years of age reported, all developed tumor recurrence. In the children reported from the Children's Hospital of Philadelphia, in a consecutive series of biopsied tumors, the mean age was only six years, with a five-year survival rate of approximately 60 percent. The operative mortality rate was zero, and the rate of severe morbidity was 3 percent. The authors believe it advisable to obtain tissue diagnosis prior to therapy in children with pineal region tumors. Neither the age, sex, CT scan, NMRI scan, nor CSF markers appear capable of differentiating between the different tumor cell types. If survival and the quality of survival is to be maximized, more information on the responses of the various tumor types to radiation therapy and chemotherapy is required. It is probable that over the next few years, there will be different chemotherapeutic regimens for each of the different tumor types. This information, required to advance therapy and improve outcome, will never be forthcoming if blind therapy is given.

References

1. Abay EO, Laws ER, Jr., Grado GL, et al: Pineal tumors in children and adolescents. Treatment by CSF shunting and radiotherapy. J Neurosurg 55:889, 1981.
2. Barrer SJ, Schut L, Sutton LN, et al: Re-operation for recurrent brain tumors in children. Child's Brain 11:375, 1984.
3. Bradfield JS, Perez CA: Pineal tumors and ectopic pinealomas. Analysis of treatment and failures. Radiology 103:399, 1972.
4. Bruce DA: Pineal III ventricle tumors in children. In: Ransohoff J (ed): Modern Techniques in Surgery/Neurosurgery. Mt. Kisco, NY, Futura Press, 1984, 32:1–8.
5. Clark K.: The occipital transtentorial approach to the pineal region. In: Schmidek HH, Sweet WH (eds): Operative Neurosurgical Techniques: Indications and Methods. New York, Grune & Stratton, 1982, pp 595–597.
6. Conway LW: Stereotaxic diagnosis and treatment of intracranial tumors including an initial experience with cryosurgery for pinealomas. J Neurosurg 38:453, 1973.
7. Dandy WE: Operative experience in cases of pineal tumors. Arch Surg 33:19, 1936.
8. Edwards MSB, Davis RL, Laurent JP: Tumor markers and cytological features of cerebrospinal fluid. Cancer 56:1773, 1985.
9. Einhorn LH, Donohue JP: Combination chemotherapy in disseminated testicular cancer. The incidence experience. Semin Oncol 6:87, 1979.
10. Fetell MR, Stein BM: Therapy of pineal region tumors. Neurology 1:185, 1984.
11. Hopkins JB, Jaffe N, Colodny A, et al: The management of testicular tumors in children. J Urol 120:96, 1978.
12. Horrax G: Treatment of tumors of the pineal body. Experience in a series of twenty-two cases. Arch Neurol Psychiatry 64:227, 1950.
13. Jenkins RDT, Simpson JK, Keen CW: Pineal and suprasellar germinomas. J Neurosurg 48:99, 1978.
14. Moser RP, Backlund EO: Stereotaxic Radiosurgery in Pineal Region Tumors. Presented at the 51st Annual Meeting of the American Association of Neurological Surgeons, Honolulu, Hawaii, April 25, 1982.
15. Ner I, Reiter RJ, Wurtman RJ: The pineal gland. Proceedings of the International Symposium. Jerusalem, November 14–17, 1977. New York, Springer-Verlag, 1978.
16. Packer RJ, Sutton LN, Rorke LB, et al: Prognostic importance of cellular differentiation in medulloblastoma of childhood. J Neurosurg 61:296, 1984.
17. Packer RJ, Sutton LN, Rorke LB, et al: Intracranial embryonal cell carcinoma. Cancer 54:520, 1984.
18. Packer RJ, Sutton LN, Rosenstock JG, et al: Pineal region tumors of childhood. Pediatrics 74:97, 1984.
19. Stein BM: Supracerebellar approach for pineal region neoplasms. In: Schmidek HH, Sweet WH (eds): Operative Neurosurgical Techniques: Indications and Methods. New York, Grune & Stratton, 1982, pp 599–607.
20. Sung DI, Harisiadis L, Chang CH: Midline pineal tumors and suprasellar germinomas: Highly curable by irradiation. Radiology 128:745, 1978.
21. Trojanowski JQ, Tascos NA, Rorke LB: Malignant pineocytoma with prominent papillary features. Cancer 50:1789, 1982.
22. Van Wagenen WP: A surgical approach for the removal of certain pineal tumors. Report of a case. Surg Gynecol Obstet 53:216, 1931.
23. Wara WM, Jenkin RDT, Evans A, et al: Tumors of the pineal and suprasellar region: Children's Cancer Study Group treatment results. 1960–1975. Cancer 43:689, 1979.
24. Wood JH, Zimmerman RA, Bruce DA, et al: Assessment and management of pineal region and related tumors. Surg Neurol 16:192, 1981.
25. Zimmerman RA, Bilaniuk LT, Wood JH, et al: Computed tomography of pineal, parapineal and histologically related tumors. Radiology 137:669, 1980.

36
METASTATIC TUMORS

Mark S. O'Brien, M.D.
Antonio Prats, M.D.

Brain metastases in children are rare. In adults, the overall frequency of intracranial metastases reported from autopsy studies ranges from 12 to 35 percent. In a study of 217 children dying of cancer, Vannucci and Baten[37] reported a 6 percent incidence of brain metastases. The discrepancy probably relates to the rarity of primary bronchogenic carcinoma in children as well as the biologic characteristics of the common childhood neoplasms.

The most common primary tumors causing brain metastases in children include Wilms's tumor, rhabdomyosarcoma, osteogenic sarcoma, and germ cell tumors.[10, 11, 31, 37] This chapter discusses some of these tumors that metastasize to the brain in children. Excluded from this chapter are the lesions that extend to the brain from contiguous structures such as skull, dura, and orbits. Pediatric lymphomatous or leukemic involvement of the central nervous system is also excluded from this discussion.

CLINICAL PRESENTATION

Metastatic disease to the brain in children, as in adults, can present with signs and symptoms that reflect increased intracranial pressure, including headaches and altered mental status, and are associated with the focal effects of the metastasis, such as hemiparesis, aphasia, sensory changes, and cranial nerve palsies.[4, 12, 25] Laurent and associates[21] reported two children with metastatic disease to the brain who presented with subarachnoid hemorrhage.

Clinical presentation differed from that found among adults in the higher incidence of seizures and in the aburpt onset of symptoms.[11] Graus and coworkers[11] reported that 36 percent of their patients developed seizures. However, in children younger than 15 years of age, seizures were the initial symptom in 50 percent of the patients.[11] Acute onset of focal deficits also appears to be more frequent in children. This usually represented hemorrhage into the tumor.[11, 24, 35] Autopsy studies revealed that 50 percent of the patients had hemorrhagic metastases.[11]

RADIOLOGIC STUDIES

Computed tomography (CT) is currently the diagnostic study of choice in the evaluation of children suspected of having metastatic disease of the brain (Fig. 36-1).[3, 8] Comparison of the pre- and the postcontrast CT characteristics of a given lesion may suggest the degree of vascularity of a tumor as well as suggest a histologic diagnosis. Chest x-ray films and, possibly, CT of the chest are also recommended, as the vast majority of children with brain metastases also have evidence of pulmonary involvement.[11, 37] Skull x-ray films may be beneficial in patients suspected of having intracerebral metastases, as they may reveal evidence of elevated intracranial pressure manifested by separation of the cranial sutures or erosion of the dorsum sellae. In children with metastatic disease to the brain from osteogenic sarcoma, skul x-ray films may reveal the calcified intracranial lesion.[5] Angiography may reveal neovascularity and will assist in excluding other lesions such as arteriovenous malformations.[5] The role of nuclear magnetic resonance imaging

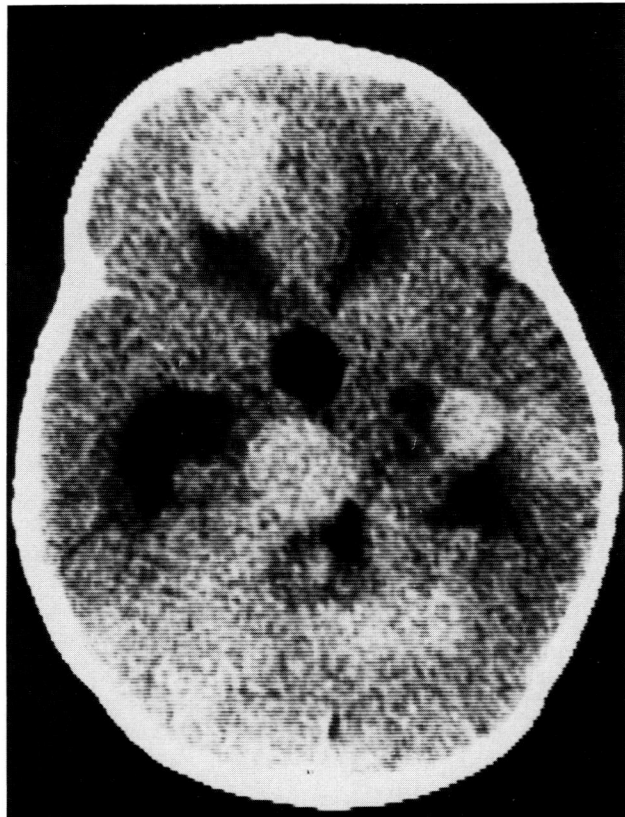

Figure 36–1. Multiple metastases in CT scan.

(NMRI) in evaluating children with brain metastases is under evaluation (Fig. 36–2).

WILMS'S TUMOR (NEPHROBLASTOMA)

Wilms's tumor is the most common malignant renal tumor in infancy and childhood, and one of the most common abdominal tumors of childhood.[13] Wilms's tumor may originate from any portion of the renal parenchyma, but usually the exact site of its inception is undetermined because of its size and the destructive nature of its growth at the time of diagnosis. The origin of this tumor is thought to be from malignant degeneration of the embryonic metamorphic blastema.[19]

Metastases of Wilms's tumor occur hematogenously as well as by direct invasion of local tissue.[23] Common sites of metastases in Wilms's tumor include the regional lymph nodes, lungs, and liver.[29] Metastasis to the brain is exceedingly rare.[2, 15, 26] However, in one study, cerebral metastases were reported in 12.9 percent of children with Wilms's tumor in postmortem examination.[37]

Case reports from the literature reveal that the patients with cerebral metastases ranged in age from four weeks to ten years, with the majority being younger than five years of age.[9, 12, 14, 26, 27, 34–37]

Multiple cerebral metastases were seen in approximately one third of the patients, and metastases occurred more frequently in females than males. The patients presented with symptoms of increased intracranial pressure, cranial nerve palsies, hemiparesis, or altered level of consciousness. The majority of the metastases were supratentorial, although brainstem metastases have been reported.[9] With the exception of two cases, there were no instances of cerebral metastases without pulmonary metastases.[9, 14] The interval between surgery for the primary tumor and the development of brain metastases ranged from 6 to 36 months.

Earlier reports described a poor prognosis for patients with brain metastases from Wilms's tumor.[14, 37] More recently, aggressive therapy, including surgery, radiation therapy, and chemotherapy, has yielded excellent results.[6, 14, 26, 27] The chemotherapeutic agents most effective in the treatment of this tumor include actinomycin D, vincristine, and doxorubicin (Adriamycin).[13]

NEUROBLASTOMA

Neuroblastoma is one of the most common extracranial solid tumors of childhood and arises from elements of the sympathetic nervous system.[16] Approximately 70 percent of these tumors occur in the

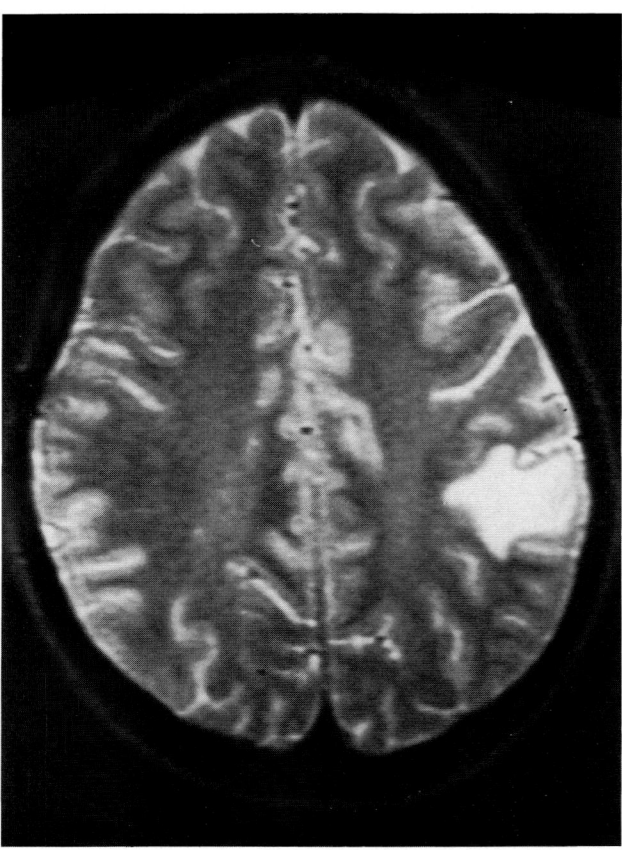

Figure 36–2. Nuclear magnetic resonance image showing brain metastasis.

mediastinum and abdomen, and the remainder occur in the neck, head, pelvis, and elsewhere.[13] Metastases to the facial bones and orbits occur frequently, and patients often present initially with periorbital ecchymosis and an associated abdominal mass.[22] Metastasis to the brain is extremely rare, and when it does occur, it usually results from extension of tumors from contiguous structures.[1, 7, 17, 30]

The reason that brain metastases are so infrequent in children with neuroblastoma appears to be the rarity of pulmonary metastases in this disease. Alpert and Mones[1] reported a seven-year-old boy with neuroblastoma metastasis to the brain parenchyma without leptomeningeal involvement. Interestingly, one of the extracranial sites of metastases reported in this child was the lung. The other reported cases of neuroblastoma with cranial metastasis had leptomeningeal involvement.[1, 7, 18, 28, 32, 33]

Treatment of brain metastases in children with neuroblastoma should be individualized, as the condition is so rare that a protocol has not been established. When feasible, surgical extirpation of the tumor should be attempted. The tumor is relatively radiosensitive; therefore, radiation therapy alone and in conjunction with chemotherapy is a viable option.[13]

OSTEOGENIC SARCOMA

Osteogenic sarcoma represents one of the most frequent primary malignant tumors of the bone. It is most frequently seen in patients between the ages of 10 to 25 years and rarely in patients older than the age of 30.[5] It most frequently arises in the distal portion of the femur, followed by proximal femur, proximal tibia, and humerus.[13] Metastases usually occur via hematogeneous spread. The tumor metastasizes primarily to the lung and other bones.[5, 13] The lung lesions are usually multiple.[13]

Metastases to the brain are rare (Fig. 36–3). In an autopsy study, cerebral metastases were seen in 1.5 percent of patients with osteogenic sarcoma. Danziger and associates[5] presented three patients with cerebral metastases from osteogenic sarcoma. All had pulmonary involvement prior to evidence of cerebral metastases.[5] The reported median interval from the diagnosis of the primary tumor to the detection of pulmonary metastases is quite short in patients with osteogenic sarcoma, indicating the aggressive nature of this tumor.[11]

After the diagnosis of osteogenic sarcoma is made, chemotherapy followed by surgery of the primary tumor forms the foundation of treatment.[20]

SUMMARY

Brain metastases in children are rare. When it does occur, it usually occurs in patients with disem-

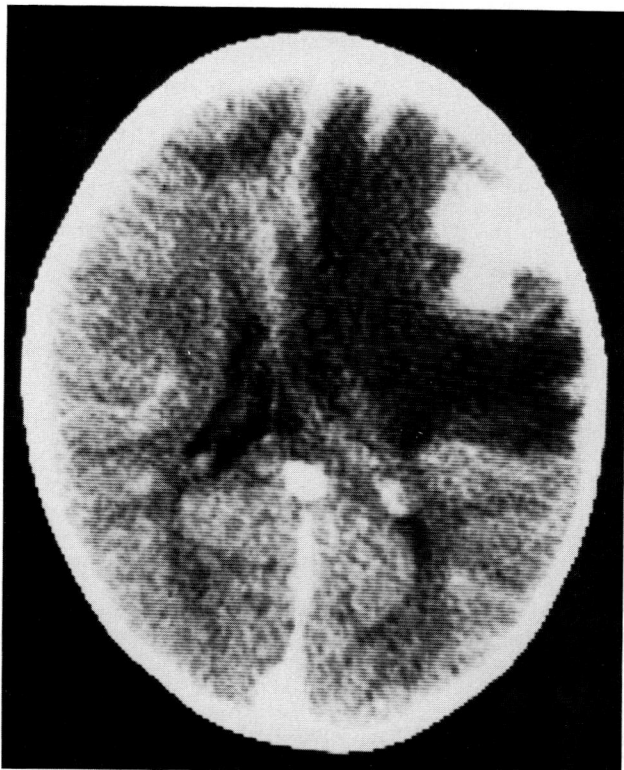

Figure 36–3. CT scan showing metastases from osteogenic sarcoma.

inated disease, especially involving the lungs. In Vannucci and Baten's study,[37] the tumors with the highest frequency of brain metastases were Wilms's tumors, osteogenic sarcomas, and rhabdomyosarcomas. In a more recent review, osteogenic sarcomas, rhabdomyosarcomas, Ewing's sarcomas, and germ cell tumors were the most common solid tumors causing brain metastases in children.[11] The lack of brain metastasis in children with neuroblastoma probably represents the rarity of pulmonary metastasis in this disease. The incidence of brain metastasis may be increasing as more aggressive treatment of disseminated disease prolongs survival of patients.

References

1. Alpert JN, Mones R: Neurologic manifestations of neuroblastoma. J Mt Sinai Hosp 36:37, 1969.
2. Bannayan GA, Huvos AC, D'Angio GJ: Effect of irradiation on the maturation of Wilms' tumor. Cancer 27:812, 1971.
3. Batnitzky S, Segall HD, Cohen ME: Radiologic guidelines in assessing children with intracranial tumors. Cancer 1:1756, 1985.
4. Bigner SH, Schold SC: The diagnosis of metastases to the central nervous system. Pathol Annu 2:89, 1984.
5. Danziger J, Wallace S, Handel SF, et al: Metastatic osteogenic sarcoma to the brain. Cancer 43:707, 1979.
6. Deutsch M, Albo V, Wollman MR: Radiotherapy for cerebral metastases in children. Int J Radiat Oncol Biol Phys 8:1441, 1982.

7. Dresler S, Harvey DG, Levisohn PM: Retroperitoneal neuroblastoma widely metastatic to the central nervous system. Ann Neurol 5:196, 1979.
8. Dyment PG, Rothner AD, Duchesneau PM, et al: Computerized tomography in the detection of intracranial metastases in children. Pediatrics 58:72, 1976.
9. Gandolfi A, Orsoni JG: Occult nephroblastoma (Wilms' tumor) presenting with symptoms of central nervous system involvement. Acta Neurol (Napoli) 34:424, 1979.
10. Gercovich FG, Luna MA, Gottlieb JA: Increased survival in sarcoma patients. Cancer 36:1843, 1975.
11. Graus F, Walker RW, Allen JC: Brain metastases in children. J Pediatr 103:558, 1983.
12. Han JS, Zee CS, Ahmadi J, et al: Intracranial metastatic Wilms' tumor in children. A report of two cases. Surg Neurol 20:157, 1983.
13. Jaffe N: Metastases in malignant childhood tumors–the role of "adjuvant" therapy and the utility of multidisciplinary treatment. Semin Oncol 4:117, 1977.
14. Kalousek DK, deChadarévian JP, Mackie GG, et al: Metastatic infantile Wilms' tumor and hydrocephalus: A case report with review of the literature. Cancer 39:1312, 1977.
15. Kapproth HJ: Wilms' tumor: A report of 45 cases and an analysis of 1351 cases reported in the world literature from 1940 to 1948. J Urol 81:633, 1959.
16. Kemshead JT, Black J: Developments in the biology of neuroblastoma: Implications for diagnosis and treatment. Dev Med Child Neurol 22:816, 1980.
17. Koizumi JH, Dal Canto MC: Retroperitoneal neuroblastoma metastatic to brain. Report of a case and review of the literature. Child's Brain 7:267, 1980.
18. Krol G, Horten, B: Neuroblastoma metastatic to the meninges. Clin Bull 8:120, 1978.
19. Lakey WH, Lieskovsky G: Tumors of the Kidney. In Kendall AR, Karafin L (eds): Goldsmith, Practice of Surgery, Urology, Vol. 2. New York, Harper and Row, 1985.
20. Lane JM, Boland PJ: Tumors of bone and cartilage. In Denton JR (ed): Goldsmith, Practice of Surgery, Orthopedics, Vol. 1. New York, Harper and Row, 1985.
21. Laurent JP, Bruce DA, Shut L: Hemorrhagic brain tumors in pediatric patients. Child's Brain 8:263, 1981.
22. Long DM, Kieffer SA, Chou SW: Tumors of the skull. In Youmans JR (ed): Tumors of the Skull, Vol. 5. Philadelphia, W. B. Saunders Co., 1982.
23. Magill HL, Strang MS: Paraspinal metastasis of Wilms' tumor visualized on bone imaging. J Nucl Med 22:481, 1981.
24. Mandybur TI: Intracranial hemorrhage caused by metastatic tumors. Neurology 27:650, 1977.
25. Markel ML, Armstrong WF, Waller BF, et al: Left atrial myxoma with multicentric recurrence and evidence of metastases. Am Heart J 111:409, 1986.
26. Mohammad AM, Meyer J, Hakami N: Long-term survival following brain metastasis of Wilms' tumor [letter]. J Pediatr 90:660, 1977.
27. Morgan SK, Buse MG: Survival following brain metastases in Wilms' tumor. Pediatrics 58:130, 1976.
28. Normann T, Havnen J, Mjolnerod O: Cushing's syndrome in an infant associated with neuroblastoma in two ectopic adrenal glands. J Pediatr Surg 6:169, 1971.
29. Pearson D, Duncan WB, Pointon RCS: Wilms' tumours. A review of 96 consecutive cases. Br J Radiol 37:154, 1964.
30. Pochedly CP: Neuroblastoma in the head and central nervous system. In Pochedly CP (ed): Neuroblastoma. Acton, MA, Publishing Sciences Group, Inc., 1976, pp 35–41.
31. Posner JB, Chernik NL: Intracranial metastases from systemic cancer. Adv Neurol 19:575, 1978.
32. Ringertz N, Lidholm SO: Mediastinal tumors and cysts. J Thorac Surg 31:458, 1956.
33. Russell DS, Rubinstein LJ: Peripheral tumors of the neurone series. In Russell DS, Rubinstein LJ (eds): Pathology of Tumors of the Nervous System. Baltimore, Williams & Wilkins, 1977, p 407.
34. Sty JR, Starshak RJ, Thorp SM: The role of brain scintigraphy in metastatic Wilms' tumor. Wis Med J 79:28, 1980.
35. Takamiya Y, Toya S, Otani M, et al: Wilms' tumor with intracranial metastases presenting with intracranial hemorrhage. Child's Nerv Syst 1:291, 1985.
36. Traggis D: Successful treatment of Wilms' tumor with intracranial metastases. Pediatric 56:472, 1975.
37. Vannucci RC, Baten M: Cerebral Metastatic disease in childhood. Neurology 24:981, 1974.

37
PEDIATRIC SKULL TUMORS

Donald H. Reigel, M.D.
Matthew R. Quigley, M.D.
Luke Lin, M.D.

OVERVIEW

Pediatric skull tumors comprise a diverse variety of clinical entities encompassing congenital inclusions, benign tumors, dysplasias, and frankly malignant lesions (Table 37–1). Their true incidence is difficult to judge because centers treating these problems are unable to estimate the population of children from which the patient originated and because many lesions are only anecdotally reported. Patients usually come to the attention of the neurosurgeon by two routes: (1) an obvious mass or lump discovered by a parent or the referring physician, and (2) an incidental x-ray finding. It is very rare that the patient exhibits signs and symptoms of intracranial pathology before the skull tumor is actually discovered.

The older literature labors over the diagnostic fine points of plain skull x-ray films. It now indicates that a computed tomography (CT) scan should be obtained to determine the following: (1) involvement of the skull tables and diploë, (2) subgaleal or soft-tissue spread, (3) intracranial extension, and (4) presence of contrast enhancement. Frequently, a firm diagnosis cannot be established by noninvasive studies; therefore, excision or at least diagnostic biopsy is warranted for most patients. The role of angiography is being re-evaluated in light of the wealth of information obtained from CT studies. Most of the older literature affirms the possible value of angiography, but this conclusion was reached prior to CT, with its ability to outline precisely the anatomy and the extent of the pathology. Angiography may still be indicated for lesions that appear vascular or may invade major sinuses.

DIFFERENTIAL DIAGNOSIS

Often, the clinical history and the skull x-ray film strongly suggest the diagnosis. An epidermoid tumor characteristically occurs as a small, lateral, supraorbital lump with x-ray lucency and sclerotic edges. But what of the six-year-old with multiple lytic lesions on skull x-ray films? Although no absolute criteria exist, a number of x-ray features assist in distinguishing malignant from benign disease.[16, 23]

1. Number of lesions. Multiplicity is not necessarily a harbinger of malignancy, but six or more lesions, especially located away from the midline, suggests an ominous diagnosis. The exception is venous lakes or pacchionian granulations, which are usually distinguished by the elevation of an intact inner table into the diploë.

2. Expansion of the diploë or widening of the diploë, with bulging of one or both intact tables, strongly suggests a benign process.

3. Ragged, undermined lesion edges are seen in malignancies.

4. Circumferential bony sclerosis occurs when benign lesions exert long-standing pressure on surrounding bone. However, metastatic neuroblastomas may mimic this finding.

5. Intralesional bone remnants are a common finding with benign tumors, the most familiar being

Table 37–1. CLASSIFICATION OF COMMON PEDIATRIC SKULL LESIONS

Acquired Disorders
Cephalohematoma
Leptomeningeal cyst

Congenital/Developmental Conditions
Encephalocele
Dermoid and epidermoid tumors
Sinus pericranii
Pacchionian granulations
Parietal foramina
Aplasia cutis congenita
Dysplasias
Fibrous dysplasia
von Recklinghausen's disease

Lymphoproliferative Disorders (Histiocytosis X)
Eosinophilic granuloma
Hand-Schüller-Christian disease
Letterer-Siwe disease

Benign Tumors
Osteoma
Hemangioma
Aneurysmal bone cyst
Chondroma
Osteoid osteoma
Ossifying fibroma
Meningioma

Malignant Tumors
Chordoma
Sarcoma
Leukemia
Lymphoma
Neuroblastoma
Fibrosarcoma

the classic "sunburst" appearance of the hemangioma.

6. Vascular channels are commonly seen with venous lakes and hemangiomas and are not associated with malignant tumors.

CT has assisted in formulating the differential diagnoses of skull tumors and has largely alleviated the need for tangential x-ray views or tomograms. The full extent and vascularity of skull tumors may be more easily appreciated by the injection of contrast material. Obvious intracranial extension and transgression of the dura identify the lesion as malignant. The unique ability of nuclear magnetic resonance imaging (NMRI) to define directly sagittal and coronal anatomy enhances surgical planning, especially at the skull base. However, bone itself produces no magnetic signal. The use of NMRI to differentiate one lesion from another has not been fully evaluated.

ACQUIRED DISORDERS

Cephalohematoma

Cephalohematoma is a subperiosteal hemorrhage of the newborn that usually occurs along the parietal convexities. It is frequently associated with forceps delivery of the infant, necessitated by high birth weight. Subperiosteal spread of the hematoma is limited by suture lines. Approximately 25 percent of these patients have an underlying fracture of the skull. X-ray films of the skull demonstrate early calcification in one to two weeks following hemorrhage, with gradual resolution in one to two months as bone modeling occurs. Occasionally, thickening and asymmetry persist (cephalohematoma deformans), simulating the x-ray film appearance of fibrous dysplasia or epidermoid tumor. In such situations, surgery is cosmetic, with cranioplasty being reserved for severe deformity.

Leptomeningeal Cyst (Growing Fracture)

Following linear skull fractures, young children occasionally develop a soft cranial mass and bone resorption along the fracture line. These defects appear as lytic lesions on x-ray film and are caused by a dural and arachnoid rent, leading to an expansile communicating cerebrospinal fluid (CSF) cyst (Fig. 37–1). The natural course is progressive enlargement of the bony defect and, in the extreme, herniation and necrosis of protruding brain. There-

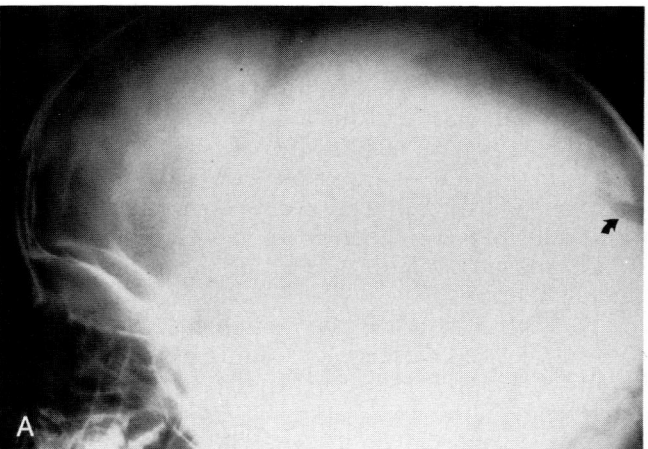 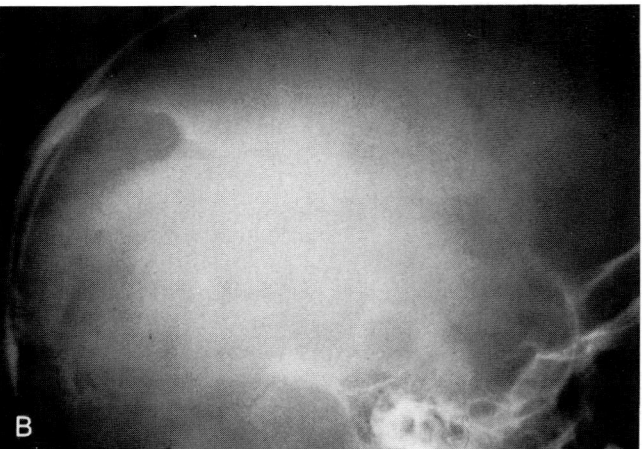

Figure 37–1. *A*, Posterior parietal skull fracture. *B*, Subsequent growing skull fracture.

fore, these lesions are best treated with surgical exposure of the defect, excision of the cyst, and closure of the intervening dural defect. All linear skull fractures in the first few years of life require follow-up until healing of the fracture can be demonstrated.

CONGENITAL/DEVELOPMENTAL CONDITIONS

Encephalocele

Encephaloceles appear at birth as midline, skin-covered herniations of cerebral tissue, CSF, or both protruding through cranial defects. They are discussed in detail in Chapter 6.

Dermoid and Epidermoid Tumors

The classic x-ray film appearance of these lesions is a round lucency with a sclerotic margin. These tumors are usually located along the supraorbital ridges. They appear as a painless lump on the skull. Midline lesions must be carefully evaluated for cutaneous stigmata or sinus tracts that may lead to an intracranial lesion. These two problems are discussed more fully in Chapter 30.

Sinus Pericranii

This is a rare condition, primarily observed during the first few years of life, but may be identified at any age.[25] The tumor consists of a mass of circulating blood adherent to the periosteum and communicating with a venous sinus through anomalous diploic veins. The unique clinical features of this lesion make diagnosis relatively easy. Usually, there is a painless fluctuant midline mass in the frontal, parietal, or occipital area. Lateral sinus pericranii have been reported in adults. Sinus pericranii spontaneously reduces when the patient assumes an upright position or following any maneuver that decreases venous pressure. X-ray films show bone thinning and, occasionally, a small lucent defect at the site of the diploic veins. This lesion may be difficult to distinguish from eosinophilic granuloma and dermoid tumor. Angiography may demonstrate extracranial venous filling. However, sinography with direct instillation of contrast solution into the lesion, with subsequent demonstration of sinus filling, may be necessary for diagnosis. Surgical treatment is recommended because of cosmetic considerations, risk of traumatic hemorrhage and air embolus, and, occasionally, symptoms of dizziness.[14] This lesion may arise following skull injury, especially in older individuals. The clinical appearance and the treatment are similar to that previously described.

Pacchionian Granulations

The normal, albeit exuberant, growth of pacchionian granulations may produce multiple small lucent areas on skull x-ray films, which usually are clustered about the sagittal sinus but may also appear in occipital, squamosal, frontal, and parietal bones. Further scrutiny discloses a thinned inner table and diploë, thus confirming the diagnosis. Larger granulations may erode the outer table. This condition requires no treatment.

Parietal Foramina

Sixty percent of skull x-ray films may show small defects in the superior parietal angles of the parietal bones through which the emissary veins pass to the calvarium. These small openings are parietal foramina.[2] Occasionally, they may achieve a large size. They are thought to result from a failure of mineralization of the membranous bone in the parietal regions (Fig. 37–2). They are not associated with skeletal anomalies and are of no clinical significance, except in the differential diagnosis of cranial defects. The enlargement of the anterior fontanelle and suture diastasis are commonly associated with parietal foramina during the first year of life. Parietal foramina should not be confused with other defects in the calvarium and such conditions as histiocytosis, epidermoid tumor, and eosinophilic granuloma.[2]

Aplasia Cutis Congenita

The congenital absence of skin and, often, underlying bone over part of the vault is termed aplasia cutis congenita.[1] The etiology of the condition is obscure. It often arises along suture lines, in conjunction with venous sinuses. The defect does not spontaneously close, and plastic surgery with occasional cranioplasty may be required.

DYSPLASIAS

Fibrous Dysplasia

This is a relatively common condition of the skeleton, appearing between 5 and 15 years of age and progressing during periods of skeletal growth. There is an accumulation of fibrous connective tissue within one or more of the bones.[1, 13] Thought to arise as a developmental mesenchymal defect, there are no hereditary associations. The literature is disparate regarding the incidence in males and females.[11] The disease is termed monostotic if only one bone is involved, and polystotic if multiple bones are affected. X-ray patterns of the lesions may be cystic or sclerotic. The former appears as a

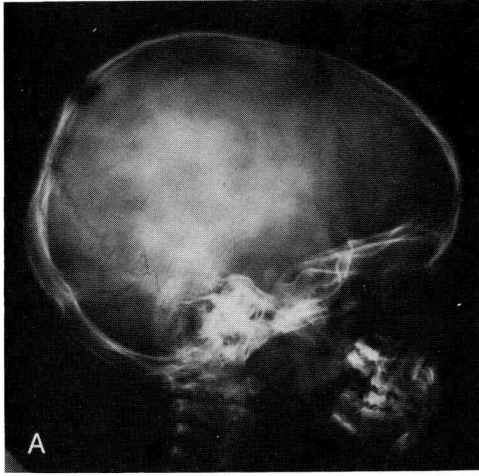
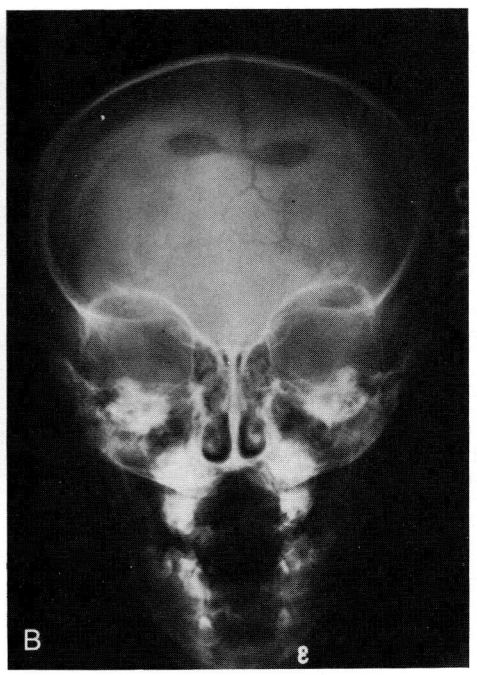

Figure 37–2. Lateral (A) and anteroposterior (B) appearances of parietal foramina.

lucent widening of the diploë, with outer table thinning and a sclerotic margin similar to an epidermoid tumor. The more common latter type demonstrates sclerosis and thickening of the anterior and middle cranial fossae, which is symmetrically centered about the sphenoid. About one third of patients with these skull changes also have long bone lesions and limb hypertrophy. The neurologic symptoms of fibrous dysplasia develop when cranial nerves (i.e., optic and auditory) are entrapped or when orbital or sellar contents are distorted, as a result of bony hypertrophy and destruction. CT scan evaluation not only aids in defining distortion but also helps differentiate fibrous dysplasia from neurofibromatosis and tuberous sclerosis.

Drugs, hormones, and radiation therapy have not altered the course of fibrous dysplasia.[13] Surgery is indicated for decompression of threatened cranial nerves and distortion of soft or nervous tissues. When contemplating resection, the surgeon should be aware of the possible intense vascularity of these tumors. Histologic examination is required to differentiate fibrous dysplasia from sarcoma, histiocytosis, osteoma, osteomyelitis, and metastasis. In the literature, confusion exists regarding the relationship among fibrous dysplasia, ossifying fibroma, and osteoma.[22, 26, 29] Some authors contend that ossifying fibroma is a monostotic form of fibrous dysplasia with identical pathology. However, others have asserted that fibrous dysplasia is a developing form of the mature benign osteoma. In any event, modern authors treat these conditions as three separate entities.

There is an undisputed association of fibrous dysplasia with subsequent sarcomatous degeneration, including osteogenic and fibrous sarcomas.[21] Although many of these patients have been previously treated with radiation for fibrous dysplasia, others have not. One should be suspicious of a sarcomatous change when exuberant growth is in a previously dormant lesion.

Von Recklinghausen's Disease

This chromosomally transmitted, mendelian dominant disease may infrequently manifest with a unilateral absence of the greater wing of the sphenoid (orbital dysplasia). The temporal lobe may not be invested with dura and then prolapses into the orbit, creating a pulsating exophthalmos. This condition must be distinguished from plexiform neurofibroma of the trigeminal nerve and optic glioma—two other causes of exophthalmos in von Recklinghausen's disease.

LYMPHOPROLIFERATIVE DISORDERS

Over the past few decades, a unified concept of reticuloendothelioses has emerged, placing eosinophilic granuloma of bone at one end and Letterer-Siwe disease at the other end of a spectrum of systemic histiocytoses involving bone, skin, and viscera.[6] Called "histiocytosis X" in the aggregate, it is believed not to be a neoplastic condition due to spontaneous regression and cellular heterogenicity, but rather a granulomatous reaction to an unknown stimulus.

The skull lesions have irregular lytic margins and may be multiple or confluent. In general, the younger child or the infant with numerous calvarial lesions is more likely to have generalized visceral involvement (Letterer-Siwe disease). The intermediate condition with skull base and skin lesions (multiple brown nodules) associated with exophthalmos, diabetes insipidus, and dwarfism is termed Hand-Schüller-Christian disease. True eosinophilic granuloma manifests only with bone lesions, characteristically in the older child of four to seven years of age, with a tender mass often limited to the skull.[17] However, the presence of other lesions must be excluded by skeletal survey.

Treatment of the single lesion is biopsy and curettage, which is almost always curative (Fig. 37-3). Multiple bone defects respond well to low doses (400 to 600 rad) of radiation. Continued observation, with frequent skeletal surveys, is required even in the child with a single lesion.[7] Prognosis is dependent primarily upon the nature of the visceral lesions, with extensive involvement foreboding an ominous outcome.

BENIGN TUMORS

Osteoma

In adult series, osteomas are frequently cited as the most common primary skull tumor, but they are less conspicuous in the pediatric population.[7] Choux and colleagues[3] found only two in a consecutive series of 36 cranial vault lesions in children, whereas Ruge and associates[19] found none in a series of 70.

Radiographically, these lesions appear as well-circumscribed, dense hyperostotic outgrowths of either table, with significant intracranial extension occasionally observed, requiring that they be differentiated from meningioma. Cranial lesions are often found in the parasagittal areas and mandible, with the nasal and mastoid sinuses also frequent sites.[24] Vault lesions appear as painless masses, whereas sinus tumors often cause obstruction and headaches. Treatment is surgical removal. A single table is removed for smaller lesions, and craniectomy is performed for larger lesions.

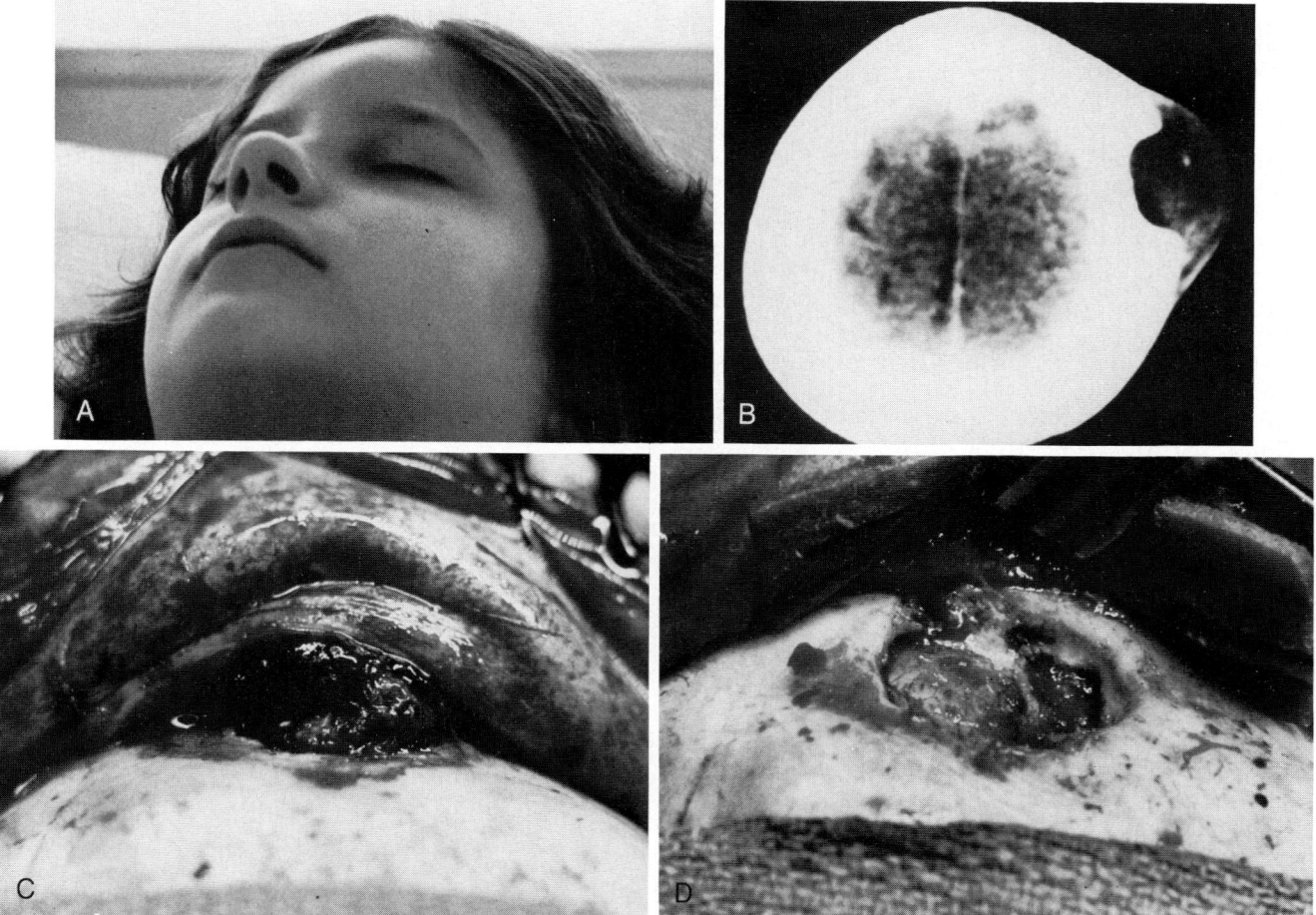

Figure 37-3. *A*, External appearance, eosinophilic granuloma. *B*, CT appearance of eosinophilic granuloma. *C*, Operative appearance of eosinophilic granuloma. *D*, Skull appearance after curettage of eosinophilic granuloma.

Hemangioma

These lesions constitute about 5 percent of pediatric calvarial masses. They are slightly tender, and approximately 25 percent of affected patients have headaches. This tumor grows between the layers of the skull, and the x-ray film may show the characteristic changes of the lesion, with an irregular margin of decreased density containing trabeculae that radiate peripherally ("sunburst"). Absence of sunburst does not exclude the diagnosis, and multiple lesions have been reported.[20] The diploë is characteristically expanded. The outer table may be eroded, and the inner table may be preserved. The typical hemangioma may be treated with excision, curettage, or both, without excessive blood loss, and is usually curative. Pathologically, these are cavernous hemangiomas.

The rare globular form of the disease may arise from the skull base and may be associated with significant intracranial extension. Selective external carotid angiography and operative external carotid occlusion have been recommended as aids for surgical removal.[20]

Aneurysmal Bone Cyst

This is an extremely uncommon lesion, with only nine cases reported in patients less than 20 years of age.[10] Usually occurring elsewhere in the skeletal system, aneurysmal bone cysts of the skull have been described in the frontal, parietal, and temporal areas. They appear as rapidly enlarging tender masses that, on x-ray film, are cystic and expansile, include both tables, and may have intracranial extension. CT reveals a multiloculated enhancing lesion, originating from the diploë, and angiography clarifies the vascular supply. Neurologic deficit and symptoms of intracranial hypertension have been described. Surgical treatment is recommended because of the risk of post-traumatic hemorrhage and intracranial extension. En bloc surgical removal is preferable, and although the lesion may adhere to the dura, it does not invade it. Removal is curative.

Chondroma

This is another rarely seen tumor, with perhaps 30 pediatric patients reported in the literature.[8] The sites of origin are the paranasal sinuses or the junction of the sphenopetrosal, petro-occipital, and spheno-occipital synchrondroses (chondroma of the synchondroses).[9] When the tumor is located extradurally, near the sella or in the middle fossa, x-ray films show a destructive calcified lesion of the sinus or skull base.[23] Presentation and symptoms are dependent upon location. Nasal tumors may cause exophthalmos and visual loss, whereas synchondrotic types involve the cranium about the caverous sinus. The differential diagnosis includes chordoma, neurinoma, craniopharyngioma, and metastatic tumor. These tumors grow relatively slowly, are susceptible to deep malignant degeneration, are radiation-resistant, and may slowly invade vital locations, producing significant deficits.[7] Therefore, operative treatment is imperative. Location may make complete removal difficult, with probable recurrence.[8, 23] Cranial chondroma may be part of a generalized chondromatosis affecting the rest of the skeleton (Ollier's disease).[27] Reported cases of cranial chondroma in young children (younger than ten years of age) are always part of a generalized chondromatosis.[7]

Osteoid Osteoma

This is a relatively common long-bone tumor that is rarely seen in the skull.[5, 23] It produces pain that may be severe and boring in nature. The x-ray film appearance is of a round, lucent defect with sclerotic margins, reminiscent of an epidermoid tumor. En bloc resection or thorough curettage is diagnostic and produces cure.

Ossifying Fibroma

Ossifying fibroma is a benign skull tumor usually arising from the mandible or maxillary sinus, with rare occurrences in the ethmoid and frontal sinuses and cranial vault.[22, 26, 29] They produce symptoms resulting from distortion of nervous tissue and foraminal compression. They usually appear as painless, enlarging masses that, on x-ray film, are lucent, with well-demarcated, thin shell-like sclerotic edges. Surgical excision is the treatment of choice, and malignant degeneration and local recurrences have been reported following subtotal removal.[22]

Meningioma

Meningiomas are rare in children and present only occasionally as skull tumors. The usual x-ray film appearance of pediatric meningioma, as in the adult, is that of an osteoblastic process associated with dilated venous channels. An unusual exception is the intraosseous or intradiploic meningioma, which may appear as a solitary lytic lesion similar to eosinophilic granuloma.[15] Complete removal is indicated for diagnosis and treatment.

MALIGNANT TUMORS

Chordoma

These unusual tumors arise at the cranial base along the clivus, from remnants of primitive notochord. In distinction to adult series, in which half of the cases involve the sacrum, most pediatric chordomas are cranial. These lesions may produce diplopia, dysphagia, nasal speech, and ataxia.[28] Radiographs demonstrate destruction of the skull base, with occasional involvement of the sphenoid and petrous bones. Coarse calcification has been described in one third of the lesions. Surgery is used as the primary treatment, with radiation therapy reserved for local disease control. A long survival can be anticipated, although fatal lung metastasis may intervene.[28]

Sarcoma

Although the most common malignant tumor of bone, it is the most rare primary tumor of the skull.[4,18,24] These rapidly growing masses produce osteolytic lesions with poorly defined margins.[4] They are treated with excision, radiation therapy, and chemotherapy. The prognosis for prolonged survival is guarded. Ewing's sarcoma and fibrosarcoma have been reported to metastasize to the skull in about 10 percent of patients.[1,9]

Leukemia

Leukemias infrequently involve the skull, in contrast with the meninges. They appear on x-ray films as multiple, lucent areas with peripheral new bone formation and are similar to the frequently metastasizing neuroblastoma.

Neuroblastoma

Neuroblastoma shows characteristic multiple, punctate lesions, with suture separation.[9]

Hodgkin's Lymphoma

Hodgkin's lymphoma may involve the skull, manifesting itself as painful lesions that radiographically may be blastic, lytic, or both. Occasional intracranial extension may mandate craniotomy for control of mass effect. The more aggressive lymphomas usually do not involve the skull.

CONCLUSION

The pediatric neurosurgeon is frequently asked to evaluate skull "lumps and bumps." The treatment of the child with a skull tumor consists of a diagnostic work-up of plain x-ray films and CT. Clinical or radiographic features may suggest a highly vascular lesion, which requires preoperative angiography. The majority of these tumors are benign but may produce significant symptoms and neurologic change. Operation is required for diagnosis and treatment. The prognosis is directly related to histologic diagnosis and location.

References

1. Bruno LA, Schut LC, Bruce BA: Pediatric tumors of cranium and meninges. In: Amador L (ed): Brain Tumors in the Young. Springfield, IL, Charles C Thomas, 1983, pp 687–722.
2. Silverman FN: Caffey's Pediatric X-ray Diagnosis, Vol. 1, 8th ed. Chicago, Year Book Pubs., 1985, p 35.
3. Choux N, Gomez A, Choux R, et al: Diagnostic and therapeutic problems concerning tumors of the vault. Child's Brain 1:207, 1975.
4. Courville CV, Deeb P, Marsh C: Notes on the pathology of cranial tumors. Bull LA Neurol Soc 27:57, 1962.
5. Prabhakar B, Reddy DR, Dayananda B: Osteoids. J Bone Joint Surg 54:146, 1972.
6. Crocker AC: The histiocytosis syndromes. In: Vaughan NC, McKay JR, Behrman RE (eds): Nelson Textbook of Pediatrics, 11th ed. Philadelphia, W. B. Saunders Co., 1979, p 1983.
7. Imagawa K, Hawashi M, Pota I, et al: Intracranial chondroma. Surg Neurol 8:268, 1977.
8. Krayenbuehl H, Yasargil MG: Cranial chondromas. Progr Neurol Surg 6:435, 1975.
9. Long DM, Kieffer SA, Chou SN: Tumors of the skull. In: Youmans JR (ed): Neurological Surgery, Vol. 5, 2nd ed. Philadelphia, W. B. Saunders Co., 1982, pp 3227–3268.
10. Luccarelli G, Fornari M: Angiography and computerized tomography in the diagnosis of aneurysmal bone cystic skull. J Neurosurg 53:113, 1980.
11. Matson DD: Tumors of the skull and meninges. In: Matson DD (ed): Neurosurgery of Infancy and Childhood. Springfield, IL, Charles C Thomas, 1969, pp 607–631.
12. Michael P: Tumors of Infancy and Childhood. Philadelphia, J. B. Lippincott, 1964.
13. Milhorat TM: Tumors of the brain, meninges and skull. In: Milhorat TH (ed): Pediatric Neurosurgery. Philadelphia, F. A. Davis, 1978, pp 211–284.
14. Ohta T, Waga S, Handa H, et al: Sinus pericranii. J Neurosurg 42:704, 1975.
15. Pearl GS, Takei Y, Parent AD, et al: Primary intraosseous meningioma presenting as a solitary osteolytic skull lesion: Case report. Neurosurgery 4:269, 1979.
16. Peterson HO, Kieffer SA: Neuroradiology. In: Baker LH (ed): Clinical Neurology. St. Louis, C. V. Mosby, 1975.
17. Rawlings CE, Wilkins RH: Solitary eosinophilic granuloma of the skull. Neurosurgery 15:55, 1984.
18. Reichenthal E, Cohen ML, Manor R, et al: Primary osteogenic sarcoma of the sellar region. J Neurosurg 55:299, 1981.
19. Ruge JR, Tomiga T, Naidich T, et al: Calvarial masses of infants and children. Neurosurgery, Vol. 22 (in press).
20. Schneider RC, Gabrioson TD, Hicks SP: Calvarial hemangioma. Neurology 23:352, 1973.
21. Schwartz T, Albert M: Malignant transformation of fibrous dysplasia. MJ Med Sci 1:35, 1964.
22. Seitz W, Olarte M, Antunes JL: Ossifying fibroma of the parietal bone. Neurosurgery 7:513, 1980.
23. Thomas JE, Baker HL: Assessment of the roentgenographic lucencies of the skull: A systematic approach. Neurology 25:99, 1975.
24. Vandenberg HJ, Conley BL: Primary tumors of the cranial bones. Surg Gynecol Obstet 90:602, 1950.
25. Vaquero J, Desola RG, Martinez R: Lateral sinus pericranii. J Neurosurg 58:139, 1983.
26. Villemure J, Meagher-Villemure K: Giant ossifying fibroma of the skull. J Neurosurg 58:602, 1983.
27. Voorhiemrm Sundaresan N: Tumors of the skull. In: Wilkins RH, Rengachary SS (eds): Neurosurgery, Vol. I. New York, McGraw-Hill, 1984, pp 984–1001.
28. Wold LE, Laws ER: Cranial chordomas in children and young adults. J Neurosurg 59:1043, 1983.
29. Yamashita J, Aoki M, Waga S, et al: Ossifying fibroma of the occipital bone. Surg Neurol 7:189, 1977.

38
INTRAMEDULLARY TUMORS OF THE SPINAL CORD

Fred J. Epstein, M.D.
Jeffrey H. Wisoff, M.D.

Intramedullary spinal cord tumors are relatively uncommon neoplasms, accounting for only 6 percent of central nervous system tumors of childhood.[1, 2, 10, 20, 26, 28] They occur most frequently between the ages of 10 and 16 and are equally divided between the sexes. Because of the rarity of these tumors, individual neurosurgeons may have relatively little experience with surgical management and long-term follow-up of afflicted patients. For this reason, there has been little impetus to modify the traditional treatment of biopsy, dural decompression, and radiation therapy, despite the recognition that after a relatively short remission serious disability or death ensues.

Over the past several years, the senior author has operated on 156 intermedullary spinal cord tumors. In most cases, a gross total excision of the neoplasm was performed. It has become clear that this surgical philosophy is compatible with neurologic recovery and, in many cases, possible permanent cure. This chapter describes this large personal experience as well as includes references to older works that will further our understanding of these relatively uncommon tumors.

PATHOLOGY

Unlike adult intramedullary tumors, of which 50 percent are ependymomas, approximately 58.7 percent of pediatric intramedullary tumors are astrocytomas. Furthermore, in pediatric patients "pure" intramedullary ependymomas represent only 28 percent of all intramedullary lesions (excluding conus medullaris or filum terminale tumors that extend into the lumbar sacral subarachnoid space).

When evaluating intramedullary lesions in children, further diagnostic considerations include "cystic lesions" (hydromyelia, syringomyelia), which have a reported incidence of 4.7 percent, and congenital tumors, with an incidence of 5.8 percent. Additional lesions include metastatic medulloblastomas, among others (e.g., dermoid tumor, intermedullary lipoma).*

There is a definite predisposition for the pediatric tumors to be rostrally located, compared with the adult tumors. A total of 46 percent of pediatric intramedullary tumors are cervical and cervicothoracic, whereas in adults, only 28 percent of these tumors occur in the cervical or cervicothoracic cord.† Intramedullary tumors generally occupy many cord segments (average, six), and rarely, the entire length of spinal cord from the cervicomedullary junction to the conus medullaris is involved.‡

CLINICAL MANIFESTATIONS

Clinical symptoms are commonly present for months, or even years, prior to neurosurgical con-

---

*References 1–4, 7–9, 15, 19, 20, 26, 28–31, 33–36, 42, 44
†References 1, 3, 8, 10, 15–17, 24–26, 34–36
‡References 1, 2, 5, 8, 15–21, 24–26, 34

sultation.* In some cases, the course may be punctuated by exacerbations and remissions that are possibly related to alterations in edema surrounding the neoplasm.[1,2] On occasion, the onset of symptoms may be associated with a trivial spinal injury. It has been suggested that in rare cases, injury may precipitate peritumoral edema and may result in the relatively rapid progression of symptoms.[2, 21, 36]

In the authors' experience, the most common early symptom was local pain along the spinal axis. Other symptoms included motor disturbance, radicular pain, paresthesia, dysesthesias, and, rarely, sphincter dysfunction.[15–18]

Weakness of the lower extremities was usually first manifested as an alteration of a previously normal gait. This was often extremely subtle and obvious only to the parent, who noted a tendency for the child to fall more frequently or to walk on the heels or the toes. In young children, there was commonly a history of being a "late walker," and in the youngest (younger than two years), there was often a history of motor regression (i.e., starting to crawl again instead of walking, or refusing to stand).

A total of 70 percent of patients experienced severe pain along the spinal axis, which was secondary to distention of the dural tube and was most acute in the bony segments directly over the tumor. Characteristically, the pain was worse in the recumbent position, as venous congestion further distended the dural tube and resulted in typical night pains. It was common to discover that patients had a long-standing history of taking analgesics, including narcotics, after a nondiagnostic orthopedic evaluation.[1, 2, 15, 18, 35]

Radicular pain occurred in 10 percent of patients and was usually limited to one or two cervical or lumbar dermatomes, similar to root pain from a variety of disease processes.[36]

Painful dysesthesias occurred in 10 percent of patients and were generally described as painful hot or cold sensations in one or more extremities. In rare circumstances, this was the primary symptom and was not associated with objective signs of neurologic dysfunction.[1, 21, 24]

Paresthesias were occasionally associated with the dysesthetic pain, and both of these symptoms were more common with neoplasms in the cervical spinal cord than with those in the thoracic spinal cord.

Cervical Tumors

The most common early symptoms were nuchal pain and head tilt with torticollis. Mild upper extremity monoparesis was the next most common symptom and was often extremely subtle during the early stages of the illness. Very often, in young children, the first manifestation of weakness was switching "handedness" in right-handed and left-handed patients. Neoplasms in the caudal cervical spinal cord commonly caused weakness and atrophy of the intrinsic muscles of the hand, in contradistinction to tumors rostral to C5, which were less likely to cause significant weakness until relatively late in the clinical course. Interestingly, weakness of the lower extremities only evolved months or, rarely, two to three years after the first symptoms, and bowel and bladder dysfunction was rarely present at the time of primary diagnosis.[1, 2, 8, 15, 21, 34, 36]

Sensory abnormalities were generally limited to one upper extremity, and a discrete sensory level was only noted very late in the course of the disease and, then, only in association with severe neurologic disability.[15, 27, 36]

In most patients, there was increased reflex activity in the lower extremities, with or without extensor plantar signs and clonus.

Thoracic Tumors

Mild scoliosis was the most common early sign of an intramedullary thoracic cord neoplasm. Pain and paraspinal muscle spasm commonly occurred before there were objective signs of neurologic dysfunction, and were commonly assumed to be secondary to the evolving scoliosis. Insidious progressive motor weakness in the lower extremities was first manifested by awkwardness and, only later, by frequent falls and an obvious limp. Early sensory abnormalities were uncommon, although dysesthesias and paresthesias were occasionally present. Increased reflexes and extensor plantar signs, with or without clonus, occurred relatively early in the neurologic course.*

A presenting complaint of bowel and bladder dysfunction was most unusual and was diagnostic of neoplasm extending into the conus medullaris. In general, these symptoms evolved only late in the clinical course if the tumor was rostral to T10.[1, 2, 8, 15, 34, 36]

Hydrocephalus

Increased intracranial pressure may complicate the clinical manifestation of intramedullary tumors in as many as 12.5 percent of patients. The computerized tomography (CT) scan may disclose a normal or markedly dilated ventricular system. Although the etiology of the increased pressure has not been established, some authors have noted a dense arachnoiditis at the outlets of the fourth ventricle, while others have maintained that the greatly elevated cerebrospinal fluid (CSF) pro-

---

*References 1, 2, 8, 13, 15–17, 27, 31, 36, 39

*References 1–3, 8, 15–17, 21, 27, 34–36

tein level interferes with normal circulatory dynamics.[2, 8, 27]

Rarely, severely increased intracranial pressure in the absence of other neurologic signs may be the presenting sign of an intramedullary tumor. It must be suspected if the CSF protein level is markedly elevated, in the absence of demonstrable intracranial pathology.

NEURODIAGNOSTIC STUDIES

Spinal cord tumors may be divided into two general categories: holocord and focal.

Holocord Astrocytomas

"Holocord" widening occurred in 60 percent of pediatric patients and was manifested by expansion of the entire spinal cord from the medulla or cervicomedullary junction to the conus medullaris. In most of these patients, the tumors were astrocytomas, although there were occasional ependymomas that had an identical appearance.[15–18, 32]

These neoplasms were almost invariably cystic, and the solid component of the neoplasm spanned a variable length of the cord and was associated with huge, non-neoplastic rostral and caudal cysts that expanded the central canal above and below the tumor.

Plain spinal x-ray films commonly disclosed a diffusely widened spinal canal with relatively localized erosion or flattening of the pedicles. Whereas the former was secondary to long-standing expansion of the entire spinal cord, the latter occurred only adjacent to the solid component of the neoplasm.[1, 2, 8, 15–18]

Although there were occasional early case reports of holocord widening, its relative frequency was probably not recognized because of the tendency to terminate the neurodiagnostic study when a lumbar myelogram disclosed a complete block secondary to an intramedullary neoplasm.[2, 5] In many patients, it was necessary to perform a cervical puncture to identify the rostral extent of cord widening. It was subsequently recognized that although it was not apparent on the myelogram, a small amount of metrizamide almost invariably trickles past the block and is obvious on the immediate or delayed spinal CT scan. Therefore, this scan defines the rostral extent of the expanded cord.[12, 15–18] It is for this reason that CT of the spine is an invaluable adjunct to the neurodiagnostic evaluation of spinal cord tumors.

A 24-hour delayed spinal CT scan was often helpful, since rostral, caudal, and, occasionally, intratumoral cysts were identified as the metrizamide diffused within them.

Holocord expansion caused by a spinal cord tumor may be confused with hydromyelia, and it is important that this differential diagnosis be firmly established prior to surgery. There are five major observations[15] that contribute to making the correct diagnosis:

1. Plain spine x-ray films often disclose erosion of pedicles adjacent to a tumor, while this is rarely present in hydromyelia. Both of these entities may be associated with a diffusely widened spinal canal.

2. While 95 percent of spinal cord tumors are associated with a complete subarachnoid block, there is, very rarely, an obstruction to the flow of metrizamide in the presence of hydromyelia. Even in the rare absence of a complete myelographic block, a spinal cord tumor is associated with some distinct focal widening, whereas hydromyelia usually causes diffuse widening of the spinal cord without one area being significantly more widened than another.

3. Hydromyelia is invariably associated with an Arnold-Chiari I malformation, and for this reason, it is essential that, in the presence of any diagnostic uncertainty, the contrast-enhanced study include the cervicomedullary junction.

4. In the presence of hydromyelia, the delayed metrizamide-enhanced spinal CT scan discloses homogeneous enhancement of the entire hydromyelic cavity, while cystic tumors have relatively localized collections of intracyst contrast material.

5. Nuclear magnetic resonance imaging (NMRI) discloses an extensive intramedullary cyst associated with an Arnold-Chiari I malformation.

Focal Tumors

Focal spinal cord neoplasms were generally four to eight segments in length and were commonly associated with flattening of pedicles immediately adjacent to the neoplasm. In some cases, plain film changes were as precise as the myelogram for tumor localization (though obviously never a substitute).

Focal tumors were associated with a total subarachnoid block in 90 percent of cases, and for this reason, immediate and delayed CT scans were necessary to define the rostral extent of cord expansion. Intratumor cysts were rarely present in the patient who had not previously had surgery and radiation therapy.

Patients who had received a full course of spinal radiation therapy (4500 rad) commonly had multiple cysts within the tumor that were obvious on the delayed CT scan or on ultrasonography (see later).[15, 32]

Nuclear Magnetic Resonance Imaging

It has become evident that NMRI (Fig. 38–1) will relegate most invasive neurodiagnostic studies to history. The NMRI scan provides an excellent image of intramedullary neoplasms, and it is often unnec-

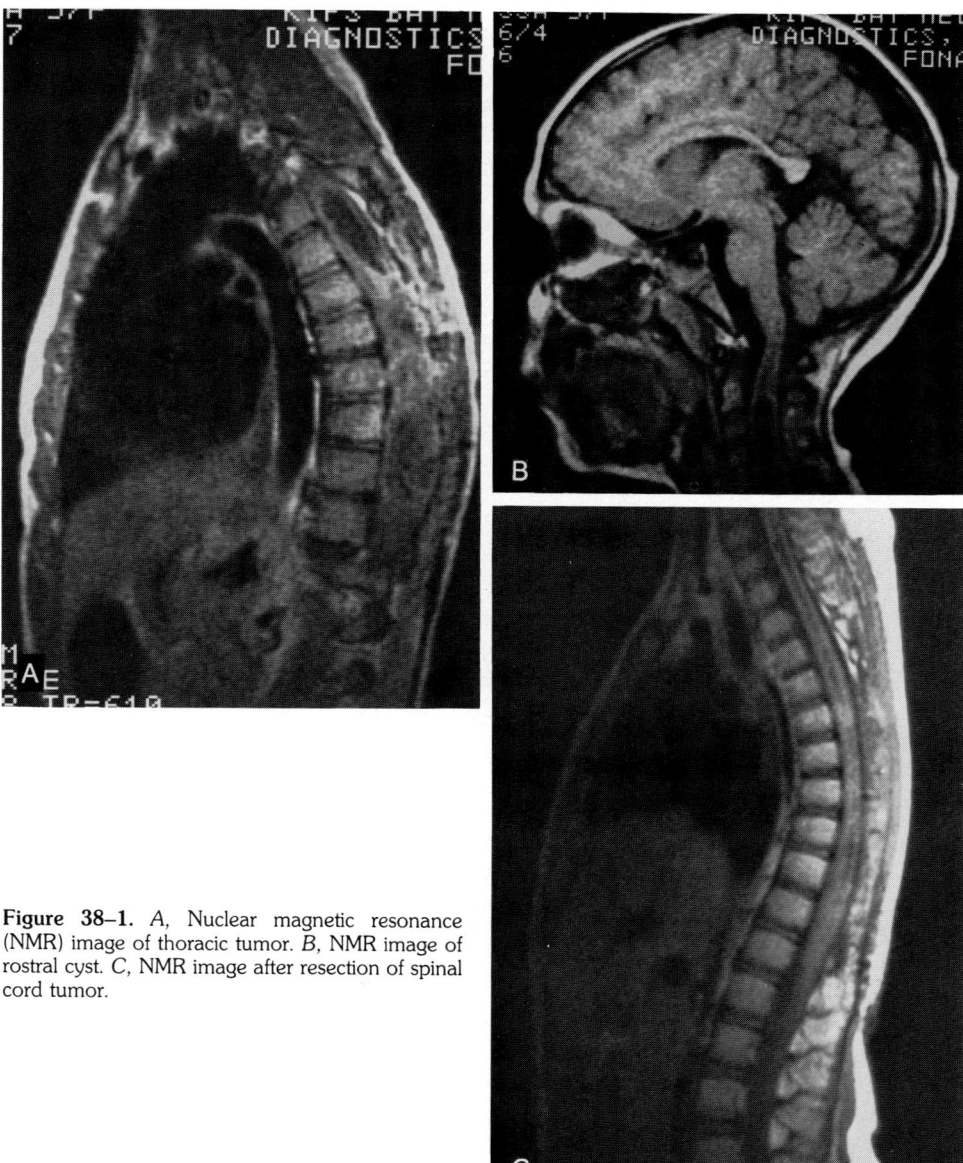

Figure 38–1. *A,* Nuclear magnetic resonance (NMR) image of thoracic tumor. *B,* NMR image of rostral cyst. *C,* NMR image after resection of spinal cord tumor.

essary to carry out other studies if the scan is satisfactory. It is essential to obtain a midsagittal view; this may occasionally be impossible in the presence of severe scoliosis.

Transcutaneous Ultrasonography

In patients who have had an earlier laminectomy, transcutaneous ultrasonography may be employed to visualize the spinal cord and the neoplasm. Utilizing this technique (real-time unit with triple frequency: 3.5 and 7.5 MHz), the cord may be studied in both sagittal and transverse projections, and the presence of significant expansion will be immediately obvious.[15, 18, 32]

Transcutaneous ultrasonography may be more informative than conventional myelography or metrizamide-enhanced spine CT scanning, as it gives a direct view of the interior of the spinal cord. In occasional cases, the tumor may be echogenic, affording a dramatic view of the neoplasm and its relationship to the spinal cord. The presence of cysts either within the tumor or in relation to the rostral and caudal poles of the neoplasm is evident. Eighteen months or longer following radiation therapy, there are commonly multiple intratumor cysts that are similar in appearance to Swiss cheese. The technique is limited by the length of the laminectomy, and it is not possible to visualize the spinal cord rostral or caudal to the laminectomy defect.[32]

TREATMENT

Elsberg[13] and Elsberg and Beer[14] first advocated radical removal of intramedullary tumors in classic reports in which a two-stage procedure was described. At the first surgery, a long, midline posterior myelotomy overlying the tumor was performed, following which the dura was not closed. One week later, the wound was reopened, and a large volume of tumor was extruded through the myelotomy, facilitating the establishment of a clear plane of cleavage and total tumor excision. Since that time, Elsberg's underlying thesis concerning the feasibility of total tumor removal has been established by many neurosurgeons, although utilization of the operating microscope and contemporary instrument systems has obviated the need for a two-stage procedure.*

Surgical exploration is mandatory for any child with a progressively symptomatic intramedullary mass. There is no justification for giving radiation therapy without obtaining a definitive tissue diagnosis. Furthermore, in most situations, surgery should be directed toward total or radical removal of the tumor; there is no acceptable rationale for intending only to obtain a biopsy specimen and then automatically administering a full course of postoperative radiation therapy.

SURGERY

The contemporary neurosurgeon must have a clear understanding of the necessity of pursuing radical or even total excision when technically possible. Ependymomas are clearly demarcated from adjacent normal cord and, therefore, in most circumstances, may be totally extirpated. Astrocytomas have an interface between the tumor and the normal spinal cord that serves as a glia-tumor interface facilitating total removal.[16]

When dealing with an intramedullary congenital tumor (dermoid, epidermoid), it is safest to evacuate its contents while leaving the cyst wall, which is often inseparable from normal neural tissue, intact.

It is desirable to carry out a limited laminectomy over the solid component of the neoplasm but not to unnecessarily extend it rostrally or caudally.

In the authors' first surgical experience with "holocord" widening, a total laminectomy from C1–T12 was carried out. It was subsequently recognized that it was not necessary to expose the spinal cord over the rostral and caudal cysts. For this reason, it was important to define as accurately as possible the location of the solid component of the neoplasm vis-a-vis the cysts.

The approximate location of the solid component of the neoplasm may be estimated on the basis of the clinical and radiographic findings.

---

*References 1, 5, 8, 15–18, 20, 22, 30, 31, 39, 43

Clinical Indications of Tumor Location in the Presence of Holocord Expansion

In the presence of holocord widening associated with a cystic astrocytoma, it is the solid component of the neoplasm that is responsible for primary neurologic dysfunction, whereas the rostral and caudal cysts that expand the remainder of the spinal cord remain asymptomatic in the early stages of the disease.

Therefore, neurologic symptoms in one or both upper extremities in the presence of holocord widening suggests that the solid component of the neoplasm is within the cervical cord.

Conversely, progressive scoliosis, neurologic dysfunction, or both limited to the lower extremities are strongly suggestive of solid neoplasm within the thoracic cord, while bowel and bladder dysfunction indicate extension of the neoplasm into the conus medullaris.

In the authors' experience, the presence of normal bowel and bladder function, and an expanded conus, are invariably associated with a cyst.

Spinal cord ependymomas do not adhere to this clinical pattern, as they may expand any length of the spinal cord, with a relative paucity of signs and symptoms referable to the segmental involvement. It is tempting to speculate that this is directly related to the primary anatomic location of the tumor in the region of the central canal, which causes very gradual compression of adjacent neural structures as the tumor increases in volume. This may be analogous to the rostral and caudal cystic components of the spinal cord astrocytomas, which are also in the region of the central canal and asymptomatic at the time of primary diagnosis. The origin of the solid component of the astrocytoma is probably relatively asymmetric and may cause symptoms as a result of both compression and infiltration of adjacent neural tissues.

Radiologic Indications of Tumor Location in the Presence of Holocord Expansion

While the entire spinal canal may be widened in the presence of a "holocord" astrocytoma, erosion of pedicles occurs only immediately adjacent to the solid component of the neoplasm (Fig. 38–2). In addition, the myelogram and myelo-CT scan disclose a disproportionate widening adjacent to the midportion of the neoplasm (most commonly associated with total subarachnoid block).

Finally, the delayed metrizamide-enhanced spinal CT scan may disclose the rostral and caudal tumor-cyst junction as the contrast diffuses into the latter.

Surgical Instrumentation

Spinal cord tumors are firm, often contain microscopic foci of calcium, and only rarely have a cleav-

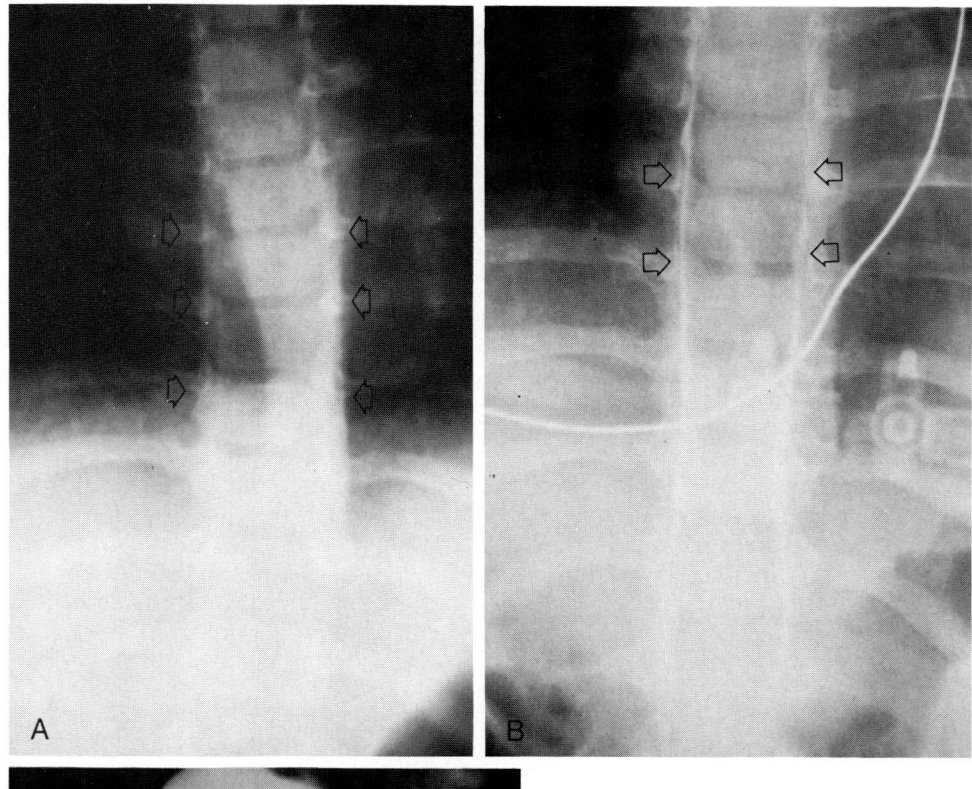

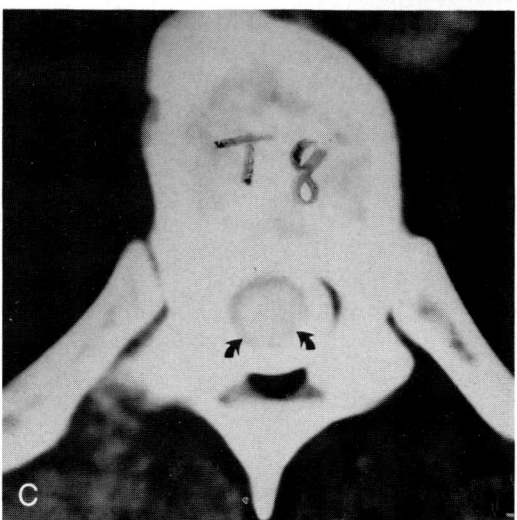

Figure 38–2. A, Thoracic spine x-ray, AP view. Note pedicular flattening (arrows) corresponding to solid tumor. B, Metrizamide-enhanced myelogram. Maximal narrowing of dye column (arrows) indicates solid tumor. C, Delayed metrizamide-enhanced CT scan. Note intramedullary cyst (arrows).

age plane to facilitate an en bloc resection. In the majority of cases it is necessary to remove the tumor from inside out, until the almost invariably present glia-tumor interface is recognized as a change in color and consistency between the tumor and adjacent normal neural tissues.

In the past, neurosurgeons were limited to traditional suction-cautery techniques for removal of neoplasms. These techniques were often satisfactory for brain tumors; however, they were extremely hazardous with tumors of the spinal cord. This was because of the heat and movement transmitted through the tumor to the adjacent normal spinal cord, which was invariably firmly adherent to it. As a result of these technical limitations, there was a significant morbidity associated with intramedullary spinal cord surgery.

The development and application of the Cavitron ultrasonic aspirator (CUSA) system was a significant improvement over the conventional systems, and made a major contribution to spinal cord surgery.[15–18] It is important to describe briefly the CUSA in order to appreciate fully its impact on intramedullary spinal cord surgery.

The CUSA system incorporates three major systems at the handpiece to provide maximum efficiency in removing tissue. The three systems are

1. Vibration. The surgical tip vibrates longitudi-

nally, thereby fragmenting tissue in contact with its distal annular end. The level of vibration is adjustable.

2. Irrigation. Sterile irrigating solution is routed from an intravenous equipment source hanging from the console to the coaxial space between the outer surface of the surgical tip and the inner surface of the flue. The fluid exits near the tip, enters the operating field, and suspends the fragmented particles.

3. Suction. A suction pump contained in the console applies suction to the hollow surgical tip. Fluid and particulate matter are aspirated at the distal end of the tip and subsequently are deposited in a cannister. The suction available at the tip is adjustable from 0 to 24 mm of mercury (0–24 mm Hg).

The ultrasonic dissecting system is capable of discrete removal of a broad range of tissue. It is important to emphasize that the primary value of ultrasonic dissection is the fragmentation of tissue by the vibrating tip of the handpiece. If it were possible to observe the operation of the instrument in slow motion, one would see the following: (1) tissue fragmentation within 1 ml of the vibrating tip, (2) suspension of fragmented tissue in the irrigation, (3) aspiration of the tissue-irrigation solution.

Because the suction removes an emulsion of tissue and irrigation solution, there is no movement of adjacent tissue. This is an important divergence from conventional suction-cautery technique in which there is a great deal of transmitted movement.

Laboratory studies of the CUSA system have demonstrated that normal electric conduction in neural tissue is maintained beyond a 1 ml radius of the vibrating instrument tip. For this reason, dissection with the ultrasonic instrument may be carried out immediately adjacent to vital structures, with little attendant risk.[15, 18]

The CUSA is the ideal instrument to rapidly debulk and remove all but residual fragments of spinal cord neoplasm. The neurosurgical laser is ideal for removing the residual fragments, as it may be employed with great precision along the length of the glia-tumor interface.

Although the laser may be employed in place of the CUSA, it is extremely tedious and time-consuming to use when the lesion is a very voluminous intramedullary neoplasm. In addition, the resulting laser "char" makes it difficult to recognize the glia-tumor interface and mandates frequent interruptions of the ongoing dissection so that the blackened tissues can be gently removed with a small-caliber suction.

Surgical Technique

In patients who have not been previously operated on, an osteoplastic laminectomy is carried out. This permits replacement of the bone that is a nidus for subsequent osteogenesis and posterior fusion. Replacement of the bone does not prevent the postsurgical evolution of spinal deformity but offers protection against future local trauma.

Even following careful consideration of the clinical and neuroradiologic examinations, it is not possible to be certain that the laminectomy is of sufficient length to expose the entirety of the solid component of the neoplasm. For this reason, transdural ultrasonography is utilized to define further the location of the tumor vis-a-vis the bone removal.

After laminectomy is carried out, the wound is filled with saline, and the head of the transducer probe is placed into gentle contact with the dura. Utilizing this technique, the spinal cord is viewed in both sagittal and transverse sections. The rostral and caudal limits of the tumor as well as the presence or absence of associated cysts are immediately obvious. Occasionally, an echogenic tumor provides a striking ultrasound image; however, most commonly, the solid component of the neoplasm is only manifest as a widened spinal cord (Fig. 38–3).

If the laminectomy is not sufficiently long to expose the entirety of the solid component of the neoplasm, it is lengthened, segment by segment, until ultrasonography discloses that the entire tumor mass is exposed. Only at this juncture is the dura opened. This is limited to the area overlying the expanded spinal cord—it is not extended rostrally or caudally over normal spinal cord. In addition, it is not necessary to open the dura widely over the rostral or caudal cyst, as these are easily drained as the solid component of the neoplasm is excised.

It is important to emphasize that the "swollen" spinal cord is commonly rotated and distorted, and it is essential that careful inspection identify normal landmarks prior to placing the myelotomy. Since the posterior median raphe is generally obliterated, the only sure way of recognizing the posterior midline is by identifying the dorsal root entry zones bilaterally. Rotation of the spinal cord may occasionally make this difficult, and even surprising, in terms of the distorted location of the midline. In any event, this is important, as otherwise it is possible that the myelotomy may be placed away from the median raphe and may sever multiple nerves along the dorsal root entry zone (Fig. 38–4A).

In the presence of holocord widening associated with rostral and caudal cysts, the ultrasound image will have clearly defined the junction of cyst and neoplasm over the rostral and caudal poles of the tumor. It is in the "junctional" regions that the midline myelotomy is started.

The carbon dioxide laser utilized at 6 to 8 watts is an ideal instrument for placing the myelotomy, as the cord is incised and hemostasis obtained simultaneously. Although neurosurgeons are loath to interrupt blood vessels on the surface of the

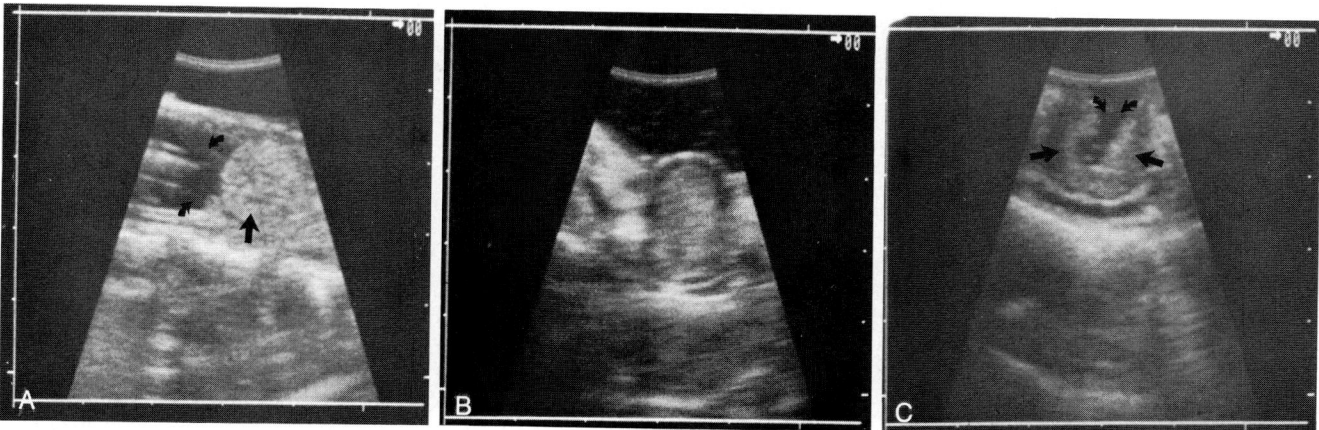

Figure 38–3. Intraoperative ultrasonography. *A*, Sagittal view prior to dural opening demonstrates solid tumor (large arrow) and polar cyst (small arrows). *B*, Transverse view. Solid tumor expands spinal cord and obliterates subarachnoid space. *C*, Transverse view, after resection. Note intramedullary cavity (curved arrows) and normal spinal cord (straight arrows).

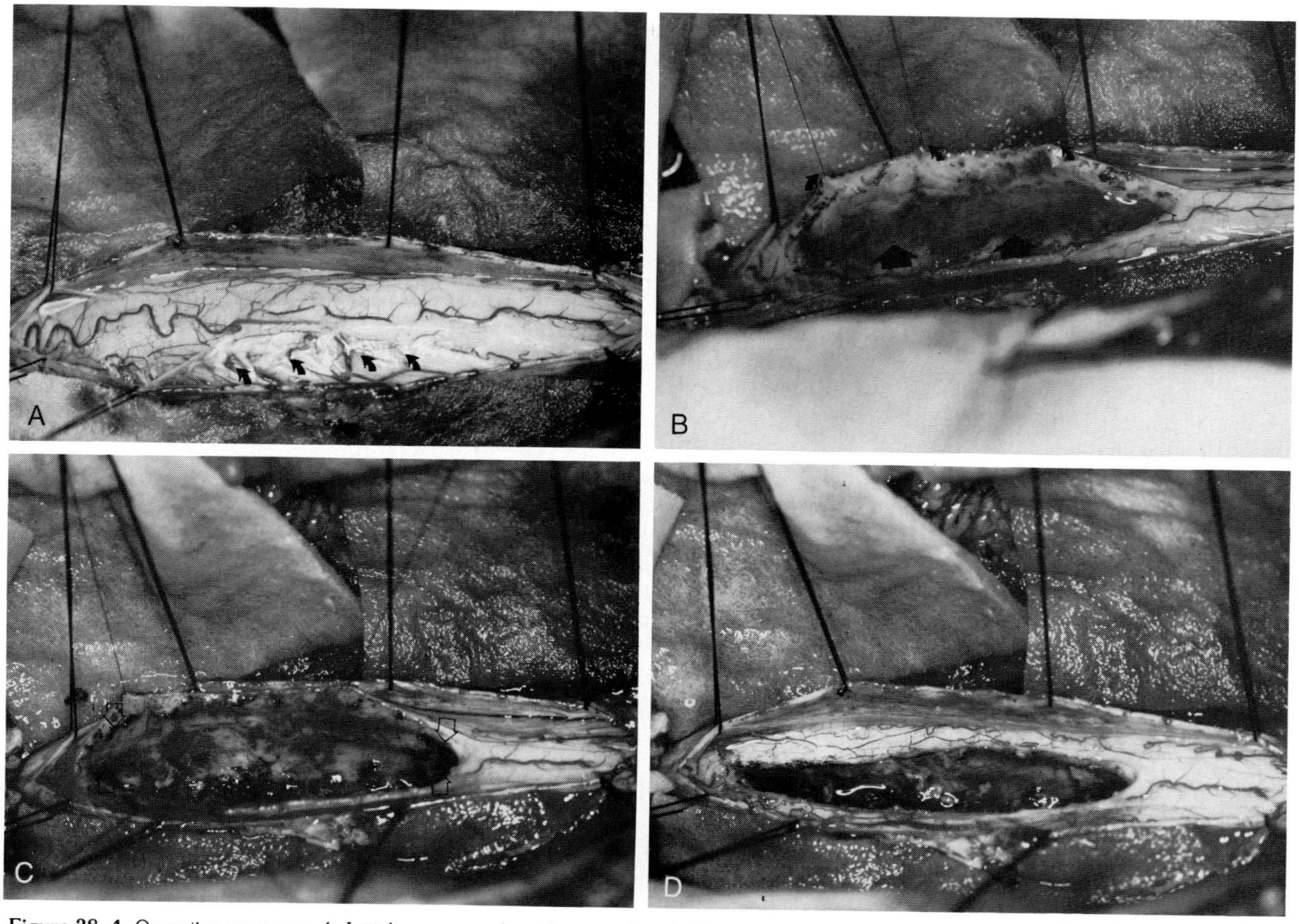

Figure 38–4. Operative exposure. *A*, Initial exposure of swollen spinal cord. Note rotation of cord with obliteration of normal landmarks. Dorsal roots (arrows) are exposed bilaterally to identify midline. *B*, Myelotomy completed. Pial traction sutures in place (small arrows). Tumor (large arrows) and caudal cyst (open arrows) exposed. *C*, Tumor resected. Note large intramedullary cavity with rostral and caudal cysts (open arrows). *D*, Pial sutures removed. Subarachnoid space re-expanded.

spinal cord, it is tedious and time-consuming to preserve these vascular channels. They are not at all essential to the preservation of neurologic function and are almost inevitably disrupted during the course of the procedure, even if primarily preserved.

After the cyst is entered, inspection of the cavity localizes the rostral or caudal neoplasm that extends into it. In most cases, it is not necessary to extend the myelotomy over the cyst, since it is easily drained as either pole of the neoplasm is identified and removed. Because the cyst fluid is produced by the tumor, it is unlikely to reaccumulate following gross total excision of the neoplasm.

After identifying the rostral and caudal cyst-tumor junctions, the myelotomy is continued over the midline of the cord between the previously placed incisions. Following completion of the myelotomy, there is usually 1 to 2 mm of white matter, overlying the neoplasm, that is removed with the laser or bipolar cautery and a very fine suction. Most astrocytomas are gray or pink and may be distinguished from adjacent white matter.

At this juncture, it is essential that pia traction sutures be utilized to open the myelotomy incision and further expose the intramedullary tumor. It is satisfactory to utilize any fine suture material, and it is the authors' practice simply to "hang" small clamps on the sutures rather than to suture the pia to adjacent tissues (Fig. 38–4B).

It must be emphasized that in the presence of an astrocytoma, there must be no effort to define a plane of cleavage around the tumor. These neoplasms must be removed from the inside out, until a glia-tumor interface is recognized by the change in color and consistency of the adjacent tissues. There is rarely a true plane of dissection, and futile efforts to define its presence result only in unnecessary retraction and manipulation of functioning neural tissue.

Ependymomas have a distinct plane of cleavage between the tumor and the adjacent neural tissue. Small tumors may occasionally be removed in one piece, whereas the more common bulky tumors must be excised bit by bit. In the latter cases, it is hazardous to attempt to carry out an en bloc excision, as there will invariably be excessive manipulation of adjacent neural tissue. In these cases, the centrum of the tumor must be debulked with the CUSA or the laser, following which the residual fragments may be removed along the cleavage plane. In all these cases, the entirety of the residual cavity is lined by normal-appearing white matter.

In the presence of cystic holocord neoplasms, tumor removal is initiated at either the rostral or the caudal pole of the neoplasm, in the region of the tumor-cyst junction.

As tumor excision continues, it is helpful to recognize that the anterior extent of the neoplasm is only very rarely ventral to the anterior wall of cyst. The bulk of the tumor is most often within the posterior two thirds of the spinal cord (as viewed in cross-section), and the general dimensions of the tumor may be roughly conceptualized following inspection of the rostral and caudal cysts (Fig. 38–4C).

The excision of the solid noncystic astrocytoma is initiated in the midportion rather than the rostral or caudal pole of the neoplasm. This is because there is no clear rostral or caudal demarcation of the tumor, as occurs when there are rostral and caudal cysts. In addition, the poles of the neoplasm are the least voluminous, and for this reason, removal of this part of the neoplasm may be the most hazardous because normal neural tissue may be easily disrupted.

The CUSA is utilized to remove the bulk of the neoplasm, following which the carbon dioxide laser is used to vaporize the visible remaining fragments. The dura is closed primarily, as it is unnecessary to utilize a dural substitute for decompression if tumor excision has been grossly complete (Fig. 38–4D).

Intramedullary Lipomas

Intramedullary lipomas are rare congenital tumors that are most commonly located in the thoracic spinal cord (Fig. 38–5). These tumors are not neoplasms, and they increase in size and in relation to fatty tissue elsewhere in the body. Myelopathic signs and symptoms evolve slowly and generally are first manifest during rapid growth spurts or after excessive weight gain.

The NMRI scan or the spinal CT scan are diagnostic of intramedullary lipomas. Therefore, there is usually no preoperative uncertainty as to the etiology of the lesion.

The goal of surgery is to carry out subtotal excision of the lipoma and a dural decompression. There must be no effort to excise totally this tumor, as it is intimately adherent and intertwined with adjacent functional neural tissues.

The carbon dioxide laser is an excellent instrument to debulk the lipoma, as the high water content of the fatty tissue is vaporized, thereby shrinking the mass. This is accomplished with no surgical trauma to adjacent tissue, as the tumor gradually "melts."

Debulking the lipoma often results in significant or complete neurologic recovery. This is often permanent, as the lipoma is unlikely to grow in the absence of alterations of body fat content.

Sensory Evoked Potential Monitoring

Sensory evoked potentials are monitored throughout the majority of the operative procedures. This monitoring is only valuable if the information is immediately available and is utilized by the surgeon to modify the operative dissection.

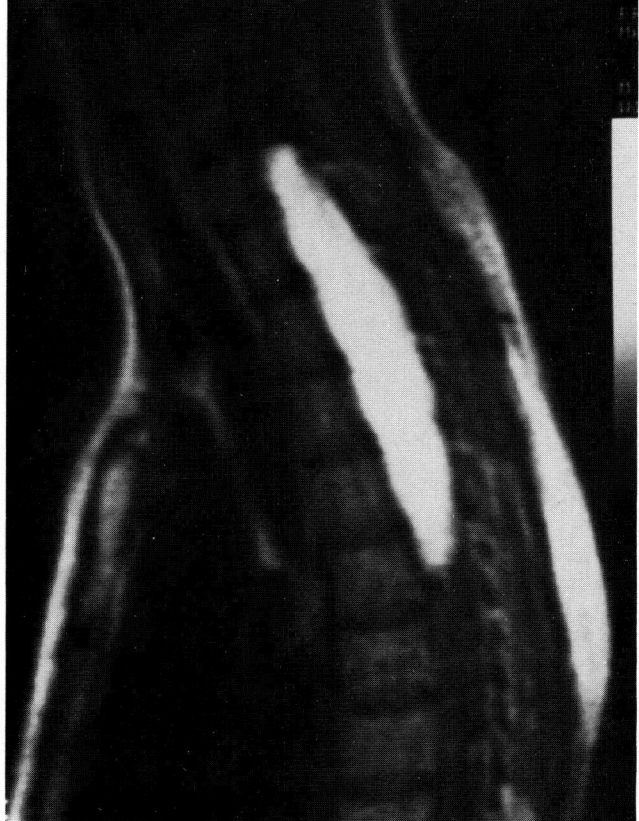

Figure 38-5. NMR image of intramedullary lipoma. Increased signal on T1.

Therefore, it is essential that the data be continuously updated and communicated. Information that is updated every two minutes only informs the surgeon that some event in the dissection has already occurred at some unknown time and, therefore, allows neither corrective steps nor assessment as to the responsible manipulation.

The conventional averaging systems such as the Tracor and the Nicolet are capable only of updating information every two minutes and require an evoked-potential amplitude in the order of 0.25 μV. Since evoked potentials (EP) from a spinal cord compressed by tumor are often less than 0.10 μV in amplitude, these instruments are not helpful surgical adjuncts for intramedullary spinal cord surgery.[18]

This is a quite different situation from scoliosis surgery or spinal cord angiography. In these situations, more conventional monitoring systems may provide valuable information inasmuch as after the straightening of the spine or the injection of contrast media, the surgeon may pause to be updated on the status of the spinal cord. The hiatus in time is not important inasmuch as the event and its place in time is well-established. Since neither of these procedures is expected to affect adversely electric conductivity, if electric changes are observed, it may be advisable for the orthopedist to release the instrumentation or for the angiographer to delay further instillation of contrast material until there is electric recovery.

In the authors' most recent experience, monitoring has been performed with the Cordis Brain-State Analyzer, which utilizes a new technique known as optimized digital filtering for averaging the evoked potential. This is a highly sensitive instrument that can update information as fast as every five to ten seconds and can detect an evoked potential smaller than 0.10 μV. For this reason, there is a continuous stream of information in real-time, and it is simple to relate this to the ongoing surgical procedure. Both brainstem (far field) and somatosensory (near field) evoked potentials are used for intraoperative monitoring. Only the near field potentials are effective when the cord is very compromised.

Several clinical correlations have been made using the Cordis Brain-State Analyzer. Placement of pia traction sutures commonly results in transient decrements in the amplitude of potentials, which probably occur as a result of movement of the posterior columns. Usually, the potential recovers within a few minutes. If it does not, the suture is removed and is placed in another location, under less tension.

If the dissection is inadvertently extended beyond the poles of the tumor, as is possible when there are no rostral or caudal cysts, there is a dramatic decrease in amplitude and an increase in latency of the evoked potential. This is most probably secondary to manipulation of the posterior columns that are in their normal anatomic position and indicates that a normal cord is being disrupted.

When the laser is employed for more than 20 seconds at one time, there is often an adverse, probably thermal effect that is manifested by a decrease in amplitude and an increase in latency. When this occurs, the dissection is temporarily interrupted, and the cord is irrigated with cool Ringer's solution. In most cases, electric activity returns to baseline within 30 to 90 seconds.

In some cases, there is deterioration of evoked potentials as the dissection is directed toward tumor removal in specific locations. When this occurs, the manipulation is temporarily interrupted, and the electric activity permitted to recover. It is very common to start and then to stop the procedure many times during the course of tumor removal.

Improved electric conductivity following tumor removal was invariably associated with a benign postoperative course. Impaired activity as compared with the preoperative baseline was not uncommon, and it was not necessarily associated with neurologic morbidity. Nevertheless, the majority of patients with deteriorated activity have had transiently greater neurologic dysfunction. However, in most circumstances, this function ultimately has recovered. In one patient, all electric activity was lost, and postoperatively, there was complete absence of the sense of position of the lower extremities.

In summary, the Cordis Brain-State Analyzer gives meaningful information, which the authors have employed to modify the surgical dissection. It is too early in our experience to state that it is an indispensable adjunct, but clearly, the information is relevant and quickly available and is easily translated into surgical action.

POTENTIAL SURGICAL PITFALLS

Missing Rostral or Caudal Tumor Fragment

In cases in which the entire spinal cord was expanded (holocord astrocytomas), it was a consistent finding that the neoplasm was associated with a rostral and a caudal cyst that extended up and down the central canal but did not contain neoplasm. In three patients, a large intratumor cyst was confused with a rostral cyst, and the tumor removal was prematurely terminated on the assumption that the superior part of the tumor had been removed. In these patients, the symptoms recurred three months, six months, and 18 months postoperatively as the cysts re-formed. The symptoms were rapidly evolving scoliosis in two patients, and paraspinal and cervical pain in one. In all patients, re-exploration disclosed only residual tumor that had been neglected as a direct result of misinterpreting a large tumor cyst for a rostral or caudal cyst. It is essential that when cysts are identified over the poles of the tumor, they be opened up widely enough to be certain that this is the cyst that is extending above or below the tumor, and not a cyst within the tumor. The former are lined by white matter, whereas cysts that occur within the neoplasm are lined by tumor tissue.

Intraoperative ultrasonography may also help differentiate the rostral and caudal cysts from the intratumor cyst. The former symmetrically expand the cord, occupy two thirds of the diameter, and are smooth-walled. Intratumor cysts are eccentric and asymmetric, are of varying volume, and often have irregular walls (Fig. 38–6).

Anterior Subarachnoid Spinal Fluid Loculation

In six patients, there has been dramatic posterior extrusion of the spinal cord through the dural opening at some time during the tumor dissection. This was associated with a deterioration of brainstem evoked potentials, and the authors initially misinterpreted this as acute spinal cord swelling. The authors now recognize that it is not uncommon for cerebrospinal fluid to become loculated anterior to the spinal cord and to result in its posterior displacement. It is effectively dealt with by retraction of the lateral margin of the spinal cord and puncturing the cyst. It has been a consistent finding that this intraoperative problem has occurred only in patients who have had previous surgery and in whom there are dense adhesions between the lateral spinal cord and the dural tube. It seems that the anterior subarachnoid space does not communicate freely with the posterior subarachnoid space, and this may be responsible for the hydrodynamics that promote this intraoperative problem.

One patient in this series had a huge tumor in the lower thoracic cord. Although the patient was neurologically stable immediately after surgery, one week later the patient became paraplegic. The CT scan disclosed that the spinal cord had extruded from the spinal canal. During surgery, there was a huge anterior loculation of cerebrospinal fluid that had displaced the spinal cord posteriorly through the dural decompression, and the cord had become incarcerated on the rostral and caudal dura, with secondary infarction. Retrospectively, it was apparent that the dura had been excised at the time of the first operation, and it had not been closed at the time of the tumor resection. This permitted the trapped anterior subarachnoid compartment to displace the cord out of the spinal canal, with subsequent infarction. As a result of this experience, the authors do not leave the dura open under any circumstances, and if it has been previously excised, a suitable dural substitute is used.

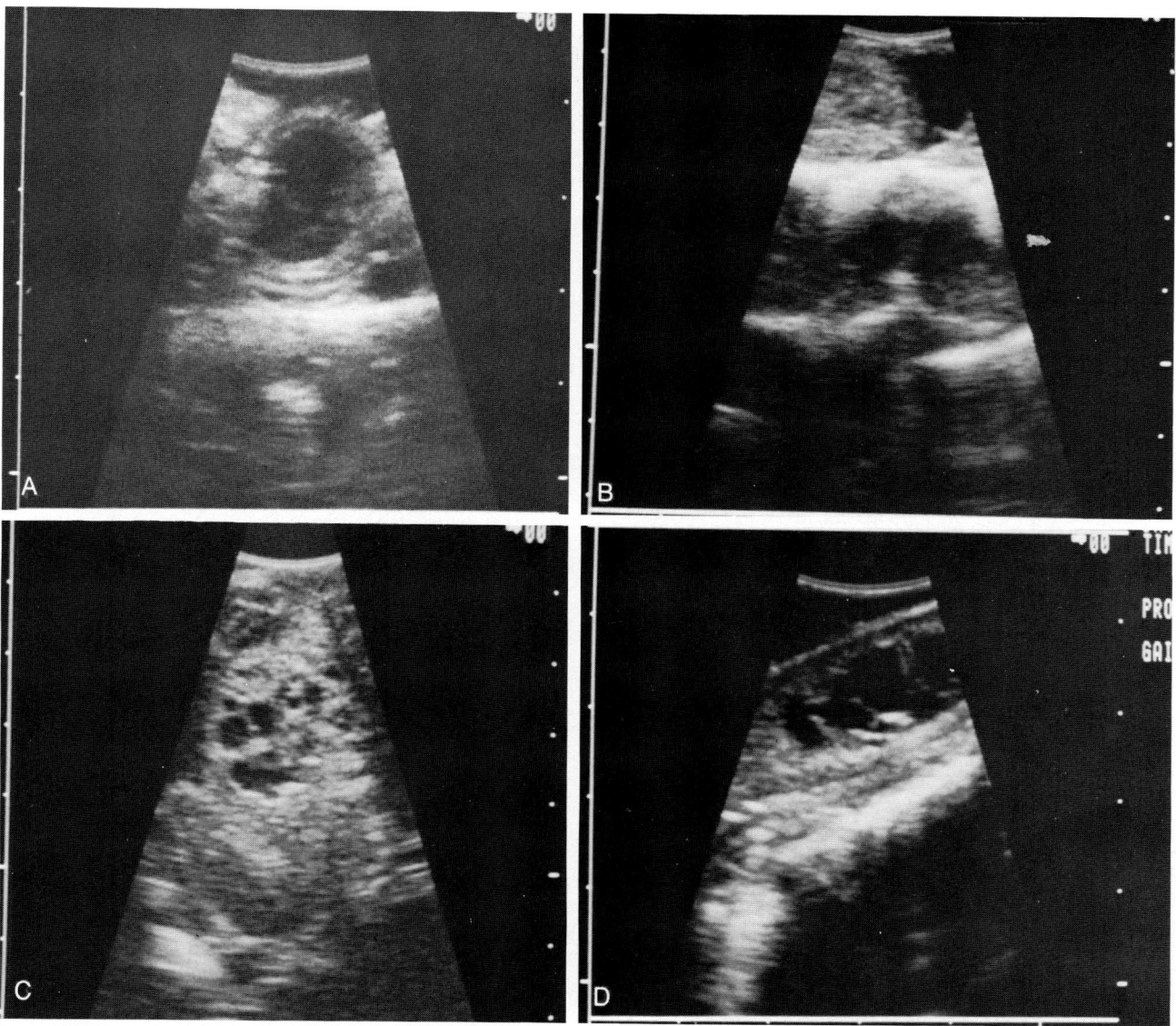

Figure 38–6. Ultrasonography of polar cyst. A, Transverse view. B, Sagittal view. Intramural cyst has "Swiss cheese" appearance. C, Transverse view. D, Sagittal view.

Postoperative Neurologic Morbidity Related to Segmental Location of the Neoplasm

Postoperative neurologic morbidity may be correlated with the segments of the spinal cord that are involved with the neoplasm. Whereas an extensive dissection may be carried out with little risk in those segments of the spinal cord that are largely white matter, this does not seem to be the case in the lowest segments, where gray matter is most abundant.

Dissections within the cervical spinal cord are associated with little morbidity, though it is not uncommon to note some anterior horn cell dysfunction as manifested by atrophy of one or more muscle groups of an upper extremity. When this has occurred, it has been permanent.

Dissections extending from the junction of the cervical and thoracic regions to T9 are associated with remarkably little neurologic morbidity.

Tumors that are located in the lower spinal cord segments, from T9 to T12, have the greatest incidence of significant postoperative neurologic morbidity. This is because neoplasms in the conus medullaris or just above it compress or infiltrate gray matter, whereas tumors that occur in more rostral regions of the spinal cord compress white matter tracts. Therefore, the resultant signs and symptoms are based on pathologic anatomy and pathophysiology that is specific to the segmental location of the neoplasm.

Whereas an extensive intramedullary dissection may be carried out with relative impunity in white matter in the rostral cord, this is not the case in the gray matter in the region of the conus medullaris, and the surgeon must be aware of these technical limitations.

Significant preoperative sphincteric dysfunction suggests that the tumor is extending into the conus medullaris, as this rarely occurs if the tumor is rostral to T12. Conversely, the absence of bowel and bladder problems suggests that the tumor does not extend into the conus medullaris, though it may be asymptomatically expanded by a caudal cyst.

If there is not preoperative bowel and bladder dysfunction, it will occur postoperatively when the conus medullaris is disrupted. Therefore, it is essential that the myelotomy not be extended, as this invariably results in sphincter dysfunction that may be permanent.

Intraoperative ultrasonography is invaluable, as it clearly discloses the location of the conus medullaris, which may not be obvious to the surgeon as a result of distortion and rotation as well as superimposed neural elements.

It is important that the patient be advised that at least a temporary increase in neurologic dysfunction is to be expected with surgery in this area, and the authors would assume that long-term or permanent morbidity will also be significant.

Dural Substitutes

In the course of operating on 78 patients who had undergone previous surgery, the authors have had the opportunity to re-explore a variety of dural substitutes (e.g., Gelfilm, Cargile membrane, cadaver dura, Silastic). Also, in many patients, the dura was simply left open.

It has been a consistent observation that all biologic material acts as a nidus for proliferation of fibrous tissue. At the time of re-exploration, there were dense adhesions between the spinal cord, the pseudodura that replaced the biologic membrane, and the deep muscle superficial to it. As a result, the dissection was invariably tedious and prolonged. In addition, the normal anatomic landmarks along the posterior surface of the spinal cord were distorted, and there were adhesions along the lateral margins of the cord, fixing it to the dural tube.

In patients in whom Silastic was used as a dural substitute, there were no adhesions and only minimal thickening of the leptomeninges immediately beneath the Silastic (Fig. 38–7).

These observations are not intended to imply that the use of biologic materials is contraindicated or in any way deleterious to neurologic function. It is only suggested that in a patient in whom there is a likelihood of future surgery, Silastic will invariably facilitate that procedure, whereas the biologic materials will make it more difficult.

Wound Closure

Patients who have been previously irradiated are at high risk for wound dehiscence and cerebrospinal fluid fistula. In the first 14 previously irradiated patients operated on in this series, nine had problems with wound healing, and five developed men-

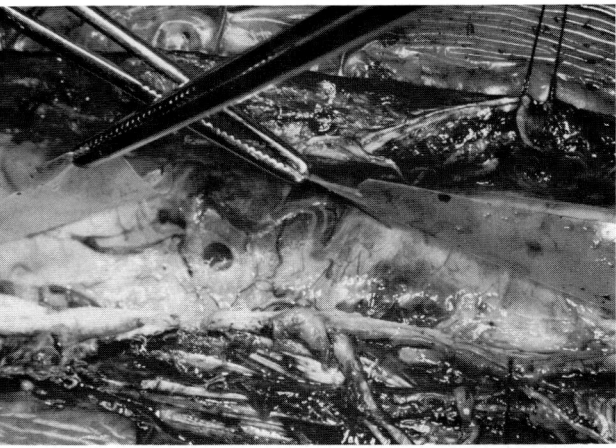

Figure 38–7. Silastic duraplasty. Note absence of adherence to spinal cord.

ingitis. Since that experience, the authors have utilized plastic surgical expertise, and muscle transposition from areas outside of the radiation fields. Although this is time-consuming, and the dissection is extensive, it has eliminated serious complications referable to wound healing. The authors view this as indispensable to procedures being carried out under these circumstances.

DISCUSSION

There are a number of important observations that are clearly relevant in terms of understanding the biology of this group of neoplasms as well as recommending proper surgical management. It has been a consistent observation that in the presence of holocord expansion, the solid component of the astrocytoma is often not as extensive as myelography alone suggests. Indeed, the actual location of the neoplasm may be in those segments of the spinal cord that correspond to neurologic dysfunction. The lack of significant neurologic dysfunction relating to spinal segments that were distended with fluid is probably directly related to the anatomic location of the cyst within the center of the cord as compared with the solid component of the neoplasm, which was relatively diffuse.

The presence of cysts that were similar in appearance to those associated with cystic astrocytoma of the cerebellum suggests that many astrocytomas are congenital tumors that have their inception sometime during gestation. The fluid produced by the tumor extends up and down the spinal cord in the region of least resistance, that is, the central canal.

One might also speculate that in some cases the classic symptoms of syringomyelia may, in fact, be a late manifestation of such a cyst in which the tumor has either involuted or is not anatomically obvious. Perhaps the centrally located cyst may gradually expand over many years and compress the surrounding cord. In this regard, it is significant that a few patients with holocord widening had exceedingly small neoplasms (between 1.5 and 3 cm) that were mistakenly diagnosed as syringomyelia or hydromyelia. The authors' experience would suggest that the presence of xanthochromic cyst fluid is pathognomonic of an associated neoplasm, whereas clear fluid is diagnostic of hydromyelia.

It is the authors' perspective that the presence of a widened spinal cord from the cervicomedullary junction to the conus medullaris, which is associated with a relatively slowly evolving neurologic deficit, is indicative of a very slowly growing tumor that may have a good long-term prognosis and should be treated aggressively.

Nevertheless, it must be emphasized that despite gross total tumor excisions, it would be naive to assume that residual tumor fragments were not commonly left in situ. The authors have hypothesized that in some patients the fragments may remain dormant or may involute in a way similar to what has been noted to occur in many astrocytomas of the cerebellum. However, whether or not this is reality or "wish-fulfillment" will only be known many years from now, following long-term follow-up and retrospective analysis.

In most cases of holocord tumor, the initial complaint was a weak arm, or a mildly weak leg, and associated pain somewhere along the spinal axis. The signs and symptoms were consistently relatively minor, when compared with the apparently diffuse nature of the pathologic process. It is perfectly understandable that neurosurgeons faced with this clinical dilemma have been most concerned about inflicting a greater neurologic deficit as a result of extensive dissection within a rather well-functioning spinal cord. This rationale has been used for a temporizing surgical approach, consisting of a limited laminectomy and biopsy and relying on radiation therapy to control tumor growth. Unfortunately, the natural history of these tumors, with radiation therapy, is slow deterioration and eventual severe neurologic disability or death.

The outcome following radical resection of these tumors was directly related to the patient's preoperative neurologic status. Although a transient increase in weakness or sensory loss was commonly present during the immediate postoperative period, only a few patients had a significant permanent increase in neurologic deficit following surgery. Patients with paraparesis or quadriparesis, who were ambulatory before surgery, had neurologic improvement over several weeks. The group with severe deficits preoperatively rarely made any significant improvement, although their downhill course abated.

There is no evidence that radiation cures benign astrocytomas of the spinal cord, and there is abundant evidence that it has a deleterious effect on the immature developing nervous system. Spinal cord neoplasms should be recognized as potentially excisable lesions, with radiation therapy being reserved for possible adjunctive use if there is a recurrence. At that time, it might be employed following a second radical surgical resection.[1, 8, 15–17, 22, 23, 26]

Intramedullary spinal cord astrocytomas are occasionally highly malignant. In these cases, the clinical course is rapid, and radical surgery has not significantly improved the dismal prognosis. Unlike cranial glioblastomas, those that occurred in the spinal cord disseminated over the entire neuraxis within six months of primary surgery.[11] For this reason, the authors now routinely employ total neuraxis irradiation in the presence of a malignant tumor.

Children who have undergone extensive laminectomy and, in addition, have denervation of the paravertebral muscles from tumor infiltration of anterior horn cells as well as operative muscle retraction are at risk for developing severe spinal deformities as they pass through periods of rapid growth. Close collaboration with a pediatric orthopedic surgeon experienced with kyphoscoliosis is essential in following these patients.[6, 37, 41]

SUMMARY

The senior author has carried out gross total excision of intramedullary spinal neoplasms in 156 consecutive patients. This experience has led to the following conclusions:

1. Holocord widening occurs in 60 percent of cases and is diagnostic of a cystic astrocytoma.
2. Radical tumor excision is compatible with partial or total recovery of neurologic function.
3. The success of surgery is directly related to the preoperative neurologic status of the patient. Paralysis or near paralysis was never improved, while mild to moderate preoperative neurologic dysfunction often improved.
4. While this experience has established the efficacy of radical surgery, there is no information to suggest the duration of remission, or the likelihood of a permanent cure. This will become known only at the time of retrospective analysis, many years from now.

References

1. Anderson FM, Carson MU: Spinal cord tumors in children. A review of the subject and representation of twenty-one cases. J Pediatr 43:190, 1953.
2. Arseni C, Horvath L, Illiescu D: Intraspinal tumors in children. Psychiatr Neurol Neurochir 70:123, 1967.
3. Banna M, Gryspaerat GL: Review article: Intraspinal tumors in children (excluding dysraphism). Radiology 22:17, 1971.
4. Bertrand B: Dynamic factors in the evolution of syringomyelia and syringobulbia. Clin Neurosurg 20:322, 1973.
5. Cairns H, Riddoch G: Observation in the treatment of ependymal gliomas of the spinal cord. Brain 14:117, 1931.

6. Catell HS, Clark GL, Jr.: Cervical kyphosis and instability following multiple laminectomies in children. J Bone Joint Surg 49:713, 1967.
7. Conway LW: Hydrodynamic studies in syringomyelia. J Neurosurg 27:501, 1967.
8. Coxe WS: Tumors of the spinal canal in children. Am Surg 27:62, 1961.
9. Craig J, Mitchell A: Spinal tumors in childhood. Arch Dis Child 6:11, 1931.
10. DeSousa AL, Kalseech JE, Mealey J, Jr., et al: Intraspinal tumors in children: A review of 31 cases. J Neurosurg 51:437, 1979.
11. Eden K: Dissemination after gliomas of the spinal cord in the leptomeninges. Brain 61:298, 1938.
12. Ellertsson AB, Greitz T: Myelocystographic and fluorescein studies to demonstrate communication between intramedullary cysts and the cerebrospinal fluid space. Acta Neurol Scand 45:418, 1969.
13. Elsberg CA: Diagnosis and Treatment of Surgical Diseases of the Spinal Cord and its Membranes. Philadelphia, W. B. Saunders Co., 1916, pp 288–289.
14. Elsberg CA, Beer R: The operability of intramedullary tumors of the spinal cord. A report of two operations with remarks upon the extrusion of intraspinal tumors. Am J Med Sci 142:636, 1911.
15. Epstein F: Spinal cord astrocytomas of childhood. In: Symon L (ed): Advances and Technical Standards in Neurosurgery, Vol. 13. Vienna, Springer-Verlag, 1986.
16. Epstein F, Epstein N: Surgical management of "holo-cord" intramedullary spinal cord astrocytomas in children. J Neurosurg 54:829, 1981.
17. Epstein F, Epstein N: Surgical treatment of spinal cord astrocytomas of childhood: A series of 19 patients. J Neurosurg 57:685, 1982.
18. Epstein F, Ragavendra N, John R, et al: Spinal cord astrocytomas of childhood, surgical adjuncts and pitfalls. In: Humphreys RP (ed): Concepts in Pediatric Neurosurgery, Vol. 5. Basel, Karger, 1985, pp 224–238.
19. Gardner WJ, Angel J: The mechanism of syringomyelia and its surgical correction. Clin Neurosurg 6:131, 1959.
20. Garrido E, Stein BM: Microsurgical removal of intramedullary spinal cord tumors. Surg Neurol 7:214, 1977.
21. Grant FC, Austin GM: The diagnosis, treatment and prognosis of tumors affecting the spinal cord in children. J Neurosurg 13:535, 1956.
22. Greenwood J: Surgical removal of intramedullary tumors. J Neurosurg 26:276, 1967.
23. Guidetti B: Intramedullary tumors of the spinal cord. Acta Neurochir 17:7, 1967.
24. Haft H, Ransohoff J, Carter S: Spinal cord tumors in children. Pediatrics 23:1152, 1959.
25. Hamby WB: Tumors in the spinal canal in childhood. J Neuropathol Exp Neurol 3:347, 1944.
26. Ingraham FD: Intraspinal tumors in infancy and childhood. Am J Surg 39:342, 1938.
27. Kernohan JW, Woltman HW, Adson AW: A review of 51 cases with an attempt at histological classification. Arch Neurol Psychiatry 25:679, 1931.
28. Kopelson G, Linggood RM, Kleinman GM, et al: Management of intramedullary spinal cord tumors. Radiology 135:473, 1980.
29. Love JG: Syringomyelia: A look at surgical therapy. J Neurosurg 24:714, 1966.
30. Mork SJ, Liken AC: Ependymoma: A follow-up study of 101 cases. Cancer 40:907, 1977.
31. Pool JL: The surgery of spinal cord tumors. Clin Neurosurg 17:310, 1970.
32. Raghavendra BN, Epstein FJ, McCleary L: The use of intraoperative ultrasound in the localization of intramedullary spinal cord tumors of childhood. Am J Neuroradiol 5:395, 1984.
33. Rasmussen TB, Kernohan JW, Adson AW: Pathologic classification with surgical consideration of intraspinal tumors. Ann Surg 3:513, 1940.
34. Reimer R, Onofrio BM: Astrocytomas of the spinal cord in children and adolescents. J Neurosurg 63:669, 1985.
35. Richardson FL: A report of 16 tumors of the spinal cord in children: The importance of spinal ridigity as an early sign of disease. J Pediatr 57:42, 1960.
36. Shenkin HA, Alpers BJ: Clinical and pathological features of gliomas of the spinal cord. Arch Neurol Psychiatry 52:87, 1944.
37. Sim FH, Svien HJ, Bicket WH, et al: Swan neck deformity following extensive laminectomy J Bone Joint Surg 49:564, 1967.
38. Singounas EG, Karvounis PC: Terminal ventriculostomy in syringomyelia. Acta Neurochir (Vienna) 46:293, 1979.
39. Stookey B: Tumors of the spinal cord in childhood. Am J Dis Child 36:1184, 1928.
40. Svien HJ, Thelen EP, Keith HM: Intraspinal tumors in children. JAMA 155:959, 1954.
41. Tachdjian MO, Matson DD: Orthopedic aspects of intraspinal tumors in infants and children. J Bone Joint Surg 47:223, 1965.
42. Wetzel N, David L: Surgical treatment of syringomyelia. Arch Surg 68:570, 1954.
43. Woltman HW, Kernohan JW, Adson AW, et al: Intramedullary tumors of the spinal cord and gliomas of the intradural portion of the filum terminale. Arch Neurol Psychiatry 65:378, 1951.
44. WorsterDrough C, Wakeley LPG, Shafar J: The surgical treatment of syringomyelia. Br J Surg 29:56, 1941.

39
EXTRAMEDULLARY SPINAL TUMORS

David M. Klein, M.D.

This chapter is concerned with extramedullary spinal neoplasms, both intradural and extradural, including paraspinal and vertebral growths that can encroach upon the neural canal in childhood. Intramedullary tumors and masses produced by developmental abnormality are considered elsewhere.

Intraspinal tumors are sufficiently rare in childhood that large experiences are seldom reported. Those series that do appear must be reviewed carefully, since they frequently include significant numbers of developmental anomalies and, even, disk protrusions.[11, 37] Although mixing such diverse entities can skew statistical conclusions, it is still possible to discern some general characteristics common to these lesions. DiLorenzo and associates[11] collected and analyzed 1234 cases of pediatric spinal neoplasm, including 56 personal cases. Not all the collected reports provide the same sorts of information. Using data from four studies, they found an average ratio of pediatric spinal to intracranial growths of 1 to 6.7. The ratio of pediatric spinal tumors to those in all age groups was 1 to 12, including ten reported series. Of the pediatric tumors, 31.4 percent were intramedullary, 24.4 percent were intradural and extramedullary, and 43.0 percent were extradural, with 1 percent transdural. During the first 15 years of life, tumors most frequently presented in the first year (12 percent), probably reflecting a large proportion of developmental masses that have been included and that are discovered in infancy.

SIGNS AND SYMPTOMS

Pain is the commonest presenting symptom of spinal tumor in adults, and subtle differences in the nature of the presenting pain are classically considered to be characteristic of the tumor's location.[21, 47] Early localized spine pain and tenderness predominate in extradural tumors; radicular pain suggests an intradural extramedullary location; and diffuse distal pain and tingling is said to be characteristic of direct spinal cord involvement. Motor symptoms usually develop later. In contrast, pain is not reported by infants who are nonverbal, and children may be unable to describe sensory differences. Changes in motor function can also be quite difficult to detect during infancy, even when severe. As a consequence, pediatric spinal tumors are frequently identified late in their course of development, with motor symptoms and findings more commonly presenting than sensory changes and with neurologic deficits often advanced by the time they are recognized.[9, 14, 22, 25, 29] There may be "nonverbal expressions of pain," such as refusal to walk or move, limitations in back motion, and irritability.[18] Among presenting symptoms in children, the commonest are weakness, then back pain, followed by bowel and bladder symptoms, spine deformity, and sensory disturbance. The commonest physical findings are reflex changes and motor deficit, then sensory changes. Paravertebral muscle spasm, torticollis, scoliosis, and spine tenderness are found less often.[22, 29] Paraspinal tumor masses may be directly palpable.

Episodes of subarachnoid hemorrhage are occasionally reported and can originate from a variety of tumors, the most common being primary or metastatic ependymoma, and neurinoma.[12, 22, 23] Both intradural and extradural spinal tumors have been associated with hydrocephalus and increased intracranial pressure, presumably resulting from increased cerebrospinal fluid (CSF) viscosity or from obstruction of CSF pathways by tumor seeding. If the spinal tumor is not recognized and is not dealt with first, shunting of this hydrocephalus can produce sudden deterioration in spinal cord function, probably because of increased impaction of the tumor against the spinal cord as CSF is drained.[24, 31, 42]

DIFFERENTIAL DIAGNOSIS

A wide range of signs and symptoms results in an extensive list of conditions with which these tumors may be confused. Chronic illness, generalized weakness, and irritability may suggest cerebral palsy, motor neuron disease, chronic malnutrition, or even functional disorders. Radicular chest or abdominal pain can mimic visceral disease. Symptoms of disseminated subarachnoid tumor can resemble those of meningitis. Presentation by subarachnoid hemorrhage or hydrocephalus, as noted earlier, can divert attention to acute intracranial possibilities. A diagnosis of idiopathic scoliosis is applied to many children, delaying discovery of an underlying tumor. Because falls are so common in childhood, an onset of back pain frequently seems to follow minor injury. In fact, incidental trauma can produce hemorrhage into an existing spinal tumor, producing a sudden increase in pain and immobility and, thus, reinforcing the impression that the injury is totally responsible for the symptoms.

Neuroblastoma and ganglioneuroma are associated with some unique and deceptive symptoms among spinal tumors. Fever is seen in 23 percent of patients.[17] Diarrhea is occasionally reported. A syndrome of ataxia, myoclonic jerks, and opsoclonus may appear, either many weeks before or concurrent with tumor presentation.[17, 45] This picture may suggest posterior fossa tumor, particularly if the neuroblastoma has not yet appeared elsewhere. The association of these symptoms with neuroblastoma is poorly understood. The manifestations differ from the cerebellar ataxia seen in adults with distant nonspecific malignancy, a phenomenon that is otherwise not observed in children. It is of historical interest to note that one of the earliest descriptions of this specific syndrome in neuroblastoma is that of Foster Kennedy, in a paper authored by Cushing and Wolbach in 1927.[7]

Among diagnostic possibilities, spinal tumor is more likely to be overlooked than to be considered too often. A high index of suspicion should be maintained, and the possibility of intraspinal tumor promptly investigated.

DIAGNOSTIC STUDIES

Nuclear magnetic resonance imaging (NMRI) is probably the best single screening procedure for masses within the neural canal. It provides excellent detail and is noninvasive. With NMRI, the entire length of the neural canal can be visualized in sagittal sections, which then can be supplemented by transverse or coronal views, as needed. In the clinic of the Children's Hospital of Buffalo, NMRI is eliminating the need for survey myelography in many cases. However, it is inadequate for the study of bone detail and must be used in conjunction with computed tomography (CT) or plain x-ray films.

Plain x-ray films of the spine show changes in approximately 50 to 70 percent of cases.[9, 22, 25, 29] Widening of pedicles, scalloping of posterior vertebral bodies, and increased anteroposterior canal diameter can indicate the presence of a long-standing mass within the canal (Fig. 39–1). Abnormal calcifications, spine deformity, congenital defects,

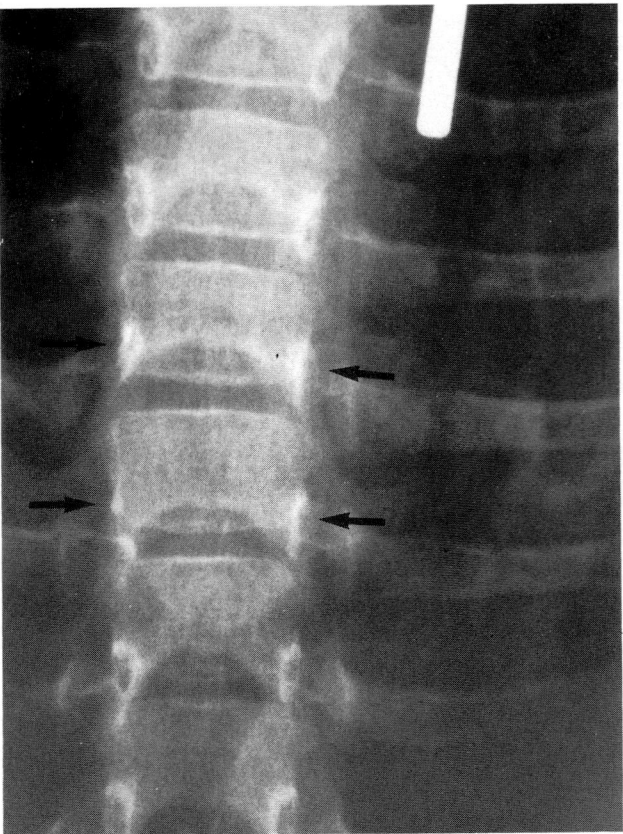

Figure 39–1. Erosion of pedicles and widened intrapedicular distance in an eight-year-old girl with intraspinal schwannoma.

erosions, enlargement of neural foramina, and paraspinal masses can be visualized (Fig. 39–2). The entire spinal column should be imaged, so that multiple lesions or associated congenital anomalies can be found. X-ray films of the chest and abdomen should be made when paraspinal extension is suspected.

Transverse CT sections provide a special dimension in the study of vertebral and paravertebral abnormalities as well as of masses within the neural canal. It is helpful to compare CT cuts made before and after intravenous contrast injection with similar sections after the injection of intrathecal contrast material (metrizamide myelography). This aids in the separate appreciation of calcification, tumor vascularity, and intraspinal encroachments.

Radionuclide bone scans are useful in detecting multiple lesions. Bone scans also aid in locating small growths that produce poorly localized pain, when these are obscured by overlapping bone shadows. Once identified, these lesions can be studied by more specific tomography.

In neuroblastoma, levels of circulating catecholamines may be elevated, as are their metabolites in the 24-hour urine specimen. Vanillylmandelic acid (VMA) and homovanillic acid (HVA) assays are commonly done. Serum ferritin may also be increased.

Myelography should be done with a water-soluble agent that does not require removal, and the procedure should not be performed until all preliminary studies are completed and reviewed. If indicated, surgery is arranged to follow the myelogram promptly, so that the spinal fluid decompression produced by thecal puncture does not increase impaction of the tumor against the spinal cord, causing an advance in deficit. In smaller children, surgery is planned to follow myelography, with the patient being kept under anesthesia. If the subarachnoid space cannot be entered by lumbar puncture (if no CSF backflow is obtained) or if a total block to upward flow is demonstrated on initial myelographic films, a cisternal puncture is made, and contrast material is injected from above. This ensures that multiple lesions or the full length of a single lesion is properly appreciated. NMRI and CT scans are carefully studied before a commitment is made to myelography. This helps in planning the myelogram and the surgery to follow. Attending physicians, house staff, and radiologists should be warned against performing incidental spinal punctures.

INTRADURAL EXTRAMEDULLARY TUMORS

When developmental masses and exophytic intramedullary tumors are not considered, by far the commonest intradural lesions in children are metastatic, the result of seeding through CSF pathways. This is in striking contrast to the situation in adults, in whom more than half of intradural tumors are meningiomas or nerve sheath tumors and are benign.

Meningiomas and Nerve Sheath Tumors

The origin of nerve sheath tumors remains in dispute, and the nomenclature (neurofibromas, neurinomas, schwannomas, neurilemomas) is confusing. In order to simplify discussion, the term "nerve sheath tumors" will be used here to refer to all growths arising from peripheral nerve or nerve root sheaths, whether intradural or extradural and whether associated with neurofibromatosis or not.

Among 1322 intraspinal tumors occurring in patients of all ages, Sloof and associates[44] at the Mayo Clinic found 29 percent to be nerve sheath tumors and 25.5 percent to be meningiomas. A total of 85 percent of the meningiomas and 62 percent of the nerve sheath tumors were totally intradural. Nerve sheath tumors were most common in the cervical and lumbar regions and in males, whereas meningiomas were most common in the thoracic area, and approximately 80 percent of these tumors were in females. In contrast, Fortuna and coworkers[16] found 136 nerve sheath tumors (10.9 percent) and 54 meningiomas (4.3 percent) among 1242 pediatric tumors in collected reports. A total of 63 percent of childhood nerve sheath tumors were in males, and there was a similar preponderance with meningiomas, contrary to the adult statistics. The duration of symptoms prior to discovery averaged between

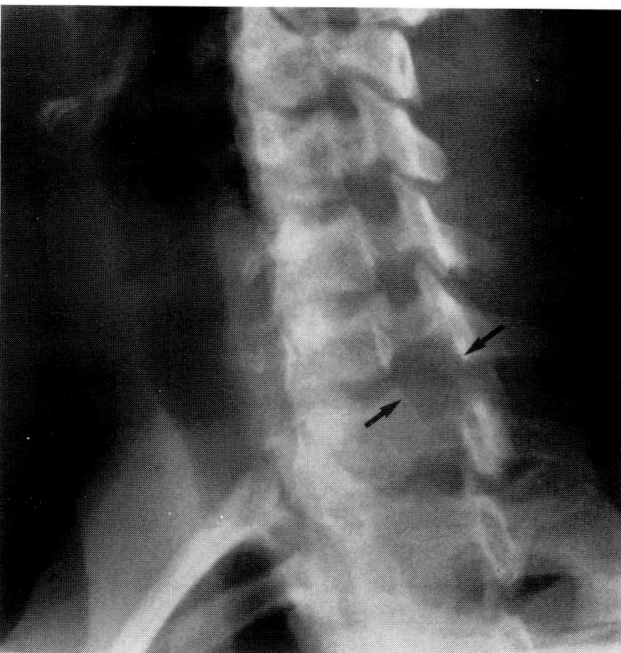

Figure 39–2. Oblique view of the cervical spine in a 15-year-old boy demonstrates an enlarged C6–7 foramen produced by a dumbbell tumor at this level.

9 and 12 months for these tumors in children, compared with several years in adults. Among children, both of these tumors were most likely to appear between the ages of 10 and 15 years, and both tumors were frequently associated with multiple neurofibromatosis (von Recklinghausen's disease) in these children. Since these tumors more often appear in the older child, it is not surprising to find that 70 percent of meningiomas and 79.5 percent of nerve sheath tumors in this series presented first with pain rather than paresis. Of 45 pediatric nerve sheath tumors, 52 percent were intradural, 29 percent were extradural, and 19 percent were transdural ("dumbbell" configuration).[16] Dumbbell meningiomas have not been reported in children. Therefore, continuity with any extradural extension is suggestive of nerve sheath tumor. Enlargement of neural foramina also suggests nerve sheath tumor, but this enlargement can be seen in neurofibromatosis without the presence of tumor. Because of the strong association of multiple lesions with neurofibromatosis, a careful search for multiple lesions should be made whenever an intraspinal tumor is suspected to be a meningioma or a nerve sheath tumor. Meningioma more often shows calcification.

The treatment of choice is laminectomy and total tumor removal, if this is possible. Extensive foraminotomy and, at times, secondary paraspinal exploration may be necessary to extirpate dumbbell tumors. Nerve sheath tumors are not radiosensitive; there have been mixed results in the experience with radiation therapy in a few cases of spinal meningiomas in children.[9, 28] As with their intracranial counterparts, spinal meningiomas in this age group can show malignant degeneration. Nerve sheath tumors can also undergo malignant change, particularly in adolescents with von Recklinghausen's disease.

Case 1

A nine-year-old girl was admitted to the Children's Hospital of Buffalo for evaluation of gradually increasing weakness and clumsiness in all extremities. The problem was vaguely attributed to a fall she sustained while rollerskating three months earlier. There was no headache, neck pain, or subjective sensory loss. The patient's mother had neurofibromatosis.

Examination showed a swayback posture and generalized weakness with rapid fatigue of all muscle groups. The weakness in the upper extremities seemed worse in distal than proximal muscle groups, while lower-extremity weakness was not localized. She shuffled and stumbled when walking, without lateralization. All deep tendon reflexes were reduced in amplitude. Plantar responses were extensor bilaterally. There was bilateral hypalgesia to pinprick in C5 and C6 dermatomes. Multiple café-au-lait spots and several depigmented areas were found on the skin. The spine showed no tenderness or limitation of motion.

Spinal x-ray films showed an enlargement of the C6–7 foramina bilaterally. Sagittal NMRI spinal survey revealed an extramedullary mass encroaching on the spinal cord at the C1–4 level, and coronal sections were then made to further delineate the lesion. Transverse CT sections through the area showed the mass to be calcific and the surrounding bone structures to be uninvolved (Fig. 39–3). A diagnosis of en plaque meningioma at C1–4 was made from this combination of images, and the diagnosis was confirmed at surgery. Additional preoperative studies, including radionuclide bone scan, cranial CT and NMRI, and metrizamide-enhanced myelogram done one hour prior to laminectomy showed no other tumors. Therefore, the bone abnormalities at C6–7 were judged to be dysplastic, in association with neurofibromatosis.

Prompt neurologic improvement followed tumor removal. The child is being followed carefully for any sign of secondary cervical spine deformity.

Metastases to the Subarachnoid Space

Metastases from distant malignancy to the spinal subarachnoid space are rare at any age, but seeding along the CSF pathways from primary intracranial tumors, so-called drop metastases, are common in childhood. A high incidence of implantable tumor, such as ependymoma and medulloblastoma, and their location within ventricles or cisterns appear to be significant factors. Deutsch and Reigel[10] found 44 percent of children with newly diagnosed medulloblastomas to have asymptomatic spinal cord involvement on myelogram. Svien and colleagues[49] found an incidence of 31.6 percent of such spinal metastases in patients dying of ependymomas.

Other primitive neuroectodermal tumors, germinomas, and choroid plexus papillomas also frequently seed in this fashion. Drop metastases are reported in children with low-grade cerebellar astrocytomas, cerebral and brainstem glioblastomas, oligodendrogliomas, neuroblastomas, retinoblastomas, lymphomas, and rhabdomyosarcomas.[3, 13, 15, 38, 43, 46, 50] Myxopapillary ependymoma, an intramedullary spinal tumor of childhood, can spread upward through the CSF system.[5, 8] Not all such metastases follow surgical disturbance of the tumor. Many are asymptomatic and are found on incidental routine myelogram. In other cases, these lesions may be the mode by which the primary brain tumor presents. Pezeshkpour and associates[34] report 18 such cases from the files of the Armed Forces Institute of Pathology. Although the age distribution in their tumor registry is not stated, it is interesting to note that 9 of these 18 cases were in patients younger than 18 years age. Eight of the pediatric patients had primitive neuroectodermal tumors, and one had a germinoma. Back pain, neck pain, and weakness were predominant symptoms.[34]

Most metastases of this type are multiple (Fig. 39–4). They are more frequently found over the dorsal than the ventral surface of the cord. Occa-

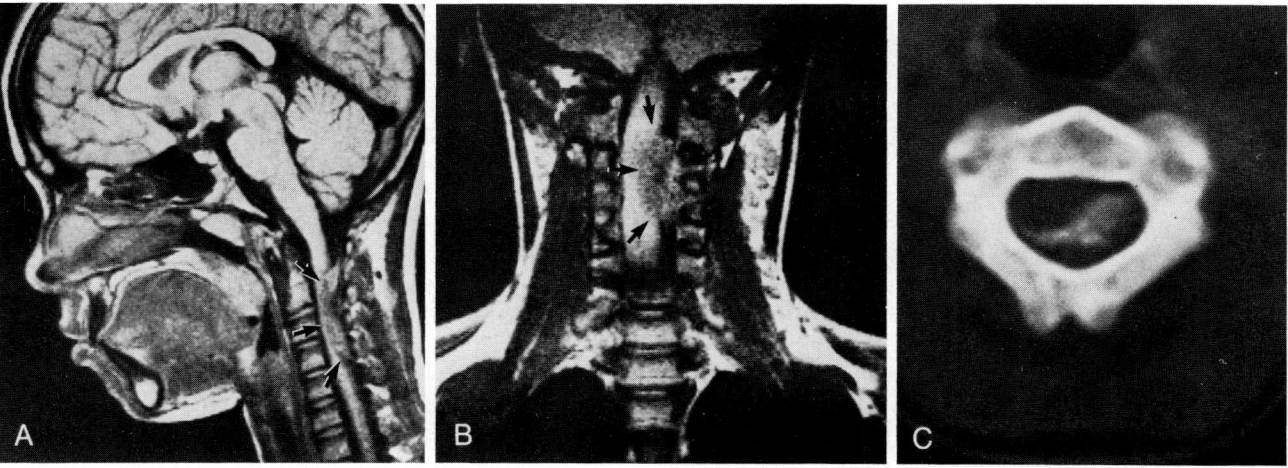

Figure 39–3. Neuroimaging results in case 1 (see text). A and B, Midsagittal and coronal nuclear magnetic resonance (NMR) imaging sections show a mass lesion deflecting the spinal cord anteriorly and to the right. The coronal section clearly shows the tumor's broad-based attachment to spinal dura and adjacent soft tissues. C, CT sections without contrast injection demonstrate that the mass is diffusely calcified and is probably extramedullary, since it outlines the displaced spinal cord discretely. It does not appear to involve surrounding bone.

sionally, the tumor encases the spinal cord over several segments, producing an appearance of cord widening on myelogram, rather than one of discrete nodulation. CSF cytology is not always positive. The use of serial transverse CT sections in conjunction with metrizamide injection can improve the detection of both types of tumor.

Since these metastases may call for changes in treatment, surgical exploration can be indicated for solitary lesions whose nature is uncertain. Surgery can also be helpful in rare instances of solitary subarachnoid metastasis refractory to other treatments and producing advancing neurologic impairment.

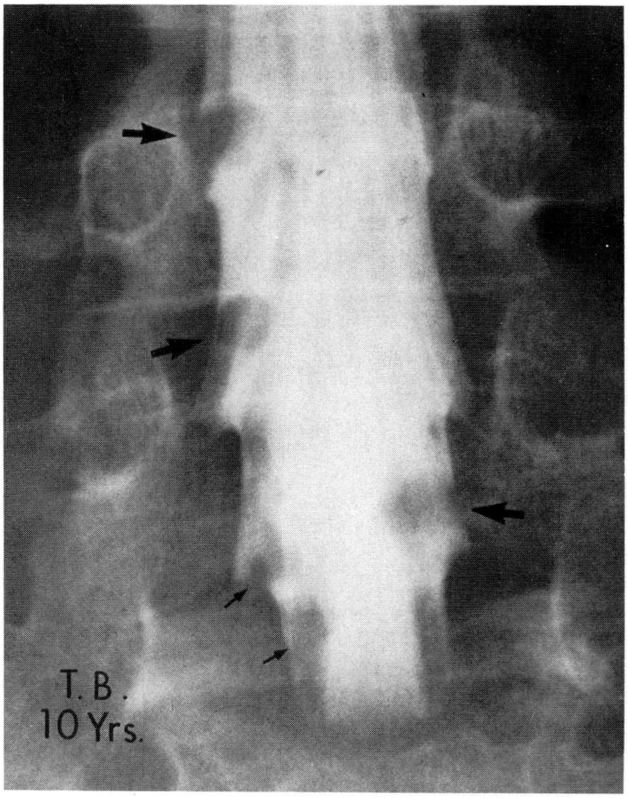

EXTRADURAL ENCROACHMENT

Primary Tumors of Bone

Of the many tumors originating in bone, few are sufficiently common in the pediatric spine to warrant discussion here. The common denominator among such tumors is the ability to encroach upon the neural canal and its contents.

Osteoblastomas

This benign tumor is characteristically encountered in children and particularly in adolescents. The tumor is commoner in males and in posterior vertebral elements. X-ray films show mottled areas of expansion that are both lytic and sclerotic, enlarging normal vertebral elements and spreading into surrounding soft tissues (Fig. 39–5). Gross tumor tissue is soft, solid, somewhat granular, and highly vascular. Even subtotal excision is usually curative, and recurrence should inspire a careful review of histology for the possibility of malignancy.

Aneurysmal Bone Cysts

This condition is probably not neoplastic. The etiology is unknown. It is characterized by the development of a solitary cystic mass, whose thin calcific walls are continuous with adjacent bony cortex. The central cavity is filled with liquid blood, a meshwork of fibro-osseous tissue, giant cells, and

Figure 39–4. Subarachnoid "drop metastases," from supratentorial ependymoma. Metrizamide-enhanced myelogram.

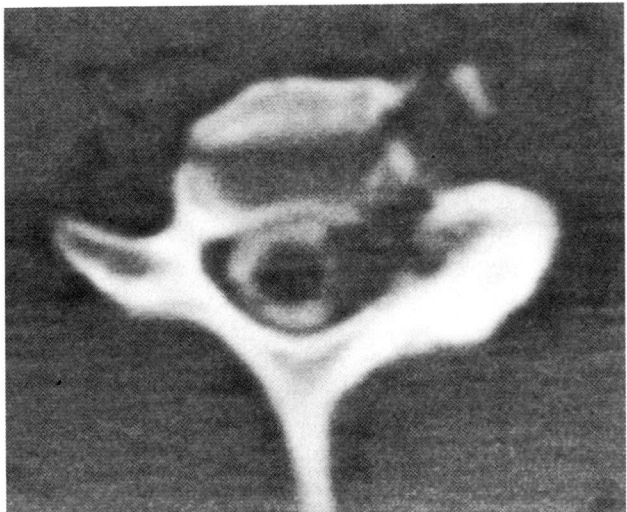

Figure 39–5. Benign osteoblastoma in a 16-year-old boy with cervicobrachial pain. CT following metrizamide-enhanced myelogram demonstrates cross-sectional extent of the expansile lesion in the lamina and pedicle, the partially calcified soft tumor in the extradural space, and the extent of dural compression. Gross total removal of the epidural mass and involved bone can result in cure.

phagocytes. The cyst resembles osteoblastoma in its adolescent predominance, localized expansion, and frequency in posterior spinal elements. Radiographically there is a "blow-out" expansion of normal bone into a paper-thin calcific wall containing occasional trabeculae (Fig. 39–6). CT is particularly helpful in identifying cyst margins and the hemorrhagic central content.[41] In a collection of 71 patients for whom there was adequate information, Hay and associates[19] reported local pain to be the presenting symptom in 72 percent, and a palpable mass in 23 percent. A total of 29 percent had evidence of spinal cord compression, and 18 percent had evidence of root compression.[19] A sudden increase in symptoms or neurologic deficit may be seen, apparently as a result of acute expansion; therefore, treatment should be carried out promptly after this diagnosis is made.[1]

Treatment is by excision or fenestration of the cystic cavity and thorough curettement of its contents, a procedure that is characteristically accompanied by profuse hemorrhage. This usually responds to packing and pressure for a few minutes. Where removal or curettement is incomplete, radiation therapy has been used effectively. Recurrences generally present within 12 months after treatment.[1] However, patients should be followed carefully beyond this time, since vertebral collapse or spine deformity can develop after these lesions heal.

Chordomas

Chordoma probably arises from notochordal remnants. It is occasionally reported in children, developing in the sacrococcygeal area, where it can enlarge to encroach upon the neural canal. The tumor produces slowly advancing signs and symptoms of cauda equina compression. Destruction of bony architecture is seen on x-ray films. CT scanning has been the most helpful imaging technique in delineating the bony involvement. NMRI is useful in assessing extension into soft tissues and in providing a view of the tumor in the sagittal plane.[33] The preferred treatment is total excision. Radiation therapy has been of benefit where resection is incomplete. The tumor grows slowly, and recurrences may appear even after many years. Metastases do occur and may precede surgical intervention. Chemotherapy has not been helpful.[32, 39, 48]

Secondary Epidural Tumors

Secondary tumors encroaching upon the epidural space include blood-borne metastases to adjacent bone, ingrowth of tumors primarily involving paraspinal structures, and those uncommon metastases appearing to develop directly within the dura or epidural tissues. Approximately 3 percent of children with systemic cancer develop spinal cord

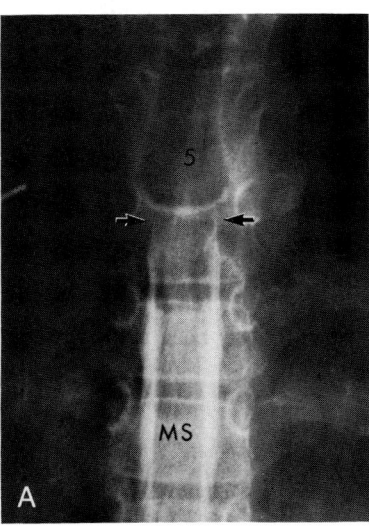
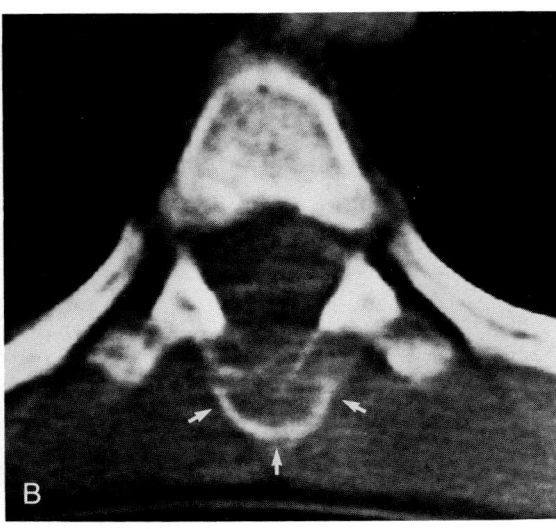

Figure 39–6. An aneurysmal bone cyst producing acute paraplegia in a seven-year-old boy. *A,* Metrizamide-enhanced myelogram shows a total block to upward flow (arrows) just below the cystlike lesion seen at T5. *B,* A CT section following metrizamide injection shows no contrast material passing into the affected level, where the neural canal is filled by the lesion. The shell-like "cyst" wall can be appreciated, expanded in the posterior vertebral elements. Emergency laminectomy was followed by excellent neurologic recovery.

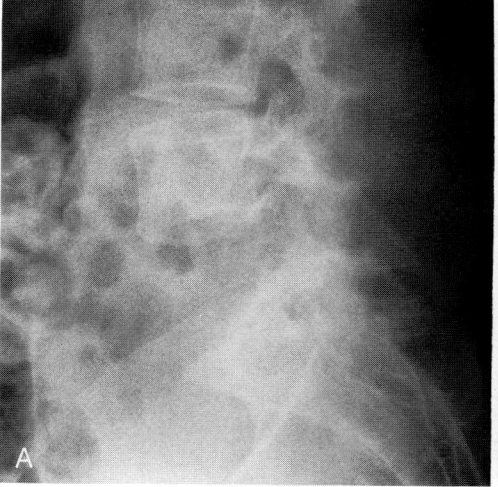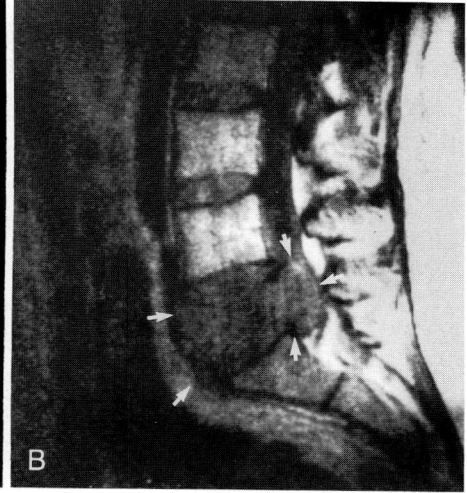

Figure 39–7. Osteosarcoma of the femur, metastatic to the lumbar spine. *A*, Plain lateral x-ray film shows almost complete erosion of L5 body. *B*, Sagittal NMR image provides better appreciation of the tumor's extent and explains the patient's radicular pain.

compression by tumor, almost all of this by epidural encroachment. Sarcomas, neuroblastomas, lymphomas, and leukemias are most common, in that general order of frequency.[6, 27]

Sarcomas

Ewing's sarcoma and osteogenic sarcoma usually originate in long bones. Metastases to the spine are infrequent and generally occur in the late stages of these diseases (Fig. 39–7). Rhabdomyosarcoma, which is the most common soft-tissue malignancy in infants and children, frequently originates in "parameningeal" sites, including the orbit, nasopharynx, middle ear, mastoid, and infratemporal fossa. Primary tumors are also common in the genitourinary tract, retroperitoneal tissues, and the extremities. The tumor can extend directly into the neural canal from paraspinal locations, may metastasize through the blood stream, and is also observed to spread through the subarachnoid pathways from parameningeal sites of origin (Fig. 39–8).[17, 38] The outlook for these tumors is usually quite poor by the time they have spread to the spinal column.

Neuroblastomas and Ganglioneuromas

This unique spectrum of tumors, derived from the autonomic nervous system, is important in infancy and childhood. Neuroblastoma is the most common intra-abdominal malignancy in children, with approximately half of these arising from the adrenal gland and half from other intra-abdominal sites, including paravertebral sympathetic ganglia and autonomic primordia buried in other organs. Approximately 14 percent originate in the thorax. About 0.3 percent seem to develop directly from primordia in the extradural space.[17] These tumors range from highly malignant neuroblastomas to benign and sessile ganglioneuromas, and intermediate grades may be of mixed histology. Neuroblas-

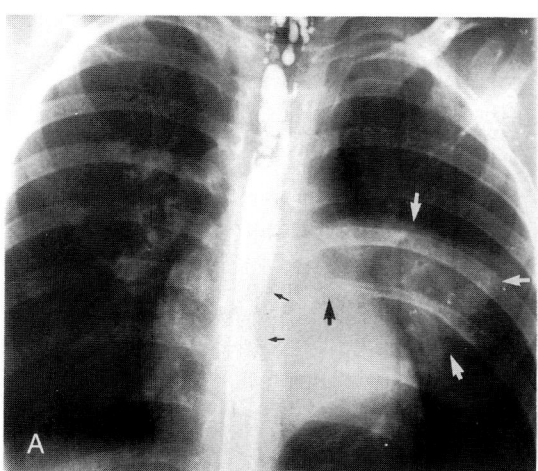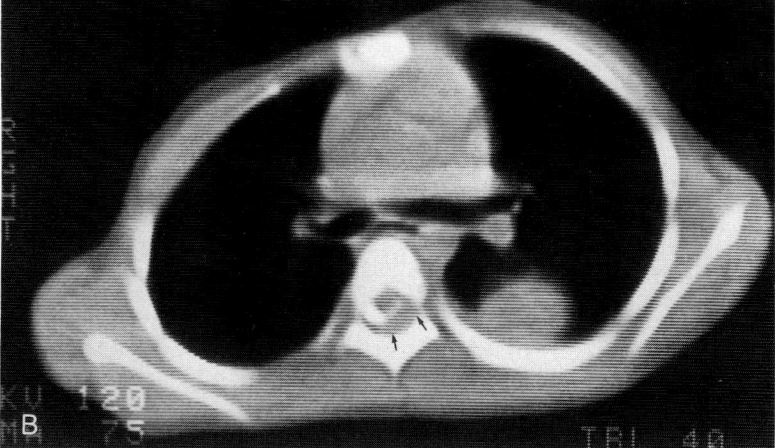

Figure 39–8. Mediastinal tumors with secondary extradural encroachment can be demonstrated by several techniques. *A*, Neuroblastoma with typical chest mass (white arrows) and rib erosion (large black arrow), growing into neural canal (small black arrows). *B*, Rhabdomyosarcoma of the left posterior chest wall is seen on CT following metrizamide-enhanced myelogram to be compressing dural contents contralaterally. In both cases, extradural encroachment was symptomatic at the time it was identified.

toma shows the unique ability to undergo maturation toward ganglioneuroma, either spontaneously or following radiation therapy and chemotherapy. Tumor maturation or involution may involve the primary tumor or metastases, and since histologic maturity is associated with superior survival, prognosis is considered more favorable for patients whose tumors contain mature ganglion cells. The outlook is considerably better with presentation earlier in infancy rather than later in childhood.

Because these tumors commonly originate in the sympathetic chain, they frequently grow in a dumbbell configuration as they extend through vertebral foramina into the epidural space. Therefore, skeletal changes can include not only those ordinarily seen with chronic intraspinal masses but also erosion of rib heads and vertebral transverse processes, and enlargement of vertebral foramina (Fig. 39–8). The tumor occasionally shows punctate or arcuate calcifications. Infants and children with demonstrated paraspinal tumors frequently have an asymptomatic extension of tumor into the neural canal. Armstrong and associates[2] found neural symptoms in only 6 of 11 patients (55 percent) who subsequently had positive myelograms. Any child found to harbor a paraspinal mass of unknown origin should have CT and NMRI sections made through the involved area, and myelography should be performed thereafter if additional information is called for.

Treatment

Just as in adults, current evidence suggests that compressive epidural tumors in children do as well with radiation therapy and chemotherapy alone as with surgical decompression followed by these modalities.[4, 6, 27, 35, 51] Chemotherapy alone has been suggested as an alternative to laminectomy and irradiation, but this method remains to be proved.[20] For neuroblastoma, prognosis seems to be more clearly related to the age at onset and the stage to which the disease has spread than it is to the extent of any surgery performed.[17, 35, 51] Nonetheless, many authorities still advocate as complete a removal of tumor as is possible in this condition, and the intraspinal portion of this tumor can lend itself to gross total removal in many instances.

When staged removal of a dumbbell tumor is indicated, it is generally best to attack the intraspinal portion first, leaving a marker at the lateral-most extent of the dissection. This avoids traction on tumor tissue and neural structures that can produce covert epidural hemorrhage, if dissection is first made in the paraspinal area. Surgery for epidural tumor is otherwise limited to situations in which the diagnosis is not known, the tumor is not sensitive to other treatment modalities, or neurologic deterioration progresses in the face of such treatment. Surgery in these cases must be tailored to achieve optimal decompression of the spinal cord. Laminectomy per se is frequently inadequate; a lateral or anterior spinal approach may be necessary to provide significant relief. At the same time, care must be taken to ensure satisfactory spinal stability and posture. In a growing child, instrumentation over many spinal segments should be avoided if possible; stabilization by fusion over short segments is preferable.

NEUROSURGICAL MANAGEMENT

Classic laminectomy for intradural tumors is best performed with the patient prone. For any position elected, careful attention must be given to the use of warming blankets and the interposition of padding over bony prominences, particularly with paralyzed extremities. In infants, when a horseshoe facerest is used rather than skull pin fixation, the face should also be carefully padded. Adhesive-backed sheets of plastic sponge are convenient for this purpose and can be cut to fit over the entire face, leaving exit space for oral and nasal tubes. Magnification, extradural ultrasonic exploration, and continuous monitoring of spinal evoked potentials can be helpful. Whenever possible, surgery is carefully planned in conjunction with the pediatric oncologist and orthopedist, for optimal results appropriate to long-term prognosis.

SECONDARY SPINAL DEFORMITY

The child who has been treated for intraspinal tumor is at significant risk for the development of spinal deformity and must be observed carefully for this on a long-term basis. Axial deformity may be a direct consequence of vertebral involvement by tumor, it may result from asymmetric paralysis, or it may follow laminectomy or irradiation. Associated congenital anomalies may also be significant.

Growth can be arrested in immature cartilage and bone by irradiation. When delivered symmetrically to an entire vertebra, radiation arrests growth evenly in all areas, producing a dwarfed vertebral body, without significant deformity. On the other hand, radiation delivered to one side of the vertebral column inhibits growth there, so that this area is foreshortened relative to the contralateral vertebral column. Deformity therefore progresses most during periods of rapid growth and may not become significant until adolescence. Deformity is reported to occur in 70 to 75 percent of children after spinal irradiation for Wilms's tumor or neuroblastoma, when these patients have had no spinal surgery performed.[26, 30, 40]

Laminectomy alone may give rise to significant deformity in children. Yasuoka and associates[52] reviewed the records of 58 patients younger than 25 years of age undergoing multilevel laminectomy for conditions ordinarily not associated with spinal deformity. Deformity developed in 46 percent of patients younger than 15 years of age and in only 6 percent of those older than this age. An abnormality was noted in 100 percent of the children after cervical laminectomy, in 36 percent after thoracic laminectomy, and in no patients following lumbar laminectomy.[52] The deformities that develop after laminectomies are usually kyphotic, with anterior vertebral wedging. Increased mobility and anterior subluxation are also found on x-ray films. Raimondi and associates[36] have suggested that laminectomy destroys posterior supporting structures that are essential to the maintenance of neuromuscular balance. They believe that the problem can be prevented by the removal of a free laminar flap over the intraspinal lesion, with replacement of this flap of attached posterior elements at the conclusion of intraspinal surgery.[36] The long-term efficacy of this technique remains to be determined.

References

1. Ameli NO, Abbassioun K, Saleh H, et al: Aneurysmal bone cysts of the spine. J Neurosurg 63:685, 1985.
2. Armstrong EA, Harwood-Nash D, Ritz CR, et al: CT of neuroblastomas and ganglioneuromas in children. Am J Roentgenol 139:571, 1982.
3. Arseni C, Horvath L, Carp N, et al: Spinal dissemination following operation on cerebral oligodendroglioma. Acta Neurochir 37:125, 1977.
4. Baten M, Vannucci RC: Intraspinal metastatic disease in childhood cancer. J Pediatr 90:207, 1977.
5. Chan HS, Becker LE, Hoffman HJ, et al: Myxopapillary ependymoma of the filum terminale and cauda equina in childhood: Report of seven cases and review of the literature. Neurosurgery 14:204, 1984.
6. Ch'ien LT, Kalwinsky DK, Peterson G, et al: Metastatic epidural tumors in children. Med Pediatr Oncol 10:455, 1982.
7. Cushing H, Wolbach SB: The transformation of a malignant paravertebral sympathicoblastoma into a benign ganglioneuroma. Am J Pathol 3:203, 1927.
8. Davis C, Barnard RO: Malignant behavior of myxopapillary ependymoma. Report of three cases. J Neurosurg 62:925, 1985.
9. DeSousa AL, Kalsbeck JE, Mealey J, et al: Intraspinal tumors in children. J Neurosurg 51:437, 1979.
10. Deutsch M, Reigel DH: Myelography and cytology in the treatment of medulloblastoma. Int J Radiat Oncol Biol Phys 7:721, 1981.
11. DiLorenzo N, Giuffre R, Fortuna A: Primary spinal neoplasms in childhood: Analysis of 1234 published cases (including 56 personal cases) by pathology, sex, age and site. Differences from the situation in adults. Neurochirurgia 25:153, 1982.
12. Djindjian M, Djindjian R, Houdart R, et al: Subarachnoid hemorrhage due to intraspinal tumors. Surg Neurol 9:223, 1978.
13. Erlich SS, Davis RL: Spinal subarachnoid metastasis from primary intracranial glioblastoma multiforme. Cancer 42:2854, 1978.
14. Farwell JR, Dohrmann GJ: Intraspinal neoplasms in children. Paraplegia 15:262, 1977–78.
15. Firsching R, Schroder R, Koning W, et al: Spinale abtropfmetastase beim cerebralen glioblastom/gliosarkom. Nervenarzt 56:629, 1985.
16. Fortuna A, Nolletti A, Nardi P, et al: Spinal neurinomas and meningiomas in children. Acta Neurochir 55:329, 1981.
17. Green DM: Diagnosis and Management of Malignant Solid Tumors in Infants and Children. Boston, Martinus Nijhoff, 1985.
18. Hahn YS, McLone DG: Pain in children with spinal cord tumors. Child's Brain 11:36, 1984.
19. Hay MC, Paterson D, Taylor TKF: Aneurysmal bone cysts of the spine. J Bone Joint Surg 60:406, 1978.
20. Hayes FA, Thompson EI, Hvizdala E, et al: Chemotherapy as an alternative to laminectomy and radiation in the management of epidural tumor. J Pediatr 104:221, 1984.
21. Haymaker W: Bing's Local Diagnosis in Neurological Diseases. St. Louis, C. V. Mosby, 1976.
22. Hendrick EB: Spinal cord tumors in children. In: Youmans JR (ed): Neurological Surgery. Philadelphia, W. B. Saunders Co., 1982, pp 3215–3221.
23. Iob I, Andrioli GC, Rigobello L, et al: An unusual onset of a spinal cord tumour: Subarachnoid bleeding and papilloedema. Case report. Neurochirurgia 23:112, 1980.
24. Jooma R, Hayward RD: Upward spinal coning: Impaction of occult spinal tumours following relief of hydrocephalus. J Neurol Neurosurg Psychiatry 47:386, 1984.
25. Jorgensen J, Niels O, Poulsen JO: Intraspinal tumors in the first two decades of life. Acta Orthop Scand 47:391, 1976.
26. Katzman H, Waugh T, Berdon W: Skeletal changes following irradiation of childhood tumors. J Bone Joint Surg 51:825, 1969.
27. Lewis DW, Packer RJ, Raney B, et al: Incidence, presentation and outcome of spinal cord disease in children with systemic cancer. Pediatrics 78:438, 1986.
28. Liu HC, DeArmond SJ, Edwards MSB: An unusual spinal meningioma in a child: Case report. Neurosurgery 17:313, 1985.
29. Matson DD: Neurosurgery of Infancy and Childhood. Springfield, IL, Charles C Thomas, 1969.
30. Mayfield JK, Riseborough EJ, Jaffe N, et al: Spinal deformity in children treated for neuroblastoma. J Bone Joint Surg 63:183, 1981.
31. Oi S, Raimondi AJ: Hydrocephalus associated with intraspinal neoplasms in childhood. Am J Dis Child 135:1122, 1981.
32. O'Neill P, Bell BA, Miller JD, et al: Fifty years of experience with chordomas in southeast Scotland. Neurosurgery 16:166, 1985.
33. Pettersson H, Hudson T, Hamlin D, et al: Magnetic resonance imaging of sacrococcygeal tumors. Acta Radiol [Diagn](Stockh) 26:161, 1985.
34. Pezeshkpour GH, Henry JM, Armbrustmacher VW: Spinal metastases. A rare mode of presentation of brain tumors. Cancer 54:353, 1984.
35. Punt J, Pritchard J, Pincott JR, et al: Neuroblastoma: A review of 21 cases presenting with spinal cord compression. Cancer 45:3095, 1980.
36. Raimondi AJ, Gutierrez FA, DiRocco C: Laminotomy and total reconstruction of the posterior spinal arch for spinal canal surgery in childhood. J Neurosurg 45:555, 1976.
37. Rand RW, Rand CW: Intraspinal Tumors of Childhood. Springfield, IL, Charles C Thomas, 1960.
38. Raney RB: Spinal cord "drop metastases" from head and neck rhabdomyosarcoma: Proceedings of the tumor board of the Children's Hospital of Philadelphia. Med Pediatr Oncol 4:3, 1978.
39. Rich TA, Schiller A, Suit HD, et al: Clinical and pathological review of 48 cases of chordoma. Cancer 56:182, 1985.
40. Riseborough EJ, Grabias SL, Burton RL, et al: Skeletal alterations following irradiation for Wilms's tumor. J Bone Joint Surg 58:526, 1976.
41. Schaffer L, Kranzler LI, Siqueira EB: Aneurysmal bone cyst of the spine. A case report. Spine 10:390, 1985.
42. Schijman E, Zuccaro G, Monges JA: Spinal tumors and hydrocephalus. Child's Brain 8:401, 1981.
43. Shapiro K, Shulman K: Spinal cord seeding from cerebellar astrocytomas. Child's Brain 2:177, 1976.
44. Sloof JL, Kernohan JW, MacCarty CS: Primary Intramedullary Tumors of the Spinal Cord and Filum Terminale. Philadelphia, W. B. Saunders Co., 1964.

45. Solomon GE, Chutorian AM: Opsoclonus and occult neuroblastoma. N Engl J Med 279:475, 1968.
46. Stanley P, Senac MO, Segall HD: Intraspinal seeding from intracranial tumors in children. AJR 144:157, 1985.
47. Stern WE: Localization and diagnosis of spinal cord tumors. Clin Neurosurg 25:480, 1978.
48. Sundaresan N, Galicich JH, Chu FCH, et al: Spinal chordomas. J Neurosurg 50:312, 1979.
49. Svien H, Gates EM, Kernohan JW: Spinal subarachnoid implantation associated with ependymoma. Arch Neurol Psychiatry 62:847, 1949.
50. Tomita T: Asymptomatic leptomeningeal dissemination of tumor to the spinal cord: Report of three cases. Neurosurgery 14:323, 1984.
51. Traggis DG, Filler RM, Druckman H, et al: Prognosis for children with neuroblastoma presenting with paralysis. J Pediatr Surg 12:419, 1977.
52. Yasuoka S, Peterson HA, MacCarty CS: Incidence of spinal column deformity after multilevel laminectomy in children and adults. J Neurosurg 57:441, 1982.

40
PHAKOMATOSES: SURGICAL CONSIDERATIONS

Luis Schut, M.D.
Ann-Christine Duhaime, M.D.
Leslie N. Sutton, M.D.

The phakomatoses, or neurocutaneous syndromes, are a group of genetic disorders having in common neurologic, ocular, and dermatologic manifestations. The term "phakomatosis" was used by van der Hoeve in 1923 to link various conditions in which birth marks, eye lesions, and tumors are found.[56] Since that time, the list of syndromes showing these features has lengthened, as has our understanding of the genetics and pathophysiology of each entity.

The phakomatoses are of interest to the neurosurgeon for several reasons. First, clues to the genesis, etiology, and biology of central nervous system (CNS) lesions, particularly tumors, can be garnered from the study of diseases in which they can be predicted to occur at a high frequency. Second, indications and goals for surgery may be different in a case of a neurocutaneous disorder than in a sporadic case. Finally, an understanding of the natural history and genetics of the disease is critical to the care of the patient as well as the family. This is particularly true in children, as these diseases tend to be progressive. Thus, the diagnosis of a genetic neurocutaneous disorder may not be obvious unless a high index of suspicion is maintained.

NEUROFIBROMATOSIS

The most common of the phakomatoses, neurofibromatosis (NF), is an autosomal dominant disorder occurring in 1 in 3000 births. Approximately half of all patients have a positive family history, suggesting a relatively high new mutation rate.[10] Whether a "maternal effect" exists, resulting in an increased disease severity in the offspring of affected mothers, remains disputed.[21, 27, 46]

Frederick Daniel von Recklinghausen introduced the term "multiple neurofibromatosis" in 1882 in a description of two patients with cutaneous neurofibromas and suggested that the tumors were composed of nervous elements.[58] It is currently believed that the disease is a disorder of neuroectodermal and mesodermal tissues in which dysplasia and neoplasia occur. Since many of the affected tissues, including nerve cells, glia, Schwann's cells, melanocytes, and some visceral or endocrine organs, are derived from the embryonic neural crest, it has been postulated that neurofibromatosis represents a disorder of neural crest differentiation. The "neurocristopathy" theory of Boland[6] and Weston[61] is an attempt to relate the findings in this disease to abnormalities in migration, cellular regulation, and cell-to-cell interactions among neural crest tissues. In addition, abnormalities in nerve growth factor, both during tissue differentiation and later in life, has been postulated as an etiologic factor in the disease.[27, 30] The yet incompletely understood relationship between a genetic defect in cell regulation and the occurrence of malignancy remains an intriguing window into cancer mechanisms in general.

Two forms of neurofibromatosis have been described, although considerable overlap is seen between the types. The peripheral form is characterized by numerous cutaneous tumors and café-au-lait spots, while the central form consists of multiple CNS tumors, particularly bilateral acoustic neuromas. These two distinct but related types of neurofibromatosis have been hypothesized to represent different alleles at a single gene focus.[27] The precise genetics of these diseases are not yet fully understood.

Clinical Manifestations in Children

Because neurofibromatosis is a disease with variable penetrance and varied manifestations, the diagnosis in a given individual may be difficult. This is particularly true in children because the cutaneous stigmata often occur later in life. Nonetheless, the most common cutaneous finding is the well-known café-au-lait spot. In adults the so-called "Crowe criteria" can be applied so that the presence of six or more spots of least 1.5 cm in diameter is considered diagnostic of the disease.[9] For children, the Whitehouse modification makes five or more spots of at least 0.5 cm diagnostic.[62] Axillary freckling may also be seen.

Neurofibromas are benign tumors containing Schwann's cells, fibroblasts, collagen, and other elements.[48] In children, they are usually sessile, subcutaneous masses but increase in size and number with puberty and pregnancy and often become pedunculated. These tumors undergo malignant degeneration, resulting in malignant schwannoma or neurogenic sarcoma in 2 to 29 percent of patients, most often in the adult population.[22]

Congenital neurofibromas are often of the plexiform type and have a propensity for the periorbital region. They are progressive and usually highly vascular lesions that present an enormous cosmetic and surgical challenge. Staged subtotal resections may be of some benefit, but the lesions are not curable and recurrence is the rule.[64] A pigmented plexiform neurofibroma of the neck or trunk that extends into the midline often indicates involvement of the spinal cord.[46] Large intrathoracic or intra-abdominal neurofibromas, as well as ganglioneuromas, may extend into the spinal canal, and nuclear magnetic resonance imaging (NMRI) can be used to assess this (Fig. 40–1). If significant cord compression is present, posterior decompression may be required before further tumor debulking is performed.

The most common eye lesions in children with NF include Lisch's nodules, orbital osseous dysplasia, and buphthalmos. Lisch's nodules are gelatinous, hamartomatous elevations of the iris and can be seen grossly or by slit-lamp examination. While they are present in almost all post pubertal peripheral neurofibromatosis patients, they are less common in early childhood but can be considered confirmatory of NF, when found.

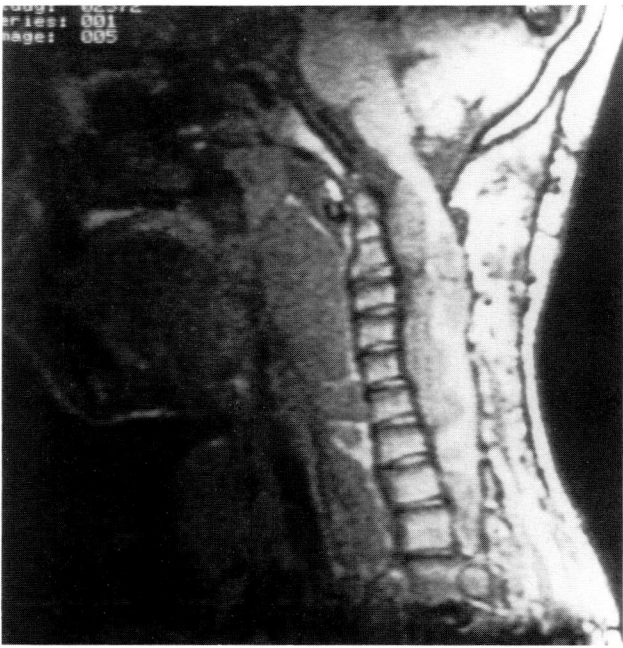

Figure 40–1. Nuclear magnetic resonance (NMR) image of large multiple spinal neurofibromatoses.

Dysplasia of the posterior superior wall of the orbit (sphenoid wings and frontal bone) leads to pulsatile exophthalmos and may be the presenting sign of NF in an infant or a young child. The defect is easily distinguished from other forms of proptosis by computed tomography (CT) scan (Fig. 40–2) and may be corrected by reconstructive surgery, most often using rib grafts.

Buphthalmos, or ox eye, may also be seen early in life. This is an enlargement of the globe resulting from glaucoma that is usually unilateral. This finding commonly occurs in patients with facial involvement and, when seen in combination with asymmetric facial hypertrophy and plexiform NF of the eyelid, is known as François's syndrome.[16] Preservation of useful vision in the involved eye is particularly important, since visual pathway tumors may compromise the opposite eye in the future.

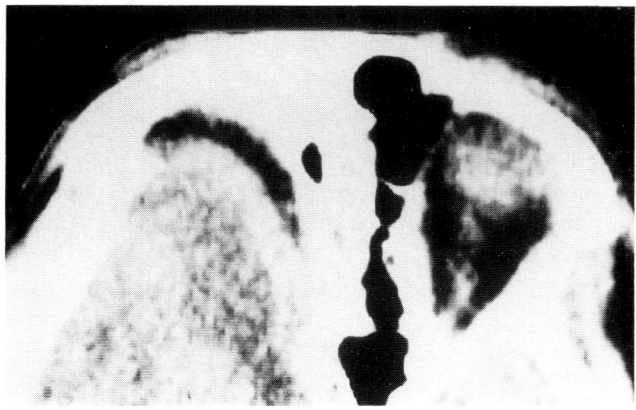

Figure 40–2. Congenital dysplasia of the sphenoid wing.

Skeletal lesions can present at birth and include congenital bowing and pseudoarthrosis, most often affecting the tibia. Segmental hypertrophy of the extremities and vertebral scalloping in association with tumors or meningoceles may occur. The most common skeletal manifestation of NF is scoliosis. This usually presents during late childhood and may be related to mesodermal dysplasia or neurogenic factors. A severe kyphoscoliosis of the cervicothoracic region is particularly characteristic and requires early aggressive surgical treatment if severe deformity and neurologic compromise are to be avoided.[7, 46]

CNS Manifestations

Neoplasms of the brain, spinal cord, cranial nerves, nerve roots, and meningeal coverings all occur with increased frequency in NF. The disease is sufficiently common that a careful history and physical examination pertinent to the diagnosis of NF should be a routine part of the work-up of any child with a brain tumor, particularly in those types less common in childhood, such as meningiomas or acoustic neuromas.

The CNS in neurofibromatosis is characterized pathologically by disorganization and the presence of hamartomas, heterotopias, and low-grade neoplasms. Such abnormal architecture may result in the syndromes of aqueductal stenosis, syringomyelia, and central precocious puberty. The latter condition can be treated medically.[32] Macrocephaly may be seen in three fourths of patients with NF.[21, 62] Developmental delay is found in about one fifth of patients,[13, 18] and an additional 20 percent may show hyperactivity or learning disability.[46]

The use of NMRI has proved quite valuable in the evaluation of these patients, for it has demonstrated in vivo the extraordinary and previously unsuspected range of abnormalities in the NF brain (Fig. 40–3). However, many completely asymptomatic lesions are also found, raising the dilemma of how to manage incidentally found focal brain lesions. It has been the authors' policy to biopsy only symptomatic lesions. The remainder have been assumed to represent hamartomas or low-grade gliomas, which can be followed closely for clinical or radiographic evidence of progression. Likewise, radiation therapy for lesions in which surgery is contraindicated is also reserved for symptomatic or markedly enlarging lesions.

The most characteristic childhood tumor associated with NF is the optic chiasmatic glioma. Anterior visual pathway tumors have been estimated to occur in 15 percent of patients with NF, and two thirds of these may be asymptomatic and may not be detected on ophthalmic examination.[34] While the mean age of patients with optic nerve tumors ranges in the early twenties, chiasmatic tumors occur most often in the first decade of life. Some authors believe

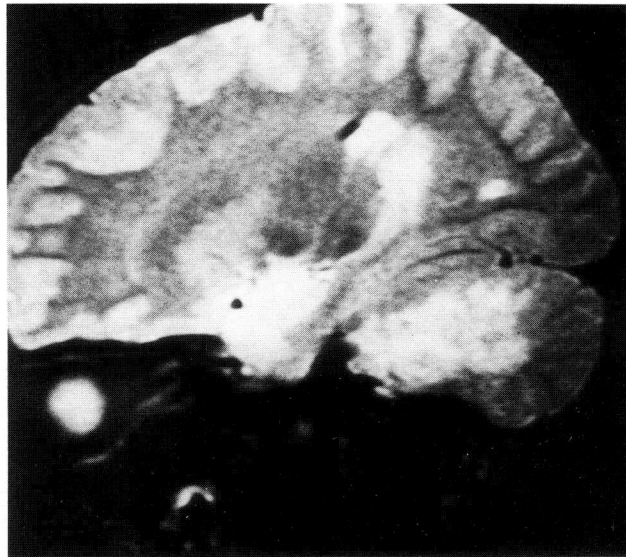

Figure 40–3. NMR image of a child with neurofibromatosis.

that virtually all optic gliomas represent a manifestation of NF, and when isolated, such a tumor is a forme fruste of the disease.

CT scan is the first diagnostic test of choice for evaluation of optic chiasmatic glioma. A pattern of "streaking" along the visual pathway may be seen. NMRI is often more sensitive in detecting this feature and may be performed when CT is equivocal. Biopsy is reserved for patients without known NF who have masses in which this feature is not seen and for whom the diagnosis is uncertain. Once the diagnosis is established, asymptomatic or stable patients are followed with serial studies. Patients with significant clinical or radiographic progression are currently treated at the Children's Hospital of Philadelphia with chemotherapy (doxorubicin and vincristine) if they are younger than five years, and with radiation if they are older than five years. Isolated optic nerve tumors are removed for cosmetic indications only.[44]

Bilateral acoustic neuromas (schwannomas) are the sine qua non of the so-called central form of NF. These tumors may also occur variably in the peripheral form. The central form usually presents in adolescence. While the clinical manifestations of NF are quite variable among family members with the peripheral form, all affected members of a family with central NF have bilateral acoustic neuromas.[37] They may also have skin manifestations, but these are often subtle.

The role and the timing of surgery in bilateral acoustic neurofibromatosis is controversial. Some reports recommend frequent screening and early surgery on small asymptomatic lesions, as this is felt to offer the greatest chance of tumor removal with preservation of hearing and facial function.[27, 37] Others recommend that surgery be reserved for large tumors causing brainstem compression or progressive hearing or cranial nerve dysfunction, since surgery often results in loss of these functions, which, when bilateral, is extremely debilitating.[38] Treatment obviously must be individualized for each patient, taking into account the capabilities and experience of the particular center providing care.

Gliomas of all grades can occur in the cerebrum, brainstem, and spinal cord with increased frequency in NF, as do ependymomas, meningiomas, schwannomas, and dumbbell spinal neurofibromas. In a recent series of 121 children younger than 18 years of age with NF, 14 percent had brain tumors.[3] A loss of developmental milestones or a new symptom of pain should prompt a search for such neoplasms in children or their relatives with NF. Lateral thoracic meningoceles are characteristic in this disease and may mimic a spinal neoplasm, from which it may be differentiated by myelography. These usually require no specific treatment.[47,49]

Other Neoplasms

Tumors of other neural crest cell derivatives that occur in association with NF include pheochromocytoma and neuroblastoma. Neurofibromas and gangliogliomas may arise from the visceral neural plexus. Non-neural crest tumors that occur more commonly than would be expected include leukemia, sarcoma, and Wilms's tumor, and NF is considered to be the most common single gene defect associated with childhood cancer.[40]

Prognosis

Neurofibromatosis is a variable but progressive disease. Unfortunately, an early mild course does not predict a smaller likelihood of serious problems in the future for a given patient.[46] The risks of CNS tumors, malignant transformation, and other cancers increase with age. These patients require a comprehensive approach to recognize early signs of complications and to help deal with the enormous psychologic burden of a progressively disfiguring and disabling disease. Research is ongoing to try to elucidate how genetic and environmental factors interact, in an attempt to slow progression and improve treatment over that currently available.

TUBEROUS SCLEROSIS

While tuberous sclerosis (TS) is inherited as an autosomal dominant trait, the majority of cases are thought to be sporadic.[37] Next to neurofibromatosis, it is the phakomatosis most likely to be seen by the neurosurgeon and has a prevalence of about 1 in 10,000.[63] Also known as Bourneville's disease, tuberous sclerosis most often becomes manifest in childhood with progressive symptoms involving the skin, viscera, and nervous system.

The most typical early skin lesions are the so-called "ash leaf spots." These are small, hypopigmented areas that often have an ash leaf or thumbprint shape, with one end rounded and the other tapered. The spots are usually present at birth and may be accentuated in pale individuals by ultraviolet light. In a few patients, ash leaf spots first appear later in childhood.[43]

Facial angiofibromas, or "adenoma sebaceum," appear in a butterfly distribution by middle childhood and occur in 90 percent of patients with tuberous sclerosis. When severe, the raised nodules may obscure vision and may bleed when traumatized. These lesions can be treated with shave excision[29] or with the carbon dioxide laser.[2]

Other skin manifestations of TS include café-au-lait spots; areas of subepidermal fibrosis (shagreen, or sharkskin, patches), which are most often located in the lumbosacral area; and subungual fibromas of the fingers and toes, presenting by adolescence.

The eye lesions of TS consist of hamartomas in the retina, which are most often asymptomatic (Fig. 40–4). Hamartomas may also be found in the visceral organs. The lungs may show cystic, or "honeycomb," changes. Angiomyolipomas of the kidneys are benign tumors occurring in a high percentage of patients with TS. When large, they may interfere with renal function. Cardiac rhabdomyomas occur in up to half of patients and sometimes prompt the diagnosis of TS in infancy.

It is the CNS lesion, however, which most often brings patients with TS to medical attention, and the disease is described classically as including the triad of characteristic skin lesions, seizures, and mental retardation. The pathologic substrate for the neurologic symptoms and that for which the disease is named is the subependymal nodule, or "tuber." These benign hamartomatous lesions are multiple and occur at the lining of the lateral and third ventricles. They can be seen on CT scan or sometimes by ultrasonography at birth.[33] The tubers are usually calcified, protrude into the ventricle ("candle guttering"), and do not enhance with contrast material. Pathologically, the subependymal lesions consist of glial nodules. Cortical tubers are similar lesions that occur at the brain surface and are felt to represent aberrant populations of cells that failed to migrate or differentiate properly.[25] Abnormal cell surface factors may play a role in the formation of these lesions. The presence of subependymal and subpial tubers illustrates the intrinsic disorganization of the brain in tuberous sclerosis, which most likely accounts for the tendency toward slow intellect and seizures. As would be predicted, these two clinical features are not entirely independent. While 80 percent of TS patients with seizures develop them by age five, those who have onset of seizures before age two have a higher incidence of retarda-

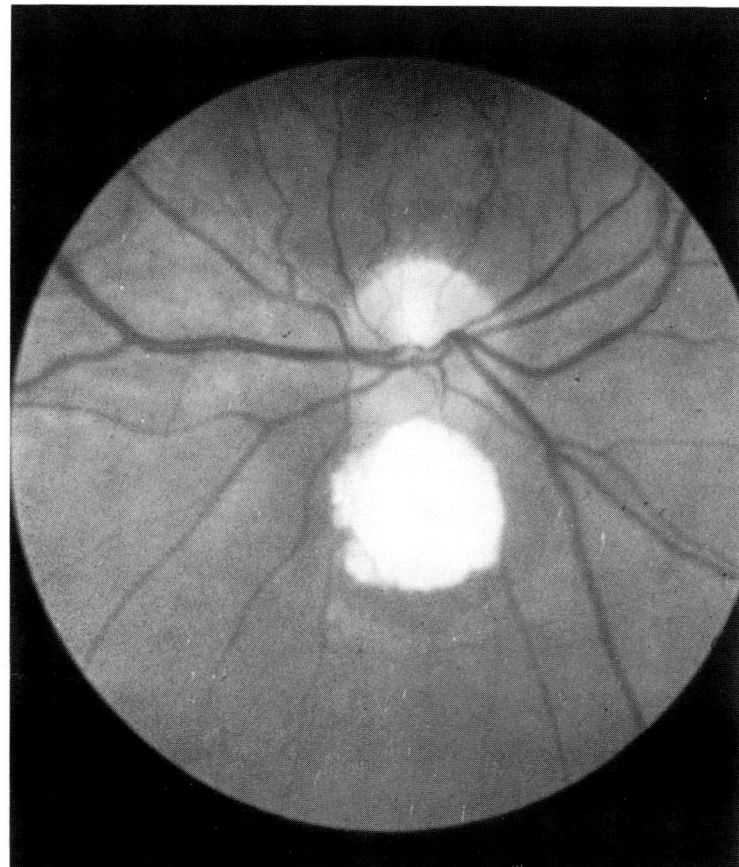

Figure 40–4. Retinal hamartoma in tuberous sclerosis.

tion. Conversely, patients without seizures are likely to be intellectually normal.[63]

Occasionally, a patient has a single prominent cortical tuber that corresponds to a seizure focus. Biopsy of cortical tubers is not routinely necessary, since, unlike the subependymal nodules, these lesions are not associated with tumor formation. However, resection may be indicated in cases of intractable seizures. Because of the diffuse nature of the disease, improved control and not elimination of seizures is the goal of surgery.

Low-density areas in the cortex and in white matter are seen on CT scan in patients with TS and have been attributed to demyelination.[14] Uncalcified tubers may also appear as hypodense areas and can be differentiated from demyelination when indicated by NMRI.[11]

The characteristic brain tumor in tuberous sclerosis is the subependymal giant cell tumor, which is reported to occur in 7 to 23 percent of patients.[14, 28, 39] These lesions are believed to arise from a subependymal tuber and nearly always occur at the foramen of Monro. Pathologically, these are usually giant cell astrocytomas, though other histologic types have been described.[5, 28, 33, 39]

Tumors usually present with headache or other indications of increased intracranial pressure when hydrocephalus develops from ventricular obstruction. CT scans show an isodense soft-tissue mass associated with calcifications that enhances brightly with contrast material (Fig. 40–5). While an enhancing mass in a patient with TS must be considered a tumor, when asymptomatic the mass may be followed using serial scans, with surgery reserved for symptomatic lesions.[39]

Most giant cell tumors can be approached transcallosally. While in some tumors, intense vascularity may limit resection, the Cavitron ultrasonic aspirator may be extremely useful in reducing the mass of the tumor. Large vessels often occur on the ventricular surface and at the site of attachment of the tumor to the lateral ventricular wall. Therefore, if the intraventricular portion of the tumor can be debulked internally, with care taken to protect the normal ependymal surface and choroid plexus, this problem may be minimized. The goal of surgery is to establish free communication between the anterior and posterior compartments of the lateral ventricles, and between the lateral and third ventricles, thus relieving obstruction. In some cases, shunting may also be necessary, but if communication has been established, a single shunt, rather than multiple shunts into various compartments, will suffice.

While these tumors tend to grow slowly and behave in a benign fashion, they may recur and cause progressive symptoms. Radiation therapy has

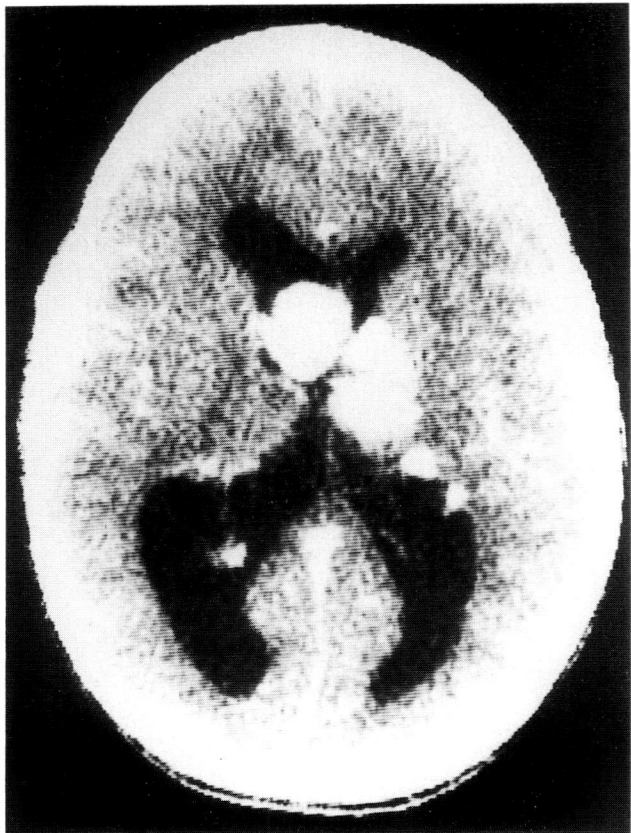

Figure 40–5. CT scan of intraventricular tumor in tuberous sclerosis.

been used to control tumor growth but has met with limited success.[28] Reoperation may be indicated for progressive disease.

STURGE-WEBER SYNDROME

This disorder, also known as encephalotrigeminal angiomatosis, is classified with the phakomatoses because of involvement of the skin, eyes, and nervous system. However, it is unlike the other syndromes in that it occurs sporadically, and the genetics remain unknown. The characteristic skin lesion in the Sturge-Weber syndrome is a facial port-wine stain, or nevus flammeus, which is present at birth. Only those nevi that include the ophthalmic trigeminal distribution (i.e., the upper eyelid and forehead) are associated with the syndrome. This group comprises about 40 percent of all children with facial port-wine stains.[12]

The brain lesion associated with this disorder is an ipsilateral pial venous angiomatous malformation that most often involves the occipital or parietooccipital lobe. Pathologically, the lesion is characterized by calcification in the outer cortical zone of the brain parenchyma surrounding the abnormal vessels. Microscopic intravascular calcifications are also seen. Eye findings in this syndrome include unilateral glaucoma, which is the most common, as well as buphthalmos and retinal angiomas.

Radiographically, the cortical calcifications in this syndrome can be discerned on plain skull film as wavy double lines, the so-called "tramtrack" sign. CT scan is even more sensitive in demonstrating the vascular malformation. This is particularly true in infants, in whom calcification may be minimal. Surrounding brain atrophy can also be seen by CT (Fig. 40–6). Arteriography shows a lack of cortical vein visualization beneath the affected cortex, enlargement of the deep draining veins, and nonfilling of the sagittal sinus.[17]

The disease is characterized clinically by seizures, hemiparesis, hemiatrophy, visual field defects, and, sometimes, retardation. Seizures usually begin in infancy and early childhood. As with tuberous sclerosis, early seizure onset is correlated with poorer prognosis for intellectual development. The progression of neurologic problems is typically described as stepwise, with each prolonged seizure episode followed by an incomplete recovery to baseline. It has been proposed that sequential cortical vessel thrombosis may explain the clinical deterioration as well as the angiographic findings.[17]

Treatment for the Sturge-Weber disease is primarily medical, with control of seizures the goal. Antiplatelet medications have also been suggested as a preventive measure for presumed cortical thrombosis, but outcome comparisons with the variable natural history of the disease are difficult to assess. Medical control of seizures may become

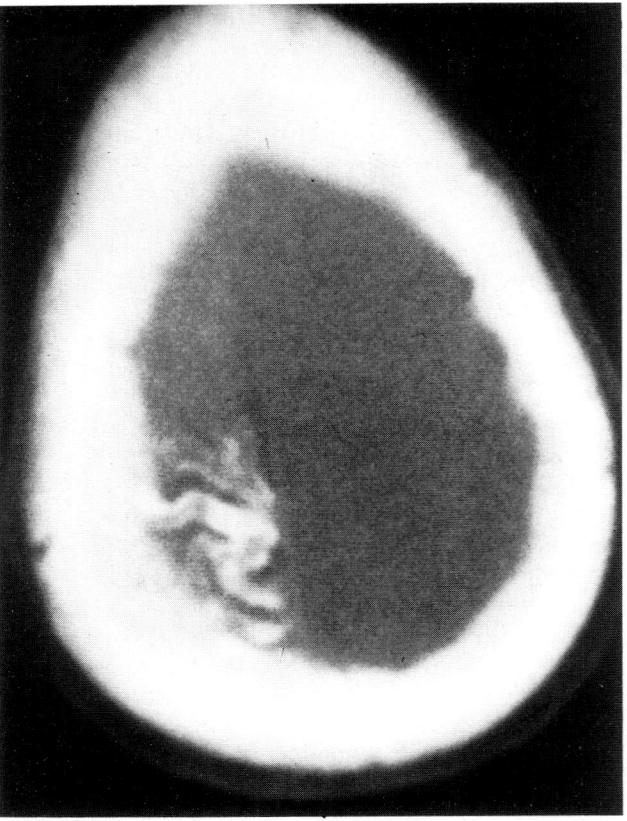

Figure 40–6. CT scan in a patient with Sturge-Weber syndrome.

more difficult with time, and refractoriness to maximum medications may occur. In light of the poor outlook for patients with large lesions and early onset of seizures, both with respect to seizure control and neurologic function, early aggressive surgery has been proposed by some authors.[20, 57] Hemispherectomy, hemidecortication, or lobectomy has been performed for this condition. These procedures seem to be tolerated best with respect to preservation of function when they are done in the first few months of life. Good seizure control, minimal hemiparesis, and normal intelligence have been reported. The procedure is not without risk, and the role of surgery in the management of Sturge-Weber disease remains controversial.

VON HIPPEL–LINDAU DISEASE

Cerebellar and other CNS hemangioblastomas, angiomatosis retinae, and various visceral cysts and tumors constitute the syndrome known as von Hippel–Lindau disease. While isolated cerebellar hemangioblastomas in children have been reported,[45] the disease usually presents in adulthood. It is transmitted as an autosomal dominant trait with variable penetrance. A positive family history is found in about 20 percent of patients. The diagnosis is made by the presence of two or more separate characteristic lesions in a given individual or by a single lesion with a positive family history.[8]

The retinal hemangiomas in von Hippel–Lindau disease occur in 60 percent of patients.[24, 37] They appear as small vascular blotches with a feeding artery and draining vein. Because of an abnormal absence of tight junctions in the capillaries of the angioma, leakage of blood into and beneath the retina can occur. Retinal detachment and visual loss may result, and this sometimes is the presenting symptom of the disease.[26] The retinal lesions can be treated with the laser or other forms of coagulation therapy. Glaucoma may also occur in association with angiomatosis retinae.[24]

The most common visceral lesions in von Hippel–Lindau disease are pheochromocytoma and renal cysts and tumors. Pheochromocytoma may be bilateral, and hypertension in a patient with the syndrome is highly suggestive. The work-up includes measurement of urine vanillylmandelic acid (VMA) and plasma catecholamines and careful body CT including the course of the sympathetic chain in the abdomen and thorax.

The renal lesions in von Hippel–Lindau disease occur in two thirds of patients and range from simple cysts to malignant hypernephroma. The risk of malignant progression of a cystic kidney lesion increases with age, and renal cell carcinoma is present in 25 to 38 percent of all patients.[8] It is the leading cause of death in von Hippel–Lindau disease. Management of the kidney lesions is controversial, ranging from a conservative approach to bilateral prophylactic nephrectomies.

Other visceral lesions include angiomas, cysts, and adenomas of the pancreas, liver, spleen, lung, epididymis, and ovary. These lesions are usually asymptomatic.

The most characteristic CNS lesion in von Hippel–Lindau disease is the cerebellar hemangioblastoma. These lesions occur in 35 to 60 percent of patients and are usually said to be more common in males.[24] When the same tumor occurs sporadically, it is usually in the older individual, whereas it is most common in young adults when associated with von Hippel–Lindau disease. These are benign tumors characterized histologically by abundant capillaries, reticulin stroma, and "pseudoxanthoma" cells. They are cystic in 60 percent of patients. An increased hematocrit is frequently seen in association with hemangioblastomas and is presumed to be a consequence of an erythropoietic factor elaborated by the tumor. Hematocrits tend to return to normal after tumor removal.

On CT scan, hemangioblastomas appear as cystic or isodense lesions that are well delineated and enhance uniformly in the solid portion with contrast material. Multiple lesions may be present, and angiography has been reported to be more sensitive in finding accessible asymptomatic lesions, which the surgeon can then remove prophylactically during an operation for larger, symptomatic lesions.[11] Angiography may also better show the location of the nodule in a cystic lesion and the vascular supply in a solid mass. At present, preoperative angiography is still recommended, though improved imaging with CT or NMRI may make this unnecessary.

Complete resection of a hemangioblastoma is curative. In a cystic lesion, the mural nodule must be removed, or the cyst will recur. Radiation therapy for subtotally removed or recurrent lesions has been reported to be beneficial.[52]

Hemangioblastomas may also occur in the spinal cord, brainstem, and cerebral hemispheres. The brainstem lesions are most common in the medulla, specifically the area postrema, and these may be difficult to remove completely. Spinal cord lesions are also associated with a syrinx cavity. These tend to be located dorsally in the cord and can be removed surgically. In a patient undergoing vertebral angiography for a posterior fossa lesion, cervical hemangioblastomas may be seen if neck films are also obtained.[51]

Since this disease is progressive, patients with von Hippel–Lindau disease should undergo screening on a routine basis, including CT scans of the head and body, specific renal imaging studies such as intravenous pyelogram (IVP) or angiograms, ophthalmic examinations, renal function tests, and measurement of urinary VMA. Genetic counseling and routine screening of adult relatives who are at risk should also be part of the treatment plan.

ATAXIA TELANGIECTASIA

Also known as Louis-Bar syndrome, after the description by Denise Louis-Bar in 1941,[36] ataxia telangiectasia is a fascinating disorder that links genetics, neurologic degeneration, immunology, aging, and cancer. It is unique among the phakomatoses in that it is transmitted as an autosomal recessive trait. The disease itself is rare, occurring in 2 to 3 per 100,000 births, but with a gene frequency estimated to occur in 1 percent of the population.[53] For this reason, ataxia telangiectasia has generated much interest among epidemiologists, geneticists, oncologists, and others seeking to understand the relationship between a faulty gene and the occurrence of more common degenerative and malignant diseases in the population at large.

As with many neurocutaneous disorders, the characteristic external lesions are not usually present at birth. The first to appear are the conjunctival telangiectasias. These are bilateral and progressively more pronounced throughout childhood.[35] Finer telangiectasias appear over the ears, neck, face, and antecubital and popliteal fossa and increase with exposure or irritation. Premature graying and thinning of the hair, loss of skin elasticity and subcutaneous fat, and seborrheic dermatitis are manifestations akin to accelerated aging and have been described as progeric.

These and other features of the disease are thought to be consequences of the underlying genetic abnormality in ataxia telangiectasia. The chromosomes of patients with the disease show increased rates of spontaneous breakage and are more sensitive to agents inducing chromosomal instability. It is thus classified, along with several other conditions, among the so-called clastogenic disorders, which are hypothesized to result from a defect in DNA repair. Other related characteristic features of the disease include immunodeficiency, radiation sensitivity, and an increased incidence of neoplasia. The immune disorder includes impaired synthesis of immunoglobulins A and E (IgA and IgE), with an increased incidence of recurrent sinopulmonary infections, which are the commonest cause of death.[23] Radiosensitivity has lead to fatalities in patients with ataxia telangiectasia treated with conventional doses of radiation.[54] Whether heterozygotes are also at increased risk remains controversial.[31] The increased risk of cancer in homozygotes, particularly lymphoreticular malignancies, has been well documented and has been estimated to occur in 10 to 38 percent of ataxia telangiectasia patients.[35, 41] Morrell and colleagues[41] studied 263 patients and found a 61-fold cancer excess for white patients and 184-fold excess for black patients with the disease. A total of 87 percent of the cancers were lymphomas or leukemias.[41] Next to infection, malignancy is the commonest cause of death in ataxia telangiectasia. The cancer risk of a heterozygote with the gene has been estimated to be several times that of the normal population[53] and may account for a large proportion of cancer deaths in younger individuals.

A persistence of fetal proteins in the serum is characteristic of ataxia telangiectasia. This feature has been hypothesized to result from a defect in differentiation of specific cell populations, but its exact cause remains unknown. An elevated serum level of alpha-fetoprotein is present in essentially all patients with the disease but is not found in heterozygotes.[59]

The principal neurologic manifestations of the disorder are ataxia and choreoathetosis. Affected children appear normal in infancy. Ataxia usually becomes obvious by age two, as mobility increases, along with a cerebellar type of dysarthria. Athethosis occurs a bit later. Intellect is preserved, but development may plateau as the child becomes progressively disabled. However, intelligence may be superficially masked by the characteristic dull, sad-looking face that is also thought to be a manifestation of the cerebellar disorder. The personality has been described as placid. Disturbances of eye movement are manifestations of oculomotor apraxia. The children have a characteristic posture, with a tendency to hunch and drop the head. Strength, however, remains normal until late in the disease. Reflexes become absent in adolescence, and toes remain downgoing. Sensation is usually normal.[4, 23, 35]

The major neuropathologic feature of ataxia telangiectasia is atrophy of the cerebellum, with diffuse cell loss most marked in the vermis. Reactive gliosis is present. Brainstem and spinal cord demyelination, cell loss, and gliosis are also found. CT scan shows a nonspecific pattern of cerebellar atrophy.

The prognosis in ataxia telangiectasia is poor. Most patients are wheelchair-bound by adolescence. While survival beyond the teens was formerly considered rare, more recent reports document longer survival.[41] Supportive care, physical therapy, and prevention and treatment of infections have been the mainstays of therapy, as no specific intervention has yet been found for the underlying pathologic lesion.

INCONTINENTIA PIGMENTI

Also known as Bloch-Sulzberger syndrome, this rare disorder has been postulated to be transmitted by a sex-linked dominant gene. There is a strong female predominance in the disease. Affected patients present at infancy with the first of three stages of skin changes, which is characterized by vesiculobullous lesions affecting the trunk, extremities, and scalp, but sparing the face. It is accompanied by peripheral eosinophilia. The second stage, usually lasting for several months, is marked by verrucous lesions, in a similar distribution. In the third stage, tan or gray macules in a whorled or streaked pattern appear. These generally resolve at puberty.

A variety of ocular findings have been reported, including intraocular masses described as pseudogliomas, optic atrophy, and uveitis.[1] Developmental defects of teeth and bones are sometimes found, suggesting a disorder of ectodermal derivatives. The CNS is involved in about half of patients, with symptoms including seizures, ataxia, and mental retardation, the latter being reported in about 15 percent.[42] As in other phakomatoses, early seizure onset is correlated with a poor intellectual outcome.

CT scan in incontinentia pigmenti may show various patterns of brain atrophy and areas of low density.[1] Pathologically, the brain shows the effects of acute hemorrhagic encephalopathy and atrophy, as well as some features suggestive of abnormal migration of fetal nervous elements.

The disease progression in incontinentia pigmenti is quite variable, with some patients dying in early childhood and others having a more benign course characterized by typical skin lesions but only mild CNS involvement.

SUMMARY

A working familiarity with the phakomatoses is essential for the neurosurgeon encountering young patients and their families. Complete care and planning for the future is greatly aided when the neurosurgeon is prepared for the development of new clinical manifestations of the disorder. Pertinent questions and examinations for cutaneous stigmata, ophthalmologic consultation, and careful family history should be a routine part of the evaluation of all children with CNS tumors. A high index of suspicion should be maintained for other signs and symptoms that might be consistent with the diagnosis of a neurocutaneous syndrome.

References

1. Avrahami E, Harel S, Jurgenson U, et al: Computed tomographic demonstration of brain changes in incontinentia pigmenti. Am J Dis Child 139:372, 1985.
2. Bellack G, Shapshay SM: Management of facial angiofibromas in tuberous sclerosis: Use of the carbon dioxide laser. Otolaryngol Head Neck Surg 94:37, 1986.
3. Blatt J, Jaffe R, Deutsch M, et al: Neurofibromatosis and childhood tumors. Cancer 57:1225, 1986.
4. Boder E, Sedgwick RF: Ataxia telangiectasia. A familial syndrome of progressive cerebellar ataxia, oculocutaneous telangiectasia and frequent pulmonary infection. Pediatrics 21:526, 1958.
5. Boesel CP, Paulson GW, Kosnick FJ, et al: Brain hamartomas and tumors associated with tuberous sclerosis. Neurosurgery 4:410, 1979.
6. Boland R: Neurofibromatosis—the quintessential neurocristopathy: Pathogenetic concepts and relationships. In: Riccardi VM, Mulvihill JJ (eds): Neurofibromatosis (von Recklinghausen's Disease). Advances in Neurology, Vol. 29. New York, Raven Press, 1981, pp 67–75.
7. Chaglassian JH, Riseborough EG, Hall JE: Neurofibromatosis scoliosis: Natural history and results of treatment in thirty-seven cases. J Bone Joint Surg 58:695, 1976.
8. Cohen ML, Duffner PK: Von Hippel-Lindau disease. In: Hoffman HJ, Epstein F (eds): Disorders of the Developing Nervous System: Diagnosis and Treatment. Boston, MA, Blackwell Scientific Pubs., 1986.
9. Crowe FW, Schull WJ: Diagnostic importance of café-au-lait spots in neurofibromatosis. Arch Intern Med 91:758, 1953.
10. Crowe FW, Schull J, Need JV: A clinical, pathological and genetic study of multiple neurofibromatosis. Springfield, IL, Charles C Thomas, 1956.
11. Curatolo P, Cusmai R, Pruna D: Tuberous sclerosis: Diagnostic and prognostic problems. Pediatr Neurosci 12:123, 1985–86.
12. Enjolras O, Riche MD, Merland JJ: Facial port-wine stains and Sturge-Weber syndrome. Pediatrics 76:48, 1985.
13. Fienman NL, Yakovac WC: Neurofibromatosis in childhood. J Pediatr 76:339, 1970.
14. Fitz CC: Tuberous sclerosis. In: Hoffman HJ, Epstein F (eds): Disorders of the Developing Nervous System: Diagnosis and Treatment. Boston, MA, Blackwell Scientific Pubs., 1986.
15. Flinter FA, Neville BG: Examining the parents of children with tuberous sclerosis. Lancet 2:1167, 1986.
16. Francois J: Ocular aspects of the phakomatoses. In: Vinken PJ, Bruyn GW (eds): Handbook of Clinical Neurology, Vol. 14. New York, American Elsevier, 1972, pp 619–667.
17. Garcia JC, Roach ES, McLean WT: Recurrent thrombotic deterioration in the Sturge-Weber syndrome. Child's Brain 8:427, 1981.
18. Griffith BH, McKinney P, Monroe CW, et al: Von Recklinghausen's disease in childhood. Plast Reconstr Surg 47:647, 1972.
19. Hoff JT, Ray BS: Cerebral hemangioblastoma occurring in a patient with von Hippel-Lindau disease. J Neurosurg 28:365, 1968.
20. Hoffman HJ, Hendrick EB, Dennise M, et al: Hemispherectomy for Sturge-Weber syndrome. Child's Brain 5:233, 1979.
21. Holt J: Neurofibromatosis in children. Am J Roentgenol 130:615, 1978.
22. Hope DG, Mulvihill JJ: Malignancy in neurofibromatosis. In: Riccardi VM, Mulvihill JJ (eds): Neurofibromatosis (von Recklinghausen's Disease). Advances in Neurology, Vol. 29. New York, Raven Press, 1981, pp 33–56.
23. Hosking G: Ataxia telangiectasis. Annotations. Dev Med Child Neurol 24:77, 1982.
24. Hubschmann OR, Vijayanathan T, Countee RW: Von Hippel-Lindau disease with multiple manifestations: Diagnosis and management. Neurosurgery 8:92, 1981.
25. Huttenlocher PR, Heydemann PT: Fine structure of cortical tubers in tuberous sclerosis: A Golgi study. Ann Neurol 16:595, 1984.
26. Jakobiec FA, Font RL, Johnson FB: Angiomatosis retinae: An ultrastructural study and lipid analysis. Cancer 38:2042, 1976.
27. Kanter W, Eldridge K, Fabricant R, et al: Central neurofibromatosis with bilateral acoustic neuroma: Genetic, clinical and biochemical distinctions from peripheral neurofibromatosis. Neurology 30:851, 1980.
28. Kapp JP, Paulson GW, Odom G: Brain tumors with tuberous sclerosis. J Neurosurg 26:191, 1967.
29. Kavanagh KT, Cosby WN: Shave excision and dermabrasion of midline angiofibroma in tuberous sclerosis. Arch Otolaryngol Head Neck Surg 112:886, 1986.
30. Kessler JA, Cochard P, Black IB: Neural crest differentiation and response to nerve growth factor in murine embryos. In: Riccardi VM, Mulvihill JJ (eds): Neurofibromatosis (von Recklinghausen's Disease). Advances in Neurology, Vol. 29. New York, Raven Press, 1981, pp 115–123.
31. Radiosensitivity and the clinician. Lancet 2:23, 1985.
32. Laue L, Comite F, Hench K, et al: Central precocious puberty in neurofibromatosis: Treatment with lutenizing hormone releasing hormone analogue. Am J Dis Child 139:1097, 1985.

33. Legge M, Sauerbrei E, MacDonald A: Intracranial tuberous sclerosis in infancy. Radiology 153:667, 1984.
34. Lewis RA, Gerson LP, Axelson KA, et al: Von Recklinghausen's neurofibromatosis. 1. Incidence of optic glioma. Ophthalmology 91:929, 1984.
35. Logan WJ: Ataxia telangiectasia. In: Hoffman HJ, Epstein F (eds): Disorders of the Developing Nervous System: Diagnosis and Treatment. Boston, MA, Blackwell Scientific Pubs., 1986, pp 635–651.
36. Louis-Barr D: Sur un syndrome progressif comprenant des telangiectasies capillaires cutanées et conjunctivals symmetrique, a disposition naevoide et des troubles cérébelleux. Confina Neurol 4:32, 1941. Quoted in Logan WJ: Ataxia telangiectasia. In: Hoffman HJ, Epstein F (eds): Disorders of the Developing Nervous System: Diagnosis and Treatment. Boston, MA, Blackwell Scientific Pubs., 1986, pp 635–641.
37. Martuza RL: Neurofibromatosis and other phakomatoses. In: Wilkins RH, Rengachary SS (eds): Neurosurgery. New York, McGraw-Hill, 1985.
38. Martuza RL, Ojemann RG: Bilateral acoustic neuromas: Clinical aspects, pathogenesis and treatment. Neurosurgery 10:1, 1982.
39. McLaurin RL, Towbin RB: Tuberous sclerosis: Diagnostic and surgical considerations. Pediatr Neurosci 12:43, 1985–86.
40. Meadows A, Coutifaris C, Obringer A, et al: Variable expression of the neurofibromatosis gene: Considerations in diagnosis and treatment of children with cancer. Presented at International Society of Pediatric Oncology, XIIth meeting, Marseilles, France, 1981.
41. Morrell D, Cromartie E, Swift M: Mortality and cancer incidence in 263 patients with ataxia-telangiectasia. JNCI 77:89, 1986.
42. O'Brien JE, Feingold M: Incontinentia pigmenti. A longitudinal study. Am J Dis Child 139:711, 1985.
43. Oppenheimer EY, Rosman NP, Dooling EC: The late appearance of hypopigmented maculae in tuberous sclerosis. Am J Dis Child 139:408, 1985.
44. Packer RJ, Rosenstock JG, Bilaniuk LT, et al: Chiasmatic hypothalamic/thalamic gliomas in childhood: Efficacy of treatment with chemotherapy alone. Ann Neurol 16:402, 1984.
45. Pasztor A, Sztenak L, Dobronyi I, et al: Angioblastoma of the posterior fossa in children. J Pediatr Neurosci 1:281, 1985.
46. Riccardi VM: von Recklinghausen neurofibromatosis. N Engl J Med 305:1617, 1981.
47. Robinson RG: Intrathoracic meningocele and neurofibromatosis. Br J Surg 51:432, 1964.
48. Rubinstein LJ: Tumors of the Central Nervous System. Washington, DC, Armed Forces Institute of Pathology, 1972.
49. Salerno NR, Edeiken J: Vertebral scalloping in neurofibromatosis. Radiology 97:509, 1970.
50. Schut L, Duhaime AC, Rorke L, et al: Von Recklinghausen's disease. In: Hoffman HJ, Epstein F (eds): Disorders of the Developing Nervous System: Diagnosis and Treatment. Boston, MA, Blackwell Scientific Pubs., 1986, pp 591–605.
51. Seeger JF, Burke DP, Knake JE, et al: Computed tomographic and angiographic evaluation of hemangioblastomas. Radiology 138:65, 1981.
52. Sung DK, Chang CH, Harisiadis L: Cerebellar hemangioblastoma. Cancer 49:553, 1982.
53. Swift M, Sholman L, Perry M, et al: Malignant neoplasms in the families of patients with ataxia-telangiectasia. Cancer 76:209, 1976.
54. Taylor AMR, Harnden DG, Arlett CA, et al: Ataxia-telangiectasia: A human mutation with abnormal radiation sensitivity. Nature 258:427, 1975.
55. Tsuchida T, Kamata K, Kawamata M, et al: Brain tumors in tuberous sclerosis. Report of 4 cases. Child's Brain 8:271, 1981.
56. Van der Hoeve J: Eye diseases in tuberous sclerosis of the brain and in Recklinghausen disease. Trans Ophthalmol Soc UK 43:534, 1923.
57. Venes JL: Sturge-Weber syndrome. In: Hoffman HJ, Epstein F (eds): Disorders of the Developing Nervous System: Diagnosis and Treatment. Boston, MA, Blackwell Scientific Pubs., 1986, pp 617–623.
58. von Recklinghausen F: Uber die multipen fibrome der haut une ihre beziehung zuden multiplen neuromen. Berlin, A Hirschwald, 1882.
59. Waldmann TA, McIntire KR: Serum alpha-fetoprotein levels in patients with ataxia-telangiectasia. Lancet 2:1112, 1972.
60. Weichert KA, Dire MS, Benton C, et al: Macrocranium and neurofibromatosis. Radiology 107:163, 1973.
61. Weston J: The regulation of normal and abnormal neural crest cell development. In: Riccardi VM, Mulvihill JJ (eds): Neurofibromatosis (von Recklinghausen's Disease). Advances in Neurology, Vol. 29. New York, Raven Press, 1981, pp 77–95.
62. Whitehouse D: Diagnostic value of the café-au-lait spot in children. Arch Dis Child 41:316, 1966.
63. Wiederholt WC, Gomez MR, Kurland LT: Incidence and prevalence of tuberous sclerosis in Rochester, Minnesota, 1950 through 1982. Neurology 35:600, 1985.
64. Zimmerman RA, Bilaniuk LT, Metzger RA, et al: Computed tomography of orbital facial neurofibromatosis. Radiology 146:113, 1983.

41
POSTSURGERY MANAGEMENT OF CHILDREN WITH BRAIN TUMORS

Roger J. Packer, M.D.

Surgery, albeit of extreme importance, is only the first step in the treatment of children with brain tumors. Optimal management of patients with primary childhood central nervous system (CNS) tumors requires a multidisciplinary, comprehensive approach. More than one half of all children with brain tumors can now be expected to be alive and free of disease five years following diagnosis, many apparently cured of their illness, after the appropriate use of surgery, radiotherapy, and chemotherapy.[36] However, such therapies can also cause significant neurologic sequelae, and their use requires an understanding of the biology of the tumor, its pattern of growth, the extent of the tumor at diagnosis, the tumor's probable response to each modality of treatment, and the possible toxicities of treatment. This chapter reviews general aspects of postsurgical management of children with brain tumors and how comprehensive treatment plans can be applied to improve outcome for patients with brain tumors.

GENERAL ASPECTS OF POSTSURGICAL TREATMENT

Postsurgical Staging Studies

Based on symptoms at the time of diagnosis, the histologic features of the tumor, and the results of postsurgical evaluations for the extent of residual disease at the primary tumor site and at distant CNS sites, it is often possible to stratify children with brain tumors into risk groups. This stratification can then be used to determine the need for a particular type of therapy. It is also crucial to the appropriate evaluation of the efficacy of newer forms of treatment.

Assessment of the extent of residual disease at the primary disease site, after surgery, has been objectively possible only since the introduction of computed tomography (CT) in the mid 1970's.[62] Neurosurgical determination of residual disease is helpful but not very reliable. The presence of enhancing masses on the postoperative CT is usually taken as evidence of residual tumor. Enhancing regions at the rim of the operative bed are more difficult to evaluate, as they may represent either residual tumor or postoperative damage to the surrounding brain.[8] It has been suggested that performing CT within the first 48 hours after surgery may obviate this problem, on the contention that tissue damaged at the time of surgery will not enhance in the first two to three days postoperatively, whereas residual tumor will.[8] However, this has not been conclusively proved, and it is often difficult to obtain CT scans on patients, who may be medically unstable, within the first 48 hours after surgery. Another area in which CT assessment of residual disease is less than optimal is in the evaluation of lesions that infiltrate the brain parenchyma, especially the brainstem.[48] CT may show no residual disease, even when the surgeon knows that infiltrating tumor was left behind. In these situations, surgical observations are more useful than CT findings.

It was originally hoped that nuclear magnetic resonance imaging (NMRI), with its better visualization of the posterior fossa and its ability to image in multiple planar orientations, would overcome the limitations of CT in the assessment of residual disease.[37, 48] However, it is now clear that NMRI demonstrates postsurgical changes never appreciated on CT, and in most cases, postoperative distinction between surgically induced change and residual disease is virtually impossible on NMRI.[47] It seems that in the forseeable future, CT performed with and without contrast enhancement will remain the gold standard for the evaluation of residual disease after surgery. It should be performed within the first week after surgery (earlier if possible) in all children with brain tumors (Table 41–1).

Primary CNS tumors in childhood are much more likely to disseminate to distant neuroaxis sites than are tumors in adults.[42] Leptomeningeal disease at the time of diagnosis occurs in as many as 10 percent of all children with CNS tumors and is especially common in patients with primitive neuroectodermal tumors (PNETs), including medulloblastoma, occurring both in and outside the posterior fossa, and germ cell tumors.[42] In the vast majority of patients, such dissemination is asymptomatic at the time of diagnosis or is overshadowed by symptoms caused by the tumor at the primary disease site. Failure to diagnose dissemination may result in disease relapse in untreated areas and increased neurologic morbidity.

Many patients with leptomeningeal disease are not correctly diagnosed when analysis of cerebrospinal fluid for the presence of tumor cells is the only technique used to assess tumor extent.[42] Myelography has shown lump disease, despite negative cytology, in as many as 50 percent of newly diagnosed patients with PNETs.[40, 42] The role of NMRI in the evaluation of subarachnoid disease dissemination is unclear, but preliminary results suggest that NMRI will not be sensitive to small areas of subarachnoid spread, especially in the cauda equina area.[49] The use of paramagnetic intravenous agents may render NMRI more helpful in the future in such evaluations. At present, concurrent cerebrospinal fluid cytologic examination and myelography is indicated within the first 14 days postoperatively, prior to the initiation of further therapy, in children at high risk for leptomeningeal spread; the patients included are those with PNETs, germ cell tumors, and anaplastic gliomas (Table 41–1). The significance of tumor cells found in the cerebrospinal fluid during the first 10 to 14 days postoperatively is unclear, as it is conceivable that these cells were shed at the time of surgery rather than being representative of preoperative disseminated disease. A repeat spinal tap at 21 days is indicated in all patients with negative myelograms and malignant tumor cells found in the cerebrospinal fluid in the first 14 days after surgery. A repeat cerebrospinal fluid sample that is still positive for tumor cells should be taken as proof of disseminated disease.

The need for other tests to assess the extent of disease, postoperatively, is less well established. Bone scans and bone marrow aspirates have been recommended for all children with PNET of the posterior fossa, but their yield is low, and their need inconclusive.[2] Tumor markers, such as the polyamines, seem better suited to follow the course of illness than to determine the extent of disease at diagnosis.[14, 52]

Radiotherapy

Radiotherapy increases the duration of survival and the rate of cure for children with many types of CNS malignancies.[27] Radiotherapy for children with brain tumors is primarily delivered by external beam techniques, utilizing photon beam irradiation produced by linear accelerators (x-rays) or cobalt teletherapy equipment (gamma-irradiation). For some types of CNS tumors that rarely spread outside their primary site, local radiotherapy results in long-term tumor control. Doses in the 5000 to 5500 cGy range, delivered as 180 to 200 cGy per dose per day, once daily, have been most successfully used and do not cause a high incidence of radionecrosis to the surrounding normal brain.[27] However, for those types of childhood CNS tumors that frequently disseminate to the neuroaxis, including most of the malignant childhood brain tumors, local radiotherapy alone infrequently results in long-term disease control.[11] Craniospinal radiotherapy, in doses between 3600 and 4000 cGy, supplemented with local radiotherapy to a total dose of 5000 to 5500 cGy at the primary tumor site, has resulted in improved tumor control (see Table 41–2).[25, 32, 34, 60, 61] In the majority of cases, this extensive neuroaxis irradiation is given "presymptomatically" in an attempt to irradicate tumor that, although not measurable, is believed to have disseminated prior to diagnosis.

Whole brain irradiation has been incriminated as causing significant neurocognitive and neuroendocrinologic sequelae.[12, 13, 54, 63] However, without such therapy, the chance for disease control in tumors, such as PNET and anaplastic gliomas of the posterior fossa, is markedly lessened.[32, 34, 60, 61] It is not known what total dose or volume of irradiation is "safe" in a child of any age, and it is unlikely that a totally safe dose exists within the ranges needed to control tumor. Age clearly does seem to be a crucial factor, as younger children are prone to

Table 41–1. POSTSURGICAL STAGING AND SURVEILLANCE STUDIES

Tumor Type	Initial Postoperative Evaluation	Six Weeks Post-Treatment Evaluation
PNET	CT; myelogram	CT; myelogram
Low-grade glioma (any site)	CT (or NMRI)	CT; myelogram*
Anaplastic glioma of cortex	CT; ? myelogram	CT; myelogram*
Anaplastic glioma of posterior fossa	CT; myelogram	CT; myelogram*
Brainstem gliomas	NMRI (CT if NMRI not available)	NMRI
Ependymomas (all grades, locations)	CT; myelogram	CT; myelogram*
Germ cell tumors	CT; myelogram; CSF tumor markers (alpha-fetoprotein; HCG)	CT; myelogram*; CSF tumor markers

*Only if initial myelogram or cerebrospinal fluid cytology is positive.
HCG, human chorionic gonadotrophin; CSF, cerebrospinal fluid.

suffer more severe sequelae, believed to be due primarily to their more immature central nervous system.[12]

Various means have been employed in an attempt to increase the efficacy, while not increasing the toxicity, of radiotherapy. Agents that enhance the effect of radiotherapy have not yet been shown to be of efficacy.[15, 31] The direct implantation of radioactive substances into the tumor may be useful, in the future, for children who have locally aggressive tumors with low proclivities to disseminate to the neuroaxis.[22] Similarly, the use of hyperfractionated radiotherapy, delivering radiation in lower individual doses, two or more times daily, may improve local tumor control.[64] By using this treatment approach, a higher dose of radiation can be delivered theoretically without causing increased damage to the surrounding normal brain.

Chemotherapy

Initially employed almost exclusively in children with recurrent disease, chemotherapy has recently been shown to play a significant role in the management of newly diagnosed patients with PNET of the posterior fossa and anaplastic gliomas of childhood when given with and after radiotherapy (Table 41–2).[2, 15, 31] Prospective multicentered trials have shown that certain subsets of children with PNETs of the posterior fossa and cortical anaplastic gliomas seem to benefit from the addition of lomustine (CCNU), vincristine, and prednisone after radiotherapy.[2, 16, 33, 42] Preliminary trials with other drug combinations have also suggested benefit. Various chemotherapeutic approaches are now being actively evaluated in newly diagnosed patients, including (1) the use of multiagent chemotherapy (the most adventurous being the 8-drugs-in-one-day regimen), in an attempt to overcome tumor heterogenity in both cellular make-up and response to treatment, and (2) preradiation chemotherapy, in an attempt to overcome microvascular changes caused by radiation that might adversely affect delivery of the drug to the tumor and possibly potentiate the effects of radiotherapy.[2, 5, 31]

As experiences with chemotherapeutic agents have grown and more effective drugs or drug regimens are developed, chemotherapy has been increasingly used in the very young child with a brain tumor, since radiotherapy is most likely to cause severe, irreversible brain damage in such patients.[66] However, the safety of most drugs with regard to the immature brain has not been established. Actinomycin D and vincristine have been successfully used in children younger than five years of age with chiasmatic gliomas.[55] MOPP chemotherapy, which is composed of Mustargen (nitrogen mustard), Oncovin (vincristine), procarbazine, and prednisone, has been shown to be somewhat effective against a variety of brain tumors in children younger than three years of age.[66] Cis-platinum–containing drug regimens have at least delayed the need for immediate radiotherapy in children younger than two years of age with PNET.[42] It is yet unclear which tumors in these very young children respond to chemotherapy, and if therapy is effective, whether tumor control will be perma-

Table 41–2. POSTOPERATIVE TREATMENT OF CHILDHOOD TUMORS

Type	Local Radiotherapy	Craniospinal Plus Local Radiotherapy	Adjuvant Chemotherapy
PNET		X	X (in certain subsets of patients)
Low-grade glioma	? (in subtotally resected tumors)		
Anaplastic glioma of cortex	X		X
Aplastic glioma of posterior fossa		X	?
Brainstem gliomas	X		
Low-grade ependymomas	X		?
Anaplastic ependymomas		X	?
Germ cell tumors		X	?
Craniopharyngiomas	X (in subtotally resected tumors)		

nent or transient and then require the use of radiotherapy.

SURVEILLANCE TESTING FOR RECURRENT DISEASE

A gray area in the postsurgical management of children with brain tumors is how frequently children should be re-evaluated for disease recurrence and what means should be employed in these evaluations.[28] Asymptomatic local disease recurrence does occur, and it seems logical, although it is unproved, that treating recurrence earlier will improve outcome. It has been recommended that neurologic evaluation and CT scanning be performed at regular intervals after diagnosis; more frequently in malignant lesions, and less frequently in slower-growing tumors. The schema arbitrary used at the Children's Hospital of Philadelphia is presented in Table 41-3.

Whether NMRI can replace CT in surveillance evaluations is speculative. Although NMRI is safer than CT, it is conceivable that early local disease recurrence could be obscured by postsurgical changes on NMRI and would be diagnosed earlier by CT. However, for infiltrating lesions, such as brainstem gliomas, NMRI has already proved superior to CT in the evaluation of disease recurrence.[48] Routine cerebrospinal fluid cytology and myelography have also been recommended as routine tests after CT. However, their yield has not been high enough, in the author's opinion, to recommend their routine use in patients with negative studies at diagnosis, and these tests should be reserved for patients with initially positive myelograms or cerebrospinal fluid cytologies.[28] Cerebrospinal fluid tumor markers such as the polyamines for patients with PNETs and human chorionic gonadotrophin (HCG) and alpha-fetoprotein for patients with mixed germ cell tumors may also be useful adjuncts in following patients for disease recurrence.[14, 46, 52]

Long-Term Sequelae

It is now well recognized that survivors of childhood brain tumors may have significant neurologic, cognitive, and endocrine residual deficits. Many of these deficits are believed to be related to treatment, although other factors, including the patient's preoperative status and postoperative course, have an impact on outcome, especially as regards intellectual function.[38]

Early reports suggested that most children who had survived primary brain tumors and received whole brain radiotherapy were retarded.[54] More recent studies have suggested that most of these patients have normal intelligence but may have significant learning disabilities.[13, 54] In addition, radiation-related cognitive changes are not static but may progress over time, with the full extent of deficits not being evident until three or more years after treatment.[13] Based on available information, it seems that all survivors of childhood CNS malignancies should undergo a complete neuropsychologic evaluation within the first year of diagnosis, to assess intellectual abilities and design appropriate educational programs. In children who have received whole brain irradiation, testing should be repeated at yearly intervals, for at least the first three years after diagnosis.

The detrimental effects of treatment on endocrine function are even more poorly characterized than are intellectual deficits.[13] Biochemical growth hormone insufficiency occurs in 67 to 100 percent of children who have received whole brain irradiation, and decreased growth velocity occurs in over one half of these patients. Thyroid and gonadotrophin function are more variably impaired. Endocrine deficits may also occur in patients treated with local radiotherapy, especially in patients with posterior fossa tumors, since radiation portals for posterior fossa tumors usually include the posterior portion of the hypothalamus.[13] Linear growth needs to be carefully followed in children with all forms of brain tumors and in any child with decelerated linear growth; endocrine evaluation is indicated. Similarly, gonadotrophin evaluation should be performed in any patient with delayed puberty. Thyroid function studies are indicated, on at least a yearly basis for the first three years after treatment, in any child who received whole brain irradiation or local irradiation that involved the hypothalamus.

POSTSURGICAL TREATMENT OF SPECIFIC TUMOR TYPES

Other chapters have dealt with the treatment of individual childhood tumors in more detail. The general principles of postoperative treatment described previously will be applied to summarize briefly postsurgical treatment for the more common forms of primary CNS tumors.

Primitive Neuroectodermal Tumors

Although PNETs may occur in any region of the central nervous system, the most extensive studies on the efficacy of antineoplastic treatment have been performed in children with posterior fossa lesions. Disagreement exists regarding whether posterior fossa PNETs (also known as medulloblastomas) should be catagorized and treated differently from PNETs in the pineal region (pineoblastomas) or cerebral cortex (central neuroblastomas).[55–57, 59] Until tumor-specific markers become available, such

Table 41–3. PROPOSED SCHEDULE OF SURVEILLANCE STUDIES FOR CHILDREN WITH BRAIN TUMORS

Tumor Type	3 mo*	6 mo	9 mo	12 mo	18 mo	24 mo	30 mo	36 mo	42 mo	48 mo
PNET	CT	CT; M[B]	CT[A]	CT; M[B]	CT	CT; M[B]	CT	CT; M[B]		CT (yearly, thereafter)
Low-grade glioma		CT or NMRI			CT or NMRI		CT or NMRI		CT or NMRI	(yearly, thereafter, if residual disease)
Anaplastic glioma	CT	CT; M[B]	CT[A]	CT; M[B]	CT	CT; M[B]	CT	CT		CT (yearly, thereafter)
Brainstem glioma	NMRI	NMRI	NMRI	NMRI	NMRI	NMRI	NMRI	NMRI	NMRI	NMRI (yearly, thereafter)
Ependymoma	CT[A]	CT; M[B]	CT[A]	CT; M[B]	CT	CT; M[B]	CT	CT; M[B]	CT	CT (yearly, thereafter)
Germ cell tumor	CT[A]	CT; M[B], TM	CT[A]	CT; M[B], TM	CT	CT; M[B], TM	CT	CT; M[B], TM	CT	CT (yearly, thereafter)

*Time noted either after diagnosis or after completion of initial treatment staging studies (see Table 41–1).
[A]Only if residual local disease is present.
[B]Only if initial myelogram is positive or if malignant cells are found in cerebrospinal fluid.
M, myelogram; TM, tumor markers (see text)

controversies cannot be settled, and for this review, all PNETs will be considered as a single entity.

After complete postoperative staging, including myelography, most patients with PNETs can be stratified into two major risk groups (Table 41-4).[2,43] It is still unsettled whether the size of the primary tumor at the time of surgery or the amount of residual disease after surgery is the more important determinant of outcome. The Chang staging system[10] has been most widely used to characterize the local extent of posterior fossa tumors at diagnosis. T_1–T_2 Chang posterior fossa PNETs are less than 3 cm in diameter and do not cause hydrocephalus, whereas T_3–T_4 Chang tumors cause internal hydrocephalus, infiltrate the brainstem, are locally disseminated, or all three. Outcome of patients with T_1–T_2 tumors is better than that of patients with T_3–T_4 lesions.[21,43] Early reports suggested that total surgical resection of PNET improved survival.[34,51] However, multivariate analyses, taking into account other factors, including the original size of the tumor and the histologic features, have failed to confirm statistically the association between extent of resection (total versus partial) and outcome. However, these studies do confirm that patients whose tumors are biopsied, but are not resected, rarely survive.[21,43] Since pineal region tumors and, to a lesser extent, cortical PNETs are less amenable to total surgical resection than posterior fossa lesions, and dissemination to other sites in the central nervous system[46] occurs readily with pineal region PNETs, most PNETs outside the posterior fossa fall into the poor-risk group.

All patients with PNETs older than three years of age at the time of diagnosis, independent of risk factors, should be treated with craniospinal and supplemental local radiotherapy.[29,32,34,51] As many as 60 percent of patients with favorable-risk characteristics can be expected to be alive and free of disease five years following diagnosis, with such treatment. A reduction in the dose of whole brain irradiation may be possible in this "average"-risk group. However, since the addition of craniospinal irradiation is probably the primary reason for the improvement in survival rates for children with PNETs, such a reduction should be done cautiously and only in completely staged patients.[65] More appropriately, such reductions should be done as part of prospective, randomized treatment trials evaluating both tumor control and long-term intellectual outcome. The addition of chemotherapy has not been shown to be of benefit in patients with favorable-risk parameters.[2]

In children with poor-risk factors, the five-year survival rate after radiotherapy alone is less than 40 percent.[2,43] In these patients, adjuvant chemotherapy with CCNU, vincristine, and prednisone has been shown to be of some benefit. In one study, children with locally extensive PNET (Chang T_3–T_4) had a 59 percent five-year disease-free survival rate after treatment with radiotherapy plus chemotherapy, as compared with 41 percent after treatment with radiotherapy alone.[2] Other drug combinations, used both prior to and after chemotherapy, also have shown efficacy in preliminary treatment trials.[33,42] Based on available information, it seems that poor-risk patients should be considered candidates for adjuvant chemotherapy, once again preferably as part of a prospective, randomized treatment trial.

In children younger than two years of age at diagnosis with PNETs, because of the potential detrimental effects of radiotherapy, treatment with chemotherapy alone or chemotherapy followed at a later time by radiotherapy should be considered. Trials using MOPP chemotherapy and cisplatin-containing treatment regimens have shown efficacy in preliminary studies.[42,66]

Ependymomas

The factors predictive of outcome and the optimal postsurgical management of children with ependymomas are far from established. Survival rates of 10 to 70 percent with similar means of treatment have been reported.[18,26,53,61] Ependymomas have a variable tendency to seed the neuroaxis. Anaplastic lesions are more likely to disseminate than are tumors arising in the posterior fossa.[42] However, based on available information, it seems that the extent of CNS disease in all children with ependymomas should be completely evaluated, and all patients should undergo postoperative myelography.

The value of radiotherapy in low-grade lesions is inconclusive, but in nonrandomized, retrospective series, reported survival rates are higher for children who have received local radiotherapy than for those patients treated with surgery alone.[61] In children with anaplastic gliomas, the best survival rates are reported in children who have received craniospinal plus supplemental radiotherapy to the primary tumor site.[61] Chemotherapy is not of proven efficacy for children with ependymomas of any histologic type but should be considered as part of

Table 41-4. STRATIFICATION OF CHILDREN WITH PNET

	Average Risk (All of the Below)	Poor Risk (Any of the Below)
Dissemination	Negative myelogram; negative cerebrospinal fluid cytology	Positive myelogram and/or positive cerebrospinal fluid cytology
Local disease	Small tumor—Chang T_1/T_2 (or ? totally resected)	Large tumor—Chang T_3/T_4 (or ? subtotally resected)
Histology	Undifferentiated	Differentiated
Age	Three years of age or older at diagnosis	Younger than three years of age at diagnosis

any randomized treatment trial. Cisplatin drugs have shown some efficacy in children with recurrent ependymomas and may be useful in newly diagnosed patients.[31]

Brainstem Gliomas

Local radiotherapy is of transient benefit in over 80 percent of children with brainstem gliomas but results in long-term disease control in probably fewer than 20 percent of patients.[35, 50] In patients with exophytic lesions at the cervicomedullary junction, which may be amenable to gross surgical resections, the role of radiotherapy is unclear.[24]

Recent work suggests that patients with brainstem gliomas can be stratified on the basis of clinical, CT, and pathologic findings into two major risk groups (Table 41–5).[1] As many as 60 percent of patients in the average risk group will be alive and free of disease five years after diagnosis and after treatment with conventionally fractionated doses of radiotherapy, with a total dose in the 5000 to 5500 cGy range.[1] Since children with one or more unfavorable criteria will rarely survive longer than 18 months following diagnosis after similar radiotherapy, more aggressive treatment regimens, even if they are potentially more neurotoxic, should be strongly considered for, and at least initially reserved for, those children with poor risk factors.

Chemotherapy has yet to be shown to be of benefit in children with brainstem gliomas.[19] Children with brainstem gliomas can develop clinically significant leptomeningeal spread early in the course of illness, and such dissemination may become an increasing problem when local disease control of malignant lesions improves.[35] However, since local disease control is so poor, extensive evaluation for dissemination at diagnosis is not warranted in children with brainstem gliomas.

Low-Grade Gliomas

The value of either radiotherapy or chemotherapy has not been well established in patients with low-grade gliomas.[6, 17, 30] There is no evidence that the addition of such therapy in lesions that are grossly resected, such as in patients with cerebellar astrocytomas, is of any benefit.[20, 21] Reported five-year survival rates for children with tumors that were partially resected, in nonrandomized series, are higher in patients who had received radiotherapy than in patients treated with surgery alone.[6, 17, 30] However, ten- and twenty-year survival rates are similar in irradiated and nonirradiated patients. When possible, a period of observation is probably indicated in those children with low-grade partially resected lesions, since for poorly understood reasons, some partially resected lesions do not grow for years, if at all. In those patients who show clinical or radiographic progression of lesions, radiotherapy is then probably indicated, if further surgery seems unlikely to be of benefit.

In young children, especially those younger than five years of age, local radiotherapy can cause significant long-term neuropsychologic deficits.[39] Treatment with actinomycin D and vincristine has been shown to be of at least short-term benefit in children with progressive chiasmatic gliomas and has delayed the need for radiotherapy.[58]

Anaplastic Gliomas of the Cerebrum

The best results, to date, in children with anaplastic cerebral gliomas have occurred after treatment with local radiotherapy and chemotherapy.[2, 16] The primary disease site is the most common site of disease failure, and at present, extensive evaluation for disease dissemination at diagnosis does not seem warranted in patients with anaplastic gliomas. However, as with patients who have brainstem gliomas, disease dissemination does occur and may be of greater concern if local disease control can be improved.

Although radiotherapy is of at least transient benefit in most patients, fewer than 15 percent of patients with anaplastic gliomas have long-lasting disease control after radiotherapy alone.[2, 16] Recently, a 40 percent five-year survival rate has been reported after treatment with radiotherapy, followed by CCNU and vincristine.[2, 16] Randomized treatment trials, attempting to confirm the benefit of this drug regimen and evaluating potentially more effective combinations, are under way. In the future, radiation implantation may also be of benefit for newly diagnosed patients.[22]

Anaplastic Gliomas of the Posterior Fossa

Anaplastic gliomas of the posterior fossa frequently disseminate to the neuroaxis, and complete postoperative staging, including myelography, is indicated in all patients.[42, 44] Craniospinal radiotherapy with supplemental local radiotherapy seems to

Table 41–5. STRATIFICATION OF CHILDREN WITH BRAINSTEM GLIOMAS

	Average Risk (All of the Below)	Poor Risk (Any of the Below)
Clinical findings at diagnosis	No cranial nerve deficits	Cranial nerve deficits
CT findings	Isodense or mixed-density mass on unenhanced CT; variable enhancement; may be exophytic; localized lesion	Hypodense mass on CT; minimal enhancement after contrast; entire brainstem involved
Histology	Low-grade glioma	Anaplastic glioma

result in the best disease control.[60] Based on information obtained from treatment trials for children with anaplastic cortical gliomas, adjuvant chemotherapy should be explored in this group of patients.[16]

Germ Cell Tumors

Germ cell tumors in childhood occur primarily in the pineal or suprasellar region.[46] Germinomas and mixed germ cell tumors (including embryonal cell carcinomas) make up the majority of tumors.[46] Both these tumor types readily disseminate to the neuroaxis, and a full extent of disease evaluation, including myelography, is indicated in all patients at the time of diagnosis.

Five-year survival rates as high as 80 percent are reported in patients with germinomas after treatment with craniospinal radiotherapy supplemented with local radiotherapy.[67] Recently, there has been an attempt to reduce the dose of craniospinal radiation in children with localized germinomas by using preradiation chemotherapy (high-dose cyclophosphamide).[4] Chemotherapy may also be of benefit in children with disseminated disease at the time of diagnosis.[4]

Patients with mixed germ cell tumors rarely experience long-term disease control after craniospinal radiotherapy and local radiotherapy.[45] Alternative means of treatment should be explored in these patients.[4, 45] One potentially beneficial approach is coupling craniospinal and local radiotherapy with chemotherapy of proven benefit in non–central nervous system germ cell tumors.

Craniopharyngiomas

The appropriate treatment for craniopharyngiomas is controversial.[7, 9, 23] However, it does seem that the addition of local radiotherapy in children with partially resected tumors is of benefit.[9] Chemotherapy has no proven role in this tumor. Since disease recurrence is almost exclusively at the primary disease site in patients with craniopharyngiomas, evaluation for disease dissemination at the time of diagnosis is not warranted.

References

1. Albright AL, Guthkelch AN, Packer RJ: Prognostic factors in pediatric brain stem gliomas. J Neurosurg 65:751, 1986.
2. Allen JC: Childhood brain tumors. Current status of clinical trials in newly diagnosed and recurrent disease. Pediatr Clin North Am 32:633, 1985.
3. Allen JC, Nelson L, Jereb B: Pre-radiation chemotherapy for newly diagnosed childhood brain tumors—a modified phase II trial. Cancer 52:2001, 1983.
4. Allen JC, Walker R, Kim JH: Pre-radiation chemotherapy for newly diagnosed central nervous system germinoma—an attempt to reduce radiotherapy dose while increasing survival. Ann Neurol 18:404, 1985.
5. Bleyer W, Milstein J, Balias F, et al: Eight-drugs-in-one-day chemotherapy for brain tumors. A new approach and rational for pre-radiation chemotherapy. Med Pediatr Oncol 11:213, 1983.
6. Bouchard J, Peirce CB: Radiation therapy in the management of neoplasms of the central nervous system, with a special note in regard to children. Twenty years experience, 1939–1958. Am J Roentgenol 84:610, 1960.
7. Bruce DA, Schut L, Rorke LB: Craniopharyngiomas in a capsule. In: Concepts in Pediatric Neurosurgery, Vol. 1. New York, S Karger, 1981, pp 29–35.
8. Cairncross JG, Pexam JHW, Rothbone MP, et al: Postoperative contrast enhancement in patients with brain tumors. Ann Neurol 17:570, 1985.
9. Cavazzuti V, Fischer EG, Welch K, et al: Neurological and psychological sequelae following different treatments of craniopharyngioma in children. J Neurosurg 59:409, 1983.
10. Chang CH, Houseplan EM, Herbert C: An operative staging system and megavoltage radiotherapeutic technique for cerebellar medulloblastoma. Radiology 93:1351, 1969.
11. Cushing H: Experience with cerebellar medulloblastoma. A critical review. Acta Pathol Microbiol Scand 7:1, 1930.
12. Danoff BF, Cowchock FS, Marquette C, et al: Assessment of the long-term effects of primary radiation therapy for brain tumors in children. Cancer 49:1580, 1982.
13. Duffner PK, Cohen ME, Thomas PRM, et al: The long-term effects of cranial irradiation in the central nervous system. Cancer 56:1841, 1985.
14. Edwards MSB, Davis RL, Laurent JP: Tumor markers and cytologic features of cerebrospinal fluid. Cancer 56:1773, 1985.
15. Edwards MS, Levin VA, Wilson CB: Brain tumor chemotherapy. An evaluation of agents in current use for Phase II and III trials. Cancer Treat Rep 64:1179, 1980.
16. Ertel I, Boesel C, Evans A, et al: Adjuvant chemotherapy of high-grade astrocytomas in children. Radiation therapy with or without CCNU, vincristine, and prednisone. Proceedings of American Society of Clinical Oncology 3:79, 1984.
17. Fazekas JT: Treatment of Grade 1 and 2 brain astrocytomas. The role of radiotherapy. Int J Radiat Oncol Biol Phys 2:661, 1977.
18. Fokes EC, Jr., Earle KM: Ependymomas: Clinical and pathological aspects. J Neurosurg 30:585, 1969.
19. Fulton DS, Levin VA, Wara WW, et al: Chemotherapy of pediatric brainstem tumors. J Neurosurg 54:715, 1981.
20. Gjerris F, Klinken L: Long-term prognosis in children with benign cerebellar astrocytoma. J Neurosurg 49:179, 1978.
21. Griffin RW, Beaufait D, Blasko JC: Cystic cerebellar astrocytoma in childhood. Cancer 44:276, 1979.
22. Gutin PM, Phillips TL, Wara WW, et al: Brachytherapy of recurrent malignant brain tumors with removable high-activity iodine—125 sources. J Neurosurg 60:61, 1984.
23. Hoffman HJ, Henrich EB, Humphreys RP: Management of craniopharyngiomas in children. J Neurosurg 47:218, 1977.
24. Hoffman JH, Becker L, Craven MA: A clinically and pathologically distinct group of benign brain stem gliomas. Neurosurgery 7:243, 1980.
25. Jereb B, Krishnaswasmi S, Ried A, et al: Radiation for medulloblastoma adjusted to prevent recurrence to the cribriform plate region. Cancer 54:602, 1984.
26. Kernohan JW, Fletcher-Kernohan EM: Ependymomas: A study of 109 cases. A Res Nerv and Ment Dis Proc 16:182, 1973.
27. Kun LE: Principles of radiation therapy. In: Cohen ME, Duffner PK (eds): Brain Tumors of Children. Principles of Diagnosis and Treatment. International Review of Child Neurology series. New York, Raven Press, 1984, pp 47–70.
28. Kun LE, D'Souza B, Tefft M: The value of surveillance testing in childhood brain tumors. Cancer 56:1818, 1984.
29. Landberg TC, Lindgren ML, Cavallin-Stahl EK, et al: Improvement in the radiotherapy of medulloblastoma, 1946–1975. Cancer 45:670, 1980.

30. Leibel SA, Sheline GE, Wara WW, et al: The role of radiation therapy in the treatment of astrocytomas. Cancer 35:1551, 1975.
31. Levin V, Edwards M, Wara W, et al: 5-fluorouracil and 1-(2-chloroethyl)-3-cyclohexyl-1-nitrosourea (CCNU) followed by hydroxyurea, misonidazole, and irradiation for brain stem gliomas: A pilot study of the Brain Tumor Research Center and the Children's Cancer Group. Neurosurgery 14:679, 1984.
32. McFarland DR, Horowitz H, Saenger EL, et al: Medulloblastoma. A review of prognosis and survival. Br J Radiol 42:198, 1969.
33. McIntosh S, Chen M, Sartain PA, et al: Adjuvant chemotherapy for medulloblastoma. Cancer 56:1316, 1985.
34. Norris DG, Bruce DA, Byrd RI, et al: Improved relapse-free survival in medulloblastoma utilizing modern techniques. Neurosurgery 9:661, 1981.
35. Packer RJ, Allen J, Deck M, et al: Brain stem glioma: Clinical manifestations of meningeal gliomatosis. Ann Neurol 14:177, 1983.
36. Packer RJ, Atkins T, Littman P, et al: Neurologic and neuropsychologic sequelae in survivors of childhood brain tumors. Proc Int Soc Pediatr Oncol 15:71, 1983.
37. Packer RJ, Batzinsky S, Cohen ME: Magnetic resonance imaging in the evaluation of intracranial tumors of childhood. Cancer 56:1767, 1985.
38. Packer RJ, Bruce DA, Atkins TA: Factors impacting on neurocognitive outcome in long-term survivors of primitive neuroectodermal tumors–medulloblastoma (PNET-MB). Ped Neurosci (in press).
39. Packer RJ, Savino PJ, Bilaniuk LT, et al: Chiasmatic gliomas of childhood: A reappraisal of natural history and effectiveness of cranial irradiation. Child's Brain 10:393, 1983.
40. Packer RJ, Siegel KR, Schut L, et al: Central nervous system spread of childhood brain tumors at diagnosis or at initial disease recurrence. In: Chapman PH (ed): Concepts in Pediatric Neurosurgery, Vol. 6. New York, S Karger, 1985, pp 16–25.
41. Packer RJ, Siegel KR, Sutton LN, et al: Leptomeningeal dissemination of primary central nervous system tumors of childhood. Ann Neurol 18:217, 1985.
42. Packer RJ, Siegel KR, Sutton LN, et al: Efficacy of combination chemotherapy with cis-platinum (CPDD), lomustine (CCNU), and vincristine (VCR) in children with primitive neuroectodermal tumors–medulloblastoma (PNET-MB) of childhood. Ann Neurol 18:394, 1985.
43. Packer RJ, Sutton LN, Rorke LB, et al: Prognostic significance of cellular differentiation in primitive neuroectodermal tumors (medulloblastoma) of childhood. J Neurosurg 61:296, 1984.
44. Packer RJ, Sutton LN, Rorke LB, et al: Oligodendroglioma of the posterior fossa in childhood. Cancer 56:195, 1985.
45. Packer RJ, Sutton LN, Rorke LB, et al: Intracranial embryonal cell carcinoma. Cancer 54:142, 1984.
46. Packer RJ, Sutton LN, Rosenstock JG, et al: Pineal region tumors of childhood. Pediatrics 74:97, 1984.
47. Packer RJ, Zimmerman RA, Bilaniuk LT: Magnetic resonance imaging (MRI) in the evaluation of treatment-related central nervous system (CNS) damage. Cancer 58:33, 1986.
48. Packer RJ, Zimmerman RA, Leurson T, et al: Nuclear magnetic resonance imaging in the evaluation of brain stem gliomas of childhood. Neurology 35:397, 1985.
49. Packer RJ, Zimmerman RA, Sutton LN, et al: Magnetic resonance imaging (MRI) of the posterior fossa and upper cervical cord. Pediatrics 76:84, 1985.
50. Panitch MS, Berg BO: Brain stem tumors of childhood and adolescence. Am J Dis Child 119:465, 1970.
51. Park TS, Hoffman HJ, Hendrich EB, et al: Medulloblastoma, clinical presentation and management. Experience at the Hospital for Sick Children, Toronto, 1950–1980. J Neurosurg 58:543, 1983.
52. Phillips PC, Kremzner LT, DeVivo DC: Cerebrospinal fluid polyamines and childhood primary brain tumors. Ann Neurol 14:372, 1983.
53. Pierre-Kahn A, Hirsch JF, Roux FX, et al: Intracranial ependymomas in childhood—survival and function results of 47 cases. Child's Brain 10:145, 1983.
54. Raimondi AJ, Tomita T: The advantages of total resection of medulloblastoma and disadvantages of whole brain postoperative radiation therapy. Child's Brain 5:50, 1979.
55. Rorke LB: Classification and grading of childhood brain tumors: Overview and statement of the problem. Cancer 56:1848, 1985.
56. Rorke LB: The cerebellar medulloblastoma and its relationship to primitive neuroectodermal tumors. J Neuropathol Exp Neurol 42:1, 1983.
57. Rorke LB, Gilles FM, Davis RL, et al: Revision of the World Health Organization classification of brain tumors for childhood brain tumors. Cancer 56:1869, 1985.
58. Rosenstock JC, Packer RJ, Bilaniuk L, et al: Chiasmatic optic glioma treated with chemotherapy: A preliminary report. J Neurosurg 63:863, 1985.
59. Rubinstein LJ: Editorial. Neuro-Oncol 3:195, 1984.
60. Salazar OM: Primary malignant cerebellar astrocytomas in children: A signal for postoperative craniospinal irradiation. Int J Radiat Oncol Biol Phys 7:1661, 1981.
61. Salazar OM, Casto-Vita M, Van Houtte D, et al: Improved survival in cases of intracranial ependymoma after radiation therapy. Late report and recommendations. J Neurosurg 59:652, 1983.
62. Segall MD, Batzinsky S, Zee C-S, et al: Computed tomography in the diagnosis of intracranial neoplasms in children. Cancer 56:1748, 1985.
63. Sheline GE: Irradiation injury of human brain. A review of clinical experience. In: Gilbert HA, Kagan AK (eds): Radiation Damage to the Nervous System: A Delayed Therapeutic Hazard. New York, Raven Press, 1980, pp 39–59.
64. Shin K, Muller P, Geggree P: Superfractionation radiation therapy in treatment of malignant astrocytoma. Cancer 52:2040, 1983.
65. Tomita T, McLone DG: Medulloblastoma in childhood: Results of radical resection and low-dose neuroaxis radiation therapy. J Neurosurg 64:38, 1986.
66. Van Eys J, Cangir A, Coady D, et al: MOPP regimen as primary chemotherapy for brain tumors in infants. J Neuro-Oncol 3:237, 1984.
67. Wara WW, Jenkins RDT, Evans A, et al: Tumors of the pineal and suprasellar regions: Children's Cancer Study Group treatment results, 1960–1975. Cancer 43:698, 1979.

42
MANAGEMENT OF RECURRENT DISEASE

Jeffrey C. Allen, M.D.

The therapeutic approaches to the management of recurrent primary brain tumors are guided by the anticipated tumor biology. For patients with recurrent low-grade tumors in accessible locations, maximum surgical resection is usually the best option. Regional radiotherapy may be added if it has not been previously administered and long-term survival is a realistic goal. However, once a recurrent or progressive malignant brain tumor is diagnosed, the prognosis is guarded and the therapeutic alternatives are more complex. The emphasis in this chapter will be on recurrent malignant primary brain tumors.

Terminating all modalities of therapy may be warranted for some patients, especially if the child has acquired devastating neurologic handicaps or the family has abandoned its enthusiasm for striving for a meaningful prolongation of life. However, most families choose some type of therapy, be it surgery, radiotherapy, or conventional or experimental chemotherapy. After treatment priorities are established and the extent of the disease is assessed, therapy usually begins with surgery, followed by a standard chemotherapy regimen, if applicable. If further disease progression or recurrence is subsequently encountered, more experimental approaches may be undertaken, usually in the form of drug therapy. Such experimental therapy should be administered in the context of controlled clinical trials that monitor toxicity as well as efficacy.

Approximately 600 to 800 children develop malignant brain tumors in the United States each year, at least half of whom do not respond to primary therapy. The analysis of this patient population should help validate better ways of treating other children with newly diagnosed disease.

DIAGNOSIS OF RECURRENT DISEASE

The suspicion of a recurrent brain tumor usually arises in one of two ways: as an incidental subclinical finding on a routine, interval neurodiagnostic study or when a neurodiagnostic study is obtained following a change in behavior or neurologic function. When reasonable doubt prevails with regard to the presence of progressive or recurrent disease on a CT scan, several strategies may be employed. A conservative approach includes watchful waiting and rescanning in two to three months to confirm the progressive nature of the lesion. The more aggressive approach leads to early surgical intervention. If the tumor has metastasized or, for other reasons, a debulking procedure is considered of questionable value, nonsurgical therapy may be offered forthwith.

Neurodiagnostic Studies

The present generation of computed tomography (CT) and magnetic resonance imaging (MRI) scanners allow the clinician to survey the anatomy of the brain and spinal cord with uncanny detail. What resolution the CT scan loses in posterior fossa studies is compensated for by the MRI scan, with its axial and sagittal views. The presence of new areas of enhancement on a CT scan in the original tumor bed or in the ventricles or subarachnoid space is highly suggestive of recurrent disease. Interval changes on MRI are not as easily interpretable. The significance of tissue abnormalities on the T2-weighted images of the MRI scan are incompletely understood. For newly diagnosed patients, MRI is an excellent screen for pathology. Following surgery, MRI may imperfectly differentiate between surgical trauma, reactive changes, and recurrent disease. Thus, it is impractical to rely solely on MRI to confirm a recurrence.

The presence of subclinical or clinical intracerebral hemorrhage is suggestive of recurrent disease, especially when it arises within the original tumor bed. Malignant childhood tumors have a relatively high predisposition to spontaneous hemorrhage.[17] Following prior conventional radiotherapy, there is less than a 5 percent likelihood that a new contrast-enhancing mass is secondary to radiation necrosis alone, rather than recurrent disease. Pure radiation necrosis may enhance on CT, simulating a recurrent brain tumor but is more likely to occur following new therapy, such as the interstitial implantation of radioactive seeds. Brain necrosis may also follow intra-arterial chemotherapy.

Myelography is the most reliable method of confirming subarachnoid metastases. This test should be performed in evaluating the extent of disease, once intracranial recurrence of a malignant brain tumor is confirmed. Myelograms should be performed routinely in patients with primitive neuroectodermal tumors, such as medulloblastoma and pineoblastoma, and selectively in patients with malignant gliomas.[3] Large, subclinical spinal or clinical metastases may require irradiation independent of chemotherapy. The cerebrospinal fluid (CSF) cytologic examination should also be obtained at least once from the lumbar space and, if possible, from within the ventricles if a shunt with a reservoir is in place. There is hope that MRI may be used to screen for subarachnoid spinal metastases, but there is insufficient experience in this matter to defer routine myelography. The use of gadolinium may allow tumors to enhance on MRI.

It is useful to include a bone marrow aspirate as a routine diagnostic test in children with recurrent central nervous system (CNS) primitive neuroectodermal tumors. Bone marrow aspirates may be positive in 5 percent of such patients.[16] However, in a selected population of patients with diffuse CNS metastases, the incidence may rise to 25 to 30 percent, regardless of whether a systemic shunt exists.

Thus, once a suspicion of recurrent disease prevails, the child should receive a battery of neurodiagnostic tests to assess the extent of disease. The identification of "evaluable" disease is useful as a tool against which to measure a response to therapy. Subclinical disease, such as large spinal metastases, may be encountered, requiring urgent intervention. As a rule, prognosis is inversely related to the magnitude of metastatic and local disease.

Clinical Presentations

The signs of recurrent disease, when present, are rarely subtle and usually correlate with the location of the recurrent disease on neurodiagnostic tests. However, problems arise in a number of circumstances. Seizures most often herald other signs of recurrent intracerebral or subarachnoid disease but also occur as a consequence of surgically induced trauma. However, relative refractiveness to prior anticonvulsant therapy is highly suggestive of recurrent disease. Subtle personality changes may indicate recurrent frontal lobe disease or a diffuse neoplastic process such as gliomatosis cerebri or leptomeningeal metastases but can also be a manifestation of a side effect of radiotherapy or chemotherapy. The occurrence of hydrocephalus may reflect further expansion of a midline tumor or leptomeningeal metastases, but a symptomatic communicating hydrocephalus may also develop following surgery, especially in the posterior fossa.

Constitutional changes such as increased lethargy and vomiting are frequently symptoms of raised intracranial pressure related to recurrent disease but are also common symptoms of the radiation somnolence syndrome. This syndrome may follow within one to three months of a therapeutic course of radiotherapy. Increased steroid dependency over time is frequently a sign of recurrent disease but may also occur as a sign of postradiation encephalopathy. The presence of multifocal neurologic signs or symptoms is highly suggestive of leptomeningeal metastases, especially if radicular symptoms or back pain prevails.

Thus, the use of clinical signs and symptoms alone to diagnose a recurrent brain tumor is hazardous, and the ultimate decision should rest on the evaluation of all facts at hand, clinical, histologic, and neurodiagnostic.

MANAGEMENT

Supportive Care

For children symptomatic from recurrent brain tumors, there are several temporizing measures that may relieve symptoms and improve the child's sense of well-being, especially when the family has decided to forego any attempt at aggressive therapy. Corticosteroids often provide weeks of relief of symptoms secondary to cerebral edema, such as raised intracranial pressure and focal neurologic signs, and may often attenuate radicular pain secondary to leptomeningeal metastases. Unfortunately, the steroid dose often has to be escalated to maintain a certain level of relief, and the side effects of corticosteroids are proportional to the dose and the duration of therapy. Such side effects include the disfigurement of appearance, especially bothersome to teenagers who are prone to develop acne and hirsutism in addition to plethoric fascies, a predisposition toward hypertension, diabetes mellitus, opportunistic infections, and, frequently, an undesirable personality alteration accompanied by hyperphagia, irritability, insomnia, and depression. Once a child becomes steroid-dependent, it is very difficult to wean him or her off the drug.

Other useful drugs for the terminal illness include nighttime sedation to give not only the child but also the parents a chance to rest. Pain or headache is usually not part of the symptom complex of a brain tumor unless there is uncontrolled raised intracranial pressure or leptomeningeal spread. Narcotic analgesics should not be spared in spite of some of their undesirable side effects such as constipation, piloerection, chills, and sedation. The latter effect is often desirable. The short-acting narcotics such as hydromophone hydrochloride (Dilaudid) and codeine have a more rapid onset of action and are less sedating but need to be given every three to four hours. At nighttime, a longer-acting drug such as levorphanol tartrate (Levo-Dromoran) or methadone may be added to the regimen. Tachyphylaxis (which results in the need to escalate the dose for the same clinical effect) will be slower to evolve with oral rather than intravenous administration. Focal radiotherapy should be used in an attempt to prevent a myelopathy or to relieve pain.

A child with a terminal illness is often better off at home. Many pediatric cancer centers offer the services of a "home care team" to help bring a complex array of medical, social, and emotional care to the child and the family in more familiar surroundings.

Surgical Intervention

Surgical confirmation of recurrent disease is required when there is any doubt about the nature of the process identified on a neurodiagnostic study, before further radiotherapy or chemotherapy is offered. When there is an extended interval (i.e., beyond five to ten years) between the initial diagnosis and the suspicion of recurrence, surgery is indicated to exclude a second primary tumor.

The neurosurgeon also must assume the role of an oncologist. This includes performing, whenever possible, a maximum debulking of the tumor within the limits of safety to create less of a tumor burden for subsequent therapies. Surgery rapidly relieves symptoms and stabilizes the patients and may serve to minimize some of the side effects of subsequent therapy.

There is little question that a child suffering from a recurring low-grade, localized brain or spinal cord tumor will benefit repeatedly from surgical debulking. For such tumors, surgery may be the only attractive treatment alternative, and many years of high-quality living may ensue between surgical procedures. Of less certain value is the role of surgery in malignant tumors or those that have spread to other locations.

Surgical debulking should primarily be considered as a prelude to other treatment modalities such as chemotherapy. Since chemotherapy manifests its effects more slowly, surgical debulking provides time for other modalities to work. The number of surgical procedures offered to the patient is related to the functional status of the child, the anticipated morbidity of the procedure, the degree of enthusiasm for continuation of care expressed by the family, and, most important, the degree of optimism shared by the medical team for the next available nonsurgical treatment modality.

Chemotherapy

Chemotherapy may be considered in two categories: conventional and experimental. Over the past 10 to 15 years, a number of studies have demonstrated a role for the traditional chemotherapy agents usually given in specific combinations to patients with recurrent primary brain tumors.[7] Two useful regimens are (1) procarbazine, lomustine (CCNU), and vincristine (PCV)[10] and (2) Mustargen (nitrogen mustard), Oncovin (vincristine), procarbazine, and prednisone (MOPP).[10] Both of these regimens have been reported to induce remissions in 25 to 50 percent of patients with such tumors as medulloblastoma and malignant astrocytoma for an average of 6 to 12 months. The toxicity of these regimens is well characterized, is usually tolerable, and consists primarily of early emesis and delayed hematologic depression. Vincristine also causes a progressive axonal peripheral neuropathy over time, with unpleasant paresthesias and distal muscle atrophy and weakness.

These regimens may be given initially unless there are more compelling phase II studies available. When these conventional chemotherapy regimens have already been tried without enduring success, there often prevails a desire to undertake a more experimental approach, usually in the context of clinical drug trials.

Clinical Trials[2]

A phase I trial assesses dose-related toxicity. Usually, a new drug with promise in a laboratory study is taken through a dose-escalation study in which the maximum tolerable dose (MTD) is determined according to a standardized toxicity-rating scale. The dose selected for the subsequent phase II, response-oriented trial is usually 20 to 30 percent less than the MTD. The phase II trial accepts patients in reasonably good health with measurable or evaluable disease on a neurodiagnostic study. Interval therapy is provided until disease progression or unacceptable toxicity is encountered. A CT or MRI scan is repeated at regular intervals after every two courses of therapy, usually every two to three months to determine the degree (complete, partial, minimal, or stable) and the duration of response or whether progressive disease emerges. The phase II trial must be disease-oriented, whereas the phase I trial may include patients with a variety of solid tumors.[1]

If nine consecutive patients with a specific type of recurrent brain tumor fail to achieve an objective response to a particular experimental therapy, it may be concluded with a 95 percent certainty that the true response rate is likely to be less than 30 percent. The trial is usually abandoned for this particular disease when this situation arises but may be continued for other tumors. If one or more responses are encountered, at least 15 patients are studied to determine more accurately the true response rate for a particular disease.

A patient may participate in several different phase II trials. However, it may become increasingly difficult to determine the importance of negative outcomes in patients who are heavily pretreated, who have highly resistant disease, and who may not tolerate the planned dose of chemotherapy. For this reason, most phase II trials attempt to preselect patients who have received minimal prior chemotherapy.

A phase III study is conducted in newly diagnosed patients where the end points are the duration of the disease-free state and total survival. Usually, one or more experimental treatments are selected from prior promising phase II studies and are added to the best available conventional treatment. The new modalities have recently consisted of single or multiple drug regimens in the cooperative children's cancer group trials, Children's Cancer Study Group (CCSG) and Pediatric Oncology Group (POG). Patients are randomized to either the conventional (control) or the experimental group.

Experimental Chemotherapy

Platinum analogues are effective in a number of childhood brain tumors. Cisplatin is the oldest and the first drug to be studied in this class. High activity has been reported in recurrent medulloblastoma and malignant cerebral astrocytoma when cisplatin was administered in high doses (120mg/m^2) with pre- and postmannitol enforced diuresis, and calcium and magnesium supplements.[2] Unfortunately, the otic and renal toxicity are dose-related, and the emetic properties are severe. The otic toxicity consisting of high-tone hearing loss is also cumulative.

Thus, newer platinum analogues such as carboplatin are currently under investigation in the cooperative groups (CCSG and POG) and at Memorial Sloan Kettering Cancer Center.[5] Carboplatin appears to be as potent as cisplatin, without its undesirable side effects and the need for large fluid volumes and diuresis. The MTD is significantly higher (five to six times) because of the absence of renal and otic toxicity. The CCSG and POG studies utilize a dose of 560mg/m^2, given as an IV short infusion over one to one and a half hours every four to six weeks. The Memorial Sloan Kettering study uses a weekly x4 IV regimen, at a weekly dose of 175 mg/m^2. The Memorial Sloan Kettering study has documented a 45 percent response rate for a median of ten months in patients with medulloblastoma.[5]

DNA-binding drugs seem to be particularly effective for brain tumors. These include drugs such as the nitrosoureas, platinum analogues, and cyclophosphamide derivatives such as nitrogen mustard and iphosphamide,[6] given with intravenous Mesna, a drug that reduces the risk of hemorrhagic cystitis common to this class of agents. This latter regimen is currently under investigation by the CCSG.

A novel type of phase II trial may be conducted in newly diagnosed patients, using the strategy of neoadjuvant or preradiation chemotherapy. Several courses of an experimental regimen are given prior to radiotherapy in newly diagnosed patients with evaluable disease. This approach can be used in poor-risk patients and may serve as well to increase the resectability of partially resected tumors.[4] The CCSG is using this strategy in its phase III medulloblastoma and malignant astrocytoma protocols.

Once single drugs have been shown to be effective for a particular tumor, the next type of phase II trial could consist of this drug in combination with others. Theoretical advantages to combination therapy include interdrug synergism and the delay in the development of tumor resistance. The better tolerated drug combinations include agents with different types of organ toxicity, to the extent possible.

One novel approach to multiagent chemotherapy is to administer many drugs over a short interval. It was felt from prior trials in clinical and laboratory settings that the administration of many drugs over a short interval would be less toxic than if the drugs were individually spaced over several days or weeks. This "8 in 1" (eight-drugs-in-one-day) regimen includes the drugs vincristine, CCNU, procarbazine, hydroxyurea, methylprednisolone, cisplatin, cyclophosphamide, and cytosine arabinoside for patients with primitive neuroectodermal tumors. Preliminary results in phase II trials have been encouraging for medulloblastoma and malignant cerebral astrocytomas, and the regimen has been rapidly advanced to phase III trials by the Children's Cancer Study Group (CCSG).[2]

All the chemotherapy trials previously mentioned involve the administration of drugs by either the intravenous or the oral route. There is a compelling pharmacokinetic rationale to administering drugs, especially those with high-lipid solubility and a short biologic half life, via a cerebral artery, if the brain tumor is confined to the distribution of a single cerebral artery. Extensive clinical studies in adults with high-grade astrocytomas have shown that the therapy can often produce objective remissions with or without prior blood-brain barrier disruption.[11, 19] However, there is a high incidence of treatment-related morbidity, especially with nitrosoureas, including injury to the ipsilateral eye, cerebrovascular embolic events, a delayed leukoencephalopathy, and, occasionally, disease recurrence outside the distribution of the injected artery. Since the relative therapeutic advantage of this technique over intravenous administration has not been firmly established in adults, regional arterial perfusion studies in children with brain tumors should be undertaken with caution.

Thus, the present thrust of chemotherapy research in this field of pediatric neuro-oncology appears to be the conduct of phase II trials with a single-agent, intravenously administered chemotherapy drug. Subsequently, various drugs are put together in rational combinations when chemotherapy toxicity and the mode of action are nonoverlapping.

Newer Therapeutic Modalities

Brachytherapy. Brachytherapy, or interstitial radiotherapy, is used primarily in adult carcinomas (e.g., prostate, lung, rectal). It involves the placement of small radioactive seeds within and around a localized tumor. The seeds emit radiation continually at a low-dose rate. Usually, very high doses (greater than 10,000 rad) can be administered to the central core of the tumor, and the dose rapidly falls off with distance. The ultimate effect is "slow surgery."

This technique has been used in Europe for primary brain tumors for many years, but only recently has it been more widely applied in the United States, both in patients with recurrent and newly diagnosed primary brain tumors.[12] Although remissions have been achieved in recurrent low-grade and high-grade tumors, clinically significant radionecrosis within the treatment field and disease recurrence outside the treatment field appear to be its major drawbacks. Interstitial implants may be more advantageous for patients with recurrent low-grade unresectable tumors rather than those with highly malignant ones capable of geographic spread or dissemination. For newly diagnosed malignant gliomas, a combination of implants plus external photon irradiation may be desirable.

Monoclonal Antibodies. With the development of monoclonal antibody (MAB) technology, there exists an intense search for brain tumor antigens against which "restricted," or tumor-specific, MABs may be formed.[18] These antigens should not only be specific for an individual's tumor, thereby avoiding cross-reactivity to normal host tissue, but also common to similar tumors arising in other patients. Highly restricted MABs thus produced may be utilized for diagnostic and therapeutic purposes. An additional problem, unique to CNS tumors, is the delivery of MABs to a brain tumor, resulting from the impediment to entry offered by the blood-brain barrier. An attempt to augment delivery, using intra-arterial mannitol appears effective.

Several lines of research are currently being undertaken primarily at a laboratory level. Efforts to conjugate MABs to toxins such as radioisotopes and chemicals (ricin or chemotherapy drugs) may produce a class of potent cytotoxic agents with high specificity. Radiolabeled MABs can be used for imaging.

The majority of MABs developed to date reflect shared organ and tumor antigens (CNS and lymphoid tumors and CNS and fetal tissue). The immunizing tissues have usually been derived from melanoma and glial cell lines or human fetal brain. Specific MABs have reacted to groups of neuroectodermal tumors such as melanomas, neuroblastomas, and gliomas. MABs have also been produced to various structural components of neural tissue such as glial fibrillary acidic protein (GFAP), vimentin, and neuron-specific enolase, but these MABs are neither tumor- nor CNS-specific.[18]

Biologic Response Modifiers. An ever-expanding series of hormones derived from mononuclear cells have been recently identified. These lymphokines have widespread biologic effects. Well-known lymphokines such as interferon and the interleukins are considered biologic response modifiers. These lymphokines may have powerful effects on not only other mononuclear cells but also tumor cells. However, they have only become of practical importance recently, as a result of their availability in relatively large quantities. With the advent of recombinant DNA technology, genes coding for these hormones have been isolated and inserted into bacteria, thereby permitting rapid production of the hormones in pure form and in relatively large amounts sufficient for not only laboratory but also clinical research.[8]

Interferons are a class of lymphoid hormones initially generated from virus-infected lymphocytes. Alpha-interferon (IFN-alpha) results from such an event; IFN-beta is derived from virus-infected mesenchymal cells; and IFN-gamma is derived from antigenically stimulated lymphocytes. Interferons as a group have been demonstrated to have antiproliferative effects in vitro against certain glioma cell lines.[9]

Clinical interferon studies are currently under way in brain tumor patients with IFN-alpha and IFN-beta, as either single agents or in combination with other cytotoxic therapy. The systemic toxicity of IFN-alpha has been dose-limiting, consisting primarily of fever, myalgia, somnolence, and confusion. INF-beta appears to be less toxic. Objective and clinical responses in brain tumor patients have already been observed to several interferons alone.[13]

A combination of interleukin-2 (IL-2) and lymphokine-activated killer (LAK) cells has been recently employed at the National Cancer Institute (NCI) in adults with various forms of metastatic solid and lymphoid cancers, with remarkably favorable results.[20] IL-2 induces certain host lymphoid cells to proliferate and attack tumor cells. Usually, a patient with systemic cancer undergoes leukophoresis, and a relatively large quantity of white cells are harvested, cultured, and expanded in vitro in the presence of IL-2 for several days, thereby producing LAK cells. These LAK cells require the continued presence of IL-2 for their viability. When the LAK cells are reinfused into the patient after three to four days of incubation, IL-2 must also be administered at regular intervals in high concentration.

Using this approach, remissions of short duration have been observed, especially in lung metastases in several types of adult cancers. Unfortunately, the systemic toxicity of IL-2 is considerable, with the majority of patients experiencing pulmonary edema and requiring intensive care unit (ICU) care. Phase I to II trials are currently under way in several other centers to confirm these preliminary observations. Two other preliminary studies have been reported in adults with recurrent malignant gliomas, employing intratumoral injections of LAK cells with or without IL-2.[14, 15]

The ultimate role for these and other biologic response modifiers will probably be as adjuvant therapy in combination with other cytotoxic agents such as chemotherapy. They appear to be most effective against minimal residual disease and may also be used in combination with other lymphokines. A major problem for this modality, as for chemotherapy, may be the impediment posed by the blood-brain barrier. Thus, direct intratumoral or intrathecal injection may be required.

To conclude this section, in spite of the rarity of childhood brain tumors as a whole (1200 cases/year), advancements are occurring on several fronts. The hope for the future is the optimum application of proven modalities such as surgery and radiotherapy, in conjunction with more experimental approaches such as chemotherapy and, possibly, combinations of biologic response modifiers. Monoclonal antibodies appear to be in a more formative stage of development. The experience with patients who have recurrent disease is a precious resource. One must consider, not only for the particular patient but for others to come, the importance of exploring new treatment modalities in the context of phase I and II clinical trials.

References

1. Allen J: The design and conduct of clinical brain tumor trials. Cancer 56:1827, 1986.
2. Allen J, Bloom J, Ertel I, et al: Brain tumors in children: Current cooperative and institutional chemotherapy trials in newly diagnosed and recurrent disease. Semin Oncol 13:110, 1986.
3. Allen J, Epstein F: Medulloblastoma and other primary CNS malignant neuroectodermal tumors: The effect of age and extent of disease on prognosis. J Neurosurg 57:446, 1982.
4. Allen J, Helson L, Jereb B: Pre-radiation chemotherapy for newly diagnosed childhood brain tumors—a modified phase II trial. Cancer 52:2001, 1983.
5. Allen JC, Walker R, Luks E, et al: Carboplatin and recurrent childhood brain tumors. J Clin Oncol 5:459, 1987.
6. Antman K, Montella D, Rosenbaum C: Phase II trial of ifosfamide with mesna in previously treated metastatic sarcoma. Cancer Treat Rep 69:499, 1985.
7. Bloom H, Thorton-Jones H: Adjuvant chemotherapy for medulloblastoma: The multicentre controlled trial of the International Society of Pediatric Oncology (SIOP), from the Proceedings of the 13th International Congress on Chemotherapy, 1983.
8. Bullard D, Gillespie G, Mehaley S, et al: Immunology of human gliomas. Sem in Oncol 13:94, 1986.
9. Cook A, Carter W, Nidzgerski F, et al: Human brain tumor–derived cell lines: Growth rate reduced by human fibroblast interferon. Science 219:881, 1983.
10. Edwards M, Levin V, Wilson C: Brain tumor chemotherapy: An evaluation of agents in current use for phase II and III trials. Cancer Treat Rep 64:1179, 1980.
11. Greenberg H, Enswinger W, Chandler W, et al: Intra-arterial BCNU chemotherapy for the treatment of malignant gliomas of the central nervous system. J Neurosurg 61:423, 1984.
12. Gutin P, Phillips T, Wara W, et al: Brachytherapy of recurrent malignant brain tumors with removable high-activity iodine-125 sources. J Neurosurg 60:60, 1984.
13. Hirakowa K, Veda S, Nakagawa Y, et al: Effect of human leukocyte interferon on malignant brain tumors. Cancer 51:1976, 1983.
14. Jacobs S, Wilson D, Kornblith P: In vitro killing of tumor glioblastoma by interleukin-2–activated autologous lymphocytes. J Neurosurg 64:114, 1986.
15. Jacobs S, Wilson D, Kornblith P, et al: Interleukin-2 and autologous lymphokine-activated killer cell treatment of malignant glioma: Phase I trial. Cancer Res 46:2101, 1986.
16. Kleinman G, Hochberg F, Richardson E: Systemic metastases from medulloblastoma. Cancer 48:2296, 1981.
17. Laurent J, Bruce D, Schut L, et al: Hemorrhagic brain tumors in pediatric patients. Child's Brain 8:263, 1981.
18. Lee Y, Bigner D: Aspects of immunobiology and immunotherapy and uses of monoclonal antibodies and biologic immune modifiers in human gliomas. Neurol Clin 3:901, 1985.
19. Neuwelt E, Frankel E, Diehl J, et al: Monitoring of methotrexate delivery in patients with malignant brain tumors after osmotic blood-brain barrier disruption. Ann Intern Med 94:449, 1981.
20. Rosenberg S, Lotze M, Muul L: Observations on the systemic administration of autologous lymphokine-activated killer cells and recombinant interleukin-2 in patients with metastatic cancer. N Engl J Med 313:1485, 1985.

V Infections

43
SUPPURATIVE CRANIAL AND INTRACRANIAL INFECTIONS

William R. Cheek, M.D.
John P. Laurent, M.D.

The treatment of suppurative cranial and intracranial infections continues to be a challenge, although the overall incidence of these disorders in the United States has undoubtedly decreased since the advent of antibiotics. Improved diagnostic methods and more sophisticated techniques of culturing purulent material have influenced certain aspects of management and have improved results.[97] The importance of early recognition of these infections cannot be overemphasized; the basic therapeutic principles of identification of the infectious agent and the administration of appropriate antibiotics in amounts sufficient to achieve systemic sterilization must be observed.

BRAIN ABSCESS

Brain abscess, fortunately, is not common in children. A busy neurosurgical service will see only one to three brain-abscess patients in the pediatric age group in a year.[2, 6, 42, 56, 93, 112] The development of antibiotics appears to have decreased the incidence of brain abscess,[60, 63] but agreement on this point is not universal.[2, 112] The reduction in incidence is logically attributed to a decrease, due to the general use of antibiotics, in the number of patients with sinusitis, mastoiditis, and otitis,[60] all of which are frequently associated with the development of brain abscess. Significant reduction in intracranial complications secondary to otitic infection following the development of antibiotics has been well documented by Proctor;[83] however, the incidence of brain abscess increased in his series relative to the total incidence of complications.

There are a variety of causes of brain abscesses: (1) contiguous infection, such as sinusitis or mastoiditis, by direct extension or propagation through venous channels; (2) direct introduction via penetrating wounds; (3) hematogenous spread from a distant focus of infection or hematogenous origin without known infection elsewhere, as is frequently the case with congenital heart disease; (4) intracranial abscess formation as a result of an infected dermoid tumor in the frontal lobe or the cerebellum.

The pathologic characteristics of the mature lesion in children do not differ significantly from those in adults. Initially, the organism produces an inflammatory reaction consisting of congestion and an outpouring of polymorphonuclear leukocytes, toxic changes in the neurons, and perivascular infiltration of the polymorphonuclear leukocytes. Next, the involved tissues become necrotic, and necrosis is accompanied by liquefaction and pus formation. The brain then attempts to wall off the necrotic purulent material; since fibroblasts in the brain arise from the vessels, this reaction occurs most effectively in the gray matter, where the fibroblasts are most common. This wall, composed of fibroblasts, capillaries, and collagen, is similar to granulation tissue elsewhere in the body and becomes thicker and more fibrous as collagen deposition increases.

Edema and swollen glial elements appear in the brain tissue surrounding the capsule.

As the lesion matures over the space of a few weeks, astrocytes proliferate and produce a gliotic zone external to the fibrous capsule (Fig. 43–1). Grant,[34] in a clinical study of patients with brain abscess during the preantibiotic era, demonstrated the presence of a capsule in every patient after a period of six weeks. Brain abscesses in children tend to be larger lesions characterized by thinner walls and the presence of more edema in the surrounding brain tissue than is the case in adults.[2] Pathologic differences have not been documented.[29]

Brain abscess is a rare occurrence in infants and, prior to the development of antibiotics, was always fatal.[94] More recent reports by Munslow, Stovall, Price, et al[73] and Hoffman, Hendrick, and Hiscox[40] have shown gram-negative organisms to be the cause of these large lesions, but the source is unknown. Infants are believed to be susceptible to gram-negative brain abscess because the M-fraction of immunoglobulins does not cross the placenta. Because infants do not develop paranasal sinuses and mastoid air cells until the age of 1 year, infection in these areas is not a source of brain abscess in young infants. Idriss, Gutman, and Kronfol[42] have reported meningitis to be frequently associated with these abscesses. The failure of the infection to become well encapsulated, together with the dearth of clinical signs, accounts for the large size of the lesion when the diagnosis is made.[40, 73] The rare disorder of pyocephalus in newborns is secondary to cerebral abscess 50 percent of the time.[43]

The incidence of brain abscess in the past has been stated to be 4 to 7 percent in children with congenital heart disease.[58, 75, 104] The early correction of congenital cardiac lesions in recent years has undoubtedly played a role in reducing the incidence in these children. A child with congenital heart disease and symptoms of stroke should be evaluated for possible brain abscess.[50] Brain abscesses from this source almost never occur in infants under 2 years of age. Tetralogy of Fallot that has not been totally corrected surgically is the most common underlying cardiac anomaly.[59, 104, 106] A right-to-left shunt is always present, causing bypass of the pulmonary bed and allowing circulating bacteria direct access to the cerebral circulation. Although the majority of these children are cyanotic, the first reported cure was that of a girl with noncyanotic disease.[100] Decreased oxygen saturation to the brain and focal encephalomalacia may set the stage for focal infection,[59] but since these conditions occur with other diseases such as sickle cell disease, which has no particular propensity to brain abscess,[84] the right-to-left shunt is the primary etiologic factor. Studies of acute bacteremia support this reasoning.[110] Brain abscess has also occurred in a child with right-to-left shunt caused by pulmonary arteriovenous aneurysm.[66] Subacute bacterial endocarditis is rarely a factor in brain abscess.

Any area of the brain may become involved but the brainstem only rarely.[21, 89] Hematogenous lesions are usually located in the distribution of the middle cerebral artery,[2, 24, 64] while those secondary to otitic or sinus infection are invariably in adjacent areas of the brain, that is, the temporal lobe or the frontal lobe, respectively.[2, 93, 96] Direct penetration of the dura can be caused by many types of wounds, and the abscess may not form for such a prolonged period that the initial injury will be unknown or forgotten.[67] Minor wounds around the eye should be examined carefully since puncture of the orbital roof in a child requires little force.[26, 68]

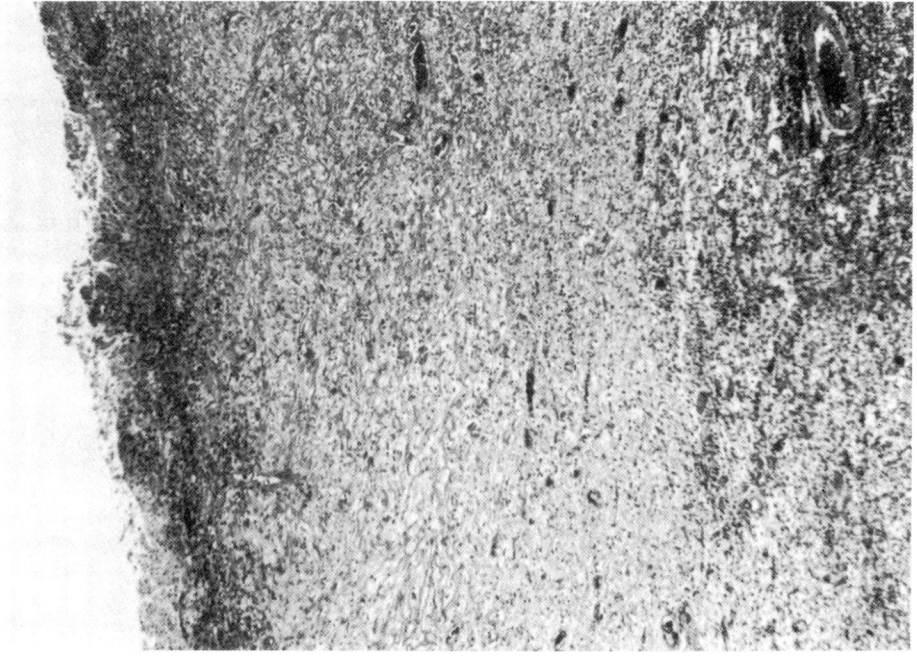

Figure 43–1. Photomicrograph of a section of the wall of a brain abscess, showing the different layers. To the left is that portion of the lining next to the cavity (× 50).

Clinical Features

Awareness of brain abscess as a possibility is extremely important, since early diagnosis is the best way to achieve low morbidity and mortality. The clinical picture in infants consists of an enlarging head and full fontanelle without localizing neurologic signs. Fever is seldom present but, should such a lesion exist, the peripheral white blood cell count will be 18,000/mm^3 or greater.[40, 42] Infants usually do not have a history of infection.

In older children, the presence of cyanotic heart disease or a history of one of the following conditions should alert the physician to the possibility of brain abscess: (1) purulent infection such as sinusitis, mastoiditis, or chronic otitis media; (2) penetrating head wound, even in the remote past;[67, 68] (3) nasal or occipital dermal sinus tract; (4) esophageal stricture and subsequent dilations.[49] The primary infection may have been treated with antibiotics and no longer be present. Fever is usually a symptom at some phase of the illness[24, 42, 105] and should suggest the possibility of brain abscess. The interval between the primary infection and abscess formation may be of many months' duration but is usually one to four weeks.[59, 93] The early symptoms are those common to many infectious processes: malaise, fever, irritability, lethargy, and anorexia. Although these symptoms are usually present at some phase of the illness,[6, 64] their absence does not rule out brain abscess. By the time a child with a brain abscess is hospitalized, the peripheral white blood cell count is usually greater than 10,000/mm^3 and the sedimentation rate is almost always elevated.[24, 42, 64, 84] Blood cultures are invariably negative.[42, 64]

Neurologic signs and symptoms are related to increased intracranial pressure and secondary to focal effects of the mass. Headache, vomiting, and diminished level of consciousness are the most common symptoms.[2, 24, 42, 59, 60, 64, 112] Because of the frequent presence of considerable cerebral edema adjacent to the lesion and the relatively late stage of the disease at which the child is first seen, coma may deepen rapidly. The level of consciousness is particularly related to outcome in patients with brain abscess, and if it is deteriorating, examination and diagnostic tests must be performed on an emergency basis.[24, 42, 101] These symptoms may be present regardless of the location of the lesion and may be the only symptoms. Focal neurologic symptoms may be noted in more than half of the patients,[24, 59, 84] and seizures may occur in 20 to 50 percent.[1, 64, 101] Specific neurologic findings are related to location of the abscess and usually are not pronounced. Partial aphasia, mild or moderate hemiparesis, and partial visual-field defects are the most common localizing signs. The seizures may have a lateralizing feature. Careful search must be made for foci of infection in the ears, paranasal sinuses, and chest; the scalp must be inspected for a sinus tract. Lumbar puncture should not be performed in a patient with symptoms suggestive of brain abscess as any information obtained would not be diagnostic for brain abscess. Cultures will be negative unless the capsule has ruptured into the cerebrospinal fluid. Protein, sugar, and cell count can be normal,[59, 112] and any abnormal findings have no characteristic pattern.[23, 84] The risk of herniation with this procedure is too great to justify its use.[64, 69, 77, 93, 112]

Diagnosis

Following the history and examination, skull roentgenograms will facilitate the search for evidence of recent or old head trauma, signs of increased intracranial pressure, or the presence of gas within the brain (Fig. 43–2).[80, 92] Computed tomography (CT) with bone and soft-tissue windows, if readily available, may show this same type of information, but a fracture may be missed. Appropriate plain x-ray films to localize a focus of infection in the sinuses, chest, or mastoids should be obtained. If the patient's condition permits, an electroencephalogram will frequently show characteristic delta waves in the area of the abscess[24, 56, 59, 64] and can be helpful in distinguishing brain abscess from encephalopathy, encephalitis, or cerebral infarction.

A radionuclide scan with technetium-99 has been helpful in the past in localization, but the findings are not as specific as those obtained with CT or nuclear magnetic resonance imaging (NMRI). A radionuclide scan can become normal when the patient is under treatment for an encapsulated lesion.[70] A major disadvantage of visualization with gallium-67 is the 48-hour waiting period between injection and scanning.[109]

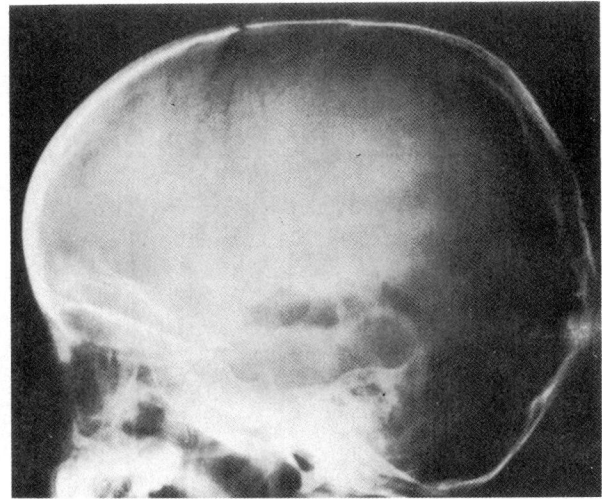

Figure 43–2. Lateral skull x-ray film of a three-year-old boy with gas in a right temporal lobe abscess due to *Clostridium perfringens*. Pieces of pencil were found in the abscess.

Prior to the advent of CT scanning, angiography and air studies were the ultimate localization procedures.[59, 60, 112] Mass effect from vessel displacement was the usual finding in angiograms of patients with brain abscess, but in a small percentage, increased vascularity in the capsule could be seen.[76]

A CT scan is currently the most readily available definitive diagnostic procedure. With this test an abscess can be diagnosed and localized with a high degree of accuracy[74, 116] in less than 30 minutes. In addition, multiple abscesses and daughter abscesses can be seen clearly[76, 102, 116] and the amount of edema assessed. The fact that the evolution from cerebritis to abscess formation can be followed[74] facilitates the timing of surgery. The CT scan should be performed with and without intravenous contrast material (Fig. 43–3). A bolus of meglumine iothalamate, 3 ml/kg of body weight, up to a maximum of 100 cc, can be used. In all patients the CT scan shows decreased attenuation in the lesion area without contrast enhancement, and in 80 to 90 percent shows a ring with enhancement on the initial study.[76, 82] The correlation of this ring with capsule formation is not yet completely known.[25, 31]

Recent clinical data show that administration of steroids to a patient whose lesion is in the cerebritis stage may result in definite reduction in contrast enhancement. Contrast enhancement in well-encapsulated lesions is not reduced.[11] Increased uptake of contrast material by the ependyma may indicate the presence of ventriculitis and signal the need for appropriate therapy.[76] NMRI has also been very helpful in the diagnosis of brain abscess and related infections of the intracranial space.[22] This technique outlines areas of edema particularly well (Fig. 43–4).

Instillation of radiopaque substances is now unnecessary in following the progress of the lesion during treatment. Real-time ultrasonography is also useful in neonates with an open fontanelle;[35, 51] it can be done easily and quickly in the nursery and repeated as necesssary in assessing progress.[79] CT or NMRI scanning should be done immediately on any child in whom brain abscess is a possibility or on any infant with an enlarging head and full fontanelle. At the present time CT scanning is preferable to NMRI in following the progress of a brain-abscess capsule as reflected by the size of the ring enhancement. This may not be the case in the future as experience with NMRI increases.

Treatment

In the main, treatment of brain abscess still consists of surgery for diagnostic culture and therapeutic evacuation of the purulent material[14] followed by administration of systemic antibiotic therapy appropriate to the organisms cultured. If diagnosed during the cerebritic stage, the disease may be cured by antibiotic therapy.[36] Cure of abscess has been reported increasingly in the last few years without surgery[7, 10, 32, 45, 107] but this mode of therapy must be used with caution and only while carefully monitoring with CT or NMRI in a hospital setting.[48] With these cautions in mind, cure of multiple abscesses without surgical diagnosis can now be accomplished in some cases.[5, 10, 88] Clinical and experimental evidence in the past has shown the relative ineffectiveness of antibiotics in killing bacteria in suppurative lesions even though apparently adequate levels of drugs are present.[9, 99] Recent experience at Texas Children's Hospital and other institutions indicates that it may be possible to cure a significant percentage of patients with brain abscess without surgery (Fig. 43–5). The organisms should be cultured for optimal antibiotic therapy, and aspiration of the lesion may be required,[16, 32] even if reduction of mass effect is not considered critical. In cases in which positive cultures can be obtained from blood or sinus drainage, direct aspiration may be obviated.

Surgical treatment is required with (1) a stuporous or comatose patient, (2) deteriorating neurologic status, (3) marked mass effect on CT scan or NMRI, (4) failure of lesions to improve with one to two weeks of antibiotic therapy, or (5) the need to obtain organisms for culture. There are three surgical op-

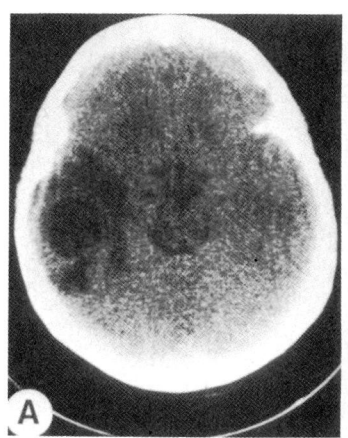
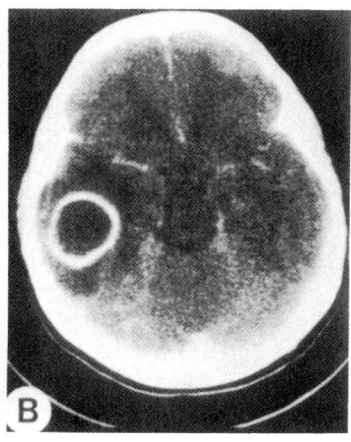

Figure 43–3. CT scan in a ten-year-old boy. *A*, Before contrast injection. *B*, After contrast injection. Note edema surrounding the abscess and typical ring enhancement after contrast injection.

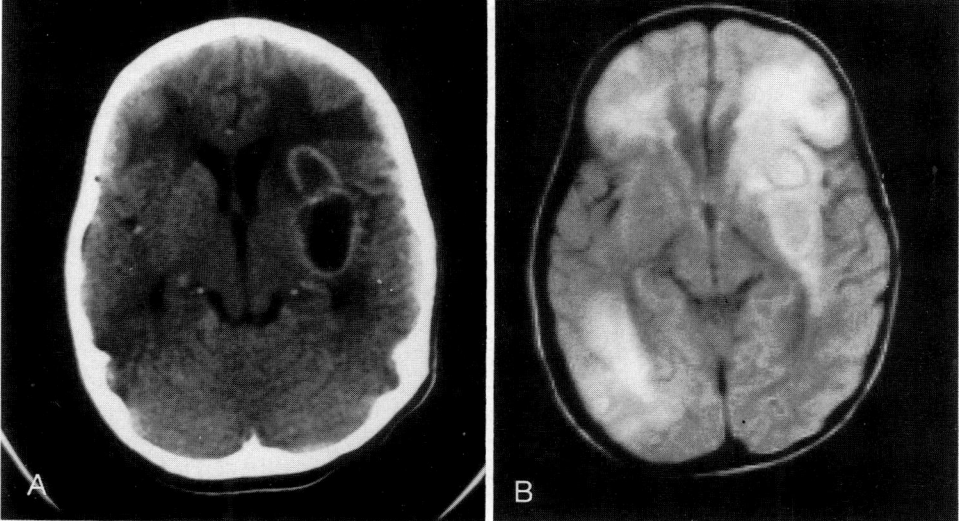

Figure 43–4. CT scan (A) and nuclear magnetic resonance image (B) made within 24 hours on a brain abscess patient. Note areas of edema.

tions—catheter drainage, single or multiple tapping, and excision.

Catheter drainage is the oldest successful method[57] and continues to be used with good results.[34, 72, 95] It consists of making a burr hole over the most insensitive portion of the cortex where the abscess is superficial, opening the dura, and making a small cortical incision. The abscess is palpated with a brain cannula and punctured with a small soft catheter (No. 10 French) over a stylet. The catheter is anchored loosely with a suture through the scalp. Pus usually flows spontaneously from the tube. Gentle aspiration with a syringe can be performed at the operating table and saline irrigation used to help empty the cavity. Instillation of local antibiotics is unnecessary[27] if the organism is sensitive to an antibiotic that perfuses well into the brain from the blood. The catheter is left in place for about seven days until drainage ceases and is then removed. This method is best suited for supratentorial lesions that are relatively near the surface.

Tapping is usually done through a burr hole also and has been a useful method since Dandy first described it in 1926.[20] It is preferred for evacuating deep collections or those in sensitive areas,[3, 44] as well as those in children with congenital heart disease.[84] With the sophisticated methods of localization and follow-up currently available (CT and NMRI)[19] and antibiotic therapy, tapping may be the treatment of choice for any brain abscess requiring surgery.[37] The procedure can sometimes be performed under local anesthesia, and a single aspiration is frequently all that is required.[20, 64] Every child should be followed up with a CT scan or NMRI. Tapping may be repeated should material reaccumulate. Current stereotaxic techniques together with intraoperative ultrasound make extremely ac-

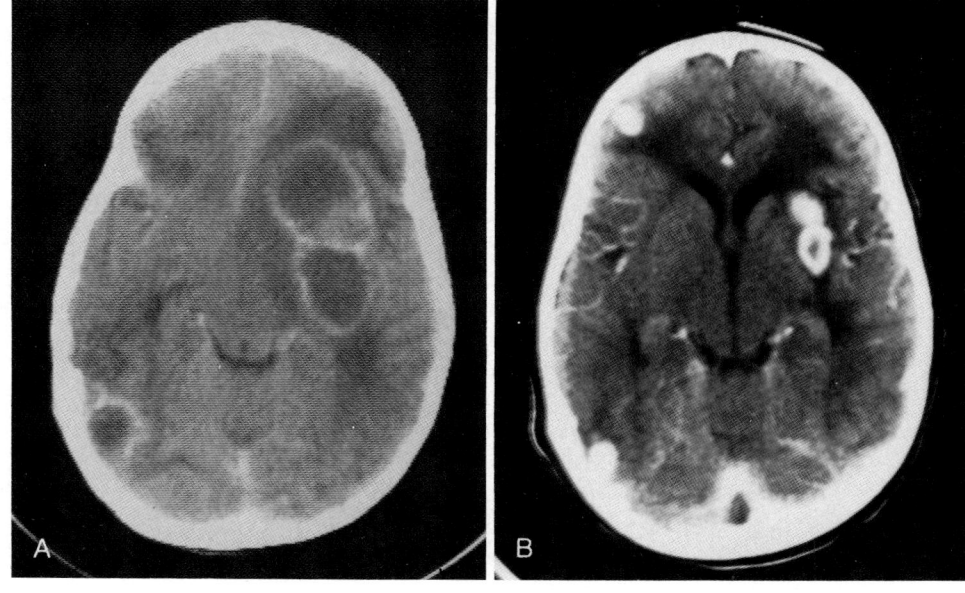

Figure 43–5. CT scans of multiple brain abscesses at time of diagnosis (A) and after two months of antibiotic therapy (B). No surgical drainage was performed.

curate placement of the cannula or catheter possible even for lesions in deep or critical areas.[12, 108]

Excision of the entire abscess is best accomplished after encapsulation, but removal of deep lesions or those in critical areas of the cortex is not advisable. Except in abscesses containing gas, the advantages of excision over the other two methods are open to serious question.[1, 30, 54, 69] Excision allows removal of the gas-containing lesion as well as identification and closure of any extracranial communication.[115] Damage to surrounding brain from the dissection may increase morbidity;[44] certainly if excision is carried out, dissection must be done carefully to cause only minimal trauma to the surrounding brain. Surrounding white matter should not be resected as was advised in the past.[52]

Excision is performed in the manner usual for removing a mass lesion. The bone opening is centered over the most superficial part of the abscess, and a cortical incision is made through the closest silent area. The capsule can be palpated with a blunt cannula to localize the lesion if intraoperative ultrasound is not available. Intraoperative ultrasound helps in localizing the abscess and directing a cannula into its center. The lesion is resected intact if possible.

If the lesion is large, deflating it by aspiration prior to removal may be advisable to decrease trauma to the surrounding brain. When resection is completed, the area is irrigated copiously with saline, and the wound closed as it would be following removal of any other intracranial mass. No drain is left in the brain. Good results can be achieved by resection,[2, 112] but atrophy on follow-up CT scan has been reported.[91] Any focus of infection elsewhere must be eradicated as soon as possible by appropriate therapy.

Regardless of the surgical treatment contemplated, as soon as the possibility of a brain abscess arises, the patient should be started on dexamethasone, to reduce cerebral edema, and antibiotics. With appropriate antibiotic coverage, dexamethasone can be given in the usual doses without increasing the risk of spreading the infection. If the organism is unknown prior to surgery because a culturable focus of infection such as mastoiditis or sinusitis is not present, antistaphylococcal penicillin, penicillin, and chloramphenicol may each be started in doses appropriate to the treatment of meningitis. Other regimens such as those employing cephalosporins along with Flagyl may be used as long as all the suspected organisms are covered. Pretreatment with antibiotics[93] probably accounts for some of the 15 to 40 percent of sterile cultures of abscess contents[1, 44, 64] but is still mandatory. When laboratory information is available regarding organism sensitivities, the antibiotic regimen can be altered appropriately. If a high rate of positive findings is expected, material from the abscess must be cultured meticulously for aerobes, anaerobes, and fungi as soon as possible. Systemic antibiotics should be continued for three to six weeks, depending on clinical response. With intensive antibiotic therapy, rupture of the abscess into the ventricular system need not be fatal; however, rupture can be avoided if the abscess is drained early. Treatment of brain abscess fails because of late recognition and inadequate antibiotic therapy.[30] Anticonvulsant medication should be given to all patients.

Results

The long-term results cannot be expected to be as good in infants as in older children. The enormous size of abscesses in infants and relatively poor host resistance make for greater brain damage; additionally, almost all of these infants have hydrocephalus.[17, 40, 73] Early recognition and referral for neurosurgical treatment improve the prognosis.[103] Mortality in older children can be reduced to nearly zero with early diagnosis, intensive antibiotic therapy, and treatment, if indicated, with surgical drainage or excision. The neurosurgeon must be prepared to perform emergency surgery if the level of consciousness is poor or deteriorating, since the death rate in comatose patients is high.[2, 113] This approach will also decrease morbidity, which tends to be greater in children than in adults.[18, 78]

One must remember that every brain abscess causes some degree of destruction of brain tissue. An increasing number of survivors experience seizures as time passes (up to 72 percent). The seizures are not related to age, type of surgical treatment, site of abscess (except for the cerebellum), or residual neurologic deficit. The presence or absence of seizures preoperatively does not necessarily predict that a patient will develop seizures postoperatively.[53] The interval between treatment and seizure development is longest in children who are under 10 years of age. The seizures usually occur infrequently and can be controlled by anticonvulsant medication, which should be given prophylactically to all patients.[46, 104] A follow-up electroencephalogram in brain-abscess patients with seizures almost invariably shows a localized sharp and slow wave complex.

SUBDURAL EMPYEMA

Subdural empyema of the intracranial space is an uncommon disorder that occurs principally in children and adolescents. The incidence is approximately one-fifth that of brain abscess.[8] It is usually secondary to paranasal sinus or middle-ear infection, but may also be a complication of purulent scalp infection or osteomyelitis of the skull or may be secondary to a hematogenous infection in a subdural hematoma. The pathway from contiguous infection is usually through infected venous chan-

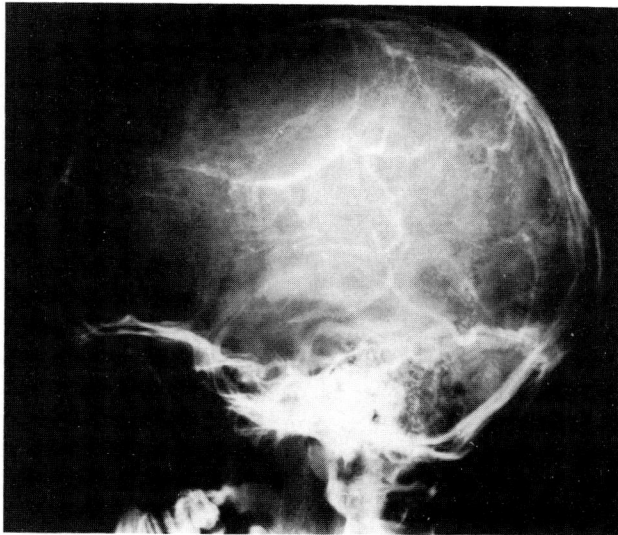

Figure 43-6. Left lateral angiogram of a 12-year-old boy with subdural empyema. Note hypervascular rim.

nels or a bone defect. The collections are located most often over the frontoparietal convexities and may involve the interhemispheric space; spread to bilateral or posterior fossa is rare.

These lesions may become very large before they are diagnosed. In patients with subdural empyema who also have meningitis, brain abscess, or extradural abscess, the prognosis worsens. Signs and symptoms consist of headache, vomiting, signs of infection, and nuchal rigidity.[65] The history may be as long as six months. Sedimentation rate and peripheral white blood cell count are elevated. Infants have increasing head size and bulging fontanelle; seizures are common.[85] Focal signs may develop late in the disease process, often accompanied by a deteriorating level of consciousness, indicating the need for rapid institution of treatment. If symptoms are suggestive of subdural empyema, spinal puncture should not be done because of the danger of precipitating brain herniation. The fluid will not be of diagnostic value, showing only elevated protein and pleocytosis, usually of lymphocytes.

The diagnosis of a subdural collection can be made by CT scanning or angiography (Fig. 43-6), although CT findings may be subtle early in the disease.[71, 87] An interhemispheric spread should be noted, as should the presence of a brain abscess. The empyema can be seen easily on CT scan as an extracerebral mass and any interhemispheric spread can be readily observed. The injection of contrast medium enhances the cortical membrane (Fig. 43-7). Lateral displacement of the pericallosal and callosomarginal branches on the anteroposterior angiogram indicates the existence of an interhemispheric collection. Plain skull roentgenograms may reveal sinusitis, mastoiditis, or skull osteomyelitis.

Treatment consists of an antibiotic regimen similar to that for brain abscess, and administration of local antibiotics is usually not necessary.[8] The patient is given steroids to control increased intracranial pressure and anticonvulsants to prevent seizures. A focus of infection identified elsewhere should be eradicated as soon as possible.

Virtually all cases of subdural empyema must be surgically drained.[4, 39, 47, 85, 98] Evacuation and irrigation through multiple burr holes are adequate if the pus is thin and there is no interhemispheric collection. If the pus is thick or an interhemispheric collection is present, a craniotomy should be performed and the infected material removed as completely as possible. Drains are usually not necessary, but irrigating catheters may be left in the subdural space for a few days.

At the time of surgery, pus should be taken in an airtight container directly to the bacteriology laboratory for gram stain and culture. Isolation of anaerobic organisms is particularly important since these bacteria are frequently present in paranasal sinus infection.[114] Mortality was formerly 40 percent[33] but widespread use of CT scanning for early diagnosis has reduced it to 10 to 13 percent.[39, 98, 117] A few cases diagnosed early have been reported cured with antibiotics alone.[62, 90]

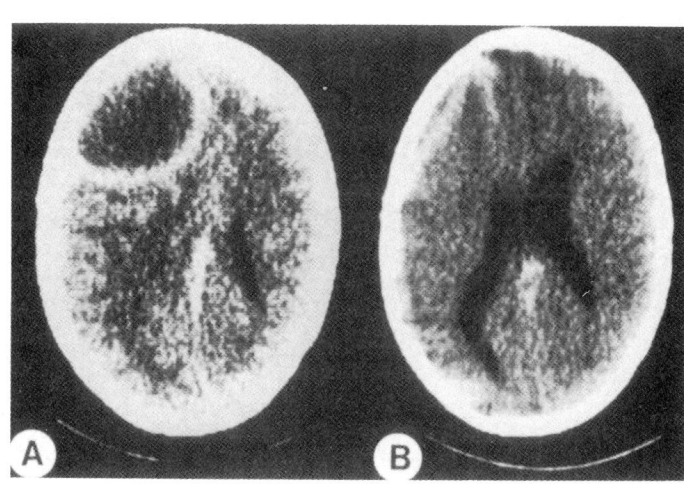

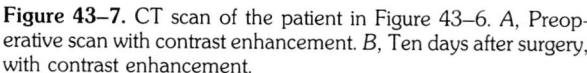

Figure 43-7. CT scan of the patient in Figure 43-6. A, Preoperative scan with contrast enhancement. B, Ten days after surgery, with contrast enhancement.

Complications such as cortical thrombophlebitis, brain abscess, and meningitis decrease the success rate. Early diagnosis and therapy, along with meticulous attention to bacteriologic studies, should improve the prognosis. After surgery, a follow-up CT scan should be obtained to rule out the presence of an intracerebral abscess not seen on the initial examination. Seizure incidence in long-term survivors is about 26 percent;[38] anticonvulsants should be continued for at least two years after surgery. If no seizures have occurred after this time and if electroencephalography shows no epileptogenic focus, the patient can be taken off anticonvulsant medication on a trial basis.

EPIDURAL ABSCESS

Epidural intracranial abscess is almost always secondary to or associated with another infection such as mastoiditis, sinusitis, postoperative flap infection, or osteomyelitis of the skull (Fig. 43–8). It may also result from infection of compound wounds of the head. A purulent extradural collection without osteomyelitis of the skull is rare.[111] Increased intracranial pressure from this lesion alone is uncommon as the mass effect is usually not great, but it can be associated with subdural empyema or brain abscess, both of which must be ruled out in all patients by CT or NMRI scanning. Epidural abscess serves as a focus of infection and may cause septicemia, which cannot be successfully treated until the epidural infection is eradicated. Plain skull roentgenograms often show osteomyelitis or air in the subdural space.[111]

The patient frequently manifests few specific clinical signs except those due to infection, such as fever or malaise. The number of peripheral white blood cells is increased. Local findings of scalp redness, swelling, and tenderness, together with focal headache secondary to sinus infection, mastoiditis, or skull osteomyelitis, are usually present. If neurologic signs and symptoms do occur, they usually appear late in the course of the disease and when a large lesion is present.

Therapy consists of evacuation of the epidural collection through burr holes or by craniectomy if osteomyelitis is present. All epidural granulations should be removed as thoroughly as possible.[111] A catheter drain may be left in the epidural space for the first few days and is desirable if the cavity is large. The bone should be treated as described in the following section. Associated sinusitis or brain abscess must be treated promptly.

In patients with frontal sinusitis and associated epidural abscess the latter can sometimes be adequately drained through an opening made in the posterior sinus wall during surgical exploration of the sinus. The antibiotics used in the initial treatment of brain abscess should be started when epidural abscess is first thought to be present. Cultures for aerobes, anaerobes, and fungi should be done carefully so that appropriate drugs can be selected. Follow-up CT scans until the patient recovers will allow monitoring of the progress of the lesion and detection of the presence of the more serious brain abscess or subdural empyema.

OSTEOMYELITIS OF THE SKULL

Osteomyelitis of the skull is most commonly a complication of a compound skull wound following either surgery or trauma. It may also occur in the frontal bone secondary to sinus infection or in the parietal and temporal bones from ear infection.[28] Osteomyelitis may develop in the skull of a newborn as a complication of an infected scalp wound

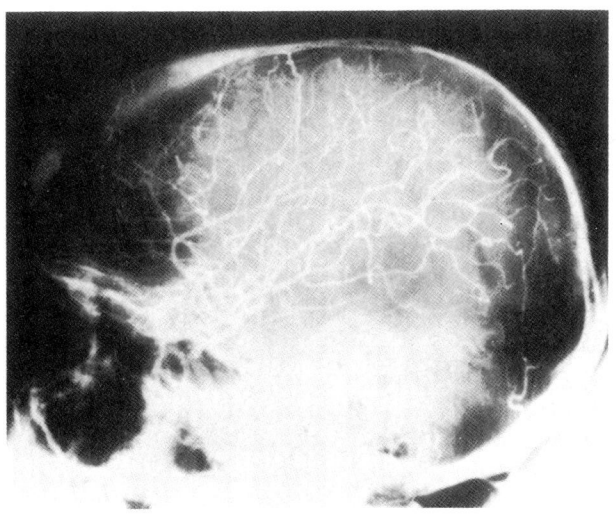

Figure 43–8. Left lateral angiogram of 15-year-old boy with frontal osteomyelitis and epidural abscess.

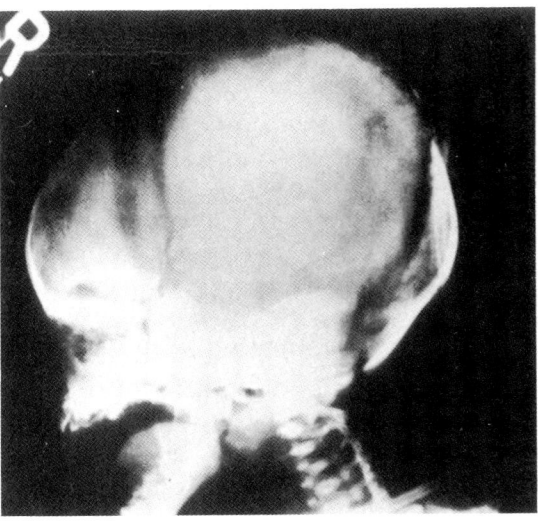

Figure 43–9. Typical "moth-eaten" appearance of osteomyelitis of the skull.

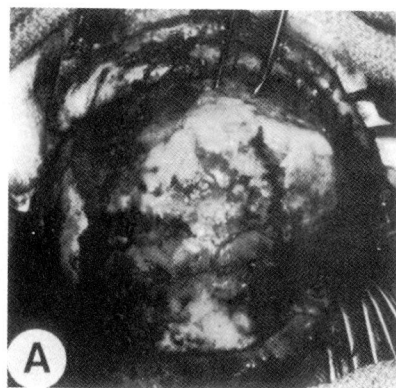 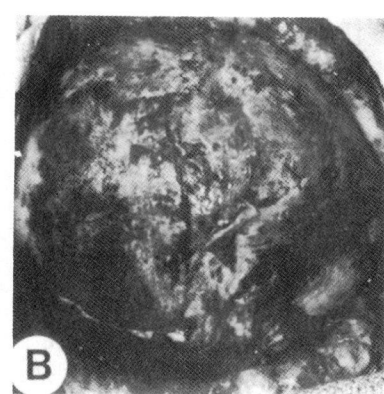

Figure 43–10. Ten-day-old girl with extensive staphylococcal osteomyelitis of the skull. A, Before débridement. Note forceps pointing to infected granulations. B, After débridement. Well-vascularized bone was preserved. The wound subsequently healed without incident.

from use of forceps or secondary to intrauterine monitoring.[13, 55, 81] Rarely it occurs opportunistically in a child with a suppressed immune mechanism and may be due to fungus.[86]

Clinical signs consist of local heat, swelling, tenderness, and redness. In the postsurgical period, poor healing of the suture line or a draining sinus of the wound may signal the problem. The patient may not have fever.[61] If the infection is severe, the patient will have high fever and suffer prostration, and peripheral white blood cells will be elevated. In this last situation, blood cultures are indicated. *Staphylococcus aureus* is the organism most commonly associated with postsurgical and post-traumatic wounds. The disease may progress rapidly if an epidural abscess is also present.[28] Meningitis almost never occurs unless the dura is open from previous surgery or has been lacerated from a compound wound.

X-ray examination of the skull may show no change for the first 10 to 14 days. Then, the classic picture is of a "moth-eaten" appearance (Fig. 43–9). Radionuclide scan with technetium-labeled organic phosphate[41] shows changes as soon as the infection is present; scalp artifact is not a problem with current scintillation cameras. CT scanning can detect bony changes and determine if any intracranial collection of pus is present.

Treatment consists of débridement of the area and antibiotic therapy, usually for a prolonged period.[15] In a postsurgical wound, the bone flap must be removed while preserving the pericranium. Poorly vascularized and infected bone surrounding the craniotomy must be removed back to a well-vascularized bone margin. It is rarely necessary to remove bone other than that already devitalized, that is, the flap or a sequestrum, if surgical treatment is prompt and antibiotic therapy adequate. Infected granulation tissue should be curetted away and any epidural abscess treated as described above with care taken not to penetrate the dura. The removal of any infected granulation tissue attached to the skull and producing bone destruction should stop the process, making removal of the underlying bone unnecessary (Fig. 43–10). The wound is copiously irrigated with saline solution throughout the procedure and is closed in one layer with nylon or stainless-steel sutures. A drain may be left in place for 24 hours. Administration of local antibiotics is usually not indicated. These same principles are used in treating skull osteomyelitis arising from other causes. Early débridement should resolve the process rapidly. Cranioplasty should be delayed for at least six months.

References

1. von Alphen HAM, Dreissen JJR: Brain abscess and subdural empyema. J Neurol Neurosurg Psychiatry 39:481, 1976.
2. Arseni C, Horvath L, Dumitrescu L: Cerebral abscesses in children. Acta Neurochir 14:197, 1966.
3. Ballantine HT Jr, White JC: Brain abscess. N Engl J Med 248:14, 1953.
4. Bannister G, Williams B, Smith S: Treatment of subdural empyema. J Neurosurg 55:82, 1981.
5. Barsoum AH, Lewis HC, Cannillo KL: Nonoperative treatment of multiple brain abscesses. Surg Neurol 16:283 1981.
6. Beller AJ, Sahar A, Praiss I: Brain abscess. J Neurol Neurosurg Psychiatry 36:757, 1973.
7. Berg B, Franklin G, Cunco R, et al: Neurosurgical cure of brain abscess: Early diagnosis and followup with computerized tomography. Ann Neurol 3:474, 1978.
8. Bhandari YS, Sarkari NBS: Subdural empyema: A review of 37 cases. J Neurosurg 32:35, 1970.
9. Black P, Graybill RJ, Charache P: Penetration of brain abscess by systemically administered antibiotics. J Neurosurg 38:705, 1973.
10. Boom WH, Tuazon CU: Successful treatment of multiple brain abscesses with antibiotics alone. Rev Infect Dis 7:189, 1985.
11. Britt RH, Enzmann DR: Clinical stages of human brain abscesses on serial CT scans after contrast infusion. J Neurosurg 59:972, 1983.
12. Broggi G, Franzini A, Peluchetti D, et al: Treatment of deep brain abscesses by stereotactic implantation of an intracavity device for evacuation and local application of antibiotics. Acta Neurochir 76:94, 1985.
13. Brook I: Osteomyelitis and bacteremia caused by *Bacteroides fragilis*: A complication of fetal monitoring. Clin Pediatr 19:639, 1980.
14. Bruszkiewicz J, Doron Y, Peyser E, et al: Brain abscess and its surgical management. Surg Neurol 18:7, 1982.
15. Bullitt E, Lehman RA: Osteomyelitis of the skull. Surg Neurol 11:163, 1979.
16. Burke LP, Ho SU, Cerullo LJ, et al: Multiple brain abscesses. Surg Neurol 16:452, 1981.

17. Butler NR, Barrie H, Paine KWE: Cerebral abscess as a complication of neonatal sepsis. Arch Dis Child 32:461, 1951.
18. Carey ME, Chou SM, French LA: Long-term neurological residua in patients surviving brain abscess with surgery. J Neurosurg 34:652, 1971.
19. Coin CG, Hucks-Follis AG, Mehegan CC: Computed tomographically guided percutaneous transmastoid drainage of a cerebellar abscess. Surg Neurol 20:387, 1983.
20. Dandy WE: Treatment of chronic abscess of the brain by tapping. JAMA 87:1477, 1926.
21. Danziger J, Allen KL, Block S: Brain stem abscess in children. J Neurosurg 40:391, 1974.
22. Davidson HD, Steiner RE: Magnetic resonance imaging in infections of the central nervous system. Am J Neurol Rad 6:499, 1985.
23. DeVio DC: Cerebral abscess in children. Dev Med Child Neurol 13:800, 1971.
24. Eberhard SJ: Diagnosis of brain abscess in infants and children: A retrospective study of 26 cases. N C Med J 30:363, 1969.
25. Enzmann DR, Britt RH, Yeager AS: Experimental brain abscess evolution; computed tomographic and neuropathologic correlation. Radiology 133:113, 1979.
26. Fanning WL, Willett LR, Phillips CF, et al: Puncture wound of the eyelid causing brain abscess. J Trauma 16:919, 1976.
27. Fischer EG, McLennon JE, Suyuki Y: Cerebral abscesses in children. Am J Dis Child 135:746, 1981.
28. French LA, Chou SN: Osteomyelitis of the skull and epidural space. In: Gurdjian ES (ed): Cranial and Intracranial Suppuration. Springfield, IL, Charles C Thomas, 1969, pp 59–72.
29. Friede RL: Developmental Neuropathology. New York, Springer-Verlag, 1975, pp 175–176.
30. Garfield J: Management of supratentorial intracranial abscess. Br Med J 2:7, 1969.
31. Garvey G: Current concepts of bacterial infections of the central nervous system. Bacterial meningitis and bacterial brain abscess. J Neurosurg 59:735, 1983.
32. George B, Roux F, Pillon M, et al: Relevance of antibiotics in the treatment of brain abscesses. Report of a case with eight simultaneous brain abscesses treated and cured medically. Acta Neurochir 47:285, 1979.
33. Glasauer FE, Coots D, Levy LF, et al: Subdural empyema in Africans in Rhodesia. Neurosurgery 3:385, 1978.
34. Grant FC: The mortality from abscess of the brain. JAMA 99:550, 1932.
35. Gray PH, O'Reilly C: Neonatal *Proteus mirabilis* meningitis and cerebral abscess: Diagnosis by real-time ultrasound. J Clin Ultrasound 12:441, 1984.
36. Heineman HS, Braude AJ, Osterholm JL: Intracranial suppurative disease. JAMA 218:1542, 1971.
37. Hirsch JF, Roux FX, Sante-Rose C, et al: Brain abscess in childhood. A study of 34 cases treated by puncture and antibiotics. Child's Brain 10:251, 1983.
38. Hitchock E, Andreadis A: Subdural empyema: A review of 29 cases. J Neurol Neurosurg Psychiatry 27:422, 1964.
39. Hockley AD, Williams B: Surgical management of subdural empyema. Child's Brain 10:294, 1983.
40. Hoffman HJ, Hendrick EB, Hiscox JL: Cerebral abscess in early infancy. J Neurosurg 33:172, 1970.
41. Humphreys RP, Gilday DL, Ash JM, et al: Radiopharmaceutical bone scanning in pediatric neurosurgery. Child's Brain 5:249, 1979.
42. Idriss ZH, Gutman LT, Kronfol NM: Brain abscesses in infants and children. Clin Pediatr 17:738, 1978.
43. Izquierdo JM, Sanz F, Coca JM, et al: Pyocephalus of the newborn child. Child's Brain 4:129, 1978.
44. Jooma O, Pennybacker JB, Tutton GK: Brain abscess: Aspiration, drainage, or excision. J Neurol Neurosurg Psychiatry 14:308, 1951.
45. Keren G, Tyrrel DL: Nonsurgical treatment of brain abscesses: report of two cases. Pediatr Infect Dis 3:331, 1984.
46. Kerr FWL, King RB, Meagher JN: Brain abscess: A study of 47 consecutive cases. JAMA 168:868, 1958.
47. Khan M, Griebel R: Subdural empyema: A retrospective study of 15 patients. Can J Surg 27:283, 1984.
48. Kobrine AI, David DO, Rizzoli HV: Multiple abscesses of the brain: Case report. J Neurosurg 54:93, 1981.
49. Kolter R, Schild JA, Holinger PH: Delayed CNS complications. Laryngoscope 85:1379, 1975.
50. Kurlan R, Griggs RC: Cyanotic congenital heart disease with suspected stroke. Should all patients receive antibiotics? Arch Neurol 40:209, 1983.
51. Lam AH, Berry A, de Silva M, et al: Intracranial *Serratia* infection in preterm newborn infants. Am J Neurol Radiol 5:447, 1984.
52. Le Beau J: Radical surgery and penicillin in brain abscess. J Neurosurg 3:359, 1946.
53. Legg NJ, Gupta PC, Scott DF: Epilepsy following cerebral abscess. Brain 96:259, 1973.
54. Liske E, Weikers NJ: Changing aspects of brain abscesses. Neurology 14:294, 1964.
55. Listinsky JL, Wood BP, Ekholm SE: Parietal osteomyelitis and epidural abscess: A delayed complication of fetal monitoring. Pediatr Radiol 16:150, 1986.
56. Loeser E, Scheinberg L: Brain abscesses: A review of 99 cases. Neurology 7:601, 1957.
57. Macewen W: Pyogenic Infective Diseases of the Brain and Spinal Cord. Glasgow, James Maclehose & Sons, 1893.
58. Maronde RF: Brain abscess and congenital heart disease. Ann Intern Med 33:602, 1950.
59. Matson DD, Salam M: Brain abscess in congenital heart disease. Pediatrics 27:772, 1961.
60. Matson DD: Brain abscess. In: Matson DD (ed): Neurosurgery of Infancy and Childhood. Springfield, IL, Charles C Thomas, 1969, pp 708–715.
61. Matson DD: Osteomyelitis. In: Matson DD (ed): Neurosurgery of Infancy and Childhood. Springfield, IL, Charles C Thomas, 1969, pp 701–704.
62. Mauser HW, Ravijst RA, Elderson A, et al: Nonsurgical treatment of subdural empyema: Case report. J Neurosurg 63:128, 1985.
63. McClelland CJ, Craig BF, Crockard HA: Brain abscesses in Northern Ireland. J Neurol Neurosurg Psychiatry 41:1043, 1978.
64. McGreal DA: Brain abscesses in children. Can Med Assoc J 86:261, 1962.
65. McLaurin RL: Subdural infection. In: Gurdjian ES (ed): Cranial and Intracranial Suppuration. Springfield, IL, Charles C Thomas, 1969, pp 73–88.
66. Meachan WF, Scott HW: Congenital pulmonary arteriovenous aneurysm complicated by *Bacteroides* abscess of brain. Ann Surg 147:404, 1958.
67. Mikhael MA, Mattar AG: Case report: Chronic graphite granulomatous abscess simulating a brain tumor. J Comput Assist Tomogr 1:513, 1977.
68. Miller CF, Brodkey JS, Colombi BJ: The danger of intracranial wood. Surg Neurol 7:95, 1977.
69. Morgan H, Wood MW, Murphey F: Experience with 88 consecutive cases of brain abscess. J Neurosurg 38:698, 1973.
70. Morte PD, Brannon WL, Furlow TW Jr: Case report: Evolution of cerebral abscess. Disparity between radionuclide and CT scans. Postgrad Med 63:226, 1978.
71. Moseley IF, Kendall BE: Radiology of intracranial empyemas, with special reference to computed tomography. Neuroradiology 26:333, 1984.
72. Mount L: Conservative surgical therapy of brain abscesses. J Neurosurg 7:385, 1960.
73. Munslow RA, Stovall VS, Price RD, et al: Brain abscess in infants. J Pediatr 51:74, 1957.
74. New PFJ, Davis KR, Ballantine HT: Computed tomography in cerebral abscess. Radiology 121:641, 1976.
75. Newton EJ: Hematogenous brain abscess in cyanotic congenital heart disease. Q J Med 25:201, 1956.

76. Nielsen H, Gyldensted C: Computed tomography in the diagnosis of cerebral abscess. Neuroradiology 12:201, 1977.
77. Nielsen H: Cerebral abscess in children. Neuropediatrics 14:76, 1983.
78. Nielson H, Harmsen A, Gyldensted C: Cerebral abscess. A long-term follow-up. Acta Neurol Scand 67:330, 1983.
79. Nielsen HC, Shannon K: Use of ultrasonography for diagnosis and management of neonatal brain abscess. Pediatr Infect Dis 2:460, 1983.
80. Norrell H, Howieson J: Gas-containing brain abscess. Am J Roentgenol 109:273, 1970.
81. Overturf GD, Balfour G: Osteomyelitis and sepsis: Severe complications of fetal monitoring. Pediatrics 55:244, 1975.
82. Price H, Danziger A: The role of computerized tomography in the diagnosis and management of intracranial abscess. Clin Radiol 29:571, 1978.
83. Proctor CA: Intracranial complications of otitic origin. Laryngoscope 76:288, 1966.
84. Raimondi AJ, Matsumoto S, Miller RA: Brain abscess in children with congenital heart disease. J Neurosurg 23:588, 1965.
85. Rao S, Dinakar I: Subdural empyema in infants. Indian J Pediatr 38:358, 1971.
86. Reinig JW, Hungerford GD, Mohrmann ME, et al: Case report 268. Diagnosis: cryptococcal osteomyelitis of the calvaria. Skeletal Radiol 11:221, 1984.
87. Renaudin JW, Frazee J: Subdural empyema—importance of early diagnosis. Neurosurgery 7:477, 1980.
88. Rennels MB, Woodward C, Robinson WL, et al: Medical cure of apparent brain abscesses. Pediatrics 72:220, 1983.
89. Robert CM Jr, Stern WE, Brown WJ, et al: Brain stem abscess treated surgically. Surg Neurol 3:153, 1975.
90. Rosazza A, de Tribolet N, Deonna T: Nonsurgical treatment of interhemispheric subdural empyemas. Helv Paediatr Acta 34:577, 1979.
91. Rousseaux M, Lesoin F, Destee A, et al: Long term sequelae of hemispheric abscesses as a function of the treatment. Acta Neurochir 74:61, 1985.
92. Russel JA, Taylor JC: Circumscribed gas-gangrene abscess of the brain. Br J Surg 50:434, 1963.
93. Samson DS, Clark K: A current review of brain abscess. Am J Med 54:201, 1973.
94. Sanford HM: Abscess of the brain in infants under 12 months of age. Am J Dis Child 35:256, 1928.
95. Selker RG: Intracranial abscess: Treatment by continuous catheter drainage. Child's Brain 1:368, 1975.
96. Shaw MD, Russell JA: Cerebellar abscess: A review of 47 cases. J Neurol Neurosurg Psychiatry 38:429, 1975.
97. Small M, Dale BA: Intracranial suppuration 1968–1982, a 15 year review. Clin Otolaryngol 9:315, 1984.
98. Smith HP, Hendrick EB: Subdural empyema and epidural abscess in children. J Neurosurg 58:392, 1983.
99. Smith MR, Wood WB: An experimental analysis of curative action of penicillin in acute bacterial infections. J Exp Med 103:509, 1956.
100. Smolik EA, Blattner RJ, Heys FM: Brain abscess associated with congenital heart disease. JAMA 130:145, 1946.
101. Snyder BD, Farmer TW: Brain abscess in children. South Med J 64:687, 1971.
102. Stephanov S: Experience with multiloculated brain abscesses. J Neurosurg 49:199, 1978.
103. Sutton DL, Ouvrier RA: Cerebral abscess in the under-6-month age group. Arch Dis Child 58:901, 1983.
104. Taussig HB, Crocetti A, Eshaghpour E, et al: Long-time observations on the Blalock-Taussig Operation. III: Common complications. Johns Hopkins Med J 129:274, 1971.
105. Torales A, Franco FR, Calderson E: Intracranial abscesses in children. Bol Med Hosp Infant Mex 35:33, 1978.
106. Tyler HR, Clark DB: Incidence of neurological complication in congenital heart disease. Arch Neurol Psychiatry 77:17, 1957.
107. Vaquero J, Cabezudo JM, Leunda G: Nonsurgical resolution of a brain stem abscess: Case report. J Neurosurg 53:726, 1980.
108. Walsh PR, Larson SJ, Rytel MW, et al: Stereotactic aspiration of deep cerebral abscesses after CT-directed labeling. Appl Neurophysiol 43:205, 1980.
109. Waxman AD, Siemsen JK: Gallium scanning in cerebral and cranial infections. Am J Roentgenol 127:309, 1976.
110. Wood WB, Smith MR, Perry WD, et al: Studies on the cellular immunology of acute bacteremia. J Exp Med 94:521, 1951.
111. Woodhall B: Osteomyelitis and epi-, extra- and subdural abscesses. In: Clinical Neurosurgery, Vol. 16. Baltimore, Williams & Wilkins, 1967, pp 239–255.
112. Wright RL, Ballantine HT: Management of brain abscess in children and adolescents. Am J Dis Child 114:113, 1967.
113. Yang SY: Brain abscess: a review of 400 cases. J Neurosurg 55:794, 1981.
114. Yoshikawa TT, Chow AW, Guze LB: Role of anaerobic bacteria in subdural empyema: Report of 4 cases and review of 327 cases from the English literature. Am J Med 58:99, 1975.
115. Young RF, Frazee J: Gas within intracranial abscess cavities: An indication for surgical excision. Ann Neurol 16:35, 1984.
116. Zimmerman RA, Patel S, Bilaniuk LT: Demonstration of purulent bacterial intracranial infections by computed tomography. Am J Roentgenol 127:155, 1976.
117. Zimmerman RD, Leeds NE, Danziger A: Subdural empyema: CT findings. Radiology 150:417, 1984.

44
SPINAL INFECTIONS

William R. Cheek, M.D.
John P. Laurent, M.D.

Although infections involving the spine are not common in children,[20] they do occasionally occur, involving the bony structures, the intervertebral disks, the spinal canal, or the spinal cord. A spinal infection may be suppurative or not; symptoms may be nonspecific unless direct or indirect involvement compromises neural function. Diagnosis has been made easier by modern imaging techniques but the clinician must be alert to the possibility of spinal infection. Surgical therapy is not always required.

SPINAL-CORD ABSCESS

Abscess in the spinal cord occurs much more rarely than brain abscess. By 1977, only 15 cases in children had been reported.[22] Spinal-cord abscess may occur from direct spread, as in the case of a dermal sinus tract. More frequently, it is metastatic from hematogenous or lymphatic routes.[1] On occasion no primary source can be determined. Spinal-cord abscess is usually single but may be multiple. It occurs most frequently in the thoracic cord but may be at any level and may involve the entire length of the cord.

The pathology is similar to that of brain abscess, and histologic findings depend upon the stage of the disease. The most common organisms recovered are staphylococcus and streptococcus, but many others, including fungi, have been cultured. Occasionally, multiple organisms are found, and sterile abscesses have also been reported.[22] The cerebrospinal fluid (CSF) findings are usually nonspecific, but organisms are sometimes found, especially if there is an associated meningitis. Abscesses arising from contiguous spread are almost always at the adjacent level of the cord.

Signs and symptoms depend on the level, size, and chronicity of the lesion. There are usually signs of infection, such as fever and elevated peripheral white blood cell count; indications may be present of a primary infection elsewhere, such as mastoiditis or endocarditis, or the child may have the symptoms of meningitis, such as headache, vomiting, and nuchal rigidity. Some children experience prolonged backache before the onset of other symptoms.

In all cases treated surgically paraparesis or paraplegia had developed before diagnosis. This complication may occur suddenly; if paralysis is complete, and especially if the onset was rapid, the prognosis is worse. If spinal-cord abscess is suspected, a nuclear magnetic resonance imaging (NMRI) scan of the spine should be carried out immediately. A computed tomography (CT) myelogram should be performed if NMRI scanning is not available. Surgical exploration should then be performed as an emergency measure.

Laminectomy is done at the appropriate level followed by aspiration of the cord at its widest point, using a 25-gauge needle inserted into the midline of the dorsal aspect of the cord. When pus is recovered, a dorsal midline myelotomy is made, just large enough to evacuate the purulent material. Cultures are sent for aerobes, anaerobes, and fungi. The wound is copiously irrigated with Ringer's solution and closed in the usual fashion. If the cavity is extensive, a drain can be left in place and brought out through the wound; the drain is removed in 24 to 48 hours.

Appropriate antibiotics are administered intravenously, and treatment should proceed as it would for brain abscess. Prior to the development of antibiotics, only two of nine children with this diagnosis survived, but from 1948 to 1977, in all six cases reported children with spinal-cord abscess survived. With the clinician's alertness to the possibility of spinal-cord abscess, current diagnostic imaging techniques, prompt surgical drainage, and adequate antibiotic therapy, the prognosis should continue to improve.

SPINAL EPIDURAL ABSCESS

Although spinal epidural abscess is rare in children,[13, 14] it is a most important spinal infection from the neurosurgical standpoint. It occurs most frequently in the midthoracic or lower lumbar region.[3] The pus collects dorsally since the dura adheres ventrally to the posterior longitudinal ligament from C1 to S2.[13] *Staphylococcus aureus* is the most common causative organism,[14] although many others have been cultured. The organism spreads into the epidural space hematogenously, except in cases in which there is a penetrating wound.[13] An antecedent infection may have been present in the latter case or a history of trauma may be obtained.[14]

Rankin and Flathow[24] described the classic symptomatic progression in 1946: spinal ache followed by root pain, impaired cord function, and finally paraplegia. This course is generally invariable in adults, but children often demonstrate no clear-cut syndrome.[14] Fever and irritability are usually present. A child will sometimes limp.[3] Rigidity of the spine and evidence of pain on movement are common in infants, and lower-extremity weakness or paralysis is usually present before the diagnosis is made. Back pain may not be present in older children,[14] but hip pain can be prominent.[11] Sufficient radicular inflammation may cause abdominal pain and spinal ileus mimicking an acute abdomen.[27] Peripheral white blood cell count may be increased and the sedimentation rate elevated. Blood cultures are frequently negative.

Once the epidural abscess is suspected, the workup should progress on an emergency basis. Plain radiographs are nonrevealing except rarely, when associated osteomyelitis of the vertebra is present.[13] Spinal CT scanning may establish the diagnosis,[21] but intrathecal-contrast injection should be used if there is any question, especially in the presence of a neurological deficit.[6] The agent may have to be introduced via cisternal or C1–C2 puncture because of the level of the abscess. Direct puncture of the abscess by spinal needle may yield pus for culture. Spinal-fluid findings are nondiagnostic. When the diagnosis of spinal epidural abscess is established, surgical decompression should be carried out immediately[3, 13, 23, 28] unless an absolute contraindication exists.

Results are best in those patients with a slow course and if surgery is done before significant neurological deficit occurs. A limited laminectomy[14] is the procedure of choice in a child since it may prevent the development of kyphoscoliosis later. In many cases the pus can be removed by irrigation of the epidural space through a limited opening.[9] If adequate evacuation of pus cannot be accomplished in this way and if multiple laminae must be removed, an en bloc removal of the laminae is advised, with débridement of the epidural space and replacement of the laminae as described by Hulme and Dott.[16]

A drain should be left in the epidural space for 24 to 48 hours. Cultures for aerobes, anaerobes, fungi, and tuberculosis should be obtained at the operating table. Following surgery appropriate intravenous antibiotics must be continued until the child is afebrile, the peripheral white blood cell count normal, and the sedimentation rate less than 20 mm/hr; these changes will take several weeks. Local irrigation with antibiotics after surgery is unnecessary. With early diagnosis and surgical drainage before serious neurologic deficit occurs, the prognosis should be good in most cases.[28]

SPONDYLITIS

Pyogenic vertebral osteomyelitis is no longer common in children.[5, 18] Characteristically caused by *Staphylococcus aureus*, it produces suppurative destruction of the vertebral body and can involve vertebrae at any level. Radiographic changes occur within two weeks of onset. Thoracic and lumbar lesions cause abdominal symptomatology and pain,[5] while the initial symptom in cervical disease may be torticollis.[29] Spondylitis is not of neurosurgical interest unless a collection of epidural pus produces cord compression. Treatment should be under the guidance of an orthopedic surgeon.

Because tuberculous spondylitis continues to be seen occasionally in the United States, the causative organism of spondylitis in a child must be established by blood culture or biopsy of the lesion. If *Staphylococcus aureus* or other pathogen cannot be cultured, a skin test for tuberculosis, a chest x-ray, and sputum and urine samples for AFB smear and culture should be obtained.

Tuberculous spondylitis in children frequently causes cord compression,[2] producing partial or complete paraplegia. Diagnosis of epidural involvement and accurate localization is now readily accomplished with CT scanning.[17] Early operation via an anterior approach[2, 18] is probably advisable in all cases but especially in those with neurologic involvement.

Posterior decompression, i.e., laminectomy, is contraindicated since tuberculosis of the spine is an anterior disease. Laminectomy can increase spinal deformity and instability[18] and can aggravate the

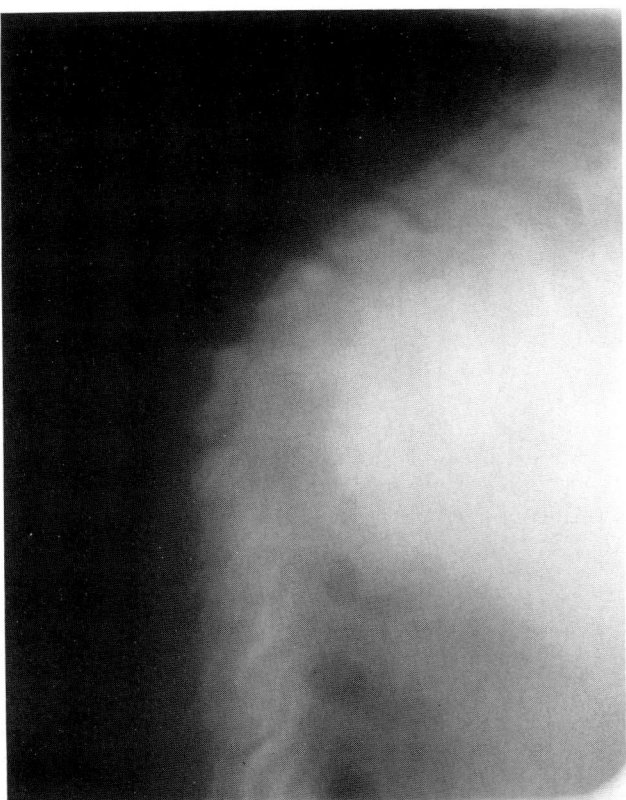

Figure 44–1. Tomogram showing marked kyphosis resulting from tuberculous spondylitis.

neurologic deficit. Any surgical exploration should be under the supervision of an orthopedic surgeon as fusion will almost certainly be required for stabilization (Fig. 44–1). Neurologic deficit tends to occur slowly over a long period of time; hence, recovery of function is usually good and may continue to improve for up to 24 months after surgery.[2]

DISKITIS

Diskitis is an inflammation of the intervertebral disk without suppuration. Children with diskitis have low-grade fever, an elevated sedimentation rate, spinal pain, and radiographic changes, which consist of a narrowing of the disk space along with irregularity and haziness of the vertebral end-plate (Fig. 44–2). There may be a history of previous infection or trauma. Young children will refuse to walk or even sit if the pain is severe enough. Older children frequently complain of back or lower-extremity pain, but abdominal pain[15] is also common. Diskitis is most commonly located in the lumbar spine, followed by the thoracic spine, and, rarely, the cervical area.[15, 19]

The cause of diskitis is debatable, although bacterial infection is most likely. The blood supply to the intervertebral disk is abundant below the age of 20 years[12] and may be responsible for the hematogenous spread of bacteria to the disks of children. Many cases have yielded positive cultures from biopsy, either open or needle, but not the majority.[26] The organism cultured is usually *Staphylococcus aureus*, although unusual causes have been found.[8, 10] Some clinicians advise reserving biopsy for those cases that do not respond to routine treatment or in which tuberculosis may be present.[25]

The diagnosis is based on the clinical symptoms noted above and on radiographic changes. CT scan is useful in evaluating early or atypical cases.[4] Treatment consists primarily of bedrest and immobilization. Antistaphylococcal drugs may hasten clinical improvement.[19]

The disease is of interest to neurosurgeons in the differential diagnosis of other spine disorders that might produce cord compression, i.e., tumor or epidural abscess. The prognosis is usually very good, with significant spine deformity a rare occurrence.[19, 25, 26]

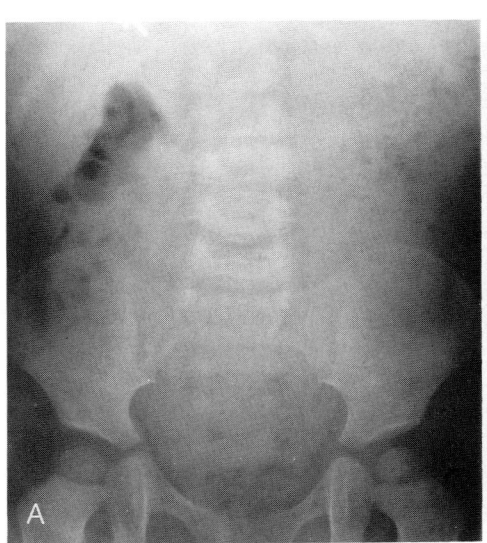
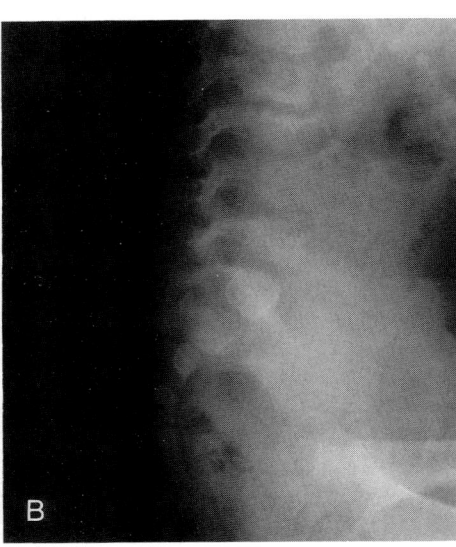

Figure 44–2. Anteroposterior (A) and lateral (B) radiographs showing typical changes of discitis at L2–L3.

CONGENITAL DERMAL SINUS

These tubular tracts are dysraphic defects that communicate from the spine to the deeper layers, sometimes all the way to the spinal cord. They are dealt with in detail elsewhere in this volume. For this section it is important to emphasize the following: (1) The skin opening is in the midline and may be tiny and difficult to see. Although it can occur from the upper cervical region to the midsacrum, it is most commonly found in the lumbar or lumbosacral area. (2) Intraspinal infectious complications can be severe and produce permanent neurologic sequelae. (3) The lesion should be excised in toto as soon as it is diagnosed.[7]

References

1. Arty PK: Abscess within the spinal cord: Review of literature and report of three cases. Arch Neurol Psychol 51:533, 1944.
2. Bailey HL, Gabriel M, Hodgson AR, et al: Tuberculosis of the spine in children. J Bone Joint Surg 54:1633, 1972.
3. Baker CJ: Primary spinal epidural abscess. Am J Dis Child 121:337, 1971.
4. Berger PE: Childhood diskitis: Computed tomographic findings. Radiology 149:701, 1983.
5. Bolivar R, Kohl S, Pickering LK: Vertebral osteomyelitis in children: Report of four cases. Pediatrics 62:549, 1978.
6. Burke DR, Brant-Zawadzki M: CT of pyogenic spine infection. Neuroradiology 27:131, 1985.
7. Cheek WR, Laurent JP: Dermal sinus tracts. In: Chapman PH (ed): Concepts in Pediatric Neurosurgery, Vol. 6. Basel, S Karger, 1985, pp 63–75.
8. Claesson B, Flasen E, Kjellman B: Kingella kingae infections: A review and a presentation of data from ten Swedish cases. Scand J Infect Dis 17:233, 1985.
9. de Villiers JC, Cluver PF: Spinal epidural abscess in children. S Afr J Surg 16:149, 1978.
10. Diament MJ, Weller M, Bernstein R: Candida infection in a premature infant presenting as discitis. Pediatr Radiol 12:96, 1982.
11. Donowitz LG, Cole WQ, Lohr JA: Acute spinal epidural abscess presenting as hip pain. Pediatr Infect Dis 2:44, 1983.
12. Doyle JR: Narrowing of the intervertebral disc space in children. J Bone Joint Surg 42A:1191, 1960.
13. Enberg RN, Kaplan RJ: Spinal epidural abscess in children. Clin Pediatr 13:247, 1974.
14. Fischer EG, Greene CS, Winston KR: Spinal epidural abscess in children. Neurosurgery 9:257, 1981.
15. Galil A, Gorodischer R, Bar-Ziv J, et al: Intervertebral disc infection (discitis) in childhood. Eur J Pediatr 139:66, 1982.
16. Hulme A, Dott NM: Spinal epidural abscess. Br Med J 1:64, 1954.
17. LaBerge JM, Brant-Zawadzki M: Evaluation of Pott's disease with computed tomography. Neuroradiology 26:429, 1984.
18. La Rocca H: Pyogenic spondylitis. In: Rothman RH, Simeone FA (eds): The Spine. Philadelphia, W. B. Saunders Co., 1982, pp 758–765.
19. LaRocca H: Intervertebral disc space inflammation in children. In: Rothman RH, Simeone FA (eds): The Spine. Philadelphia, W. B. Saunders Co., 1982, pp 766–767.
20. LaRocca H: Spinal sepsis. In: Rothman RH, Simeone FA (eds): The Spine. Philadelphia, W. B. Saunders Co., 1982, pp 757–774.
21. Leys D, Lesoin F, Viaud C, et al: Decreased morbidity from acute bacterial spinal epidural abscesses using computed tomography and nonsurgical treatment in selected patients. Ann Neurol 17:350, 1985.
22. Menezes AH, Graf CJ, Perret GE: Spinal cord abscess: A review. Surg Neurol 8:461, 1977.
23. Phillips GE, Jefferson A: Acute spinal epidural abscess. Observations from fourteen cases. Postgrad Med J 55:712, 1979.
24. Rankin RM, Flothow PG: Pyogenic infection of the spinal epidural space. West J Surg 54:320, 1946.
25. Scoles P, Quinn TP: Intervertebral discitis in children and adolescents. Clin Orthoped 162:31, 1982.
26. Spiegel PG, Kengla KW, Isaason AS, et al: Intervertebral disc space inflammation in children. J Bone Joint Surg 54A:284, 1972.
27. Tyson GW, Grant A, Strachan WE: Spinal epidural abscess presenting as acute abdomen in a child. Br J Surg 66:3, 1979.
28. Verner EF, Musher DM: Spinal epidural abscess. Med Clin North Am 69:375, 1985.
29. Visudhiphan P, Chiemchanya A, Somburanasin R, et al: Torticollis as the presenting sign in cervical spine infection and tumor. Clin Pediatr 21:71, 1982.

45
NEUROCYSTICERCOSIS

Fernando Rueda-Franco, M.D.

EPIDEMIOLOGY

Neurocysticercosis (NCC) is a common neurologic disease in many developing countries.[6, 10, 23] In a 1979 study by Flisser and colleagues,[8] it was noted that 1.9 percent of all general autopsy patients in Mexico were infected with cysticercosis at the time of death, but inasmuch as in many patients cerebral cysts may be resorbed and may disappear completely, the number of people infected at some time in their lives is much greater than the 1.9 percent figure reported. NCC is a major health problem in view of its prevalence, which may reach 3.6 percent of the population in some regions.[4] NCC is prevalent in Central and South America, India, Northern China, Indonesia, and Eastern Europe and in some regions of South Africa.[13] Massive immigration from endemic areas is making NCC a common disease in countries that were previously free of it.[24] The most typical example of this phenomenon is the increased number of cases of NCC that are now reported from the southwestern United States.[14] Cysticercosis is now one of the most common causes of seizures and of hydrocephalus among the Hispanic population in places such as Los Angeles, California.[1, 15, 30] However, the incidence of NCC in children is less than in adults. The largest series reported dealt mostly with adult patients, and in the mixed reports, patients younger than 15 years of age constitute only 2 to 10 percent of the patients. Up to the present time, the largest series published on cerebral cysticercosis in children are the ones by López-Hernández and Garaizar,[11] with 89 cases, and by Thomson and associates,[33] with 61 patients.

PARASITOLOGY AND PATHOGENESIS

Cysticercosis is infection with the larval stage of the cestode *Taenia solium* (pork tapeworm), and humans are the only known definitive hosts of the adult worm. In 1947, Stoll[31] estimated that about 2.5 million people in the world were infected with *T. solium*. The gravid proglottids of *T. solium* are passed in the stool, and in areas with poor sanitation, the ova contaminate the soil and the vegetation. If pigs are allowed free access to the contaminated areas, infestation of ova results in larval infestation of the pig's muscle, eye, and brain (the larval, or cysticercus, stage of the life cycle). Consumption by the human of undercooked "measly" pork results in the development of adult tapeworm in the human gastrointestinal tract. Humans develop cysticercus infestation by ingestion of either ova-contaminated vegetation or water or by autoinfestation by anus-hand-mouth contact, but this is the least common way of infestation. The contention that mature proglottids may regurgitate into the stomach and let ova loose after digestion has never been proved (internal autoinfection.) Children in endemic areas are at high risk because of poor personal hygiene, poor sanitation, frequent presentation of pica, and the presence of free-roaming pigs. The already stressed fact that NCC is less common in children than it is in adults may be explained in part by the extended interval between exposure and expression of illness.[18]

Once infestation has occurred, the oncosphere (larval form) may invade a variety of tissues, but the central nervous system is the most frequent and important and, in some cases, may be the only tissue invaded. Maturation of the oncosphere into the cysticercus requires 10 to 12 weeks, but symptoms may not appear for several months or years or may never be present at all. Death of the cysticerci occurs approximately 18 months or longer after the initial infestation, and the resultant breakdown products are accountable for the inflammatory response that produces the neurologic syndromes.

PATHOLOGY

The presence of parasites in human tissues triggers an immunologic inflammatory response that varies not only from individual to individual but also from tissue to tissue. A thorough description of the pathology and morbid anatomy of NCC is important to understand and correlate the clinical, radiologic, and immunologic findings. The identification of cysticerci is an important step in the diagnosis, especially when dealing with brain biopsies. The inexperienced pathologist may erroneously diagnose a colloid cyst for a cysticercus if he or she has been told that the specimen comes from the third ventricle. Light microscopy examination with a scanning lens allows proper identification of rudimentary strobila and a scolex formed by a rostellum with four suckers and some twenty pairs of hooks arranged as a crown (Fig. 45–1).

In order to be able to identify the scolex in a histologic preparation, serial sections are needed. The scolex appears as a more compact structure, very similar to the membrane, and the hooks appear as an anhistous cornified semitransparent structure. According to Escobar[5] the cysticerci evolve in several stages throughout their lifetime in the brain. The earliest stage is the vesicular one, in which the parasite appears to be formed by a very thin, friable, translucent whitish membrane. Inside, bathed in transparent fluid is the invaginated larva. When the parasite begins to show degenerative changes, the transparent fluid inside the cyst is replaced by a jellylike, whitish material. The larva may still be found, and this is the so-called colloidal stage. In the third stage, the cyst begins to reduce in size, the wall becomes thicker, and its contents are transformed into coarse granules owing to mineralization with calcium salts. This is the granular nodular stage. Finally comes the nodular calcified stage. The parasite has a small size, about one half or one fourth of the original cysticercus. Whether all cysticerci follow the sequence just described or pass very rapidly to the final stage is not known, since this sequence has not been followed in an experimental model.

The cysticerci almost always produce an inflammatory reaction around them, composed of a conglomerate of round mononuclear lymphocytic and plasma cells. Another important fact in NCC is the vascular reaction. Vasculitis is a common finding around the parasite: the vessels show thickening of the adventitia, with fibrosis of the media, and endothelial hyperplasia. In large arteries (e.g., basilar artery), atheromalike deposits may appear at the endothelial level, and they tend to reduce the lumen.

In the nervous tissue, the most common finding is a secondary astrocytic gliosis. The neurons in the area are usually affected in variable degrees and tend to undergo degenerative changes. When NCC is located in the meningeal compartment, especially at the base of the brain, rostral to the brainstem, or in the sylvian fissure, one can see the so-called racemose form of cysticercosis, in which the vesicles tend to be multiloculated and joined together to form conglomerates. In a few of the cases with cysticerci at the base of the brain, a very severe and strong thickening of the leptomeninges develops in such a way that it forms a thick layer of granulomatous tissue that covers the entire basal surface of the brain. It has exactly the same appearance as tuberculous meningitis. The most common form of ventricular cysticercosis is that of a single parasite in the fourth ventricle that may be free-floating in the cerebrospinal fluid (CSF) or attached to the ependymal walls. The parenchymal form of NCC is usually found in the gray matter, because of the richer vascularization of this area. The number of parasites may reach several hundreds, but commonly, one finds only a scattered few. Intraspinal cysticercosis, which is very rare, can be subarachnoid or parenchymal. No case of intraspinal cysticercosis has been reported in children. The mixed forms of NCC are seen quite often. The most common is that of meningeal and ventricular infestation.

CLINICAL MANIFESTATIONS

The clinical symptoms and signs of NCC are extremely variable, and the diagnosis must be con-

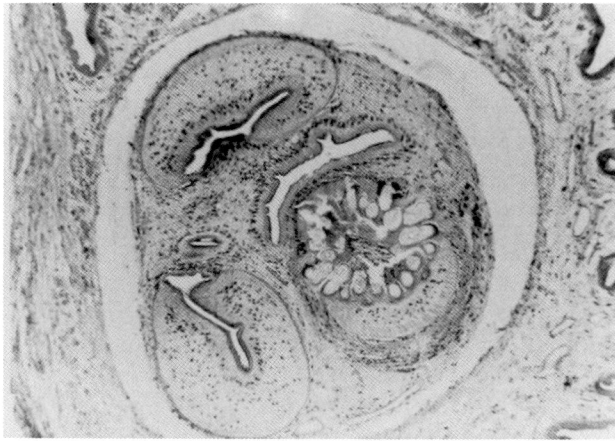

Figure 45–1. Microphotography of a scolex with two suckers and the rostellar hooks (H & E × 200).

sidered in any patient presenting from an endemic area with neurologic symptoms. The manifold clinical pictures seen in NCC are dependent on the following factors: The sites and the number of infesting larvae, the reaction to the larvae by host tissues, and the possibility of recurrent bouts of larval infestation or larval breakdown.

There have been several recent attempts to make a classification of NCC,[27, 30, 34] but inasmuch as all of these papers are based on mixed series that include both children and adults, the author prefers, on the grounds of clinicopathologic correlations, to describe the spectrum of this illness in children as follows:

Parenchymal Involvement. This is the most common form in children and may appear in either an acute or a chronic fashion. The lesion can be single, multiple, or diffuse. The *acute diffuse parenchymatous* disease, the so-called cysticercotic encephalitic syndrome,[11] presents with generalized cerebral edema, in many cases severe enough to cause an acute rise in intracranial pressure, with deterioration of consciousness, cerebral shifts, and multiple encephalitic symptoms (e.g., seizures). The reason for the higher prevalence of cerebral edema in children is unknown. *Acute focal parenchymatous* disease presents with localized, patchy edema or a cystic formation. The symptoms depend on the area involved and may manifest as either seizures or signs and symptoms of deficit (e.g., paralysis). *Chronic focal parenchymatous* disease presents with intracranial calcified cysts, which may or may not produce symptoms.

Meningeal Involvement. This form most commonly affects the base of the brain, with the development of the multicystic or racemose form, with a basal adhesive arachnoiditis, or both. In any case, the patient usually presents with a syndrome of increased intracranial pressure, obstructive or communicating hydrocephalus, and, eventually, cranial nerve involvement, particularly nerves II, V, VI, and VII. Vasculitic lesions are common in this variety of NCC.

Ventricular Involvement. This form occurs when the parasite reaches the ventricular system via the choroid plexus or ruptures through the ependymal lining and enlarges to become multicystic or racemose. The cysts may be adherent or free-floating. They commonly lodge in the fourth ventricle,[12, 22] producing intermittent acute obstructive hydrocephalus, which may result in loss of consciousness and posture brought on by sudden changes in head position (Osterwald-Bruns syndrome).[3]

Mixed Forms. These are usually a combination of parenchymal and meningeal forms, with a rather protean clinical picture.

Intraspinal Involvement. No case has been reported in children as yet, but it may occur and would present as an intramedullary mass lesion or in a form of arachnoiditis and vasculitis.

RADIOLOGIC DIAGNOSIS

Before the introduction of computed tomography (CT), the radiologic diagnosis of NCC was based on plain skull x-ray films and contrast studies such as pneumoencephalograms, ventriculograms, and cerebral angiograms. The accuracy of these methods is poor in comparison with that of CT. Furthermore, CT has the advantage of clearly establishing the topographic localization of the parasite in a single study. Also it has permitted us to learn more about the natural history of neurocysticercosis. In children, CT allowed the description of the hitherto undescribed form of the disease "acute encephalitic cysticercosis."[21]

CT is the most important tool for the recognition of NCC. With CT, one can see the different clinicopathologic varieties of the illness.

Parenchymatous Localization. This is the most common kind of infestation in children. There are three well-identified forms: calcified granulomas; single or multiple intracerebral cysts, mostly in the supratentorial compartment; and the diffuse "encephalitic" form. The calcifications may be single or multiple and may vary in size and location. Because of the greater sensitivity of CT, they can be detected in the scans before they are evident on plain skull x-ray films (Fig. 45–2).

The cyst may be single or multiple and varies in size. The single large form of the racemose variety produces compression and distortion of the intracranial structures, as do cystic tumors or other space-occupying lesions such as meningeal cysts and abscesses. Usually, these lesions do not enhance by an intravenous injection of contrast medium.

Acute encephalitic cysticercosis is an entity found in children. On CT, one can see multiple nodules of variable size and distribution, which enhance with contrast medium and are accompanied by diffuse, generalized edema with small collapsed ventricles (Fig. 45–3).

Meningeal Localization. In the acute form of arachnoiditis, enhancement of the basal meninges is evident only in those patients in whom there is an inflammatory reaction. This anatomopathologic form produces hydrocephalus in a large number of patients as a result of alterations in CSF absorption. One can also see different changes consequent to vasculitis.

Intraventricular Localization. In this form of NCC, sometimes it is necessary to do the CT scan with injection of contrast material into the ventricles, in order to demonstrate the exact location of the cyst and whether it is free-floating or attached to the ventricular walls. The time-honored neuroradiologic contrast studies such as pneumoencephalography, ventriculography, and cerebral angiography are used only when CT is not available or when there is a special indication (e.g., vasculitis of the

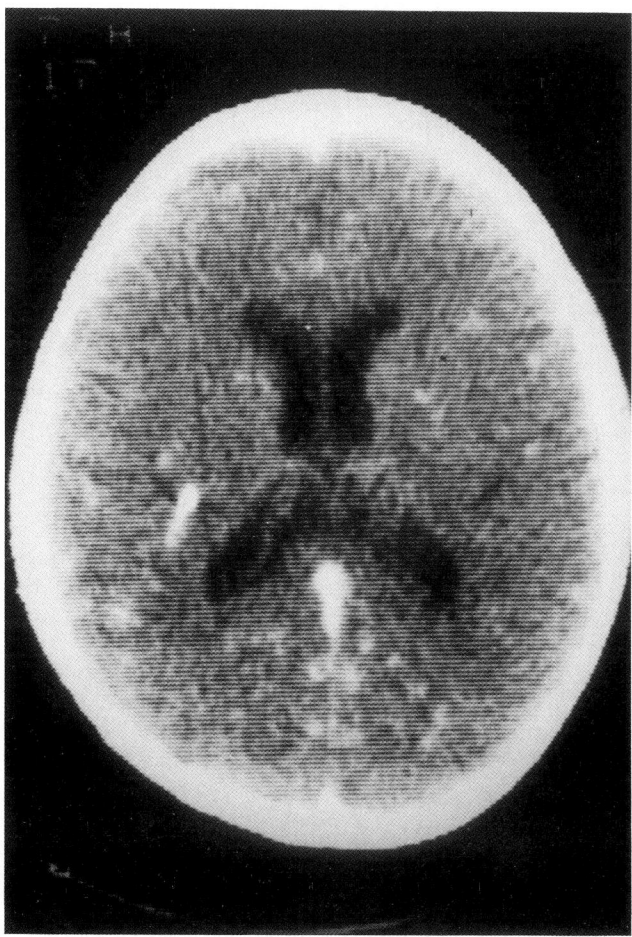

Figure 45-2. CT scan in a nine-year-old boy with numerous calcified lesions on both hemispheres.

cosis than in the parenchymal form. For example, McCormick and colleagues[14] reported that only 66 of 113 patients had a positive IHA. In meningitis, the test was positive in 79.6 percent. However, only 46.9 percent of patients without meningitis had positive IHAs. In patients with inactive parenchymal forms of NCC, CSF may be normal. However, in patients with the meningeal form, the ventricular form, or both, there is an inflammatory reaction, with elevation of cells, mononuclear lymphocytes, and, in very few cases, eosinophils. There is an increase in the protein content and a moderate tendency of glucose levels to decrease.

TREATMENT

The two treatment approaches to NCC are medical and surgical. Until recently, the *medical treatment* was aimed at alleviating symptoms. Its goal was to control seizures and, in cases of increased intracranial pressure, to reduce edema by the use of steroids such as dexamethasone as well as osmotic

gross arteries or migrating intraventricular cysts) (Fig. 45-4).

IMMUNOLOGIC TESTS

Immunologic tests for cysticercosis are suboptimal. Nieto[17] used the complement-fixation test with an extract of cysticercus antigen. It is used in CSF. A modification of that test, the indirect hemagglutination assay (IHA), was developed in the early 1960's and is now used by the Centers for Disease Control (CDC).[14] Another test is the enzyme-linked immunosorbent assay (ELISA), which measures specific antibodies to cysticercus antigen, in both serum and CSF. Immunoelectrophoresis as well as radioimmunoassay has also been used.[8] The most recent test was developed by Miller and coworkers.[16] This new method measures specific IgG antibodies in serum and in CSF, using a solid-phase radioimmunoassay in which cysticercus antigen is linked to a cellulose disk. Binding of antibodies to the disk is quantified. It is generally accepted that all these tests are more prone to be positive in cases of cysticercal meningitis or intraventricular cysticer-

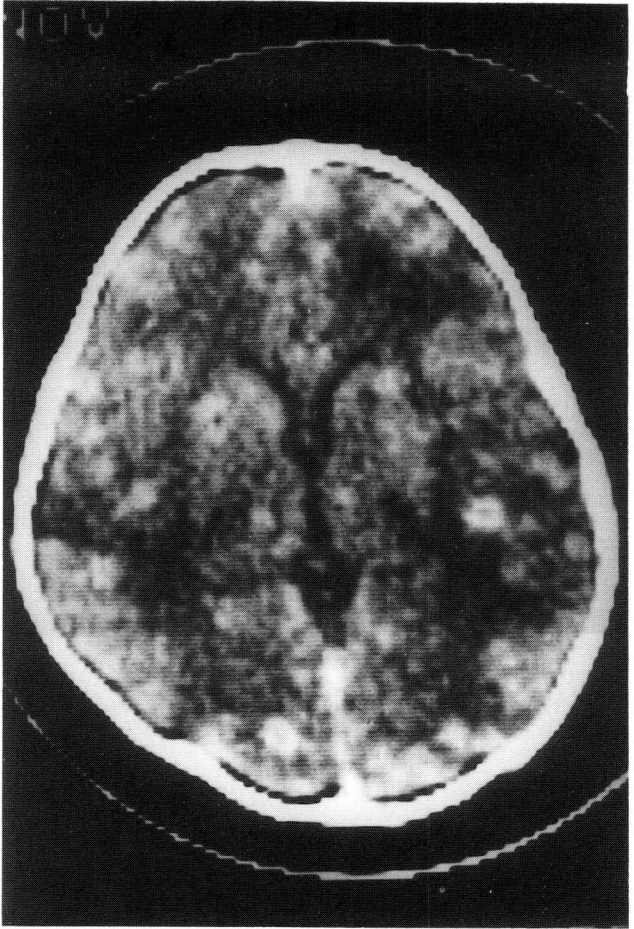

Figure 45-3. CT scan in a six-year-old boy with cysticercotic encephalitic syndrome. The CT with contrast medium shows multiple, ringlike enhanced lesions; edema in the white matter; and collapsed ventricles.

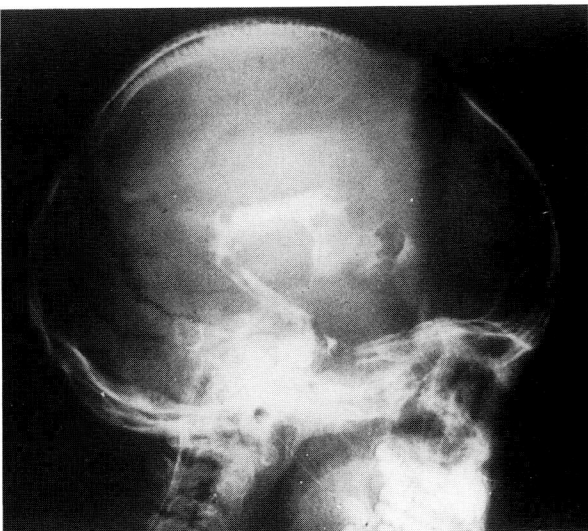

Figure 45–4. Iodoventriculogram showing multiple intraventricular cysts as rounded lesions.

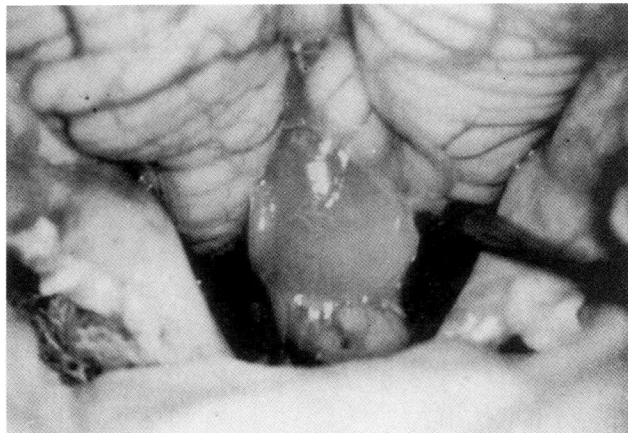

Figure 45–5. Cysticercus in the fourth ventricle, exposed through a suboccipital craniectomy, ready for its removal.

diuretics (mannitol or urea). In 1980, Robles and Chavarría[20] in Mexico obtained a beneficial response in a six-year-old boy with NCC treated with a pyrazinoisoquinoline 2-(cyclohexylcarbonyl)-1,2,3,6,7,11b-hexahydro-4H-pyrazinol[2,1,a]isoquinolin-4-one, which is now known as praziquantel.[25] Later, this finding was confirmed by other reports.[2, 19, 29, 32] However, most of these studies include a variety of forms of NCC, such as those characterized by parenchymal calcifications, cysts, hydrocephalus, and intracranial hypertension, and for that reason subjective evaluation was the rule. At present, the best conducted trial for praziquantel is the one by Sotelo and associates[26] at the National Institute of Neurology and Neurosurgery, Mexico City. The first part of the study was published in 1984,[26] and the second one in 1985.[28] In this study, 35 patients with active NCC were treated with praziquantel and were followed for one year. After therapy, CT and CSF analysis showed that 91 percent of patients with parenchymal cysts improved, but only 47 percent of the patients with chronic arachnoiditis had remission. The treatment consisted of a daily dose of 50 mg/kg of body weight for two weeks.

Unfortunately, there is not yet a similar trial conducted in children.

The *surgical treatment* of NCC can be divided into palliative and curative.[7, 9, 30] Various clinical manifestations of NCC and their surgical indications are listed.

- Cases of focal seizures, with or without generalization of fits, that are resistant to medical treatment. In these cases, surgical resection of the cysticercus or cysticerci improves or even cures the patient.
- In the case of racemose cysticercus that behaves as a tumoral mass, compressing and displacing the adjacent neural tissue, the extirpation or drainage of the cyst is indicated. This alleviates the compression of neighboring structures and, at times, increased intracranial pressure.
- In cases of impairment of vision resulting from adhesive arachnoiditis in the chiasmatic area, a craniotomy to free adhesions or to decompress the structures in the visual pathway is useful.
- In the event of an intraventricular cyst that blocks the CSF pathways, producing hydrocephalus and intracranial hypertension, the extirpation of the blocking cyst, when accessible, re-establishes the free circulation of the CSF (Fig. 45–5).
- In cases of hydrocephalus secondary to basal meningitis, a shunt is mandatory.
- In cases of acute encephalitic cysticercosis with increased intracranial pressure and slit ventricles that are resistant to medical treatment, subtemporal decompressive craniectomies are indicated. At times, internal decompression involving the thorough resection of brain tissue, mainly in the temporal lobe, is necessary.

Surgery is not always indicated in NCC and does not effect a complete cure in every case in which it is performed. Occasionally, surgery can partially and temporarily relieve intracranial hypertension and, sometimes, focal epilepsy caused by a cortical cysticercus.

Experience indicates that even in the case of CSF shunts, the catheter will sooner or later become occluded, necessitating further surgical intervention.

In conclusion, at present, the sanitary engineering and public health approach will have the widest influence in eliminating this disease.[30]

References

1. Apuzzo MLJ, Dobkin W, Zee C-S, et al: Surgical considerations in treatment of intraventricular cysticercosis. An analysis of 45 cases. J Neurosurg 60:400, 1984.

2. Botero D, Castaño S: Treatment of cysticercosis with praziquantel in Colombia. Am J Trop Med Hyg 31:811, 1982.
3. Bruns L: Neuropathologischen Demostrationen. Neurologisches Zentralblatt 25:265, 1906.
4. Costero I: Tratado de Anatomia Patologica. Mexico, D. F. Editorial Atlante, 1946, pp 1485–1495.
5. Escobar A: The pathology of neurocysticercosis. In: Palacios E, Rodriguez-Carbajal J, Taveras JM (eds): Cysticercosis of the Central Nervous System. Springfield, IL, Charles C Thomas, 1983, pp 27–54.
6. Escobar A, Nieto D: Cysticercosis. In: Minkler J (ed): Pathology of the Nervous System, Vol. 3. New York, McGraw-Hill Book Co., 1972, pp 2507–2515.
7. Escobedo F, Gonzalez-Mariscal G, Revuelta R, et al: Surgical treatment of cerebral cysticercosis. In: Flisser A, Willms K, Laclette J, et al (eds): Cysticercosis. Present State of Knowledge and Perspectives. New York, Academic Press, 1982, pp 201–205.
8. Flisser A, Pérez-Montfort R, Larralde C: The immunology of human and animal cysticercosis. Clin Exp Immunol 39:27, 1980.
9. Locke GE, Byrd SE, Zant JD: Cerebral cysticercosis: Surgical considerations. Bull Clin Neurosci 48:93, 1983.
10. Lombardo L, Mateos JH: Cerebral cysticercosis in Mexico. Neurology (Minneap) 11:824, 1961.
11. López-Hernández A, Garaizar C: Manifestations of infantile cerebral cysticercosis. In: Palacios E, Rodriguez-Carbajal J, Taveras JM (eds): Cysticercosis of the Central Nervous System. Springfield, IL, Charles C Thomas, 1983, pp 69–83.
12. Loyo M, Kleriga E, Estañol B: Fouth ventricular cysticercosis. Neurosurgery 7:456, 1980.
13. Mahajan RC: Geographical distribution of human cysticercosis. In: Flisser A, Willms K, Laclette J, et al (eds): Cysticercosis. Present State of Knowledge and Perspectives. New York, Academic Press, 1982, pp 39–46.
14. McCormick GF, Zee C-S, Heiden J: Cysticercosis cerebri: Review of 127 cases. Arch Neurol 39:534, 1982.
15. Miller BL, Goldberg MA, Heiner D, et al: Cerebral cysticercosis. An overview. Bull Clin Neurosci 48:2, 1983.
16. Miller B, Goldberg MA, Heiner D, et al: A new immunologic test for CNS cysticercosis. Neurology (Cleveland) 34:695, 1984.
17. Nieto D: Cysticercosis of the central nervous system: Diagnosis by means of the spinal fluid complement fixation test. Neurology (Minneap) 6:725, 1956.
18. Perry AK, Byrd SE, Locke GE: Cerebral cysticercosis. Paediatrics 66:967, 1980.
19. Robles C: Tratamiento médico de la cisticercosis cerebral. Salud Pública Mex 23:443, 1981.
20. Robles C, Chavarría M: Un caso de cisticercosis cerebral curado medicamente. Gac Med Mex 116:65, 1980.
21. Rodriguez-Carbajal J, Palacios E, Zee C-S: Neuroradiology of cysticercosis of the central nervous system. In: Palacios E, Rodriguez-Carbajal J, Taveras JM (eds): Cysticercosis of the Central Nervous System. Springfield, IL, Charles C Thomas, 1983, pp 101–143.
22. Salazar A, Sotelo J, Martinez H, et al: Differential diagnosis between ventriculitis and fouth ventricle cyst in neurocysticercosis. J Neurosurg 59:660, 1983.
23. Schenone H, Ramirez R, Rojas A: Aspectos epidemiológicos de la neurocisticercosis en America Latina. Bol Chil Parasitol 28:61, 1973.
24. Schultz TS, Ascherl GF, Jr.: Cerebral cysticercosis occurrence in the immigrant population. Neurosurgery 3:164, 1978.
25. Seubert J, Pohlke R, Loebich F: Synthesis and properties of praziquantel, a novel broad-spectrum antihelminthic with excellent activity against schistosomes and cestodes. Experientia 33:1036, 1977.
26. Sotelo J, Escobedo F, Rodriguez-Carbajal J, et al: Therapy of parenchymal brain cysticercosis with praziquantel. N Engl J Med 310:1001, 1984.
27. Sotelo J, Guerrero V, Rubio F: Neurocysticercosis: A new classification based on active and inactive forms. A study of 753 cases. Arch Intern Med 145:442, 1985.
28. Sotelo J, Torres B, Rubio Donnadieu F, et al: Praziquantel in the treatment of neurocysticercosis: Long-term follow-up. Neurology (Cleveland) 35:752, 1985.
29. Spina-Franca A, Nobrega JPS, Livramento JA, et al: Administration of praziquantel in neurocysticercosis. Tropenmed Parasitol 33:1, 1982.
30. Stern WE: Neurosurgical considerations of cysticercosis of the central nervous system. J Neurosurg 55:382, 1981.
31. Stoll NR: This wormy world. J Parasitol 33:1, 1947.
32. Thomas H, Andrews P, Mehlhorn H: New results of the effect of praziquantel in experimental cysticercosis. Am J Trop Med Hyg 31:803, 1982.
33. Thomson AJ, De Villiers JC, Moosa A, et al: Cerebral cysticercosis in children in South Africa. Ann Trop Paediatr 4:67, 1984.
34. Zenteno-Alanis GH: A classification of human cysticercosis. In: Flisser A, Willms K, Laclette J, et al (eds): Cysticercosis. Present State of Knowledge and Perspectives. New York, Academic Press, 1982, pp 107–126.

VI Vascular Diseases

46
STROKES IN CHILDREN

R. Michael Scott, M.D.
Kenneth L. Renkens, Jr., M.D.

In this chapter, the major causes of stroke in children are reviewed, with special attention directed to those of neurosurgical importance, such as moyamoya disease. Certain causes of pediatric stroke such as aneurysm and arteriovenous malformation (AVM) rupture and bleeding dyscrasias are discussed in other chapters in this text and will not be reviewed here.

HISTORY

The first generally acknowledged report of stroke in children was by Thomas Willis in 1667.[65] Multiple reports of "pediatric hemiplegia" were subsequently presented in the latter part of the nineteenth century without regard for etiology. Osler,[38] Sachs,[44] and Freud[14] all reported series of pediatric patients with strokes. In a landmark paper in 1927, Ford and Schaffer[13] described the etiology, outcome, and quality of survival in a series of children with strokes[13] and began the modern era of the evaluation of the child with stroke.

INCIDENCE

The general incidence of stroke in children is not known with certainty. A survey in a Rochester, Minnesota, population of children younger than 15 years of age detected an incidence of cerebrovascular disease, including both ischemic stroke and subarachnoid or intracerebral hemorrhage, of 2.52 per 100,000 population.[46] Banker's pediatric autopsy series reported that 8.7 percent of the patients had died of complications of cerebrovascular disease,[2] but the most common cause of death was hemorrhage secondary to bleeding from an AVM rather than occlusive cerebrovascular disease.

NEONATAL STROKES

The etiology of fixed neurologic deficits noted at birth or detected shortly thereafter has been disputed for many years. Suggested etiologies have included perinatal asphyxia and trauma, as well as in utero arterial occlusions probably secondary to embolization.[3] Other possible etiologies for this so-called hemiplegic cerebral palsy include disseminated intravascular coagulation, respiratory distress syndrome, infection, and congenital heart disease. Clinically, these children are often hypotonic at presentation but may also have brainstem symptoms including hypotension, apnea, and bradycardia. CT scanning may not detect the perinatal or neonatal stroke until the second week of life.[25]

ARTERIOSCLEROSIS

Premature cardiac or cerebrovascular atherosclerosis may be an occasional etiologic factor in a child presenting with stroke. The most common laboratory findings in this group of children are low levels of high-density lipoprotein cholesterol (C-HDL) and high levels of triglycerides, with the mechanism of cerebrovascular atherosclerosis thought to be related to lipoprotein-mediated endothelial damage and thrombus formation.[9] A more unusual cause is homocystinuria,[5] atherosclerosis being caused by homocystine-related endothelial cell injury and cell detachment. The treatment in both syndromes is directed toward correcting the metabolic abnormalities by the appropriate dietary measures and the administration of antiplatelet and cholesterol-lowering agents, although there is very little literature on the efficacy of any of these medications in children.

CEREBRAL ARTERITIS

Stroke in children may occur from cerebral arteritis due to a variety of causes: (1) collagen vascular disease, particularly lupus erythematosis,[32] and (2) following infections, such as cat scratch disease[49] or *Mycoplasma* upper respiratory tract infections.[30] CT scans show areas of infarction, and cerebral arteriography demonstrates segmental arteritis. Treatment of these children is directed toward the underlying cause of the arteritis, with steroids often prescribed empirically in hopes of reducing the inflammatory component of the demonstrated arterial changes.

FIBROMUSCULAR DYSPLASIA

Fibromuscular dysplasia has been implicated as the cause of an ischemic stroke occurring in a child.[23] There is controversy regarding the appropriate treatment of this syndrome in adults, but most authorities favor medical treatment with antiplatelet agents. Rarely, surgery to dilate the stenotic segment of the internal carotid may be indicated[34]; extracranial to intracranial bypass[53] and balloon catheter angioplasty[33] have also been proposed.

SICKLE CELL ANEMIA

Strokes occur in approximately 20 percent of patients with sickle cell disease, and children with this illness have a high risk for cerebral infarction. In one third of such patients, neurologic symptoms have their onset before the age of five. Strokes usually occur because of progressive occlusive disease of the major vessels of the circle of Willis—probably as a result of intravascular sickling in the vasa vasorum of these arteries leading to arterial wall damage and stenosis,[54] or as a result of reduction in brain capillary flow as a direct consequence of sickling. Typically, the strokes in children with SS disease are marked by acute hemiparesis and seizures, and long-term neurologic deficits, mental retardation, or both often occur. Although there seems to be no predictive factor indicating the sickler at risk to develop stroke,[40] an initial stroke is followed by a subsequent one in two thirds of patients, with 80 percent of the recurrences occurring within three years of the first stroke. Hyperventilation may trigger stroke by inducing cerebral arteriolar constriction and a decrease in cerebral blood flow, and those factors known to induce sickling, such as fever, infection, dehydration, and surgery, also may lead to stroke in susceptible patients.

Treatment includes increasing intravascular volume with fluids, correction of metabolic acidosis, administration of oxygen, and transfusion of packed red cells. Heparinization has been advocated but is unproven. Hypertransfusion to decrease the level of hemoglobin S to less than 30 percent has been reported to stop the progression of intracranial stenoses and to reduce the incidence of stroke recurrence,[43] although this therapy risks such effects as progressive iron accumulation in body tissues and sensitization to red cell antigens.

CARDIAC DISEASE

Strokes may occur in children with either congenital or acquired heart disease.[7] In children with left-to-right shunts, emboli from bacterial endocarditis may lead to acute stroke, although this cause of stroke in children is becoming less frequent with the widespread use of prophylactic antibiotics in children at risk. Mycotic aneurysms may occur in these children as well; their diagnosis and treatment are discussed elsewhere in this text. Stroke may also occur in this group of children because of the combination of dehydration, fever, and polycythemia, with vascular thromboses occurring most often in the distribution of the middle cerebral artery territory. Mitral valve prolapse has also been reported as a cause of stroke in children,[42] although the incidence and the cause of stroke in patients so affected remain unclear.

EXTRACRANIAL ARTERIAL DISSECTION

Dissection of the carotid or vertebral arteries may occur spontaneously or secondary to trauma,[35] with ischemic deficits resulting from emboli from the site of dissection or reduced cerebral blood flow from the narrowed vessel caliber. The site of carotid dissection is most commonly between C2 and the skull base; in children, the vessel is most commonly injured at this site by contusion or puncture from a sharp object such as a pencil entering the open mouth. The development of symptoms may occur hours or days following the trauma, with the injury presumably leading to dissection of the vessel, eventual development of thrombus, and, finally, cerebral embolization leading to symptoms. There may be a history of headache; facial, neck, or scalp pain; and an associated Horner's syndrome noted by the patient or examiner, resulting from injury to the sympathetic plexus around the internal carotid artery. Onset may be spontaneous and unrelated to trauma, but this is quite rare in children. The diagnosis should be suspected if a neurologic deficit develops in a child who has a history of trauma but who has a normal CT or a CT abnormality that does not account for the clinical deficit. Angiography establishes the diagnosis, demonstrating a long-tapering segment of stenosis (the so-called "string" sign); there is frequently an associated aneurysmal pouch at the most distal cervical extracranial carotid.

The treatment of such dissections remains controversial, but since the evidence seems to point clearly to thrombus formation and subsequent embolization as the cause of neurologic symptoms, the authors favor the use of anticoagulation with heparin initially and, then, conversion to sodium warfarin (Coumadin) for a period of six months. Follow-up angiography frequently discloses healing of the dissection. Recurring symptoms during treatment may necessitate surgical therapy such as direct carotid surgery with resection and grafting of the injured section of vessel or extracranial to intracranial arterial bypass and ligation of the internal carotid artery.[15]

MIGRAINE

Migraine is usually a benign disease in children, but there are reports of infarcts documented by CT as occurring in children with variants of the classic disorder, particularly in the vertebrobasilar distribution.[10] The etiology of these permanent deficits is unknown but is presumably related to changes in vessel caliber and reactivity during the migraine attack.

MOYAMOYA DISEASE

Moyamoya disease is a chronic occlusive cerebrovascular disease characterized by progressive stenosis of the distal internal carotid and basilar arteries and their branches, with concomitant enlargement of perforating arteries at the base of the brain to form the so-called moyamoya vessels. These unusual, dilated vessels presumably serve to provide collateral flow to the ischemic cerebral hemispheres. The word "moyamoya" in Japanese means "something hazy, like a puff of cigarette smoke drifting in the air" and is the term coined by Suzuki in 1969[59] to describe the angiographic appearance of the dilated collateral vessels seen in this disorder. The disease, which was initially described in Japan, is now recognized worldwide, with about half of the case reports in the literature occurring in other cultures.[57]

The etiology of the disorder is unknown. There is a familial incidence in Japan of 7 percent,[19] and the disease has occurred in identical twins.[67] There is an association with other hereditary diseases such as neurofibromatosis[22, 45, 60] and sickle cell anemia.[48, 54] Acquired moyamoya disease is seen following infectious diseases of the central nervous system, including tuberculous meningitis[26] and leptospirosis[66]; following radiation therapy to the brain[41, 50]; in Fanconi's anemia,[8] Down's syndrome,[39] connective tissue diseases,[12, 51, 63] and renal artery stenosis with hypertension[11]; and in patients with type I glycogenosis,[56] craniopharyngioma,[64] and optic glioma.[36] The common factor in all patients with the syndrome is an ongoing progressive occlusive process of the supraclinoid carotid artery and its bifurcation, with the gradual development of the moyamoya collateral pathways. The posterior circulation becomes involved in many cases as the disease progresses.[31] The histopathologic findings are nonspecific and include intimal hyperplasia and disordered or redundant internal elastic lamina in the stenotic proximal vessels. The moyamoya vessels themselves can either be normal or show attenuation of the elastic lamina, fibrin deposition with resultant thrombi, and microaneurysm formation. There are usually no inflammatory cells present.

The angiographic progression of moyamoya disease has been well-described in the literature and has been divided into six stages by Suzuki[59] (Figs. 46–1 and 46–2). Matsushima and Inaba[29] correlated the angiographic staging proposed by Suzuki with clinical presentations and noted that symptoms occur when there is an imbalance between the spontaneously developing collaterals from the moyamoya vasculature, skull base, dura, and leptomeninges and the ischemia of the brain caused by the proximal occlusive disease process. The rate of progression of the disease process is difficult to predict, but it is generally thought that the disease has a progressive phase during which the occlusions occur and the collaterals develop, and a stable phase when all collaterals are fully developed, the occlusive process is completed, and ischemic attacks disappear. Clinical disease progression may be erratic and episodic, with neurologic events and deficits building up over decades, or fulminant, with multiple bilateral strokes occurring within a period of several months.[47] Prognosis has been felt to be related to age of onset of symptoms, with a poorer prognosis related to onset in patients younger than six years of age.[24] Angiographically, prognosis appears directly related to the extent of proximal occlusive disease, with extension into the proximal posterior cerebral arteries and bilateral or dominant hemisphere disease carrying a relatively poor prognosis.

The most common clinical presentation in children is recurrent episodes of cerebral ischemia and stroke, as opposed to the adult presentation or intracranial hemorrhage, which can be intraventric-

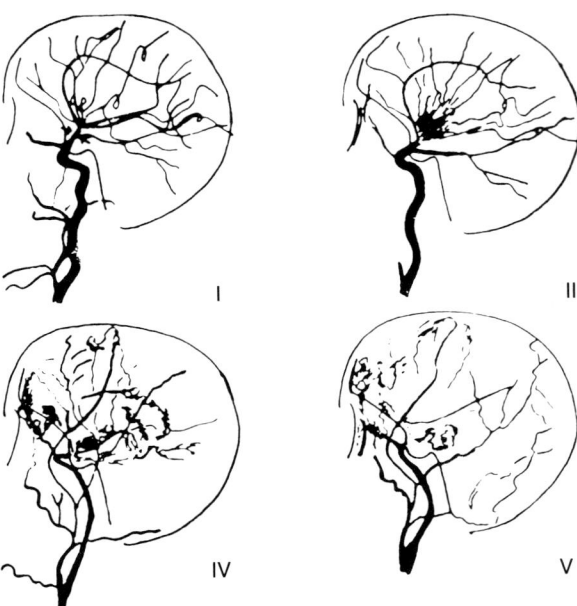
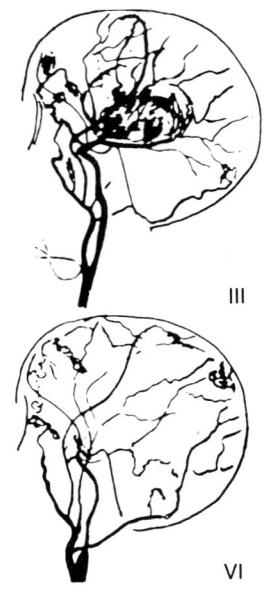

Figure 46–1. Angiographic progression of moyamoya disease (according to Suzuki). The characteristic "puff of smoke" occurs in stage 3. (Reprinted with permission of the publisher, from Surgical Neurology, vol. 4, p. 359, 1975; Copyright © 1975 by Elsevier Science Publishing Company, Inc., New York.)

ular, intracerebral, or subarachnoid.[58] Headache, stroke, and seizures were the most characteristic presenting signs and symptoms in series of children from both Japan and the western hemisphere.[37, 68] In six patients with moyamoya disease younger than 12 years of age seen by one of the authors (RMS), the initial signs were transient ischemic attacks (TIAs) in three children and strokes in three.

The diagnostic evaluation of these children begins with a CT scan, which in some cases may demonstrate the blush of the enlarged moyamoya vessels on contrast enhancement[61] or small infarcts in various distributions (Fig. 46–3). The electroencephalogram (EEG) shows interesting changes during and after hyperventilation, termed the "rebuild-up phenomenon." During hyperventilation, there is a build-up of high-voltage, slow waves that disappear after termination of hyperventilation; 20 to 60 seconds later there is a return of high-voltage, slow waves. Karasawa and associates[18] attributed these changes to the vasoconstrictive effect of hyperventilation on cerebral blood flow in the normal vessels over the cortical surface. The second slow wave effect is thought to be due to ischemia deep in the brain, secondary to a "steal" from the deep moyamoya collateral vessels to the now dilated cortical vessels, following the termination of hyperventilation. Although other tests have been proposed to evaluate these children, such as radioisotope scanning[24] and cerebral blood flow studies,[62] cerebral angiography is the definitive test, for obvious reasons. It is important to perform selective internal and external carotid artery injections, in order to determine the presence of pre-existing collateral

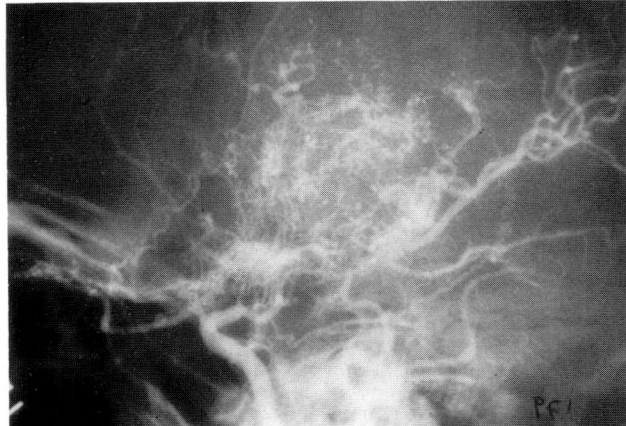

Figure 46–2. Stages 3–4 of moyamoya disease in a 15-year-old girl. There is severe stenosis of the anterior and middle cerebral arteries, and branches of the posterior cerebral arteries, with a prominent moyamoya pattern. (Reprinted with permission of the publisher, from Chapman PH (ed): Concepts in Pediatric Neurosurgery, vol. 6. Basel, S. Karger, 1985.)

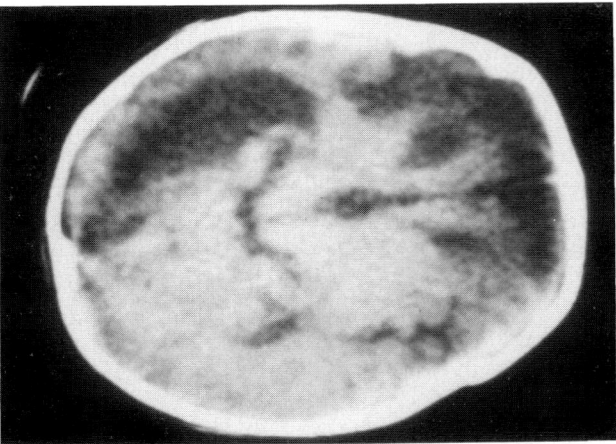

Figure 46–3. CT scan in an 11-month-old girl, demonstrating at least three infarcts in various distributions, secondary to progressing moyamoya disease.

flow from the carotid artery external system and to determine if surgical therapy might be helpful.

No medical therapy (e.g., steroids, vasodilators, low molecular weight dextran, antiplatelet agents, and anticoagulants) has been proved to be an effective treatment in this condition, and in the child with symptoms and the appropriate angiographic anatomy, a surgical procedure should be considered. Anesthetic management is extremely important when any surgical procedure is carried out in a child with moyamoya disease. The anesthesiologist should be made aware that hyperventilation during induction must specifically be avoided because of its potential to worsen neurologic deficts in these children who already have compromised cerebral blood flow.[55]

Most surgical procedures to treat moyamoya disease, with the exception of attempts to denervate the cerebral vasculature proposed by Suzuki and colleagues,[58] have been designed to augment transdural collaterals that are already a part of the ongoing moyamoya process. Superficial temporal to middle cerebral artery bypass, initially carried out by Yasargil in a child with moyamoya disease,[21] can very effectively increase hemisphere collateral flow.[4, 17, 57] However, there are significant technical problems in carrying out this procedure in children. The donor and the recipient vessels are often extremely small, pre-existing leptomeningeal collateral flow may be disturbed when the middle cerebral branch is temporarily occluded, and extensive opening of the dura, necessary to find a suitable recipient vessel, may disturb pre-existing transdural collateral.

Other operative techniques have depended on the natural tendency of the ischemic brain to form collateral flow from any available source. The encephalomyosynangiosis (EMS), described by Henschen,[16] involves the placement of the inner surface of the temporalis muscle directly on the brain surface, following an extensive temporal craniotomy. No series describing this procedure in patients with moyamoya disease treated in the western hemisphere has been published, although recent reports from Japan have documented improved clinical status and dramatic postoperative angiographic results.[20, 28] Complications related to the procedure include transient focal seizures and chronic subdural hematomas; the alteration in skull configuration following the relocation of the temporalis may be disfiguring. The large skin incision and dural flap required for the procedure have the potential to interrupt a number of pre-existing collaterals to the brain from the dura, and this procedure would seem to have limited application in the treatment of children with moyamoya disease in the West.

It is apparent from the literature that a less dramatic stimulus than the EMS can induce collateral vessels in the appropriate patient. Ausman and coworkers[1] noted this process in a patient in whom the bone flap was not replaced following a bypass from the superficial temporal artery (STA) to the middle cerebral artery (MCA), and the authors have noted similar phenomena (Fig. 46–4). Spetzler and colleagues[52] noted multiple transdural collaterals occurring six weeks after an intact superficial temporal artery was sutured to the arachnoid in a patient with no satisfactory recipient vessel at the time of an intended STA-MCA anastomosis. Matsushima and colleagues[27] transposed the intact superficial temporal artery with a strip of attached galea to a narrow dural opening beneath a linear craniotomy in hopes of promoting transdural collateral formation, naming their procedure "encephalo-duro-arterio-synangiosis (EDAS)." Subsequent papers by Matsushima and coworkers[28, 29] have demonstrated dramatic enlargement of the donor vessel, increased transdural collateral formation, and other favorable changes such as a decrease in moyamoya vessels and increased middle cerebral artery filling. Clinical and EEG improvement was also noted, although intellectual function appeared unchanged.

The advantages of this surgical technique are that (1) it is simple, (2) both hemispheres can be operated on during a single procedure, (3) there is no temporary occlusion of middle cerebral artery branches, (4) there are multiple donor arteries available, including the occipital artery and both divisions of the superficial temporal artery, and (5) the craniotomy can be planned to avoid disruption of pre-existing transdural collaterals. In Matsushima's original description of the procedure, the arachnoid membrane was left intact, but the authors as well as others[37] have found that failure to open the arachnoid widely may hinder the development of

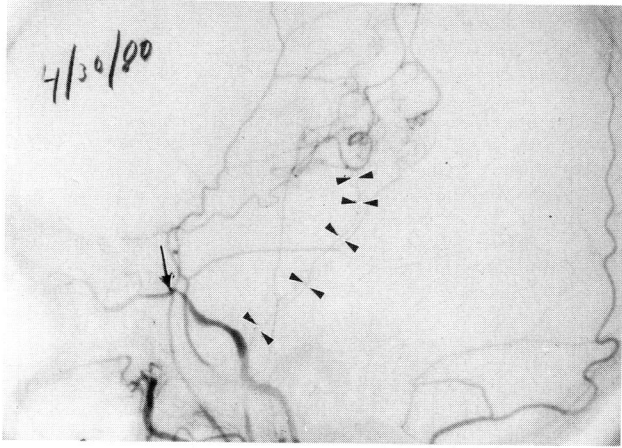

Figure 46–4. Arteriogram two years after STA to MCA bypass in an adult with occlusion of the supraclinoid carotid artery (arrow). The superficial temporal artery (arrowheads) has atrophied, and the ischemic brain is now vascularized by extensive transdural collaterals from meningeal and other scalp vessels. (Reprinted by permission of the publisher, Barnett HJM, Stein BM, Mohr JP, Yatsu FM (eds.): Stroke: Pathophysiology, Diagnosis, and Management. New York, Churchill Livingstone, 1986, p. 1223.)

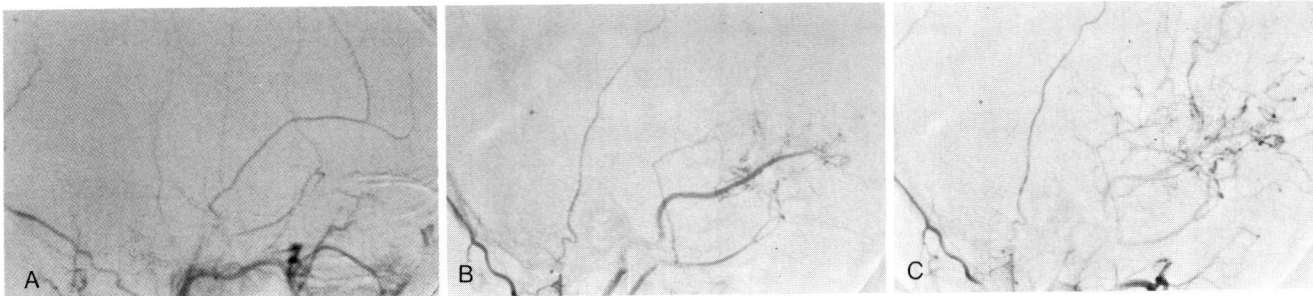

Figure 46–5. Successful EDAS procedure, with arachnoid opened and scalp vessel sutured directly to the pia. A, Preoperative external carotid arteriogram demonstrating small-caliber, superficial temporal vessels. B and C, Arteriograms six months after surgery, demonstrating marked hypertrophy of superficial temporal artery and extensive collateralization of the right hemisphere.

collaterals, which probably explains the failure of the EDAS procedure in the case reported by Cahan.[6] The authors have modified Matsushima's procedure by widely opening the arachnoid and suturing the vessel with the attached galeal strip directly to the pia with 8-0 or 10-0 suture; postoperative arteriograms have demonstrated a very satisfactory increase in transdural collateral flow to the operated hemisphere (Fig. 46–5).

References

1. Ausman JI, Moore J, Chou SN: Spontaneous cerebral revascularization in a patient with STA-MCA anastomosis. J Neurosurg 44:84, 1985.
2. Banker BQ: Cerebral vascular disease in infancy and childhood. I. Occlusive vascular diseases. J Neuropathol Exp Neurol 20:127, 1961.
3. Barmada MA, Moossy J, Schuman RM: Cerebral infarcts with arterial occlusion in neonates. Ann Neurol 6:495, 1979.
4. Boone SC, Sampson DS: Observations on Moyamoya disease: Case treated with superficial temporal–middle cerebral artery anastomosis. Surg Neurol 9:189, 1978.
5. Brattstorm LE, Hardebo JE, Hultberg BL: Moderate homocysteinemia. A possible risk factor for arteriosclerotic cerebrovascular disease. Stroke 15:1012, 1984.
6. Cahan LD: Failure of encephalo-duro-arterio-synangiosis procedure in moyamoya disease. Pediatr Neurosci 12:58, 1985–86.
7. Chugani HT, Menkes JH: Neurologic manifestations of systemic disease. In: Menkes MD (ed): The Textbook of Child Neurology. Philadelphia, Lea & Febiger, 1985, pp 720–763.
8. Cohen N, Berant M, Simon J: Moyamoya and Fanconi's anemia. Pediatrics 65:804, 1980.
9. Daniels SR, Bates S, Lukin RR, et al: Cerebrovascular arteriopathy (arteriosclerosis) and ischemic childhood stroke. Stroke 13:360, 1982.
10. Dunn DW: Vertebrobasilar occlusive disease and childhood migraine. Pediatr Neurol 1:252, 1985.
11. Ellison PH, Largent JA, Popp AJ: Moyamoya disease associated with renal artery stenosis. Arch Neurol 38:467, 1981.
12. Ferris FJ, Levine HL: Cerebral arteritis: Classification. Radiology 109:327, 1973.
13. Ford FR, Schaffer AJ: The etiology of infantile acquired hemiplegia. AMA Arch Neurol Psychiatry 18:323, 1927.
14. Freud S: Die Infantile Cerebrallahmung. Vienna, Holder, 1897.
15. Gratzl O, Schmeidek P, Steinhoff H: Extra-intra-cranial arterial bypass in patients with occlusion of cerebral arteries due to trauma and tumor. In: Handa H (ed): Microneurosurgery. Baltimore, University Park Press, 1980, pp 68–80.
16. Henschen C: Operative revaskularisation des zirkulatorisch geschadigten Gehirns durch Auflage gestielter Muskellappen (Encephalo-Myo-Synangiose). Langenbecks Arch Chir 264:392, 1950.
17. Karasawa J, Kikuchi H, Furuse S, et al: Treatment of moyamoya disease with STA-MCA anastomosis. J Neurosurg 49:679, 1978.
18. Karasawa J, Kikuchi H, Takahashi N, et al: Electroencephalographic study of "moyamoya" disease in children: Pre- and postsurgical EEG changes and its pathophysiology (in Japanese). Rinsho Noha 22:527, 1980.
19. Kitahara T, Ariga N, Yamaura A, et al: Familial occurrence of moyamoya disease: Report of three Japanese families. J Neurol Neurosurg Psychiatry 42:208, 1979.
20. Kobayaski K, Takeuchi S, Tsuchida T, et al: Encephalo-myo-synangiosis (EMS) in moyamoya disease with special reference to postoperative angiography. Neurol Med Chir (Tokyo) 21:1229, 1981.
21. Krayenbuhl HA: The moyamoya syndrome and the neurosurgeon. Surg Neurol 4:353, 1975.
22. Lamas E, Diez Lobato R, Caballo A, et al: Multiple intracranial arterial occlusions (moyamoya disease) in patients with neurofibromatosis. One case report with autopsy. Acta Neurochir 45:133, 1978.
23. Llorens-Terol J, Sole-Llenas J, Tura A: Stroke due to fibromuscular hyperplasia of the internal carotid artery. Acta Paediatr Scand 72:299, 1983.
24. Maki Y, Nakada Y, Nose T, et al: Clinical and radioscopic follow-up study of "moyamoya." Child's Brain 2:257, 1976.
25. Mannino FL, Trauner DA: Strokes in neonates. J Pediatr 102:605, 1983.
26. Mathew NT, Abraham J, Chandy J: Cerebral angiographic features in tuberculous meningitis. Neurology 20:1015, 1970.
27. Matsushima Y, Fukai N, Tanaka K, et al: A new surgical treatment of moyamoya disease in children. A preliminary report. Surg Neurol 15:313, 1981.
28. Matsushima Y, Inaba Y: Moyamoya disease in children and its surgical treatment. Child's Brain 11:155, 1984.
29. Matsushima Y, Inaba Y: The specificity of the collaterals to the brain through the study and surgical treatment of moyamoya disease. Stroke 17:117, 1986.
30. Maytal J, Resnick TJ: A TIA-like syndrome associated with Mycoplasma pneumoniae infection. Pediatr Neurol 1:308, 1985.
31. Miyamoto S, Kikuchi H, Karasawa J, et al: Study of the posterior circulation in moyamoya disease. J Neurosurg 61:1032, 1984.
32. Moore P, Cupps TR: Neurological complications of vasculitis. Ann Neurol 14:155, 1983.
33. Mullen S, Duda EE, Patronas NJ: Some examples of balloon technology in neurosurgery. J Neurosurg 52:321, 1980.
34. Ojemann RG, Crowell RM: Surgical Management of Cerebrovascular Disease. Baltimore, Williams & Wilkins, 1983, pp 107–110.
35. Ojemann RG, Crowell RM: Surgical Management of Cerebrovascular Disease. Baltimore, Williams & Wilkins, 1983, pp 111–121.

36. Okuno T, Prensky AL, Gado M: The moyamoya syndrome associated with irradiation of an optic glioma in children: Report of two cases and review of the literature. Pediatr Neurol 1:311, 1985.
37. Olds MV, Hoffman HJ: Moyamoya: Experience at the Hospital for Sick Children, Toronto. Presented at the 13th Annual Meeting, Section of Pediatric Neurological Surgeons of the American Association of Neurological Surgeons. Salt Lake City, Utah, December 13, 1984.
38. Osler W: The Cerebral Palsies of Children: A Clinical Study from the Infirmary for Nervous Diseases. Philadelphia, Blakiston & Co., 1889, pp 1–55.
39. Pearson E, Lenn NJ, Cail WS: Moyamoya and other causes of stroke in patients with Down's syndrome. Pediatr Neurol 1:174, 1985.
40. Powars D, Wilson B, Imbus C, et al: The natural history of stroke in sickle cell disease. Am J Med 65:461, 1978.
41. Rajakulasingam K, Cerullo LJ, Raimondi AJ: Childhood moyamoya syndrome. Postradiation pathogenesis. Child's Brain 5:467, 1979.
42. Rice CPG, Boughner DR, Stiller C, et al: Familial stroke syndrome associated with mitral valve prolapse. Ann Neurol 7:130, 1980.
43. Russell MO, Goldberg HI, Hodson A, et al: Effect of transfusion therapy on arteriographic abnormalities and recurrence of stroke in sickle cell disease. Blood 63:162, 1984.
44. Sachs B, Peterson F: A study of cerebral palsies of early life, based upon an analysis of one hundred and forty cases. J Nerv Ment Dis 17:295, 1890.
45. Salyer WR, Salyer DC: The vascular lesions of neurofibromatosis. Angiology 25:510, 1974.
46. Schoenberg BS, Mellinger JF, Schoenberg DG: Cerebrovascular disease in infants and children: A study of incidence, clinical features, and survival. Neurology 28:763, 1978.
47. Scott RM: Surgical treatment of moyamoya syndrome in children. In: Chapman PH (ed): Concepts in Pediatric Neurosurgery, Vol. 6. New York, S Karger, 1985, pp 198–212.
48. Seeler RA, Royal JE, Powe L, et al: Moyamoya in children with sickle cell anemia and cerebrovascular occlusion. J Pediatr 93:808, 1978.
49. Selby G, Walker GL: Cerebral arteritis in cat-scratch disease. Neurology 29:1413, 1979.
50. Servo A, Puranen M: Moyamoya syndrome as a complication of radiation therapy. J Neurosurg 48:1026, 1978.
51. Silverstein A, Hollin S: Occlusion of the supraclinoid portion of the internal carotid artery. Neurology 13:679, 1963.
52. Spetzler RF, Roski RA, Kopaniky DR: Alternative superficial temporal artery to middle cerebral artery revascularization procedure. Neurosurgery 7:484, 1980.
53. Stephens HW, Jr.: Microvascular anastomosis and carotid artery ligation for fibromuscular hyperplasia and carotid artery aneurysm. In: Fein JM, Reichman OH (eds): Microvascular Anastomosis for Carotid Ischemia. New York, Springer-Verlag, 1974, pp 307–316.
54. Stockman JA, Nigro DO, Mishkin MM, et al: Occlusions of large cerebral vessels in sickle cell anemia. N Engl J Med 287:846, 1972.
55. Sumikawa K, Nagai H: Moyamoya disease and anesthesia. Anesthesia 58:204, 1983.
56. Sunder TR: Moyamoya disease in a patient with Type I glycogenosis. Arch Neurol 38:251, 1981.
57. Suzuki J, Kodama N: Moyamoya disease—a review. Stroke 14:104, 1983.
58. Suzuki J, Takaku A, Kodama N, et al: An attempt to treat cerebrovascular "moyamoya" disease in children. Child's Brain 1:193, 1975.
59. Suzuki J, Takaku A: Cerebral vascular "moyamoya" disease. A disease showing abnormal net-like vessels of brain. Arch Neurol 20:288, 1969.
60. Taboada D, Alonso A, Moreno J, et al: Occlusion of the cerebral arteries in von Recklinghausen's disease. Neuroradiology 18:281, 1979.
61. Takahashi M, Miyauchi T, Kowada M: Computed tomography of moyamoya disease: Demonstration of occluded arteries and collateral vessels as important diagnostic signs. Radiology 134:671, 1980.
62. Takeuchi S, Tanaka R, Ishii R, et al: Cerebral hemodynamics in patients with moyamoya disease. A study of regional cerebral blood flow by the Xe-133 inhalation method. Surg Neurol 23:468, 1985.
63. Trevor RP, Sondheimer FK, Fessel WJ, et al: Angiographic demonstration of major cerebral vessel occlusion in systemic lupus erythematosus. Neuroradiology 4:202, 1972.
64. Tsuji N, Kuriyama T, Iwamoto N, et al: Moyamoya disease associated with craniopharyngioma. Surg Neurol 21:588, 1984.
65. Willis T: Pathologiae Cerebri et Nervosi Generis Specimen. In quo Agitur de Morbis Convulsivis, et de Scorbuto. Oxonii, excudebat Guil Hall, impensis Ja, Allestry, 1667, p 49.
66. Ximin L, Zuzhong R, Zhuan C, et al: Moyamoya disease caused by leptospiral cerebral arteritis. Chinese Med J 93:599, 1980.
67. Yamada H, Nakamura S, Kageyama N: Moyamoya disease in monovular twins. J Neurosurg 53:109, 1980.
68. Yamashiro Y, Takahashi H, Takahashi K: Cerebrovascular moyamoya disease. Eur J Pediatr 142:44, 1984.

47
ARTERIOVENOUS MALFORMATIONS OF THE BRAIN

Robin P. Humphreys, M.D.

The problem of stroke in children was put into perspective by the 1973 Report of the Joint Committee for Stroke Facilities.[10] Children can suffer either ischemic or hemorrhagic cerebrovascular events, but on a basis that differs from those occurrences in adults. While the clinical and grading phenomena of hemorrhagic stroke in children, the subject of this chapter, may be similar in adults and children, the causation, definition, and remarkable recuperative powers of the pediatric brain distinguish the child who has suffered a hemorrhagic ictus.

Intracranial arterial aneurysms and arteriovenous malformations (AVM) are collectively though not exclusively the commonest causes of spontaneous subarachnoid hemorrhage/intraventricular hemorrhage (SAH/IVH). In adults, a ruptured saccular aneurysm would be 6.5 times more likely than an AVM to account for that hemorrhage.[23] It is a moot point whether the ratio is reversed in children. Hourihan and associates[15] in a review of 167 patients aged 20 years and younger note that in twice as many, SAH was caused by aneurysm rather than AVM. Their paper includes the work of other authors studying the problem of pediatric SAH.[21, 23, 38] In a total review of 478 such patients, ruptured aneurysm accounts for 40 percent of children's SAH and AVM for 26 percent; no lesion was defined in 31 percent. That such has been cumulative experience might appear to be at odds with the results of the cooperative study, in which 33 percent of AVMs associated with hemorrhage occurred before age 20 years. This finding contrasts with that of only 1.5 percent of intracranial aneurysms becoming symptomatic in that same period.[23, 35]

The material to be reviewed in this chapter is taken from the experience at the Hospital for Sick Children (HSC), Toronto, from 1954 to 1985. This hospital serves as a widespread referral base exclusively for the care of children up to age 18 years; the statistics reflect the general population needs. With regard to SAH as the presenting symptom, 26 of 35 (74 percent) of our aneurysm patients bled from that lesion, and 78 (77 percent) children with AVM suffered spontaneous intracranial bleeding. In the author's experience, therefore, rupture of an AVM is three times more likely to be the cause of the SAH/IVH than is a burst aneurysm.[17]

It remains a mystery why these two vascular lesions, allegedly related to some congenital malfeasance, are not more flamboyant during childhood and adolescent years. At HSC, there has been no case of an incidental aneurysm or AVM defined by arteriography or computed tomography (CT) performed for other reasons. Nor have there been many children with a conglomerate of vascular problems. The Cooperative Study contained 37 patients with co-existing angiomatous malformations and one or more aneurysms.[35] Hayashi and co-workers[13] reviewed 73 patients with AVM associated with aneurysm and noted that only two patients were below the age of 10 years. Ostergaard has recently added two more children with saccular aneurysm attendant to the AVM.[32] In the HSC series, there were no children with an admixture of aneurysm and AVM, but there was one child who had bilateral symmetric internal carotid artery aneurysms and another with a pontine AVM in association with a facial, orbital, and dural vascular malformation. A third child had an extensive spinal cord AVM associated with a small and similar lesion in the right temporal lobe.[14]

Of 453 intracranial angiomatous malformations entered into the Cooperative Study, almost 20 percent were diagnosed before the age of 20 years.[35] Hence, the AVM, although of congenital origin, does not necessarily declare itself at birth nor in the early childhood years. The fact that most lesions become symptomatic between the ages of 20 and 40 years suggests a latency in the malformation's usual evolution.[35] While there is a certain age bias in the reporting of series from predominantly adult units, we have observed that of approximately 10,000 cerebral arteriograms performed in our hospital for whatever reason, not one incidental aneurysm nor AVM has been uncovered, although three of the AVMs to be reported were incidental necropsy findings in children.[12]

Matson declared the AVM "the most frequent abnormality of intracranial circulation in childhood," and reported on his experience with 34 patients.[26] Since then, a number of reports have examined the problem of symptomatic AVM in children under 19 years of age.* This chapter will consider 105 children with AVM of the brain who were admitted to HSC from 1954 to 1985. Only those cases of AVM confirmed by arteriography, histopathological analysis of operative or necropsy tissues, or both, have been entered into the study. Children with Galenic, cavernous, and venous malformations have been excluded from this review. The 105 patients reported comprise 101 studied for specific neurological symptoms, three who died of other causes and whose AVM was discovered unruptured at necropsy, and one girl whose pontine AVM was detected in follow-up study of an extensive cranio-orbital vascular malformation.

EMBRYOGENESIS AND PATHOLOGY

The classical AVM is presumed to represent a structural defect in the formation of the primitive arteriolar–capillary network normally interposed between brain arteries and veins. The stimulus, timing, and early architectural deficiencies in such malformations are not entirely clear. Padget believed that most of the malformations occur before the 40-mm embryo length, that is, before the arterial walls thicken, notwithstanding that it is after this time when the late histologic changes in the walls of the vessels convert them into the final adult form.[33]

The pathological analysis of resected AVM specimens does not provide much additional information about the causation of AVM. The tangled arteriovenous communications because of their low resistance attract exaggerated blood flow. Given enough time, the malformations do have the capacity to expand their bulk by enlarging and increasing the tortuosity of the feeding and draining channels. The number of fistulous connections, however, likely does not change, and some lesions (such as those of the brainstem) may always remain small.[5]

The conglomeration of turgid, tortuous vessels covered by opacified and thickened arachnoid on the brain's surface is easily recognizable as the classic AVM. Sometimes the malformation is hidden in a sulcus or the subcortical tissues, and served by a straightened, dilated anomalous artery, which acts as its only surface hallmark. The nearby cerebral convolutions show variable degrees of atrophy, and there may be local rusty staining from previous hemorrhage. The tough texture of the adjacent gray and white matter is due to gliosis, which permits dissection of the lesion through its relatively inert tissue.

While some malformations are globular in shape, most describe a course to the subjacent ventricle in an inverted wedge-shaped fashion (Fig. 47–1). The component vessels show variation in their numbers, caliber, and the thickness of their walls. Venous tortuosity, intimal thickening, arteriolization of veins, and evidence of hemorrhage and neuronal loss are indicative of the long-standing hemodynamic consequences within the malformation. In almost all circumstances is there microscopic evidence of previous hemorrhage, with hemosiderin-laden macrophages.[27, 42] Elastic and muscle fibers in the arteries are altered; the media vary in thickness and substantial thinning of some vessels can result in aneurysmal dilatation of the structure.[31, 36, 42] But those vessels with marked saccular dilatations are venous in origin.[27] Even the knowledge that some arteries show focal absence of elastic lamina does not isolate the primary vascular fault.

Given that the stage may be set by 60 days' gestation for maldevelopment of a portion of the cerebrovascular tree, it is remarkable that the typical AVM does not declare itself except with symptoms. While ruptured AVM is the commonest cause of hemorrhagic stroke in children, most AVMs become symptomatic between 20 and 40 years of age.[35] Nor has there been any convincing evidence concerning the cause—hypertension, strenuous activity, and head trauma—of bleeding from a malformation.[27] It is tempting to believe therefore that whatever the

---
*References 1, 2, 9, 15, 19, 20, 29, 30, 38, 39, 43

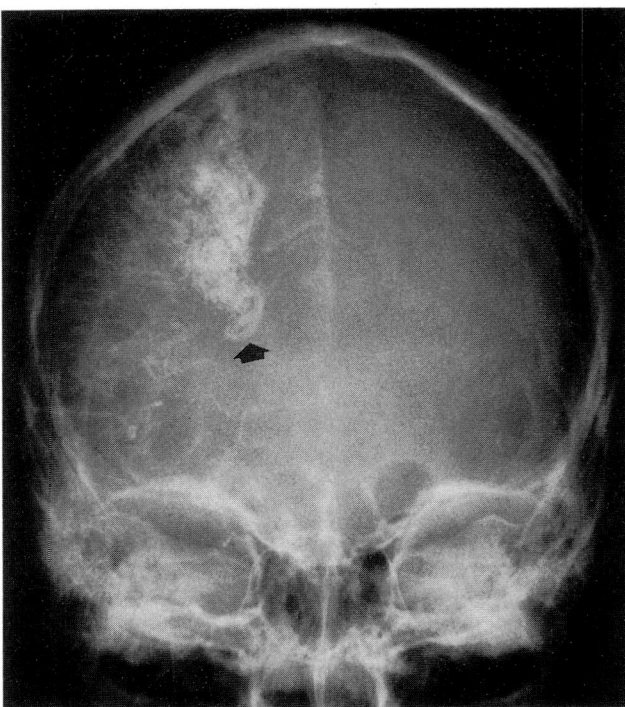

Figure 47–1. This midhemisphere malformation has a characteristic wedge-shaped outline as it reaches to the deep ventricular wall. Note the supplying, or draining, vessel (arrow) that lies partly in the ventricle and is tangled on the choroid plexus.

early embryologic fault, there are substantial postnatal and delayed factors that influence the development and declaration of the cerebral AVM.

NATURAL HISTORY

The criteria for patient selection for AVM therapy are still the subject of controversy. Matched trials of nonsurgical and surgical management programs for patients with cerebral AVM have understandably not been reported. Papers by Forster,[7] Schatz and Botterell,[37] Svien and McRae,[41] and Troupp[44, 45] have analyzed nonsurgical treatment methods. It is to be recalled that these experiences were gathered at a time when surgical and anesthetic techniques were not as precise as those available currently, and that the patients relegated to a nonsurgical program were often those whose lesions were considered inoperable. But, with advances in surgical and anesthetic technology, the indications for and success with surgery have broadened. It is argued, however, that the improved results depend more importantly on the selection criteria and only marginally on surgical technique.[34] The matter is now further complicated by additional treatment options—proton-beam irradiation, stereotactic cryosurgery, and glue-and-balloon embolization.

If a decision is made not to operate on a patient's cerebral AVM, then what is the risk to that patient? Repeat hemorrhage, the major threat, varies from 6 to 33 percent during the first year at least and diminishes thereafter, especially beyond the fourth year.[7, 11, 41] The expected mortality from a repeat hemorrhage is 6 percent.[41] Graf and associates[11] identify as the patient at greatest risk (for first or subsequent bleed) a woman whose symptoms include seizures related to a small (less than 3.0 cm) AVM located in the right temporal region. Pelletteri and colleagues[34] have taken the predictions in a different direction and determined that the most favorable risk profile for operation on a cerebral AVM exists in a woman under 40 years, with a small, superficial AVM in a silent area, whose presenting symptom is SAH but who is neurologically normal. Luessenhop and colleagues[25] also state that the "natural risk" of AVMs less than 4.0 cm in diameter exceeds that of the surgical risk, and these lesions should be excised. The debate continues but it may never be possible to determine unequivocally what is the right treatment policy.

There are no figures available that document the natural history of cerebral AVMs in children. The present study, however, which agrees with that of others, indicates that children are more liable to hemorrhage (77 percent risk) from their malformations than adults (68 percent risk), and that there is a threat of repeat hemorrhage.[9, 30] Celli and associates[3] state that the effects of hemorrhage are worse on patients under 15 years of age, and that children have a higher frequency (than adults) of intraparenchymal hematomas and intraventricular bleeding. More important, the fate of a child with an unexcised AVM is worse than that of an adult as there is a statistically higher risk of bleeding (32 percent at 10 years), especially in patients with a nonhemorrhagic onset.

If it is agreed that the surgical treatment of cerebral AVMs, if undertaken, should as Drake states, "carry a very low mortality and morbidity, certainly lower than that of the natural history," then surgical care for children's AVMs is recommended.[5, 9, 24, 39, 46] For not only is there a greater risk of hemorrhage as the first symptom in children, but also the mortality from that hemorrhage in the HSC series is 24 percent, substantially greater than the 6–10 percent rate quoted for adults.[31, 35] The HSC surgical mortality is 8 percent and represents patients who were grade 4 or 5 category at the time of emergency measures to evacuate a clot or place an external ventricular drain. Surgical treatment of children's AVMs thus adheres to Drake's principle. It also supports Matson's stance on surgical care, recommended because "there is expectation of many years in which these lesions may enlarge and cause increasing disability and, the resiliency of the cerebral circulation is better."[26]

INITIAL CLINICAL ASSESSMENT

Symptoms

The symptoms of a cerebral AVM, whenever they appear, are representative of the structural defects in the vessels of the malformation, and the sump effect of the direct arteriovenous shunting. Perhaps the progressive biological activity of the malformation accounts for a greater percentage of children (than adults) suffering intracranial bleeding from the lesions, whereas relatively larger numbers of adults display the presumed ischemic symptoms of headache, dementia, and slowly progressive neurological dysfunction. It is not always clear at operation nor with histopathological examination of excised tissues just where the hemorrhage originated. Certainly, there are deficiencies in some vessel walls possibly making them liable to rupture, yet others of the abnormal channels are thickened.[42] However, it appears to be true that it is the smaller AVMs that bleed, and that generally there is less violent parenchymal disruption following AVM hemorrhage than with burst aneurysm.[47]

Spontaneous subarachnoid or more frequently intracerebral/intraventricular bleeding are the commonest causes of symptoms experienced by children.[26, 30, 39] In our review, 78 patients (78/101 = 77 percent) experienced spontaneous intracranial hemorrhage as determined by the syndrome of headache, with bloody spinal fluid or blood clot recognized on CT or recovered at operation or autopsy (Table 47–1). The ictus is often explosive, when the previously well child screams out about sudden headache. It has again been confirmed that a surprising number of AVMs bleed during periods of quietude or even during sleep.[23] In a few instances when the child has subsequently fallen from bed, the lingering coma has been erroneously ascribed to a head injury. Not surprisingly therefore, the subarachnoid grading reflects the critical nature of the child at the time of first assessment (Table 47–2). Altered consciousness, meningism, and appropriate lateralized motor and sensory signs are present. Rapidly deepening stupor usually occurs when blood bursts into the ventricular system.

Children seem liable to repeated hemorrhage.[9, 30, 39] While it was not possible to determine in the present review the number of children who suffered more than one hemorrhage, there was in almost every examination of surgical AVM tissues evidence (hemosiderin free or in histiocytes) of previous hemorrhage. That earlier occurrence could have been silent or perhaps manifest by the "warning leak," which historically has preceded the present ictus by weeks or months.

Epilepsy, which presumably results from gliosis of brain because of chronic ischemia adjacent to the arteriovenous shunt occurs as a presenting symptom in 20 to 67 percent of adult patients with AVM.[22, 26, 28, 35] The proper management for a patient who has had one or two convulsions from an AVM and exclusive of SAH challenges treatment decisions. Recent reports indicate, however, that better than 70 percent of patients with epilepsy related to AVM will remain seizure-free (or "nearly so") when the associated epileptogenic tissue is excised.[22, 34] Moreover, the child with seizures has a diminished threat of future hemorrhage when the AVM is excised.[6] While "acute" seizures occurred at the time of, or shortly after the hemorrhage in 14 of our children, "chronic" seizures were the presenting problem in only 16 (15 percent) patients.

Of the remaining 11 children who had neither hemorrhage nor epilepsy in their profile, four had presenting symptoms of delayed development or signs of cerebral ischemia, two of congestive heart failure, one of chronic headache, and four of incidental malformations (Table 47–1).

Investigations

When a child is seen with the typical headache–hemorrhage ictus, the surgeon should directly proceed with computed tomography (CT) and cerebral arteriography. Lumbar puncture serves no useful purpose and may be dangerous.[16] The CT head scan will outline the blood clot and calcification if present, and on enhanced study may detail the dilated feeding and draining vascular channels and large blood-containing varices. It will thus provide a clue to the site and side of the brain to be studied first with cerebral arteriography.

By means of selective internal carotid and vertebral artery injections, the numbers and location of the arterial feeders can be examined by arteriography. The numbers of arterial contributors can be determined by properly timed sequential films processed with subtraction techniques. Seldom is a malformation served by only one arterial channel. There may be only one *major* artery contributing to the lesion, but the surgeon should anticipate any

Table 47–1. AVM—MODE OF PRESENTATION—HOSPITAL FOR SICK CHILDREN†

Symptom	No. of Patients
Hemorrhage	78
Chronic epilepsy	16
Delayed development/ischemia	4
Congestive heart failure	2
Headache	1
Incidental*	4
	105

*Three cases at postmortem, and one as a result of craniofacial evaluation for complex facial vascular malformation.
†n = 105 patients

Table 47–2. BOTTERELL GRADING OF 78 CHILDREN WITH INTRACRANIAL HEMORRAGE FROM AVM

Grade	No. of Patients
1	11
2	17
3	25
4	13
5	12

number of minor vessels coming from pial or deep perforating sources (Fig. 47–2).

On the other hand, the venous drainage in a child's AVM is frequently through a solitary channel via either a large cortical vein or the deep venous system, and is usually precisely defined on arteriography (Fig. 47–3). The geography of the lesion is carefully studied on the arteriogram and its operability thus determined. If operation proceeds, then the surgeon must be able to match the vascular findings at craniotomy with those on the arteriogram.

Some vascular malformations are angiographically "cryptic" and are thus not demonstrated on angiography.[4] These lesions, often in the distribution of the middle cerebral artery are usually small and there is evidence of a recent or old hemorrhagic history. Meticulous processing of the pathologic material uncovers the vascular malformation. There were five such cases in the present series.

The arteriograms and other examinations performed on children in the HSC review did not demonstrate more than one parenchymal lesion. Table 47–3 outlines the location of the malformations in this review. As a rule, 90 percent of the malformations found are supratentorial, most frequently within the distribution of the middle cerebral artery.[35, 36] But any intracranial artery can be associated with the malformation (hence the advisability of total cerebral arteriography to study all components of the identified lesion), and in the HSC study, 22 patients (21 percent) had malformations located below the tentorium, and these have been documented in another communication.[18]

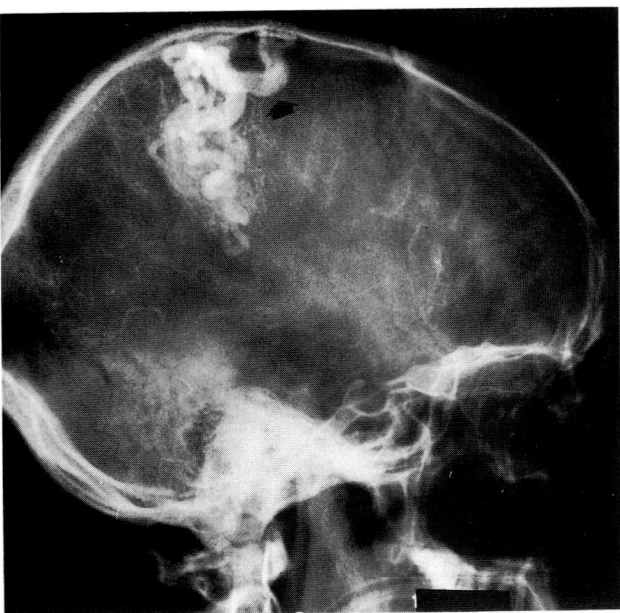

Figure 47–3. In this girl's nondominant hemisphere AVM, there was only one major draining vein (arrow), which must be preserved to the end of the dissection.

PREOPERATIVE MANAGEMENT

The luxury of a planned, elective operation for a child with a ruptured AVM may not always be realized. Inasmuch as the presenting symptom of 77 per cent of the lesions is spontaneous intracranial hemorrhage, urgent neurodiagnostic assessments and operative care are usually undertaken to identify and release the associated clot. AVM surgery can be tedious and protracted and is therefore not ideally begun as an emergent procedure late at night. Thus, if only subarachnoid hemorrhage has occurred, or if the intracerebral hemorrhage is small and the patient's condition stable, interval surgery may be staged after a few days' wait. During that time, the child is monitored carefully by a "subarachnoid routine" in an intensive-care unit. Cerebral vasospasm is seldom a problem in children with AVMs, but rebleeding during the interval frequently is. Thus antispasm, antihypertensive pharmacologic measures are not required, but drug and nursing care for the restless or bored child will

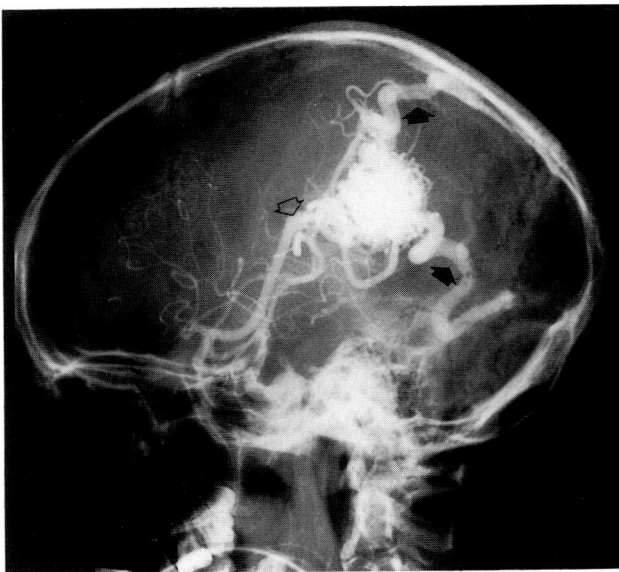

Figure 47–2. The large dominant Rolandic malformation is served principally by branches of the middle cerebral artery (open arrow), but there will be multiple associated feeding arteries, some of them deep at the ependymal layer. Of interest, this boy has at least two large draining veins (black arrows) (cf. Fig. 47–3).

Table 47–3. LOCATION OF CEREBRAL AVMs

Location	No. of Patients
Supratentorial (79%)	
Cerebral hemisphere/centrum	73
Basal ganglion	6
Intraventricular	3
Corpus callosum	1
Infratentorial (21%)	
Cerebellum	11
Brainstem	11

be a challenge. If the operation can possibly be delayed for three to seven days after the hemorrhage, then the surgeon will be rewarded with a properly prepared patient whose relaxed brain contains a liquifying hematoma.

There is not the same urgency for the 24 percent of patients whose presenting symptom is other than spontaneous hemorrhage. This group has been investigated in a traditional fashion for headaches, seizures, developmental delay, and the malformation has been discovered during the testing or even during elective surgery.[4] The clinical challenge will be to determine in advance whether surgical obliteration of the malformation will influence the headache, seizure, or developmental problem and whether, therefore, it should even be undertaken.[45, 48]

SURGERY

The ideal treatment for a brain AVM is total excision.[5, 8] Excision has now been achieved in almost all eloquent regions of brain (motor, basal ganglia, brainstem) as well as in less critical areas. Thus, except for lesions that penetrate the brainstem or basal ganglia, it is not so much the anatomical location of the lesion in the child that restrains the surgeon as it is the lesion's size. As large, lush and thirsty AVMs are not common in children, and as it is usually the small malformations that produce hemorrhage, then paradoxically it may be the small, awkwardly positioned AVM that will present the greatest challenge to the surgeon.[47] Lesions that are about 1.0 cm across and located adjacent to or within a ventricle or positioned deeply along the medial face of the hemisphere can be difficult to isolate, particularly if the hemorrhage has been in a direction away from the malformation.

Moreover, the lateral-hemispheral AVM may not always be found classically curled on the cortex. Instead, it may be hidden subcortically and bear as its only surface landmark an unusually straightened feeding artery running a nonanatomical course, or a red draining vein striking out toward an adjacent venous sinus. The most reliable surface markings are the veins because, regardless of their origin, all at some point, cross the surface.[40]

Surgical management of a child with an AVM requires all of the major anesthetic and pharmacologic techniques currently available. Curiously, AVMs are less likely to bleed during surgery from their original site of hemorrhage than are aneurysms, and thus the various vascular coils and varices can be gently manipulated aside. When bleeding does occur, it tends to be less torrential than with aneurysm rupture, and the bleeding usually represents transgression into the malformation itself. This bleeding can be controlled with gentle packing while dissection proceeds at a more remote site.

The operating microscope is often though not always an ally—it may be a disadvantage to the surgeon working upon large-convexity or cerebellar lesions. In these circumstances, the surgeon may lose sight of the perimeter of the AVM when working with the lowest magnifications. Magnifying loupes and a fiber-optic headlight can thus provide more mobility, permitting the surgeon to stay at the margin of the malformation, in its glial plane. A parenchymal clot if present can create much autodissection of the AVM. After the clot is removed, the surgeon will recognize the AVM hanging like a chandelier from the wall or roof of the clot cavity. Sometimes however, the clot can be located "downstream" from the AVM, which often is isolated before the hematoma is reached.

The dissection proceeds with microinstruments in an organized circumferential fashion about the malformation, preserving until the end one or two major draining veins. As a rule, the feeding and draining vessels run a straight course to and from the malformation but become coiled within it. These vessels can be freed by dissection along the long axis and isolation with a blunt hook before applying the bipolar coagulation forceps. It is not unusual for an accompanying artery or vein to be hidden immediately deep to the vessel about to be severed, and manipulation with the blunt hook will bring this surreptitious neighbor into view for coagulation too. Such is frequently the case with the major draining vein, which may obscure otherwise inconsequential arteries running beneath it or feeding it.[40]

Most AVMs describe a wedge or torpedo profile toward the adjacent ventricle (Fig. 47–1) and the surgeon should not be content that a total excision has been achieved until the ventricular wall has been visualized. Once the malformation dissection has been completed, bleeding will cease in its bed and the brain is considerably relaxed. If operation has been decided upon, then the surgeon should be satisfied with nothing less than total excision, even if two stages are necessary to achieve it. Proximal-vessel ligation can be dangerous and is an inadequate solution; subtotal excision is messy and the shunt remains served by newly recruited contributors.

The embolization of particulate material into the feeding channels of AVMs has been advocated during the past 20 years. While these techniques have been used for patients with dural and extracranial vascular malformations in our hospital, they have not been tried in the cerebral lesions.

POSTOPERATIVE CARE AND RESULTS

The child's biologic plasticity is such that the degree of postoperative recovery can be as complete and gratifying as the preoperative deterioration was rapid and dramatic. The experienced surgeon who attempts total excision of the malformation will usually know if that goal has been achieved at the conclusion of the first craniotomy. If there is some doubt about the completeness of excision, especially after prolonged surgery, and if the operative region is neither bleeding nor swelling, then it may be advisable to close the wound, allow the child to recover, and study the situation further with repeat arteriography. One or two strategically placed metallic hemostatic clips will permit identification of the area of surgery and serve as coordinates for the further radiologic and surgical examination of the malformation that remains.

Whether one or two procedures are required to obliterate the lesion, the surgeon cannot be satisfied that total excision has been achieved until postoperative arteriography confirms it (Fig. 47–4). Arteriography also happens to show a diminished size of the proximal contributing arteries.[1] Thereafter, convalescence depends only on the child's rehabilitation needs, if any. Prophylactic anticonvulsant medication will usually be required for six to 24 months following AVM excision.

In the HSC series, 101 patients were treated (four children with incidental malformations have been excluded). Twenty-three children received nonsurgical treatment, and 13 died (57 percent mortality). A majority of this group (9/14) were grade 5 category at the time of admission. There were 78 patients who were operated upon and any one or a combination of complete or incomplete AVM removal, obliteration of feeders, evacuation of hematoma, or shunting procedures achieved. In 51 patients, the malformation was completely removed at the first operation, and in another six at a second procedure. Six patients in the group treated by surgery died (8 percent mortality), all of whom were grade 4 or 5 at the time of first assessment. All patients who died suffered hemorrhage; thus, the mortality from the bleed, regardless of the method of treatment, is 24 percent (19/78).

A chronic seizure disorder was the reason for neurological evaluation in 16 patients. All but one of these children were operated upon, and three had a lingering convulsive problem during the follow-up period. None had an AVM associated with hematoma. There is thus a 20 percent (3/15) risk of postoperative epilepsy in patients whose only presenting symptom is an established seizure disorder related to an AVM. Fourteen patients had acute seizures most related to their hemorrhages, and only one (7 percent) had lingering postoperative epilepsy. Paradoxically, six patients who had been

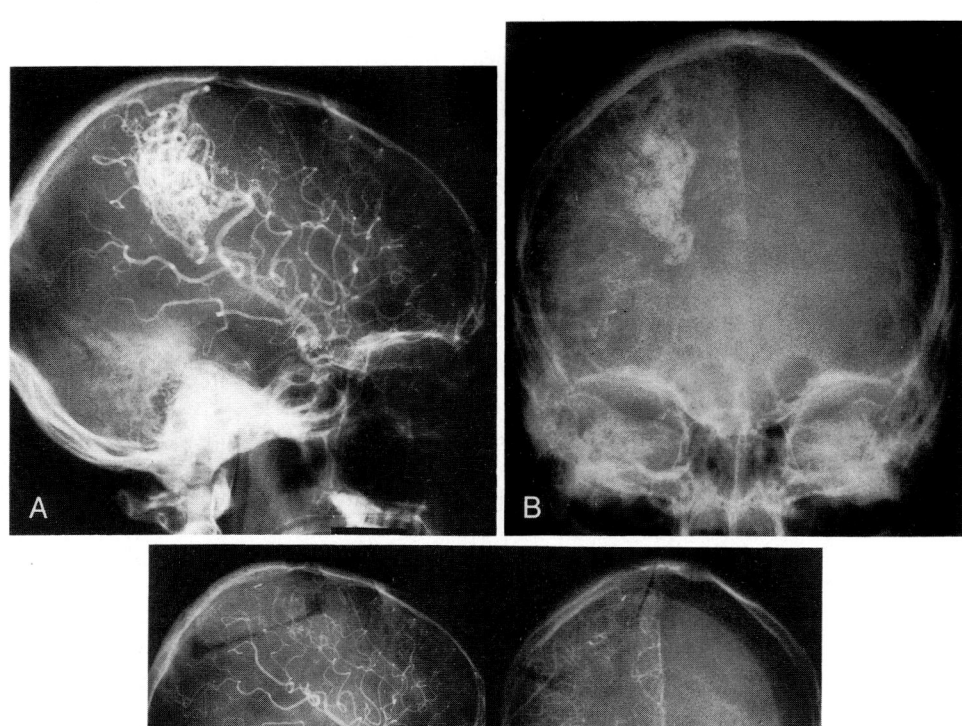

Figure 47–4. This right frontoparietal AVM is fed primarily by a branch of the middle cerebral artery (A) as well as the deep choroidal supply (B). C, These postresection arteriograms, taken ten days later, confirmed complete excision of the malformation, and a somewhat smaller caliber of the middle cerebral artery.

Table 47-4. RESULTS OF TREATMENT—81 CHILDREN TREATED FOR CEREBRAL AVM

	Grading	Nonsurgical Treatment	Surgical Treatment
I	Neurologically intact	4	45
II	Focal neurological deficit without limitation of activity or epilepsy	2	15
III	Partially disabled, with focal deficit or mild retardation	1	10
IV	Totally disabled	0	0
	Lost to follow-up	3	1

operated upon and who did not have any seizure disturbances before surgery were subject to this malady during the follow-up period. All six patients had intracerebral clots.

Except for those patients with incidental malformations and those who have died, there are 82 children available for follow-up examination nine months to 15 years after treatment. One of these patients died suddenly at home five years after "total" resection of his AVM. Neither the completeness of resection nor the ultimate cause of death is known. The results of care in the remaining 81 patients are listed in Table 47-4.

Five children were not treated because their AVMs were either deemed nonresectable (one throughout the dominant motor strip, two in the basal ganglia, and one in pons) or asymptomatic (minor cardiomegaly and objective bruit). Four of these children remain normal, and the fifth, a teenage boy, suffers infrequent seizures, his only symptom from the rolandic lesion. Of the 71 children who were operated upon, 45 (63 percent) were neurologically intact following surgery.

CONCLUSION

Hemorrhagic stroke, at least in this review, is more likely to be due to bleeding from an arteriovenous malformation than a ruptured intracranial aneurysm. This process, which also distinguishes the child from the adult is characterized by a number of other differentiations. More children bleed from their malformations and fewer suffer chronic seizures than do adults. In that regard, there are remarkable similarities between the HSC review and that of Gerosa and coworkers.[9] The latter authors also indicate that 28 percent of children suffer overt repeat hemorrhage, and the HSC study concludes that the mortality rate from any hemorrhage is 24 percent. As with intracranial aneurysms, AVMs in children can be scattered throughout the brain, often in awkward locations. There are an unusual number (21 percent) located below the tentorium. Wherever possible, total excision of the malformation must be attempted, with the expectation that the child's brain vasculature may be resilient to operative intrusion. Sixty-four percent of children receiving surgical care can be expected to be neurologically intact following surgery. The surgical mortality of 8 percent is influenced by the severity of the SAH/IVH, as all patients were clinical grade 4 or 5. Hence, with regard to arteriovenous malformations, Matson's exhortation is still valid, 12 years later.[26]

References

1. Amacher AL, Allcock JM, Drake CG: Cerebral angiomas: The sequelae of surgical treatment. J Neurosurg 37:571, 1972.
2. Bruce DA, Schut L: Arteriovenous malformations in children. Child's Brain 8:232, 1981.
3. Celli P, Ferrante L, Palma L, et al: Cerebral arteriovenous malformations in children. Clinical features and outcome of treatment in children and in adults. Surg Neurol 22:43, 1984.
4. Cohen HCM, Tucker WS, Humphreys RP, et al: Angiographically cryptic histologically verified cerebrovascular malformations. Neurosurgery 10:704, 1982.
5. Drake CG: Cerebral arteriovenous malformations: Considerations for and experience with surgical treatment in 166 cases. Clin Neurosurg 26:145, 1979.
6. Epstein N, Epstein F: Arteriovenous malformation presenting as a first seizure in a 13-year-old child: Surgical indications. Neurosurgery 7:391, 1980.
7. Forster DMC, Steiner L, Hakanson S: Arteriovenous malformation of the brain. A long-term clinical study. J Neurosurg 37:562, 1972.
8. French L, Seljeskog EL: Arteriovenous malformations of the brain. In: Youmans JR (ed): Neurological Surgery, Vol. 2. Philadelphia, W. B. Saunders Co., 1973, pp 827–836.
9. Gerosa MA, Cappellotto P, Licata C, et al: Cerebral arteriovenous malformations in children (56 cases). Child's Brain 8:356, 1981.
10. Gold AP, Challenor YB, Gilles FH, et al: Report of the Joint Committee for Stroke Facilities. IX. Strokes in children (Part I). Stroke 4:835, 1973.
11. Graf CJ, Perret GE, Torner JC: Bleeding from cerebral arteriovenous malformations as part of their natural history. J Neurosurgery 58:331, 1983.
12. Harwood-Nash DC, Fitz CR: Neuroradiology in Infants and Children, Vol. 3. St. Louis, C. V. Mosby Co., 1976, pp 907, 913–939, 1164.
13. Hayashi S, Arimoto T, Itakura T, et al: The association of intracranial aneurysms and arteriovenous malformations of the brain. Case report. J Neurosurg 55:971, 1981.
14. Hoffman HJ, Mohr G, Kusunoki T: Multiple arteriovenous malformations of spinal cord and brain in a child. Case report. Child's Brain 2:317, 1976.
15. Hourihan M, Gates PC, McAllister VL: Subarachnoid hemorrhage in childhood and adolescence. J Neurosurg 60:1163, 1984.
16. Humphreys RP: Computed tomography and the early diagnostic lumbar puncture. Can Med Assoc J 121:150, 1979.
17. Humphreys RP: Special article—hemorrhagic stroke in childhood. Riv Neuroscienze Pediatriche 2:1, 1986.
18. Humphreys RP: Infratentorial arteriovenous malformations. In: Edwards MSB, Hoffman HJ (eds): Cerebrovascular Disease in Childhood and Adolescence. Baltimore, Williams & Wilkins, 1988.
19. Kelly JJ, Jr., Mellinger JF, Sundt TM, Jr.: Intracranial arteriovenous malformations in childhood. Ann Neurol 3:338, 1978.
20. Laine E, Dhellemmes P, Clarisse C: Supratentorial arteriovenous malformations in children except aneurysm of the vein of Galen. Child's Brain 8:63, 1981.
21. Laitinen L: Arteriella aneuryusm med subarachnoidal-blodning hos barn. Nord Med 71:329, 1964.
22. LeBlanc R, Feindel W, Ethier R: Epilepsy from cerebral arteriovenous malformations. Can J Neurol Sci 10:91, 1983.

23. Locksley HB: Report on the Cooperative Study of Intracranial Aneurysms and Subarachnoid Hemorrhage. Section V, Part I. Natural history of subarachnoid hemorrhage, intracranial aneurysms and arteriovenous malformations. Based on 6,368 cases in the Cooperative Study. J Neurosurg 25:219, 1966.
24. Luessenhop AJ: Operative treatment of arteriovenous malformation of the brain. *In*: Morley TP (ed): Current Controversies in Neurosurgery. Philadelphia, W. B. Saunders Co., 1967, pp 203–209.
25. Luessenhop AJ, Rosa L: Cerebral arteriovenous malformations. Indications for and results of surgery, and the role of intravascular techniques. J Neurosurg 60:14, 1984.
26. Matson DD: Neurosurgery of Infancy and Childhood, 2nd ed. Springfield, IL, Charles C Thomas, 1969, pp 749–766.
27. McCormick WF: Pathology of vascular malformations of the brain. *In*: Wilson CB, Stein BM (eds): Intracranial Arteriovenous Malformations. Baltimore, Williams & Wilkins, 1984, pp 44–63.
28. Mohr JP: Neurological manifestations and factors related to the therapeutic decisions. *In*: Wilson CB, Stein BM (eds): Intracranial Arteriovenous Malformations. Baltimore, Williams & Wilkins, 1984, pp 1–11.
29. Monges J, Jaimovich R, Cragnaz RJ: Vascular malformations in children. Bol Asoc Argentina Neurocir 30:41, 1981.
30. Mori K, Murata T, Hasimoto N, et al: Clinical analysis of arteriovenous malformations in children. Child's Brain 6:13, 1980.
31. Northfield DWC: The Surgery of the Central Nervous System: A Textbook for Postgraduate Students. Oxford, Blackwell Scientific Publications, 1973, pp 402–420.
32. Ostergaard JR: Association of intracranial aneurysm and arteriovenous malformation in childhood. Neurosurgery 14:358, 1984.
33. Padget DH: The cranial venous system in man in reference to development, adult configuration and relation to the arteries. Am J Anat 98:307, 1956.
34. Pellettieri L, Carlsson C-A, Grevsten S, et al: Surgical versus conservative treatment of intracranial arteriovenous malformations. Acta Neurochir (Suppl) 29:1, 1980.
35. Perret G, Nishioka H: Report of the Cooperative Study of Intracranial Aneurysms and Subarachnoid Hemorrhage. Section VI. Arteriovenous malformations. An analysis of 545 cases of craniocerebral arteriovenous malformations and fistulae reported to the Cooperative Study. J Neurosurg 25:467, 1966.
36. Russell DS, Rubinstein LJ: Pathology of Tumors of the Nervous System, 4th ed. London, Edward Arnold Publishers Ltd, 1977, pp 136–138.
37. Schatz SW, Botterell EH: The natural history of arteriovenous malformations. *In*: Milliken C (ed): Cerebrovascular Disease, Proceedings of the Association of Research in Nervous and Mental Diseases, Vol. 41. Baltimore, Williams & Wilkins, 1974, pp 180–187.
38. Sedzimir CB, Robinson J: Intracranial hemorrhage in children and adolescents. J Neurosurg 38:269, 1973.
39. So SC: Cerebral arteriovenous malformations in children. Child's Brain 4:242, 1978.
40. Stein BM: General techniques for the surgical removal of arteriovenous malformations. *In*: Wilson CB, Stein BM (eds): Intracranial Arteriovenous Malformations. Baltimore, Williams & Wilkins, 1984, pp 143–155.
41. Svien HJ, McRae JA: Arteriovenous anomalies of the brain. Fate of patients not having definitive surgery. J Neurosurg 23:23, 1965.
42. Takashima S, Becker LE: Neuropathology of cerebral arteriovenous malformations in children. J Neurol Neurosurg Psychiatry 43:380, 1980.
43. Tiyaworabun S, Kramer HH, Lim DP, et al: Cerebral arteriovenous malformations in children: Clinical analysis and followup results. Child's Brain 8:232, 1981.
44. Troupp H, Marttila I, Halonen V: Arteriovenous malformations of the brain: Prognosis without operation. Acta Neurochir 22:125, 1970.
45. Troupp H: Arteriovenous malformations of the brain: What are the indications for operation? *In*: Morley TP (ed): Current Controversies in Neurosurgery. Philadelphia, W. B. Saunders Co., 1967, pp 210–216.
46. Trumpy JH, Eldevik P: Intracranial arteriovenous malformations: Conservative or surgical treatment. Surg Neurol 8:171, 1977.
47. Waltimo O: The relationship of size, density and localization of intracranial arteriovenous malformations to the type of initial symptom. J Neurol Sci 19:13, 1973.
48. Wilson CB, Sang UH, Dominque J: Microsurgical treatment of intracranial vascular malformations. J Neurosurg 51:446, 1979.

48
HEMOPHILIA AND OTHER COAGULOPATHIES

Kerry R. Crone, M.D.
Robin P. Humphreys, M.D.

Perhaps more than any other surgical practitioner, the neurosurgeon is obsessive about hemostasis and the consequences of even trivial amounts of bleeding during an operation. The rigid confines of the skull and spinal skeleton allow for minimum accumulations of blood without disastrous sequelae. Hemostasis involves three basic elements—the integrity of the blood vessel wall, the presence and function of circulating platelets, and coagulation factors.

Hemorrhage occurring as a consequence of a coagulation disorder usually implies an abnormality of the plasma coagulation factors or platelets, their numbers, or function. Owen and Bowie state, "the most tragic instances of untoward bleeding in surgery are those in which there was a pre-existent hemostatic failure that was unsuspected," but, that said, surgeons often need to be gently reminded that the commonest cause of hemorrhage during or following an operation results from mechanical faults directly related to the conduct of that operation.[36]

It is not the authors' intention in this chapter to examine those hemorrhagic events that arise from an operation. Rather we will review the management of hemorrhage that occurs within the nervous system because of a dysfunction (perhaps undefined) in the normal coagulation cycle. Furthermore, only those conditions occurring in children will be examined, so that secondary central nervous system (CNS) hemorrhage arising as the result of anticoagulation therapy, a very uncommon prescription in children, will not be considered.

CLINICAL PRESENTATION

When planning an operation on the child's nervous system, it is not often that the neurosurgeon must seek out the easiest "screening test of all"[36] namely a history of previous bleeding disorder in the patient or family. As will be appreciated, it is a rare circumstance in which the pediatric neurosurgeon unexpectedly encounters bleeding during operation that relates to a heretofore undiagnosed coagulation disorder.

Instead, there are one or two explanations for a child's bleeding problem during an operation. These relate to mechanical factors in which normal vascular channels in normal position have been violated and prove troublesome, or in which the surgeon has encountered blood vessels that, because of abnormality or unusual location, are responsible for the annoying bleeding.

By rather marked contrast, patients with traditional coagulation disorders have frequently had that disorder precisely defined. They arrive in the operating room with a diagnosis and an extensive regimen of replacement therapy that is to be administered during operation. Seldom is there any "middle ground" between these two extremes.

Children who suffer a confirmed coagulation defect or a blood-cell condition that predisposes to a coagulopathy generally are at low but real risk of secondary hemorrhage within the central nervous system. Such bleeding is the leading cause of death among hemophiliacs and patients with idiopathic thrombocytopenic purpura.[19, 41] When that hemorrhage occurs, it is often a flamboyant event. Even subarachnoid hemorrhage suffered after minor head trauma in children with diagnosed hemophilia produces severe headache, which may take more than a few days to resolve. Regrettably, the spontaneous hemorrhagic ictus that strikes a child with hemophilia, leukemia, or idiopathic thrombocytopenic purpura can be devastating. Many of these events occur while the child is hospitalized and receiving care for the primary blood disorder. Even when such ideal conditions permit expeditious treatment to salvage the nervous system, a substantial number of children will perish from the hemorrhage. And many of those who survive will be disabled from the destructive effects of the hemorrhage on brain parenchyma.

HEMOPHILIA

Hemophilia was first described by Rabbi Simon Ben Gamliel in the Talmud in the second century A.D.[29] At a much later date, it may have been responsible for pivotal changes in Russian history. Alexis, the son of the Russian czar Nicholas II and Alexandra, suffered from hemophilia, and his mother in her angst prevailed upon the debauched "holy man" Rasputin. As Kerensky was subsequently to note, "if there had been no Rasputin, there would have been no Lenin."[23]

Hemophilia was first described in medical literature by Otto in 1803,[29] and the first report of intracranial hemorrhage in a probable hemophiliac was made in 1819.[43] It was not unusual through the first half of the 20th century to read of the numerous diagnostic and therapeutic frustrations with the neurologic consequences of hemophilia.[47]

By the mid-1950's treatment programs improved when detailed knowledge of the particular deficiencies in the hemophiliac states became available. Subsequently fractionated replacement products were developed for quick and precise re-establishment of procoagulant activity.

Physiology

Factors VIII and IX are part of the intrinsic prothrombin activation system. Factor IX (having been activated by factor XI) then reacts with factor VIII, the resulting product bringing about activation of factor X, which in a subsequent chain of activating events brings about the generation of thrombin.

Hemophilia is the most common hereditary bleeding abnormality, with an incidence of 0.72 to 0.8 per 10,000.[2, 29] Hemophilia A (factor VIII deficiency) and hemophilia B (factor IX deficiency), sometimes known as Christmas disease, are transmitted as X-linked recessive characteristics. Christmas disease is one fifth as common as hemophilia A.

Biggs[2] notes that many hemophiliacs have observed that their bleeding seems to come in phases and can be worse at certain times of the year. During the quiescent phases, the hemophiliac may sustain certain strain or trauma without serious consequences, whereas the same or lesser injury during a "bad" phase may lead to bleeding and admission to a hospital for several weeks. Kerr[24] has recorded the circumstances of four hemophiliac boxers, none of whom had required medical attention for injury received during a total of 144 bouts.

The diagnosis of hemophilia is based on the history of prolonged and excessive bleeding in a male patient with or without the appropriate family history, and the finding, on laboratory testing, of a reduced amount of factor VIII or IX in his blood. The whole-blood clotting time is not a sensitive test of factor VIII or IX deficiencies, though the prothrombin consumption test is a little more selective for this deficiency.[2]

The normal levels of factors VIII and IX range from 50 to 150 percent, and the hemophiliac state is classified as follows: severe (VIII, less than 1 percent); moderate (VIII, 1 to 5 percent); and mild (VIII, greater than 5 percent). A level of 30 percent is safe for major surgery. There are no rigid guidelines concerning replacement therapy for hemophiliacs who sustain head trauma and minor subarachnoid bleeding. However, those patients who will require surgical relief of intracranial hematoma will also need treatment with cryoprecipitate or factor VIII concentrate. Each packet of cryoprecipitate contains an amount of factor VIII equivalent to that found in one unit of blood, and is administered at the rate of one packet per 5 kg of body weight. Patients with factor IX deficiency used to be treated with fresh frozen plasma but now receive concentrations of the factor in a commercial form—Konyne (Cutter Laboratories Inc., Berkeley, California).

Intracranial Hemorrhage

Intracranial hemorrhage is the most dreaded complication in hemophiliacs with an annual occurrence risk in such patients of 2 to 3.5 percent.[17] It is the leading cause of death and accounts for about one third of all deaths in hemophiliacs.[29] There may not be a distinct relationship between head trauma and intracranial bleeding episodes in a hemophiliac. Trauma is the overt cause of intracranial bleeding in 50 to 60 percent of patients, but the absence of such a history does not exclude intracranial hemorrhage.[29, 43] While the provocation for intracranial bleeding may be unrecognized, the neurologic phenomena, if they develop, will be a factor of the site of hemorrhage, the rapidity of its formation, and the effectiveness with which replacement substances can be quickly administered.

Martinowitz and coworkers[29] and Eyster and associates[11] have commented upon the indolent nature of bleeding in hemophiliacs after even minor trauma, which differs from the briefer symptom-free interval encountered in nonhemophiliac patients with post-traumatic intracranial hemorrhage. Fujino and coworkers[15] hypothesize that such may occur because trivial trauma or infarction of unknown cause results in minor bleeding or oozing, which is controlled by transient hemostasis, but delayed "rebleeding" occurs that provokes brain edema and then subsequent massive bleeding. Intracranial bleeding may occur in any one of the usual sites—extradural, subdural, subarachnoid, intracerebral, and intraventricular.

The hemophiliac who experiences sudden spontaneous headache may seek neurosurgical advice. Does one presume that headache equates with subarachnoid bleeding in a hemophiliac? Is lumbar puncture required to confirm bloody cerebrospinal fluid? Will the presence of bloody spinal fluid then influence subsequent decisions to provide replacement therapy? The patient's history, degree of meningismus, and procoagulant levels must influence the clinical diagnosis and decision regarding treatment and the value of diagnostic lumbar puncture. Despite the assurances of some authors about the safety of lumbar puncture, one need have only a single tragedy with this technique to question its validity.[7, 43] Lumbar puncture cannot provide any information additional to that available with computed tomographic (CT) scanning and is therefore outmoded in the assessment of the hemophiliac who experiences severe headache.[20, 29]

The crux of patient management depends upon the interwoven actions of hematologist and surgeon. The former must establish with certainty the diagnosis of the clotting disorder, assay the factor level, and where applicable (particularly for any patient to be subjected to major surgery) identify the presence of inhibitor to the missing procoagulant (a problem in about 10 percent of hemophiliacs). With this knowledge the hematologist can secure the replacement substitute and schedule its administration. For the hemophiliac who suffers head trauma, there must be immediate replacement of the missing factor calculated to raise the plasma level about 50 percent.[29] For those patients with normal CT scans or those who show evidence of subarachnoid hemorrhage only, repeated doses of replacement therapy are given to maintain plasma factor levels between 30 and 50 percent during the period of observation. A repeat CT scan should be obtained to search out *delayed* and more vigorous intracranial bleeding.

Obviously then, the neurosurgeon might best be advised to leave the coagulation worries to the hematologist and treat the intracranial bleeding just as in any other individual. However, hematoma evacuation must always remain a prime consideration because of the known ability of hemophiliacs to intermittently bleed around the clot despite adequate replacement therapy.[29] After a proper neurological evaluation of the hemophiliac, the surgeon will follow customary management plans for patients with concussion or subarachnoid hemorrhage. Alternatively, if the usual signs of a progressively expanding mass are present, and if the surgeon has confirmed this diagnosis with CT, then the surgeon and the hematologist must schedule their treatment in tandem. One half hour after a loading dose of the replacement factor has been given, a sample of blood is assayed for the deficient factor. The result of this test determines whether it is safe to proceed with surgery. Once factor VIII or IX levels have been therapeutically re-established, surgical evacuation of the clot is the mandatory course of action for patients with accumulating hematoma. The average half-life of factor VIII in vivo is 6 to 14 hours. A minimum of 15 units of replacement factor per kilogram, therefore, is required every 12 hours to keep the therapeutic level between 30 and 60 percent.[40] The usual neurosurgical techniques and support pharmacotherapy measures are used; there are no special "tricks" that the surgeon needs.

In 1948 Paillas, Boudouresques, and Tamelet first reported the relief by surgery of an intracranial hematoma in a hemophiliac patient.[37] Originally surgical techniques to control bleeding were, of necessity, ingenious. By the late 1950s, plasma treatment and then the specific use of cryoprecipitate were offered to the hemophiliac, and in the early 1960s a series of articles reported experience with the treatment of intracranial hematoma in children and adults.* More recently, the use of antifibrinolytic agents has been recommended as part of the treatment regimen because of the reduced rate of rebleeding in these patients.[29]

It is entirely feasible for a surgeon, therefore, to evacuate a life-threatening intracranial hematoma or even operate electively on any other intracranial process in a hemophiliac, when this action is performed in concert with that of the hematologist.[28] Despite the advances of the past 30 years, however, many hemophiliacs who have suffered intracranial bleeding are left with severe neurologic residua—hemiparesis, visual and speech defects, epilepsy, retardation, and hydrocephalus.

Fujino and colleagues[15] reviewed 108 hemophiliacs younger than 15 years of age and encountered intracranial bleeding 13 times in nine cases. There were six subdural hematomas and four subarachnoid hemorrhages and two children with intracerebral hematomas and one child with intraventricular hemorrhage. Five of the patients underwent

---

*References 8, 12, 13, 16, 21, 32, 33, 35, 39, 42–45

surgery, and it is of interest that none died; 30 percent, however, showed residual neurological deficits. Eyster and associates[11] have reported on 71 hemorrhages into the central nervous system among 2,500 hemophiliacs over a 12-year period. Sixty-five were in children younger than three years of age, and in only half these cases was there evidence of trauma. In half of these, the bleeding-related symptoms appeared after an interval of four or more days. Again, a substantial mortality of 34 percent is confirmed. It is suggested that replacement therapy continue for 10 to 14 days.

Intraspinal Hemorrhage

As expected intraspinal hemorrhage is uncommon in hemophiliacs. Trauma precipitates bleeding in about one third of the cases and three quarters of patients have extramedullary bleeding. The treatment principles are those basic to the hematologic care of the hemophiliac and the neurosurgical care of the patient with an intraspinal mass.

Peripheral Nerve Lesions

Virtually all peripheral nerve lesions in hemophilia are due to external compression of or traction on the nerve, particularly related to hemorrhage within closed tissue spaces such as the forearm or anterior compartment of the leg. Characteristically the femoral, ulnar, median, sciatic, or a cutaneous nerve of the thigh is involved.[17] The syndrome is one of acute and often painful radiculopathy, perhaps associated with visible swelling and ecchymosis. The detection of the peripheral nerve lesion however, may be masked by the muscle atrophy, areflexia, and contractures related to recurrent hemarthrosis and intramuscular bleeding. Lutschg and Vassella[27] urge prompt recognition and treatment of hemorrhage in "areas that could involve peripheral nerves." They believe such treatment is especially important in patients with hemorrhage in the iliopsoas muscle producing groin pain and for whom immediate replacement therapy is recommended. After appropriate replacement therapy has been given, the surgeon may consider evacuation of the hematoma or fasciotomy. Rehabilitation is difficult and prolonged.

LEUKEMIC HEMORRHAGE

One of the penalties of successful chemotherapeutic treatment of acute childhood leukemia has been a marked rise in the neurologic manifestations of this disease. As the drug treatment of leukemia became more effective between 1948 and 1960, the incidence of central nervous system (CNS) manifestations increased from 4 to 40 percent, and it is now stated that over one-half of children with acute leukemia can be expected to have neurologic involvement.[10, 38] The type of CNS lesion may be quite variable, but the neurosurgeon's advice is most likely to be sought at the time of an acute and major neurologic event related to intracranial hemorrhage.

The latter has traditionally been the explanation for a leukemic patient's sudden death. In 1960 intracranial hemorrhage was found to be responsible for 49 percent of deaths in an autopsy series of acute leukemia patients.[18] Hemorrhage may result from either the associated severe thrombocytopenia, or infiltration of white matter of the brain with leukemic cells. The latter plug small cerebral arteries and subsequently spread through the vessel walls, which become weakened and eventually rupture into the cerebral parenchyma.

A leukemic patient who suddenly develops the clinical phenomena of a hemorrhagic stroke has usually suffered spontaneous intracranial bleeding. The CT examination will quickly certify the presence, site, and extent of the suspect intracranial bleeding in leukemic patients. The neurosurgeon can then accurately elucidate a prognosis for the disrupted cerebrum, and the hematologist can assemble this information in an overview of the patient's primary illness and likely survival from it.

IDIOPATHIC THROMBOCYTOPENIA PURPURA (ITP)

Idiopathic thrombocytopenia purpura (ITP) is an acquired hemorrhagic disorder common in children. The condition is frequently preceded by an infection. The diagnosis is suggested by the presence of thrombocytopenia, absence of associated hematologic changes other than those due to hemorrhage and infection, and absence of associated systemic illness except for infection. Bone-marrow sampling is essential for proper documentation and should demonstrate abundant megakaryocytes with normal erythroid and myeloid cells.

In most children the presenting symptoms include a petechial rash and a history of increased bruisability. When the diagnosis of ITP is confirmed, the sole form of management in this mild form of ITP is restriction of physical activity until platelet counts return to normal, usually within a few weeks. About 80 percent of patients with the acute form recover spontaneously in the first few months of illness.

Intracranial hemorrhage represents the most serious complication of ITP occurring in 1 to 4 per cent of patients.[41] Although parenchymal hemorrhages are the most common, bleeding may instead be subdural or subarachnoid in location. In 1976, Humphreys and colleagues[19] reviewed their experience with intracranial hemorrhage complicating

ITP. Prompt diagnosis followed by aggressive management was recommended for an apparent favorable outcome. During the subsequent decade, eight additional cases have appeared in the English-language literature.[14, 25, 48, 49] Review of these previous cases combined with additional experience at the Hospital for Sick Children prompted a critical appraisal of factors that affected outcome.[6]

Nineteen cases of ITP have been complicated by an intracranial hemorrhage. Cerebral bleeding in these children was documented by angiography, computed tomography, or postmortem examination. In addition to the intracranial bleeding, active hemorrhage was present at other sites at the time of diagnosis in eight of these patients. Seven of the latter died. Four of five children who were comatose when first seen died. As a result of these observations, a schematic is proposed to facilitate management of these severely ill children (Fig. 48–1).

First the diagnosis of ITP if not previously established must be confirmed by bone-marrow aspiration. Any patient in whom intracranial hemorrhage is suspected must be examined by computed tomography. Emergency splenectomy is carried out in all patients who have evidence of intracranial bleeding. After platelet transfusion, a craniotomy is immediately performed in those patients who are neurologically impaired with parenchymal hemorrhage or who demonstrate evidence of active bleeding at other sites in addition to the parenchymal hemorrhage.

Although careful observation is necessary of patients with intracranial hemorrhage who are neurologically normal and who are without evidence of active bleeding at other sites, craniotomy should follow at any time when neurologic deterioration occurs. Traditional methods to reduce cerebral edema should be used in all these patients.

A favorable outcome can be expected in at least 50 percent of patients so treated. Active bleeding at other sites of the body appears to worsen the prognosis, as does severely impaired consciousness at the time of an intracranial hemorrhage.

VITAMIN-K DEFICIENCY

Vitamin K is an essential component for the conversion of precursor proteins into proteins with coagulant activity (factors II, VII, IX, and X). Reported conditions responsible for vitamin-K deficiency in infants and neonates include maternal drug ingestion, inadequate exogenous intake, reduced endogenous production, and malabsorption of fat, each of which has been associated with intracranial bleeding.[3, 26, 30, 34] Vitamin-K deficiency may produce such bleeding in both acutely ill and healthy appearing neonates.

Although a broad spectrum of clinical presentations has been described, in most infants the presenting symptoms are sudden pallor, irritability, seizures, and progressive neurologic deterioration

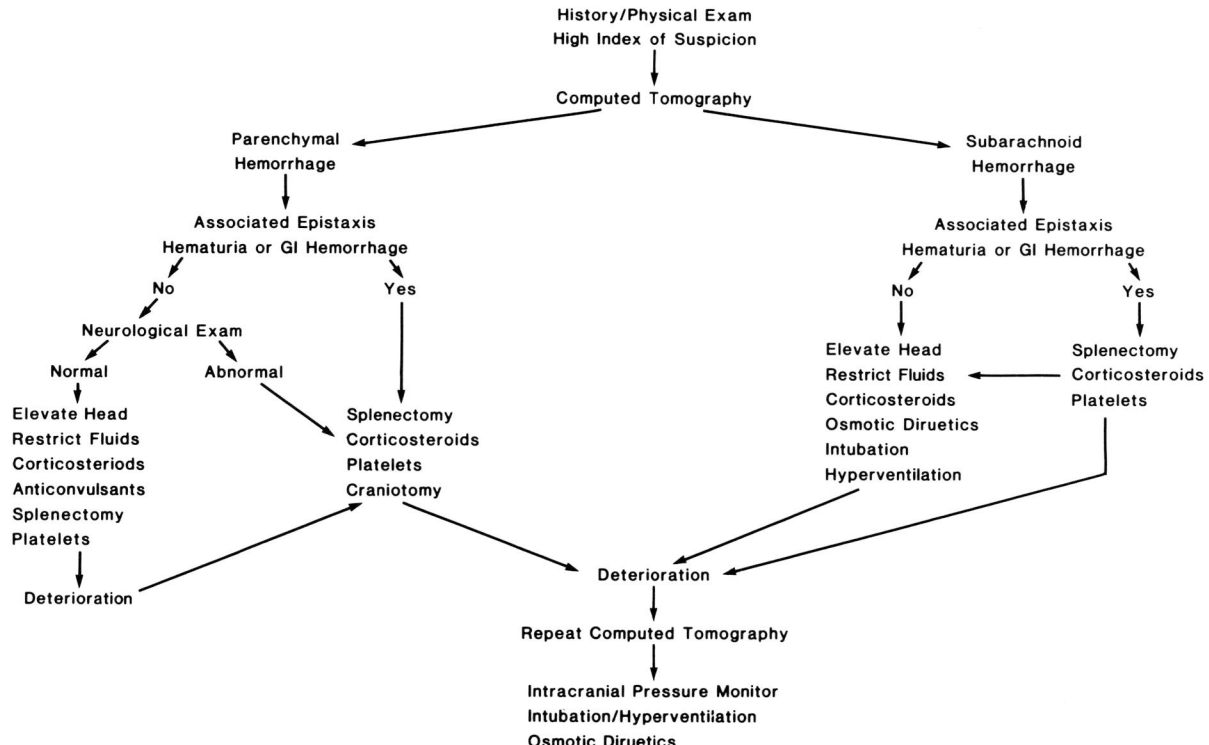

Figure 48–1. Management of intracranial hemorrhage in childhood ITP.

often resulting in death. Coagulation screening is essential in establishing the diagnosis. Deficiency of vitamin K produces prolongation of the prothrombin time (PT) and partial thromboplastin time (PTT) without appreciable change in either platelets or fibrin-degradation products.

Administration of vitamin K will correct the coagulation abnormality, and this correction further helps to establish the diagnosis. Simultaneous administration of fresh frozen plasma is essential if immediate surgical intervention is necessary.

Hematologic and gastroenterologic consultations will be helpful to investigate cases of intracranial bleeding resulting from vitamin-K deficiency. Since 1983, three cases occurring in infants younger than six months of age have been recorded at the Children's Hospital Medical Center, Cincinnati, Ohio. Underlying conditions responsible for the vitamin-K deficiency and intracranial bleeding include biliary atresia, alpha-1-antitrypsin deficiency, and acalculous cholecystitis.

DISSEMINATED INTRAVASCULAR COAGULATION (DIC)

Disseminated intravascular coagulation (DIC) with fibrinolysis is an acquired syndrome characterized by excessive intravascular consumption of clotting factors and platelets. The basic process is a stimulation of physiologic coagulation, which, as it progresses, brings about widespread intravascular blood coagulation. Coincident activation of the fibrinolytic enzyme system that clears fibrin and fibrinogen results in microvascular fibrin thromboembolism. A hypocoagulable state is produced when the accelerated consumption of platelets and clotting factors results in inadequate levels to maintain hemostasis.[22]

Disseminated intravascular coagulation is not a primary disease but represents a response to a variety of pathologic stimuli. The most common conditions initiating or predisposing children to DIC include shock, hypoxia, sepsis, trauma, and neoplasia.[5] Gram-negative microorganisms that produce endotoxin are responsible for most infectious causes of DIC. The endotoxin, a lipopolysaccharide, can initiate coagulation by activating factor XII or by increasing serum lipids, which in turn increase platelet adhesiveness and the response to adenosine diphosphate. Less common but well documented infectious causes include gram-positive bacteria, fungi, viruses, and protozoans; acute leukemia and neuroblastoma are the more common neoplastic conditions predisposing to the development of DIC in children. Tissue thromboplastin released from injured tissues has been suggested to be the initiating process in trauma.[46] As brain has a high concentration of tissue thromboplastin, DIC following cerebral injury has received recognition in recent years.[1, 4, 9] Miner and associates[31] reported a fourfold increase in mortality in children who demonstrated evidence of DIC at the time of admission.

The clinical manifestations of DIC are extremely variable. Continual oozing from venipuncture sites may be the first clinical manifestation of DIC. Coagulation studies are essential to confirm the presence of DIC and are necessary when evaluating severely traumatized patients as DIC occurs more frequently than expected. Hypofibrinogenemia, thrombocytopenia, and prolongation of the prothrombin and partial thromboplastin times are common laboratory findings in DIC. Confirmation of DIC is established through the measurement of fibrin/fibrinogen-degradation products (FDP).[36] Mild elevations of FDP may occur secondary to metabolic insults, hypoxia, ischemia, or surgical procedures, but elevations above 40 mcg/ml coupled with additional coagulation abnormalities indicate DIC. Although the use of heparin remains controversial in the management of DIC, there is general agreement that identification and treatment of precipitating factors coupled with avoidance of hypotension, anoxia, and acidosis, which are potent stimulants of DIC, are the keystones of management in this condition.[5]

SUMMARY

The formulation of potent chemotherapeutic compounds and the purification of individual elements involved in the clotting process have presented fresh challenges to the surgeon handling the neurologic consequences of the primary hematologic upset. The hematologist must still act first, but by virtue of sophisticated diagnostic CT and pharmacotherapy, the surgeon will be increasingly expected to participate in a planned management program.

References

1. Astrup T: Assay and content of tissue thromboplastin in different organs. Thromb Diath Haemorrh 14:401, 1965.
2. Biggs R: Human Blood Coagulation, Haemostasis and Thrombosis, 2nd ed. Oxford, Blackwell, 1976.
3. Bleyer WA, Skinner AL: Fatal neonatal hemorrhage after maternal anticonvulsant therapy. JAMA 235:626, 1976.
4. Clark JA, Finelli RE, Netsky MG: Disseminated intravascular coagulation following cranial trauma. J Neurosurg 52:266, 1980.
5. Colman RW, Robboy SJ, Minna JD: Disseminated intravascular coagulation: a reappraisal. Ann Rev Med 30:359, 1979.
6. Crone KR, Humphreys RP: Intracranial hemorrhage in childhood idiopathic thrombocytopenic purpura. A reappraisal (in press).
7. Curless RG, Corrigan JJ, Jr.: Headache in classical hemophilia. The risk of diagnostic procedures. Child's Brain 2:187, 1976.
8. Davies SH, Turner JW, Cumming RA, et al: Management of intracranial haemorrhage in haemophilia. Br Med J 2:1627, 1966.
9. Drayer BP, Poser CM: Disseminated intravascular coagulation and head trauma. JAMA 231:174, 1975.

10. Evans AE: Central nervous system involvement in children with acute leukemia. A study of 921 patients. Cancer 17:256, 1964.
11. Eyster ME, Gill FM, Blatt PM, et al: Central nervous system bleeding in hemophiliacs. Blood 51:1179, 1978.
12. Ferguson GG, Barton WB, Drake CG: Subdural hematoma in hemophilia: Successful treatment with cryoprecipitate. J Neurosurg 29:524, 1968.
13. Fessy BM, Meynell MJ: Haemorrhage involving the central nervous system in haemophilia: Account of the management of five cases. Br Med J 2:211, 1966.
14. Findler G, Aldor A, Hadani M, et al: Traumatic intracranial hemorrhage in children with rare coagulation disorders. J Neurosurg 57:775, 1982.
15. Fujino H, Kuwabara T, Yamashita T, et al: Intracranial hemorrhage in hemophilia of children. Child's Brain 11:213, 1984.
16. Guerth JH, Teng P, Goldenberg E: Surgery in a hemophiliac child with intracranial hemorrhage. Pediatrics 28:800, 1961.
17. Gilchrist GS, Piepgras DG: Neurologic complications in hemophilia. In: Hilgartner MW (ed): Progress in Pediatric Hematology/Oncology, Vol. I. Hemophilia in Children. Littleton, MA, Publishing Sciences Group Inc., 1976.
18. Groch SN, Sayre GP, Heck FJ: Cerebral hemorrhage in leukemia. Arch Neurol Psychiatry 2:439, 1960.
19. Humphreys RP, Hockley AD, Freedman MH, et al: Management of intracerebral hemorrhage in idiopathic thrombocytopenic purpura. Report of four cases. J Neurosurg 45:700, 1976.
20. Humphreys RP: Computed tomography and the early diagnostic lumbar puncture. Can Med Assoc J 121:150, 1979.
21. Jones RK, Knighton RS: Surgery in hemophiliacs with special reference to the central nervous system. Ann Surg 144:1029, 1956.
22. Keith RG, Mahoney LJ, Garvey MB: Disseminated intravascular coagulation: An important feature of the fat embolism syndrome. Can Med Assoc J 105:74, 1971.
23. Kerensky A: Russia and History's Turning Point. New York, Duell, Sloan and Pearce, 1965.
24. Kerr CB: Intracranial haemorrhage in haemophilia. J Neurol Neurosurg Psychiatry 27:166, 1964.
25. Kuenzlen E, Bauer J, Bertram U, et al: Fatal outcome of acute thrombocytopenic purpura associated with a viral infection in an 11-year-old child. Blut 48:363, 1984.
26. Latimer JS, Shapp HL: Alpha-1-antitrypsin deficiency in childhood. Curr Problems Pediatr: 11:1, 1980.
27. Lutschg J, Vassella F: Neurological complications in hemophilia. Acta Pediatr Scand 70:235, 1981.
28. MacGee EE: Surgical treatment of arteriovenous anomaly in a hemophiliac patient. J Neurosurg 30:289, 1969.
29. Martinowitz U, Heim M, Tadmor T, et al: Intracranial hemorrhage in patients with hemophilia. Neurosurg 18:538, 1986.
30. McNinch AW, Orme RL, Tripp JH: Hemorrhagic disease of the newborn returns. Lancet 1:1089, 1983.
31. Miner ME, Kaufman HH, Fraham SH, et al: Disseminated intravascular coagulation fibrinolytic syndrome following head injury in children: Frequency and prognostic implications. J Pediatr 100:687, 1982.
32. Moody RA, Mullen S: Factor VIII in hemophilia. Case report. J Neurosurg 29:520, 1968.
33. Myles ST, Harris CEC, Hansebout RR: Epidural hematoma in hemophilia: Successful treatment. Can Med Assoc J 104:51, 1971.
34. Nammacher MA, Willemin M: Vitamin-K deficiency in infants beyond the neonatal period. J Pediatr 76:549, 1970.
35. Olsen ER: Intracranial surgery in hemophiliacs: Report of a case and review of the literature. Arch Neurol 21:401, 1968.
36. Owen CA, Bowie EJW: Review article. Surgical hemostasis. J Neurosurg 51:137, 1979.
37. Paillas JE, Boudouresques J, Tamalet J: Les hématomes intracraniens des hémophiles. Semaine Hop Paris 24:432, 1948.
38. Pochedly C: Management of CNS leukemia in childhood: Outline of current concepts. Clin Pediatr 11:503, 1972.
39. Potter JM: Head injury and haemophilia. Acta Neurochir 13:380, 1965.
40. Raggio JR, Fleischer AS, Corley CC: Posterior fossa subdural hematoma in a hemophiliac. Neurosurgery 3:213, 1978.
41. Renaudin JW, George RP: Coagulopathies causing intracranial hemorrhage. In: Wilkins RH, Rengachary SS (eds): Neurosurgery. New York, McGraw-Hill Book Company, 1985, pp 1518–1520.
42. Seeler RA, Imana RB: Intracranial hemorrhage in patients with hemophilia. J Neurosurg 39:181, 1973.
43. Silverstein A: Intracranial bleeding in hemophilia. Arch Neurol 3:141, 1960.
44. Singer RP, Schneider RC: The successful management of intracerebral and subarachnoid hemorrhage in a hemophiliac infant. A case report. Neurology 12:293, 1962.
45. Travis RL, Mitchell OC, Youmans JR, et al: Intracranial surgery in hemophilia: Use of potent antihemophilic factor concentrate. Am Surg 34:602, 1968.
46. Van Der Sande JJ, Veltkamp JJ, Boekhout-Mussert RJ, et al: Head injury and coagulation disorders. Neurosurgery 49:357, 1978.
47. Wilson, cited by Silverstein A: Intracranial bleeding in hemophilia. Arch Neurol 3:141, 1960.
48. Woerner SJ, Abildgaard CF, French BN: Intracranial hemorrhage in children with idiopathic thrombocytopenia purpura. Pediatrics 67:453, 1981.
49. Zerella JT, Martin LW, Lampkin BC: Emergency splenectomy for idiopathic thrombocytopenia purpura in children. J Pediatr Surg 13:243, 1978.

49
INTERVENTIONAL NEURORADIOLOGY

Jeffrey H. Wisoff, M.D.
Alex Berenstein, M.D.
Fred Epstein, M.D.

Recent advances in microsurgical technique and neuroanesthetic care have permitted contemporary neurosurgeons to extirpate the majority of cerebral and spinal vascular malformations. Unfortunately, a significant proportion of pediatric malformations are not amenable to surgical excision. The development of interventional neuroradiologic techniques has provided an effective alternative treatment regimen for these children. The authors' experience over the past eight years in treating 83 pediatric patients with a variety of vascular lesions of the central nervous system with embolization forms the basis of this chapter (Tables 49–1 through 49–4).

TECHNICAL CONSIDERATIONS

A variety of interventional techniques are available for the treatment of different vascular lesions (Tables 49–5 and 49–6). Catheters with detachable balloons may be used to occlude arteriovenous fistulas and large feeding vessels or to trap a segment of a vessel. Flexible flow-guided microcatheters can reach small distal arteries for the controlled injection of fluid embolic agents, such as isobutyl cyanoacrylate (IBCA), to occlude feeding arteries or to obliterate the nidus of an arteriovenous malformation (AVM). Particulate emboli of gelatin sponge, polyvinyl alcohol foam, or silicone pellets may be flow-directed to reduce the size of a racemose AVM or to decrease the blood supply to a hypervascular tumor.[1,2]

For the most part, the best results in intracranial lesions have been obtained using flow-guided mi-

Table 49–1. PEDIATRIC FISTULAS AND ANEURYSMS—TREATMENT BY EMBOLIZATION

Diagnosis	No. of Patients	No. of Embolizations	Angiogram Only
CCF	5	6	—
I.C. fistula	5	5	1
E.C. fistula	2	3	1
Scalp AVMs	2	2	—
Aneurysms	3	4	—
TOTAL	17	20	2

CCF, carotid-cavernous fistula; IC, internal carotid; EC, external carotid

Table 49–2. PEDIATRIC NEUROEMBOLIZATION—BRAIN AVMs

Diagnosis	No. of Patients	No. of Embolizations	Angiogram Only
Vein of Galen	25	40	11
Midline (thalamic, basal ganglia)	6	10	1
Supratentorial	10	8	6
Bilateral	3	5	1
Cerebellar	1	3	—
Brainstem	1	3	—
Corpus callosum	1	—	1
TOTAL	47	69	20

Table 49-3. PEDIATRIC SPINAL VASCULAR LESIONS

Diagnosis	No. of Patients	No. of Embolizations	Angiogram Only
AVMs	5	9	1
Tumors or Hemangiomas	4	5	—
TOTAL	9	14	1

croballoon catheters with a calibrated leak balloon and IBCA as the embolic agent. At the beginning of the authors' experience, the original Kerber Silastic tubing and balloons were used;[3] frequently technical difficulties were encountered. The use of a latex balloon with a calibrated leak, attached or ligated to no. 2 French Silastic tubing,[4] with the employment of pressure chambers[5] has significantly advanced delivery system capabilities. The IBCA mixture consists of 1 cc of IBCA, 0.2 to 0.8 cc of Pantopaque (iophendylate), and 1 gm of tantalum powder for digital angiography (2 gm of tantalum powder is needed with routine fluoroscopy).[6] The Pantopaque retards polymerization time. A lesser amount, or none, is used for closing high-flow fistulas, whereas a larger amount is added when a parenchymatous or angiomatous network has to be closed to allow for greater penetration of the abnormal angioarchitecture.

Silicone spheres as flow-directed particles were used as the sole embolic agent in the beginning of the authors' experience. Currently, they are utilized when superselective catheterization of small perforators cannot be achieved. In general, spheres only occlude feeders and are less effective than liquid agents. Detachable balloons are reserved for obliteration of large fistulas or proximal occlusion of a major feeder.

Accurate radiographic guidance of the microcatheters requires high-quality fluoroscopy with biplane or C-arm angiographic capability. Video recording and electronic fluoroscopic subtraction are extremely helpful in the real-time monitoring of catheter position and the deposition of embolic material. To minimize the dose of contrast material administered while maintaining the ability to document periodically and angiographically the extent of malformation obliteration, the authors have routinely used digital subtraction angiography.

In the young child, maintaining vascular access for multiple, staged embolizations has been a recurring problem. Initially, all children had surgical arteriotomy; however, as these patients returned

Table 49-4. PEDIATRIC TUMORS EMBOLIZED

Diagnosis	No. of Patients	No. of Embolizations	Angiogram Only
Meningiomas	4	4	—
Neurinomas	3	2	1
Others	2	2	—
Malignant gliomas	1	BCNU infusion	—
TOTAL	10	9	1

Table 49-5. CATHETERS

Conventional Catheters
  Tapered
  Nontapered
  Berenstein superselective catheter
Balloon Catheters
  Single-lumen flow-guided
    ("calibrated leak balloon catheter")
  Double-lumen balloon catheter
  Detachable balloon catheter
Coaxial Catheter System
  (Using conventional or balloon catheter)

for additional treatment, the surgically exposed vessels were either thrombosed, or significant fibrosis was encountered. A technique of percutaneous graduated dilatation of the artery has been developed. The authors employ progressive vessel dilatation, starting with a no. 3 French introducer sheath and progressing to a no. 4 French, a no. 5 French, and finally a no. 6 French introducer sheath. In the patients who have had percutaneous catheterization of the femoral vessels using this system, the arteries have been preserved and were reused in multiple subsequent embolizations. Neonates may still require arteriotomy if the umbilical vessels cannot accommodate the catheter.

Direct surgical carotid puncture had been attempted in early cases; however, the catheterization of the carotid arteries, the manipulations of the vessels, and the short length of the neck made the direct carotid route extremely difficult. In addition, the diminished blood flow through the carotid artery prevented flow-guided movement of the microcatheter. Future development of a "chimney" type access that would permit leaving a device subcutaneously with an end-to-side anastomosis to a major artery may eliminate this problem.

CLINICAL CONSIDERATIONS

To optimize patient care, a multidisciplinary team including neuroradiologists, neurosurgeons, neurologists, anesthesiologists, and pediatricians is es-

Table 49-6. EMBOLIC AGENTS

Absorbable
  Gelfoam
  Autologous blood clot
  Microfibrillar collagen
  Oxidized cellulose
Nonabsorbable Solids
  Polyvinyl alcohol foam
  Silicone spheres
  Stainless-steel coils
  Dura mater
Nonabsorbable Liquids
  Isobutyl cyanoacrylate (IBCA)
  Silicone fluid mixture
  Ethyl alcohol
Opacifying Agents
  Tantalum powder
  Pantopaque (retards IBCA polymerization)

sential. Meticulous pretreatment radiographic and clinical planning is needed to minimize the inherent risk of embolizing lesions of the brain and the spinal cord. When the patient's condition permits, diagnostic radiographic studies should be performed at a separate sitting, to allow adequate time for analysis of the lesion and selection of appropriate catheters and embolic agents and to limit contrast dye toxicity.

Medical considerations must include (1) limits on contrast and fluid load; (2) electrolyte balance; (3) potential need for exchange transfusion; (4) management of congestive heart failure (including potential need for emergent phlebotomy during the embolization); and (5) the effect of embolization on any associated systemic anomalies. Real-time neurophysiologic monitoring of evoked potentials or computerized electroencephalography (EEG) may be required to assess the patient's tolerance to embolization.

Although the aim of any vascular occlusive procedure is the selective obliteration of abnormal "angioarchitecture" or vascular nidus while preserving normal blood supply to adjacent structures, the embolization techniques utilized and the therapeutic goals may differ, depending on the pathologic lesion and the patient's clinical status. When used as a surgical adjunct, preoperative embolization may eliminate deep, inaccessible feeding vessels, making operative dissection less extensive. Intraoperative embolization can be employed to occlude deep feeders or to avoid dissection in inaccessible areas. Both techniques can convert an inoperable lesion into one that may be surgically extirpated. In other patients, following surgical ligation of superficial feeders, small, deep vessels may increase in size and become accessible for embolization.

Embolization may be the primary or sole therapeutic modality for obliteration of a malformation and is especially effective for occluding large high-flow fistulas. Reduction of flow through a malformation may eliminate a "steal" phenomena, reverse ischemic symptoms and venous hypertension, or in neonates with secondary high-output congestive heart failure, ameliorate the hemodynamic state.

CEREBRAL ARTERIOVENOUS MALFORMATIONS

The goal of all forms of treatment for arteriovenous malformations (AVMs) is complete obliteration or excision of the lesion, since there is no evidence to indicate that partial resection or subtotal embolization protects against hemorrhage. Embolization may be used preoperatively or as an intraoperative adjunct in patients with lesions not initially resectable because of size or location of feeding arteries. In unresectable cases, palliative embolization may be performed for the control of intractable seizures and headaches and for the relief of neurologic deficit related to ischemia of adjacent brain resulting from steal phenomena or venous hypertension. Even when embolization is used as the sole modality, the intent should be complete obliteration of the nidus whenever possible. On occasion, subtotal embolization of the vascular nidus results in progressive thrombosis, with ultimate obliteration of the lesion.

Particulate Agents

Silastic or silicone pellets can reduce the size of a large AVM sufficiently to allow safer and easier operative excision. In unresectable cases, palliative embolization may redistribute blood flow to ischemic brain. These pellets are usually injected through a no. 6 or 7 French introducer catheter that is positioned proximally in the internal carotid or vertebral artery. Successful embolization depends on a large vascular steal phenomena, with a large ratio of arterial to venous vessels (Fig. 49-1).

Complications of particulate embolization include subclinical pulmonary embolization from pellets migrating through to the venous side and neurologic impairment from occlusion of normal vessels. Rarely, rapid occlusion of the abnormal vascular bed leads to a breakthrough in normal cerebrovascular autoregulation, with secondary cerebral swelling and hemorrhage. For this reason, patients with large malformations should be treated in stages to guard against this complication.

FLUID EMBOLIC AGENTS

The major disadvantage of particulate embolization has been the lack of control over the deposition of the embolic material, with the risk of inadvertent occlusion of normal vessels. Currently, superselective catheterization and embolization with low-viscosity fluid embolic agents is the technique used for the majority of malformations. Small flexible, flow-guided balloon-tip catheters are maneuvered through the tortuous distal branches of the internal carotid or vertebral artery to deposit the embolic material directly into the feeding vessel. Successful embolization with IBCA depends on placing the tip of the catheter just proximal to the nidus of the AVM, beyond normal vessels. Ideally, the polymerization time of the IBCA will be retarded by the addition of iophendylate, so that the nidus as well as the feeding vessel will be occluded (Fig. 49-2). Rapid withdrawal of the balloon catheter after injection is required to prevent gluing of the catheter into the intravascular cast. The major danger is excessive prolongation of the polymerization time, with passage of the IBCA into the venous side of the AVM. Venous occlusion may result in progressive venous thrombosis, edema, and hemorrhage, with a catastrophic outcome.

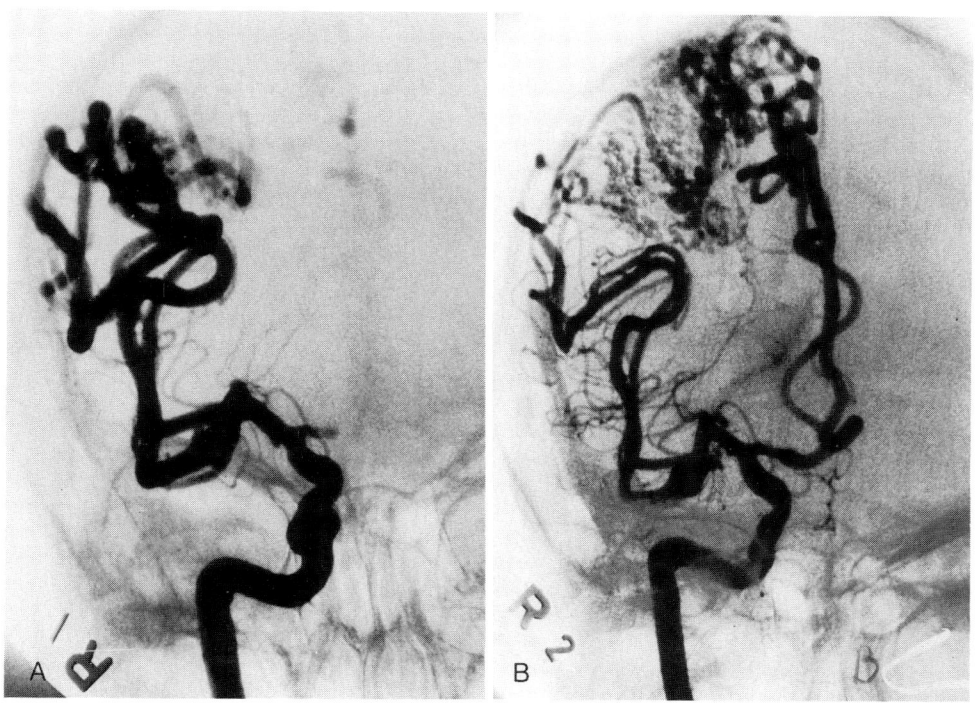

Figure 49–1. The use of silicone spheres. A, Frontal subtraction angiogram of the right internal carotid artery in early arterial phase demonstrates preferential flow toward the middle cerebral artery territory. Multiple branches of the middle cerebral artery are hypertrophied. There is poor opacification of normal arteries. There is only flash filling of the anterior cerebral artery. B, After multiple silicone spheres were introduced via the right internal carotid artery for embolization. Note diminution in the caliber of the abnormal middle cerebral artery. There is now filling of the malformation primarily from the anterior cerebral artery as well as opacification of multiple normal middle cerebral artery branches.

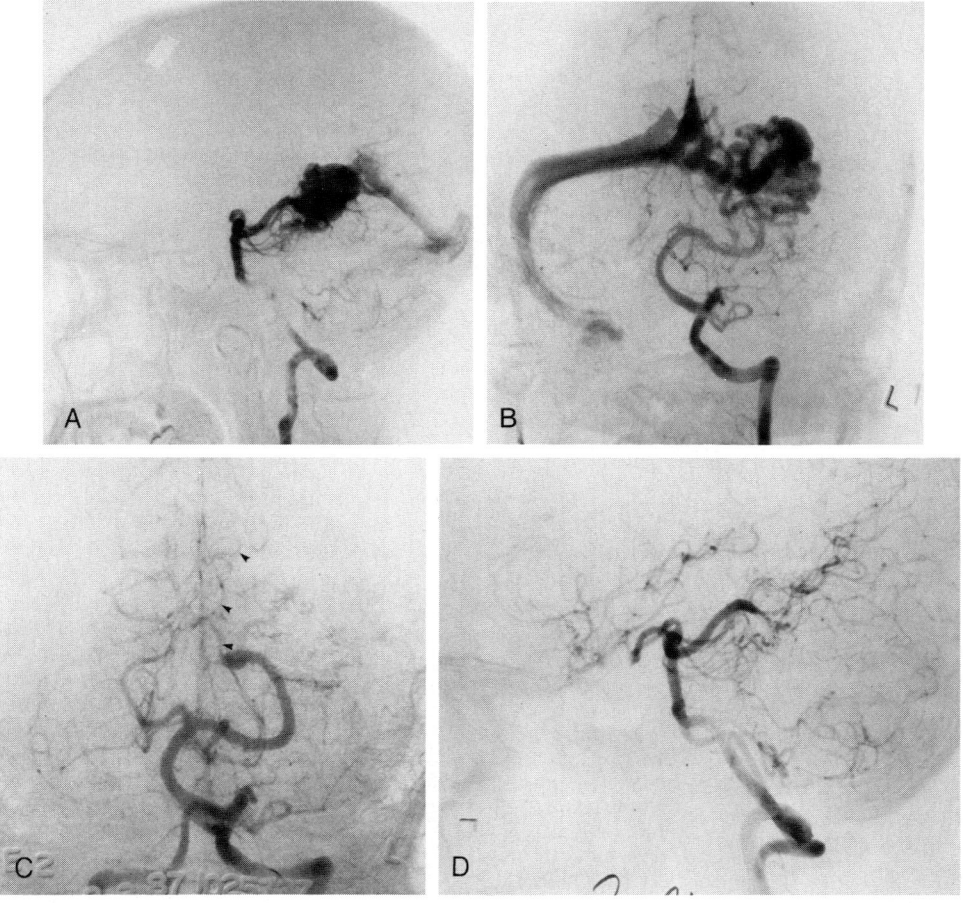

Figure 49–2. An 18-year-old male with an arteriovenous malformation (AVM) in the distribution of the left posterior cerebral artery. A, Lateral subtraction angiogram of the left vertebral artery demonstrates a vascular malformation supplied by the left posterior cerebral artery. B, Frontal subtraction angiogram demonstrates the malformation with prominent venous drainage toward the vein of Galen and transverse sinus of the contralateral side. Frontal (C) and lateral (D) subtraction angiograms after embolization. Note occlusion of the malformation, with preservation of the calcarine branch (arrowheads). There was no disturbance of visual function.

While cure with embolization alone is uncommon, sequential, staged embolizations are extremely useful in managing large lesions. Deep vascular supply may be eliminated, and with the subsequent decrease in the size of the nidus, surgical excision may be considered. Large, resectable lesions may be "staged" by partial embolization, obviating the need for multiple operative procedures in patients at risk for postresection perfusion breakthrough (Fig. 49–3). Unfortunately, while partial AVM obliteration may ameliorate symptoms, there is no evidence that it will protect against hemorrhage.

CAROTID CAVERNOUS FISTULAS

While large single-hole fistulas may occur anywhere, the most common location is between the internal carotid artery and the cavernous sinus. In children, this occurs most often as a post-traumatic event and usually consists of only one or two large holes between the artery and the sinus. Traditional surgical treatment requires both open craniotomy and exposure of the cervical internal carotid artery, with trapping of the intervening segment of intracavernous carotid.[8]

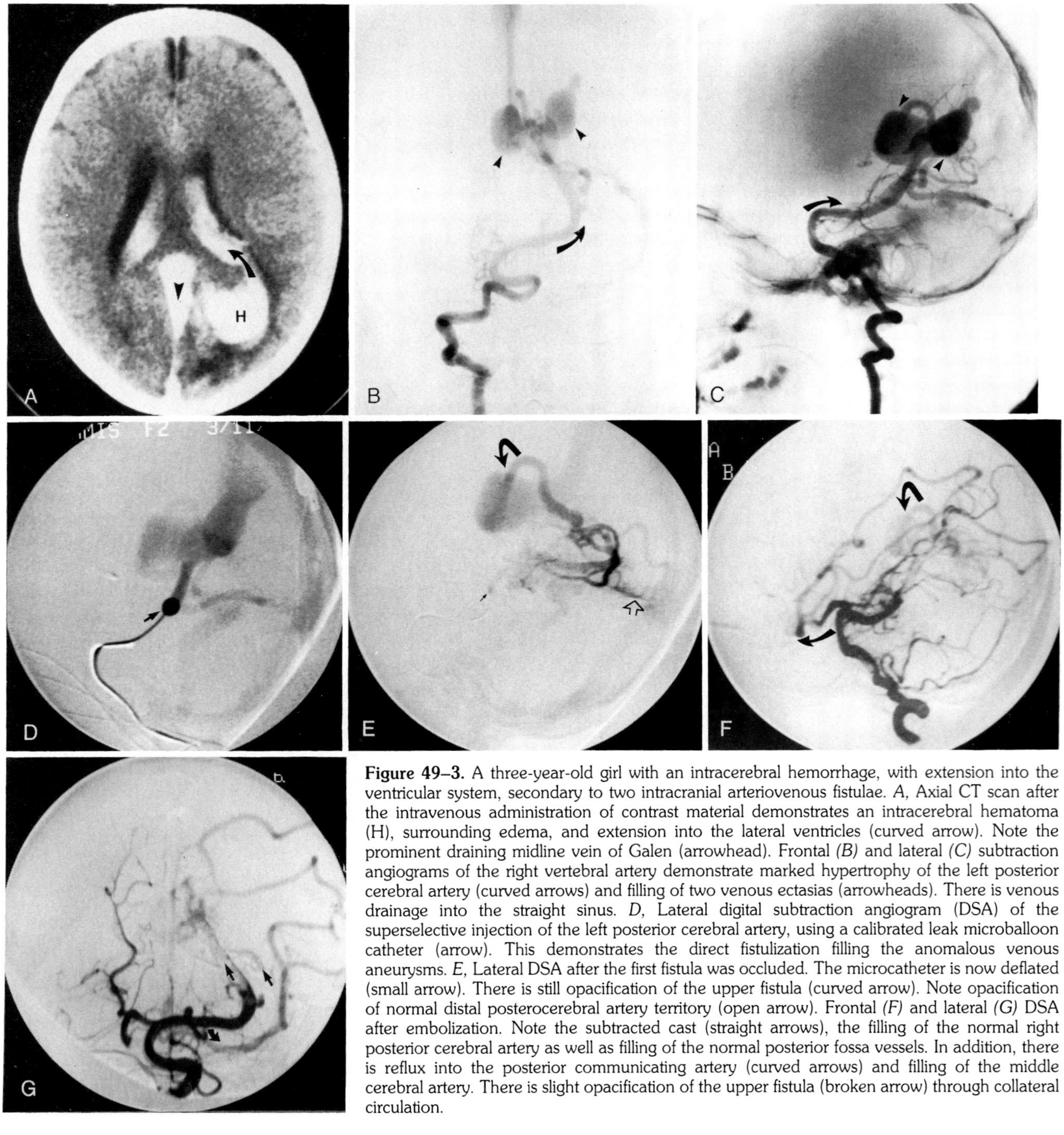

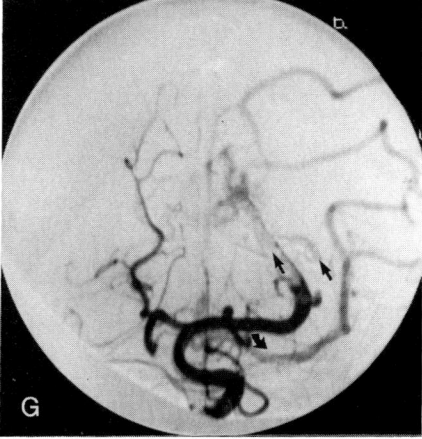

Figure 49–3. A three-year-old girl with an intracerebral hemorrhage, with extension into the ventricular system, secondary to two intracranial arteriovenous fistulae. A, Axial CT scan after the intravenous administration of contrast material demonstrates an intracerebral hematoma (H), surrounding edema, and extension into the lateral ventricles (curved arrow). Note the prominent draining midline vein of Galen (arrowhead). Frontal (B) and lateral (C) subtraction angiograms of the right vertebral artery demonstrate marked hypertrophy of the left posterior cerebral artery (curved arrows) and filling of two venous ectasias (arrowheads). There is venous drainage into the straight sinus. D, Lateral digital subtraction angiogram (DSA) of the superselective injection of the left posterior cerebral artery, using a calibrated leak microballoon catheter (arrow). This demonstrates the direct fistulization filling the anomalous venous aneurysms. E, Lateral DSA after the first fistula was occluded. The microcatheter is now deflated (small arrow). There is still opacification of the upper fistula (curved arrow). Note opacification of normal distal posterocerebral artery territory (open arrow). Frontal (F) and lateral (G) DSA after embolization. Note the subtracted cast (straight arrows), the filling of the normal right posterior cerebral artery as well as filling of the normal posterior fossa vessels. In addition, there is reflux into the posterior communicating artery (curved arrows) and filling of the middle cerebral artery. There is slight opacification of the upper fistula (broken arrow) through collateral circulation.

Balloon embolization techniques are aimed at fistula closure, with preservation of normal arterial flow. Fistula closure may be achieved by percutaneous transarterial or transvenous routes.[9-14] Rarely in patients with tortuous or anomalous vessels, the balloons may be introduced through an operative approach.

The technique entails percutaneous insertion of a coaxial detachable balloon assembly. Systemic heparinization and preoperative salicylate platelet inhibition can be used to prevent thromboembolic complications. The balloon catheter is fluoroscopically flow-guided within the carotid artery, through the fistula into the cavernous sinus. The balloon is inflated with iso-osmotic metrizamide to occlude the fistula. After fistula closure and confirmation of carotid patency by angiography, a coaxial detaching catheter is advanced over the balloon base to release it within the cavernous sinus. Secondary sinus thrombosis occurs over several days, ensuring permanent fistula obliteration (Fig. 49-4). When catheterization of the sinus cannot be achieved, trapping of the fistula may be performed by placement of balloons just distal and then proximal to the fistula, in the intracavernous carotid, provided the patient has previously been shown to tolerate carotid occlusion.

Virtually all the authors' patients have had a dramatic response to treatment.[15] Cranial nerve palsies related to neural compression by the balloon within the sinus may occur. This complication has, in the authors' experience, resolved over three to six weeks. Asymptomatic pseudoaneurysms frequently occur. Patients with pain or persistent nerve palsies from a pseudoaneurysm may have the pseudoaneurysm occluded at a subsequent sitting, usually with carotid sacrifice (none of the authors' patients have required treatment for pseudoaneurysm).[16]

VEIN OF GALEN MALFORMATIONS

Several authors have suggested the use of embolization as primary or adjunctive therapy in the management of vein of Galen malformations.[17-19] There are several theoretical advantages to the use of interventional techniques in these patients. Since the malformations are usually varices with direct arteriovenous fistulas, obliteration of the feeders leads to progressive shrinkage of the aneurysm, obviating the need to excise the lesion. Ischemic symptoms can be reversed by selective occlusion of the major arteriovenous (AV) fistulas, avoiding operative trauma to already compromised brain. The neonate with a precarious cardiovascular status can have obliteration of the hemodynamically significant portion of the malformation without cardiac arrest or the need for hypotensive anesthetic technique.

Our current treatment strategy is based upon whether the patient presents with severe congestive heart failure (CHF) (usually a neonate in extremis) or with ischemic deficits (as an infant or older child). The primary goal in the neonate is obliteration of the major portion of the fistula, to allow resolution of the CHF. Since these patients cannot tolerate a significant volume or contrast load and usually have compromised renal function, angiography is limited

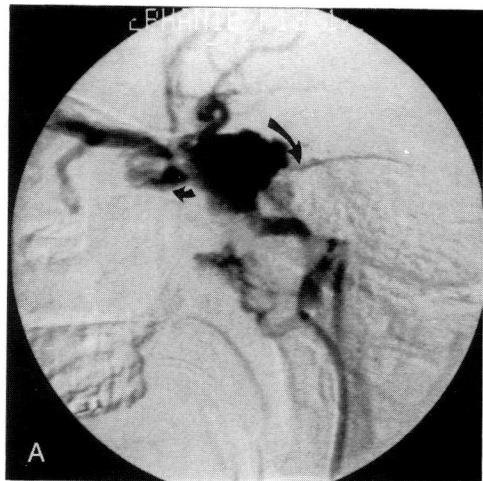

Figure 49-4. Traumatic carotid cavernous fistula. A, Lateral digital subtraction angiogram (DSA) of the left internal carotid artery demonstrates a traumatic internal carotid to cavernous sinus fistula filling the ophthalmic vein (small curved arrow) anteriorly and filling of the aneurysmally dilated posterior superior compartment of the cavernous sinus (large curved arrow) draining into the superior and inferior petrosal sinus. B, Lateral common carotid angiogram after a detachable balloon (arrow) is subtracted and is occluding the fistula, with preservation of the internal carotid artery flow.

to selective and superselective studies of the vertebrobasilar system. The majority of the hemodynamically significant feeders are visualized by these studies. At the same sitting, the major fistulas are occluded with IBCA (Fig. 49–5). Meticulous attention to the patient's cardiac, renal, and hepatic function and coagulation parameters is essential. Closure of the major fistulas may result in acute volume overload; emergency phlebotomy may be required within minutes of fistula closure. When a lengthy procedure is anticipated, with multiple injections of contrast material, exchange transfusion may be used to accommodate the increased required contrast or volume load.

Usually, cardiac function and urinary output are improved by the end of the initial embolization, with resolution of hepatic dysfunction over several days. If CHF persists, additional embolization is performed within several days. The patients are restudied at six to nine months to determine whether to proceed with further staged embolizations or to attempt surgical obliteration. The prohibitive morbidity and mortality with conventional surgical care have been dramatically altered by this approach.

In infants and older children, the predominent clinical presentation has been developmental delays or neurologic deterioration secondary to ischemia from steal phenomena and chronic venous hypertension. Serial CT scans in untreated infants have demonstrated progressive cortical atrophy and dystrophic calcifications. In these patients, embolization may be used as a surgical adjunct or as the sole therapeutic modality. When a large anterior cerebral artery supply to the vein of Galen malformation exists, it is technically simple to surgically clip these vessels, increasing the "sump" of the deeper feeders and rendering them more accessible for subsequent embolization to complete the obliteration of the lesion. Children who underwent subtotal surgical obliteration as infants and subsequently present with progressive ischemic encephalopathy can have the remainder of the malformation embolized. Alternatively, newly diagnosed

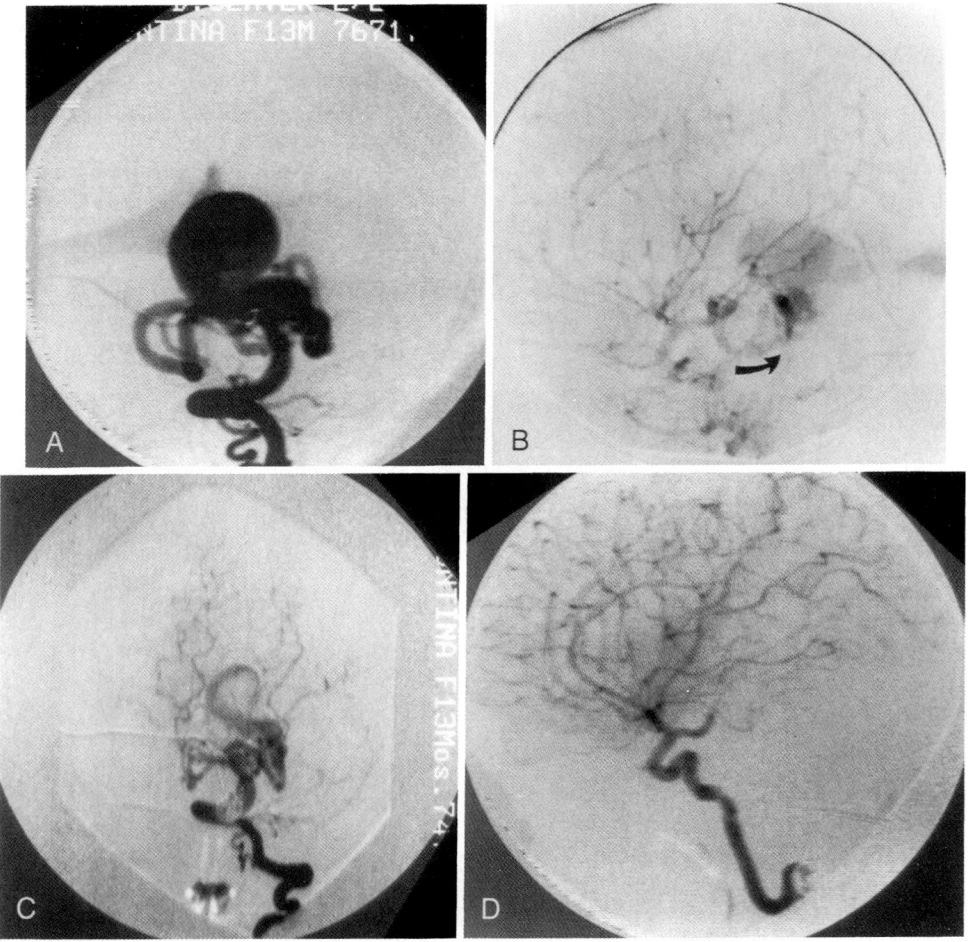

Figure 49–5. A 13-month-old infant with a midline arteriovenous malformation draining into the vein of Galen. *A,* Frontal DSA of the left vertebral artery demonstrates a high-flow arteriovenous malformation, with evidence of fistulization into the vein of Galen. *B,* Lateral DSA of the left common carotid artery demonstrates filling of the malformation via the posterior communicating artery (curved arrow). *C,* DSA after two depositions of isobutyl cyanoacrylate (IBCA) demonstrates slight opacification of the vein. Note the significant opacification of normal arteries compared with that in *A*. *D,* Lateral DSA of the left internal carotid artery demonstrates the stump of the posterior communicating artery without opacification of the malformation.

patients may have sequential staged embolizations to obliterate completely, or nearly completely, the lesion, with resolution of the patient's clinical signs and symptoms, thus obviating the need for surgery.

Thirty-eight separate embolizations were performed on 20 patients with vein of Galen malformations. There were six instances of technical complications, including failure to enter the vascular system, inability to perform superselective angiography, and asymptomatic migration of emboli to the venous system; none of these events resulted in any morbidity. Significant complications from infarction of deep structures by aberrant emboli occurred in two patients, both of whom made a complete recovery over several months. The first two patients that the authors treated died of uncontrolled heart failure; the authors were using only particulate embolization at that time. Two of the subsequent 18 patients have died; in both cases, there was massive migration of bucrylate through a high-flow fistula into the venous circulation, resulting in massive, fatal pulmonary embolization.

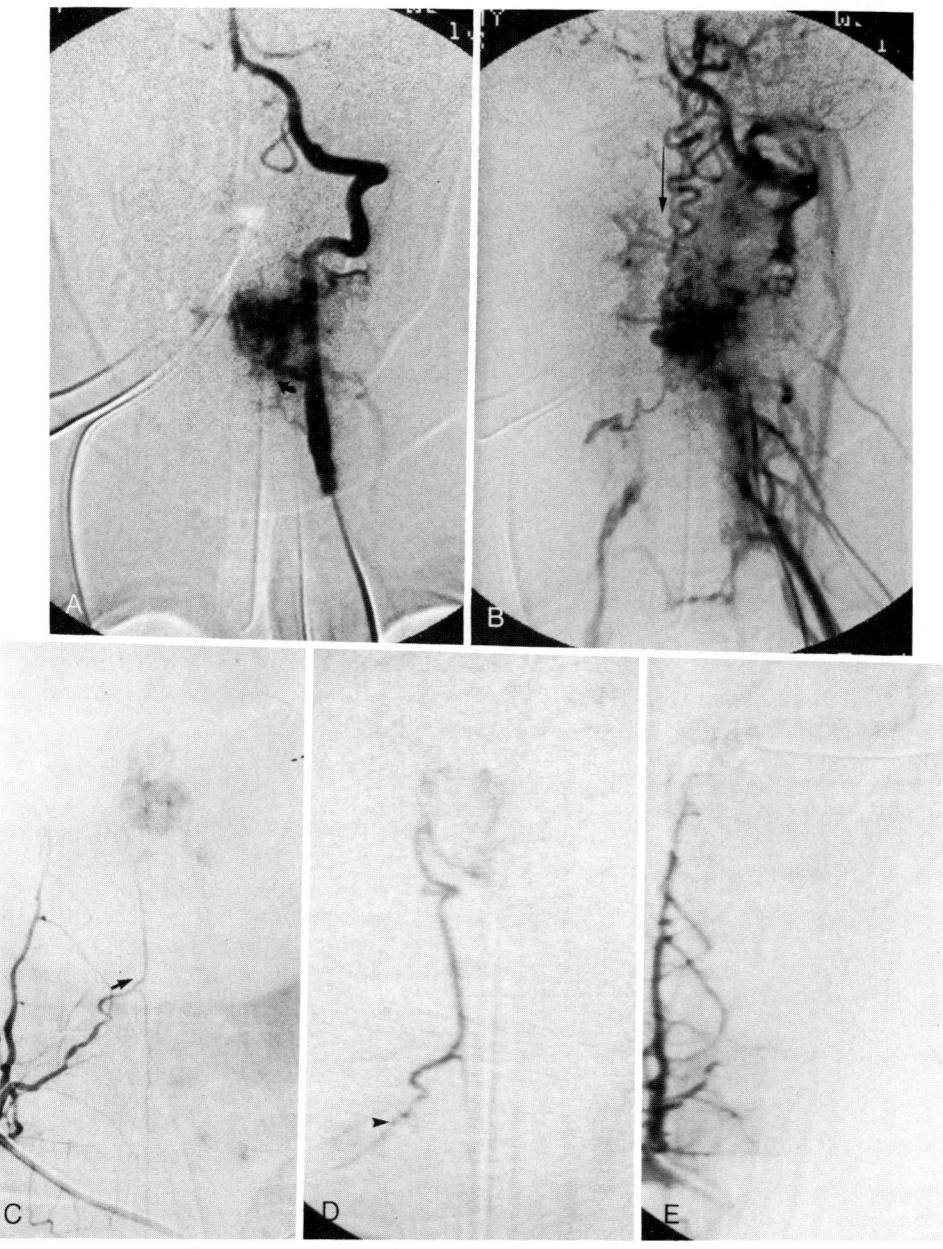

Figure 49–6. Intramedullary spinal cord arteriovenous malformation in a nine-year-old child with multiple subarachnoid hemorrhages. Frontal DSA of the left vertebral artery in the early arterial phase (A) and late-phase (B) demonstrates an intramedullary arteriovenous malformation supplied by the artery of the cervical enlargement (curved arrow, A) as well as the anterior spinal artery from above (long arrow, B). C, Frontal subtraction angiogram of the right thyrocervical trunk demonstrates the artery of C6 originating from this pedicle and supplying the anterior spinal artery (arrow). There is supply to the malformation from the ascending limb. D, Frontal DSA with a microcatheter (arrowhead). Using flow-control, multiple particles of polyvinyl alcohol foam (PVA) were injected, while somatosensory evoked potentials were monitored, producing devascularization of the nidus of the malformation. E, Frontal DSA at the end of the embolization in D demonstrates no filling of the malformation.

Illustration continued on following page

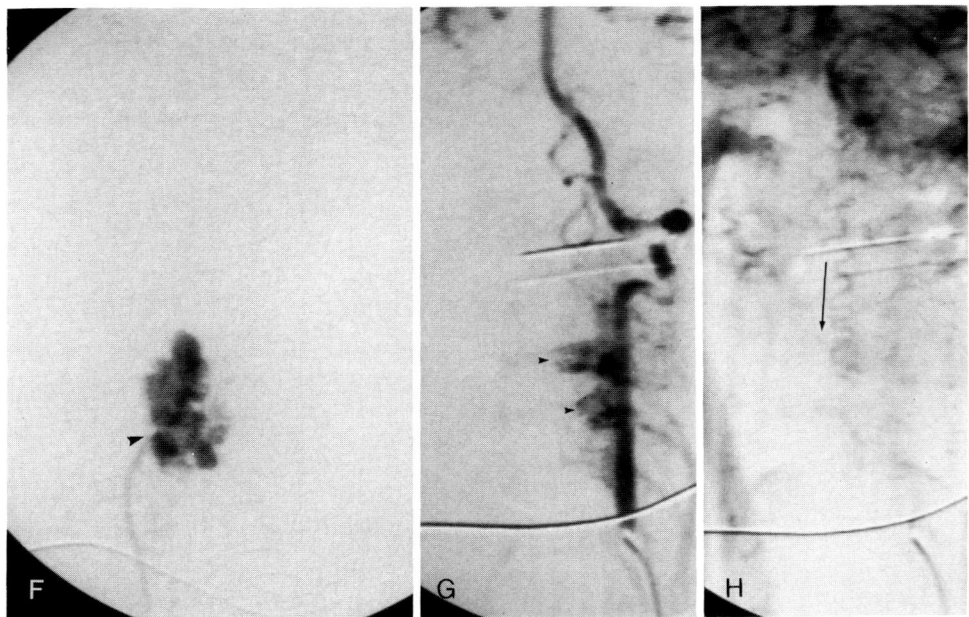

Figure 49-6 *Continued F*, Lateral DSA after catheterization of the artery of the cervical enlargement within the malformation itself (arrowhead). Note filling of the malformation with multiple ectatic and dilated venous structures and no filling of normal tissue. 75 mg of amobarbital sodium were injected superselectively in this position. No abnormality in clinical or SEP monitoring was noted, for which this pedicle was embolized with IBCA. *G*, Frontal DSA in the midarterial phase demonstrates no opacification of the malformation. There is filling of two hemivertebra (arrowheads). *H*, Late-phase demonstrates the anterior spinal artery but no filling of the malformation (compare with *A* and *B*).

Meticulous attention to polymerization time of the IBCA is required to guard against this catastrophic outcome.

SPINAL CORD ARTERIOVENOUS MALFORMATION

Pediatric vascular malformations of the spinal cord are rare lesions. They usually are high-flow fistulas or AVMs that present clinically with subarachnoid hemorrhage. Often, these lesions are primarily intramedullary and are not amenable to surgical excision.

The embolization techniques utilized depend on the anatomic disposition of the lesion; frequently a combination of embolic agents and different catheters is needed (Fig. 49-6). Metameric (segmental) lesions are particularly difficult to manage and may require multiple, staged procedures. Preoperative particulate embolization may be used as a preoperative adjunct in lesions involving bone, to decrease the overall vascularity and to permit biopsy or surgical excision, with minimal blood loss.

HYPERVASCULAR TUMORS

Childhood brain tumors with a prominent attachment to dura or bone may be quite hypervascular, with a significant blood supply through the external carotid circulation. These tumors exhibit extremely aggressive behavior and extend beyond the bony calvarium into facial structures.[19, 20] Recent experience with radical embolization of these tumors with 95 percent ethanol has yielded promising early results. Ethanol has provided both devascularization and a cytotoxic effect, with apparent arrest of tumor growth for up to four years. Although long-term follow-up is lacking, embolic techniques may ultimately play an important role in the management of certain pediatric tumors.

SUMMARY

At the present time, interventional neuroradiologic techniques are in the process of evolution. Although important advances have been made over the past decade, these procedures are not without significant risk and should be reserved for situations that are not amenable to more conventional treatment. An experienced team combining neuroradiologic and clinical expertise is essential for the proper management of these patients. Future advances in the understanding of functional vascular anatomy, combined with the development of increasingly sophisticated catheters and embolic agents will propel us to establish new treatment techniques for today's difficult problems.

References

1. Berenstein A, Kricheff II: Catheter and material selection for transarterial embolization: Technical considerations. I. Radiology 132:619, 1979.

2. Berenstein A, Kricheff II: Catheter and material selection for transarterial embolization: Technical considerations. II. Radiology 132:631, 1979.
3. Berenstein A, Kricheff II, Ransohoff J: Carotid cavernous fistulas. Intraarterial treatment. AJNR 1:449, 1980.
4. Berenstein A, Young W, Ransohoff J, et al: Somatosensory evoked potentials during spinal angiography and therapeutic transvascular embolization. J Neurosurg 6:777, 1984.
5. Cromwell LD, Kerber CW: Modification of cyanoacrylate for therapeutic embolization: Preliminary experience. Am J Roentgenol 132:799, 1979.
6. Debrun G, Lacour P, Caron JP, et al: Detachable balloon and calibrated leak balloon technique in the treatment of cerebral vascular lesions. J Neurosurg 49:635, 1978.
7. Debrun G, Lacour P, Vinuela F, et al: Treatment of 54 traumatic carotid cavernous fistulas. J Neurosurg 55:678, 1981.
8. Debrun G, Vinuela, F: A new calibrated leak latex balloon. Presented at the Second Symposium on Embolization, Park City, Utah, 1981.
9. Hamby W: Carotid cavernous fistula. Springfield, IL, Charles C Thomas, 1966, pp 71–106.
10. Heishima G: A new silicone detachable balloon. Presented at the Second International Symposium on Embolization. Park City, Utah, 1981.
11. Hoffman HJ, Chuang S, Hendrick EB, et al: Aneurysms of the vein of Galen. J Neurosurg 57:316, 1982.
12. Kerber C: Balloon catheter with a calibrated leak: A new system for superselective angiography and occlusive catheter therapy. Radiology 120:547, 1976.
13. Kupersmith M, Berenstein A, Flamm E, et al: Neuro-ophthalmologic abnormalities and intravascular therapy of traumatic carotid cavernous fistulas (submitted for publication).
14. Lasjaunias P, Berenstein A: Interventional Neuroradiology. New York, Springer-Verlag, 1986.
15. Manelfe C, Berenstein A: Treatment of carotid cavernous fistulas by venous approach. J Neuroradiol 7:13, 1980.
16. Mullan S: Treatment of carotid cavernous fistulas by cavernous sinus occlusion. J Neurosurg 50:131, 1979.
17. Pevsner PH: Microballoon catheter for superselective angiography and therapeutic occlusion. Am J Roentgenol 128:225, 1977.
18. Sano K, Wakai S, Ochiai C, et al: Characteristics of intracranial meningiomas of childhood. Child's Brain 8:98, 1981.
19. Servinenko FA: Balloon catheterization and occlusion of a major cerebral vessel. J Neurosurg 41:125, 1974.
20. Ventureyra ECG, Ivan LP, Nabavi N: Deep-seated giant arteriovenous malformations in infancy. Surg Neurol 10:365, 1978.
21. Wisoff J, Berenstein A: Interventional Neuroradiology. *In:* Edwards MSB, Hoffman HJ (eds): Cerebrovascular Disease in Childhood and Adolescence (in press).

# VII Miscellaneous Diseases

50
EPILEPSY SURGERY IN CHILDHOOD

John K. Vries, M.D.
Patricia K. Crumrine, M.D.
Richard M. Dasheiff, M.D.

Epilepsy is a paroxysmal disorder of the nervous system brought about by abnormal discharges from groups of neurons in the brain. It is characterized by combinations of psychic experiences, altered consciousness, automatic or convulsive movements, and autonomic phenomena. Descriptions of major and minor epileptic seizures as well as the relationship between head injury and epilepsy are found in the Hippocratic writings of the fifth century BC.[43, 79] Modern descriptions of epilepsy date from the work of Hughlings Jackson, who classified epilepsy into generalized and partial forms.[46] This notion is still central in the classification scheme adopted by the International League against Epilepsy in 1981.[12] Effective drug treatment for epilepsy emerged in the earlier part of this century, with the introduction of phenobarbital in 1912 and phenytoin in 1937. Subsequently, dozens of antiepileptic drugs have been marketed abroad and in the United States.[90] However, a significant number of epilepsy patients remain refractory to medical therapy.[11, 72] That many of these patients may be cured by surgery will be the topic of this chapter.

Epilepsy is a common disorder throughout the world. This has been documented in epidemiologic studies over the past 50 years from the United States, England, Iceland, Japan, Norway, Israel, Africa, and the Mariana Islands.* These studies show an incidence that ranges from a low of 17.3 cases per 100,000 population to a high of 48.7 per 100,000. They show a prevalence ranging from 2.32 cases per 1000 population to 8.0 per 1000. The most thorough study in the United States was conducted by Hauser and Kurland.[41] They performed a detailed survey of the population of Rochester, Minnesota, from 1935 to 1967, with respect to age, sex, and seizure type. Using a population figure of 240,000,000 for the United States, the incidence and prevalence figures from this study predict 116,880 new cases of epilepsy per year, with a total epilepsy population of 1,368,000. The study also predicts that more than half the epilepsy population will suffer from partial seizures. Applying the therapeutic failure rates documented by Rodin to the total epileptic population indicates that 200,000 to 300,000 patients in this country suffer from uncontrolled seizures.[72] Rodin's figures also show that the majority of these therapeutic failures are in the partial seizure category, with complex partial seizures being the most common subtype.

There has been an increased realization in recent years that most patients who suffer from intractable seizure disorders have the onset of this process in childhood. Ounsted and coworkers[64] estimated that 10 percent of all seizures in childhood were complex partial seizures. In 100 children with this disorder, they found a median age of five years and four months. Glaser and Dixon[35] put the figure for com-

---

*References 3, 5, 10, 34, 38, 41, 49, 51–54, 74.

plex partial seizures much higher. They estimated that 30 percent of all childhood seizures fell into this category. In a follow-up study of 74 Danish patients who had undergone temporal lobectomy for intractable complex partial epilepsy, Jensen[48] found that 90 percent of the seizure disorders had originated before the age of 20, and 49 percent had originated before the age of ten. Falconer[27] reported that 46 percent of his temporal lobectomy patients had seizure onset in the first decade of life. These findings have major implications in formulating therapeutic strategies for children with epilepsy. It is becoming increasingly recognized that uncontrolled seizure disorders in childhood have a devastating effect on development, socialization, and education. Several studies of school-age children with epilepsy who were educated in normal schools demonstrate below-average intelligence in 31 to 69 percent.[42, 44] Behavior disturbances were seen in 21 percent of one of the populations.[44] It is also clear that prolonged antiepileptic drug therapy has adverse effects on cognition, memory, behavior, and motor development in a significant number of children.[73] These facts make a strong case for considering surgical intervention in children with intractable partial seizure disorders. Further evidence for this viewpoint is provided by the study of Vaernet,[81] who showed that 61 percent of patients who underwent temporal lobectomy for intractable complex partial seizures between the ages of 4 and 17 were functioning normally in long-term follow-up. Only 30 percent of patients between the ages of 17 and 56 who underwent this operation had similar results.[81]

HISTORICAL SURVEY OF EPILEPSY SURGERY

Focal Excision

The earliest known surgical procedure was cranial trephination. According to many authorities, this was performed for the relief of epilepsy.[84] In his monograph "On the Sacred Disease," Hippocrates gave directions for trephination of the skull, on the side opposite the focal seizure, to relieve "phlegm" producing the seizure disorder.[43] The concepts that form the basis for modern epilepsy surgery, however, did not emerge until the latter part of the nineteenth century. The most important of these were the principles of cortical localization expounded by Dax, Bouillard, and Broca, the observations by Jackson of the march of convulsive seizures, and the demonstration by Fritsch and Hitzig that electric stimulation of the cerebral cortex could elicit movements from the opposite extremities.[84] Also important was the development of anesthesia and asepsis. The first craniotomies for epilepsy in the modern era were performed by Sir Victor Horsley. In 1886, in an article entitled "Brain Surgery," he described three patients in whom a local subpial excision of scar tissue led to a cure of epilepsy.[45, 45a] Following World War I, Foerster and Penfield[31] reported success in treating 12 patients with long-standing epilepsy by excision of damaged brain tissue. Most of the injuries resulted from gunshot wounds or birth trauma. They formulated the theory that the contraction of cicatricial tissue in the area of injury was responsible for the epileptic process.[31] Penfield continued this work in Montreal, performing the first temporal lobectomy for focal epilepsy in 1928. By 1950, Penfield had collected a series of 68 patients treated with temporal lobectomy, with a 55 percent success rate for relief of seizures.[67]

The invention of electroencephalography by Berger in 1929 provided the basis for the next advances in the understanding and treatment of epilepsy.[4] In 1938, Gibbs reported a characteristic 4–6 per second EEG pattern associated with seizure disorders with illusional and hallucinatory components. He coined the term "psychomotor epilepsy" to describe this class of patients.[33] Shortly thereafter, Jasper and Kershman[47] determined that the majority of these patients have abnormal spiking activity in the anterior temporal lobe, and that this activity tends to be unilateral. Bailey built on these findings to introduce intraoperative electroencephalography.[2] He became one of the first advocates of epilepsy surgery based on electric findings alone. This position was soon adopted by Green,[36] Morris,[62] and Penfield.[66] From there, it was taken up by Guillaume,[39] Paillas,[65] deVet,[17] Obrador,[63] and Falconer.[29]

The center formed by Falconer became the major center for epilepsy surgery in Europe for the next two decades. Falconer altered the technique of temporal lobectomy, introducing the concept of en bloc resection including the amygdala and the anterior hippocampus. Pathologic examination of these complete specimens extended the understanding of the pathologic changes in temporal lobe epilepsy. Rasmussen, who has one of the largest personal experiences with temporal lobectomy in the world, noted that 10 percent of all epilepsy surgery in the 1930's involved the temporal lobe. By the 1940's, this had risen to 25 percent. By the 1950's, it had reached 50 percent, and today it accounts for two thirds of all cases.[68] In 1975, Jensen surveyed temporal lobectomy around the world and found 2282 published cases.[48] At follow-up, two thirds of the patients were free or nearly free of seizures. Moreover, one half the patients who were mentally abnormal prior to surgery had returned to normal. It is now well established that focal cortical excision in properly selected cases can lead to cure of epilepsy, without major morbidity. This is particularly true for complex partial seizure disorders associated with unilateral temporal lobe abnormalities.

Corpus Callosum Section

In 1940, Erickson[25] published the results of his research in the monkey on the spread of epileptic discharges from one hemisphere to the other. He concluded that the spread occurs largely if not entirely through the corpus callosum.[25] In that same year, Van Wagenen and Herren[83] reported the first human commissurotomy for epilepsy. They based the operation on the observation that patients with epilepsy who also had progressive lesions involving the corpus callosum experienced a decreased level of seizures. They eventually performed 26 corpus callosum sections. Most of the operations were performed in two stages. Four of the reported cases also had section of one fornix, and one had division of the anterior commissure. There appeared to be significant improvement in the seizure disorders in all these patients, although the follow-up for these patients was only a few months. In 1944, Akelaitis[1] studied the first group of Van Wagenen's patients and concluded that corpus callosum section had no major effect on cognitive function. Bogen began to perform this operation for epilepsy in 1962.[6, 8] Over the next decade, he performed 15 callosotomies. The results in ten of these cases are reported in a 1975 paper.[9] Bogen's operation was systematic and extensive. He divided the entire corpus callosum, the dorsal and ventral hippocampal commissures, the anterior commissure, and the massa intermedia. Many of his patients had stormy postoperative courses but good long-term results with respect to seizure control. All patients still required antiepileptic medication, but the frequency of atonic spells, generalized tonic-clonic seizures, and absence attacks was reduced by more than 90 percent, and some patients were seizure free. Many of Bogen's patients were studied by Gazzaniga and Sperry,[32] providing much of the information in the literature about the "split-brain" syndrome. All of Bogen's earlier patients displayed a disconnection syndrome when carefully tested. Toward the end of his series, he treated two patients, in whom he limited the callosal section to the anterior two thirds. In these patients, careful neuropsychologic testing revealed no measurable dysfunction.[71] He concluded that sparing the splenium of the corpus callosum was all that was necessary to prevent a disconnection syndrome. In 1971, Luessenhop and coworkers[57] selected four children with intractable seizure disorders and unilateral brain damage for corpus callosum section. The results were good, and they suggested this operation as an alternative to hemispherectomy.

In the 1970's, corpus callosum section was popularized by Wilson, who performed 20 operations in two series.[88, 89] In the last few years, the operation has gained increasing acceptance as a legitimate tool in the surgical treatment of epilepsy. In 1986, at the International Conference on the Surgical Treatment of Epilepsy at Palm Desert, 120 cases of corpus callosum section from centers around the world were discussed in a workshop.[20] Although there was no uniformity in approach, technique, or indications, several common themes emerged. Most centers performed an anterior two-thirds section as part of a two-stage operation. Frequently, the second part of the operation was not deemed necessary. Few clinical effects are apparent from anterior two-thirds callosotomies. Most patients were significantly improved, with respect to generalized seizures. This is particularly true for patients with atonic spells, and patients with partial seizures that became secondarily generalized. Some patients were rendered seizure free, but most continued to require antiepileptic medication and had occasional seizures. There was a consensus that the operation should be reserved for those intractable patients who were not candidates for focal excision. It was clear that corpus callosum section could benefit properly selected patients in the childhood epilepsy group.

THE NATURAL HISTORY OF EPILEPSY IN CHILDHOOD

It is well-known that a significant percentage of children with epilepsy "outgrow" their seizure disorders. This was well documented in a recent study by Thurston and coworkers,[80] who withdrew anticonvulsant medication from 148 children who had been seizure free on a long-term basis. Only 28 percent of the children experienced recurrent seizures over a follow-up period ranging from 15 to 23 years. However, the seizure type, in a large percentage of the recurrent patients, was "Jacksonian" or "psychomotor." This study does not address the group of childhood seizure disorders that were never well controlled.

A similar recurrence (31 percent) was found by Emerson and colleagues[19] in a population of 68 children withdrawn from medication after a mean seizure-free interval of 4.9 years.[59] These authors noted that risk of recurrence was greatest in those patients with seizure onset before two years of age, with many generalized seizures before control was established, and with a paroxysmal pattern on the electroencephalogram before medication was discontinued. We know from the work of Rodin[72] that most of these patients suffer from partial seizures.

The good prognosis for patients with epilepsy who are treated with medications is repeatedly being re-evaluated, and the results are disturbing. Excellent studies by Elwes and associates[18] and Mattson and coworkers[59] have found that only 39 percent of adults can achieve complete seizure control after one year of treatment. Even in the most favorable childhood epilepsy—pure absence (petit mal)—20 percent of the patients persist in having seizures into adulthood. In children with tonic-clonic or other types of seizures as well as absence, up to 90 percent have medically refractory epilepsy into adulthood.[61] Deonna and associates[15] studied 107 neurologically normal children with partial seizures. The syndrome of benign partial epilepsy of children with rolandic spikes was clearly identified, and its uniformly benign final prognosis was confirmed in 95 percent of the patients. However, the number of children with all other types of partial seizures who remained seizure free for five years was less than 30 percent. Despite the use of the latest antiepileptic drugs combined with sound medical management, many patients remain intractable. Reynolds and colleagues[71] have reviewed the subject of why epilepsy becomes intractable and note that the course is set in the first two years of treatment. Dasheiff and associates[13] have extended this work by evaluating the efficacy of second-line antiepileptic drugs in the treatment of patients who have failed first-line antiepileptic drugs. The majority of these patients failed on second-line drugs. Based on this study, Dasheiff recommends that suitable patients with partial epilepsy be referred for surgical evaluation after failing the first-line drugs, and that second-line drugs be reserved for nonsurgical candidates.

The most thorough study of children who are potential candidates for epilepsy surgery was conducted by Lindsay and coworkers.[56] They selected 100 patients with temporal lobe epilepsy from a clinic population of 1000 seizure patients in 1948. This group of patients has been continuously followed to the present day. Ten patients in this series had severe neurologic handicaps from infancy and were never considered for surgery. Thirty-two patients experienced spontaneous remission of seizures. In 78 percent of these patients, the remission occurred before the age of 13. All but two had remitted before age 16. Of the remaining 45, 16 were rejected for surgery because of technical reasons, and 13 underwent surgery. Most of the patients undergoing surgery had anterior temporal lobectomy. A high percentage of the patients not undergoing surgery developed severe psychiatric or behavioral disturbances. None of them made a spontaneous epileptic, social, psychiatric, or personality recovery. All of the 13 patients who underwent surgery made significant recoveries with respect to seizure control and socialization. Nine of these patients were gainfully employed on a long-term basis.

The psychiatric problems associated with epilepsy in children are considerable. In a study of 50 children younger than 17 years of age with intractable seizure disorders, Lindsay and colleagues[55] showed that major behavioral disorders had occurred in 44 patients. Following surgical treatment, none of these patients developed psychiatric problems as adults. Thirty-four were seizure-free, and 49 of the 50 had made demonstrable gains traceable to their surgery. The psychiatric implications of uncontrolled complex partial seizures are further documented by the study of 100 consecutive adult candidates for temporal lobectomy.[78] Taylor[78] found only 13 patients in this group with a normal mental state. Thirty were neurotic, 48 were psychopathic, 16 were psychotic, and 5 had "epileptic personality." Postoperatively, 32 patients were considered to have a normal mental state. These studies of adult patients suggest that abnormalities of mental status may be identifiable in early childhood, indicating those who are less likely to benefit from surgery. They also indicate that surgical intervention in properly selected patients can reverse this process.

SURGICAL EPILEPSY SERIES IN CHILDREN

Falconer[26] was the earliest advocate of temporal lobectomy in childhood for the treatment of temporal lobe epilepsy. In a 1970 paper, he reviewed the cases of nine children in a series of 100 temporal lobectomy patients. He noted that these patients as well as the majority of his adult patients had the onset of their disease during the first decade of life. Many had an onset below five years of age. The favorable results in his surgical series and the correlation between good seizure control and lower age at the time of operation led him to advocate temporal lobectomy at 10 to 12 years of age for those patients with refractory temporal lobe seizures.[28, 30]

A number of surgeons and institutions followed the lead of Falconer to extend temporal lobe surgery to childhood epilepsy patients. These included Rasmussen at Montreal, Vaernet at Copenhagen, Green at Phoenix, the Mayo Clinic group, and the group at the Hospital for Sick Children in Toronto.[14, 20, 37, 60, 69, 81] A summary of the results of these groups is shown in Table 50–1. Relief of seizures was obtained in three fourths of all patients treated. The younger patients also experienced an improvement in behavior and social adaptation in general. This is best documented in Vaernet's series, where 24 of 33 patients had significant behavioral disturbances before surgery, but 61 percent went on to good social adjustment and gainful employment on long-term follow-up.

Table 50–1. EPILEPSY SURGERY SERIES IN CHILDHOOD

Series	Total Cases	Number Controlled	Success (%)
Falconer	40	31	77
Rasmussen	72	53	73
Vaernet	33	27	82
Green	32	26	81
Mayo Clinic	50	39	78
Toronto	41	30	75
TOTAL	268	206	77

One of the main challenges in childhood epilepsy is to identify those patients who are medically intractable before puberty and to evaluate them in a comprehensive fashion to determine if they are candidates for surgery. If surgery can be accomplished before the completion of puberty, the outcome with respect to seizure control, socialization, and personality development appears favorable. Children should be considered medically intractable after a four-year period, using appropriate antiepileptic drugs with documented compliance, and with evidence that the antiepileptic drugs have been pushed individually, or in combination, to toxicity. Criteria for the selection of children for surgery are similar to those currently used for adults:

1. Documentation of intractability for four years or longer.
2. Failure to control seizures with aggressive medical management.
3. Impairment of cognition, behavior, socialization, or all three.
4. Documentation of typical seizures with surface, depth, or grid electrodes.

In 1983, a decision was made to establish an epilepsy center at the University of Pittsburgh to serve the needs of patients with intractable epilepsy in the tri-state region surrounding the city of Pittsburgh. This effort was undertaken as a joint venture between the Departments of Adult and Pediatric Neurology, and the Department of Neurosurgery. Overall sponsorship for the program was provided by the Office of the Senior Vice President for the Health Sciences at the University. In 1984, the program became operational, evaluating six patients. In 1985, the capacity had increased to 12 patients per year. By 1986, extensive protocols were established covering all phases of evaluation and treatment of intractable epilepsy. The Center currently has the capacity to evaluate 24 patients per year. When all phases of construction are complete, this capacity will rise to 48 per year.

The protocols that have been developed reflect the evaluation and treatment philosophies of the authors of this chapter. These philosophies are based largely on the material presented in the previous sections of this chapter. The salient points are

- Surgical treatment for intractable seizures should be instituted as early as possible. Surgery before the age of 12 is desirable if focality and intractability can be determined.
- Young patients with significant behavioral or psychiatric problems should not be excluded from surgical evaluation.
- Surgical decisions should be based primarily on depth electrode studies. Patients should be thoroughly screened by noninvasive CCTV/EEG recordings, neuropsychologic test batteries, and neuroradiologic investigation prior to invasive recording.
- The Center will concentrate on two types of seizure patients at the present time. The first group consists of patients with complex partial seizures of temporal or frontal lobe origin. The second group consists of patients with no clear-cut focus who are suffering from atonic spells or secondary generalization of partial seizures. The former group will be considered for anterior temporal lobectomy and frontal lobectomy. The latter group will be considered for corpus callosum section.
- All surgery will be done under general anesthesia (without intraoperative electrocorticography) following preoperative carotid amobarbital (Amytal) tests to assess speech dominance and memory function.
- The Center will strive to improve the efficiency of the evaluation protocols as technology evolves, to decrease the waiting time for the program and to lower patient and hospital costs.

These principles have been incorporated into a staged protocol that goes from phase 0 to phase IV. Phase 0 covers evaluation in the outpatient department. Phase I involves neuroradiologic screening, neuropsychologic testing, and CCTV/EEG evaluation. Phase II involves invasive monitoring, usually with stereotaxically placed depth electrodes. Phase III is surgical treatment. Phase IV consists of follow-up neuropsychologic assessment, and re-evaluation of the need for antiepileptic drugs. Selected patients may be considered for further surgery under special circumstances.

The Phase 0 Evaluation

Patients referred to the Center are first evaluated as outpatients. A careful history, physical examination, and neurologic examination are performed to establish a baseline and to identify any causative factors for the seizure disorder. An attempt is made to establish a close relationship with the patient through direct contact and through follow-up contact by a nurse clinician. This provides means for assessing psychosocial factors, adjustment, and compliance. Antiepileptic medications are carefully reviewed and an attempt is made to establish seizure control by optimizing levels of appropriate medications, using pharmacokinetic studies. Patients are often hospitalized for assessment of their antiepileptic drugs. Peak, trough, free, and bound levels are obtained, and doses are adjusted accordingly.

Patients who have not had satisfactory trials with all of the major antiepileptic drugs are systematically treated with these medications to see if control can be achieved. Patients with uncontrolled seizures for more than one year under optimal therapy are considered for the phase I waiting list. There is a waiting period of one to two years before a phase I work-up can be initiated. This provides time for additional manipulation of medications, and it gives more time to establish a rapport with the patient and the family, which is necessary to undertaking an epilepsy surgery work-up.

Phase I Evaluation

A phase I evaluation begins with a neuroradiologic investigation to identify structural lesions. Each patient receives a nuclear magnetic resonance imaging (NMRI) scan with extensive coronal cuts to evaluate the temporal lobes, the orbitofrontal cortex, and the insulae. This is supplemented by axial and parasagittal cuts. If the study shows no abnormalities, further studies are not done. If there is a question regarding the NMRI scan, complementary information is sought from a computed tomography (CT) scan, and a cerebral blood flow study is done using the nonradioactive xenon technique.[40, 91] Blood-flow abnormalities analogous to regions of hypometabolism on deoxyglucose positron emission tomography (PET) are sought.[21, 23]

Extensive neuropsychologic testing is performed during phase I. The purpose is to determine the general level of function of the individual as a baseline, to gather specific information about dysfunction that may have localizing value, and to assess language.

The mainstay of phase I is prolonged CCTV/EEG recording. Recording is carried out until at least one typical seizure can be captured on videotape for analysis. It is preferable to obtain this seizure without having to adjust the patient's antiepileptic drug regimen. An important part of this testing is to evaluate properly the results for the presence of pseudoseizures. The incidence of pseudoseizures in patients with true epileptic seizures is significant, and their detection can be quite difficult.[16, 50] It is essential that the Center rule out pseudoseizures as the cause of medical intractability before proceeding to invasive studies. Analysis of interictal activity also provides guidance for the next phase of evaluation. The recording facilities used for this phase of the work-up are shown in Figure 50–1.

Phase II Evaluation

The majority of patients entering phase II have complex partial seizures with a suspected focus in the temporal or frontal lobe. Depth electrodes suitable for screening the mesial temporal lobe, the orbitofrontal cortex, and the supplementary motor area are inserted stereotaxically, using the technique published by Lunsford and associates.[58] Patients are first weaned from any medication that could interfere with blood coagulation, such as valproic acid. Typically, four electrodes are employed. They consist of stainless-steel, flexible, twisted wires with

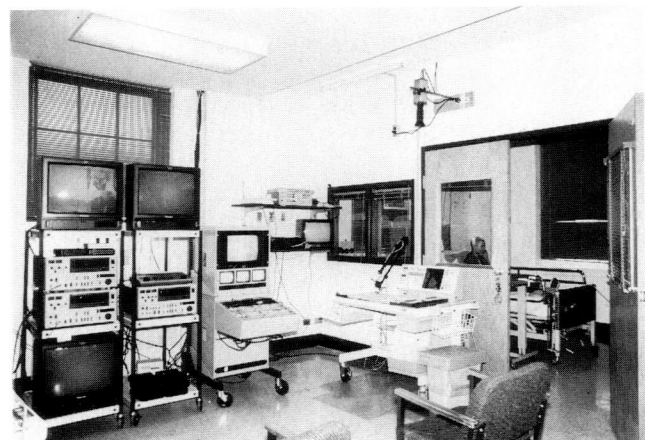

Figure 50–1. CCTV/EEG recording suite. The patient and the EEG trace are recorded by television cameras. The output is displayed on a color monitor as a split-screen image. The split-screen images are stored on video tape for review.

six active contacts at 0.5 or 1 cm intervals. One of these electrodes is shown in Figure 50–2. The procedure is carried out with the patient under general anesthesia. The stereotaxic frame employed is the Leksell frame. A CT stereotaxic operating room incorporating a GE 8800 scanner provides the means to insert the electrodes and immediately check for proper position and for the possibility of intracranial hematoma. A picture of the operating room set-up is shown in Figure 50–3. The temporal electrodes are inserted from an occipital approach. The anteriormost electrode is placed in the amygdala. The remainder of the electrode chain parallels the hippocampal formation. The approach is similar to that employed by Spencer and colleagues.[77] The insertion technique is shown in Figure 50–4. The frontal electrodes are placed at the level of the coronal suture. The distal electrodes record from the orbitofronal cortex. The proximal electrodes parallel the supplementary motor cortex. The position of the

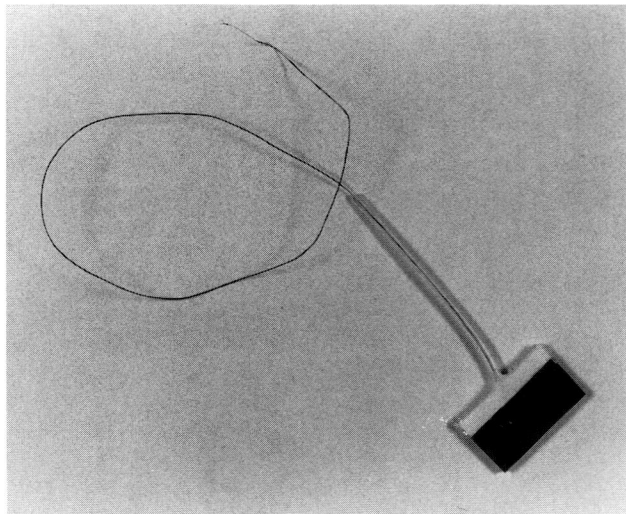

Figure 50–2. Depth electrode with six active contacts at 1-cm intervals.

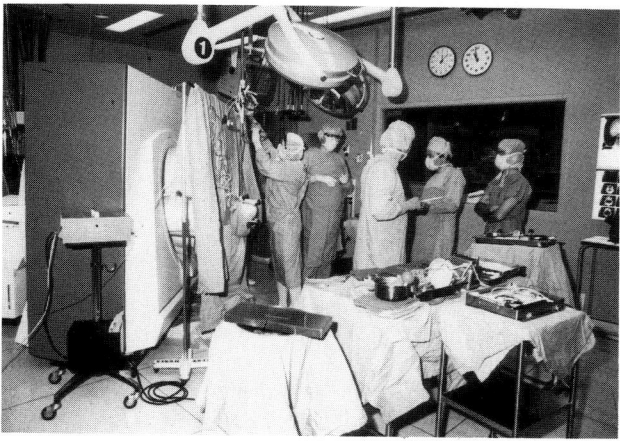

Figure 50–3. CT stereotaxic operating room. A GE 8800 CT scanner is used to determine the coordinates for the depth electrodes. It is also used postoperatively to check placement and to screen for intracranial bleeding.

temporal electrode chains in a postoperative CT cut is shown in Figure 50–5. Recordings are carried out from the depth electrodes on a daily basis until enough seizures have been captured for accurate analysis. Again, it is optimal not to taper the patient off all antiepileptic drugs, as this may produce seizures from brain areas not normally involved in the habitual seizures.[22] This point is contested by others.[76] Nevertheless, there is a clear risk for inducing convulsive seizures and status epilepticus when withdrawing antiepileptic drugs in these patients. Independent of whether drugs are tapered, it seems to take two to six weeks of recording to obtain a reliable database for surgical decisions. Figure 50–6 shows the appearance of a complex partial seizure recorded from depth electrodes.

After a sufficient number of seizures have been analyzed, additional tests are employed to investigate abnormalities in brain tissue excitability, as proposed by Engel and associates.[24] These include thiopental sodium activation and afterdischarge thresholds.

The thiopental sodium test is performed by a neuroanesthesiologist. Twenty-five mg boluses of thiopental are injected intravenously every 30 seconds until the corneal reflex is lost, or the patient becomes hypoxic or hypotensive. The authors have had no complications from this test, and the usual dose has ranged from 300 mg to 1000 mg. The EEG is monitored using depth electrodes. Barbiturates normally produce fast activity (beta) in the EEG. The absence of this physiologic response in a temporal or frontal lobe implies focal cerebral dysfunction. This dysfunction has been associated with the focal pathology accompanying epilepsy. The thiopental may also induce activation of focal interictal

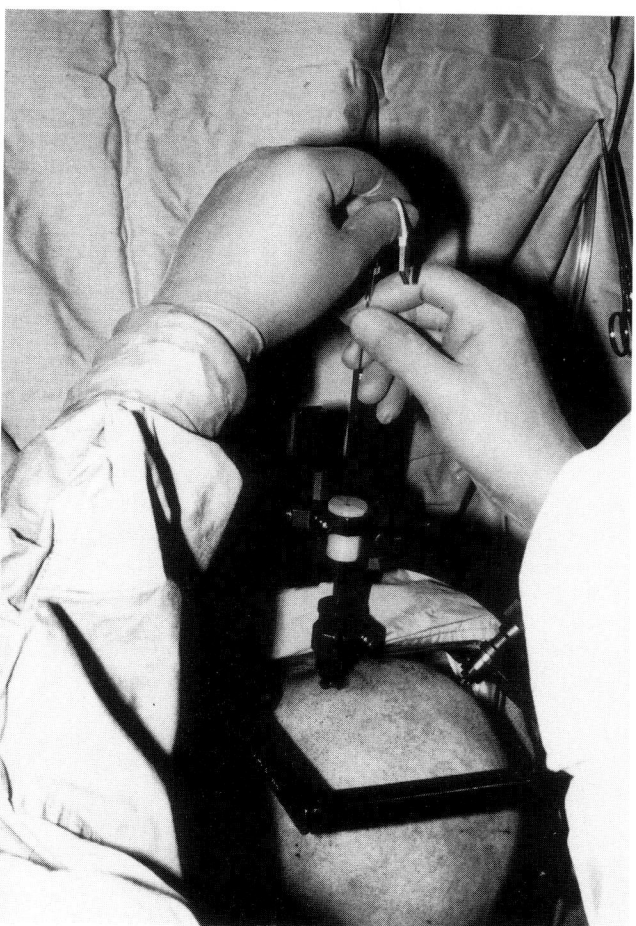

Figure 50–4. Stereotaxic insertion of temporal depth electrodes, using an occipital approach. The electrode is introduced through a twist drill hole.

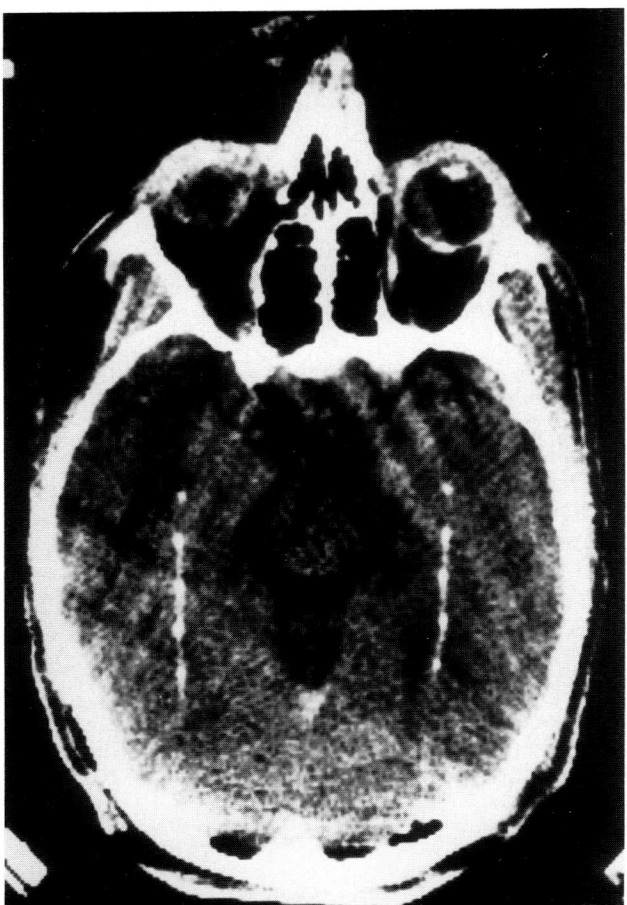

Figure 50–5. Axial CT cut showing the temporal depth electrode chains. The first recording contact is placed in the region of the amygdala. The posterior contacts parallel the hippocampal formation.

epileptiform activity. This abnormal excitation has also been associated with the epileptic focus.

Electric stimulation of normal brain can produce a limited electrographic seizure. This is termed an afterdischarge. The threshold for producing such afterdischarges varies throughout the brain and is lowest in the hippocampus. The purpose of the afterdischarge threshold test is to determine the relative thresholds in homologous regions. The side with the higher threshold has been associated with focal pathology that may be the cause, or result, of the epileptic region. The usual paradigm uses 1 msec biphasic square wave pulses, 10 or 30 hertz, 10 sec in duration, applied between adjacent contacts on the depth electrode. The voltage is stepped from 5 to 10 to 14 volts after each negative response. The impedance between contacts usually runs between 40 to 60 Kohms. When an afterdischarge is obtained, the next pair may be stimulated with only a short rest. Asymmetries between homologous regions are best evaluated when afterdischarges can be elicited bilaterally. Although the absence of an afterdischarge may reflect an abnormally high threshold, it can also result from technical factors.

The intracarotid sodium amobarbital test is performed on all patients older than ten years of age, prior to temporal lobe surgery. The interpretation of the results concerning memory, however, remains controversial. No two centers around the world do the test the same way, and even the evaluation of lateralization of language is not standard.[70] However, all centers do agree that the test is essential and that it can provide unique information of pivotal importance to the therapeutic decision-making process.

Phase III Evaluation

Patients are selected as candidates for surgery, based on laterality and localization of ictal seizure activity. Ideally, all seizure activity should originate in the same lobe on the same side of the brain. Candidates who have a preponderance of activity on one side and one lobe are also considered if the ancillary information is consistent with the predominant site. Patients who are clearly multifocal or nonlocalized are considered for corpus callosum section if generalized seizures constitute a major component of their seizure disorder.

Operative Indications

Anterior Temporal Lobectomy

Anterior temporal lobectomy is one of the most common and successful operations performed for intractable seizures.[48] The main indications for this operation at the Center are depth electrode recordings of ictal events (complex partial seizures) that have a unilateral anterior temporal lobe onset. Patients are also considered for this operation if the majority of ictal events (two thirds) originate on one side, or if all activity originates on one side and at least half originates in the anterior temporal lobe. In these latter cases, confirmatory evidence localizing the seizure disorder must be obtained from ancillary tests. These tests include analysis of interictal discharge patterns, neuropsychologic testing, neuroradiologic imaging, and the thiopental and afterdischarge threshold tests. All potential candidates are subjected to a carotid amobarbital test. The main function of this test is to demonstrate that memory function will be supported by the remaining temporal lobe. If memory function is not adequately supported, the operation is not performed. In special cases, a limited operation confined to the temporal neocortex is considered in patients who have failed this test.[85]

Frontal Lobectomy

Frontal lobectomy is the next most common operation for intractable seizures. Approximately 10 to 20 percent of complex partial seizures with or without secondary generalization originate in the

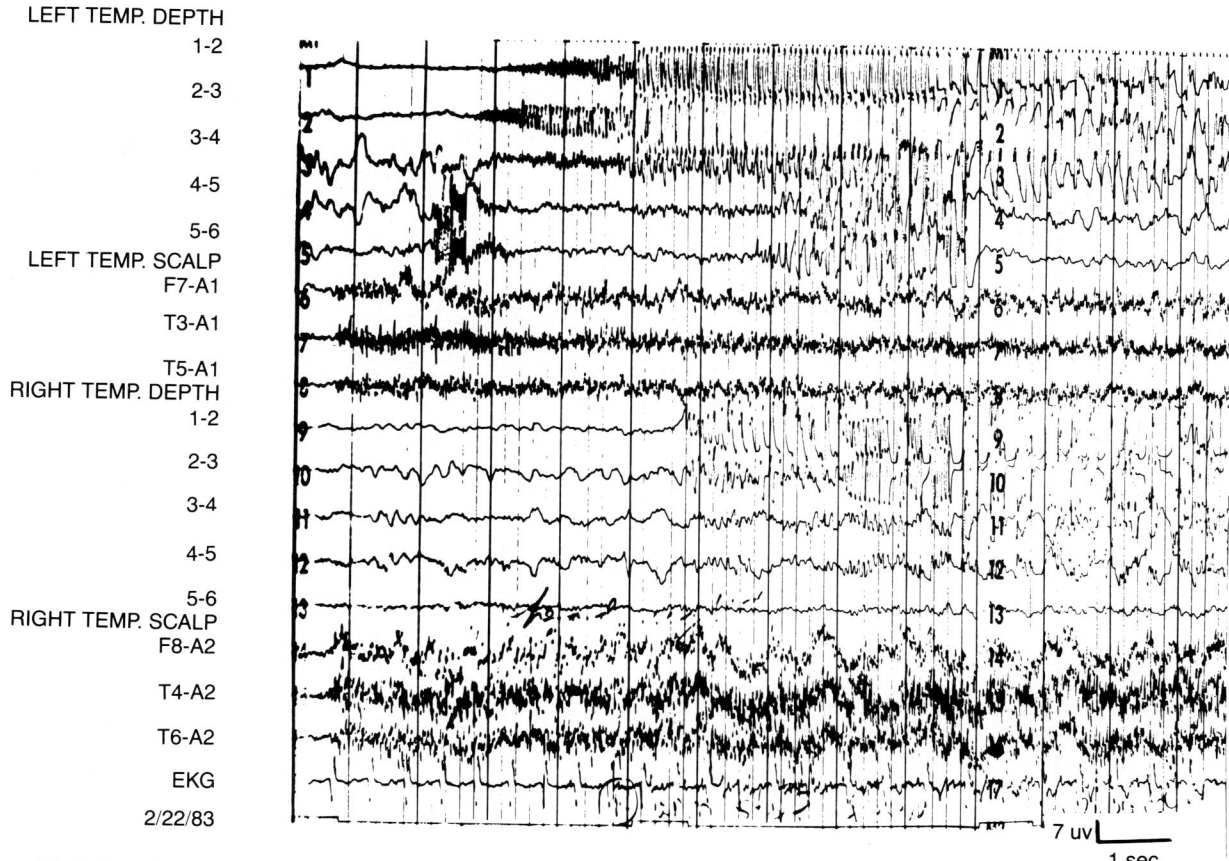

Figure 50–6. Complex partial seizure recorded from depth electrodes. The seizure begins in the anterior contacts of the left temporal electrode. It is not seen in the simultaneous EEG tracings from the scalp. It spreads to the right temporal depth electrode several seconds later. At this point, the patient experienced his typical complex partial seizure.

frontal lobe.[87] The main indication for this operation is also depth electrode recordings of ictal events showing that the seizures originate from the same side and the same lobe. Patients having a predominance of seizures (two thirds) from one side are considered for operation using the same ancillary methods described for temporal lobectomy. Patients with unilateral ictal activity with an even distribution between the frontal lobe and the temporal lobe are offered temporal lobectomy with the possibility of frontal lobe surgery at a later date.

A special circumstance exists for seizure disorders that originate in the frontal lobes because of the rich interconnection of the frontal lobes by pathways through the corpus callosum that support rapid spread of electric activity. This tends to make unilateral ictal activity look like bilateral synchronous activity. In some cases, this problem can be resolved by weighing the evidence provided by the ancillary studies. When this is not the case, the authors have resorted to anterior section of the corpus callosum followed by re-evaluation with depth electrodes after six months to one year, if the seizures fail to resolve. The objective is to perform an operation that may benefit the seizure disorder as well as isolate the focus. This approach has been taken by Wada[82] and by Williamson.[86]

Corpus Callosum Section

Corpus callosum section is reserved for those patients who are either multifocal or unlocalized following depth electrode evaluation, who are suffering major morbidity from the generalized components of their seizure disorders. Particular emphasis is placed on selecting patients who have atonic spells resulting in frequent injury, or patients with complex partial seizures who have frequent secondary generalization. The fact that control of generalized seizures might result in worsening of partial seizures is carefully considered.[75] Corpus callosum section is performed as a two-stage operation. The first stage consists of an anterior two-thirds callosotomy. Patients are considered for completion of callosotomy 12 to 18 months later if their seizure disorders are not significantly improved.

Operative Technique

Anterior Temporal Lobectomy

Anterior temporal lobectomy is carried out with the patient under general anesthesia and with the patient's head secured in a headholder in the lateral position. The operation is performed through a large question-mark incision similar to that used by Falconer.[29] A large osteoplastic frontotemporal bone flap is employed to gain access to the anterior temporal lobe. The dura is opened to provide access from the temporal pole to the vein of Labbé. The temporal lobectomy begins by marking a point on the middle temporal gyrus that is 5 cm from the temporal tip if the operation is on the side of speech dominance, and 5.5 cm if it is not on the side of speech dominance. Serial coronal NMRI scan cuts through the temporal lobe are reviewed to facilitate this marking. A vertical pial incision is made in the middle temporal gyrus at the site of this mark and carried inferiorly beneath the temporal lobe to within 1 cm of the incisura. A parallel incision is made 1 cm anterior to this incision. The intervening cerebral tissue is removed by suction to create a 1-cm "corridor" in the temporal lobe. The lateral ventricle is next identified by working from interior to superior in this corridor. This portion is done under the operating microscope. The presence of the corridor makes retractors unnecessary and ensures easy identification of the lateral horn. Once the ventricle is identified, a pathway from the ventricle to the sylvian fissure that slants forward at an angle of 45 degrees is mapped on the temporal lobe surface. The forward slant spares the posterior portion of the superior temporal gyrus, providing greater safety with respect to postoperative speech impairment. A pial incision that follows this pathway is carried to the sylvian fissure and then anteriorly to the limen insulae. An attempt is made to preserve a thin layer of brain tissue over the middle cerebral vessels for protection. The pes hippocampus is then divided with a blunt knife, and the temporal lobe is separated by opening the choroidal fissure to the amygdala, then joining the incision at the limen by resecting the amygdala by suction. If the operation requires any retraction in a superior or medial direction to open the choroidal fissure, the operation is carried lateral to the pes hippocampus, and the neocortex is removed as a separate specimen. The amygdala and hippocampus are then removed by suction. The appearance of a typical temporal lobe resection site is shown in Figure 50–7.

Frontal Lobectomy

Frontal lobectomy is carried out with the patient under general anesthesia and in the supine position. A large, bicoronal incision and a unilateral free bone flap are used to gain access to the frontal lobe. After opening a mesially based dural flap, the mesial surface of the frontal lobe is mobilized using the operating microscope. Frequently, there are significant adhesions due to multiple bouts of trauma, and the cingulate gyri are often adherent. The anterior cerebral and callosomarginal arteries as well as the corpus callosum are identified. A pial incision is next outlined on the surface of the frontal lobe, extending from the region of the coronal suture to the region of the anterior sylvian fissure. This incision is deepened by suction passing just anterior to the frontal horn of the lateral ventricle. It is then developed inferiorly beneath the frontal lobe, paralleling the sphenoid wing. The surface and inferior incisions are joined mesially, sparing the anterior cerebral and callosomarginal arteries. The olfactory bulb on the operated side is sacrificed. The remaining white matter is divided by suction, and the specimen is removed en bloc. The extent of the operation is shown in the postoperative NMRI scan in Figure 50–8.

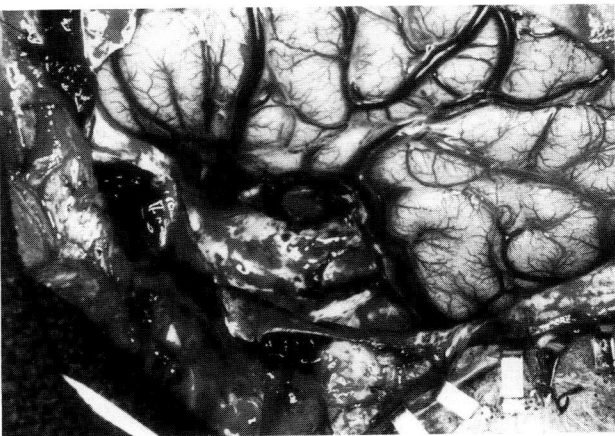

Figure 50–7. Temporal lobe resection site. The resection has been carried posteriorly to the vein of Labbé. The amygdala and the anterior hippocampal formation have been included in the mesial portion of the resection.

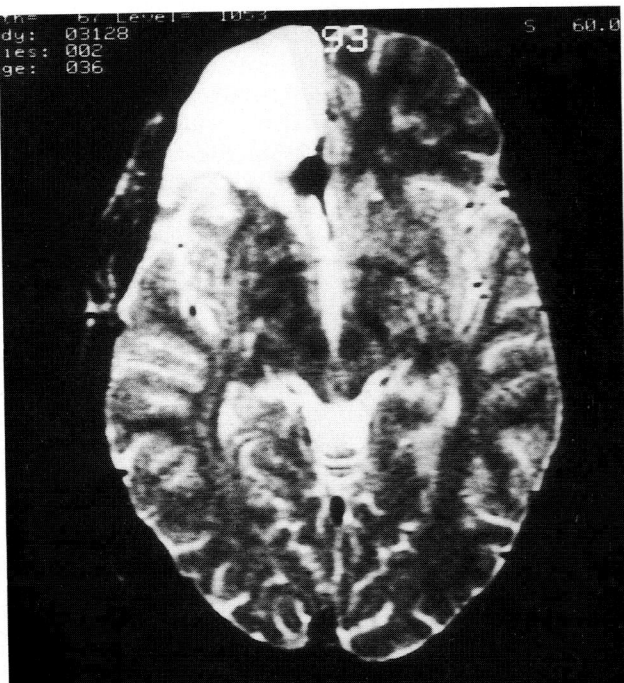

Figure 50–8. Axial cut from a nuclear magnetic resonance (NMR) image showing the extent of a typical frontal lobe resection for epilepsy. Posteriorly, the resection extends to the level of the coronal suture. It includes all of the orbitofrontal cortex.

Corpus Callosum Section

Anterior Callosal Section. Anterior callosal section is carried out with the patient in the supine position and under general anesthesia. A bicoronal incision and a square bone flap whose posterior margin lies on the coronal suture is used for exposure. The mesial surface of the hemisphere is first mobilized using the operating microscope and gentle lateral retraction. The adhesions between the hemispheres are dissected until both anterior cerebral arteries and the corpus callosum are identified. An incision is then made in the corpus callosum, at the level of the foramen of Monro, with a blunt knife entering the lateral ventricle. This incision is carried posteriorly between the anterior cerebral arteries to the level of the trigone of the lateral ventricle. It is then carried anteriorly to the rostrum of the corpus callosum. At this point, the incision is continued lateral to the anterior cerebral artery until the rostrum is divided to the point opposite where the forniceal column becomes the anterior lip of the foramen of Monro. The problems related to opening the lateral ventricle described by Wilson have not been experienced by the author.[89]

Posterior Callosal Section. Posterior callosal section is carried out with the patient under general anesthesia and in the prone position. A "reverse bicoronal incision" and a square bone flap whose anterior margin is at the level of the vein of Trolard are used for exposure. A mesially based dural flap is developed to gain access to the mesial surface of the hemisphere. The interhemispheric adhesions are dissected in a fashion similar to that described for anterior callosal section. The splenium of the corpus callosum is then divided between the pericallosal arteries until the vein of Galen is fully exposed. A combination of blunt knife and suction dissection is employed. The vein of Galen is then traced forward until the internal cerebral veins are identified. The posterior third ventricle is entered by dissecting between these veins. The division of the corpus callosum is then carried forward to the

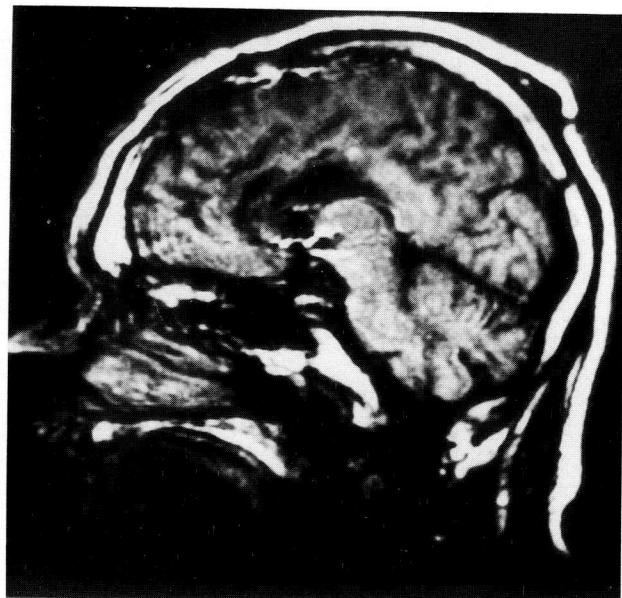

Figure 50–9. Midline cut from an NMR scan on a patient who has undergone an anterior corpus callosum section.

level where the forniceal columns come together in the roof of the third ventricle. The postoperative appearance of the NMRI scan of a patient who underwent an anterior corpus callosum section is shown in Figure 50–9.

Phase IV Evaluation

Patients are admitted to the hospital one month after surgery for an intensive follow-up evaluation that includes neuropsychologic testing, speech evaluation, a scalp EEG, an NMRI scan, and antiepileptic blood levels. Those patients who are completely free of seizures including auras are started on a six-month taper off their antiepileptic medications. Medication is immediately reinstituted if seizures occur. Long-term follow-up is handled in the out-

Table 50–2. EARLY PROTOCOL EVALUATIONS FOR INTRACTABLE SEIZURES

Name	Age/Sex	Depth	Amytal	Operation	Outcome
J.P.	8 M	+		Not offered	
K.S.	9 M			Focal excision	Seizure free
E.A.	9 M			Focal excision	Improved
K.C.	11 M			Focal excision	Seizure free
S.H.	14 F		+	Temp. lobectomy	Seizure free
D.L.	17 F			Focal excision	Improved
D.B.	20 M	+		Temp. lobectomy	Seizure free
T.S.	23 M	+	+	Temp. lobectomy	Improved
G.B.	23 M	+		Not offered	
T.G.	24 M		+	Temp. lobectomy	Seizure free
A.M.	25 M	+		Ant. callosotomy	Improved
R.C.	21 M			Not offered	
A.Z.	30 M		+	AP callosotomy	Improved
J.C.	32 F	+	+	Temp. lobectomy	Seizure free
T.K.	43 M	+		Not offered	
R.M.	30 M	+		Not offered	

Table 50-3. RECENT PROTOCOL EVALUATIONS FOR INTRACTABLE SEIZURES

Name	Age/Sex	Depth	Thiopental	Stimulation	Amytal	Operation	Outcome
G.M.	31 M	+	+		++	Temp. lobectomy	Too Recent
J.M.	32 F	+	+	+	+	Temp. lobectomy	Seizure free
L.K.	25 M	++	+		+	Frontal lobectomy	Improved
T.G.	33 M	+	+		+	Temp. lobectomy	Seizure free
G.B.	29 M	+	+	+		Not offered	
A.R.	22 F	++	+		+	Ant. callosotomy	Not improved
L.R.	9 F					Not offered	
J.H.	14 M	+	+	+	+	Frontal lobectomy	Too recent
T.G.	16 F	+	+	+	+	Temp. lobectomy	Too recent
C.E.	36 M	+	+	+	+	Temp. lobectomy	Too recent

patient program similar to the phase 0 protocol. Patients are initially seen on a monthly basis. When the clinical picture is stable, follow-up continues at three-month intervals. It is important to maintain close contact with the patient and the family during the first three months after surgery. Patients are reluctant to report adverse affects of surgery or recurrent seizure activity. A self-limited but significant postsurgical depression is also common. It is important to provide full social service support following surgery as patients try to readjust to freedom from a condition that has produced lifelong disability.

PRELIMINARY RESULTS

A total of 26 patients have undergone protocol evaluations for intractable seizure disorders since the University of Pittsburgh Epilepsy Center was established. Because the Center is new, long-term follow-up is not available. The 26 patients represent a mixture of children and adults. All but two of these patients had onset of epilepsy in childhood. The first 16 patients went through an abbreviated version of the full protocol. A summary of their evaluations is presented in Table 50-2. A total of 12 operations were performed on 11 patients. The early results appear to be comparable to the results presented for the series in Table 50-2.

For the last six months, the full protocol workups outlined in this chapter have been carried out. A total of ten evaluations leading to eight operations have been carried out. A summary of these patients is shown in Table 50-3.

CONCLUSIONS

It is the long range goal of the Center to push the age for evaluation and treatment into the 10 to 12 range. It is clear from the medical literature that the opportunity to cure intractable seizure disorders with surgery decreases with older patients. Furthermore, it seems that the greatest chance to reverse personality disorders and socialization problems is with early surgery. Finally, adequate criteria for identifying these patients have been established. Children who have early onset of seizures that are not responsive to adequate dosages of appropriate antiepileptic medications are likely to remain intractable. The majority of children who undergo spontaneous remission of seizures do so before the age of 13. As many as one third of these children are cured by surgery, sparing them a lifetime of misery. The authors feel that there is adequate evidence to justify an aggressive approach to the treatment of childhood epilepsy. The challenge that lies ahead is to develop safer, cheaper, and quicker methods for evaluating children with intractable seizure disorders for surgery.

References

1. Akelaitis AJ: A study of gnosis, praxis and language following section of the corpus callosum and anterior commissure. J Neurosurg 1:94, 1944.
2. Bailey P, Gibbs FA: The surgical treatment of psychomotor epilepsy. JAMA 145:365, 1951.
3. Baldwin R, Davens E, Harris VG: The epilepsy program in public health. Am J Public Health 43:452, 1953.
4. Berger H: Uber das Elektroenkephalogramm des Menschen. Arch Psychiat Nervenkr 87:527, 1929.
5. Bird AV, Heinz HJ, Klintworth G: Convulsive disorders in Bantu mine workers. Epilepsia 3:175, 1962.
6. Bogen JE, Fisher ED, Vogel PJ: Cerebral commissurotomy. A second case report. JAMA 194:1328, 1965.
7. Bogen JE, Gordon HW, Sperry RW: Absence of deconnection syndrome in two patients with partial section of the neocommissures. Brain 94:327, 1971.
8. Bogen JE, Vogel PJ: Cerebral commissurotomy in man. Bull Los Angeles Neurol Soc 27:169, 1962.
9. Bogen JE, Vogel PJ: Neurologic status in the long-term following complete commissurotomy. In: Michel F, Schott B (eds): Les syndromes de disconnexion calleuse chez l'homme. Lyon, Lyon Hop Neurol, 1975, p 227.
10. Brewis M, Poskanzer D, Rolland C: Neurological disease in an English city. Acta Neurol Scand 42:1, 1966.
11. Coatsworth JJ: Studies on the clinical efficacy of marketed antiepileptic drugs. In: NINDS monograph no. 12. Washington, DC, U.S. Government Printing Office, 1971.
12. Commission on classification and terminology of the International League against Epilepsy: Proposal for revised clinical and electroencephalographic classification of epileptic seizures. Epilepsia 22:489, 1981.
13. Dasheiff RM, McNamara D, Dickinson L: Efficacy of second-line antiepileptic drugs in the treatment of patients with medically refractive complex partial seizures. Epilepsia 27:124, 1986.
14. Davidson S, Falconer MA: Outcome of surgery in forty children with temporal lobe epilepsy. Lancet 1:1260, 1975.
15. Deonna T, Ziegler AL, Despland PA, et al: Partial epilepsy

in neurologically normal children: Clinical syndromes and prognosis. Epilepsia 27:241, 1986.
16. Desai BT, Porter RJ, Penry JK: Psychogenic seizures. A study of 42 attacks in six patients, with intensive monitoring. Arch Neurol 39:202, 1982.
17. deVet AC: Temporal epilepsy, c.q. psychomotor epilepsy. Experiences and present-day conceptions. Schweiz Arch Neurol Neurochir Psychiatr 111:453, 1972.
18. Elwes RDS, Johnson AL, Shorvon SD, et al: The prognosis for seizure control in newly diagnosed epilepsy. N Engl J Med 311:944, 1984.
19. Emerson R, D'Souza BJ, Vining EP, et al: Stopping medication in children with epilepsy: Predictors of outcome. N Engl J Med 304:1125, 1981.
20. Engel J, Jr.: Surgical Management of the Epilepsies. New York, Raven Press, 1986.
21. Engel J, Jr., Brown WJ, Kuhl DE, et al: Pathological findings underlying focal temporal lobe hypometabolism in partial epilepsy. Ann Neurol 12:512, 1982.
22. Engel J, Jr., Crandall PH: Falsely localizing ictal onsets with depth EEG telemetry during anticonvulsant withdrawal. Epilepsia 24:344, 1983.
23. Engel J, Jr., Kuhl DE, Phelps ME, et al: Interictal cerebral glucose metabolism in partial epilepsy and its relation to EEG changes. Ann Neurol 12:510, 1982.
24. Engel J, Jr., Rausch R, Lieb JP, et al: Correlation of criteria used for localizing epileptic foci in patients considered for surgical therapy of epilepsy. Ann Neurol 9:215, 1981.
25. Erickson TC: Spread of the epileptic discharge. Arch Neurol Psychiatry 43:429, 1940.
26. Falconer MA: Significance of surgery for temporal lobe epilepsy in childhood and adolescence. J Neurosurg 33:233, 1970.
27. Falconer MA: Genetic and related aetiologic factors in temporal lobe epilepsy. A review. Epilepsia 12:13, 1971.
28. Falconer MA: Temporal lobe epilepsy in children and its surgical treatment. Med J Aust 1:1117, 1972.
29. Falconer MA, Hill D, Meyer A, et al: Treatment of temporal-lobe epilepsy by temporal lobectomy. A survey of findings and results. Lancet 268:827, 1955.
30. Falconer MA, Serafetinides EA: A follow-up study of surgery in temporal lobe epilepsy. J Neurol Neurosurg Psychiatry 26:154, 1963.
31. Foerster O, Penfield W: The structural basis of traumatic epilepsy and results of radical operation. Brain 53:99, 1930.
32. Gazzaniga MS, Bogen JE, Sperry RW: Some functional effects of sectioning the cerebral commissures in man. Proc Natl Acad Sci USA 48:1765, 1962.
33. Gibbs FA, Gibbs EL, Lennox WG: The likeness of cortical dysrhythmias of schizophrenia and psychomotor epilepsy. Am J Psychiatry 95:255, 1938.
34. Giel R: The problem of epilepsy in Ethiopia. Trop Geogr Med 22:439, 1970.
35. Glaser HG, Dixon MS: Psychomotor seizures in childhood. Neurology 6:646, 1956.
36. Green JR, Duisberg REH, McGrath WB: Focal epilepsy of psychomotor type. A preliminary report of observations on the effects of surgical therapy. J Neurosurg 8:157, 1951.
37. Green JR, Pootrakul A: Surgical aspects of the treatment of epilepsy during childhood and adolescence. Ariz Med 39:35, 1982.
38. Gudmundsson G: Epilepsy in Iceland: A clinical and epidemiological investigation. Acta Informatica Neurol Scand 43:1, 1966.
39. Guillaume J, Mazard G: Indications et resultats du traitement chirurgical des epilepsies temporales. Sem Hop Paris 32:2013, 1956.
40. Gur D, Good WF, Wolfson SK, Jr., et al: In vivo mapping of local cerebral blood flow by xenon-enhanced computed tomography. Science 215:1267, 1982.
41. Hauser WA, Kurland LT: The epidemiology of epilepsy in Rochester, Minnesota, 1935 through 1967. Epilepsia 16:1, 1975.
42. Henderson P: Epilepsy in school children. Br J Prev Soc Med 7:9, 1953.
43. Hippocrates: The sacred disease. In: Chadwick J, Mann WN (eds): Medical Works of Hippocrates. Oxford, Blackwell, 1950, p 189.
44. Holdsworth L, Whitmore K: A study of children with epilepsy attending ordinary schools. Dev Med Child Neurol 16:746, 1974.
45. Horsley V: Remarks on surgery of the central nervous system. Br Med J 2:1286, 1890.
45a. Horsley V: Brain surgery. Br Med J 2:670, 1886.
46. Jackson JH: On epilepsy and epileptiform convulsions. In: Taylor JA (ed): Selected Writings of J. Hughlings Jackson, Vol. 1. London, Hodder and Stoughton, 1931, p 500.
47. Jasper H, Kershman J: Electroencephalographic classification of the epilepsies. Arch Neurol Psychiatry 45:903, 1941.
48. Jensen I: Temporal lobe epilepsy: Types of seizures, age, and surgical results. Acta Neurol Scand 53:335, 1976.
49. Krohn W: A study of epilepsy in northern Norway, its frequency and character. Acta Psychiatry Neurol Scand 36:215, 1961.
50. Krumholz A, Niedermeyer E: Psychogenic seizures: A clinical study with follow-up data. Neurology 33:498, 1983.
51. Kurland LT: The incidence and prevalence of convulsive disorders in a small urban community. Epilepsia 1:143, 1959.
52. Leibowitz U, Alter M: Epilepsy in Jerusalem, Israel. Epilepsia 9:87, 1968.
53. Lessell S, Torres JM, Kurland LT: Seizure disorders in a Guamanian village. Arch Neurol (Chic) 7:37, 1962.
54. Levy LF, Forbes JI, Parirenyatwa T: Epilepsy in Africans. Central African J Med 10:241, 1964.
55. Lindsay J, Glaser G, Richards P, et al: Developmental aspects of focal epilepsies of childhood treated by neurosurgery. Dev Med Child Neurol 26:574, 1984.
56. Lindsay J, Ounsted C, Richards P: Long-term outcome in children with temporal lobe seizures. V: Indications and contraindications for neurosurgery. Dev Med Child Neurol 26:25, 1984.
57. Luessenhop AJ, Dela Cruz TD, Fenichel GM: Surgical disconnection of the cerebral hemispheres for intractable seizures. Results in infancy and childhood. JAMA 213:1630, 1970.
58. Lunsford LD, Latchaw RE, Vries JK: Stereotactic implantation of deep brain electrodes using computed tomography. Neurosurgery 13:280, 1983.
59. Mattson RH, Joyce JA, Collins JF, et al: Comparison of carbamazepine, phenobarbital, phenytoin, and primidone in partial and secondarily generalized tonic-clonic seizures. N Engl J Med 313:145, 1985.
60. Meyer FB, Marsh WR, Laws ER, Jr., et al: Temporal lobectomy in children with epilepsy. J Neurosurg 64:371, 1986.
61. Mirsky AF, Duncan CC, Myslobodsky MS: Petit mal epilepsy: A review and integration of recent information. J Clin Neurophysiol 3:179, 1986.
62. Morris AA: Temporal lobectomy with removal of uncus, hippocampus, and amygdala. Results for psychomotor epilepsy three to nine years after operation. Arch Neurol Psychiatry 76:479, 1956.
63. Obrador S: Personal experience in the surgical treatment of epilepsy. J Neurosurg 10:52, 1953.
64. Ounsted C, Lindsay J, Norman R: Biological Factors in Temporal Lobe Epilepsy. London, Heinemann, 1966.
65. Paillas JE, Gastaut H, Vigorouroux R, et al: Correlations anatomo-electro-cliniques dans l'epilepsie temporale: a propos des resultats obtenus chez 38 operes. Neurochirurgia 10:477, 1964.
66. Penfield W, Baldwin M: Temporal lobe seizures and the technic of subtotal temporal lobectomy. Ann Surg 136:625, 1952.
67. Penfield W, Flanigin H: Surgical therapy of temporal lobe seizures. Arch Neurol Psychiatry 64:491, 1950.
68. Rasmussen T: Surgical treatment of patients with complex partial seizures. In: Penry JK, Daly DD (eds): Complex Partial

Seizures and Their Treatment (Advances in Neurology, Vol. 2). New York, Raven Press, 1975, pp 415–449.
69. Rasmussen T: Surgical aspects of the treatment of epilepsy. *In*: Blaw M, Rapin I, Kinsbourne M (eds): Topics in Child Neurology. New York, Spectrum Publications, 1977, pp 143–57.
70. Rausch R: The neuropsychological evaluation. *In*: Engel J, Jr. (ed): Surgical Treatment of the Epilepsies. New York, Raven Press, 1986, (in press).
71. Reynolds EH, Elwes RDC, Shorvon SD: Why does epilepsy become intractable? Prevention of chronic epilepsy. Lancet 2:952, 1983.
72. Rodin EA: The Prognosis of Patients with Epilepsy. Springfield, IL, Charles C Thomas, 1968.
73. Sackellares JC: Pharmacologic management of epilepsy in childhood. *In*: Dreifuss FE (ed): Pediatric Epileptology. Littleton, MA, John Wright, 1983, pp 231–260.
74. Sato S: The epidemiological and clinico-statistical study of epilepsy in Niigata City. Part 2. The epidemiological study of epilepsy in Niigata City. Clin Neurol (Tokyo) 4:413, 1964.
75. Spencer SS, Spencer DD, Glaser GH, et al: More intense focal seizure types after callosal section: The role of inhibition. Ann Neurol 16:686, 1984.
76. Spencer SS, Spencer DD, Williamson PD, et al: Ictal effects of anticonvulsant medication withdrawal in epileptic patients. Epilepsia 22:297, 1981.
77. Spencer SS, Spencer DD, Williamson PD, et al: The localizing value of depth electroencephalography in 32 patients with refractory epilepsy. Ann Neurol 12:248, 1982.
78. Taylor DC: Mental state and temporal lobe epilepsy. A correlative account of 100 patients treated surgically. Epilepsia 13:727, 1972.
79. Temkin O: The Falling Sickness. Baltimore, Johns Hopkins Press, 1945, p 380.
80. Thurston JH, Thurston DI, O'Leary J: Prognosis in childhood epilepsy. Follow-up study of 148 cases in which therapy had been suspended after prolonged anticonvulsant control. N Engl J Med 286:170, 1972.
81. Vaernet K: Temporal lobotomy in children and young adults. Advances in Epileptology. The XIVth Epilepsy international symposium, New York, 1983, pp 255–261.
82. Wada J: Personal communication, 1986.
83. Van Wagenen WP, Herren RY: Surgical division of commissural pathways in the corpus callosum. Acta Neurol Psychiatr 44:740, 1940.
84. Walker AE: A History of Neurological Surgery. Baltimore, Williams & Wilkins, 1951.
85. Wieser HG: Electroclinical Features of the Psychomotor Seizure. New York, Butterworths, 1983.
86. Williamson PD: Corpus callosum section for intractable epilepsy. Criteria for patient selection. *In*: Reeves AG (ed): Epilepsy and the Corpus Callosum. New York, Plenum Press, 1985, pp 243–257.
87. Williamson PD, Spencer DD, Spencer SS, et al: Complex partial seizures of frontal lobe origin. Ann Neurol 18:497, 1985.
88. Wilson DH, Reeves A, Gazzaniga M: Division of the corpus callosum for uncontrollable epilepsy. Neurology 28:649, 1978.
89. Wilson DH, Reeves AG, Gazzaniga MS: "Central" commissurotomy for intractable generalized epilepsy: Series two. Neurology 32:687, 1982.
90. Woodbury DM, Penry JK, Pippinger CE: Antiepileptic Drugs. New York, Raven Press, 1982.
91. Yonas H, Good WF, Gur D, et al: Mapping cerebral blood flow by xenon-enhanced computed tomography: Clinical experience. Radiology 152:435, 1984.

51
HEMISPHERECTOMY FOR INTRACTABLE EPILEPSY

Harold J. Hoffman, M.D., B.Sc. (Med.)
Corey Raffel, M.D., Ph.D.

Hemispherectomy was first performed by Dandy in 1928, when he removed one hemisphere in a patient with a glioma.[8] The use of hemispherectomy for the control of intractable seizures in children was first described by McKenzie in 1938.[31] By 1950, 41 hemispherectomies had been reported in the world literature at which time Krynauw's report on the successful use of hemispherectomy in 12 patients with intractable epilepsy served as the stimulus for increasing the popularity of the operation.[19] This report clearly demonstrated the benefit of removal of the atrophic hemisphere in children with infantile hemiplegia and intractable seizures with associated behavioral disturbances. Subsequently, large series of patients undergoing hemispherectomy were reported with encouraging results.[23, 30, 32]

Alexander and Norman in their studies on Sturge-Weber disease showed that if seizures began in infancy, then by later childhood the patient would be institutionalized because of dementia and hemiplegia and would likely die in status epilepticus at a relatively early age.[2]

In our institution we therefore began doing hemispherectomies on infants with hemispheral Sturge-Weber disease early in infancy.[16] We were pleased to find that not only did this deal with the seizure disorder, but the early treatment resulted in a higher IQ and better neurologic function.[16]

INDICATIONS FOR HEMISPHERECTOMY

The indications for hemispherectomy are different in infants and young children than in older children. In infants and young children, the indications are (1) a structural lesion involving only one hemisphere in its entirety, (2) epilepsy that is refractory to medical management, (3) seizures originating in the abnormal hemisphere. In infants with hemispheric involvement demonstrated on a contrast-enhanced computed tomography (CT) scan, hemispherectomy should be performed early in those whose seizures have onset in the first months of life. In older children hemispherectomy is indicated for those conditions in which (1) the patient has seizures refractory to medical management, (2) the seizure foci are present in more than one lobe in only one hemisphere, (3) there is a gross structural lesion affecting only one hemisphere, (4) the patient has a contralateral hemiparesis, (5) speech is subserved by the unaffected hemisphere, as determined by an intracarotid amobarbital (Wada) test, (6) the patient's IQ is above 60.

At the Hospital for Sick Children, we have performed hemispherectomies in infants for the past two decades. We believe that early surgery prevents the appearance of independent seizure foci in the unaffected hemisphere due to the constant stimulation originating in the affected hemisphere (kindling). This constant abnormal stimulation may also be the cause of the behavioral disturbances and loss of intellect seen in patients who have not undergone surgery.

PREOPERATIVE EVALUATION

The preoperative evaluation of children who are potential candidates for hemispherectomy consists of two parts. The structural abnormality of the abnormal hemisphere must be identified. CT scanning is the study of choice for evaluating patients with uncontrolled seizures. The CT scan will demonstrate abnormalities of the brain parenchyma, occult neoplasms, or vascular malformations. Magnetic resonance imaging (MRI) provides additional anatomical information of exquisite detail. Other imaging studies—plain films, angiography—are rarely needed.

After the structural lesion has been identified, a careful investigation of the seizure foci must be performed. One must establish that the foci are restricted to one hemisphere. Initially a routine EEG is done to identify the seizure focus. If there are abnormal electrical discharges in the structurally normal hemisphere, an intracarotid injection of amobarbital into the internal carotid artery feeding the abnormal hemisphere will abolish the seizure activity in the normal hemisphere as well as in the abnormal hemisphere, if this is only mirror activity. Seizure activity in the normal hemisphere that continues after amobaribital injection on the abnormal side indicates that there is independent seizure activity on the normal side. Furthermore, the amobarbital test will localize speech in the child over five years of age.

TECHNIQUE OF HEMISPHERECTOMY

Hemispherectomy en bloc has proven in our hands to be a more satisfactory technique than piecemeal removal of brain tissue, particularly in the Sturge-Weber syndrome where the pial vascular malformation leads to unnecessary bleeding in multiple lobectomies.

In order to carry out an en bloc removal, a large frontoparietal bone flap is turned and the dura is opened. The Sylvian fissure is exposed and the bifurcation of the internal carotid is dissected free. The anterior and middle cerebral arteries are then clipped and divided, to allow for reduction of blood supply to the affected hemisphere. One can thus quite safely approach the parasagittal draining veins and divide them after bipolar coagulation.

The hemisphere can then be retracted away from the falx, thus exposing the corpus callosum, which is transsected, allowing entry into the lateral ventricle. The incision is then carried from just above the caudate nucleus through the central white matter and through putamen down to the temporal horn. The incision in corpus callosum is extended anteriorly to the genu and the rostrum and is carried through the frontal-lobe cortex immediately in front of the optic chiasm and optic nerve. The incision is then carried down through the medial portion of the temporal lobe taking the hippocampus and uncus. The draining veins under the temporal lobe and over the medial side of the occipital lobe are now occluded and divided, as in the posterior cerebral artery as it enters the calcarine sulcus just beyond its origin. The splenium of the corpus callosum is now divided. The entire cerebral cortex is then removed en bloc leaving basal ganglia and thalamus. Care is taken to leave the foramen of Monro open to allow for irrigation of the hemicranium by cerebrospinal fluid (CSF) (Fig. 51–1).

RESULTS OF HEMISPHERECTOMY AT THE HOSPITAL FOR SICK CHILDREN

Patients with one of three lesions—Sturge-Weber syndrome, infantile hemiplegia or unilateral megalencephaly—have been candidates for hemispherectomy at our institution.

Sturge-Weber Syndrome

The Sturge-Weber syndrome, or encephalotrigeminal angiomatosis, was first described by Sturge in 1879, who reported a case of epilepsy associated

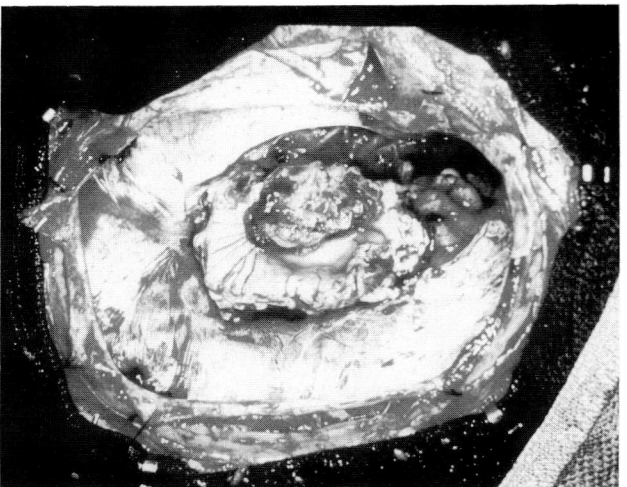

Figure 51–1. Surgical field after hemispherectomy, demonstrating empty hemicalvarium.

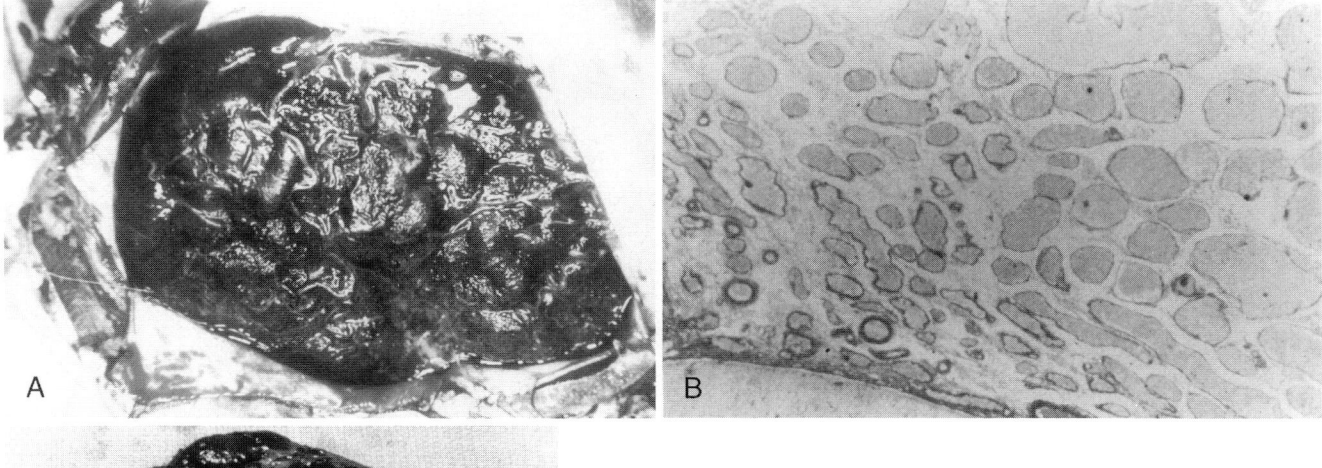
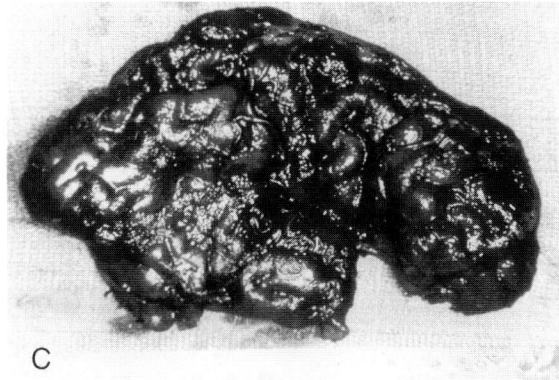

Figure 51–2. Intraoperative photograph showing the surface of the affected hemisphere in a patient with Sturge-Weber syndrome. Note the myriad vessels in the pia. B, Histologic section through the leptomeninges and cortex of a specimen from a patient with Sturge-Weber syndrome. The layers of abnormal pial vessels are easily seen. C, Surgical specimen demonstrating en bloc removal of the left hemisphere in a patient with Sturge-Weber syndrome.

with a venous malformation of the leptomeninges and a port-wine nevus of the face.[26] Weber described the characteristic "tram track" calcification seen on plain skull radiographs of affected children over two or three years of age.[28, 29] Krabbe demonstrated in 1934 that the mineral deposits were in the cortex and not within the venous malformation.[18] Associated glaucoma and buphthalmos have been described in up to 28 percent of affected patients.[2] The intracranial pathology is usually on the side of the port-wine nevus, but may be bilateral.[5]

The intracranial lesion is a pial arteriovenous malformation. It gives rise to capillaries and small veins that form multilayered channels in the subarachnoid space (Fig. 51–2). These vessels penetrate the cortex and enter the white matter. The studies of Alexander and associates have demonstrated decreased blood flow in the brain beneath the malformation.[1] The resulting hypoxia results in cell death followed by calcification. The deposition of mineral in the cortex can be seen histologically as early as 1 month of age and the amount of calcium increases with age[11] (Fig. 51–3). Calcium is also found in the white matter and around intraparenchymal blood vessels. Associated with the calcification, there is gliosis of the underlying white matter, again as early as one month of age.

The characteristic tram track calcification is not seen on radiographs of patients under two years of age. In the older child, these findings are pathognomonic and are associated with a smaller hemicranium on the affected side.

CT scanning is currently the radiographic study of choice.[5, 11] In infancy, calcification and atrophy of the affected side are noted. With the injection of intravenous contrast, the affected hemisphere shows diffuse enhancement under the angioma (Fig. 51–4). Bilateral disease is easily detected.

Early in the disease, an EEG will reveal only slowing in the affected hemisphere. As the child

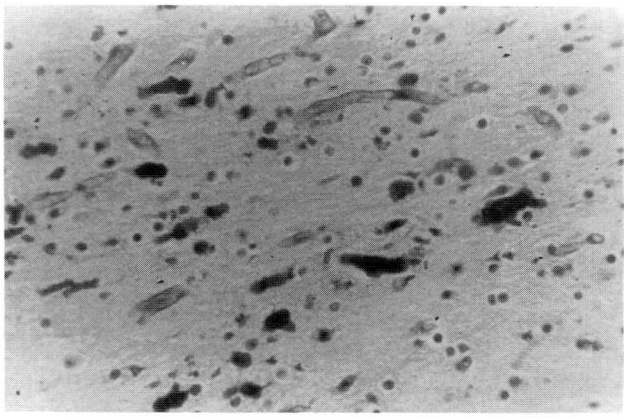

Figure 51–3. Histologic section through the cortex of a patient with Sturge-Weber syndrome, hemispherectomized at age three months. Calcification is already apparent.

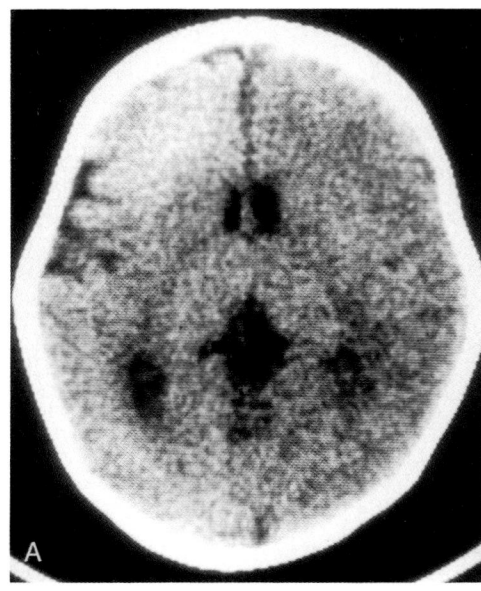 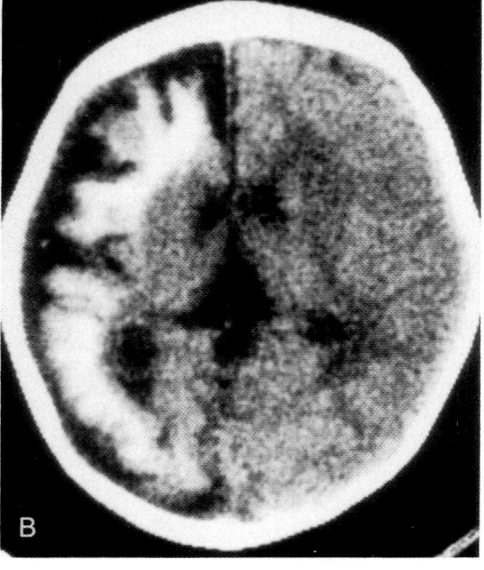

Figure 51–4. Serial CT scans of a patient with Sturge-Weber syndrome (A) at age one month. B, At age 12 months. Note the progressive cerebral atrophy and calcification in this infant.

increases in age, epileptiform discharges appear on the involved side, which may be mirrored on the uninvolved side.

The natural history of a patient born with the Sturge-Weber syndrome has been poorly studied. However, the study of Alexander and Norman showed that if a patient began to have seizures in infancy, the patient would be institutionalized by later childhood with mental retardation and hemiplegia[2] (Fig. 51–4). Most of the patients in their study died at an early age of status epilepticus or its complications.

In many patients with Sturge-Weber syndrome, the characteristic tram track calcifications are seen only in the occipital region. This finding led early workers to confine surgical treatment of the disease to occipital lobectomy, with mixed results.[6, 13, 14, 24, 33]

Falconer carried out the first hemispherectomy for the treatment of uncontrolled epilepsy in a patient with Sturge-Weber syndrome.[22] He reported the results of hemispherectomy in five such patients in 1959;[12] all of his patients had disease affecting the entire hemisphere, all were treated with en bloc hemispherectomy, and all were treated after infancy. All of the patients were rendered seizure-free. The four younger patients improved intellectually, but still had IQs ranging from 53 to 66. The fifth patient, operated upon at age 16 years remained grossly retarded with an IQ of 30.

Because the natural progression of Sturge-Weber syndrome leads to progressive loss of intelligence,[2] and because hemispherectomy gives better seizure control than lobectomy, infants with this disease who have seizures and unilateral hemispheral involvement have been treated by hemispherectomy at the Hospital for Sick Children.

Twelve patients with Sturge-Weber syndrome have undergone hemispherectomy at the Hospital for Sick Children (Fig. 51–4); seven of these have been the subject of a previous report.[16] One patient had his operation at age seven years although he had had uncontrolled seizures since the age of nine months. At presentation, he had a marked hemiparesis and an IQ of 58. Postoperatively, he has remained seizure free for 15 years; his intelligence has remained unchanged. The other eleven patients all underwent hemispherectomy at 1 year of age or younger (range 3 months to 12 months). Seven of the eleven patients have a normal IQ (greater than 80). Two of the patients have moderate developmental delay (IQ currently 70 to 80) and two patients are markedly retarded (IQ < 70). Eight of the patients are seizure-free on no anticonvulsant medication, two patients are having occasional seizures on multidrug regimens, and two patients continue to have seizures frequently despite attempts at control with multiple anticonvulsant medications. These two patients are severely retarded. Three of the patients required shunting procedures, two for hydrocephalus and one for bilateral subdural hygromas. The patient with hygromas and one of the patients with hydrocephalus are the two severely retarded children who continue to have seizures. None of the patients have had significant late deterioration despite a follow-up from three to 22 years.

In summary, we believe that children with Sturge-Weber syndrome that causes seizures in infancy can have a pial arteriovenous malformation overlying the majority of the affected hemisphere, unlike children with the more restricted posterior parietal–occipital venous malformation who develop seizures later in life. Our results show that seizure control can be obtained with hemispherectomy and that if hemispherectomy is performed before 1 year of age a normal IQ can result.

Infantile Hemiplegia

Infantile hemiplegia is a term used to describe children with a hemiplegia from many differing causes. At the Hospital for Sick Children, the term is reserved for infants whose symptoms include hemiplegia and evidence of infarction in the territory of the middle cerebral artery or evidence of diffuse venous infarction of the hemisphere. The patients fall into two categories: 1) those with perinatal trauma or hypoxia and 2) those with an acute febrile illness in early childhood, accompanied by seizures.[15, 32] The pathology of the condition is either cystic infarction of the middle cerebral artery territory in the congenital cases, or diffuse infarction and gliosis in the acquired cases[32] (Fig. 51–5).

In the past, children with infantile hemiplegia and medically refractory seizures have been treated with hemispherectomy. Large series have been reported with excellent seizure control in up to 85 percent of cases.[23, 32] At the Hospital for Sick Children, hemispherectomy for infantile hemiplegia has given good results. As previously reported,[15] only two of 13 patients had seizures postoperatively, and these are controlled with medication. Eight of 13 had improved overall IQ scores. All patients had improvement in personality. There was one perioperative death related to an undetected congenital heart defect. The youngest patient in this series was 2.5 years old at the time of operation.

At the Hospital for Sick Children, fewer hemispherectomies for infantile hemiplegia have been performed in recent years, we believe because medical management of the seizure disorder has been improved. Also, recent reports in the literature have suggested that anterior corpus callosotomy is effective in reducing seizures in this disorder.[3]

Unilateral Megalencephaly

Unilateral megalencephaly is a syndrome of diffuse enlargement of one hemisphere. Children with this disorder have seizures during the first few months of life. The seizure activity is confined to the large hemisphere, and there is a contralateral hemiplegia. The pathology in this disorder consists of a mild to severe derangement of glia and neurons with increases in the absolute numbers of both.[4, 9, 27] Untreated, the patients die in late infancy.[27]

Three patients with unilateral megalencephaly have undergone cortical resection for intractable epilepsy at the Hospital for Sick Children. All had the onset of seizures in the first days to weeks of life. The seizures in all three proved refractory to medical therapy with combinations of multiple anticonvulsant drugs. EEG recordings showed diffuse, poorly organized activity with multifocal sharp waves in the affected hemispheres of two patients; in the third patient the abnormal recordings were limited to the right frontal region. CT scanning documented the unilateral megalencephaly in all patients.

The first patient to undergo hemispherectomy was five months old at the time of surgery. He was already developmentally delayed and remained so after surgery although he had no further seizures. He was institutionalized and died at age five years of pneumonia.

The second patient underwent a right temporal lobectomy at seven months of age as intraoperative EEG recordings suggested that most of the seizure foci were contained in this location. Unfortunately, she continued to have intractable seizures postoperatively. She therefore underwent a right hemispherectomy as a second procedure soon after the first. Intraoperative complications led to massive bleeding and the patient died on the fourth day after surgery.

The third patient, who seemed to have the abnormal tissue restricted to the right frontal lobe underwent an extensive right frontal lobectomy at age three years, eight months. At age four years, the patient continues to have two to three seizures

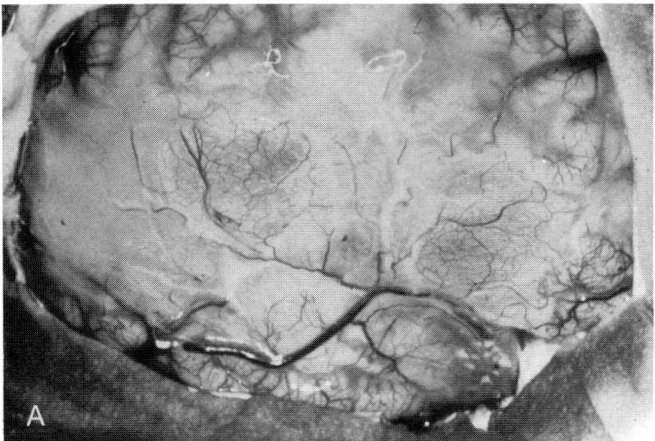
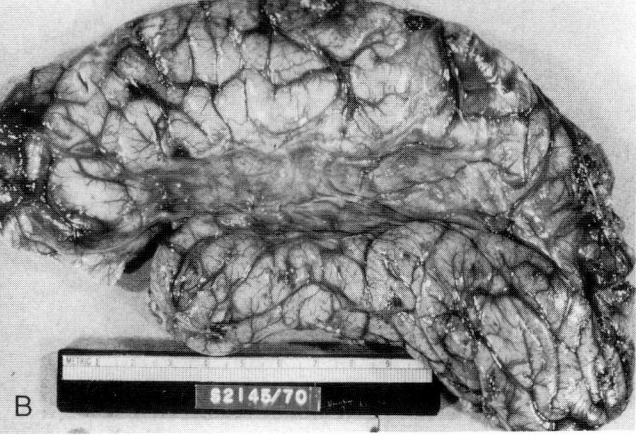

Figure 51–5. *A*, Intraoperative photograph showing the surface of the affected hemisphere in a patient with infantile hemiplegia. Note the loss of normal brain topography. *B*, Surgical specimen demonstrating en bloc removal of the left hemisphere in a patient with infantile hemiplegia. Note the loss of brain substance in the frontal and parietal lobes.

per week on anticonvulsants. He functions at a 2.5-year-old level.

The Hospital for Sick Children experience with hemispherectomy for unilateral megalencephaly is too small at the current time to come to definitive conclusions. In light of the lethal nature of the underlying malformation, it seems further attempts at surgical resection of the abnormal hemisphere are warranted.

COMPLICATIONS

The initial enthusiasm for hemispherectomy brought about by the excellent results in seizure control has been tempered by late, unexpected complications. The patients are susceptible to death from minor head injury.[20] In some patients, a delayed deterioration in intelligence years after the operation frequently leading to death has been noted.[7] In Wilson's series of 50 cases of hemispherectomy over a 15-year period, 11 patients had delayed deterioration due to late accumulated effects of recurrent hemorrhage into the evacuated hemicranium.[32] Rasmussen reported similar complications in nine of 27 total hemispherectomy patients.[23] In both series, pathologic examination of the brain revealed diffuse hemosiderin deposits involving the ventricular system and remaining hemisphere in addition to evidence of chronic and acute subdural hematomas. In light of this complication, Rasmussen has advocated subtotal hemispherectomy, in which the deafferented occipital or frontal lobe or both are left in place.[23] In his series, the incidence of late complications decreased to two in 40 when this modification in technique was used. However, seizure control was not as good in this second group.[23]

At the Hospital for Sick Children, we have not encountered the late complications of hemispherectomy listed above, we believe because we perform the operation in infancy in many of our patients. The remaining hemisphere grows to fill the space of the removed hemisphere, so that the large empty space seen with later surgery is not present (Fig. 51–6). For this reason, we recommend hemispherectomy in appropriate patients at the earliest possible time.

Patients who undergo hemispherectomy with a pre-existing hemiparesis rarely have increased weakness postoperatively. Usually there is a worsening in sensory function.[32] If no pre-existing hemiparesis is present, it is our experience that the resulting weakness is least when the operation is performed early in infancy. All patients have a complete homonymous hemianopia after the operation. Careful examination of higher cortical functioning has shown that while basic visuospatial skills are mastered by patients with right hemispherectomy, these patients do not acquire advanced skills in this area.[17,25] Similarly, careful

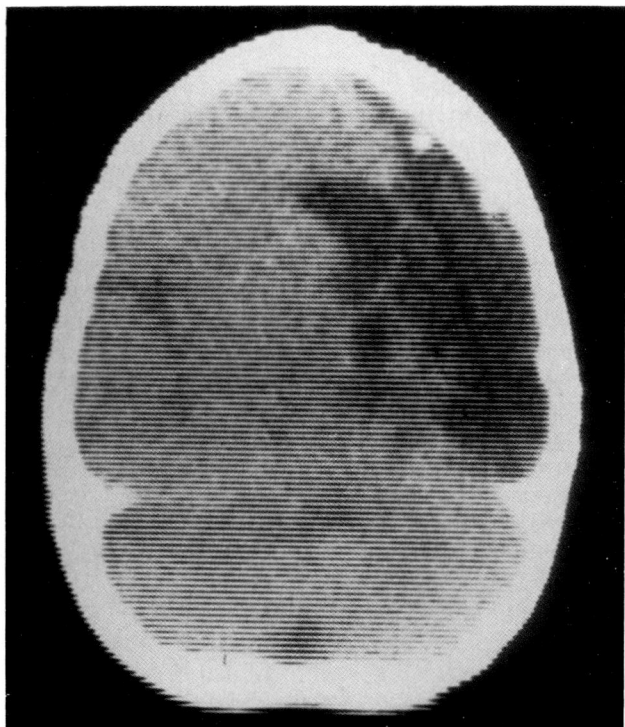

Figure 51–6. Postoperative CT scan one year after hemispherectomy at age three months. Note the shift of the normal left hemisphere across the midline, with significant filling of the right hemicalvarium.

testing of patients with left hemispherectomies reveals subtle speech deficits when compared with patients with right hemispherectomies.[10] The younger the patient at the time of hemispherectomy, the smaller the deficit appears on testing; these deficits are not disabling.

One must note that the cognitive and speech deficits noted are more severe in patients undergoing hemispherectomy after infancy. Early hemispherectomy, as advocated at this hospital, leads to lesser or undetectable deficits.

CONCLUSION

Hemispherectomy deserves a place in the list of surgical procedures for epilepsy. This operation is indicated for structural lesions resulting in epileptic foci involving more than one lobe of only one hemisphere. Seizure control is usually achieved; behavioral improvement may also be seen. If the procedure is performed during infancy, significant neurologic deficits are avoided, late complications are rare, and most importantly, the relentlessly progressive loss of intellect that occurs in candidate children may be avoided.

References

1. Alexander GL, Cooper R, Crow HJ: EEG, ECOG and oxygen availability in the cortex of a case of the Sturge-Weber

syndrome. Electroencephalog Clin Neurophysiol 14:284, 1962.
2. Alexander GL, Normal RM: The Sturge-Weber Syndrome. Bristol, John Wright, 1960.
3. Avila JO, Raovany J, Huck FR, et al: Anterior callosotomy as a substitute for hemispherectomy. Acta Neurochir (Suppl) 30:137, 1980.
4. Bignami A, Palladini G, Zappella M: Unilateral megalencephaly with nerve cell hypertrophy. Brain Res 9:103, 1968.
5. Boltshauser E, Wilson J, Hoare RD: Sturge-Weber syndrome with bilateral intracranial calcification. J Neurol Neurosurg Psychiatry 39:429, 1976.
6. Broager B, Hertze H: An electroencephalographically localized focus in a case of Sturge-Weber syndrome extirpated with good result. Acta Psychiat Neurol 24:1, 1949.
7. Carmichael EA: The current status of hemispherectomy for infantile hemiplegia. Clin Proc Child Hosp Wash 22:285, 1966.
8. Dandy WE: Removal of right cerebral hemisphere for certain tumors with hemiplegia. JAMA 90:823, 1928.
9. Davis RL, Nelson E: Unilateral ganglioglioma in a tuberosclerotic brain. J Neuropathol Exp Neurol 20:571, 1961.
10. Dennis M, Kohn B: Comprehension of syntax in infantile hemiplegics after cerebral hemidecortication: Left-hemisphere superiority. Brain and Language 2:472, 1975.
11. Enzmann DR, Hayward RW, Norman D, et al: Cranial computed tomographic scan appearance of Sturge-Weber disease. Unusual Presentation. Radiology 122:721, 1977.
12. Falconer MA, Rushworth RG: Treatment of encephalotrigeminal angiomatosis (Sturge-Weber disease) by hemispherectomy. Arch Dis Child 35:433, 1960.
13. Green JR, Foster J, Berens DL: Encephalotrigeminal angiomatosis (Sturge-Weber syndrome). Am J Roentgenol 64:391, 1950.
14. Goscinski I, Kunicki A: Surgical treatment of Sturge-Weber syndrome. Acta Med Polowa 13:229, 1972.
15. Hendrick EB, Hoffman JR, Hudson AR: Hemispherectomy in children. Clin Neurosurg 16:315, 1969.
16. Hoffman HJ, Hendrick EB, Dennis M, et al: Hemispherectomy for Sturge-Weber syndrome. Child's Brain 5:233, 1979.
17. Kohn B, Dennis M: Selective impairment of visuo-spatial abilities in infantile hemiplegics after right cerebral hemidecortication. Neurol Psychol 12:505, 1974.
18. Krabbe K: Facial and meningeal angiomatosis associated with calcifications of the brain cortex. Arch Neurol Psychiatry 32:737, 1934.
19. Krynauw RA: Infantile hempiplegia treated by removing one cerebral hemisphere. J Neurol Neurosurg Psychiatry 13:243, 1950.
20. Laine E, Pruvot P, Osson D: Résultats éloignés de l'hémisphérectomie dans les cas d'hémiatrophie cérébrale infantile génératrice d'epilepsie. Neuro-Chirurgie 10:507, 1964.
21. Maki Y, Semba A: Computed tomography of Sturge-Weber disease. Child's Brain 5:51, 1979.
22. Polani PE: Encephalotrigeminal angiomatosis (Sturge-Weber syndrome) treated by removal of affected cerebral hemisphere. Proc R Soc Med 45:860, 1952.
23. Rasmussen T: Hemispherectomy revisited. Can J Neurol Sci 10:71, 1983.
24. Rasmussen T, Mathieson G, LeBlanc F: Surgical therapy of typical and forme fruste variety of the Sturge-Weber syndrome. Arch Suis Neurol Neurochir Psychiatry (Suppl 2) 3:393, 1972.
25. Smith A: Nondominant hemispherectomy. Neurology 19:442, 1969.
26. Sturge WA: A case of partial epilepsy, apparently due to one of the vasosmotor centers of the brain. Trans Clin Soc Lond 12:162, 1879.
27. Townsend JJ, Nielson SL, Malamuo N: Unilateral megalencephaly: Hamartoma or neoplasm? Neurology 25:448, 1975.
28. Weber PF: Right-sided hemi-atrophy resulting from right-sided congenital hemiplegia with a morbid condition of the left side of the brain, revealed by radiograms. J Neurol Psychopathol 3:134, 1922.
29. Weber PF: A note on the association of extensive hemangiomatous naevus of the skin with cerebral (meningeal) hemangioma, especially cases of facial vascular naevus with contralateral hemiplegia. Proc R Soc Med 22:431, 1929.
30. White HH: Cerebral hemispherectomy in the treatment of infantile hemiplegia. Confinir Neurol 21:1, 1961.
31. Williams DJ, Scott JW: The functional responses of the sympathetic nervous system of man following hemidecortication. J Neurol Psychiatry 2:313, 1939.
32. Wilson PJE: Cerebral hemispherectomy for infantile hemiplegia. A Report of 50 Cases. Brain 93:174, 1970.
33. Wocjan J, Biozinski J: Surgical treatment of some cases of Sturge-Weber syndrome. Neurol Neurochir Pol 2:63, 1968.

52
MOVEMENT DISORDERS AND SPASTICITY

Sanford J. Larson, M.D., Ph.D.

Spinal-cord injury is uncommon in children, and with the exception of dystonia musculorum deformans, the treatable progressive disorders of involuntary movement are restricted to adults. Therefore, the treatment of spasticity and involuntary movements in children is almost exclusively the treatment of cerebral palsy.

The term "cerebral palsy" encompasses a group of disorders characterized by abnormalities of posture and movement, present from birth and persistent throughout life. Although the abnormal postures and movements may be modified to some extent by maturation and training, the basic physiologic and anatomic deficits persist without change. The physiologic abnormalities, however, have not been quantitatively defined, and the anatomic spectrum extends from brains that appear normal to those that are severely malformed.

The etiologic factors are similarly variable. Although antenatal or perinatal events such as anoxia, physical injury, and kernicterus have been considered to be the major causes of cerebral palsy, there is evidence that many cases are a result of genetically determined maldevelopment or arrested development.[1,20,33] As in other disorders of involuntary movement, clinical findings often cannot be correlated with an anatomic substrate.

Since it has not been possible to describe patients with cerebral palsy on anatomic or quantitative physiologic grounds, the dominant clinical manifestation has been used as a basis for classification. The most commonly used terms include spastic quadriplegia (double hemiplegia), spastic diplegia (lower limbs more severely affected than the upper limbs), spastic paraplegia, and athetosis (double athetosis). While some patients are almost exclusively spastic and others athetoid, most display a mixture, with one functional abnormality being dominant.

Because classification and definition of physiologic abnormalities fluctuates and is significantly influenced by emotional factors, and because overall performance usually improves with increasing age, the evaluation of treatment has been difficult. It is safe to say, however, that pharmacologic treatment has been ineffective. Physical therapy has been useful in limiting contractures and improving gait in patients with spasticity but has had little effect on ultimate function in patients with athetosis.[36] Surgical treatment has largely been equated with orthopedic operations such as arthrodesis, osteotomy, and tenotomy.

Both physical therapy and orthopedic surgery are attempts at adaptation to a fixed physiologic abnormality. Neurosurgical treatment, although not widely applied, represents an effort toward modification of this abnormality with a view to releasing function obscured by the spasticity or athetosis. Neurosurgical treatment has had three major directions: interruption of motor pathways, of sensory pathways, and of cerebellothalamocortical pathways.

INTERRUPTION OF MOTOR PATHWAYS

Horsley was perhaps the first to treat athetosis by resection of motor cortex that had been identified by electric stimulation.[28] Following surgery, the patient had not only paralysis of the contralateral upper limb but also a profound reduction in sensory perception. From these deficits Horsley concluded that the percentral gyrus was essential for perception of sensation, although it is likely that the resection was more extensive than anticipated. In any event, the patient recovered some sensory perception and motor function, but the involuntary movements were almost completely obliterated. A number of years later, this procedure was revived.[8,9] On the basis of the hypothesis that involuntary movements were generated in premotor cortex and transmitted over extrapyramidal corticifugal pathways, attempts were made to spare area 4.

In these operations, however, the resection had been carried down to the lateral ventricle, and the patient had severe postoperative weakness suggesting that motor as well as premotor fibers were involved. Nevertheless, involuntary movements were satisfactorily relieved, and the motor function that reappeared after several weeks was unimpeded by involuntary movements and was, therefore, significantly more useful than prior to operation.

These operations could only be applied unilaterally, however, and for involuntary movements of the upper limb. To improve function in those patients with bilateral involvement of upper and lower limbs, Putnam advocated anterior cordotomy to interrupt tracts considered extrapyramidal such as the reticulospinal, tectospinal, and vestibulospinal.[38,39] This procedure was performed at a single stage bilaterally at the C-2 and C-3 levels. Following surgery, most patients had a profound quadriparesis, indicating corticospinal-tract involvement, with loss of sphincter control and difficulty with ventilation. After several weeks, motor function recovered substantially, and involuntary movements returned but not with the preoperative intensity.

Although the net effect of these operations on motor pathways was positive, these techniques were not widely applied and were eventually abandoned.

INTERRUPTION OF AFFERENT PATHWAYS

The treatment of spasticity by dorsal rhizotomy is effective but in patients with cerebral palsy, total deafferentiation of a limb is unacceptable. Consequently, subtotal rhizotomy has been applied, particularly for spastic diplegia. In these procedures, either two thirds or three fourths of each root is divided or the afferent fibers involved in the stretch reflex are identified electrophysiologically and are cut.[18,19] After lumbar rhizotomy, spasticity has been reported to be substantially decreased in the lower limbs and to a lesser extent in the upper limbs.

Although communication with many of the patients who had undergone these procedures was difficult, sensory perception was apparently not significantly affected. Subtotal rhizotomy has also been done to relieve spasticity in the upper limbs and has been effective without producing a significant sensory deficit.[2,22] Bilateral dorsal rhizotomy of C-1 through C-3 has been performed in an effort to abolish tonic neck reflexes, and the severity of spasticity and involuntary movements have been reduced in the upper and lower limbs.[26] The improvement, although significant, was not substantial. Complications were minimal.

When the procedure was extended to include C-4, C-5, and C-6, however, more than 50 percent of patients had respiratory problems.[22] Other operations designed to interrupt afferent pathways have included the creation of stereotactic lesions in the thalamocortical radiation.[16] Although involuntary movements were reduced and permanent significant loss of sensory perception was not observed, the improvement appeared related to the degree of sensory deficit observed immediately following surgery.

The reduction of spasticity and of involuntary movements without disabling sensory loss after a considerable interruption of afferent pathways reflects the redundancy of the nervous system and the relative crudeness of the clinical evaluation and suggests that involuntary movements depend upon intact afferent pathways.[3,15,29]

INTERRUPTION OF CEREBELLOTHALAMOCORTICAL CIRCUITS

The gratifying results of stereotactic procedures directed at the globus pallidus and the ventrolateral nucleus of the thalamus in patients with Parkinson's disease and other dyskinesias led to the application of these operations to patients with cerebral palsy.[11,34] But except in the case of the relatively few almost purely athetoid patients with cerebral palsy, relief from involuntary movements and posture was not nearly as striking as in dystonia musculorum deformans, and the effect upon spasticity was not significant.[11,24]

Because of the known hypotonia associated with large cerebellar lesions or with lesions of the dentate nucleus or superior cerebellar peduncle, attention was directed to the cerebellum. Schneider reported delayed but substantial bilateral reduction in spasticity following extensive unilateral cerebellar resection in a patient with cerebral palsy.[41] He indicated, however, that this procedure could probably not be widely applied because of difficulty in determining precisely how much cerebellum should be resected to achieve a satisfactory reduction of spasticity without an undesirable degree of hypotonia. Subsequently, stereotactic dentatotomy was introduced and considered relatively effective, but the postoperative improvement, although significant, was not sufficient to be worthwhile.[21, 24, 25, 42]

The application of electric current to the cerebellum for relief of involuntary movements and spasticity was proposed by Cooper.[12, 13] Others have also observed reduction in spasticity and in severity of involuntary movements associated with cerebellar stimulation.[31, 38, 43, 44]

The major problem associated with evaluation of the effects of cerebellar stimulation in cerebral palsy, and this is true of all types of treatment of this disorder, is that the observed changes are difficult to express quantitatively. The temporal variation in severity and the significant influence of emotional stress upon spasticity and involuntary movements compound the problem.

Recording of somatosensory evoked potentials, however, while not necessarily related to changes in spasticity or involuntary movements, nevertheless represents an objective and quantitative means of assessing the effects of application of current to the cerebellum. In both humans and monkeys, the amount of current required to produce a functional change is approximately the same as that required to produce a significant reduction in amplitude of the somatosensory evoked potential.[27, 30, 31, 40, 43, 44] Application of current to the animal cerebellum at intensities similar to that used clinically is associated with the applied current.[4-6]

Furthermore, Purkinje cells remote from the locus of applied current are driven at latencies suggestive of activation by axon collaterals of inferior olivary neurons. The latter factor may account for the changes observed in both involuntary movements and evoked potentials with directly effective application of current to only a relatively small proportion of the cerebellar neuronal population.[30] Since the dentate and other cerebellar subcortical neurons have a tonic facilitatory effect on those neurons with which they synapse,[17] an increase in Purkinje cell activity would have a dysfacilitatory effect. Consequently, the improvement in spasticity and involuntary movements and the reduction in somatosensory evoked potential amplitude could well be causally related.

Questions have been raised regarding the safety of cerebellar stimulation, and damage to the cerebellar cortex associated with application of current has been reported.[7, 14] Evidence, however, is available that currents applied at levels sufficient to reduce spasticity, involuntary movements, and the amplitude of evoked potentials do not produce significant injury.[27, 30, 31] Neuronal loss observed has been superficial and related to mechanical injury.

When currents were applied through the cerebellum from negative electrodes on one surface to positive electrodes on another substantially greater effects were observed as compared with application through electrodes of alternate polarity, and the levels of current were well below those found to cause neuronal damage.[31, 40] Furthermore, in those patients who have shown significant clinical changes and significant reduction in evoked potential associated with currents, the amount of current required to produce these changes has not increased with the passage of time, as would be expected with progressive injury to the cerebellum.[31]

As indicated previously, the major problem associated with evaluation of the treatment given patients with cerebral palsy is the lack of objective, quantitative means of assessment of physiological function. The systems that have been employed for this purpose evaluate functional improvement related to education, both physical and intellectual. In many patients with cerebral palsy, useful function may be present but masked by spasticity and involuntary movements. If these impediments can be relieved, then education should be more effective.

In children who already have neuromuscular disability, the imposition of an additional deficit associated with an anatomic lesion is undesirable. There is evidence that the effects of thalamotomy and dentatotomy can be reversibly reproduced by cerebellar stimulation and without significant anatomic damage. Despite the encouraging results that have been reported, quantitative, objective means of assessing neurologic disability must be developed and used over extended periods of time to determine the use of the cerebellar stimulation.[23, 32, 37, 44]

We have conducted periodic evaluations in patients with cerebral palsy in whom cerebellar-implant systems have been placed. Although the data have not been formally tabulated and analyzed, it appears that the initial significant relief of spasticity has not been maintained over the long term in most patients. The most favorable results have come in those individuals whose major problem was athetoid involuntary movements. Significant modification of movement has been maintained in a number of patients over an extended period of time.

In most instances, however, the modification of involuntary movement with implant systems using a subcutaneous receiver and transcutaneous transmission from an antenna and external transmitter is associated with a number of problems that preclude extensive application. These include difficulty in maintaining accurate relationship between the antenna and the subcutaneous receiver, breakage of the subcutaneous wires, and difficulty in maintaining an optimum level of current application.

These problems are magnified where the home setting is less than ideal, and particularly in an institutional environment. As compared with a cardiac pacemaker, the substantially larger current requirements for the cerebellar-implant systems make a totally implanted system impractical.

For the time being, at least, until better methods of patient selection are developed and battery technology improves, cerebellar stimulation does not appear to be a widely applicable method of treatment for the patient with cerebral palsy.

The association of prematurity and cerebral palsy is well known. With the development of neonatal intensive-care units, increasing numbers of prematurely born children survive, and, therefore, an increasing number of patients with cerebral palsy can be anticipated.

Although the various surgical procedures employed have been shown to have some beneficial effect, all involve tissue destruction. Therapeutic application of current to various portions of the nervous system is in its infancy; however, this technique whether applied to the cerebellum or other portions of the nervous system, has the advantage of reversibility and minimal anatomic disruption. Consequently, continued efforts in this direction appear justified.

References

1. Alexander L: The fundamental types of histopathologic changes encountered in cases of athetosis and paralysis agitans. Res Publ Assoc Res Nerv Ment Dis 21:334, 1942.
2. Benedetti A, Carbonin C, Columbo F: Extended posterior cervical rhizotomy for severe spastic syndromes with dyskinesias. Appl Neurophysiol 40:41, 1978.
3. Bertrand C: Anatomy and physiology of extrapyramidal diseases. J Neurosurg 24:233, 1966.
4. Bilof R, Boehmer R, Sances A, Jr., et al: On the relationship between cerebellar cortical current application and the underlying cellular activity. Proc 29th Ann Conf Eng Med Biol 18:450, 1976.
5. Boehmer RD: Distribution of applied electrical current in the cerebellum and its effect on Purkinje cell activity. Ph.D. Dissertation, Marquette University, Milwaukee, WI, April 1979.
6. Boehmer RD, Bilof RM, Sances A, Jr., et al: Recording from Purkinje cells during cerebellar stimulation. Proc 14th Ann AAMI Mtg, Las Vegas, May 20-24, 1979, p 30.
7. Brown WJ, Babb TL, Soper HV, et al: Tissue reaction to long-term electrical stimulation of the cerebellum in monkeys. J Neurosurg 47:366, 1977.
8. Bucy PC, Buchanan DN: Athetosis. Brain 55:479, 1932.
9. Bucy PC, Case TJ: Athetosis-II. Surgical treatment of unilateral athetosis. Arch Neurol Psychiatry 37:983, 1937.
10. Carpenter MB: Athetosis and the basal ganglia. Arch Neurol Psychiatry 63:875, 1950.
11. Cooper IS: Involuntary Movement Disorders. New York, Harper & Row, 1969, p 410.
12. Cooper IS, Riklan M, Amin I, et al: Chronic cerebellar stimulation in cerebral palsy. Arch Neurol 26:744, 1976.
13. Cooper IS, Riklan M, Tabaddor K, et al: A long-term follow-up study of chronic cerebellar stimulation for cerebral palsy. *In*: Cooper IS (ed): Cerebellar Stimulation in Man. New York, Raven Press, 1978, pp 59-99.
14. Dauth GW, Defendin R, Gilman S, et al: Long-term surface stimulation of the cerebellum in the monkey—I. Light microscopic, electrophysiologic and clinical observations. Surg Neurol 7:377, 1977.
15. Denny-Brown D: The Basal Ganglia. London, Oxford University Press, 1962.
16. Dierssen G: Treatment of dystonic and athetoid symptoms by lesions in the sensory portion of the internal capsule. Confin Neurol 26:404, 1966.
17. Eccles JF, Ito M, Szentagothai J: The Cerebellum as a Neuronal Machine. New York, Springer-Verlag, 1967, p 335.
18. Fasano VA, Broggi G, Barolat-Romana G, et al: Surgical treatment of spasticity in cerebral palsy. Child's Brain 4:289, 1978.
19. Fasano VA, Barolat-Romana G, Zeme S, et al: Electrophysiological assessment of spinal circuits in spasticity by dorsal root stimulation. Neurosurgery 4:146, 1979.
20. Ford FR: Diseases of the Nervous System in Infancy, Childhood, and Adolescence, 6th ed. Springfield, IL, Charles C Thomas, 1973.
21. Fraioli B, Guidetti B: Effects of stereotactic lesions of the dentate nucleus of the cerebellum in man. Appl Neurophysiol 38:81, 1975.
22. Fraioli B, Nucci F, Baldassarre L: Bilateral cervical posterior rhizotomy: Effects on dystonia and athetosis on respiration and other autonomic functions. Appl Neurophysiol 40:26, 1978.
23. Harris GF, Sances A, Jr., Ackmann JJ, et al: Biomechanical quantification of passive resistance to motion in patients with cerebral palsy: Before and after cerebellar implant. Proc 2nd Ann Mtg of the Amer Soc of Biomechanics, Ann Arbor, MI, Oct 25-27, 1978.
24. Heimburger RF, Whitlock CC: Stereotaxic destruction of the human dentate nucleus. Confin Neurol 26:346, 1965.
25. Heimburger RF: The role of the cerebellar nuclei in spasticity. Confin Neurol 32:105, 1970.
26. Heimburger RF, Slominski A, Griswold P: Cervical posterior rhizotomy for reducing spasticity in cerebral palsy. J Neurosurg 39:30, 1973.
27. Hemmy DC, Larson SJ, Sances A, Jr., et al: The effect of cerebellar stimulation on focal seizure activity and spasticity in monkeys. J Neurosurg 46:648, 1977.
28. Horsley V: The function of the so-called motor area of the brain. Br Med J 2:121, 1909.
29. Larson SJ, Sances A, Jr.: The specific somatosensory system and dyskinesia. Arch Neurol 18:543, 1968.
30. Larson SJ, Sances A, Jr., Cusick JF, et al: Cerebellar implant studies. IEEE Trans Biomed Eng 23:319, 1976.
31. Larson SJ, Sances A, Jr., Hemmy DC, et al: Physiological and histological effects of cerebellar stimulation. Appl Neurophysiol 40:160, 1978.
32. Larson SJ, Harris GF, Millar EA, et al: Quantitative evaluation of cerebellar stimulation. Proc 14th Ann AAMI Mtg, Las Vegas, May 20-24, 1979, p 158.
33. Miller JQ: Lissencephaly in two siblings. Neurology 13:841, 1963.
34. Mundinger F, Riechert T, Disselhoff J: Long-term results of stereotaxic operations on extrapyramidal hyperkinesia (excluding Parkinsonism). Confin Neurol 32:71, 1970.
35. Narabayashi H: Stereotaxic surgery for athetosis or the spastic state of cerebral palsy. Confin Neurol 22:364, 1962.
36. Paine R: On the treatment of cerebral palsy: The outcome of 177 patients, 74 totally untreated. Pediatrics 29:605, 1962.
37. Penn RD, Gottlieb GL, Agarwal GC: Cerebellar stimulation in man: Quantitative changes in spasticity. J Neurosurg 48:779, 1978.
38. Putnam TJ: Treatment of athetosis and dystonia by section of extrapyramidal motor tracts. Arch Neurol Psychiatry 29:504, 1933.
39. Putnam TJ: Results of treatment of athetosis by section of

extrapyramidal tracts in the spinal cord. Arch Neurol Psychiatry 39:258, 1938.
40. Sances A, Jr., Larson SJ, Myklebust J, et al: Evaluation of electrode configurations in cerebellar implants. Appl Neurophysiol 40:141, 1978.
41. Schneider RC, Crosby EC: The interplay between cerebral hemispheres and cerebellum in relation to tonus and movements. J Neurosurg 20:188, 1963.
42. Siegfried J, Esslen E, Gretener U, et al: Functional anatomy of the dentate nucleus in the light of stereotaxic operations. Confin Neurol 32:1, 1970.
43. Upton AR, Cooper IS: Some neurophysiological effects of cerebellar stimulation in man. Can J Neurol Sci 3:237, 1976.
44. Wong PKH, Hoffman HJ, Froese AB, et al: Cerebellar stimulation in the management of cerebral palsy: Clinical and physiological studies. Neurosurgery 5:217, 1979.

53
STEREOTAXIC PROCEDURES IN CHILDREN

Bruce B. Storrs, M.D.

Stereotaxic procedures have traditionally not been included in the armamentarium of the neurosurgeon dealing with the problems of children. The inclusion of a section dedicated to this topic in a textbook devoted to pediatric neurosurgery reflects the changing face of pediatric neurosurgery and its desire to explore all modalities in the care of children.

The search for more precise methods of localizing structures and pathologic processes within the brain has been a constant theme since the beginnings of neurosurgery. The standard study of skull and brain topography was dramatically changed by the introduction of ventriculography in the early twentieth century. The subsequent development of pneumography, angiography, ultrasonography, computerized tomography (CT), and nuclear magnetic resonance imaging (NMRI) has had a dramatic effect on our ability to identify structure and abnormal processes. A desire for a method of accurate guidance to these targets is a natural outgrowth of the flood of information currently available.

The first efforts at external guidance began long before this century's explosion of imaging information. These early efforts culminated in the achievements of Horsley and Clarke, who, in 1908, successfully developed an external guidance apparatus for the precise placement of probes into the deep cerebellar nuclei of experimental animals.[1]

The stereotaxic apparatus continued to be primarily a laboratory tool until the landmark operation in 1947 when Spiegel and Wycis, refining Horsley and Clarke's technique with the addition of ventriculography, used their stereotaxic apparatus to benefit a human patient with mental disease.[9] In the first few years following this breakthrough, stereotaxic procedures were limited to the control of behavioral disorders. With the development of high-quality atlases of deep anatomy, the goals of stereotaxic procedures widened to include the treatment of intractable pain, the treatment of movement and posture disorders, and the refinement of procedures for disorders of emotion and behavior.[7, 8, 11]

Stereotaxic neurosurgery attained worldwide acceptance and a large body of experience was gained with these procedures. Contributions were truly international in scope. Nashold in his 1970 report estimates the worldwide volume at 40,000 cases for the ten-year period 1960–1970.[4]

The development of new imaging procedures has drastically changed the basis of stereotaxic neurosurgery. The classical stereotaxic procedures were performed relying on calculations made from positive-contrast ventriculography and extrapolated to the patient using stereotaxic atlases derived from pooled data. The obvious shortcomings of this system are variations in individual anatomy and the mechanical problems of parallax and magnification error. These sources of error were minimized by meticulous technique and the verification of probe location by stimulation or recording techniques.

The introduction of the computerized axial tomogram to clinical practice brought a new level of sophistication and accuracy to the imaging of normal and pathological anatomy in the nervous system. This new technique piqued the interest of those interested in stereotaxic neurosurgery because for the first time the area of interest could be visualized on the same study that could potentially provide the localizing coordinates. An additional benefit was that CT scans eliminated many of the intrinsic errors in the ventriculographic technique.

Efforts to join the CT scan information with stereotaxic technique proceeded in two general directions. The first was the adaptation of an accurate, successful, and popular stereotaxic system to the CT scan.[3] The Leksell apparatus was modified and used successfully in many centers, and the transition to CT-guided stereotaxic neurosurgery was eased by using a frame already familiar to many neurosurgeons.[2] The second direction was the development of an entirely new instrument conceived with CT and NMRI compatability as a basic design principle.

THE STEREOTAXIC SYSTEM

A multidisciplinary effort at the University of Utah, led by Theodore S. Roberts, produced the innovative Brown-Roberts-Wells stereotaxic frame.[6] This stereotaxic system was developed to utilize data generated by standard CT scanners. These data, in the form of "x" and "y" coordinates, are translated into three-dimensional coordinates by the use of a computer program contained in a small portable computer. Data acquisition is simple and rapid. The instrument has the ability to place a probe at any specified intracerebral target with ± 1-mm accuracy.

The mechanical foundation for this instrument is the base ring, which is affixed to the skull with metallic pins. Exact rectilinear placement is not necessary and the base ring is not attached to the CT table (Fig. 53–1).

A circular localizing device of nine composite rods arranged in vertical and oblique fashion is secured to the base ring prior to scanning (Fig. 53–2). CT scanning is then performed in the standard manner. A single CT slice containing the desired target and a cross section of all nine localizing rods is all that is necessary to provide the raw data for CT stereotaxis. Using the region-of-interest cursor (ROI) the "x" and "y" coordinates of the nine localizing rods and the target(s) are determined and verified (Fig. 53–3).

The patient may be removed from the CT suite at this time. The raw data are entered into the menu-driven stereotaxic program contained within the portable computer.

An elective skull entry point may be entered into the program using the phantom to determine the "x," "y," and "z" coordinates of this point (Figs. 53–4 and 53–5). As an alternative, the closest skull point to the target may be selected using a program alternative.

The program is then run. Running time is less than 30 sec. The program then produces numbers for the four adjustable settings on the stereotaxic arc as well as the depth of the target(s). The target position as well as the approach parameters are verified on the phantom (Fig. 53–5), the frame is sterilized, and the procedure is carried out. These preliminary steps are the same for all stereotaxically directed procedures.

The proliferation of the CT scan and NMRI as imaging tools has brought central nervous system lesions to attention at a size much smaller than would have been detected using previous imaging techniques. The pediatric age group, already plagued by brain tumor as its most frequent solid tumor, bears the brunt of increased and earlier discovery. The discovery of smaller and more deeply placed tumors raises questions regarding

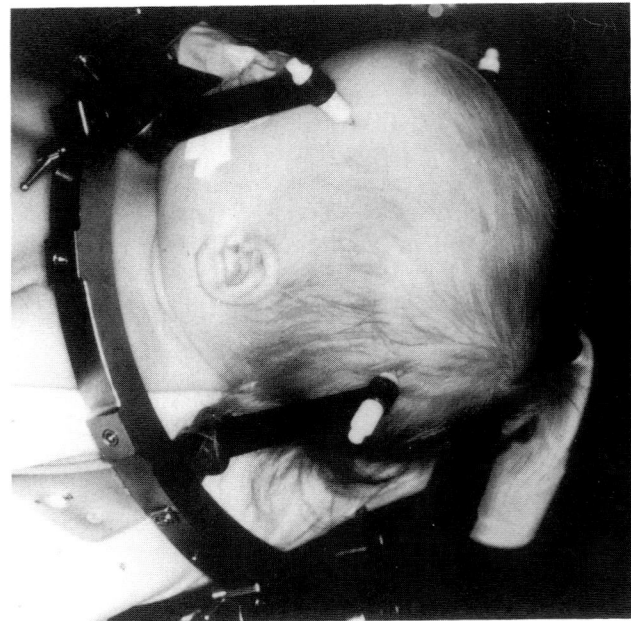

Figure 53–1. Patient with base ring in place. Note composite pins to reduce artifact.

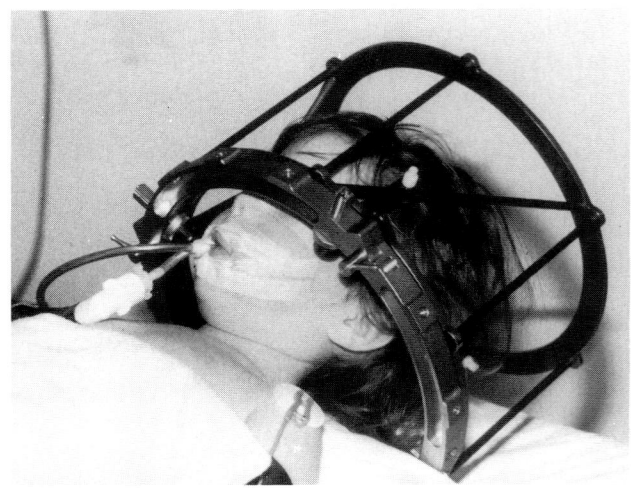

Figure 53–2. Localizing device attached to base ring.

STEREOTAXIC PROCEDURES IN CHILDREN 563

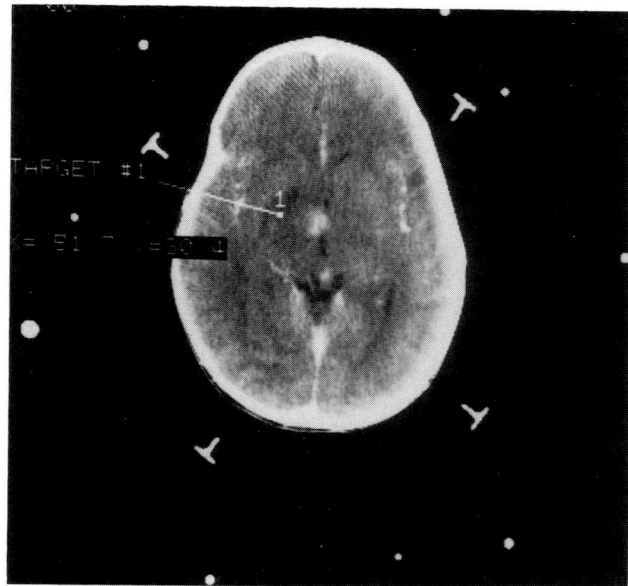

Figure 53–3. CT scan slice containing nine localizing rods in cross section and target(s).

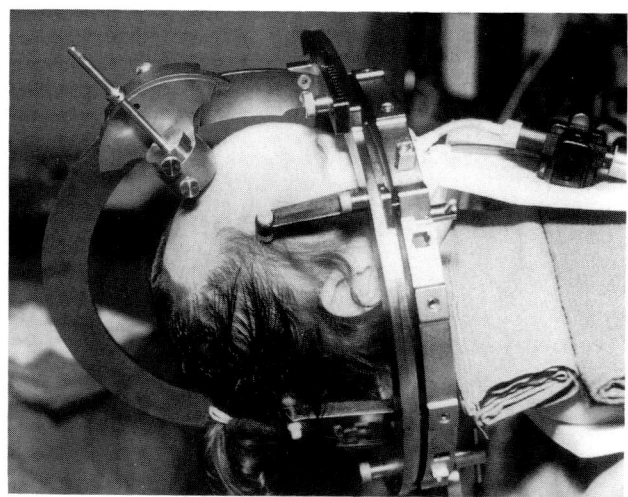

Figure 53–4. Determination of elective skull entry point coordinates.

Figure 53–5. Verification of calculations using phantom.

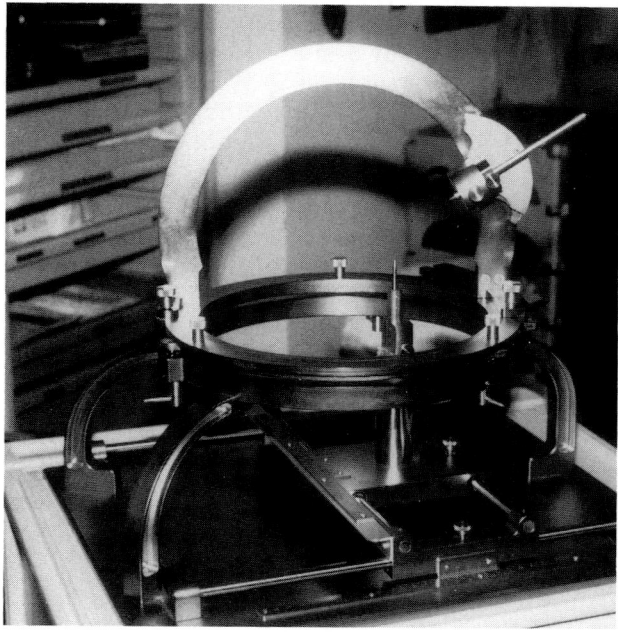

therapy. Tissue diagnosis is often an essential component of the therapeutic decision.

The stereotaxic frame allows these small lesions to be approached for diagnostic biopsy, or the frame may be used as a guidance instrument for resection with limited exploration and retraction of normal brain.[5, 10, 12] The initial experience in children using the B-R-W frame was that of biopsy and or guidance.[5] With the development of experience in the capabilities of the system new procedures were added: stereotaxic puncture and drainage of brain abscesses, stereotaxic placement of shunt catheters in deep arachnoid cysts, and stereotaxic placement of radioactive materials for brachytherapy.[10]

During the period 1983–1986 at the Primary Children's Hospital, Salt Lake City, Utah, stereotaxic technique was used to treat or evaluate 26 children. Twenty underwent biopsy of a mass lesion. Nine did not require subsequent craniotomy; six of these nine patients had pontine gliomas, two had thrombosed arteriovenous malformations, and one had a pineal-suprasellar germinoma.

Of the 11 who had subsequent craniotomies, the final pathologic diagnosis agreed with the biopsy in all cases. Sample size did not interfere with the ability to make a diagnosis. Six miscellaneous procedures were performed. Brain abscess puncture and drainage were performed on two, intracerebral hematoma drainage on two, and placement of shunt catheters in deep arachnoid cysts on two.

There were no surgical complications in this group of children. All procedures were performed under general anesthesia induced in the CT suite. The average time in the CT suite, including anesthesia time, was less than 1 hr. After the initial data acquisition portion, all patients were transported to the operating room for the open part of the procedure.

Follow-up CT scans were performed on all patients within 8 hr of completion of the procedure, which served to verify the biopsy site in those not requiring craniotomy and provided a postoperative assessment opportunity in the others. There were no hemorrhages beyond the boundary of the biopsy sites. The biopsy site was identified by a small amount of air or blood seen on the unenhanced scan.

CONCLUSION

The application of the new generation of stereotaxic techniques to the problems of children is straightforward and beneficial. The ability to biopsy small, deep, or perilously located lesions and to be guided to them with no wasted effort or dangerous exploration is of unquestionable benefit.

The future of stereotaxic applications is a bright one. Current projects in radiation brachytherapy, the investigation and treatment of epilepsy, and the transplantation of brain tissue in heredodegenerative diseases all require the precision and guidance of stereotaxic systems. Advances in these areas are the frontiers for stereotaxic neurosurgery in children.

References

1. Horsley V, Clarke RH: The structure and function of the cerebellum examined by a new method. Brain 31:45, 1908.
2. Leksell L: A stereotaxic apparatus for intracerebral surgery. Acta Chir Scand 99:229, 1949.
3. Leksell L, Jernberg B: Stereotaxis and tomography. A technical note with 6 figures. Acta Neurochir 52:1, 1980.
4. Nashold BS Jr: Stereotactic neurosurgery: The present and future. Am Surg 36:85, 1970.
5. Nauta HJ, Briner RP, Eisenberg HM: Computed tomogram–guided stereotaxic brain biopsy in the pediatric patient. Pediatr Neurosci 12:63, 1985.
6. Roberts TS, Brown R: Technical and clinical aspects of C.T.-directed stereotaxis. Appl Neurophysiol 43:170, 1980.
7. Schaltenbrand G, Bailey P: Introduction to Stereotaxis with an Atlas of the Human Brain. Stuttgart, Thieme, 1959.
8. Spiegel EA, Wycis HT: Stereoencephalotomy. New York, Grune & Stratton, 1962.
9. Spiegel EA, Wycis HT, Marks M, et al: Stereotaxic apparatus for operations on the human brain. Science 106:349, 1947.
10. Storrs BB, Walker ML: Use of a C.T.-guided stereotaxic apparatus in pediatric neurosurgery. Humphreys RP (ed): Concepts in Pediatric Neurosurgery, Vol. 5. New York, S Karger, 1985, pp 214–223.
11. Talairach J, David M, Tournoux P, et al: Atlas d'anatomie stereotaxique. Paris, Masson, 1957.
12. Thomas DG, Davis CH, Ingram S, et al: Stereotaxic biopsy of the brain under M.R. imaging control. AJNR 7:161, 1986.

54
PEDIATRIC NEUROANESTHESIA AND INTENSIVE CARE

D. Ryan Cook, M.D.

Pediatric neuroanesthesia requires awareness both of the anatomic, physiologic, pharmacologic, and psychologic characteristics of the infant or child as they relate to anesthesia, and of the special problems of the neurosurgical patient. The anesthetist must be knowledgeable in both these special areas to provide optimal anesthesia care. The pediatric neuroanesthetist, for example, must provide (1) anesthesia for infants with myelomeningocele, hydrocephalus, or craniosynostosis; (2) anesthesia for neurodiagnostic procedures; (3) anesthesia for patients with intracranial tumors or vascular malformations; (4) anesthesia for noncranial procedures; and (5) neural intensive-care unit support for the head-injured or comatose patient.

Recent review articles,[63] monographs, and books[36, 39, 55] have surveyed the anesthetic care of the adult neurosurgical patient. The purpose of this chapter is to provide an overview of the pediatric aspects of neuroanesthesia and intensive care.

Planning the anesthetic management of the pediatric neurosurgical patient may best be accomplished by placing the patient at some point on an imaginary grid, of which one coordinate is a scale of the nature and severity of the neurosurgical problem, and the other, the age and psychologic maturity of the patient. Many neurosurgical procedures present minimal problems in anesthetic management. Similarly, in all but infants and very young children, the management of a major craniotomy, for example, differs little from that of the adult. Table 54–1 reviews procedures performed at the Children's Hospital of Pittsburgh.

Although the foregoing seems to belabor the obvious, it is intended to forestall an unfortunate tendency toward over-reacting in the management of many of these patients, that is, to endow all children with the physiologic limitations of the infant, or, on the other hand, to consider all these patients, simply because they are "neurosurgical," as high risks requiring specialized techniques. Careful preoperative evaluation in the manner suggested places the patient and the patient's problem in proper perspective.

PHYSIOLOGIC AND PHARMACOLOGIC FACTORS THAT INFLUENCE ANESTHESIA IN THE INFANT

Physiologic Factors

The head of the young infant is large and poorly supported on the trunk by a short, weak neck. The tongue is large and the teeth, of course, have not developed. To maintain a patent airway in the unconscious infant, the head is extended largely by arching the back. The head, particularly in the child with hydrocephalus, should be stabilized during anesthesia by placing the crown of the head in a head ring. The body of the child with severe hydrocephalus can be supported on several blankets in order to maintain the airway and to facilitate endotracheal intubation. Heat loss from the large head

Table 54–1. NEUROSURGICAL PROCEDURES: PERFORMED UNDER GENERAL ANESTHESIA (CHILDREN'S HOSPITAL OF PITTSBURGH 1978/1979 AND 1985/1986)

Operative Procedures	78/79	85/86
Insertion intracranial monitor (isolated procedure)	33	2
Craniotomy for subdural or epidural bleeding	15	6
Craniotomy for tumor/vascular	45	35
Elevation depressed skull fracture	18	10
Repair encephalocele	3	—
Repair meningomyelocele	13	30
Craniectomy (synostosis)	14	30
Shunt/shunt revision	230	100
Lumbar/cervical laminectomy	18	32

can be minimized prior to surgery by the use of a stocking cap or a plastic bag.

The infant larynx is funnel-shaped, the narrowest portion being not at the glottis but at the cricoid ring below the glottis. In the infant, the diameter of the airway at the cricoid ring, thus, determines the size of the endotracheal tube that may be passed. The larnyx, which is small in the absolute sense, is easily obstructed by edema. For this reason, the author is reluctant to perform endotracheal anesthesia on consecutive days.

The various lung volumes and capacities are generally comparable with those of an adult on a percentage basis (Table 54–2). Lung compliance is low in the newborn, since it is a function of the size of the patient, but distensibility of the infant's lung is comparable with that of the adult on a unit per body weight basis. The same pressures are required to inflate the lungs of the infant and the adult to achieve a tidal volume. The functional respiratory surface area of the infant's lung is small per unit of lung volume or body weight.

The breathing of the newborn is largely diaphragmatic, the intercostal muscles being relatively ineffective. The ribs lie in an almost horizontal position, and the sternum offers little fixation against diaphragmatic contraction. Sternal and suprasternal retraction, therefore, is common in exaggerated breathing. The pattern of normal respiration is shallow and frequently irregular. Oxygen consumption per kilogram in the infant is nearly twice that of the adult (6.2 mg/kg/min); therefore, the infant must move twice the amount of air per kilogram. This increased work is accomplished mainly through an increased respiratory rate that is nearly double that of the adult. Because of the relatively greater effort required to achieve normal respiration, the infant's ventilation is easily compromised by drugs, hypothermia, or hypoxia.

The cardiovascular system of the infant functions at lower pressures and at higher pulse rates than those of the adult. Both pulse and blood pressure are quite labile and may increase markedly with crying, straining, or even minor stimuli. On the other hand, the heart is particularly sensitive to vagal stimulus, and the rate may slow alarmingly with hypoxia or certain parasympathomimetic drugs. Normal cardiovascular values are given in Table 54–3. Cardiovascular compensation in response to blood loss or hypovolemia is accomplished mainly through intense vasoconstriction. Circulatory collapse, when it occurs, develops suddenly and without the premonitory signs usually seen in the adult.

Homeostasis of Body Heat

The infant, who has a relatively large surface area per unit of weight, is unable to maintain normal body temperature in a cool environment. Diminished muscle tone and peripheral vasodilatation caused by general anesthetics and muscle relaxants further contribute to the risk of hypothermia. Ideally, therefore, the temperature of the operating room itself should be increased to 25–27°C. During preparation for surgery, the infant should be kept as closely covered as possible with blankets. A transparent plastic bag that encloses the body except for the head and neck makes an effective device to prevent heat loss. A circulating warm-water mattress covered with a single layer of drapes should be used. The mattress temperature should be carefully monitored and maintained at no more than 37°C to prevent burns. Radiant heat lamps are also very effective in reducing heat loss. Anesthetic gases should be heated and humidified if nonre-

Table 54–2. NORMAL VALUES FOR LUNG FUNCTIONS

	Newborn	Adult
FRC (ml)	75	3030
VC (ml)	100	4620
$\dot{V}_E$ (ml/min)	550	6000
$\dot{V}_T$ (ml)	17	500
f (frequency)	34	12
$\dot{V}_A$ (ml/min)	385	4140
V_D (ml)	7.5	150
C_l (ml/cm H_2O)	5	163
Peak flow rates (l/min)	10	457
R (cm H_2O/l/sec)	29	2

Table 54–3. NORMAL CARDIOVASCULAR VALUES FOR INFANTS AND ADULTS

Comparison	Newborn	Adult
SA (m^2)	0.25	1.75
Weight (kg)	3.2	70
Arterial BP (mm Hg)	70/40	120/80
Rate (l/min)	120/140	70
Cardiac output (l/min)	0.5/0.6	5–6.0
Stroke vol (cc/beat)	4–6	60–80
Total peripheral resistance	+++	+
Circulation time arm to eye (sec)	10.2 (5–14)	10 (70–15.6)

breathing techniques are used. Antiseptic solutions used for surgical preparation should be warmed.

The danger of hypothermia is best seen at the conclusion of anesthesia and surgery, when such patients normally can be expected once again to maintain their own airways and to sustain normal spontaneous ventilation. Hypothermic infants, however, remain lethargic and have poor muscle tone and, thus, are less able to rewarm themselves. Spontaneous ventilation is depressed or nonexistent. The additive effects of hypoventilation, hypoxia, and the hypothermia itself engender both metabolic and respiratory acidosis. The acidosis, in turn, leads to less forceful myocardial contraction and, if not treated, to circulatory collapse. These hazards of cold stress underline the importance of careful temperature monitoring and efforts to prevent heat loss during anesthesia. In the event the body temperature does fall more than a degree, active measures for rewarming and respiratory support must be instituted in the operating room until temperature returns to normal.

Pharmacologic Differences

The young infant, especially during the neonatal period, differs from the adult in the quantitative responses to many anesthetic drugs and adjuncts.[18] During the first several months of life, there are rapid physical growth and rapid maturation and change in the factors involved in the uptake, distribution, redistribution, metabolism, and excretion of drugs. Important differences in these processes between the infant and the adult have been identified to explain the young infant's altered response to many drugs. In addition, variations in penetration of the blood-brain barrier and in receptor sensitivity have been observed in infants for some anesthetics.

Several factors make the use of potent inhalation anesthetics less suitable for neonates and young infants than for older children and adults.

1. The infant requires higher alveolar anesthetic concentrations than the adult for a given surgical stimulus. For example, in infants, the minimum alveolar concentration (MAC) of halothane is 30 to 50 percent higher than that of a young adult.

2. The rate of rise of alveolar levels of inhalation anesthetic agents toward equilibrium, at constant inspired concentrations, is more rapid in infants and children than in adults. Markedly larger alveolar ventilation relative to the functional residual capacity in the neonate as compared with the adult allows more rapid equilibration of alveolar tension in the neonate than in the adult. In addition, greater perfusion and ventilation on a weight basis, the low fat and muscle content, and diversion of a greater fraction of the cardiac output to highly perfused tissues in the neonate also explain these differences in uptake.

3. Unfortunately, at equal MAC levels of halothane, myocardial contractility seems more easily depressed in the neonate than in the adult. The therapeutic ratio thus is less in the neonate. Significant hypotension and caridac arrest are more common in neonates than adults when potent anesthetics are used. Therefore, the pediatric anesthetist depends heavily upon the use of muscle relaxants and narcotics as adjuncts to nitrous oxide-oxygen anesthesia in order to eliminate or reduce the need for high concentrations of potent inhalation anesthetics.

In the neonate, differences in the size of the body fluid compartments, relatively smaller muscle mass and fat stores, and presumably greater blood flow per unit of organ weight influence the distribution of drugs to their active sites and secondary redistribution. Total body water, extracellular fluid, and body volume of the neonate are larger on a weight basis than those of an adult (Table 54–4). The initial larger volume for distribution of a parenterally administered drug may explain, in part, why neonates appear to require larger amounts of some drugs on a milligram-per-kilogram basis to produce a given effect. Differences in fat stores and muscle mass at different ages are shown in Table 54–4. Smaller muscle and fat stores provide less uptake to inactive sites and tend to keep plasma concentration higher. The smaller amount of fat tissue in neonates provides a relatively small reservoir for fat-soluble drugs. Little is known about the blood flow per unit mass of various organs in neonates.

Neonatal hepatic enzyme systems responsible for the metabolism of drugs are incompletely developed or absent. However, the activity of oxidative and reductive enzymes increases to adult levels within a few days of life. The ability of the infant to conjugate with acetate develops by one month of age, with glucuronide by two months, and with amino acids by three months. The activity of all

Table 54–4. PHARMACOLOGIC DIFFERENCES: DIFFERENCES IN BODY COMPOSITION

Body Compartment	Premature (1.5 kg)	Full Term (3.5 kg)	Adult (70 kg)
Total body water (% body weight)	83	73.0	60.0
ECF (% body weight)	62	44	20.0
Blood volume (ml/kg)	60	85–105	70
ICW (% body weight)	25	33	40
Muscle mass (% body weight)	15	20	50
Fat (% body weight)	3	12	18

Adapted from Friss-Hansen B: Body composition during growth. Pediatrics 47:264–274, 1971; reproduced by permission of Pediatrics, copyright © 1971.

these enzyme systems can be increased by known enzyme inductors such as benzpyrene or phenobarbital. Thus, the low enzyme activity for various substrates reflects lack of stimulation rather than inability of the enzyme system to be stimulated. The age from birth is important for maturation of these enzyme systems, not the duration of gestation. Premature infants and mature-born infants develop the ability to metabolize drugs to the same degree at the same time period after birth.

Since many drugs or foreign substances are simply filtered by the kidney, glomerular filtration rate (GFR) influences drug excretion and action. Inulin and thiosulfate clearances that reflect GFR are lower in newborns and young children than in adults. Volume clearance, when related to surface area, approaches adult values at about three months of age. If, on the other hand, clearance is related to weight, adult values are reached in about ten days or two weeks. The time-clearance method eliminates this choice of what basis to select. The elimination half-life for thiosulfate is about three times slower in newborns than in older children or adults; by three weeks of age, these differences disappear. The maturation of glomerular function may be related to changes in the permeability of the glomerular membrane of conversion of nonfunctional glomeruli to functional participants in the process of filtration. Proximal tubular secretion assumes adult values during the first four to five months of age.

Thus, there is rapid maturation in the infant's ability to metabolize and excrete drugs. This pharmacologic maturation combined with gradual physiologic maturation lessens the anesthetist's concerns about immaturity.

EVALUATION OF THE NEUROSURGICAL PATIENT

Assessment of the Patient

The neurosurgical patient should be evaluated in a three-step approach:

1. The neurosurgical problem itself, its nature, severity, and duration.
2. The general medical condition, especially those organ systems of particular concern to the anesthetist, for example, the state of consciousness, the airway, the cardiovascular status, ventilation, medications, and laboratory findings.
3. The patient as a candidate for anesthesia—reaction to the illness and to hospitalization, anxiety, and degree of comprehension.

Much of this information can be gleaned from the patient's record and from the surgeon, but it is incomplete without direct contact with the patient and, when possible, with the parents. Baseline values of blood pressure, pulse, temperature, respiration, level of consciousness, and focal neurologic signs, if any, should be ascertained and recorded. The level of consciousness of the response of the patient to commands, painful stimuli, and the like should be recorded.

PREOPERATIVE PREPARATION AND PREMEDICATION

Preoperative Preparation

Pediatric patients, because of their age, background, awareness, or previous hospitalization, differ widely in their reactions to a discussion of anesthesia. Parents, too, depending on their education and experience, present a wide range of responses. The child or the parent who expresses more than minimal interest in or anxiety about the anesthetic deserves honest and straightforward, if not too detailed, answers to any questions. Where no such interest is evident, detailed explanations may create anxiety where none previously existed. Ordinarily, the best policy is a simple explanation of what may be expected before induction; this reduces the element of surprise. In the case of the alert, older child, this preanesthetic discussion establishes a degree of rapport between patient and anesthetist and permits the child to identify a familiar face in the strange atmosphere of the operating room. The anesthetist may choose to show a mask and "balloon" to the child and have the child practice breathing.

In recent years, increasing emphasis has been placed on better emotional preparation of the child for anesthesia and surgery through teaching. This teaching can best be done by the anesthetist or even more efficaciously by the parents, if they are able. However, this is not always possible. Many hospitals have instituted preanesthetic group teaching sessions in which films are shown and the equipment is handled and "tried out" by the patient. The effects of this preanesthetic teaching have yet to be critically evaluated.

Preanesthetic Medication

Traditionally sedative-hypnotic, narcotic, or ataractic drugs together with a belladonna preparation are administered before anesthesia, primarily to allay anxiety but also to facilitate induction, to control secretions, and to obtund vagal reflexes evoked by anesthetic drugs and surgical stimuli. Nowhere has this been considered more important than in the pediatric age group because of the child's relative inability to cope with fear, but also because the child, and particularly the infant, is most vulnerable to vagal stimulus.

The ideal drug or combination of drugs for this purpose has not been found; preferences vary widely. Many of the most commonly used drugs have disadvantages in that they are long-acting both in onset and duration and may cause respiratory depression or undesired dizziness or restlessness. Recently, partly for these reasons and because greater emphasis has been placed on psychologic rather than pharmacologic preparation of the pediatric patient, many anesthesiologists have abandoned or greatly reduced the use of preanesthetic medication for children. Definitive studies, as mentioned previously, have yet to be devised accurately to evaluate the effectiveness of either approach.

However, even without the availability of such data, one cannot but be impressed with the quiescence or drowsiness of the properly sedated child at the time of induction of anesthesia. The fully alert, unsedated child, of course, may not manifest anxiety by crying or other untoward behavior but may nonetheless be unduly frightened. The use of preoperative medication in those patients who are not at risk because of cortical depression, or central or peripheral respiratory impairment, therefore seems justified and desirable.

Atropine and Scopolamine

Atropine or scopolamine is virtually always a part of preanesthetic medication in pediatrics. Of the two drugs, atropine is the superior vagolytic agent, and scopolamine is more effective in controlling airway secretions. The choice between the two drugs depends on the principal effect desired and, to some extent, on personal preference. Atropine is administered preoperatively to prevent the bradycardia that may be caused by certain anesthetic agents or surgical stimuli; however, it has a relatively short duration of action and is ineffective 30 minutes after intramuscular or subcutaneous injection. Therefore, it is often given intravenously at the time of the induction of anesthesia.

At the age when sedative drugs are indicated, the author prefers scopolamine to atropine because of its contribution of additional sedation, amnesia, and effective suppression of secretions in the airway. The usual dose is approximately half that of atropine.

Sedatives and Narcotics

Sleep (or quiescence) and freedom from apprehension are desirable for the child who is to undergo anesthesia and surgery; however, such a state is achieved at the price of some degree of respiratory depression. The anesthetist must decide not only the degree of sedation desired for the patient but also how much sedation the patient can "afford." The child with increased intracranial pressure, obtunded consciousness, respiratory depression from any cause, or any impairment of the airway or airway reflexes should receive no preanesthetic sedation whatsoever.

The ideal choice of sedative drugs for children remains a matter of controversy. The barbiturates are by far the most commonly used and, for the most part, are the safest. However, the child given barbiturates alone often complains of dizziness. With larger doses, the sleep induced is frequently fitful. Thus, a sleeping child may suddenly become resistive and uncooperative when aroused by being picked up, by the prick of a needle, or by the application of a mask. For this reason, narcotics (preferably morphine) are often given with the barbiturate. Diazepam, in oral doses of 0.1–0.15 mg/kg, is an excellent substitute for the barbiturate.

Many drugs and combinations of drugs have been tried, but in the author's experience, they are little better than the combination of narcotic, sedative, and scopolamine. Table 54–5 shows a dosage schedule that may be used as a guide.[53] The doses of sedative and narcotic in this table are quite conservative. Yet, with scopolamine, they provide adequate sedation in most situations. Either the narcotic or the barbiturate, however, may be safely increased several degrees or even doubled for the particularly apprehensive child, if heavier sedation is desired.

Route of Administration

Preanesthetic medication may be given orally or by rectum as well as by intramuscular injection. A number of commonly used barbiturates and sedatives are available as suppositories or flavored syrups. However, in general, the results are less satisfactory, except in the hands of those accustomed to this practice. Absorption from the rectum is uneven and unpredictable, and oral preparations may be refused or vomited. Unless the child has an intense fear of needles or requires frequent injections, the intramuscular route does not appear to be unduly traumatic and is by far the most reliable.

Table 54–5. PREOPERATIVE MEDICATION TABLE

Age	Weight (kg)	Morphine (IM) (mg)	Atropine or Scopolamine (mg)	Seconal (IM) (mg) (cc)
Premature	Under 2.5		Atr. 0.075	
0–1 month	2.6–3.5		Atr. 0.1	
2–3 months	3.6–5.5		Atr. 0.15	
4–5 months	5.6–7.0		Atr. 0.2	
6–7 months	7.1–8.5	0.5	Scop. 0.1	15 (0.3)
8–11 months	8.6–10.0	0.6	Scop. 0.1	20 (0.4)
12–18 months	10.1–11.5	0.8	Scop. 0.15	25 (0.5)
19–24 months	11.6–13.0	1.0	Scop. 0.15	30 (0.6)
2–3 years	13.1–15.0	1.5	Scop. 0.15	40 (0.8)
4–5 years	15.1–20.0	2.0	Scop. 0.15	50 (1.0)
6–8 years	20.1–30.0	3.0	Scop. 0.2	75 (1.5)
9–10 years	30.1–40.0	4.0	Scop. 0.2	75 (1.5)
11–12 years	40.1–50.0	5.0	Scop. 0.3	100 (2.0)
13–14 years	50.1–60.0	8.0	Scop. 0.3	100 (2.0)
Over 14 years	Over 60.0	10.0	Scop. 0.3	100 (2.0)

Atr., atropine; Scop. scopolamine.

Time of Injection

Sedative drugs can be effective only if sufficient time is allowed for them to achieve their full effect. The various drugs used reach their maximum effect at different times and, therefore, theoretically should be given separately. However, in most cases, this is impractical, and usually all drugs are administered at the same time. They should be given at least 45 minutes to one hour before anesthesia. It is the author's practice that each patient is called twice: one hour before operation for medication, and a second time just before anesthesia is to be begun. This requires planning and cooperation of the surgical, nursing, and anesthesia staffs. It is well worth the effort, however, since the sedation is more effective and anesthesia inductions are made easier for patient and anesthetist alike.

ANESTHETIC DRUGS AND TECHNIQUES

For most pediatric neurosurgical procedures, general endotracheal anesthesia is required. The choice of anesthetic agents and adjuncts is dictated by the nature of the neurosurgical problem and the age and associated problems of the patient. Likewise, for most procedures, controlled ventilation is mandatory, either to facilitate control of intracranial pressure or to reduce the work of breathing in infants or those in the prone position. Appropriate, intensive monitoring of the pediatric neurosurgical patient is now feasible because of satisfactory miniaturization of adult equipment.

Endotracheal Intubation

Because most neurosurgical procedures involve unusual positions, distortion of the airway, or conditions in which the anesthetist does not command access to the airway, endotracheal intubation is an indispensable part of all neurosurgical procedures. For procedures involving extreme flexion of the head and neck or other situations in which the endotracheal tube might be kinked, the author prefers wire-reinforced endotracheal tubes. Routine intubation of infants and children can be achieved with an exceedingly low incidence of laryngeal edema or other sequelae.

However, movement of the head and use of wire-reinforced tubes does increase the incidence of postintubation croup in neurosurgical patients. Trauma in intubation can be minimized by gentleness and by ensuring adequate relaxation, either with a sufficiently deep plane of anesthesia or with muscle relaxants. The choice of the proper size of endotracheal tube is of utmost importance; it should be as large as possible but should pass the glottis and cricoid without resistance. At most, there should be only a slight air leak. Table 54–6 provides a guide to proper selection. In general, the use of cuffed endotracheal tubes in children younger than ten years of age is neither necessary nor good practice.

Regulation of Cerebral Blood Flow

Although the brain accounts for about 2 percent of body weight, it receives approximately 20 percent of total cardiac output to support its relatively high metabolic rate. About 50 percent of brain energy and cerebral blood flow (CBF) requirements go into active electrophysiologic function that directs motor activity and mental function. The remainder of the energy requirement is directed toward maintenance and restoration of the ionic gradients required for the foregoing function,[92] reuptake of neurotransmitters, and transfer of metabolic substrates and wastes. Cerebral functional activity and brain metabolism are coupled to local modulation of CBF by poorly defined messenger substances. This intrinsic mechanism of CBF regulation can be modified or over-ridden by extrinsic factors affecting CBF (e.g., pH or blood gas status, cerebral perfusion pressure, and neurogenic influences). Acute brain injury or disease and pharmacologic factors can also shift the relative contribution of intrinsic and extrinsic factors regulating CBF. Extracellular hydrogen ion concentration and, to a lesser degree, potassium and calcium clearly influence CBF.[92] Other cellular metabolites, including the cyclo-oxygenase products of membrane metabolism (released by agonist-receptor interaction), also couple metabolic activity to CBF.

Neurogenic and myogenic factors can modify CBF and link localized intrinsic and global extrinsic regulating mechanisms. Cerebrovascular innervation includes contributions from cholinergic, adrenergic and serotonergic components with extracranial and intracranial origins. These neurogenic systems apparently exert their greatest influence upon larger cerebral vessels as the innervation density declines

Table 54–6. APPROXIMATE SIZE OF ENDOTRACHEAL TUBES

Age	Weight (kg)	ID (estimated) (mm)
Premature	1.0–2.3	2.5
Newborn–3 months	2.3–5.0	3.0
6 months	6	3.5
9 months	9	4.0
9 months–18 months	9–11	4.5
2 years	11–15	5
4 years	16	5.5
6 years	20	6
8 years	26	6.5
10 years	30	7

with vessel diameter.[14] Constriction of larger extracranial and intracranial cerebral vessels following sympathetic activation may actually limit CBF, while intrinsic metabolic factors dilate the smaller intracranial vessels.[102] Myogenic-related CBF responses rely upon vascular smooth muscle responses that occur without detectable changes in brain metabolic milieu.[12, 14, 31, 92, 102, 111] Myogenic factors rapidly modulate cerebral vascular resistance following minor rapid alterations in cerebral perfusion pressure. With extreme alterations in perfusion pressure, metabolic changes become more important in the autoregulatory response.

Cerebral perfusion pressure and arterial blood gases are the major extracranial factors contributing to control of CBF. Under normal conditions of autoregulation, CBF is maintained over a perfusion pressure range of about 50 to 150 mm Hg. Cerebral blood flow varies directly with arterial carbon dioxide tension (Pa_{CO_2}), and inversely with arterial oxygen tension (Pa_{O_2}). Cerebral blood flow is most sensitive to Pa_{CO_2} within the 25 mm Hg to 80 mm Hg range. Cerebral blood flow Pa_{CO_2} sensitivity is blunted below a Pa_{CO_2} of 25 mm Hg because of ischemic or hypoxic vasodilation. Cerebral vascular responsiveness to hypocapnia is attenuated or absent during elective hypotension to a mean blood pressure of 50 mm Hg.[8, 9] When hypocapnia is maintained for prolonged periods, its influence upon CBF becomes progressively attenuated as a result of CSF bicarbonate exchanges, which restore CSF acid-base balance toward a pH of 7.4.[76] Arterial oxygen tension has its greatest influence upon CBF when levels fall below 50 mm Hg, leading to intense cerebral vascular dilation. At Pa_{O_2} levels above 300 mm Hg, cerebral vasoconstriction begins to occur.

Effects of Anesthetics on Cerebral Blood Flow

Most anesthetic agents can effect direct or indirect changes in CBF either by influencing Pa_{CO_2} and Pa_{O_2}, brain metabolism, or blood pressure, or by the direct vasodilation effects of the anesthetics themselves, independent of changes in Pa_{CO_2}.[57-59, 94, 95] Anesthetic techniques can also influence cerebral venous flow, that is, cerebral venous flow can be affected by posture or surgical positioning; by positive-pressure ventilation, especially continuous positive-pressure ventilation (CPPV); and by changes in blood volume. In the patient with reduced brain compliance, such increases in CBF or retardation of cerebral venous flow can dramatically raise intracranial pressure. Since Pa_{CO_2} has such a profound effect on CBF, the specific drug effects of anesthetics on CBF can be determined only if Pa_{CO_2} is controlled. Cerebral blood flow and cerebral oxygen consumption at normocapnia have been determined for the various intravenous induction agents, narcotics, and inhalation anesthetics.[42, 56, 60-62, 66, 105-107]

Volatile agents may influence CBF via several mechanisms. The most common mechanism is by direct vasodilation. Direct vasodilation may be countered to some extent by the ability of the volatile agent to reduce cerebral metabolic rate. This may explain why isoflurane, the most metabolically depressant volatile agent, has the least effect with regard to elevating CBF. Global cerebral blood flow and cerebral metabolism rate measurements for the volatile agents (at 1 MAC) indicate the following order of decreasing potency in the elevation of CBF: halothane, enflurane, isoflurane. The potency of these agents in reducing cerebral metabolic rate is generally in reverse order. A similar potency scale emerges from studies comparing the degree of brain surface protrusion and cortical blood flows caused by volatile agents.[26, 28] At higher anesthetic concentrations, all the volatile anesthetics can significantly increase CBF. These CBF elevations are associated with an increased cerebral blood volume, which forms the basis for intracranial pressure elevations caused by volatile anesthetics. However, correlation between cerebral blood volume and intracranial pressure appears to be present only during the initial 30 minutes of anesthetic administration. Thus, factors beyond blood volume alteration may also contribute to intracranial pressure increases associated with the volatile agents. Alterations in cerebrospinal fluid secretion, absorption rates, or both may be responsible for some of the "late" intracranial pressure increases.[6, 7] Nitrous oxide can modestly increase CBF and intracranial pressure in clinical concentrations. When added to volatile agents, N_2O greatly enhances their cerebral dilation effects.[49-51]

Most of the intravenous anesthetics, with the exception of ketamine, reduce CBF and cerebral metabolic rate with a relationship that suggests that the flow-metabolism coupling remains intact. Etomidate and althesin reduce CBF and cerebral metabolic rate with the same degree of potency as the barbiturates.[10, 67] Lidocaine is slightly less potent in this respect. When intracranial hypertension is present, these potencies can be useful in considering selection of the appropriate anesthetic agents.

Intravenous induction agents such as thiopental or diazepam can be safely used in all age groups. In patients with suspected increased intracranial pressure, an intravenous induction with thiopental is preferable to an inhalation induction. When starting an infusion provokes crying and struggling, however, an inhalation induction appears to be a lesser evil than to persist with attempts at venipuncture. Unfortunately, no data exist to clarify this issue. The use of volatile agents for intracranial surgery is somewhat controversial because they increase CBF to a variable degree at normocapnia. However, when preceded by intravenous thiopen-

at central, convenient locations often remote from the sampling source. The central switching device allows gases to be sampled successively from each source for a period of 15 to 20 seconds. Each sample is analyzed, and the information is processed and stored in a computer. It is made available for display both on a centrally located screen and on one located near the sampling source. A capnographic tracing of the most recent sample is displayed as well as an alphanumeric display of inspired and end-tidal values of each gas expressed in volumes percent or torr, the respiratory rate, and the inspiratory-expiratory (I:E) ratio. Trending can be displayed as well. The computer interprets as inspired and end-tidal values those occurring at the instants of minimal and maximal carbon dioxide concentrations, respectively. Thus, the accuracy of the displayed inspired and end-tidal values depends crucially upon the faithfulness of the capnographic tracing.[103]

Temperature

The thermistor thermometer has greatly facilitated continuous temperature determination during anesthesia. The hazards of elevated temperature as well as hypothermia in the infant have already been mentioned. Temperature monitoring should be routine in virtually all surgical patients. Its importance is unquestioned in the management of all infants and in major cases at any age.

Doppler Ultrasonic Bubble Detector

Continuous-wave Doppler ultrasonography produces a characteristic signal when reflected from moving red blood cells. Since ultrasonography is much better reflected from an air-blood interface, a higher-pitched, easily recognized, and distinctly diagnostic audible signal is produced during air embolism. To monitor right heart flow, such detectors should be placed in the right third to fifth intercostal space along the sternum. The lower limit of response of such detectors is 0.25 to 0.5 ml.

Electroencephalography

In the neurosurgical patient, the electroencephalogram can be used to indicate impaired cerebral oxygenation, perfusion, or both. EEG patterns seen during anesthesia vary according to anesthetic agents, depth of anesthesia, degree of stimulation, arterial tensions of respiratory gases, body temperature, and other factors. To detect changes in EEG that indicate ischemia, hypoxia, or other threats to the functional integrity of the brain, the anesthesiologist should maintain a relatively steady state, both pharmacologically and physiologically, particularly during the most dangerous parts of the anesthesia and operation.

Evoked Potentials

Evoked potentials (EPs) are the electrophysiologic responses of the nervous system to sensory or motor stimulation. Evoked potential recording systems use summation or averaging to extract the signal of the evoked potential from background noise. The resulting waveforms are displayed as plots of voltage against time. Intraoperative monitoring of evoked potentials potentially serves three main purposes: to monitor the functional integrity of neural structures that may be at risk intraoperatively; to identify important structures such as the sensorimotor strip of the cerebral cortex, branches of the brachial plexus, and cranial or peripheral nerves; and to serve as indicators of the depth of anesthesia.

Sensory evoked potentials (SEPs) allow monitoring of the spinal cord and of both subcortical and cortical structures of the brain. SEPs are transmitted primarily in the dorsal columns, and it is clear that in partial spinal cord injury, dissociation between motor and sensory function may be seen. Dorsal nerve roots can be identified using SEPs during neurosurgical operations within the spinal canal. SEP monitoring has the relative disadvantage of reflecting primarily the function of the dorsal columns of the spinal cord, with no direct assessment of anterior cord function. Motor evoked potentials are currently being evaluated as a means of monitoring anterior segments of the spinal cord. Motor potentials recorded from the intermediolateral tract of the spinal cord are faster than the somatosensory evoked potentials transmitted by the dorsal columns. They may be more readily affected by injury to the anterior cord than are the SEPs traveling in the dorsal columns. For optimal monitoring, one would like to assess the function of anterior horn cells as well. This can be done by stimulating either the motor cortex of the brain or motor pathways in the spinal cord, then recording nerve action potentials from motor nerves or the resulting electric or mechanical activity in muscle. When motor evoked potentials are to be monitored by recording muscle activity, neuromuscular blockade must be reversed or allowed to dissipate.

Cortical SEPs are used to rapidly and accurately identify the sensorimotor strip during operations that may affect this vital structure or its blood supply. They can detect inadequate perfusion of the cerebral cortex or of subcortical structures during such procedures as carotid endarterectomy, resection of intracranial aneurysms or arteriovenous malformations, and cardiopulmonary bypass. Finally, cortical SEPs can detect generalized insults such as hypoxia that may threaten brain function intraoperatively. This last application may eventually find more widespread use for monitoring brain function during general anesthesia or in the intensive care unit.

Intraoperative monitoring of brainstem auditory evoked potentials (BAEPs) is most frequently employed for monitoring of the eighth nerve and brainstem during operations in the posterior cranial fossa, particularly those operations in the cerebellopontine angle. BAEPs are particularly valuable for detecting ischemic dysfunction of neural structures in the posterior fossa produced by surgical retractors. Retractors can then be repositioned before permanent damage is done. Because BAEPs reflect only subcortical function, they may continue to be normal even in the face of severe cortical injury.

Visual evoked potentials (VEPs) are the first evoked potentials to be used for intraoperative monitoring when sufficient stability of waveforms can be achieved in the operating room prior to critical surgical manipulations. VEPs are used to monitor perfusion of the retina and anterior visual pathways during operations that place these structures at risk. Because VEPs are exquisitely sensitive to the effects of general anesthetics, they have been suggested as an objective, quantitative monitor of the depth of anesthesia.

On some occasions, the anesthetic technique may be altered to facilitate electrophysiologic monitoring. In other cases, monitoring techniques may be modified to accommodate the anesthetic management that is best in a given situation. Accurate and timely communication with the anesthesiologist is critical to meaningful interpretation of evoked potentials recorded in the operating room. Regardless of the anesthetic technique or the method used to monitor evoked potentials, the anesthesiologist can greatly facilitate electrophysiologic monitoring by maintaining a relatively steady state, both pharmacologically and physiologically, during the phases of the operation when EP changes related to surgical manipulations are most probable. In many cases, light balanced anesthesia with nitrous oxide in oxygen; a constant infusion of thiopental, at 1–3 mg/kg/hr; low doses of narcotics; and muscle relaxants may be appropriate. Vasoactive agents are used to control cardiovascular responses to surgical stimulation. When neuromuscular blockade must be allowed to dissipate, as when the facial nerve is to be identified by observing facial twitches in response to electric stimulation within the surgical field, potent volatile halogenated agents are added to keep the patient immobile.

INTRAOPERATIVE FLUIDS AND BLOOD LOSS REPLACEMENT

Intraoperative fluid therapy may involve the initiation of fluid management or, alternatively, may be a continuation of ongoing fluid therapy. It can be as simple as replacing the deficits from the preoperative NPO (nothing by mouth) status and providing maintenance fluids, or as complex as correcting preoperative abnormal deficits, intraoperative translocated fluids, and variable blood loss in addition to providing maintenance fluids. Conceptually, it is best to consider each of these factors separately before discussing general guidelines.

NPO Deficit

Because of their high metabolic rate and water turnover, significant hypoglycemia and dehydration may occur in infants who are allowed to fast for prolonged periods of time.[20, 74, 75] The fasting period before induction of anesthesia should be adjusted by timing feeding and surgery to minimize both the risk of dehydration and the risk of aspiration. The author allows normal feedings (milk) until six to eight hours before scheduled surgery; clear fluids (i.e., glucose water) are given until two to three hours before. However, delays in the surgical schedule may place the infant at risk for hypoglycemia and dehydration. In these instances, giving fluids intravenously is prudent. The fluid deficit incurred during fasting should be replaced during anesthesia. Assuming that a healthy neonate is in water and electrolyte balance at the time oral feedings stop, the fluid deficit at the start of anesthesia can be estimated by multiplying the neonate's hourly maintenance fluid requirement by the number of hours since the last feeding. This deficit may be replaced by giving half of the calculated volume during the first hour of anesthesia and the other half over the next two hours,[48] in addition to intraoperative maintenance fluids.

Thus, in the first three hours, in a neonate having a superficial surgical procedure with minimal or no third-space losses, fluid would be given as follows:

1st hour fluids = MFR + 1/2 EFD
2nd hour fluids = MFR + 1/4 EFD
3rd hour fluids = MFR + 1/4 EFD

(estimated fluid deficit [EFD] = hours NPO × maintenance fluid requirements [MFR] [ml/kg/hr]). Five percent dextrose in quarter-normal saline (5 percent D/0.25 NS) is frequently used for maintenance fluid. Minimal deficits can be replaced more rapidly during short surgical procedures.

"Third-Space" Intraoperative Losses

Surgical trauma, blunt trauma, burns, infections, and a host of surgical conditions are associated with isotonic transfer of fluids from the extracellular fluid compartment and, to a lesser extent, from the intracellular compartment to a nonfunctional interstitial compartment.[89] This acute sequestration of edema fluid to a nonfunctional compartment has been called third-space loss. Plasma volume may be decreased. The magnitude of third-space loss varies with the surgical procedure and is usually highest in infants having intra-abdominal, intestinal surgery. In addition, failure to cover the exposed gut and the use of heat lamps may increase evaporative loss. In infants, estimated third-space loss during intra-abdominal surgery varies from 6 to 10 ml/kg/hr; in intrathoracic surgery it is less (4 to 7 ml/kg/hr); in superficial surgery or neurosurgery it is trivial (1 to 2 ml/kg/hr).[11] Translocated fluids are a finite functional loss and contribute to the magnitude of dehydration. Thus, clinical signs of the extent of dehydration may be used to estimate needed fluid replacement. Generally, lactated Ringer's (LR) solution is used to restore third-space losses.[82-84] In cases of massive volume replacement, some advocate using 5 percent albumin to restore one third to one fourth of the loss. The end-point of third-space replacement therapy is sustained adequate blood pressure (appropriate for the patient's gestational age and weight), tissue perfusion, and urine volume.

Isotonic fluid also may be translocated in hypovolemic shock. When blood is lost, some interstitial fluid moves into the central circulation to restore plasma volume, but some moves intracellularly, perhaps because of altered membrane permeability. In severe shock, intracellular fluid volume expands to as much as 6 percent of body weight. Maintaining adequate circulating volume and avoiding hypoperfusion during periods of massive volume replacement may prevent these intracellular shifts.

Conceptually, two types of fluids may be indicated. For long procedures with moderate to extensive third-space loss, 5 percent D/0.25 NS should be used for normal maintenance and balanced salt solution to compensate for third-space losses. For short surgical procedures with minimal to moderate third-space losses, one type of fluid usually suffices (e.g., 5 percent D/LR or 5 percent D/0.9 NS). These relatively hypertonic fluids are used for a dual purpose, but large volumes of 5 percent D/LR, especially given over a long time, can lead to hyperglycemia and hyperosmolality—an osmotic diuretic effect is common. This diuresis may cause cellular dehydration in the brain, leading to intracranial hemorrhage. These problems are more common in stressed infants.[27, 47] To avoid these problems, one can limit the volume of 5 percent D/LR to 15 to 20 ml/kg and then switch to lactated Ringer's solution for maintenance, alternate fluids, or insert a second intravenous catheter for replacement therapy. To mix types of fluids, consider 5 percent D/LR a substitute for the usual 5 percent D/0.25 NS used for maintenance, and then add volume of LR to achieve a total of 7 to 10 ml/kg/hr. Glucose should be maintained between 100 to 150 mg/dl; balanced salt solution used as a substitute for blood or packed red cells should not contain glucose.

Fluid Management of the Neurosurgical Patient

Adequacy of circulating vascular volume, timely replacement of fluid losses, maintenance of electrolyte balance, and control of blood glucose are important goals for all surgical patients. A meticulous approach to these problems is particularly important in patients with brain tumors or other intracranial masses, head trauma, and cerebral aneurysms. Large volumes of free water, for example, may contribute to cerebral edema; diuresis for control of brain volume may rapidly produce hypokalemia; and inadequate fluid replacement may produce marked cardiovascular instability.

Water, sodium, albumin, glucose, and mannitol move slowly across the intact blood-brain barrier. With a disrupted blood-brain barrier, there is a generalized increase in permeability and movement of water, and other molecules become a function of the hydrostatic pressure. Osmotic pressure gradients tend to be lost. Permeability to sodium increases greatly, and brain concentrations of sodium parallel plasma concentrations. Disruption of the blood-brain barrier produces a marked increase in albumin permeability. Albumin moves into gray matter, paralleling the plasma concentration. However, concentrations of albumin in the brain remain elevated as the plasma concentration falls. The effects of mannitol on brain volume rely on an intact blood-brain barrier. As larger amounts of the brain are involved in a lesion, mannitol becomes increasingly less effective. Movement of mannitol into areas with a disrupted blood-brain barrier may account for the rebound increase in ICP, seen occasionally after mannitol. Mannitol excretion into urine requires a significant amount of free water. The osmotic diuresis secondary to mannitol also increases renal losses of sodium and potassium. These losses are increased further when loop diuretics (furosemide) are given along with the mannitol.[86]

Even with an intact blood-brain barrier, large volumes of isotonic glucose solutions increase intracranial pressure (ICP).[30] Hypertonic glucose initially decreases ICP, but there will be a rebound increase in ICP as the glucose is metabolized. Outcome after severe brain ischemia of various types was poorer in animals with elevated blood glucose concentrations, compared with animals who had been fasted.[37, 80, 91, 108] The blood glucose levels in these experiments tended to be high (often greater than 500 mg/100 ml), but two of the studies[37, 80, 91, 108] suggested that mild hyperglycemia (plasma glucose concentrations greater than 200 mg/100 ml) may also prove harmful. This damage may be related to the greatly increased cerebral lactate levels that occur during some types of ischemia. Except for complete ischemia, glucose delivery continues during the ischemic period, though at a slower rate than normal. With inadequate oxygen delivery, the rate of anaerobic glycolysis greatly increases, markedly increasing lactate production.[80] Intraoperative ischemia can occur in patients undergoing neurosurgical procedures. Deliberate hypotension especially when coupled with hyperventilation can produce a critical decrease in cerebral perfusion pressure. In addition, Albin and coworkers[3] have shown that the pressure exerted by brain retractors, especially when combined with hypotension, can exceed cerebral perfusion pressure and thus produce localized cerebral ischemia. Thus, it may be prudent to avoid giving excessive amounts of glucose intraoperatively, thereby possibly avoiding the potential risk that glucose may aggravate intraoperative ischemic insults. Recently, Seiber and colleagues[88] showed that withholding glucose during craniotomies of four hours or less in duration resulted in normoglycemia as opposed to hyperglycemia when glucose was infused.

Blood Replacement

All blood loss in infants and children should be somehow replaced. Accurately measuring blood loss and accurately assessing the acceptable blood loss in the infant are vital to any replacement regimen. Weighing sponges, using calibrated miniaturized suction bottles, and visually estimating (combined with a "guess factor") will define the magnitude of the blood loss. "Davenport's law" that intraoperative blood loss under 10 percent requires no replacement and that intraoperative blood loss over 20 percent must be replaced is unsatisfactory in that it does not consider the starting blood volume, hemoglobin, or hematocrit of the patient. The concept of allowable red blood cell (RBC) loss or allowable blood loss is a preferable guide to blood replacement.[13, 35] Normovolemic hemodilution to a predetermined hematocrit can be achieved with crystalloid or colloid solutions.

Anemia is defined dynamically in infants and children, since a normal "physiologic" anemia occurs within the first several months. Cardiac output, oxygen-carrying capacity, type of anesthesia, and type of surgery are factors other than hematocrit that help define allowable blood loss. The neonate has 60 to 90 percent Hgb F, and it is not until six months of age that the adult Hgb A/Hgb F ratio is achieved. Hgb F has a high affinity for oxygen, and the oxygen dissociation curve is shifted to the left. Thus, oxygen delivery to the tissues at a given oxygen tension is decreased. As the neonate matures from one to six months, the AV oxygen content and tissue oxygen delivery progressively increase. A full-term infant's hematocrit rarely decreases below 50 percent during the first several weeks of life. It takes about three months for the hematocrit to reach its nadir at 30 percent. This decrease in hematocrit results from decreased erythropoietin production, shorter RBC survival, and increased plasma volume. In the neonate, one arbitrarily considers 40 percent the lowest acceptable hematocrit level.

There is little developmental change in platelet count in infants. However, sepsis can depress the platelet count, particularly in premature infants. Bleeding from thrombocytopenia is rare with a platelet count above 50,000; serious bleeding is usual with a platelet count below 20,000. Normal adult values for clotting factors are attained between one and 12 months of age, depending on the specific factor. Mostly vitamin K–dependent factors (factors II, VII, and X) are affected. Consequently, coagulation screens have a wider range of normal values in infants. For example, prothrombin time may vary from 13 to 20 seconds, and partial thromboplastin time between 45 and 75 seconds, in neonates. Some factor levels are lower than others in infants. While factors IX and XI may be only 28 percent of adult levels, factors V and VIII are 100 percent of adult levels.[16, 17]

Estimating Allowable Blood Loss

Several methods have been proposed for estimating allowable blood loss (ABL) from the blood volume, weight, and hematocrit.[13, 35] The formulas range from the simple to the complex, but all involve an estimate of blood volume. Blood volume is about 10 percent of body weight (100 ml/kg) in the premature infant, and about 9 percent (90 ml/kg) in the full-term newborn. The timing of umbilical cord clamping and a host of other factors influence blood volume in infants. In fact, the usual range is 85 to 115 ml/kg; 100 ml/kg is an arbitrary median. During the first few days of life, the estimated blood volume (EBV) may be more accurately determined by the formula:[11]

$$\text{EBV (ml/kg)} = \text{hematocrit (Hct)} + 50$$

These estimates can be used with the following methods to calculate allowable blood loss. In these equations, H_o is the original hematocrit, H is the lowest acceptable hematocrit, and $\bar{H}$ is the average hematocrit $(H_o + H_1)/2$; all hematocrits are decimal values (e.g., 0.6, 0.5). In the following equations, equation (1) assumes that all blood was lost and replaced as a slug. Equations (2) and (3) assume that blood loss and replacement were gradual and exponential. Although equation (3) is more accurate, it is more complex mathematically, and hence errors frequently accompany it. Therefore, for accuracy combined with simplicity equation (2) is probably best. This equation has general applicability for all age groups. The difference in allowable blood loss calculated from the three equations is small but significant in neonates. This can be illustrated by estimating the allowable blood loss for a 3-kg infant with a 100 ml/kg blood volume and an original hematocrit of 50 percent; H_1 was 40 percent.

One would transfuse blood earlier according to equations (1) and (2) than with equation (3).

Equations

(1) Oversimplified

$$ABL = Wt \times EBV \times \frac{[H_o - H_1]}{[H_o]}$$

$$ABL = 3 \text{ kg} \times \frac{100 \text{ ml}}{\text{kg}} \times \frac{[0.5 - 0.4]}{[0.5]} = 60 \text{ ml}$$

(2) Simplified exponential

$$ABL = Wt \times EBV \times \frac{[H_o - H]}{\overline{H}}$$

$$ABL = 3 \text{ kg} \times \frac{100 \text{ ml}}{\text{kg}} \times \frac{[0.5 - 0.4]}{\frac{[0.5 + 0.4]}{2}} = 66.6 \text{ ml}$$

(3) Complex exponential

$$ABL = Wt \times EBV \times [H_o - H][3 - \overline{H}]$$

$$ABL = 3 \text{ kg} \times \frac{100 \text{ ml}}{\text{kg}} \times [0.5 - 0.4]\left[3 - \frac{0.5 + 0.4}{2}\right] = 76.5 \text{ ml}$$

There is controversy over how the blood volume should be supported while the hematocrit is being allowed to decrease. Data are nonexistent, and several approaches are possible. If ongoing blood loss is replaced milliliter for milliliter with 5 percent colloid (i.e., albumin, fresh-frozen plasma), using equations (2) or (3) the hematocrit will be within 1 to 3 vol/dl of the desired level. Furman and associates[35] recommend replacing ongoing blood loss with an equal volume of lactated Ringer's solution until serum albumin concentration approaches 5 gm/dl; after this point, blood volume is maintained with 5 percent albumin until the allowable blood loss has been exceeded. Others replace blood loss with three to four times the volume of lactated Ringer's solution. Although this volume of clear fluid may be needed in patients in shock, it seems excessive in patients with well-perfused tissues. Hypoproteinemia may result.

The author replaces blood loss with volumes of crystalloid 1.5 times the measured or calculated loss. In major surgery involving one to two body cavities, intravascular albumin may be transiently depleted or translocated. If 25 percent salt-poor albumin is used to replace these losses, its hypertonicity will mobilize fluids from the extracellular compartment; if the patient's "third space" is depleted, fluid will be mobilized from the intracellular compartment, leading to intracellular dehydration. Therefore, serum albumin should be replaced with 5 percent albumin.

Blood component therapy depends on the clinical setting and the availability of various blood products. Fresh whole blood (less than four hours old) has a limited availability. The septic infant benefits from its clotting factors, platelets, and white blood cells. If predicted blood loss is greater than or equal to 40 percent of blood volume, it is helpful in supplying platelets and clotting factors. However, component therapy is usually the rule.[16, 17] Packed red blood cells have a hematocrit between 70 and 80 percent. On the average, 1 ml/kg of packed cells will increase the hematocrit by 1.5 percent. Units of packed cells can be subdivided into pediatric packs of 80 to 100 ml. The fluid of these cells is relatively hyperkalemic (K^+ 15–20 mEq/l), acidotic (pH < 7.0), and low in ionized Ca^{++}. With rapid administration each of these factors is significant.

When the amount of blood lost approaches one blood volume, labile clotting factors are greatly reduced; normal clotting requires 5 to 20 percent of factor V and 30 percent of factor VIII. All the coagulation factors except platelets are present in normal quantities in fresh-frozen plasma. The author prefers to give nearly equal volumes of fresh-frozen plasma and packed cells to patients (hematocrit = 35–40 percent) with massive blood loss (i.e., ≥ 1 blood volume). The ratio of cells to plasma can be varied to produce any desired hematocrit. The need for platelets intraoperatively may be predicted from the postoperative platelet count. Platelets can be mobilized from the spleen and bone marrow as bleeding occurs. An infant with a high preoperative count (> 250,000) may not need a platelet transfusion until two to three blood volumes are lost, whereas an infant that has a low count (< 150,000) may need platelets after only one blood volume is lost.[16, 17, 23] One platelet pack per 10 kg is usually adequate. Rapid administration of cold, citrated blood products can be hazardous; all such products obviously should be warmed before infusion. Fresh-frozen plasma (FFP) contains the greatest amount of citrate per unit volume of any blood product; rapid infusion of FFP should cause the greatest change in ionized calcium. Under most circumstances, the mobilization of calcium and hepatic metabolism of citrate are sufficiently rapid to prevent precipitous decreases in ionized calcium. However, because the infant's stores of calcium are small and because a larger fraction of his or her blood volume can be replaced more rapidly, the infant is at special risk for hypocalcemia. For example, transient decreases in ionized calcium are seen in jaundiced infants during exchange transfusion. Coté and colleagues[22] demonstrated that infusion of FFP at rates of 1 to 2.5 ml/kg/min was associated with transient decreases in Ca^{++} and with occasional significant decreases in arterial blood pressure. Equipotent doses of calcium chloride (2.5 mg/kg) or calcium gluconate (7.5 mg/kg) were efficacious in increasing Ca^{++} and in ameliorating the hemodynamic changes.[21] Empiric buffering of blood may lead to profound metabolic alkalosis as citrate loads are metabolized.

ANESTHESIA FOR NEURORADIOLOGY

Children and infants, unlike their adult counterparts, frequently require general anesthesia or heavy sedation for neuroradiologic diagnostic and therapeutic procedures. Although some of these procedures are painful, at least during part of the procedure, the principal indication for anesthesia is the inability of the young patient or combative patient to cooperate and to maintain the necessary immobility for extended periods; rigid restraints are strong stimuli for struggling and movement in infants, the semiconscious, and otherwise uncooperative patients.

A major problem common to all these procedures is that they must be performed in a location not usually designed for the administration of anesthesia and which is remote from the operating rooms and recovery facilities. All or most of the equipment must be transported to the radiology department. The situation is often further complicated by the fact that in many institutions, these facilities are shared by both adult and pediatric patients, and generally it is the pediatric patient who is the exception. Thus, the radiology staff is less likely to be able to deal with the special needs of infants and children. Finally, at the conclusion of the procedures, the anesthetized infant or child must be transported over long distances to the recovery area. Portable oxygen equipment, including a bag/mask/valve unit and a portable ECG monitor, must be available during transportation to the recovery area.

Anesthesia or Sedation

Since the anesthetic requirement for most of these procedures is minimal, the question frequently arises as to whether sedation may be substituted for formally administered general anesthesia. In the author's experience, sedation has been effective in only a small percentage of these patients—generally the older, cooperative children undergoing angiography or those undergoing studies that require immobility only for short periods of time. Difficulties encountered with sedation as a substitute for general anesthesia have been numerous. Even moderately heavy sedation with a combination of narcotics and sedatives has not provided adequate quiescence and immobility when the child was firmly restrained or placed in an unnatural position. There has been a wide and unpredictable variation in the effectiveness of the drugs even at comparable ages and dosages. The large doses of these drugs by either the intramuscular or intravenous route (or a combination of both) required to achieve quiescence have led to respiratory depression and increased arterial carbon dioxide tension and cerebrovascular dilatation. The dilatation in turn increased ICP and interfered with successful angiography. Sedation, effective or not, that was heavy enough to induce unconsciousness and respiratory depression became, in fact, a form of general anesthesia in which the anesthetist had no direct control of airway or ventilation. The effects of the sedative drugs, not all of which could be satisfactorily reversed, far outlasted the duration of the procedure. For all these reasons, endotracheal inhalation anesthesia, in the author's experience, has proved to be far safer, more flexible, and more predictable. The rare exception is the older, already cooperative child for whom "continuous sedation" may be all that is required.

Technique of Anesthesia

The type of anesthesia used for these procedures differs little in principle from that for neurosurgical patients of comparable age. The choice of anesthetic agents and relaxants is usually of secondary importance. Endotracheal intubation is mandatory, because the anesthetist may not have access to the head and because the patient may be turned into one (or more) difficult positions.

Routine monitoring of pulse, respiration, blood pressure, ECG, and temperature is essential. Special efforts to maintain normal body temperature, particularly in the very young, are essential but may prove difficult because it is frequently impossible to regulate the temperature of the room and because the use of the circulating warm-water mattress may interfere with radiography. Radiant heat lamps, wrapping of the extremities, a plastic bag about the head (when possible), and heated, humidified anesthetic gases are effective means that are available to combat heat loss.

Cerebral Angiography

The anesthetist must be aware of the volume and type of fluids used in conjunction with angiography and must adjust the administration of fluids accordingly. In general, the total volume of Hypaque Sodium (Winthrop Laboratories, New York, NY) should be limited to 4 to 6 ml/kg.

Following hyperosmolar contrast materials, there is an initial increase in blood viscosity and a decrease in hematocrit followed by a translocation of fluid that increases circulating blood pressure, cardiac output, and usually urine flow. Occasionally, anaphylactoid reactions with angioneurotic edema, hypotension, and bronchospasm may occur. In addition, severe dehydration has occurred in some patients receiving contrast material. Mass lesions of the brain associated with loss of autoregulation may be enhanced by hyperventilation, which decreases CBF to normal brain tissue; in general, however, hyperventilation results in enhanced angiograms.

Air Studies

The introduction of gas into the ventricles or subarachnoid space for air myelography, pneumoencephalography, and ventriculography complicates the use of general anesthesia. Nitrous oxide, which is often used for this type of procedure, is contraindicated because as a result of its relatively greater solubility than nitrogen in blood, it accumulates in the closed gas-filled compartments and raises their pressure.[85] The exception is, of course, when nitrous oxide itself is used by the radiologist as the contrast gas instead of air/oxygen.

The anesthetist must be aware and informed of the volumes of cerebrospinal fluid removed and the volumes of gas injected. Changes in pulse and blood pressure as fluid and gas are exchanged must be watched for, recorded, and communicated immediately to the radiologist. During all these procedures, but particularly during pneumoencephalography, the patient may have to be moved into a variety of unnatural positions that may affect the circulation and present technical problems with anesthetic and monitoring equipment attached to the patient.

Radiation Therapy

The greatest number of technical problems for the anesthetist present with the infant or child who is to undergo radiation therapy. These include problems common to the infant and the neurologic disease, the need for absolute immobility, lack of access to the patient, and, in addition, the need for daily serial anesthetics, frequently on an outpatient basis. Sedation, regardless of the combinations and doses of drugs or their route of administration, has proved unsatisfactory for radiation therapy because it does not ensure the absolute immobility required and because of the long duration of action of the drugs used. Inhalation anesthetics are unsatisfactory because of the hazards either of airway obstruction without intubation or of multiple intubations. The technical difficulties inherent in securing an intravenous infusion in a small infant on so many successive occasions virtually preclude the use of intravenously administered drugs.

The following technique, which admittedly involves a degree of compromise, has proved successful.[52] On each treatment day, the fasting infant, preferably accompanied by a parent, is brought to a quiet room adjacent to the radiation laboratory a few minutes before the scheduled treatment. When the radiation team is completely ready, the infant is given a single intramuscular injection containing atropine, 0.02 mg/kg, and ketamine, 5 mg/kg. Upon becoming quiescent, the infant is quickly taken to the laboratory and positioned by the radiation therapist and anesthetist. Monitoring equipment is attached, supplemental oxygen begun, and the patient is carefully observed for adequate airway and respiration. Radiation treatment is then begun without delay. Following treatment the infant is taken to the recovery room by the anesthetist.

Careful prior planning and communication are absolutely essential for the success of this deceptively simple technique. All necessary equipment must be available. Since the anesthetist must leave the patient during the therapy, special arrangements for remote monitoring and unobstructed viewing of the patient must be available. The radiation and anesthesia teams must thoroughly understand each other's problems. The short duration of effective anesthesia necessitates the avoidance of any delay once the injection is made. A plan for termination of therapy in the event of complications must be agreed upon.

Usually, slight increases in ketamine dosage are required with successive treatments. However, in a few cases, the infant seems to adapt to the daily routine and will remain quiescent on progressively smaller dosage. In addition to the usual anesthetic record, a simple tabular log showing date, dosage, effect, and complications should be kept to indicate these trends.

SUPPORTIVE CARE OF HEAD-INJURED PATIENTS OR POSTCRANIOTOMY PATIENTS

Many neurosurgical patients, particularly those with head injuries or following major craniotomies, may require short- or long-term respiratory care, nutrition, and long-term control of intracranial pressure. In many instances, attention to these aspects of care will decide the degree of morbidity and eventual outcome.

Respiratory Support

Intubation and ventilatory support are often required in neurosurgical patients to relieve upper airway obstruction, to maintain adequate oxygenation by protecting the lung from aspiration of secretions, to provide means for tracheobronchial toilet and artificial sighing or coughing, and to provide an adjunct to ICP control by manipulation of Pa_{CO_2}.

Table 54–7 lists major indications for intubation and ventilatory support. Sedation with intravenous thiopental, lidocaine, or small doses of narcotics can be used to diminish ICP, and muscle relaxants used to prevent coughing during endotracheal in-

Table 54-7. INDICATIONS FOR INTUBATION AND VENTILATION

Clinical signs of elevated ICP
Pulmonary insufficiency
    $Pa_{CO_2} > 45$ torr with elevated ICP
    $Pa_{O_2} < 60$ torr by face mask, $FIO_2 > 0.60$
Absent cough or gag reflexes
Anatomic airway obstruction
Spontaneous hyperventilation
    $Pa_{CO_2} < 20$ mm Hg
Progressive deterioration of neurologic status

---

tubation and during suctioning. In the absence of a basal skull fracture or rhinorrhea, nasal intubation is preferable, since it facilitates oral hygiene and nasal tubes are easier to secure. Uncuffed endotracheal tubes are adequate for ventilating children younger than nine or ten years of age.

Airway Care

Heated humidification of inspired gases through an artificial airway is indispensable in maintaining ciliary function and mucus flow, in preventing thickening of secretions, and in minimizing heat loss. Inspired gases saturated with water vapor at 32°C provide about 70 percent relative humidity when they reach body temperature in the lung; this is sufficient humidity to prevent cellular damage of the upper airways without causing unwanted heat gain or causing damage to the respiratory mucosae.[34]

Sterile endotracheal suctioning combined with re-expansion of alveoli and reoxygenation is performed routinely at least every two hours. Small amounts (0.2 to 2 ml, depending on the size of the patient) of sterile saline solution are instilled through the endotracheal tube to facilitate the removal of secretions.

Arterial P_{O_2} should be kept at 100 to 150 torr to guarantee complete hemoglobin saturation and to provide some leeway in oxygenation if a pulmonary setback should occur; ideally, inspired oxygen should be no more than 50 percent. All intubated patients should have a small amount of positive end-expiratory pressure (PEEP) (2–4 cm H_2O) to facilitate gas exchange and to maintain an adequate functional residual capacity. In high levels (greater than 8–10 cm H_2O), PEEP can occasionally raise ICP by impeding cerebral venous return.[2] Therefore, this modality should be used cautiously. Elevation of the head of the bed 30 degrees both facilitates gas exchange and helps counteract the effects of PEEP.

Mechanical Ventilation

The difference in tidal volume and respiratory rate between infants and older children makes it difficult to use the same ventilator for all age groups. In some instances, one may modify an adult ventilator for infants. On the other hand, a ventilator used exclusively for infants may be unsatisfactory for older children. An ideal pediatric ventilator should allow accurate control of a wide range of tidal volumes with small internal compliance, inspiratory and expiratory times, inspiratory flow rates, and inspired oxygen concentrations. An adjustable high-pressure relief valve should be included. There should be access to the exhalation valve to provide PEEP. In addition, there should be a mechanism to allow the patient to inspire out of phase with the mechanical ventilator (intermittent mandatory ventilation, IMV). The choice of ventilators in any intensive care unit probably should not exceed two or three types. This limitation permits technicians, nurses, and physicians to become thoroughly familiar with their use and idiosyncrasies. The inflation pressure generated by the ventilator should be monitored. Changes in the patient's lung compliance will be reflected by this pressure. Pressure alarms must be added to all ventilators to warn if pressure limits are exceeded or if minimal pressure is not reached in a definite time. The latter then serves as a disconnect alarm. This is imperative, since many patients are paralyzed to facilitate ventilator care.

Extubation requires the fulfillment of specific criteria. Table 54–8 lists the criteria using the mnemonic SOAP. *S*ecretions should be minimal; *o*xygenation should be adequate ($P_{O_2} > 65$ torr, with FIO_2 0.45, PEEP 2–4 cm H_2O); the *a*irway must be protected with presence of cough and gag reflexes; and *p*arameters must be met. The parameters should include a resolving or stable neurologic status and an inspiratory force of more than -25 cm H_2O.

Prolonged intubation, especially with the use of a ventilator, has been associated with laryngeal edema, ulceration, glottic granulomas, and subglottic stenosis. Subglottic stenosis is seen in 2 to 8 percent of patients surviving long-term endotracheal intubation.[1, 5] It is difficult to predict how long an endotracheal tube may be kept safely in place. The patient's age, duration of intubation, number of tube changes, relative tube size, use of mechanical ventilation, effective fixation of the tube, nasal or oral intubation, type and material of the tube, and presence and type of cuff all are contributing factors to glottic and subglottic injury.

Tracheostomy should be considered in infants and children when the need for intubation exceeds

---

Table 54-8. CRITERIA FOR EXTUBATION

S—Minimal Secretions
O—Adequate Oxygenation
A—Protected Airway
P—Other Parameters

one week. Ideally, all tracheostomies should be performed in the operating room, under controlled sterile conditions. The author prefers tracheostomies to be done between the second and third tracheal rings, when possible. Low tracheostomies, particularly in the infant, increase the incidence of pneumothorax and endobronchial cannulation. A longitudinal tracheal incision without a wedge-shaped flag is used.[101] Stay sutures are placed in both sides of the tracheostomy site. Tracheostomy tubes that have universal male connectors for attachment onto ventilator tubing are now available in all sizes. In children younger than ten years of age, uncuffed tracheostomy tubes are preferable.

Fluids and Nutrition

Neurosurgical patients require frequent adjustments in fluid management to maintain a mean arterial pressure of at least 60 torr and venous pressures in the low to midnormal range (4 to 8 torr). Initial fluid rates should provide one half to two thirds of the normal calculated maintenance requirements. If the perfusion pressure cannot be maintained despite adequate volume therapy, the use of vasoactive agents such as dopamine or dobutamine is indicated. In the choice and amount of fluids, neurologic function takes precedence over renal function. Central venous or pulmonary artery catheters provide important information that can be used in managing fluid therapy.

The syndrome of inappropriate antidiuretic hormone secretion (SIADH) is a clinical complex consisting of serum hyponatremia and hypo-osmolality in conjunction with a high urine sodium and osmolality. This problem frequently follows head injury and should be carefully looked for. It is normally a transient phenomenon lasting 24 to 48 hours and is, in the vast majority of cases, successfully treated by fluid restriction. In cases of severe hyponatremia (< 125 mEq/l), the use of a potent loop diuretic and hypertonic sodium chloride (NaCl) (3 N) will facilitate a more rapid correction of the hyponatremic state.

Diabetes insipidus often follows operations or injury involving the pituitary and hypothalamus. The diagnosis is based on the presence of a rising serum sodium and osmolality in association with the excretion of large volumes of dilute urine. Early after fluid resuscitation or operation, the diagnosis may be in doubt, since the large volumes of urine may represent excretion of excess water given during the operative procedure; however, in this case, the serum Na$^+$ and osmolality are generally within the normal ranges. Treatment consists of hourly replacement of urine output, using 0.2 to 0.3 NaCl solutions. If the urine output is greater than 1 percent of body weight per hour, subcutaneous aqueous vasopressin (Pitressin) is recommended. The beginning dose is one unit. Incremental doses of one unit are then added until the desired effect is seen.

Fluid losses from nasogastric drainage can be significant and, if untreated, can lead to hyponatremia and metabolic alkalosis. Such losses should be replaced with equal volumes of 0.45 N or 0.9 N saline solutions.

In the neurosurgical patient, as with any other critically ill child who is in a catabolic state, weight loss is progressive and significant. Caloric intake should be no less than 100 cal/kg of body weight for the first 10 kg, and 25 to 50 cal/kg for each subsequent kilogram of body weight. Peripheral alimentation with 10 percent dextrose and a 2.5 percent amino acid solution with vitamins should be started within 24 to 48 hours after admission to the intensive care unit. Enteral feedings of an elemental high-caloric, iso-osmolar formula can be given if the gastrointestinal system tolerates them. If the formula is not tolerated, central hyperalimentation should be instituted within five to seven days after injury. Lipid-containing solutions can be easily given peripherally, both to supplement caloric intake and to provide essential fatty acids. Liver and renal function, mineral levels, and serum triglyceride levels should be regularly checked when central hyperalimentation and lipid solutions are used. Adequate nutrition can frequently decrease morbidity associated with neurosurgical injuries and should be viewed as an integral part of the management in these patients.

SPECIFIC NEUROLOGIC THERAPY AND ICP CONTROL

The desired result of all therapy is the preservation of normal cerebral function. The ultimate success of therapy during the acute stages of neurologic injury may lie in the control of intracranial pressure. The unique volume-compliance relationship of the brain indicates that very small changes in volume can lead to very rapid and significant changes in intracranial pressure. Changes in neurologic status as determined by clinical examination can lag behind these changes in ICP by hours. For this reason, direct measurement of ICP is an essential part of therapy in severely brain-injured patients. The two most commonly used techniques are the Richmond subarachnoid screw and the intraventricular catheter. Both techniques accurately reflect intracranial pressure. The subarachnoid screw may be inserted while the child is in the intensive care unit. However, its stability requires a cranial bone that is thick enough to support the apparatus, and therefore, it is generally used only for children older than two years of age. Catheters have the added advantage of offering cerebrospinal fluid drainage capabilities but are more invasive and, therefore, are not favored in some centers.

Techniques for measuring cerebral function such as evoked potentials and bedside measurement of regional blood flow are promising adjuncts for following the course of therapy.

Blood pressure as well as ICP must be considered. The cerebral perfusion pressure is determined by the difference between the mean arterial pressure and the ICP. Thus, perfusion to the brain is diminished by either arterial hypotension or intracranial hypertension. In the normal brain, CBF remains normal until the perfusion pressure falls below 40 to 45 mm Hg. However, in damaged brain, CBF is more pressure-sensitive, and the minimal perfusion pressure may need to be higher.[31, 78] Data are not readily available concerning cerebral perfusion pressure in children. Nevertheless, it is important to maintain an adequate blood pressure (mean arterial pressure between 55 and 110 mm Hg), especially in the presence of increased ICP.

Specific treatment modalities for increased ICP include hyperventilation, corticosteroid use, osmotherapy, hypothermia, barbiturate therapy, and craniectomy. Use of each is intended to affect ICP by decreasing the volume of one or more of the three types of tissue contained in the cranium. Table 54–9 summarizes these modalities and the tissue matter each is designed to affect.

Hyperventilation

Hypocapnia with Pa_{CO_2} levels of 25 to 30 torr decreases cerebral blood volume by causing constriction of cerebral vasculature.[72, 79] How long cerebral vessels continue to constrict in the presence of hypocarbia of more than a few hours duration is unclear. It is also unclear what the effect of hypocarbia is upon regional blood flow in areas of the brain with altered or absent autoregulation.

Corticosteroids

Despite the absence of any accepted explanation of how they work, corticosteroids have enjoyed a tremendous popularity as therapeutic agents for brain injury. The indications for their use are controversial. High-dose dexamethasone (1–1.5 mg/kg/day) therapy has become popular. Initial results indicated potential advantages over conventional low-dose therapy (0.25–0.5 mg/kg/day).[29, 38] Recent studies, however, also question the efficacy of high-dose steroid therapy.[19, 40] Despite questions regarding their usefulness, steroids are often used for five to seven days following the injury and are then tapered over a similar period of time.

Osmotherapy

Treatment of cerebral edema with osmotic agents has remained an important mode of therapy. Mannitol, currently the most popular agent, is presumed to work by causing extravascular dehydration by establishing an osmotic gradient across the blood-brain barrier. A desired serum osmolality is approximately 320 mOsm/l. Small doses (0.25 gm/kg) appear to have the same desired effect as higher doses, of 1 gm/kg.[54] Continuous versus bolus therapy is controversial.

Osmotherapy has been challenged on several grounds. Brain injury in the pediatric patient appears to involve an early hyperemic phase.[15, 71] The transient hypervolemia that may occur following osmotherapy could aggravate this phase. The effectiveness of mannitol requires an intact blood-brain barrier. Disruption of this partition for whatever reason would allow the osmotic agent to escape into extravascular spaces and possibly establish a reverse osmotic gradient. This would result in a worsening of cerebral edema. For these two reasons, some people now recommend osmotherapy only as a temporizing measure, using other modes of therapy as definitive treatment.

Furosemide, a loop diuretic, may be useful in the treatment of cerebral edema.[25] It is believed to work by altering cellular ion exchange pumps, with a resulting decrease in cerebrospinal fluid production.[43] It does not work by creating a diuresis, although this may be a side effect. This diuresis should be replaced, if massive.

Hypothermia

Hypothermia lowers cerebral oxygen consumption approximately 4 to 5 percent per degree Celsius. Rapid cooling can be established with judicious use of chlorpromazine, in conjunction with a cooling blanket. Shivering should be avoided by using muscle relaxants. Mild levels of hypothermia, 31–32°C, can be a useful adjunct in the treatment of increased ICP. Levels lower than this, near 28°C, increase the risk of spontaneous ventricular arrhythmias, including ventricular fibrillation. It is debatable whether hypothermia alters the course of the treated disease, and it is not used consistently for this reason.

Table 54–9. TREATMENT MODALITY AND ALTERED TISSUE VOLUME

Blood	CSF	Brain Tissue	Cranium
Hyperventilation	Steroids	Steroids	Frontal craniectomy
Osmotherapy	Furosemide	Osmotherapy	
Barbiturates	Acetazolamide (Diamox)	Hypothermia	
	Catheter drainage	Barbiturates	
		Ca^{++} channel blockers	

Barbiturates and Calcium Channel Blockers

Barbiturates, both short-acting and moderately long-acting, may be useful agents in the treatment of increased ICP. Barbiturates appear to decrease both cerebral metabolism and CBF.[73, 77] In many centers, pentobarbital currently is being given to achieve blood levels of 2.5 to 3.5 mg/dl, in an attempt to control ICP if hyperventilation and osmotherapy have failed to do so.[81] A more controversial issue has been the proposed use of barbiturates and calcium channel blockers to preserve ischemic or hypoxic brain tissue.

It is now generally accepted that there is no place for barbiturate therapy following resuscitation from cardiac arrest or complete cerebral ischemia. Cerebral metabolic suppression by barbiturates (and other anesthetics) is seemingly not possible in the absence of an active EEG. The latter can be expected to remain isoelectric for many minutes following resuscitation. In the event of incomplete ischemia, EEG activity is usually present (albeit altered), and metabolic suppression and, hence, possibly protection can be induced with barbiturates. Barbiturates improve the brain's tolerance for the ischemic insult as judged by metabolic, electrophysiologic, and histopathologic criteria or outcome.[64, 65, 70, 93] Although barbiturate therapy offers an alternative approach to controlling ICP in head trauma, it is no better than other aggressive forms of therapy (hyperosmotic agents and hyperventilation). Barbiturates do not offer any unusual "protective" effect in head trauma.

Calcium entry blockers may produce beneficial effects during or after cerebral ischemia. They appear to have a predilection for cerebral as opposed to systemic vascular smooth muscle. Two such drugs that show promise in animal models are nimodipine and lidoflazine. Nimodipine has been reported to reduce significantly the deleterious effects of cerebral vasospasm in patients suffering from subarachnoid hemorrhage.[4] In the event of complete global ischemia (cardiac arrest), reperfusion is characterized by an immediate reactive hyperemia followed within 20 to 30 minutes by a delayed postischemic hypoperfusion state.[97] The latter contributes to the ultimate neurologic outcome. In animals, nimodipine, given either before or after the ischemic period, either prevents or attenuates this hypoperfusion state.[99, 100] In a primate study, nimodipine, given after 17 minutes of complete ischemia, significantly improved both the neurologic outcome and the histopathologic effects of the ischemic episode.[96] It is tempting to conclude that the improved outcome is accounted for by the improved blood flow. However, lidoflazine has no effect on postglobal ischemic CBF but may nonetheless improve outcome.[32] The latter studies of outcome are somewhat conflicting,[109, 110] and no primate studies have yet been reported.

Other pharmacologic interventions have been suggested or tested for possible brain "protection." These include phenytoin, naloxone, mannitol, steroids, various anesthetics (other than barbiturates and isoflurane), and compounds that might attenuate damage from free oxygen radicals during the postischemic phase. The latter includes the iron chelator, deferoxamine, which by binding available iron should partially block free radical formation. However, in a model of complete cerebral ischemia, pretreatment with deferoxamine did not alter neurologic outcome.[33] Similarly, the enzymes catalase and super oxide dismutase should minimize free radical damage but again failed to alter neurologic outcome in the same dog model.[98] An important determinant of outcome following cerebral ischemia appears to be the blood (and brain) glucose levels at the time of the ischemia. Even modest increases in glucose as produced by the preischemic infusion of a 5 percent dextrose solution (10 to 15 ml/kg) have been shown in primates to aggravate significantly neurologic outcome.[46] In that study mean preischemic glucose was 180 mg/dl versus 140 mg/dl in animals not given a dextrose solution. Clinically, it would seem prudent to avoid intraoperative infusion of glucose-containing solutions in patients who might experience a transient period of cerebral ischemia (e.g., intracranial and cerebrovascular procedures). Similarly, the intensive-care management of head trauma patients should include avoidance of hyperglycemia.

Bifrontal Craniectomy

Bifrontal craniectomy has generally been reserved for patients refractory to all other therapy. In most centers, results with this technique have been disappointing. It may be that more success could be obtained by performing this procedure at an earlier point in the course of the disease.

References

1. Abbott T: Complications of prolonged nasotracheal intubation in children. Br J Anaesth 40:347, 1968.
2. Aidinis S, Lafferty J, Shapiro H: Intracranial responses to PEEP. Anesthesiology 45:275, 1976.
3. Albin MS, Bunegin BS, Marlin A, et al: Brain retraction pressure and cerebral perfusion. Anesthesiology 53:S117, 1980.
4. Allen GS, Ahn HS, Preziosi TJ, et al: Cerebral arterial spasm—A controlled trial of nimodipine in patients with subarachnoid hemorrhage. N Engl J Med 308:619, 1983.
5. Allen T, Stevens I: Prolonged endotracheal intubation in infants and children. Br J Anaesth 37:566, 1965.
6. Artru A: Relationship between cerebral blood volume and CSF pressure during anesthesia with halothane or enflurane in dogs. Anesthesiology 58:533, 1983.
7. Artru A: Relationship between cerebral blood volume and CSF pressure during anesthesia with isoflurane or fentanyl in dogs. Anesthesiology 60:575, 1984.
8. Artru AA: Cerebral vascular responses to hypocapnia during nitroglycerin-induced hypotension. Neurosurgery 16:468, 1985.
9. Artru AA, Colley PS: Cerebral blood flow responses to hypocapnia during hypotension. Stroke 15:878, 1984.

10. Bendtsen A, Kruse BC, Madsen JB, et al: Use of a continuous infusion of althesin in neuroanesthesia. Br J Anaesth 57:369, 1985.
11. Bennett EJ: Fluid balance in the newborn. Anesthesiology 43:210, 1975.
12. Bill A, Linder J, Linder M: Sympathetic effect on cerebral blood vessels in acute arterial hypertension. Acta Physiol Scand 96:114, 1976.
13. Bourke DL, Smith TC: Estimating allowable hemodilution. Anesthesiology 41:609, 1974.
14. Briggs L, Garcia JH, Conger KA, et al: Innervation of brain intraparenchymal vessels in subhuman primates: Ultrastructural observations. Stroke 16:297, 1985.
15. Bruce D, Gennarelli T, Langfitt T: Resuscitation from coma due to head injury. Crit Care Med 6:254, 1978.
16. Buchholz DH: Blood transfusion: Merits of component therapy I. J Pediatr 84:1, 1974.
17. Buchholz DH: Blood transfusion: Merits of component therapy II. J Pediatr 84:165, 1974.
18. Cook DR: Pediatric pharmacology: A review. Drugs 12:212, 1976.
19. Cooper P, Moody S, Drone W, et al: Dexamethasone and severe head injury: A prospective double-blind study. J Neurosurg 51:307, 1979.
20. Cornblath M, Schwartz R: Disorders of Carbohydrate Metabolism in Infancy. Philadelphia, W. B. Saunders Co., 1976, pp 345–443.
21. Coté CJ, Daniels AL, Drop LJ: Comparative hemodynamic and ionized calcium effects of calcium gluconate and calcium chloride. Anesthesiology 61:A422, 1984.
22. Coté CJ, Drop LJ, Daniels AL, et al: Ionized hypocalcemia following fresh-frozen plasma administration to thermally injured children. Anesthesiology 61:A421, 1984.
23. Coté CJ, Liu LMP, Szyfelbein SK, et al: Changes in serial platelet counts following massive blood transfusion in pediatric patients. Anesthesiology 57:A409, 1982.
24. Cottrell JE, Hartung J, Giffin JP, et al: Intracranial and hemodynamic changes after succinylcholine administration in cats. Anesth Analg 52:1006, 1983.
25. Cottrell J, Robustelli A, Post K, et al: Furosemide- and mannitol-induced changes in intracranial pressure and serum osmolality and electrolyte. Anesthesiology 47:28, 1977.
26. Drummond JC, Todd MM, Toutant SM, et al: Brain surface protrusion during enflurane, halothane, and isoflurane anesthesia in cats. Anesthesiology 59:288, 1983.
27. Dweck HS, Cassady G: Glucose intolerance in infants of very low birth weight. Pediatrics 53:189, 1974.
28. Eintrei C, Leszniewski W, Carlsson C: Local application of ^{133}xenon for measurement of regional cerebral blood flow (rCBF) during halothane, enflurane, and isoflurane anesthesia in humans. Anesthesiology 63:391, 1986.
29. Faupel G, Reulen HJ, Muller D, et al: Double-blood study on the effects of steroids on severe closed head injury. In: Pappius HM, Feindel W (eds): Dynamics of Brain Edema. Berlin/Heidelberg/New York, Springer Verlag, 1976, pp 337–343.
30. Fishman RA: Effects of isotonic intravenous solutions on normal and increased intracranial pressure. Arch Neurol Psychiatry 70:350, 1953.
31. Fitch W, MacKenzie ET, Harper AM: Effects of decreasing arterial blood pressure on cerebral blood flow in the baboon; influence of sympathetic nervous system. Circ Res 37:550, 1975.
32. Fleischer JE, Lanier WL, Michenfelder JD: Effect of lidoflazine on cerebral blood flow and neurologic outcome when administered after complete cerebral ischemia in dogs. Anesthesiology 67:336, 1987.
33. Fleischer JE, Lanier WL, Milde JH, et al.: Lidoflazine does not improve neurological outcome when administered after complete cerebral ischemia in primates. J Cereb Blood Flow Metab 7:336, 1987.
34. Forbes A: Temperature, humidity, and mucus flow in the intubated trachea. Br J Anaesth 46:29, 1974.
35. Furman EB, Roman DG, Lemmer LAS, et al: Specific therapy in water, electrolyte and blood-volume replacement during pediatric surgery. Anesthesiology 42:187, 1975.
36. Geevarghese KP (ed): Anesthesia for Neurological Surgery (International Anesthesiology Clinics, Vol. 15, no 3). Boston, Little Brown, 1977.
37. Ginsberg MD, Welsh FA, Budd WW: Deleterious effect of glucose pretreatment on recovery from diffuse cerebral ischemia in the cat. I. Local cerebral blood flow and glucose utilization. Stroke 11:347, 1980.
38. Gobiet W, Bock WJ, Liesegang J, et al: Treatment of acute cerebral edema with high dose of dexamethasone. In: Becks JWF, Bosch DA, Brock M (eds): Intracranial Pressure III. Berlin/Heidelberg/New York, Springer Verlag, 1976, pp 231–235.
39. Gordon E: A Basis and Practice of Neuroanesthesia. New York, Excerpta Medica, 1975.
40. Gudeman S, Miller J, Becker D: Failure of high-dose steroid therapy to influence intracranial pressure in patients with severe head injury. J Neurosurg 51:301, 1979.
41. Halldin M, Wahlin A: Effects of succinylcholine on the intraspinal pressure. Acta Anaesthesiol Scand 3:155, 1959.
42. Jobes DR, Kennell E, Bitner R, et al: Effects of morphine–nitrous oxide anesthesia on cerebral autoregulation. Anesthesiology 42:30, 1975.
43. Kimelberg H: Glial enzymes and ion transport in brain swelling. In: Popp AJ (ed): Neural Trauma. New York, Raven Press, 1979, p 137.
44. Kochansky SW: Potential deficiencies in modifying the dinamap for use in the neonate. Anesthesiology 60:171, 1984.
45. Lanier WL, Milde JH, Michenfelder JD: Cerebral stimulation following succinylcholine in dogs. Anesthesiology 64:551, 1986.
46. Lanier WL, Stangland KJ, Scheithauer BW, et al: Effects of I.V. dextrose and head position on neurologic outcome after complete cerebral ischemia. Anesthesiology 63:A110, 1985.
47. Srinivasan G, Jain R, Pildes RS, et al.: Glucose homeostasis during anesthesia and surgery in infants. J Pediatr Surg 21:718, 1986.
48. Liu LMP: Pediatric blood and fluid therapy. In: Hershey SG (ed): Refresher Courses in Anesthesiology, Vol. 12. Philadelphia, J. B. Lippincott Co., 1984.
49. Manohar M, Parks C: Regional distribution of brain and myocardial perfusion in swine while awake and during 1.0 and 1.5 MAC isoflurane anesthesia produced with or without 50 per cent nitrous oxide. Cardiovasc Res 18:344, 1984.
50. Manohar, Parks C: Porcine brain and myocardial perfusion during enflurane anesthesia without and with nitrous oxide. J Cardovasc Pharmacol 6:1092, 1984.
51. Manohar M, Parks C: Porcine brain and myocardial blood flows during halothane-O_2 and halothane–nitrous oxide anesthesia: Comparisons with equipotent isoflurane anesthesia. Am J Vet Res 45:465, 1984.
52. Marcy JH: Commentary in "The Experts Opine." Surv Anesthesiol 24:2:124, 1980.
53. Marcy JH, Cook DR: Pediatric anesthesiology. In: Practice of Surgery, General Surgery Introduction. Hagerstown, Harper & Row, 1974.
54. Marshall L, Smith R, Rauscher L, et al: Mannitol dose requirements in brain-injured patients. J Neurosurg 48:169, 1978.
55. McComish PB, Bodley PO: Anaesthesia for Neurological Surgery. Chicago, Year Book, 1971.
56. McDowall DG: The effects of general anesthetics on cerebral blood flow and cerebral metabolism. Br J Anaesth 37:236, 1965.
57. McDowall DG: Cerebral Circulation. (International Anesthesiology Clinics, Vol. 7, no 3). Boston, Little Brown, 1969.
58. McDowall DG: Pharmacology of the cerebral circulation. Int Anesthesiol Clin 7:557, 1969.
59. McDowall DG: Fluid dynamics of the cerebral circulation. In: Scurr C, Teldman S (eds): Scientific Foundation of Anaesthesia. Chicago, Year Book, 1974.
60. McDowall DG, Harper AM: Blood flow and oxygen uptake

of the cerebral cortex of the dog during anaesthesia with different volatile agents. Acta Neurol Scand 41:146, 1965.
61. McDowall DG, Harper AM, Joacobson I: Cerebral blood flow during halothane anesthesia. Br J Anaesth 35:394, 1963.
62. Michenfelder JD, Cucchiara RF: Canine cerebral oxygen consumption during enflurane anesthesia and its modification during induced seizures. Anesthesiology 40:575, 1974.
63. Michenfelder JD, Gronert GA, Rehder K: Neuroanesthesia. Anesthesiology 30:65, 1969.
64. Michenfelder JD, Milde JH: Influence of anesthetics on metabolic, functional and pathological responses to regional cerebral ischemia. Stroke 6:405, 1975.
65. Michenfelder JD, Milde JH, Sundt TM, Jr.: Cerebral protection by barbiturate anesthesia. Arch Neurol 33:345, 1976.
66. Michenfelder JD, Theye RA: Effects of fentanyl, droperidol, and innovar on canine cerebral metabolism and blood flow. Br J Anaesth 43:630, 1971.
67. Milde LN, Milde JH, Michenfelder JD: Cerebral functional, metabolic and hemodynamic effects of etomidate in dogs. Anesthesiology 63:371, 1985.
68. Minton MD, Stirt JA, Bedford RF: Impact of prior neuromuscular blockade on the increase in intracranial pressure induced by succinylcholine (abstract). Anes Rev 12:30, 1985.
69. Minton MD, Stirt JA, Bedford RF, et al: Intracranial pressure after atracurium in neurosurgical patients. Anesth Analg 6:1113, 1985.
70. Nussmeier NA, Arlund C, Slogoff S: Neuropsychiatric complications after cardiopulmonary bypass: Cerebral protection by a barbiturate. Anesthesiology 64:171, 1986.
71. Obrist W, Gennarelli T, Langfitt T, et al: Relation of cerebral blood flow to neurological status and outcome in head-injured patients. J Neurosurg 51:292, 1979.
72. Phelps ME, Grubb RL, Ter-Pogossian MM: Correlation between $PaCO_2$ and regional blood volume by x-ray fluorescence. J Appl Physiol 35:741, 1973.
73. Pierce EC, Jr., Lambertson C, Datsch S, et al: Cerebral circulation and metabolism during thiopental anesthesia and hyperventilation in man. J Clin Invest 41:1164, 1962.
74. Pildes RS: Carbohydrate metabolism in the mother, fetus and neonate. In: Behrman RE (ed): Neonatal Perinatal Medicine. St. Louis, C. V. Mosby, 1977.
75. Pildes RS: Management of acute metabolic problems in the neonate. In: Aladjem S, Brown AK (eds): Perinatal Intensive Care. St. Louis, C. V. Mosby, 1977, pp 294–324.
76. Plum F, Siesjo BK: Recent advances in CSF physiology. Anesthesiology 42:708, 1975.
77. Price M, Price H: Effects of general anesthetics on contractile responses of rabbit aortic strips. Anesthesiology 23:16, 1962.
78. Purves MJ: Control of cerebral blood vessels: Present state of the art. Ann Neurol 3:377, 1978.
79. Reivich M: Arterial PCO_2 and cerebral hemodynamics. Am J Physiol 206:25, 1964.
80. Rhencrona S, Rosen I, Siesjo BD: Brain lactic acidosis and ischemic cell damage: I. Biochemistry and neurophysiology. J Cereb Blood Flow Metab 1:297, 1981.
81. Rockoff M, Marshall L, Shapiro H: High-dose barbiturate therapy in humans: A clinical review of 60 patients. Ann Neurol 6:194, 1979.
82. Rowe MI, Arango A: The neonatal response to massive fluid infusion. J Pediatr Surg 6:365, 1971.
83. Rowe MI, Arango A: The choice of intravenous fluid in shock resuscitation. Pediatr Clin North Am 22:269, 1975.
84. Rowe MI, Arango A: Colloid versus crystalloid resuscitation in experimental bowel obstruction. J Pediatr Surg 11:635, 1976.
85. Saidman LJ, Eger EL: Change in cerebrospinal fluid pressure during pneumoencephalography under nitrous oxide anesthesia. Anesthesiology 26:67, 1965.
86. Schettini A, Stahurski B, Young HF: Osmotic and osmotic-loop diuresis in brain surgery. Effects of plasma and CSF electrolytes and ion excretion. J Neurosurg 56:677, 1982.
87. Schieber RA: Noinvasive recognition and assessment of the failing circulation. Circulation 68:1021, 1983.
88. Seiber FE, Smith DS, Crosby L, et al: The effects of intraoperative glucose on protein metabolism and serum glucose levels in patients with supratentorial tumors. Anesthesiology 64:453, 1986.
89. Shires T, Williams J, Brown F: Acute changes in extracellular fluids associated with major surgical procedures. Ann Surg 154:803, 1961.
90. Showman A, Betts EK: Hazard of automatic non-invasive blood pressure monitoring. Anesthesiology 55:717, 1981.
91. Siemkowicz E, Gjedde A: Post-ischemic coma in rat: Effect of different pre-ischemic blood glucose levels on cerebral metabolic recovery after ischemia. Acta Physiol Scand 110:225, 1980.
92. Siesjo BK: Cerebral circulation and metabolism. J Neurosurg 60:883, 1984.
93. Smith AL, Hoff JT, Nielsen SL, et al: Barbiturate protection in acute focal cerebral ischemia. Stroke 5:127, 1974.
94. Smith AL, Neigh JL, Hoffman JC, et al: Effects of general anesthesia on autoregulation of cerebral blood flow in man. J Appl Physiol 29:665, 1970.
95. Smith AL, Wollman H: Cerebral blood flow and metabolism: Effect of anaesthetic drugs and techniques. Anesthesiology 36:378, 1972.
96. Steen PA, Gisvold SE, Milde JH, et al: Nimodipine improves outcome when given after complete cerebral ischemia in primates. Anesthesiology 62:406, 1985.
97. Steen PA, Milde JH, Michenfelder JD: Cerebral metabolic and vascular effects of barbiturate therapy following complete global ischemia. J Neurochem 31:1317, 1978.
98. Forsman M, Fleischer JE, Milde JH, et al.: Superoxide dismutase and catalase failed to improve neurologic outcome after complete cerebral ischemia in the dog. Acta Anaesth Scand 32:152, 1988.
99. Steen PA, Newberg LA, Milde JH, et al: Nimodipine improves cerebral blood flow and neurologic recovery after complete cerebral ischemia in the dog. J Cereb Blood Flow Metabol 3:38, 1983.
100. Steen PA, Newberg LA, Milde JH, et al: Cerebral blood flow and neurologic outcome when nimodipine is given after complete cerebral ischemia in the dog. J Cereb Blood Flow Metabol 4:82, 1984.
101. Stool S, Campbell J, Johnson D: Tracheostomy in children: The use of plastic tubes. J Pediatr Surg 3:402, 1968.
102. Strandgaard S, Paulson OB: Cerebral autoregulation. Stroke 15:413, 1984.
103. Swedlow DB: The role of mass spectrometry in the operating room postanesthesia recovery and intensive care unit. ASA Refresher Course Abstracts 220, 1984.
104. Sy WP: Ulnar nerve palsy possibly related to use of automatically cycled blood pressure cuff. Anesth Anal 60:687, 1981.
105. Takeshita H, Okuda Y, Sari A: The effects of ketamine on cerebral circulation and metabolism in man. Anesthesiology 36:69, 1972.
106. Theye RA, Michenfelder JD: The effect of halothane on canine cerebral metabolism. Anesthesiology 29:1113, 1968.
107. Theye RA, Michenfelder JD: The effect of nitrous oxide on canine cerebral metabolism. Anesthesiology 29:1119, 1968.
108. Todd MM, Chadwick HS, Shapiro HM: Outcome after cardiac arrest: The role of plasma glucose. Anesthesiology 55:A265, 1981.
109. Vaagenes P, Cantadore R, Safar P, et al: Effect of lidoflazine on neurologic outcome after cardiac arrest. Anesthesiology 59:A100, 1983.
110. Vaagenes P, Cantadore R, Safar P, et al: Amelioration of brain damage by lidoflazine after prolonged ventricular fibrillation cardiac arrest in dogs. Crit Care Med 12:846, 1984.
111. Vinall PE, Simeone FA: Central autoregulation: An in vitro study. Stroke 12:640, 1981.
112. Yelderman M, New W, Jr.: Evaluation of pulse oximetry. Anesthesiology 59:349, 1983.
113. Zmyslowski WP, Lena DM: Dinamap adaptation for neonatal blood pressure determination. Anesthesiology 58:583, 1983.

INDEX

Page numbers in *italics* refer to illustrations; page numbers followed by t refer to tables.

Abdominal cysts, shunt and, 226, *226*
Abscess, brain. See *Brain abscess*.
   epidural, 486, *486*
   spinal cord, 490–491
   spinal epidural, 491
Acetazolamide, CSF formation and, 162, 203, 232–233, 247–248
Achondroplasia, basilar impression in, 145, *145*
Acidosis, 567
Acoustic nerve trauma, 268
Acoustic neuroma, 455–456
Adolescent, pressure-volume index in, 242, *242*
Afterdischarge threshold test, 542
Age, cerebellar astrocytoma and, 338, 339t
   epilepsy surgery and, 538–539, 545, 554
   medulloblastoma prognosis and, 353
   neoplasm type and, 373–374
   radiation effects and, 378
Air studies, 580
Airway, 581
Albright's syndrome, 136
Alpha-fetoprotein, germ cell tumors and, 412
   prenatal, 48–49, 101
Althesin, CBF and, 571
Ambulation, hydrocephalus and, 188
   myelomeningocele and, 55, 59
   spina bifida and, 47
Amendares syndrome, 125t
Aminopterin syndrome, 126t
Amnesia, concussion and, 272
Amniotic band syndrome, 123t
Andersen-Pindborg syndrome, 126t
Anemia, 577
   subdural hematoma and, 284
Anesthesia, 565–586
   before radiologic procedure, 579–580
   blood replacement and, 577–579
   body heat homeostasis and, 566–567, 579
   CBF regulation in, 570–572
   endotracheal intubation for, 570, 570t
   evaluation for, 568
   fasting before, 575
   fluid management in, 575–579
   in astrocytoma surgery, 342
   in posterior fossa surgery, 342
   intensive care after, 580–584

Anesthesia *(Continued)*
   monitoring during, 572–575
      arterial oxygen, 573
      blood pressure, 572–573
      bubble detection, 574
      EEG, 574
      evoked potentials, 574–575
      respiration, 573–574
      temperature, 574
   pharmacologic factors in, 567–568, 567t
   physiologic factors in, 565–566, 566t
   premedication for, 568–570, 569t
Anesthetic agents, CBF and, 571–572
   infant metabolism of, 567–568
   preanesthetic, 568–570, 569t
Aneurysm, stroke and, 508–509
Aneurysmal bone cyst, skull, 426
   spine, 447–448, *448*
Angiography, anesthesia before, 579–580
   digital subtraction, in embolization, 525, *527*, *529–532*
   in arteriovenous malformations, 511–512, *512*
   in carotid artery dissection, 503
   in craniopharyngioma, 400, *400*
   in encephalocele, 99–100
   in hemispheric tumors, 376
   in hydrocephalus, 194, *194*
   in moyamoya disease, 503–504, *504*
   in pineal region tumors, 411
   in subdural empyema, 485, *485*
   in von Hippel-Lindau disease, 459
Anterior encephalocele, 98t
   repair of, 100
Antibiotics, in brain abscess, 484
   in CSF rhinorrhea, 266
   in shunt infections, 222t
   prophylactic, before shunt insertion, 222–223
      before skull fracture surgery, 265
Anticonvulsant therapy, after craniopharyngioma surgery, 404
   in brain abscess, 484
   in epilepsy, 537–538
      evaluation of, 539–540
   in intracranial hypertension, 249, 251–252
   in posttraumatic seizures, 272
   in subdural empyema, 486
   prophylactic, 295
Antley-Bixler syndrome, 126t
Anus, imperforate, 90, *90*
Apert's syndrome, 121, 123t, 125t

Aplasia cutis congenita, *261*, 423
Apnea, hydrocephalus and, 188
Arachnoid cyst, 103–105, *104*
 classification of, 103t
 clinical presentation of, 104–105
 hydrocephalus and, 184
 imaging of, 105
 incidence of, 103–104
 myelomeningocele and, 66, *67*
 outcome in, 105
 pathology of, 104
 spinal cord compression by, 323, *324*
 treatment of, 105
 vs. brain tumor, 105
 vs. hydrocephalus, 104, *104*
Arachnoid villus, CSF drainage by, 163, 174
 in hydrocephalus, 165–166
Arnold-Chiari malformation, 19, 37
 anomalies associated with, 19t
 embryogenesis of, 21–25
 embryologic timing of, 19–21, *20*, 20t, *21*
 shunt dependence in, 215–216
 I, 25, *25*
 II, myelomeningocele and, 60–61, *61–62*, 67
 III, encephalocele with, 98
Arteriovenous malformations, *194*, 508–516
 aneurysm and, 508–509
 embolization of, 526, *527*, 528, *528*, *531*, 532
  in carotid cavernous sinus fistula, 528–529, *529*
  in vein of Galen malformation, 529–532, *530*
 embryogenesis of, 509
 in Sturge-Weber syndrome, 551
 localization of, 511–512, *512*, 512t
 natural history of, 510
 pathology of, 509–510, *510*
 postoperative care in, 513–515, *514*
 preoperative management of, 512–513
 spinal cord, 531–532, *532*
 surgery in, 510–513
 symptoms of, 510–511, 511t
 treatment results in, 514–515, 515t
Arteritis, cerebral, stroke and, 502
Asphyxia, perinatal, stroke and, 233–234
Aspiration, ultrasonic. See *Ultrasonic aspiration*.
Astrocytoma, brainstem, 358t, 364–365
  cystic, 358, *359*, 360–363
 cerebellar, 338–346
  age and, 338, 339t
  clinical presentation of, 338–340, *339*
  cystic, 340, *341*
  diagnosis of, 340–341, *340*, *341*
  follow-up of, 343
  histology of, 344–345, *344*, *345*, 345t
  incidence of, 338
  management of, 341–343, *342*
   postoperative, 340–341, 343
  outcome in, 345–346
  pathology of, 344
  recurrence of, 345
 hemispheric, 378–379
 holocord, 430, 440–441
  clinical indications of, 432, *433*
  surgery in, 434, 436, 440
   pitfalls of, 438–440, *439*
  terminal vs. intratumor cyst in, 438, *439*
  vs. hydromyelia, 430
Ataxia, in astrocytoma, 339
 in medulloblastoma, 349
Ataxia telangiectasia, 460
Atherosclerosis, 501–502
Athetosis, motor pathway interuption in, 557
Atlantoaxial luxation, 312–313, *313*, *314*
Atlanto-occipital dislocation, 311–312, *312*

Atlas, formation of, 142
 fusion of, 148
 occipitalization of, 148
 pediatric, 300
 spina bifida of, *149*
 trauma to, 311–313, *312–314*
Atropine, 569, 569t
Avulsion, nerve root, 323
  brachial plexus, 308, *309*, 323
   neonatal, 326, *327*, 328–330, *328*
  scalp, 257–258
Axis, trauma to, 312–313, *313*, *314*

Bacterial infection. See also *Infection*.
 hydrocephalus and, 184
 shunt, 220–223, 222t
Baller-Gerold syndrome, 125t
Balloon catheter, 524–525, *526*
Barbiturates, in epilepsy evaluation, 541–542
 in intracranial hypertension, 249, 251–252, 584
 in posttraumatic seizures, 272
  prophylactic, 295
 preanesthetic, 569, 569t
Basal angle, 143, *143*
Basal encephalocele, 98, 98t
Basicranium, 142, *143*. See also *Craniocervical junction*.
Basilar impression, 144–147
 causes of, 143
 Chamberlain's line and, *143*
 conditions associated with, 145–146, *146*
 differential diagnosis in, 146–147
 symptoms of, 146
 treatment of, 147
Basioccipital cleft, 147
Behavior, epilepsy and, 537
 posttraumatic, 296
 shunt replacement and, 215
 tumor recurrence and, 473
Berant's syndrome, 125t
Bifrontal craniectomy, 247, *247*, 584
Biologic response modifiers, 476–477
Biopsy, in brainstem tumors, 365
 in pineal region tumors, 412
 stereotaxic, 412, 564
Birth trauma, basilar impression and, 145
 brachial plexus, 326, *327*, 328–330, *328*
 extradural hematoma and, 277–278
 intracerebral hematoma and, 287, *287*
 skull fracture and, 263–264
 spinal, 299, 301, 306, 308–309, *309*
 subdural hematoma and, 282, 283, 285
Blood-brain barrier, 159, *161*, *161*, 170, *171*
 disrupted, 576
 edema and, 250
 fluid management and, 576–577
Blood, See also *Cerebral blood flow (CBF)*.
 intracranial pressure and, 241, 248–249, 583t
 replacement of, 577–579
Blood pressure, cerebral perfusion and, 583
 edema and, 250
 monitoring of, 572–573
Blood products, 578
Blood vessels, CSF absorption by, 164
 in hydrocephalus, 166, 185
 scalp, 255–256, *256*
Body composition, infant vs. adult, 567–568, 567t
Body heat homeostasis, 566–567, 579
Bone grafts, posttraumatic, 291, *291*
Bone scan, in craniosynostosis, 107, 124
 in spinal tumor, 445

Brachial plexus root avulsion, 308, *309*, 323
  neonatal, 326, *327*, 328–330, *328*
Brachytherapy, 476
Brain, abscess of. See *Brain abscess.*
  CSF absorption by, 163–164
  CSF flow in, 171–174, *173–175*
  development of, 4–5, 5t, 16–17
  edema of. See *Edema.*
  growth of, 120, *121*
  hemorrhage location in, 231
  metastasis to. See *Metastasis.*
  penetrating wounds to, 265, *481*
  spina bifida and, 39
  tumors of. See *Brain tumors.*
  volume added to, 240–241
Brain abscess, 479–484
  causes of, 479
  clinical features of, 481
  congenital heart disease and, 480
  diagnosis of, 481–482, *481–483*
  intracranial dermoid sinus and, 102, 103, 481
  pathophysiology of, 479–480, *480*
  prognosis in, 484
  treatment of, 482–484
Brain tumors, age and, 373–374
  brainstem. See *Brainstem tumors.*
  cerebral hemisphere. See *Cerebral hemisphere tumors.*
  classification of, 336–337
  embolization of, 532
  experimental treatment of, 475–477
  follow-up of, 465t, 466, 467t
  fourth ventricle. See *Fourth ventricle, tumors of.*
  incidence of, 335, 336t
  intraventricular. See *Intraventricular tumors.*
  location of, 335–336, 336t
  neurofibromatosis and, 456
  postsurgical management of. See *Postsurgical management.*
  recurrent. See *Recurrence of disease.*
Brainstem evoked potentials, intraoperative, 361–362, 575
Brainstem tumors, 357–365
  biopsy in, 365
  cervicomedullary, 359–360, *360*, 361, 363–365
  classification of, 358t
  clinical manifestations of, 360–361
  cystic, 358, *359*, 360–363
  diffuse, 357, *358*, 364
  exophytic, 358–359, *360*, 361, 364
  focal, 358, *359*, 360, *360*, 364
  treatment of, 469, 469t
  surgical, 361–365, *362*
Brain-ventricle index, 227–228
Brown-Roberts-Wells stereotaxic frame, 562, *563*, 564
Buphthalmos, 454

Calcification, in Sturge-Weber syndrome, 551, *551, 552*
Calcium channel blockers, 584
Canalization, 4, 14–15, 74–75, *74*
  abnormal, 30
Carboplatin, 475
Cardiovascular values, 566t
Carotid artery, as embolization access, 525
  dissection of, 502–503
Carotid–cavernous sinus fistula, 294
  embolization of, 528–529, *529*
Carpenter's syndrome, 123, 123t, 125t
Catecholamines, neuroblastoma and, 445

Catheter, distal, 206–207, *208*
  for embolization, 524–525, 525t
  in brain abscess, 483
  lumbar, 206
  malfunction of, 219–220, *220*
  ventricular, 204–206, *205, 206*
Cauda equina, formation of, 4, 15–16, *15*
Caudal regression syndrome, 91
  embryogenesis of, 79–81, *80*
Cavitron ultrasonic aspirator, 433–434
  in hemispheric tumor surgery, 378
  in intraventricular tumor surgery, 384
  in spinal tumor surgery, 434
CBF. See *Cerebral blood flow (CBF).*
Central nervous system (CNS), induction of, 2–3, 10
  neurofibromatosis and, 455–456, *455*
  normal development of, 1–8, 10–17
Central venous pressure monitoring, 573
Cerebellar astrocytoma. See *Astrocytoma, cerebellar.*
Cerebellar implants, 558–559
Cerebellum, development of, 5, 6t, 16–17
  in cerebral palsy, 557–559
Cerebral blood flow (CBF), anesthesia and, 570–572
  barbiturates and, 251–252
  blood pressure and, 583
  intracranial hypertension and, 248–249
  neonatal, 230
    hemorrhage and, 232
    stroke and, 233–234
Cerebral cortex, development of, 4–5
Cerebral edema. See *Edema.*
Cerebral hemisphere tumors, 373–382
  astrocytomas as, 378–379
  clinical presentation of, 374–375, *374, 375*
  diagnosis of, 375–377, *376, 377*
  ependymomas as, 379–380, *380*
  gangliogliomas as, 380, *380*
  metastatic, 380
  oligodendrogliomas as, 379
  teratomas as, 380, *381*
  treatment of, 377–378
Cerebral infarction, perinatal, 233–235, *234*
  meningitis and, 235
Cerebral mantle, intellectual development and, *200*, 201, 227
Cerebral palsy, 556–560
  afferent pathway interruption in, 557
  cerebellothalamocortical circuit interruption in, 557–559
  motor pathway interruption in, 557
Cerebrospinal fluid (CSF), absorption of, 162–165, *165*, 241
  in hydrocephalus, 165–166
  analysis of, after tumor surgery, 464
  in medulloblastoma, 351
  in pineal region tumors, 411–412
  anatomy of, 170–171, *171*
  choroid plexus and, 159–162, *160, 161*, 370
  circulation of, 170–179, 181
    in hydrocephalus, 174–175, *176*, 177–178
    major pathways in, 172–174, *174, 175*
    minor pathways in, 172, *173*
  cysts containing, 214, *214*
  formation of, 17, 160–162, *161*
    in hydrocephalus, 166
    intracranial pressure and, 162, 239–240, 247–248
    rate of, 161–162
  in pseudotumor cerebri, 252–253
  isolated fourth ventricle and, 212–213
  leakage of, after spina bifida surgery, 47
  localization of, 266, *267*

Cerebrospinal fluid (Continued)
  leakage of, posttraumatic, 266–267, 267
  removal of, 247–248, 248
    in premature infant, 202–203, 232, 233
  shunting of. See Shunt.
  tumor markers in, 466
Cerebrotomy, in intraventricular tumors, 384–385, 386–387, 386
Chamberlain's line, 143, 143
Chemical irritants, hydrocephalus and, 184
Chemotherapy, 465–466, 465t
  cerebral artery administration of, 476
  clinical trials of, 475–476
  experimental, 475–476
  in ependymoma, 369, 469
  in germ cell tumors, 470
  in gliomas, 469–470
  in hemispheric tumors, 378
  in medulloblastoma, 352–354, 468
  in optic glioma, 397
  in pineal region tumors, 415, 468
  in recurrence, 474–476
Chiari malformation. See Arnold-Chiari malformation.
Child, brain tumors in, 335–336, 336t. See also Brain tumors.
  concussion in, 273–274
  endotracheal tube size for, 570t
  hemispherectomy in, 549–550
  hydrocephalus in, 188–189, 196
  intracranial pressure in, 238–239
  pressure-volume index in, 242, 242
  spine in, 299–300
Child abuse, subdural hematoma and, 284, 285
Chondrification, vertebral, 17
Chondroma, skull, 426
Chordoma, skull, 426–427
  spine, 448
Choriocarcinoma, pineal region, 413, 415
Choroid plexus, 159–162, 160, 161
  development of, 16–17
  papilloma of, 162
    fourth ventricle, 369–370
    intraventricular, 384–386, 385–390, 389
  removal of, 204
Christian's syndrome, 125t
Christmas disease, 518
Chromosome abnormalities, craniosynostosis and, 125t
Cisplatin, 475
Cisternography, in CSF rhinorrhea, 266, 267
  in hydrocephalus, 191
  radionuclide, 194
Clinical trials, in recurrent brain tumor, 475–476
Cloverleaf skull, 115, 118, 122, 123
  conditions accompanying, 123t
CNS. See Central nervous system (CNS).
Coagulation factors, 518, 577
  replacement of, 519
Coagulopathies, 517–523
  clinical presentation of, 517–518
  disseminated intravascular coagulation, 522
  hemophilia, 518–520
  idiopathic thrombocytopenia purpura, 520–521, 521
  leukemic, 520
  vitamin K deficiency, 521–522
Coccyx, agenesis of, 79–81, 80
Cognitive function, astrocytoma and, 346
  hydrocephalus treatment and, 201, 227–228
  myelomeningocele and, 55, 55, 58
  posttraumatic, 296
  radiation therapy and, 354, 466
  shunt replacement and, 215

Cognitive function (Continued)
  spina bifida and, 47
  Sturge-Weber syndrome and, 552
Coma, concussion and, 274
  pressure monitoring in, 246
Computed tomography, in arachnoid cyst, 105
  in astrocytoma, 340–341, 340, 341, 343
  in brain abscess, 481–482, 482, 483
  in brain tumor recurrence, 473
  in choroid plexus papilloma, 370
  in concussion, 272, 273
  in contusion, 275, 275
  in craniopharyngioma, 400
  in craniosynostosis, 107, 124
  in CSF rhinorrhea, 266
  in dermal sinus, 87, 102
  in dermoid cyst, 307, 371, 371
  in diastematomyelia, 89, 89
  in encephalocele, 99
  in ependymoma, 367, 368, 369
  in extradural hematoma, 278, 279, 280, 281
  in growing skull fracture, 294
  in hemispheric tumors, 376
  in hydrocephalus, 191, 192, 193
  in intracerebral hematoma, 288, 288
  in isolated fourth ventricle, 213, 213
  in lipomyelomeningocele, 85, 86
  in medulloblastoma, 349, 349, 351
  in metastasis, 417, 418
  in moyamoya disease, 504, 504
  in neurocysticercosis, 496–497, 497
  in neurofibromatosis, 454, 454
  in peripheral nerve injury, 323, 324
  in pineal region tumors, 411, 411
  in skull fracture, 264
  in spinal cord injury, 307, 308
  in spinal cord tumor, 430
  in spinal tumor, 445
  in Sturge-Weber syndrome, 458, 458
  in subdural empyema, 485, 485
  in subdural hematoma, 282, 282, 283, 285, 285
  in tuberous sclerosis, 457, 458
  of craniocervical junction, 144
  postoperative, 463–464, 466, 473
  stereotaxic. See Stereotaxic techniques.
Concussion, 271–274
  clinical aspects of, 272–274
  defined, 271
  mechanism of, 271–272
  prognosis in, 274
Congenital heart disease, brain abscess and, 480
Congenital malformations. See also specific malformation, e.g., Arnold-Chiari malformation.
  associated with basilar impression, 146
  associated with craniosynostosis, 125t–127t
  associated with hydrocephalus, 182–183, 183t
  associated with spina bifida, 19t, 39, 40t
Consciousness, level of, brain abscess and, 481
Contrast materials, 579
Contusion, 275–276, 275
Conus medullaris, formation of, 74
  lipoma of, resection of, 92, 93
  postoperative morbidity and, 439–440
Cor pulmonale, vascular shunt and, 439–440
Cordis Brain-State Analyzer, 437–438
Coronal synostosis, 124, 127, 128–132
Corpus callosum, glioma surgery and, 385
  section of, 537, 545, 545
    indications for, 543
Corpus cerebelli dysraphism, 26–27
Corticosteroids, in cerebral edema, 251, 583
  in contusion, 275
  in craniopharyngioma, 401, 404–405
  in pseudotumor cerebri, 253

Corticosteroids *(Continued)*
  in recurrent brain tumor, 474
  in spinal cord injury, 305
  postoperative, 583
  side effects of, 474
Counseling, 155–156
  in spina bifida, 42–43
Cranial meningocele, 98t
Cranial midline anomalies, 98t
Cranial nerve trauma, 267–268
Craniectomy, decompressive, 247, *247*, 584
  in astrocytoma, 342–343
  in craniosynostosis, 107–108
    sagittal, 108–111, *109–112*, 113–114
      bilateral parasagittal, 108, *109*
      "clam shell," 110, *110*
      "keyhole," 111–112, *112*
      pi, 110–111, *111, 112*
      single midline, 108–110, *109, 110*
      transposition, 112, *113*
      vault remodeling, 112, *113*
      vertex, 110, *111*
    simple linear, 115, *115*, 133
      in craniotelencephalic dysplasia, 117
  in ependymoma, 368–369
  in medulloblastoma, 349–351
Craniocerebral disproportion, 286
Craniocervical junction, 142–150
  anomalous bone formations at, 147
  basilar impression at, 144–147
    causes of, 144–145, *145*, 145t
    conditions associated with, 145–146, *146*
    radiography of, 146
    symptoms of, 146
    treatment of, 147
  basioccipital cleft at, 147
  congenital skull dysplasias and, 148, 148t
  embryology of, 142–143, *143*
  first sclerotome abnormalities at, 148–149, 148t, *149*
  occipital condylar hypoplasia at, 147
  occipital synchondroses at, premature closure of, 147–148
  paracondylar process at, 147
  radiologic measurements of, 143–144, *143, 144*
  trauma to, 310–313, *310, 312–314*
Craniofacial dysmorphism. See *Craniosynostosis.*
Craniofacial dyssynostosis, 125t
Craniofacial surgery, 120–141. See also *Craniosynostosis.*
  clinical evaluation for, 107, 124
  early, 107, 120–121, *121*
  in craniometaphyseal dysplasia, 137, *139*
  in coronal synostosis, 124, 127, *128–132*
  in fibrous dysplasia, 136–137, *136*
  in hydrocephalus, 137, *140*
  in hypertelorism, 134, *134, 135*, 136
  in kleeblattschädel, 122
  in multiple synostoses, 115, *116–118*, 133, *133*
  in neoplasms, 137, *140*
  in neurofibromatosis, 137, *138–139*
  in trigonocephaly, 127, 131, 133, *133*
  syndromes involved in, 121, 123–124, 125t–127t
Craniometaphyseal dysplasia, 137, *139*, 148
Craniopharyngioma, 399–408, 470
  clinical features of, 400
  follow-up of, 405, 470
  pathology of, 399
  preoperative evaluation in, 400–401, *400–402*
  radiation therapy in, 405, 407, *407*
  recurrence of, 405, 470
  surgery in, 401–405, *404–406*
Cranioplasty, posttraumatic, 290–291, *291*

Craniosynostosis, 107–119
  clinical evaluation of 107, 124
  coronal, 124, 127, *128–132*
  craniofacial dysmorphism and, 121, 123–124, 125t–127t
    kleeblattschädel, 115, *118, 122*, 123, 123t
  early repair in, 107, 120–121, *121*
  lambdoidal, 114–115, *114, 115*
    calvarial transfers in, 115, *115*
    vs. positional flattening, 115
  metopic, 127, 131, 133, *133*
  multiple, 115, *116–118*, 118, 133, *133*
  sagittal, 108–114, *109–112*
  shunting and, 224
  syndromes involved in, 121, 123–124, 125t–127t
Craniotelencephalic dysplasia, 115, *117*
Craniotomy, in hypertelorism, 134
  in subdural hematoma, 286
  repeat, 378
  supportive care after, 580–582
Cranium, development of, 6, 7t, 18
Cranium bifidum, 98t
Croup, postintubation, 570
Crouzon's syndrome, 121, *121*, 123t, 125t, *128*
  surgery in, *131, 132*
Crown-rump length, 2, 10
CSF. See *Cerebrospinal fluid (CSF).*
Cutaneous signs. See *Skin signs.*
Cyanoacrylate adhesives, 266
Cyst(s). See also specific cyst, e.g., *Arachnoid cyst.*
  abdominal, shunt and, 226, *226*
  cystic astrocytoma vs., 340, *341*
  supratentorial CSF, 214, *214*
  terminal vs. intratumor, 438, *439*
Cysticercosis. See *Neurocysticercosis.*
Cysticercotic encephalitic syndrome, 496, *497*. See also *Neurocysticercosis.*

Dandy-Walker cyst, 27, 196, *196*
Dandy-Walker malformation, 25–27, *26*
  embryogenesis of, 25–27
  hydrocephalus with, 25, *26*, 183
  surgery for, 211–212
Debulking, 474
Decubitus ulcer, in spinal cord injury, 314–315
Deferoxamine, 584
Dehydration, 575–577
Dens. See *Odontoid process.*
Dermal sinus, intracranial, 101–103, *102*
  clinical presentation of, 101–102, *102*
  dermoid cyst and, 370–371
  imaging of, 102
  incidence of, 101–102
  infection with, 102
  outcome in, 103
  pathology of, 101
  treatment of, 102–103
  spinal, 27–28, 83, 86–87, *87*, 493
    dermoid tumor and, 78, 87, *88*
    embryogenesis of, 29, *30*, 78
    surgery on, 370–371
Dermoid tumor, 423
  dermal sinus and, 78, 87, *88*, 370–371
  intracranial, 101, 102, 103
  fourth ventricle, 370–371, *370, 371*
  imaging of, 102
  inclusion, 66, *68*, 78
  pineal region, 413–414
Desmopressin, after craniopharyngioma surgery, 405
Developmental arrest theory, 21–22
Dexamethasone, 583

Diabetes, embryonic deformation and caudal suppression syndrome and, 91
Diabetes insipidus, postoperative, 583
  tumors and, 396, 400, 401, 405
Diagnosis related groups, 154
Diastematomyelia, 28, 87–90, 89
  cleft meninges in, 88–89, 89
  cutaneous signs of, 83, 88
  embryogenesis of, 30, 31, 32–33, 78–79
  myelomeningocele and, 66
Diazepam, 569
  CBF and, 571
Diet, spina bifida and, 38
Dimethyl sulfoxide, in cerebral edema, 251
Diskitis, 492, 492
Disseminated intravascular coagulation, 522
Diuretics, in cerebral edema, 251, 583
  in spinal cord injury, 305
Down's syndrome, basilar impression in, 145
"Drop" metastasis, 446–447, 447, 473
Drug(s). See also specific drugs, e.g., *Acetazolamide*.
  anesthetic, CBF and, 571–572
  infant metabolism of, 567–568
  chemotherapeutic. See *Chemotherapy*.
  clinical trials of, 475–476
  CSF formation and, 162, 247–248
  in cerebral edema, 250–252, 583–584
  in hydrocephalus, 203, 232–233
  in ischemia, 584
  muscle relaxant, 572
  preanesthetic, 568–570, 569t
Drug administration, cerebral artery, 476
  preanesthetic, 569–570
"Dumbbell" tumor, 446, 450
Dura, lacerations of, 127, 136
    expanding, 291–294, 293
    grafts on, 266
    substitutes for, 440
Dysraphism, spinal, 36–37
    occult, 27–33, 35–36

Economic factors, treatment decisions and, 153–154
Edema, causes of, 250
  fluid management and, 575–577
  intracranial hypertension and, 249–252
  postoperative, 582–584
  white matter, 177, 177
EEG. See *Electroencephalography (EEG)*.
"Eight-in-one" chemotherapeutic regimen, 475–476
Electrodes, 540–541, 540, 541
  cerebellar stimulation by, 558
Electroencephalography (EEG), in epilepsy, 540–542, 540–543
  history of, 536
  in hemispheric tumors, 376–377
  in moyamoya disease, 504
  intraoperative, 574
Electrophysiology, in peripheral nerve injury, 322
Elejalde's syndrome, 125t
Embolic agents, 524–525, 525t
  for arteriovenous malformations, 526, 527
  for hypervascular tumors, 532
Embolism, pulmonary, vascular shunt and, 224–225, 225
  therapeutic. See *Embolization*
Embolization, 524–533
  agents for, 524–525, 525t
  catheters for, 524–525, 525t
  clinical considerations in, 525–526

Embolization (Continued)
  complications of, 526, 531–532
  lesions treated by, 524t, 525t
  of arteriovenous malformations, 526, 527, 528, 528
    spinal cord, 531–532, 532
  of carotid–cavernous sinus fistula, 528–529, 529
  of hypervascular tumors, 532
  of vein of Galen malformation, 529–532, 530
  technique for, 524–525
Embryo, bilaminar, 10–11, 11
  CNS development in, 2–6, 4–6t, 10–17
    abnormal, 9t, 19–21, 19t, 20t, 75–81, 75–77, 80
  cranial development in, 6, 7t, 18
  growth stages in, 1–2, 2t, 10
    Arnold-Chiari/spina bifida complex and, 19–21, 20, 20t, 21
  meningeal development in, 8, 8t
  neurulation in, 3–4, 4t, 13–14, 14, 73, 73, 74
    abnormal, 75–79, 75–77
  spinal cord development in, 4, 5t, 6, 17, 71–75, 72–74
  trilaminar, 11–13
  vertebral development in, 6, 7t, 17–18, 72
Embryogenesis, of arachnoid cyst, 104
  of Arnold-Chiari/spina bifida complex, 19–21
    developmental arrest theory, 21–22
    hydrodynamic theory, 23–24
    neuroectodermal theory, 24
    neuroschisis theory, 24
    overgrowth theory, 22–23
    traction theory, 24–25
  of arteriovenous malformation, 509
  of basicranium, 142–143
  of Dandy-Walker malformation, 25–27
  of dermal sinus, 78
    intracranial, 101
  of diastematomyelia, 78–79
  of embryonic deformation and caudal suppression, 79–81, 80
  of encephalocele, 97
  of lipomyelomeningocele, 77–78, 77
  of myelomeningocele, 75–77, 75, 76
  of neurenteric cyst, 81
  of occult spinal dysraphism, 27–33
  of spina bifida, 38–39
  of terminal myelocystocele, 79
  of tight filum terminale syndrome, 79
Embryonal cell carcinoma, pineal region, 413, 415
Embryonic deformation and caudal supression, 91
  embryogenesis of, 79–81, 80
Employment, myelomeningocele and, 60
Empyema, subdural, 484–486, 485
Encephalocele, 97–101
  classification of, 98t
  clinical presentation of, 98–100
  hydrocephalus and, 196
  hypertelorism and, 134, 135
  incidence of, 97
  outcome in, 100–101
  prevention of, 101
  treatment of, 100
Encephalo-duro-arterio-synangiosis, 505–506, 506
Encephalomeningocele, 98t
Encephalomyosynangiosis, 505
Encephalotrigeminal angiomatosis. See *Sturge-Weber syndrome*.
Endocrine function, radiation therapy and, 466
Endocrine testing, in craniopharyngioma, 401, 405

Endotracheal intubation, 570, 570t, 579–581
  indications for, 581t
Engelmann-Camurati disease, 148
Enteric fistula, dorsal, 81
Eosinophilic granuloma, 424–425, *425*
Ependymal cyst, hydrocephalus and, 184
Ependymoblastoma, 367
Ependymoma, fourth ventricle, 366–369, 367t, *368, 369*
  hemispheric, 379–380, *379*
  intraventricular, 383–384
  metastatic to subarachnoid space, 446–447, *447*
  postoperative management of, 467t, 468–469
  prognosis in, 369
  spinal cord, 432, 436
Epidural abscess, 486, *486*
  spinal, 491
Epilepsy, 535–536. See also *Seizures*.
  arteriovenous malformations and, 511
  incidence of, 535
  natural history of, 537–538
  posttraumatic, 294–295
  surgery in, anterior temporal lobectomy, 542, 543–544, *544*
    corpus callosum section, 543, 545, *545*
    evaluation for, 538–542, 538t, *540–542*
    follow-up of, 545–546
    frontal lobectomy, 542–543, 544, *544*
    hemispherectomy, 549–560
      complications of, 554, *554*
      in infantile hemiplegia, 553, *553*
      in Sturge-Weber syndrome, 550–552, *551, 552*
      in unilateral megalencephaly, 553–554
      indications for, 549–550
      preoperative evaluation for, 550
      technique of, 550, *550*
    history of, 536–537
    indications for, 542–543
    results of, 545t, 546, 546t
  tumor and, 374, *374*
Erb's palsy, 326, *327*, 328–330, *328*
Ethacrynic acid, in cerebral edema, 251
Ethanol, as embolic agent, 532
Ethical questions. See *Medical ethics*.
Etomidate, CBF and, 571
Evoked potentials, brainstem, 361–362, 575
  cortical, 574–575
  intraoperative, 574–575
    during spinal cord surgery, 436–438
  somatosensory, in neonatal spina bifida, 42
    in tethered cord syndrome, 81
  visual, 575
Extracellular fluid, CSF and, 172
Extracellular space, brain, 160, 164, 170–171
Extradural hematoma, 277–281
  clinical presentation of, 278–279, *280, 281*
  pathophysiology of, 278, *278, 279*
  posterior fossa, 281, *281*
  prognosis in, 281
  treatment of, 279–281
Extramedullary spinal tumors, 443–452
  aneurysmal bone cyst, 447–448, *448*
  diagnosis of, 44–445, *447*
    differential, 444
  "drop" metastasis, 446–447, *447*
  "dumbbell," 446, 450
  incidence of, 443
  meningioma, 445–446
  nerve sheath, 445–446
  neuroblastoma, 449–450, *449*
  osteoblastoma, 447, *448*
  sarcoma, 449, *449*
  secondary epidural, 448–450, *449*

Extramedullary spinal tumors *(Continued)*
  signs and symptoms of, 443–444
  surgery in, 446, 450
    deformity after, 450–451
Extubation, 581, 581t
Eye signs. See also *Vision*.
  in basilar impression, 146
  in hydrocephalus, 187–188, *187*, 189
  in neurofibromatosis, 454
  in pineal region tumors, 410
  in pseudotumor cerebri, 252, 253
  in subdural hematoma, 284
  in tuberous sclerosis, 456, *457*
  in von Hippel-Lindau disease, 459

Facial nerve trauma, 268
Fairbank's syndrome, 126t
Fetus, CNS development in, 2, 5–6, 6–7t
  cranial development in, 6, 7t
  hydrocephalus in, 189, *191*, 196
  spinal cord development in, 72
  vertebral development in, 7t
FG syndrome, 125t
Fibromuscular dysplasia, stroke and, 502
Fibrous dysplasia, 136, *136*
  craniofacial surgery in, 137
  skull in, 423–424
Filum terminale, formation of, 4, 15–16, *15*, 74–75, *74*
  lipoma of, 90–91, *90*
  tight. See *Tight filum terminale syndrome*.
Fistula, enteric, dorsal, 81
"Floating forehead" technique, in coronal synostosis, 124
Fluid management, 575–579, 582
Foot, tethered cord syndrome and, 82, *84*
Foramen magnum, 143–144, *144*
  malformations of, 144–148, *145, 146*, 145t
Foramen of Luschka, congenital atresia of, 26
Foramen of Magendie, congenital atresia of, 26
Foramen of Monro, choroid plexus surgery and, 387–388
Forceps, bipolar, in choroid plexus surgery, 387
Forebrain, development of, 5
Forehead, reconstruction of, 291
Fourth ventricle, anatomy of, 366
  cannulation of, 213
  isolated, 212–213, *212, 213*
  tumor(s) of, 366–372
    choroid plexus papilloma as, 369–370
    dermoid cyst as, 370–371, *370, 371*
    ependymoma as, 366–369, 367t, *368, 369*
Fractures, compartment syndrome and, 330–331, *330*
  skull. See *Skull fractures*.
  vertebral, 300–303, *302, 303*, 309–310, *310, 311*
Frontal bossing, transposition craniectomy in, 112, *113*
Frontal lobectomy, 544, *544*
  indications for, 542–543
Frontonasal dysplasia, 125t
Furosemide, in cerebral edema, 251, 583
  in hydrocephalus, 203, 232–233
Fusion, spinal, *311*
  cervical, 309–310

Gait, in astrocytoma, 339
  in spinal cord tumor, 429
Ganglioglioma, hemispheric, 380, *380*
Ganglioneuroma, 449–450
  deceptive symptoms of, 444
Gastrulation, 11, *12*

Genetic counseling, 38
Germinal matrix hemorrhage, 184, 230–232
　hydrocephalus and, 232–233
Germinoma, *395,* 470
　pineal region, 411, 413, 415
Giant cell tumor, in tuberous sclerosis, 457–458
Glioblastoma, 365, 379
Glioma, brainstem, 469, 469t
　cerebral hemisphere, 378–379, 469
　intraventricular, 384–385, *384*
　optic, 391–398
　　biologic behavior of, 391–392
　　chiasm involvement in, 393–394, *394*
　　diagnosis of, 392, 393, 393t, 394, 396
　　hypothalamus involvement in, 394, *394–396,* 396–397
　　pathology of, 391, *392*
　　treatment of, 393–394, 396–397
　　　postoperative, 465t
　pineal region, 414, 415
Glomerular filtation rate, 568
Glucose, ischemia and, 576–577, 584
Glycerol, in intracranial hypertension, 250
Gorlin-Chaudhry-Moss syndrome, 125t
Growing skull fracture, 291–294, *292, 293,* 422–423, *422*
Growth, after craniopharyngioma surgery, 405
Guilt, parents', 42–43
Gunshot wounds, craniocerebral, 265
　peripheral nerve injury from, *332*

Hall's syndrome, 126t
Halo traction, 309, *310*
Hamartoma, in tuberous sclerosis, 456–457, *457*
Hand-Schüller-Christian disease, 425
Head injury. See also specific injury.
　barbiturates and, 584
　carotid–cavernous sinus fistula after, 294
　cranial defects after, 290–291, *291*
　hematoma after. See *Hematoma.*
　in hemophilia, 519
　neuropsychologic deficit after, 295–296
　seizures after, 294–295
　supportive care after, 580–584
Head size, infant, 186–187, *187*
Headache, in arteriovenous malformation, 511
　in astrocytoma, 339
　in hemispheric tumors, 375
　in pineal region tumors, 410
　in pseudotumor cerebri, 252, 253
　morning, 410
Health maintenance organizations, 154
Hearing, acoustic nerve trauma and, 268
Heart disease, congenital, brain abscess in, 480
　stroke and, 502
Hemangioblastoma, in von Hippel-Lindau disease, 459
Hemangioma, skull and, 426
Hematocrit, 577–578
Hematoma, 277–289
　cephalohematoma, 422
　extradural, 277–281, *278–281*
　　clinical presentation of, 278–279, *280, 281*
　　pathophysiology of, 278, *278, 279*
　　posterior fossa, 281, *281*
　　treatment of, 279–281
　hemophilia and, 519
　hygroma and, 286–287
　intracerebral, 287–289, *287, 288*
　subdural, 281–289, *282, 283, 285, 287, 288*
　　acute, 246, 281–283, *282, 283*
　　chronic, 283–286, *285*
　　　treatment of, 286

Hematoma *(Continued)*
　subdural, posterior fossa, 283
　　shunting and, 223–224, *223,* 286
　tumor and, 375
Hemimyelomeningocele, 18–19
Hemiplegia, infantile, 553, *553*
Hemispherectomy, 549–560
　complications of, 554, *554*
　in infantile hemiplegia, 553, *553*
　in Sturge-Weber syndrome, 550–552, *551, 552*
　in unilateral megalencephaly, 553–554
　indications for, 549–550
　preoperative evaluation for, 550
　technique of, 550, *550*
Hemophilia, 518–520
　intracranial hemorrhage in, 518–520
　intraspinal hemorrhage in, 520
　peripheral nerve lesions in, 520
Hemorrhage. See also *Hematoma;* and specific site.
　arteriovenous malformations and, 508–509, 510, 511
　coagulopathies and, 517–518
　hydrocephalus and, 184, 185, 201–203
　in hemophilia, 518–520
　in idiopathic thrombocytopenic purpura, 520–521
　in vitamin K deficiency, 521–522
　leukemic, 520
　posthemispherectomy, 554
　tumor and, 375
Hensen's node, 3, 11, *11*
Hernia, inguinal, shunt and, 226
Herrmann's syndrome, 126t
Hindbrain dysfunction, in myelomeningocele, 55–56, *56,* 60–61, *61*
Histiocytosis X, *396,* 424
　skull in, 425, *425*
Hodgkin's lymphoma, skull in, 427
Holocord astrocytoma, 430, 440–441
　clinical indications of, 432, *433*
　surgery in, 434, 436, 440
　　pitfalls of, 438–440, *439*
　terminal vs. intratumor cyst in, 438, *439*
Holoprosencephaly, trigonocephaly with, 131
Homocystinuria, stroke and, 502
Hootnick-Holmes syndrome, 126t
Hormone replacement, after craniopharyngioma surgery, 405
Hydranencephaly, 188, *190*
　arteriography in, 194
Hydrocephalus, 180–199
　acquired, 184–185
　acute, 181, 189
　anesthesia and, 565
　Arnold-Chiari malformation and, 19–21
　"arrested," 215
　astrocytoma and, 341–342
　choroid plexus papilloma and, 370
　clinical presentation of, 186–189, *187,* 188t, *189–191*
　　antenatal, 189, *191*
　　in infant, 186–188, *187*
　　in older child, 188–189
　communicating, 181, *192*
　　causes of, 182, 182t
　　CSF circulation in, 174–175, *176*
　　shunt independence in, 216
　compartmentalized, 211–214, *212–214*
　compensated, 181, 215
　congenital, 182t
　　causes of, 182–184
　　syndromes associated with, 182–183, 183t

Hydrocephalus (Continued)
  craniofacial surgery in, 137, 140
  craniopharyngioma and, 405, 406
  craniosynostosis and, 115, 118, 224
  CSF absorption in, 165–166
  CSF circulation in, 174–175, 176, 177–178
    compensatory, 175, 177–178, 177
  Dandy-Walker malformation with, 25, 26, 183, 211–212
  dermal sinus and, 102, 103
  diagnosis of, 189, 191, 191t, 191–194, 194–195
    differential, 188, 190
  edema with, 177–178, 177
  encephalocele and, 100
  etiology of, 181–185, 182t–184t
  evaluation of, 194–196, 200–201, 200, 202
  history of, 180–181
  in premature infant, 184, 195–196, 201–203
  incidence of, 185
  IQ and, 58, 201, 227–228
  isolated fourth ventricle in, 212–213, 212, 213
  medulloblastoma and, 349–350
  mortality from, 227
  myelomeningocele and, 56–57, 57, 182, 196
  natural history of, 196–197
  noncommunicating, 181, 192
    causes of, 182, 182t
    CSF circulation in, 175, 176
  "normal pressure," 189
  pathologic effects of, 185–186
  pineal region surgery and, 414, 414t
  posthemorrhagic, 184, 201–203, 232–233
  prognosis in, 196–197, 200–201
  progressive, 181
    causes of, 182t
  shunt dependence in, 214–216
  spina bifida surgery and, 46
  spinal tumors and, 429–430, 444
  supratentorial CSF cyst and, 214, 214
  terminology in, 181
  treatment of, 200–217. See also Shunt.
    drugs in, 203, 232–233, 247–248
    goals of, 216
    nonsurgical, 201, 232, 233
    selection for, 200–201, 200, 202
    surgical, 203–207, 205–206, 208–210, 209, 211, 233
      complications of, 219–227, 220, 221, 222t, 223, 225, 226
    in Dandy-Walker malformation, 211–212
    results of, 227–228
    shunt dependence after, 214–216
  vs. arachnoid cyst, 104, 104
  vs. hydranencephaly, 188, 190
  vs. macrocrania, 186, 187, 188, 188t, 189
  vs. subdural hematoma, 284
Hydrodynamic theory, 23–24, 27
Hydromyelia, myelomeningocele and, 61–64, 62, 63
  surgery for, 62–63
  vs. spinal cord tumor, 430
Hydrosyringomyelia, Arnold-Chiari malformation with, 25, 25
Hydrosyringomyelomeningocele, 19
Hygroma, subdural, 286–287
Hyperalimentation, 582
Hyperbaric oxygenation, in spinal cord injury, 306
Hypertelorism, 134, 134, 135, 136
Hypertension, intracranial. See Intracranial hypertension.
Hyperventilation, in extradural hematoma, 279
  in intracranial hypertension, 249, 583
  moyamoya disease and, 504, 505

Hypothalamus, craniopharyngioma and, 403
  optic chiasm tumors and, 394, 394–396, 396–397
Hypothermia, in spinal cord injury, 306
  perioperative, 566–567, 583

Idaho syndrome, 126t
Idiopathic thrombocytopenic purpura, 520–521
Imperforate anus, 90, 90
Inclusion dermoid tumor, 66, 68, 78
Incontinence, urinary. See Urinary incontinence.
Incontinentia pigmenti, 460–461
Infant, anemia in, 577
  anesthesia in, 565–568, 566t, 567t. See also Anesthesia.
  body composition in, 567t
  body heat homeostasis in, 566–567
  brain abscess in, 480
  concussion in, 272–273
  cranial development in, 7t
  drug metabolism in, 567–568
  endotracheal tube size for, 570t
  hydrocephalus in, 186–188, 187. See also Hydrocephalus.
  intracranial pressure in, 238–239
  macrocrania in, 186, 187, 188, 188t
  newborn. See Neonate.
  peripheral nerve injury in, 321–322
  premature. See Premature infant.
  pressure-volume index in, 242–243, 242
  spine in, 299–300
  vertebral development in, 7t
Infantile hemiplegia, 553, 553
Infection. See also Bacterial infection; Parasitic infection; Viral infection; and specific infection.
  after spinal bifida surgery, 46, 47
  dermal sinus and, 87, 102
  hydrocephalus and, 183–185, 195
  myelomeningocele and, 57–58
  shunt, 200–201, 220–223, 222t
    pseudocyst and, 226, 226
Informed consent, 154–155
Inguinal hernia, shunt and, 226
Injection, peripheral nerve injury from, 331–332, 331
Intellectual function, astrocytoma and, 346
  hydrocephalus treatment and, 201, 227–228
  myelomeningocele and, 55, 55, 58
  posttraumatic, 296
  radiation therapy and, 354, 466
  shunt replacement and, 215
  spina bifida and, 47
  Sturge-Weber syndrome and, 552
Intensive care, 582–584. See also Anesthesia.
  fluid management in, 582
  intracranial pressure control in, 249–252, 582–584
  nutritional, 582
  respiratory, 580–582
Interferons, 476–477
Interventional neuroradiology. See Embolization.
Intracarotid amobarbital test, 542, 550
Intracerebral hemorrhage, traumatic, 287–289, 287, 289
Intracranial dermal sinus. See Dermal sinus.
Intracranial hypertension, adult vs. child, 238
  anesthesia and, 571–572, 576–577
  blood volume and, 248–249
  CSF volume and, 247–248, 248
  dermal sinus and, 102, 103
  edema and, 249–252, 582–584
  in infant, 242–243

Intracranial hypertension *(Continued)*
  mass lesion and, 246–247, 250, 286, 374–375, *375*, 410
  mechanical ventilation and, 249, 581
  medulloblastoma surgery and, 351
  pseudotumor cerebri and, 252–253
  steady state dynamics vs., 240–242, *241*
  treatment of, 245–254, 582–584
    by blood volume reduction, 249
    by CSF removal, 247–248, *248*
    by edema reduction, 249–252, 582–584
    surgical, 246–247, *247*, 250, 584
Intracranial pressure, 238–244
  cribside measurement of, 186–187
  CSF formation and, 162, 239–240
  drugs and, 203
  increased. See *Intracranial hypertension.*
  monitoring of, 246, 247, 582–583
    in contusion, 275, 276
    in hydrocephalus, 194–195, 196
  normal, 238–239, *239*
    steady state, 239–240, *239*
  volume changes and, 240–242, *241–243*
    in infant, 242–243
Intramedullary spinal cord tumors, 428–442
  clinical manifestations of, 428–430
  diagnosis of, 430–431, *431*
  focal, 430
  holocord astrocytomas as, 430, 440–441
    clinical indications of, 432, *433*
    surgery in, 434, 436, 440
      pitfalls of, 438–440, *439*
      terminal vs. intratumor cyst in, 438, *439*
  hydrocephalus with, 429–430
  lipomas as, 436, *437*
  location of, 428
  pathology of, 428
  surgery in, 431–438, *435*
    CSF loculation during, 438
    dural substitutes in, 440
    missed tumor in, 438, *439*
    morbidity after, 439–440
    wound closure in, 440
  vs. hydromyelia, 430
Intraorbital distance, 134
Intravenous fluids, 575–577, 582
Intraventricular hemorrhage, 230–232, *231*
  arteriovenous malformations and, 508–509
  hydrocephalus and, 184, 201–203, 232–233
Intraventricular tumors, 383–390
  choroid plexus papillomas as, 385–390, *384–386*, *389*
  ependymomas as, 383–384
  glial, 384–385
  pineal region, 389–390
  third ventricle, 389–390
Intubation, endotracheal, 570, 570t
  indications for, 579–581, 581t
  nasal, 581
IQ, astrocytoma and, 345
  hydrocephalus treatment and, 201, 227–228
  myelomeningocele and, 55, *55*, 58
  posttraumatic, 296
  radiation therapy and, 354
  spina bifida and, 47
  Sturge-Weber syndrome and, 552
Ischemia, barbiturates and, 584
  calcium channel blockers and, 584
  glucose and, 576–577, 584
  in spinal cord injury, 303
  perinatal, 233–234
  tethered cord syndrome and, 81
  vein of Galen malformations and, 530

Isobutyl cyanoacrylate, in embolization, 526, *527*, 530, *530*
Isoflurane, CBF and, 571
Isosorbide, in hydrocephalus, 203, 248

Ketamine, 580
Kidney, drug metabolism by, 568
  in von Hippel-Lindau disease, 459
Kleeblattschädel, 115, *118*, *122*, 123
  conditions accompanying, 123t
Kyphectomy, 43–44, *44*, *45*, 46
Kyphosis, after laminectomy, 451, 491
  diastematomyelia and, 88
  myelomeningocele and, 44, *44*, *45*, 46, 62
  spondylitis and, 491, *492*

Laceration, dural, 127, 136
  expanding, 291–294, *293*
  scalp, 256–257
Lambdoidal synostosis, 114–115, *114*, *115*
  calvarial transfers in, 115, *115*
  vs. positional flattening, 115
Laminectomy, 305
  deformity after, 450–451
  in spinal cord abscess, 490
  in spinal epidural abscess, 491
  in spinal tumor surgery, 434, 446, 450
Larynx, of infant, 566
Laser, in brainstem tumor surgery, 362, 365
  in intraventricular tumor surgery, 384
  in lipoma surgery, 91–92, 94
  in spinal tumor surgery, 434, 436
Lateral canthal advancement, in coronal synostosis, 124, 127, *129–132*
  in kleeblattschädel, *122*
  in trigonocephaly, 133
Legal factors, 153
  nerve injury and, 321, *321*
Leptomeningeal cyst, 291–294, *292*, *293*, 422–423, *422*
Letterer-Siwe disease, 425
Leukemia, intracranial hemorrhage in, 520
  skull in, 427
Lidocaine, CBF and, 571
Lidoflazine, 584
Lipoma, 28, *28*, 36. See also *Lipomyelomeningocele.*
  embryogenesis of, 29–30, 77, *77*
  filum terminale, 90–91, *90*
  intradural, 84, *84*
  intramedullary, 436, *437*
Lipomeningocele, 36
Lipomyelocele, 84–86
  surgery for, 91–93
Lipomyelolipoma, 36
Lipomyelomeningocele, 28, 36, *37*, *83*, 84–86, *85–87*
  embryogenesis of, 29–30, 77–78, *77*
  surgery for, 91–92, *92*, *93*
Lipomyeloschisis, 36
Liver, infant, 567–568
Lobectomy, frontal, 544, *544*
  indications for, 542–543
  in astrocytoma, 378
  temporal, 536, 538
    anterior, 543–544, *544*
    indications for, 542
Lordosis, hydromyelia and, 64
Lowry's syndrome, 126t

Lumbar puncture, in hydrocephalus, 202, 232, 233
  in pseudotumor cerebri, 253
Lumboperitoneal shunt, 206
  complications of, 224
  in isolated fourth ventricle, 213
  in pseudotumor cerebri, 253
Lung function, 566, 566t
  monitoring of, 573–574
  support of, 580–582
Lymphatic system, CSF drainage by, 163
Lymphoma, skull in, 427
Lymphokines, 476–477

Macrocrania, 186, *187*, 188, 188t, *189*
Magnetic resonance imaging, nuclear. See *Nuclear magnetic resonance imaging (NMRI).*
Mannitol, 250, 576, 583
Mass lesions. See *Neoplasms.*
Mass spectrometry, 573–574
McGregor's line, 143, *144*
Mechanical ventilation, 580–582
  indications for, 581t
  intracranial hypertension and, 249, 581
Median cleft face syndrome, 134, *135*
Medical ethics, 151–157
  autonomy and, 155–156
  economic factors and, 153–154
  government and, 153
  guidelines for, 151–152
  history of, 151–152
  in spina bifida treatment, 40–41, 43, 152
  informed consent and, 154–155
  prognosis and, 156
  society and, 152–153
  surrogate role and, 156
  technology and, 152
Medulloblastoma, *192*, 347–356
  chemotherapy of, 352–353
  clinical features of, 348–349
  diagnosis of, 349, *349*, *350*
  epidemiology of, 347
  follow-up in, 466, 467t, 468, 468t
  histology of, 348, *348*
  metastatic to subarachnoid space, 446
  pathology of, 347–348
  postoperative management of, 351–353, *352*
  prognosis in, 353
  radiation therapy of, 352
  recurrence of, 354
  shunt spread of, 227
  surgery in, 349–351
  treatment sequelae in, 353–354
Megalencephaly, unilateral, 553–554
Memory, craniopharyngioma and, 401
  posttraumatic, 296
Meninges, cleft, in diastematomyelia, 88–89, *89*
  development of, 8, 8t
Meningioma, skull, 426
  spine, 445–446, *447*
Meningitis, after astrocytoma surgery, 343
  CSF leakage and, 266, 267
  dermoid cyst and, 370–371
  hydrocephalus and, 184
  intracranial dermal sinus and, 102, 103
  neonatal bacterial, 235
Meningocele, anterior, 36, 48, 91, *92*
  anterolateral, 48
  cranial, 98t
  spinal, 19, 36
  treatment of, 47–48

Metastasis, "drop," 446–447, *447*, 473
  radiography in, 417–418, *418*
  spinal cord compression by, 448–449
  to brain, 417–420
    cerebral hemisphere, 381
    clinical presentation of, 417
    from neuroblastoma, 418–419
    from osteogenic sarcoma, 419, *419*
    from Wilms' tumor, 418
  to spine, 448–450, *449*
  to subarachnoid space, 446–447, *447*, 473
Microsurgery, in peripheral nerve injury, 325, *325*
  brachial plexus, 329–330
  in scalp avulsion, 257
Metocurine, 572
Monoclonal antibodies, 476
Mortality rates, in hydrocephalus, 227
  in myelomeningocele, 54–55, *54*
  in spina bifida, 41
Motor examination, in neonatal spina bifida, 42
Movement disorders. See *Cerebral palsy.*
Moyamoya disease, 503–506, *504–506*
  diagnosis of, 504–505, *504*
  stages of, 503, *504*
  treatment of, 505–506, *505*, *506*
Multiple sutural synostoses, 115, *116–118*, 118
Muscle relaxants, 572
Myelocele, 75, *76*
Myelocystocele, terminal, 79
  surgery for, 93–94, *93*, *94*
Myelography, in medulloblastoma, 351, *352*
  in peripheral nerve injury, 322–323
  in spinal tumor, 445
  in tumor recurrence, 473
  of craniocervical junction, 144
Myelomeningocele, 18–19, 36, *36*. See also *Spina bifida.*
  ambulation and, 59
  closure of, 43–44, *44*, *45*, *46*
  embryogenesis of, 75–77, *75*, *76*
  hindbrain dysfunction with, 55–56, *56*, 60–61
  history of, 53–54
  hydrocephalus with, 46, 56–57, *57*, 182–183, 196
  infection in, 57–58
  intelligence and, 55, *55*, 58
  kyphosis with, 44, *44*, *45*, 46, 62
  late complications of, 60–64, *61–68*, 61t, 66, 68–69
  motor function and, 59
  neurophysiology of, 39–40
  prognosis in, 68–69
  shunt dependence in, 215–216
  survival in, 54–55, *54*
  urinary continence and, 59
Myeloschisis, 18, 77
Myelotomy, 434, *435*, 436
Myocutaneous reconstruction, in spina bifida, 44

Naloxone, in spinal cord injury, 306
Narcotics, in recurrent brain tumor, 474
  preanesthetic, 569, 569t
Nasal encephalocele, 98, *99*
Nasal intubation, 581
Neonatal assessment, ethical questions in, 151–157
  in encephalocele, 98–99
  in hydrocephalus, 186–188, *187*, *190*, 194–196, *195*, 200–201, *200*, *202*
  in spina bifida, 41–42
  in spinal cord injury, 308–309
  in tethered cord syndrome, 81–82

Neonate, acquired problems of, 230–236, *231*, *234*
　anemia in, 577
　anesthesia in, 565–568, 566t, 567t. See also *Anesthesia*.
　assessment of. See *Neonatal assessment*.
　bacterial meningitis in, 235
　basicranium of, *143*
　birth trauma in. See *Birth trauma*.
　body composition in, 567t
　cardiovascular values in, 566t
　cephalohematoma in, 422
　intracerebral hematoma in, 287, *287*
　lung function in, 566t
　peripheral nerve injury in, 321
　skull fracture in, 263–264
　spine in, 299, 301
　stroke in, 233–235, *234*, 501
　subdural hematoma in, 282, 283, *285*
　teratoma in, 380, *380*
　vitamin K deficiency in, 521–522
Neoplasms. See also specific neoplasm and location, e.g. *Astrocytoma; Brain tumors; Extramedullary spinal tumors*.
　craniofacial surgery and, 137, *140*
　hydrocephalus and, 184, 185
　intracranial hypertension and, 246–247, 250
　neurofibromatosis and, 456
　peripheral nerve injury and, 323, *324*
Nephritis, shunt, 221–222
Nephroblastoma, brain metastasis from, 418
Nerve root avulsion, *323*
　brachial plexus, 308, *309*, 323, 326, *327*, 328–330, *328*
Nerve root sleeves, CSF drainage into, 164–165, *165*
Nerve sheath tumors, 445–446
Nerves, peripheral. See *Peripheral nerves*.
Neural axis volume, 240–242, *241*
Neural crest, 80, *80*
　neurofibromatosis and, 453
Neural plaque, *36*, 36, 37, 39
　neurophysiology of, 39–40
Neural plate, 75–76, *75*, *76*
Neural tube, 3–5, 13–16, *14*, *15*, 73, *74*
　caudal, 4
Neurenteric canal, abnormal formation of, 32–33
Neurenteric cyst, 28–29, 91
　embryogenesis of, 30, 32, 81
Neuroblastoma, brain metastasis from, 418–419
　catecholamines and, 445
　deceptive symptoms of, 444
　skull in, 427
　spinal, 449–450, *449*
Neurocutaneous syndromes. See *Phakomatoses*.
Neurocysticercosis, 494–499
　clinical manifestations of, 495–496
　diagnosis of, 496–497, *497*, *498*
　epidemiology of, 494
　hydrocephalus and, 184–185
　immunologic tests for, 497
　pathogenesis of, 494–495
　pathology of, 495, *495*
　treatment of, 497–498, *498*
Neuroectoderm, 2–3, 13
Neuroectodermal-mesodermal spatial dyssynchrony theory, 24
Neurofibromatosis, 137, *137*, 453–456, *454*, *455*
　CNS in, 455–456, *455*
　craniofacial surgery in, 137, *138–139*
　hemispheric tumors in, 375, *376*
　in children, 454–455
　optic glioma in, 391, 392, *395*, 397

Neurofibromatosis *(Continued)*
　peripheral nerve injury and, *324*
　prognosis in, 456
　skull in, 424
　spinal tumors in, 446
Neurogenic bladder, in spina bifida, 42, 47
Neuroradiology, interventional. See *Embolization*.
Neuroschisis theory, 24
　of Dandy-Walker syndrome, 27
　of dermal sinus, 29
　of spinal dysraphism, 32
Neurulation, 3–4, 4t, 13–14, *14*, 73, *73*, *74*
　abnormal, 32, 75–79, *75–77*
Nimodipine, 584
Nitrous oxide, CBF and, 571
NMRI. See *Nuclear magnetic resonance imaging (NMRI)*.
Norepinephrine, spinal cord injury and, 305–306
Notochord, 2, 11–13, *12*, *13*, 72–73
　abnormal development of, 30, *31*, 32
　split, 31
Notochordal process, 11–12, *12*, 72, *72*
Nuclear magnetic resonance imaging (NMRI), in arachnoid cyst, *105*
　in astrocytoma, 341, *341*
　in brain abscess, 482, *483*
　in dermal sinus, 87, *102*
　in diastematomyelia, 89, *89*
　in encephalocele, 99
　in epilepsy, evaluative, 540
　　intraoperative, *544*, *545*
　in hemispheric tumors, 376, *376*
　in hydromyelia, 62, *63*
　in lipomyelomeningocele, 86, *86*
　in medulloblastoma, 349, *350*
　in metastasis, *418*
　in neurofibromatosis, 454, *454*, 455, *455*
　in pineal region tumors, 411, *411*
　in spinal cord injury, 307, *308*
　in spinal cord tumor, 430–431, *431*
　in spinal tumor, 444, *447*
　in tumor recurrence, 473
　of craniocervical junction, 144
　postoperative, 464, 466
Nurse, counseling by, 155–156
Nutrition, congenital hydrocephalus and, 184, 184t
　postoperative, 582
　spina bifida and, 38
Nystagmus, in basilar impression, 146
　in craniopharyngioma, 400
　in optic nerve tumors, 392, *393*
　see-saw, 400

Occipital bone, 142, *143*
Occipital condyle, hypoplasia of, 147
　third, 147
Occipital encephalocele, 97, *99*
　angiography in, 100
　repair of, 100
Occipital vertebra, 147
Occult spina bifida. See *Spina bifida occulta*.
Occult spinal dysraphism, 27–33, 35–36, 81–82
Odontoid process, abnormalities of, 149
　formation of, 142–143
　trauma to, 309, *310*, 312–313
Olfactory nerve trauma, 267
Oligoastrocytoma, 379
Oligodendroglioma, 379
Omental transposition, in spinal cord injury, 306

Optic chiasm tumors, 393–394, *394*
 craniopharyngioma, 400–401, *401, 402*
 hypothalamus involvement in, 394, *394–396,*
  396–397
 neurofibromatosis and, 455
 prognosis in, 396–397
Optic glioma, 391–398
 biologic behavior of, 391–392
 chiasm involvement in, 393–394, *394*
 diagnosis of, 392, *393, 394, 396*
 hypothalamus involvement in, 394, *394–396,*
  396–397
 pathology of, 391, *392*
 treatment of, 393–394, 396–397
Optic nerve trauma, 267–268
Os odontoideum, *301*
Osmotic therapy, in cerebral edema, 250–251, 583
Ossification, basicranial, 142
 cranial, 6, 7t, 18
 vertebral, 6, 7t, 17–18
Ossifying fibroma, skull, 426
Osteoblastoma, craniofacial surgery and, *140*
 spinal, 447, *448*
Osteogenic sarcoma, brain metastasis from, 419, *419*
Osteogenesis imperfecta, basilar impression in, 145
Osteoid osteoma, skull, 426
Osteoma, skull, 425–426
Osteomyelitis, skull, 486–487, *486, 487*
Osteopetrosis, 148
Osteosarcoma, metastatic to spine, 449, *449*
Osteotomy, spinal, 46
Otorrhea, CSF, posttraumatic, 267
Overgrowth theory, 22–23
Oxygen therapy, in edema, 249–250

Pacchonian granulations, 423
Pain, in spinal cord tumors, 429
 in spinal tumors, 443
 in tethered cord syndrome, 82
Pancuronium, 572
Papilledema, in hemispheric tumors, 374–375, *375*
 in hydrocephalus, 188
 in pseudotumor cerebri, 252
Papilloma, choroid plexus, 162
 fourth ventricle, 369–370
 intraventricular, *384–386, 385–390, 389*
Paracondylar process, 147
Paralysis, facial, 268
 spinal cord injury and, 307
  care in, 314–315
Paraplegia, 307
 care in, 314–315
Parasitic infections. See also *Neurocysticercosis.*
 acquired hydrocephalus and, 184–185
 congenital hydrocephalus and, 183–184, *193*
Parents, anesthetist and, 568
 autonomy of, 155–156
 counseling of, 42–43
 informed consent by, 154–155
 surrogate role of, 156
Paresis, in basilar impression, 146
Parietal foramina, 423, *424*
Pederson's syndrome, 126t
Pediatric concussion syndrome, 272–273
Penetrating trauma, cranial, 265
 abscess and, 480, *481*
 peripheral nerve, *332*
 spinal, 301
Perforation, peritoneal, shunt and, 226–227

Peripheral nerves, 318–333
 anatomy of, 318–319, *319*
 clinical examination of, 321–322
 electrophysiologic studies of, 322
 pathology of, 319–320
 physiotherapy of, 325–326
 radiology of, 322–323, *323, 324*
 surgery on, 323, *325, 325, 331, 332*
  brachial plexus, 326, *327,* 328–330, *328*
  in compartment syndrome, 330–331, *330*
  in hemophilia, 520
  in injection injuries, 331–332, *331*
  reconstructive, 326
  timing of, 320–321, *321*
Peritoneum, as distal shunt site, 206–207
 complications of, 226–227, *226*
Pfeiffer's syndrome, 121, 123t, 126t
Phakomatoses, 453–462
 ataxia telangiectasia, 460
 hemispheric tumors and, 375, *376*
 incontinentia pigmenti, 460–461
 neurofibromatosis. See *Neurofibromatosis.*
 Sturge-Weber syndrome, 458–459, *458*
  hemispherectomy in, 550–552, *551, 552*
 tuberous sclerosis, 456–458, *457, 458*
 von Hippel-Lindau disease, 459
Phenytoin, after craniopharyngioma surgery, 404
Physician, ethical decisions by. See *Medical ethics.*
Physiotherapy, in peripheral nerve injury, 325–326
Pineal gland, 409
Pineal region tumors, 389, 409–416
 biopsy in, 412
 chemotherapy of, 415
 common types of, 410t, 412t
 CSF studies in, 411–412
 diagnosis of, 411–412, *411*
 pathology of, 409–410, 412t, *414*
 presentation of, 410–411
 radiation therapy of, 415
 recurrence of, 415
 surgery in, 412–414, 414t
Pineoblastoma, 414, 415
 follow-up in, 466, 467t, 468, 468t
Pineocytoma, 414, 415
Platelet count, 577, 578
Platybasia, 144
Pleural cavity, as distal shunt site, 207
Porencephaly, growing skull fracture and, 293
 "needle," 202
PNET. See *Primitive neuroectodermal tumor (PNET).*
Positive end-expiratory pressure, 581
Posterior fossa tumors. See specific tumors.
Postsurgical management. See also *Intensive care.*
 chemotherapeutic, 465–466, 465t. See also *Chemotherapy.*
 of arteriovenous malformation, 513–515, *514*
 of astrocytoma, 343
 of brain tumor, 463–471
 of craniopharyngioma, 470
 of ependymoma, 467t, 468–469
 of glioma, 467t, 469–470, 469t
 of medulloblastoma, 351–353, *352,* 466, 467t, 468, 468t
 of PNETs, 466, 467t, 468, 468t
 of recurrence. See *Recurrence of disease.*
 of spina bifida, 46
 radiotherapeutic, 464–465, 465t. See also *Radiation therapy.*
 staging in, 463–464, 465t, 468t
 surveillance in, 465t, 466, 467t

Praziquantel, in neurocysticercosis, 498
Precocious puberty, pineal region tumors and, 409, 410
Premature infant, body composition of, 567t
   endotracheal tube size for, 570t
   hydrocephalus in, 184, 195–196, 201–203
   intraventricular hemorrhage in, 230–232, *231*
   stroke in, 234–235
Prenatal diagnosis, of arachnoid cyst, 104, *104*
   of encephalocele, 100, *101*
   of hydrocephalus, 189, *191*
   of spina bifida, 41, 48–49
Pressure-volume index, 241–242, *241*, *242*
   infant, 242–243
   varying, 242, *243*
Primitive neuroectodermal tumors (PNET), 347–356. See also *Medulloblastoma*.
   defined, 348
   of pineal region, 412, 415
   postsurgical management of, 464, 465, 466, 467t, 468, 468t
   recurrence of, 473
Primitive pit, 72, *72*
Primitive streak, 11, *11*, *12*
Proptosis, in neurofibromatosis, 454
   in optic nerve tumors, 392
Prostheses, for forehead repair, 291
   for scalp reconstruction, 260–261
Pseudoaneurysm, postembolization, 529
Pseudocyst, shunt infection and, 226, *226*
Pseudomeningocele, 322–323, *323*
   after astrocytoma, 343
"Pseudorosettes," in medulloblastoma, 348
Pseudoseizures, 540
Pseudotumor cerebri, 252–253
   pathology with, 252t
Psychoemotional factors, in epilepsy, 537
Psychosocial factors. See *Medical ethics; Quality of life.*
Pulmonary embolism, vascular shunt and, 224–225, *225*
Pulmonary function, 566, 566t
   monitoring of, 573–574
   support of, 580–582
Pulse oximetry, 573
Pulsed lumbar cisternostomy, 203
Pyknodysostosis, 148
Pyle's disease. See *Craniometaphyseal dysplasia*.

Quadriplegia, 307
Quality of life, astrocytoma and, 346
   myelomeningocele and, 58–60, 68–69
   spina bifida and, 40–41, 42–43, 47, 49

Rachischisis, 37
Radiation therapy, anesthesia before, 580
   in astrocytoma, 343
   in craniopharyngioma, 405, 407, *407*
   in ependymoma, 369
   in hemispheric tumors, 378
   in medulloblastoma, 352, 354, 468
      recurrent, 354
   in optic glioma, 397
   in pineal region tumors, 415, 468
   interstitial, 476
   late sequelae of, 353–354, 378, 464–465, 466
   postsurgical, 464–465
   spinal deformity after, 450
Radiography. See also specific modality, e.g., *Computed tomography*.
   anesthesia before, 579–580

Radiography *(Continued)*
   in arachnoid cyst, 105
   in basilar impression, 146
   in brain abscess, 481, *481*
   in concussion, 272
   in craniosynostosis, 107
   in dermal sinus, 102
   in encephalocele, 98–99
   in hemispheric tumor, 376, *377*
   in holocord astrocytoma, 432, *433*
   in metastasis, 417
   in peripheral nerve injury, 322–323
   in skull fracture, 263, *264*
   in skull osteomyelitis, *486*
   in spinal cord injury, 307
   in spinal tumor, 444–445, *444*, *445*
   of craniocervical junction, 143–144, *143*, *144*
Recurrence of disease, 472–477
   biologic response modifiers in, 476–477
   brachytherapy in, 476
   chemotherapy in, 474–476
   clinical presentation of, 473
   clinical trials in, 475–476
   diagnosis of, 472–473
   monoclonal antibodies in, 476
   supportive care in, 473–474
   surgery in, 474
Reflexes, in spinal cord injury, 307
Respiration, 566, 566t
   monitoring of, 573–574
   support of, 580–582
Resuscitation, 584
Retrogressive differentiation, 4, 15–16, *15*, 72, *72*, 74–75
   abnormal, 79
Reye's syndrome, decompressive craniectomy in, 247, *247*
Rhabdomyosarcoma, metastatic to spine, 449, *449*
Rhinorrhea, CSF, posttraumatic, 266–267, *267*
Rhizotomy, in cerebral palsy, 557
Rhombencephalon, 5, *16*
Rosenthal's fibers, 344, *344*

Sacrococcygeal teratoma, 11
Sacrum, agenesis of, 79–81, *80*
   scimitar, 91, *92*
Saethe-Chotzen syndrome, 121, 123, 126t
Sagittal craniectomy, 108–111, *109–112*, 113–114
   bilateral, 108, *109*
   "clam shell," 110, *110*
   "keyhole," 111–112, *112*
   pi, 110–111, *111*
      modified, 111, *112*
   single midline, 108, *109*, *110*
      modified, 109–110, *110*
   transposition, 112, *113*
   vault remodeling, 112, *113*
   vertex, 110, *111*
      modified, 110, *111*
Sakati's syndrome, 127t
Sarcoma, metastatic to spine, 449, *449*
   skull, 427
Scalp, 255–262
   anatomy of, 255–256
   avulsions of, 257–258
   blood supply to, 255–256, *256*
   flaps of, 257–260, *258*
   lacerations of, 256–257, 264–265
   tissue expansion in, 260–261, *260*, *261*
Schwannoma, 455
   intraspinal, *444*
Scimitar sacrum, 91, *92*

Scoliosis, diastematomyelia and, 88
  myelomeningocele and, 60–61
  neurofibromatosis and, 455
  spinal cord injury and, 315
  spinal cord tumor and, 429
  tethered cord and, 82
Scopolamine, 569, 569t
Seatbelt injuries, 301–302
Seconal, 569t
Sedatives, before radiologic procedure, 579
  preanesthetic, 569, 569t, 570
Seizures. See also *Epilepsy.*
  arteriovenous malformation and, 511
  brain abscess and, 484
  complex partial, 543
  concussion and, 272
  encephalocele and, 100
  extradural hematoma and, 279
  hydrocephalus and, 189
  metastasis and, 417
  NMRI in, 376
  posttraumatic, 294–295
  shunting and, 224
  subdural empyema and, 486
  surdural hematoma and, 284
  Sturge-Weber syndrome and, 458
  tuberous sclerosis and, 456–457
  tumors and, 374, *374*
Sensory evoked potentials, during spinal cord tumor surgery, 436–438
Sensory examination, in neonatal spina bifida, 42
Sexual function, in spina bifida, 47
Shunt, alternatives to, 201–203
  complications with, 219–227, *220, 221,* 222t, *223, 225, 226*
    shunt type and, 227
  dependence on, 214–216
  history of, 203–204
  in Dandy-Walker malformation, 211–212
  in hydrocephalus, 203–207, *205–206, 208–210, 209, 211*
    compartmentalized, 211–214, *212–214*
    patient selection for, 200–201
    placement of, 204–207, *205–206, 208, 209, 209*
    results of, 227–228
    risks vs. benefits of, 200–201, *200*
    valve system of, 209, *210,* 211
  in isolated fourth ventricle, 212–213, *212, 213*
  in subdural hematoma, 286
  in supratentorial CSF cyst, 214, *214*
  infection of, 200–201, 220–223, 222t
    pseudocyst and, 226, *226*
  intracranial dermal sinus repair and, 103
  IQ and, 58, 200, 227–228
  lumboperitoneal, 206
    complications of, 224
    in isolated fourth ventricle, 213
    in pseudotumor cerebri, 253
  malfunction of, 219–220, *220,* 221
  myelomeningocele and, 56–57, *57*
  neoplasm spread by, 227
  overdrainage from, 223–224, *223*
  preoperative, in astrocytoma, 341–342
  postoperative, in astrocytoma, 343
    in pineal region surgery, 414, 414t
  removal of, 214–216
    in infection, 222, 226
  revision of, 57, 215, 227
  seizures and, 224
  valve system of, 209–211, *210*
    malfunction of, 220

Shunt *(Continued)*
  ventriculoatrial, 207, *209*
    complications of, 224–226, *225*
    infection of, 221, 222
    vs. ventriculoperitoneal shunt, 227
  ventriculoperitoneal, 206–207, *208*
    complications of, 226–227, *226*
    infection of, 221, 222
    vs. ventriculoatrial shunt, 227
Shuntography, 220
Sickle cell anemia, stroke and, 502
Silastic dural substitute, 440
Silastic pellets, 526, *527*
Sincipital encephalocele, 97–98
  hypertelorism and, 134, *135*
Sinus pericranii, 423
Siphoning, 210–211, *210*
  slit-ventricle syndrome and, 223
Skin flaps, scalp, 257–260, *258*
Skin signs, in diastematomyelia, *83,* 88
  in intracranial dermal sinus, 101–102
  in neurofibromatosis, 454
  in Sturge-Weber syndrome, 458
  in tuberous sclerosis, 456
  of shunt infection, 220–221
  of spinal pathology, 81–82, *83*
Skull. See also *Craniofacial surgery; Craniosynostosis.*
  congenital dysplasias of, 148, 148t
  development of, 6, 7t, 18
  fractures of. See *Skull fractures.*
  osteomyelitis of, 486–487, *486, 487*
  posttraumatic defects of, 290–291, *291*
  tumors of. See *Skull tumors.*
Skull fractures, 263–270
  basal, 266
  cephalohematoma and, 422
  cranial nerve injury and, 267–268
  CSF otorrhea in, 267
  CSF rhinorrhea in, 266–267, *267*
  depressed, 263–265, *264, 265*
    extradural hematoma with, *279*
  growing, 291–294, *292, 293,* 422–423, *422*
  linear, 263, *264*
  penetrating trauma and, 265
Skull tumors, 421–427
  aplasia cutis congenita, 423
  benign, 425–426
    vs. malignant, 421–422
  cephalohematoma as, 422
  classification of, 422t
  dermoid. See *Dermoid tumors.*
  differential diagnosis of, 421–422
  dysplastic, 423–424
  encephalocele. See *Encephalocele.*
  growing skull fracture, 291–294, *292, 293,* 422–423, *422*
  lymphoproliferative disorders and, 424–425, *425*
  malignant, 426–427
  pacchonian granulations, 423
  parietal foramina, 423, *424*
  sinus pericranii, 423
Slit-ventricle syndrome, 216, 223, *223*
Somatosensory evoked potentials, in cerebral palsy, 558
  in neonatal spina bifida, 42
  in tethered cord syndrome, 81
Somites, 3–4, 13
  vertebral formation and, 17, 18, 72
Spasmus nutans, 394
Spasticity. See *Cerebral palsy.*
Speech, localization of, 542, 550
Sphenoid wing, agenesis of, 137, *137*

Spina bifida, 35–52
  anomalies associated with, 19t, 39, 40t
  bladder function in, 42
  clinical assessment of, 41–43
  combined anterior and posterior, 29
    embryogenesis of, 31, 32–33
  embryogenesis of, 38–39
  etiology of, 38
  genetics of, 38
  parent counseling in, 42–43, 49
  postoperative management in, 46
  prognosis in, 40–41, 47, 49
  treatment of, 40–41, 43–44, 44, 45, 46
    ethical questions in, 40–41, 43, 152
    postoperative, 46
    results of, 47
Spina bifida aperta, 18–19, 36
  embryogenesis of, 21–25
  embryonic timing of, 19–21, 20, 20t, 21
  incidence of, 37–38
Spina bifida cystica, 36
Spina bifida occulta, 35–36
  incidence of, 37
  of atlas, 149
Spinal cord, abscess of, 490–491
  arteriovenous malformation of, 531–532, 532
  development of, 4, 5t, 6, 17, 71–75, 72–74
  extramedullary tumors of. See *Extramedullary spinal tumors.*
  injury to. See *Spinal cord injury.*
  intramedullary tumors of. See *Intramedullary spinal cord tumors.*
  neurofibromatosis and, 454, 454
  spina bifida and, 39
Spinal cord injury, 298–317
  at birth, 299, 301, 306, 308–309, 309
  classification of, 305
  compression and, 302, 303, 303
    by arachnoid cyst, 323, 324
  diagnosis of, 306–307, 308
  incidence of, 298–299
  location of, 298–299
  long-term management of, 314–315
  mechanism of, 300–305, 302–304
  prognosis in, 307
  to craniovertebral junction, 310–313, 310–314
  treatment of, 305–306, 308–310, 311, 312
  without radiographic abnormalities, 313–314
Spinal dermal sinus. See *Dermal sinus.*
Spinal dysraphism, 36–37
  occult, 27–33, 36–36
Spinal epidural abscess, 491
Spinal meningocele, 19, 36
Spinal shock, 307
  neonatal, 308
Spine. See also *Vertebra(e).*
  cervical, 300, 300
    trauma to, 309–310, 310
  extramedullary tumors of. See *Extramedullary spinal tumors.*
  infections of, 490–493, 492
  injury to. See *Spinal cord injury.*
  pediatric, 299–300, 300
Spondylitis, 491–492, 492
Sports injuries, atlantoaxial, 312, 314
Staging, of gliomas, 469, 469t
  of PNETs, 468, 468t
  postsurgical, 463–464, 465t
Status epilepticus, evaluation, preoperative, 541
Stereotaxic techniques, 412, 561–564, 562, 563
  future applications of, 564
  history of, 561–562
  in epilepsy evaluation, 540–541, 541, 542
  operating room, 541

Stroke, 501–507
  arteriosclerosis and, 501–502
  arteriovenous malformations and. See *Arteriovenous malformations.*
  cerebral arteritis and, 502
  extracranial arterial dissection and, 502–503
  fibromuscular dysplasia and, 502
  incidence of, 501
  migraine and, 503
  moyamoya disease and, 503–506, 504–506
  perinatal, 233–235, 234, 501
    meningitis and, 235
  sickle cell anemia and, 502
Sturge-Weber syndrome, 458–459, 458
  hemispherectomy in, 550–552, 551, 552
Subarachnoid space, 171
  CSF absorption and, 162–165, 165
  in hydrocephalus, 166
  metastasis to, 446–447, 447, 473
Subdural empyema, 484–486, 485
Subdural hematoma, 281–289, 282, 283, 285, 287, 288
  acute, 246, 281–283, 282, 283
  chronic, 283–286, 285
    treatment of, 286
  posterior fossa, 283
  shunting and, 223–224, 223
Subdural hygroma, 286–287
Subpial lipoma, 84, 84
Succinylcholine, 572
Summitt's syndrome, 126t
"Sunburst" appearance, in hemangioma, 426
Sunset sign, in hydrocephalus, 187, 187
Superior sagittal sinus, CSF absorption and, 163
  in hydrocephalus, 166
Supratentorial CSF cyst, 214, 214
Surgeon, as anatomist, 318–319
  counseling by, 42–43
  ethical decisions by. See *Medical ethics.*
Surgery. See also *Anesthesia;* and specific procedure.
  coagulopathies and. See *Coagulopathies.*
  craniofacial. See *Craniofacial surgery.*
  in arachnoid cyst, 105
  in arteriovenous malformations, 510, 513
  in astrocytoma, 341–343, 342
  in brain abscess, 482–484
  in brainstem tumors, 361–365, 362, 363
  in cerebral edema, 250, 584
  in cerebral palsy, 556–560
  in choroid plexus papilloma, 370, 384–386, 385–390, 389
  in craniopharyngioma, 401–405, 404–406
  in craniosynostosis. See *Craniectomy; Craniofacial surgery.*
  in CSF rhinorrhea, 266–267
  in Dandy-Walker malformation, 211–212
  in dermoid cyst, 370–371
  in encephalocele, 100
  in ependymoma, 368–369, 383–384
  in epidural abscess, 486
    spinal, 491
  in epilepsy. See *Epilepsy.*
  in extradural hematoma, 280–281
  in glioma, 384–385
    optic, 393
  in hemispheric tumors, 377–378
  in hemophilia, 519–520
  in hydrocephalus, 203–207, 205–206, 208–210, 209, 211
  in hydromyelia, 62–63
  in intracranial mass, 246–247, 250
  in lipomyelomeningocele, 91–93, 92, 93

Surgery *(Continued)*
  in medulloblastoma, 349–351
    recurrent, 354
  in meningocele, 47–48
  in moyamoya disease, 505–506, *505, 506*
  in neurocysticercosis, 498
  in neurofibromatosis, 455–456
  in pineal region tumors, 412–414, 414t
  in posttraumatic cranial defects, 290–291, *291*
  in recurrent brain tumor, 474
  in skull fracture, 264–265
  in skull osteomyelitis, 487
  in spina bifida, 40–41, 43–44, *44, 45, 46*
    results of, 47
  in spinal cord abscess, 490–491
  in spinal cord injury, 305, 309–310, *311,* 312
  in spinal cord tumor, 431–438, *435*
    pitfalls, of, 438–440, *439*
  in spinal tumor, 446, 450
  in spondylitis, 491–492
  in Sturge-Weber syndrome, 459
  in subdural empyema, 485
  in subdural hematoma, 283
  in terminal myelocystocele, 93–94, *93, 94*
  in tethered cord syndrome, 94–95
  in tuberous sclerosis, 457–458
  in von Hippel-Lindau disease, 459
  management after. See *Postsurgical management.*
  peripheral nerve. See *Peripheral nerves, surgery on.*
  scalp. See *Scalp.*
Sutures, cranial, 107, *108.*
  premature closure of. See *Craniofacial surgery; Craniosynostosis.*
    volume expansion and, 242–243
    widened, 187
  occipital, premature closure of, 147–148
Syndrome of inappropriate antidiuretic hormone secretion (SIADH), 582
Syringobulbia, myelomeningocele and, 66, 67
Syringomyelia, basilar impression with, 146
  cystic astrocytoma and, 440–441
  hydrocephalus compensation and, 215

Taenia solium, 494–495
Temperature, monitoring of, 574
Temporal lobectomy, 536, 538
  anterior, 543–544, *544*
  indications for, 542
Teratogenesis, 38
  aminopterin and, 126t
  experimental, 2, 77
  hydrocephalus and, 184, 184t
Teratoma, hemispheric, 380, *380*
  pineal region, 413–414, *414*
  sacrococcygeal, 11
Terminal illness, 473–474
Terminal myelocystocele, 79
  surgery for, 93–94, *93, 94*
Tetanus prophylaxis, in scalp injuries, 256
Tethered cord syndrome, 28, 71–96
  anterior meningocele and, 91
  clinical features of, 81–82, *83, 84*
  dermal sinus and, 86–87, *87, 88*
  diastematomyelia and, 87–90, *89*
  embryogenesis of, 29–30, 75–81, *75–77*
  embryonic deformation and caudal repression syndrome and, 91
  lipomas and, 82, 84–86, *84–87*
    filum terminale, 90–91, *90*
  myelomeningocele repair and, 64, *64–66,* 66

Tethered cord syndrome *(Continued)*
  neurenteric cyst and, 91
  normal development vs., 4, 5t, 6, 17, 71–75, *72–74*
  pathophysiology of, 81
  retethering in, 94–95
  surgery for, 91–95, *92–94*
  tight filum terminale syndrome and, 90, *90*
Thanatophoric dwarfism, kleeblattschädel in, 123t
Therapeutic embolization. See *Embolization.*
Thiopental, CBF and, 571
Thiopental sodium test, 541–542
Third space fluid loss, 575–576
Third ventricle tumors, 389–390
Thyroid function, craniopharyngioma and, 401, 405
Thyrotropin-releasing hormone, in spinal cord injury, 306
Tight filum terminale syndrome, 71, 79, 90, *90*
  defined, 90
Tinel's sign, 322
Tissue expansion, scalp, 260–261, *260, 261*
Tonsillar herniation, basilar impression with, 145–146, *145*
  shunting and, 224
Toxoplasmosis, congenital hydrocephalus and, 183–184, *193*
Tracheostomy, 581–582
Traction theory, 24–25
Trauma. See also specific injury, e.g., *Concussion; Skull fractures.*
  basilar impressin and, 145
  birth. See *Birth trauma.*
  cranial nerve, 267–268
  craniectomy and, 114
  head. See *Head injury.*
  penetrating, 265, 301, 332
    abscess and, 480, 481
  scalp, 256–257, 264–265
  spinal cord. See *Spinal cord injury.*
  spinal tumor and, 444
Treatment sequelae, 466
  in medulloblastoma, 353–354
  of radiation therapy, 353–354, 378, 464–465, 466
Trephination, 536
Trigonocephaly, 127, 131, *133, 133*
Tuberculous spondylitis, 491–492, *492*
Tuberous sclerosis, 456–458, *457, 458*
  hemispheric tumors in, 375
D-Tubocurarine, 572
Tumors. See *Brain tumors; Extramedullary spinal tumors; Intramedullary spinal cord tumors; Metastasis; Neoplasms; Skull tumors;* and specific tumors.

Ulcer, decubitus, in spinal cord injury, 314–315
Ultrasonic aspiration, 433–434
  in hemispheric tumor surgery, 378
  in intraventricular tumor surgery, 384
  in spinal tumor surgery, 434
Ultrasonography, bubble detection by, 574
  in blood pressure monitoring, 572–573
  in brainstem tumor surgery, 363
  in hydrocephalus, 191, *193*
    treatment monitoring, 233
  in spinal cord tumor, 431
    intraoperative, 434, *435, 436*
  in subdural hematoma, 285, *285*
  in tethered cord syndrome, 86, *87*
  prenatal. See *Prenatal diagnosis.*

Uncal herniation, in extradural hematoma, 279
Unilateral megalencephaly, 553–554
Urea, in intracranial hypertension, 2509
Ureter, as distal shunt site, 207
Urinary incontinence, after spinal cord tumor surgery, 439–440
   myelomeningocele and, 59
   spina bifida and, 42, 47
   tethered cord syndrome and, 82, 95
Urokinase, in intraventricular hemorrhage, 203
Utilization review committees, 153

Vascular shunt. See *Ventriculoatrial shunt*.
Vasculitis, in neurocysticercosis, 495
   neonatal meningitis and, 235
Vasogenic edema, 250–252
Vasopressin, pseudotumor cerebri and, 252–253
Vein of Galen malformation, embolization of, 529–532, *530*
Ventilation, mechanical, 580–582
   indications for, 581t
   intracranial hypertension and, 249, 581
Ventilators, 581
Ventricle. See also *Fourth ventricle*.
   puncture of, 247
      in hydrocephalus, 202
   size of, myelomeningocele and, 57, *57*
   slit, shunt and, 216, 223, *223*
   third ventricle tumors, 389–390
Ventricle-brain index, 227–228
Ventriculitis, after spinal bifida surgery, 46, 47
   hydrocephalus and, 195
   myelomeningocele and, 57–58
Ventriculoatrial shunt, 207, *209*
   complications of, 224–226, *225*
   infection of, 221, 222
   vs. ventriculoperitoneal shunt, 227
Ventriculocisternostomy, 204
Ventriculography, anesthesia before, 580
   in hydrocephalus, 191
   radionuclide, 194
Ventriculoperitoneal shunt, 206–207, *208*
   complications of, 226–227, *226*
   infection of, 221, 222
   vs. ventriculoatrial shunt, 227

Vertebra(e). See also *Atlas; Spine*.
   development of, 6, 7t, 17–18, 72
   diastematomyelia and, 88
   first cervical sclerotome abnomalities of, 148–149, 148t, *149*
   fractures of, 300–302, *302, 303*, 309–310, *310, 311*
   in spinal tumors, 444–445, *444, 445*
   myelomeningocele and, 36
   occipital, 147
   occult abnormalities of, 35–36
   tumors of, 447–449, *448, 449*
Viral infections, congenital hydrocephalus and, 183
Vision, astrocytoma and, 340
   concussion and, 273
   craniopharyngioma and, 400, 401
   hemispheric tumors and, 375, *375*
   hydrocephalus and, 187–188, 189
   optic glioma and, 392, *392*
   optic nerve trauma and, 267–268
   posthemispherectomy, 554
   pseudotumor cerebri and, 252, 253
Visual evoked potentials, 575
Vitamin A, neural tube reopening and, 77
Vitamin K, deficiency of, 521–522
Volume replacement, 576–579, 582
Vomiting, in astrocytoma, 339
   in concussion, 272
Von Hippel-Lindau disease, 459
Von Recklinghausen's disease. See *Neurofibromatosis*.

Waardenburg's syndrome, 127t
Walking. See *Ambulation*.
Washington's syndrome, 126t
Weiss's syndrome, 126t
Wheelchair use, myelomeningocele and, 59
Wilms' tumor, brain metastasis from, 418
Wisconsin syndrome, 127t
Wounds, penetrating, 265, 301, 332
   abscess and, 480, *481*

X-rays. See *Radiography*.

Yolk-sac tumor, pineal region, 413